CARE OF THE ELDERLY
Clinical Aspects of Aging

Fourth Edition

CARE OF THE ELDERLY
Clinical Aspects of Aging
Fourth Edition

Editor

William Reichel, M.D.

Clinical Professor, Department of Community Health, Tufts University School of
Medicine, Boston, Massachusetts; Adjunct Professor, Department of Family Medicine,
Brown University School of Medicine, Memorial Hospital of Rhode Island,
Pawtucket, Rhode Island

Associate Editors

Joseph J. Gallo, M.D., M.P.H.

Assistant Professor, Department of Mental Hygiene, The Johns Hopkins School of
Hygiene and Public Health, Baltimore, Maryland

Jan Busby-Whitehead, M.D.

Associate Professor of Internal Medicine, Program on Aging, University of North Carolina
School of Medicine, Chapel Hill, North Carolina

John R. Delfs, M.D.

Director, Deaconess Center for ElderCare, Chief, Section of Geriatric Medicine,
Department of Medicine, Assistant Professor, Department of Medicine, Harvard Medical School,
Boston, Massachusetts

John B. Murphy, M.D.

Associate Professor of Family Medicine, Brown University, School of Medicine,
Memorial Hospital of Rhode Island, Pawtucket, Rhode Island

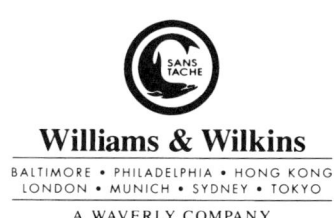

Williams & Wilkins

BALTIMORE • PHILADELPHIA • HONG KONG
LONDON • MUNICH • SYDNEY • TOKYO

A WAVERLY COMPANY

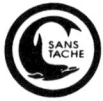

Editor: David C. Retford
Managing Editor: Molly L. Mullen
Copy Editor: Anne K. Schwartz
Designer: Wilma Rosenberger
Illustration Planner: Ray Lowman
Production Coordinator: Barbara J. Felton

Copyright © 1995
Williams & Wilkins
428 East Preston Street
Baltimore, Maryland 21202, USA

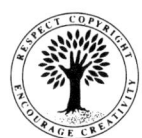

Accurate indications, adverse reactions, and dosage schedules for drugs are provided in this book, but it is possible that they may change. The reader is urged to review the package information data of the manufacturers of the medications mentioned.

Printed in the United States of America

First Edition 1978
Second Edition 1983
Third Edition 1989

Library of Congress Cataloging in Publication Data

Care of the elderly : Clinical Aspects of Aging/William Reichel, editor; associate editors, Joseph J. Gallo . . . [et al.]. — 4th ed.
   p. cm.
  Includes bibliographical references and index.
  ISBN 0-683-07209-9
  1. Geriatrics. 2. Aging. I. Reichel, William, 1937–   .
  [DNLM: 1. Geriatrics. 2. Aging. WT 100 C644 1995]
RC952C53 1995
618.97—dc20
DNLM/DLC
for Library of Congress   94-26125
                                                CIP

95 96 97 98 99
1 2 3 4 5 6 7 8 9 10

Reprints of chapter(s) may be purchased from Williams & Wilkins in quantities of 100 or more. Call Isabella Wise, Special Sales Department, (800)358-3583.

The sign in the West Virginia lunch counter read:

Don't criticize the coffee.
You may be old and weak yourself someday.

Preface to the Fourth Edition

In preparing this Fourth Edition, it was apparent that a major expansion of knowledge regarding the care of the elderly has taken place since the Third Edition was released in 1989. Examples of new areas of knowledge and skill include the use of transesophageal echocardiography for the study of heart disease; the emergence of the prostatic-specific antigen test in screening for prostatic cancer; the use of total cholesterol and HDL cholesterol and mammography in health screening of the elderly; emphasis on health-promoting behaviors in older persons, including exercise and strength training, appropriate nutritional choices, and smoking cessation; the use of tamoxifen in breast cancer; increasing use of advance directives and living wills; advances in palliative and hospice care; new proposed models of health care economics and health care reform; and the discovery of not one gene implicated in Alzheimer's disease as described in the Third Edition, but now four genes are being studied. With this information, there is heightened controversy and conflict in many of these areas. With time, we look forward to more certainty and consensus.

Since 1989, the number of medications in each of the major drug families has vastly expanded. Previously there were limited numbers of angiotensin converting enzyme inhibitors, calcium channel blockers, nonsteroidal antiinflammatory agents, and serotonin reuptake inhibitor antidepressants, and now there are multiple products. The entire book could have been devoted to the wide array of pharmacologic products available to benefit our older patients (and also capable of producing harm or side effects).

Despite all this new information and controversy, an attempt has been made to be clear and concise, to emphasize the most practical and useful information, and to focus on the older person. As in previous editions, it is again not our purpose to prepare a subspecialty treatise but rather to emphasize the care of the older person. Throughout the United States and Great Britain and around the world, government agencies, research institutions, and professional societies are all busily preparing clinical guidelines, protocols, and parameters for daily practice. Are the guidelines sensitive to the clinical and psychosocial needs of the older patient? Are special clinical aspects of care of the young-old, middle-old, and old-old being considered in formulating guidelines or parameters of care for a problem? For example, in approaching the problem of breast cancer in older patients, what guidelines should be used for radiotherapy following breast-conserving treatment, tamoxifen after surgery, or adjuvant chemotherapy in the older woman, and especially in the very frail? In the management of depression in the elderly, do we have sufficient understanding of the variegated presentations of depression in older persons, and do we know how to treat these various types? It should be recognized that textbooks have always represented the best opinion of guidelines in clinical practice. This text attempts to focus on the special clinical aspects in the care of elders, and contains concise, practical guidelines for the use of the generalist physician and other health professionals in caring for the older patient.

As in previous editions, we want to promote health care for the elderly that would mirror the health care that we will want for ourselves as we join their ranks. We again focus on compassion and respect, continuity of care, health maintenance and disease prevention, and communication skills and the doctor-elderly patient relationship. The book emphasizes the integration of the biopsychosocial model; working with family members or caregivers; excellence of care in nursing facilities and in alternatives to institutionalization; and complex ethical decision-making.

As we approach the end of the decade and the beginning of a new millennium, it is apparent that there are many challenges, such as the continuing rapid expansion of new information in diagnosis and management, and the need to be concerned that newly promulgated clinical practice guidelines address the needs of the older person. The most daunting challenge will be the existence of new information from molecular genetics, biotechnology, and the Human Genome Project, which will affect the practitioner's everyday experience, as better and better genetic screening tests identify those at risk for breast cancer, colon cancer, syndrome X, Alzheimer's disease, Huntington's disease, and many other disorders. One can envision earlier identification of those at risk for illnesses or disorders seen in older persons, identification as early as in the prenatal period, and the development of effective preventive as well as therapeutic interventions. It will be certain that this will markedly affect all medical practice, and will be an important part of the Fifth Edition.

It is hoped that this volume will enhance the practitioner's ability to understand and integrate all aspects of the health care of the older person.

William Reichel, M.D.

Acknowledgments

I am very grateful for the time, energy, and expertise contributed to this new edition by the four Associate Editors and the eight members of the Editorial Board. Their wisdom and enthusiastic hard work made this a better book with a higher standard of peer review than in previous editions.

It has been a pleasure to continue to work with members of the Williams & Wilkins editorial family who have provided support, enthusiasm, and guidance at every step along the way. I am especially grateful to Jonathan W. Pine, Jr., David Retford, and Molly L. Mullen. Their encouragement and suggestions have made the Fourth Edition a better book for the 90s. Since the First Edition in 1978, Williams & Wilkins has always shared in the vision of this multidimensional book on all aspects of aging and health care of the aged.

I want to thank four others for their review or conceptualization of portions of this book: Paula M. Minahan, M.S.W., M.P.H., of Boston; Julie Glowacki, Ph.D., of Boston; Joanne G. Schwartzberg, M.D., of Chicago; and Andrew A. White, M.D., M.A., of Beverly, Massachusetts.

Finally I want to thank Patricia L. Lynch of Tufts University School of Medicine and Barbara A. Malloy of Memorial Hospital of Rhode Island for their technical assistance. I am most grateful to June K. Harner of Boston for her masterful technical and administrative efforts in bringing the book to completion.

William Reichel, M.D.

Editorial Board

Contributors

Marilyn Adlin, M.D.
Assistant Professor
Department of Medicine
Section of Geriatrics and Gerontology
University of Wisconsin-Madison
Madison, Wisconsin

Elizabeth A. Alexander, M.D., M.S.
Professor and Associate Chair of Clinical Affairs
Department of Family Practice
College of Human Medicine
Michigan State University
East Lansing, Michigan

April L. Allison, M.A., M.P.H.
Research Associate
Department of Family Medicine
College of Medicine
Michigan State University
East Lansing, Michigan

Lodovico Balducci, M.D.
Professor of Medicine and Program Leader
Senior Adult Oncology Program
H. Lee Moffitt Cancer Center and Research Institute
University of South Florida College of Medicine
Tampa, Florida

Patricia P. Barry, M.D., M.P.H.
Associate Professor of Medicine
Chief, Geriatrics Section
Director, Home Medical Service
Boston University School of Medicine
Boston, Massachusetts

Bruce E. Beacham, M.S., M.D., F.A.C.P.
Clinical Associate Professor
Department of Dermatology
University of Maryland School of Medicine
Consultant in Dermatology
Department of Internal Medicine
Franklin Square Hospital Center
Baltimore, Maryland

B. Lynn Beattie, M.D., F.R.C.P. (C)
Professor and Head, Division of Geriatric Medicine
Department of Medicine
Vancouver Hospital and Health Sciences Center
University of British Columbia
Faculty of Medicine
Vancouver, British Columbia
Canada

Michele Frances Bellantoni, M.D.
Assistant Professor
Department of Medicine
Division of Geriatric Medicine & Gerontology
The Johns Hopkins University School of Medicine
Baltimore, Maryland

Patricia Lanoie Blanchette, M.D., M.P.H.
Professor of Medicine and Public Health
Chief, Division of Geriatric Medicine
Director, Pacific Islands Geriatric Center
John A. Burns School of Medicine
University of Hawaii at Manoa
Honolulu, Hawaii

Louis C. Breschi, M.D.
Consultant in Urology
Department of Surgery
Franklin Square Hospital Center
Baltimore, Maryland

John J. Brink, Ph.D.
Professor and Chairman
Department of Biology
Clark University
Worcester, Massachusetts

Jan Busby-Whitehead, M.D.
Associate Professor of Internal Medicine
Program on Aging
University of North Carolina
School of Medicine
Chapel Hill, North Carolina

Mary C. Ciotti, M.D.
Associate Professor
Department of Obstetrics, Gynecology, & Reproductive
  Biology
Michigan State University
East Lansing, Michigan

Jacob Climo, Ph.D.
Professor
Department of Anthropology
Michigan State University
East Lansing, Michigan

Elise M. Coletta, M.D.
Assistant Professor
Department of Family Medicine
Brown University School of Medicine
Chief of Gerontology
Department of Geriatrics & Rehabilitation
Memorial Hospital of Rhode Island
Pawtucket, Rhode Island

Dorothy H. Coons, B.S.
Research Associate
Institute of Gerontology
Associate Professor Emeritus
The University of Michigan, Ann Arbor
Formerly, Director, Alzheimer's Disease Project
    on Subjective Experiences of Families and
Director, Alzheimer's Disease Project
    on Environmental Intervention
Ann Arbor, Michigan

John Delfs, M.D.
Director, Deaconess Center for ElderCare
Chief, Section of Geriatric Medicine
Department of Medicine
New England Deaconess Hospital
Assistant Professor
Department of Medicine
Harvard Medical School
Boston, Massachusetts

Adrian S. Dobs, M.D., M.H.S.
Associate Professor of Medicine
Division of Endocrinology
The Johns Hopkins University School of Medicine
Baltimore, Maryland

David J. Doukas, M.D.
Assistant Professor
Department of Family Practice
University of Michigan Medical School
Ann Arbor, Michigan

Jay S. Duker, M.D.
Associate Professor of Ophthalmology
Director, Vitreoretinal Service
New England Eye Center
New England Medical Center
Tufts University School of Medicine
Boston, Massachusetts

Johanna Dwyer, D.Sc, R.D.
Professor Department of Medicine
Tufts University School of Medicine
U.S.D.A. Human Nutrition Research Center on Aging
Director, Frances Stern Nutrition Center
Boston, Massachusetts

John K. Erban, M.D.
Assistant Professor of Medicine
Division of Hematology/Oncology
Department of Medicine
Director, Medical Oncology Breast Cancer Program
New England Medical Center
Tufts University School of Medicine
Boston, Massachusetts

John A. Flynn, M.D.
Assistant Professor of Medicine/Rheumatology
The Johns Hopkins University School of Medicine
Baltimore, Maryland

Joseph H. Friedman, M.D.
Chief, Division of Neurology
Roger Williams Medical Center
Professor, Department of Clinical
Neurosciences (Neurology)
Director, Brown University Parkinson's
Disease & Movement Disorder Unit
Brown University School of Medicine
Providence, Rhode Island

Joseph J. Gallo, M.D., M.P.H.
Assistant Professor
Department of Mental Hygiene
The Johns Hopkins University School of Hygiene and
    Public Health
Baltimore, Maryland

Steven R. Gambert, M.D.
Professor of Medicine and Gerontology
Associate Dean for Academic Programs
New York Medical College
Valhalla, New York

R. I. Garcia, D.M.D.
Director, VA Dental Longitudinal Study
Department of Veterans Affairs Outpatient Clinic
Associate Research Professor
Department of Oral Pathology and Medicine
Tufts University School of Dental Medicine
Boston, Massachusetts

Lisa N. Geller, Ph.D.
Instructor
Department of Neurobiology
Harvard Medical School
Boston, Massachusetts

Marjorie Harvey Glassman, L.I.C.S.W., O.T.R.
Consultant in Gerontology
Boston, Massachusetts

John C. Gordon, M.D.
Consultant in Orthopedics
Franklin Square Hospital Center and St. Joseph
    Hospital
Baltimore, Maryland

David S. Greer, M.D.
Dean of Medicine Emeritus
Professor
Department of Community Health
Brown University School of Medicine
Providence, Rhode Island

Geoffrey Habershaw, D.P.M.
Chief
Section of Podiatry
New England Deaconess Hospital
Clinical Instructor
Department of Surgery
Harvard Medical School
Boston, Massachusetts

Alan W. Hackford, M.D.
Chief, Section of Colon & Rectal Surgery
New England Medical Center Hospital
Associate Professor of Surgery
Tufts University School of Medicine
Boston, Massachusetts

Warren L. Holleman, Ph.D.
Assistant Professor, Department of Family Medicine
Assistant Professor, Center for Ethics, Medicine, and
   Public Issues
Baylor College of Medicine
Houston, Texas

Renee Hollison
Research Assistant
Division of Geriatric Medicine
John A. Burns School of Medicine
University of Hawaii at Manoa
Honolulu, Hawaii

Anne L. Hume, Pharm.D.
Associate Professor
College of Pharmacy
University of Rhode Island
Adjunct Associate Professor
Department of Family Medicine
Brown University School of Medicine
Memorial Hospital of Rhode Island
Pawtucket, Rhode Island

Gerald J. Jogerst, M.D.
Assistant Professor
Department of Family Practice
University of Iowa
Iowa City, Iowa

Susan W. Lehmann, M.D.
Assistant Professor
Department of Psychiatry and Behavioral Sciences
The Johns Hopkins University School of Medicine
Baltimore, Maryland

Steven A. Levenson, M.D., C.M.D.
Director of Medical Services
Asbury Methodist Village
Gaithersburg, Maryland

Victoria Y. Louie, M.Sc., R.D.N.
Consultant Dietitian
Royal Arch Masonic Home
Columbus Residence
Vancouver, British Columbia
Canada

Thomas E. Lyons, D.P.M.
Clinical Instructor
Department of Surgery
Harvard Medical School
Department of Surgery/Podiatry
New England Deaconess Hospital
Boston, Massachusetts

Ian Maddocks, M.D., F.R.A.C.P., D.T.M.& H.
Professor of Palliative Care
The Palliative Care Unit
Flinders University of South Australia
Adelaide, South Australia

Rex L. Mahnensmith, M.D.
Associate Professor of Medicine
Clinical Director of Nephrology
Yale University School of Medicine
New Haven, Connecticut

Cynthia Mattox, M.D.
Assistant Professor
Department of Ophthalmology
New England Eye Center
New England Medical Center
Tufts University School of Medicine
Boston, Massachusetts

Laurence B. McCullough, Ph.D.
Professor of Medicine, Community Medicine, and
   Medical Ethics
Center for Ethics, Medicine, and Public Issues
Baylor College of Medicine
Houston, Texas

Thomas D. McRae, M.D.
Director of Education
Division of Geriatrics
Department of Internal Medicine
New York University School of Medicine
Chief, Geriatrics Clinic
Bellevue Hospital Center
New York, New York

Brian Merrick, M.S.W., L.I.C.S.W.
Senior Social Work Gerontologist
Deaconess ElderCare
New England Deaconess Hospital
Boston, Massachusetts

Kenneth Minaker, M.D., F.R.C.P. (C)
Associate Professor of Medicine
Division on Aging
Harvard Medical School
Director
Brockton/West Roxbury Division of the Boston Area
   Geriatric Research, Education and Clinical Center
Associate Director
Clinical Research Center
Beth Israel Hospital
Boston, Massachusetts

Vincent Mor, Ph.D.
Director, Center for Gerontology and Health
Care Research
Department of Community Health
Brown University
Providence, Rhode Island

Arthur J. Moss, M.D.
Professor of Medicine
University of Rochester School of Medicine &
 Dentistry
Rochester, New York

John B. Murphy, M.D.
Associate Professor
Department of Family Medicine
Brown University School of Medicine
Memorial Hospital of Rhode Island
Pawtucket, Rhode Island

Ted D. Nirenberg, Ph.D.
Director
Substance Abuse Treatment Center
Roger Williams Medical Center
Associate Professor of Psychiatry and Human
 Behavior
Brown University School of Medicine
Providence, Rhode Island

Richard A. Norton, M.D.
Professor of Medicine
Tufts University School of Medicine
Boston, Massachusetts

James G. O'Brien, M.D.
Professor and Senior Associate Chairman
Department of Family Practice
College of Medicine
Michigan State University
East Lansing, Michigan

Thomas F. O'Donnell, Jr., M.D.
Chief, Division of Vascular Surgery
Professor and Chairman
Department of Surgery
New England Medical Center
Tufts University School of Medicine
Boston, Massachusetts

Norma J. Owens, Pharm.D.
Associate Professor of Pharmacy Practice
College of Pharmacy
University of Rhode Island
Kingston, Rhode Island
Geriatric Clinical Pharmacy Consultant
Department of Pharmacy
Rhode Island Hospital
Providence, Rhode Island

Deborah N. Pearlman, Ph.D.
Research Fellow
Center for Gerontology & Health Care Research
Brown University
Providence, Rhode Island

Carmen A. Puliafito, M.D.
Professor and Chair of Ophthalmology
Director, New England Eye Center
New England Medical Center
Tufts University School of Medicine
Boston, Massachusetts

David L. Rabin, M.D., M.P.H.
Professor and Associate Chairman
Department of Family Medicine
Director
Division of Community Health Care Studies
Georgetown University School of Medicine
Washington, D.C.

Peter V. Rabins, M.D., M.P.H.
Professor of Psychiatry and Behavioral Sciences
The Johns Hopkins University School of Medicine
Baltimore, Maryland

William Rakowski, Ph.D.
Assistant Professor
Department of Community Health
Center for Gerontology and Health Care Research
Brown University
Providence, Rhode Island

Elias Reichel, M.D.
Assistant Professor
Department of Ophthalmology
New England Eye Center
New England Medical Center
Tufts University School of Medicine
Boston, Massachusetts

William Reichel, M.D.
Clinical Professor
Department of Community Health
Tufts University School of Medicine
Boston, Massachusetts
Adjunct Professor
Department of Family Medicine
Brown University School of Medicine
Memorial Hospital of Rhode Island
Pawtucket, Rhode Island

Rebecca B. Reilly, M.D.
Clinical Geriatrician
Internal Medicine Midwest
Omaha, Nebraska
Formerly, Fellow
Section on Geriatrics
Huffington Center on Aging
Baylor College of Medicine
Houston, Texas

Jill A. Rhymes, M.D.
Professor, Department of Medicine
Huffington Center on Aging
Baylor College of Medicine
Director, Geriatric Evaluation Unit
Department of Medicine
Houston VA Medical Center
Houston, Texas

Joel S. Schuman, M.D.
Associate Professor of Ophthalmology
New England Eye Center
New England Medical Center
Tufts University School of Medicine
Boston, Massachusetts

C. B. Sherman, M.D., M.P.H.
Director
Pulmonary Division
The Miriam Hospital
Assistant Professor
Department of Medicine
Brown University School of Medicine
Providence, Rhode Island

Rebecca A. Silliman, M.D., Ph.D.
Formerly Scientist, The Health Institute
New England Medical Center
Associate Professor of Medicine
Geriatrics Section
Boston University School of Medicine
Boston, Massachusetts

T. Skovrinski, M.D.
Staff Internist
Department of Internal Medicine
Florida Community Health Center
Fort Pierce, Florida
Formerly, Senior Medical Resident
The Miriam Hospital
Providence, Rhode Island

Laura Stanley, M.S., R.N., C.
Gerontological Nurse Practitioner
Deaconess ElderCare
New England Deaconess Hospital
Boston, Massachusetts

Michael D. Stein, M.D.
Assistant Professor
Department of Medicine
Brown University School of Medicine
Providence, Rhode Island

Thomas A. Teasdale, Dr. P.H.
Medical Statistician
Geriatrics and Extended Care Service
Veterans Affairs Medical Center
Department of Medicine and Huffington Center on
   Aging
Baylor College of Medicine
Houston, Texas

Roy Verdery, M.D., Ph.D.
Associate Professor of Medicine
Arizona Center on Aging
University of Arizona School of Medicine
Tucson, Arizona

Michael S. Vernon, M.D.
Associate Professor
Department of Family Medicine
Director, Geriatric Division
East Carolina University School of Medicine
Greenville, North Carolina

Tom J. Wachtel, M.D.
Physician-in-Charge
Division of Geriatrics
Rhode Island Hospital
Associate Professor of Community Health and
   Medicine
Brown University School of Medicine
Providence, Rhode Island

Gregg A. Warshaw, M.D.
Associate Professor
Department of Family Medicine
University of Cincinnati College of Medicine
Cincinnati, Ohio

Alan A. Wartenberg, M.D., F.A.C.P.
Medical Director
Addiction Recovery Program
Faulkner Hospital
Assistant Professor of Medicine
Tufts University School of Medicine
Boston, Massachusetts

Harold J. Welch, M.D.
Assistant Clinical Professor of Surgery
Uniformed Services
University of the Health Sciences
Bethesda, Maryland
Head, Division of Vascular Surgery
U.S. Naval Medical Center
Portsmouth, Virginia

Gilbert L. Wergowske, M.D.
Associate Professor of Medicine
Division of Geriatric Medicine
Associate Director
Pacific Islands Geriatric Education Center
John A. Burns School of Medicine
University of Hawaii at Manoa
Honolulu, Hawaii

Fredrick M. Wigley, M.D.
Associate Professor of Medicine
Director, Division of Rheumatology
The Johns Hopkins University School of Medicine
Baltimore, Maryland

Glenys O. Williams, M.D.
Professor, Department of Family Practice
College of Medicine
The University of Iowa
Iowa City, Iowa

Nancy L. Wilson, M.A., A.C.S.W.
Assistant Director for Program Development
Huffington Center on Aging
Baylor College of Medicine
Houston, Texas

Helen K. Wu, M.D.
Assistant Professor of Ophthalmology
New England Eye Center
New England Medical Center
Tufts University School of Medicine
Boston, Massachusetts

Joan Yesner, M.S.W., L.I.C.S.W.
Senior Social Work Gerontologist/Administrator
Deaconess ElderCare
New England Deaconess Hospital
Boston, Massachusetts

Milton G. Yoder, M.D., F.A.C.S.
Courtesy Staff
Clinical Instructor
Department of Otolaryngology and Head and Neck
  Surgery
The Johns Hopkins University School of Medicine
Baltimore, Maryland

Naomi E. Zack, M.S., R.N., C.
Gerontological Nurse Practitioner
ElderCare
New England Deaconess Hospital
Boston, Massachusetts

Contents

SECTION I

Care of the Elderly Patient
Evaluation, Diagnosis, and Management

SECTION II

Care of the Elderly Patient
Other Considerations

SECTION III ═══

Ethical Issues in the Elderly Patient

SECTION I

Care of the Elderly Patient
Evaluation, Diagnosis, and Management

1/ Essential Principles in the Care of the Elderly

William Reichel

A sign in a West Virginia lunch counter reads: "Don't criticize the coffee; you may be old and weak yourself someday."

As we all move forward as members of a longitudinal cohort into old age, we certainly want good health care waiting for us in our golden years. But what is good care?

ROLE OF PHYSICIAN AS INTEGRATOR OF BIOPSYCHOSOCIAL MODEL

With medical care becoming more complex and specialized and with greater reliance on technology, good care requires having a physician who provides leadership in the integration and coordination of the health care of the elderly patient. We have witnessed a century of increasing advances in research and great accomplishments in diagnostic and curative medicine, but today we are realizing that scientific reductionism is not enough. The reforms in medical education, care, and research that we have witnessed throughout this century have resulted in a tunnel vision of knowledge and skills about certain types of diseases and problems.

What society is calling out for is a physician with a commitment to the person, not just to a specific disease state or mechanism. The person is part of a family and a larger community, or sadly, there are elders who have no family and are isolated from the community. The first essential for the physician who cares for the elder is to act as an integrator of the biopsychosocial model (1, 2). To accomplish this, the physician must know the patient thoroughly. This is not to denigrate the excellence of the specialties and subspecialties that have achieved much over the past few decades. But ideal health care will exist when the patient is seen not from a single specialty point of view but with the full appreciation of other organ systems, emotional or psychosocial factors, information based on continuity over a period of time, and knowledge of the patient's family and community.

CONTINUITY OF CARE

The ideal situation is a warm and supportive relationship with the same personal physician serving as advisor, advocate, and friend as the patient moves through the labyrinth of medical care. It is unfortunate to see the many disruptions that take place in today's complex medical environment as the patient moves between office, home, hospital, specialized care units (coronary care units, intensive care units, stroke units, or oncology centers), and nursing home.

The failure of physicians to make visits as necessary in the home and in the long-term care facilities is related to several factors in the United States, including training, physician attitudes, and reimbursement systems. Our medical school and residencies for generalist physicians have been doing an increasingly better job of including the home and the nursing home as proper environments for medical education. The lack of reasonable reimbursement for visits to the home and nursing home remains a major problem. Physician attitudes have also been a problem, in that doctors in the health care system of the past few decades have been more interested in the acute aspects of care than in chronic and long-term care. These attitudes have been reinforced by the educational and reimbursement systems in place.

Wasson and associates (3) demonstrated that continuity of outpatient provider care for men aged 55 years and older resulted in more patient satisfaction, shorter hospitalizations, and fewer emergent hospital admissions. The carefully controlled study by Wasson et al. backs up, by vigorous research methodology, the value of continuity of care and its beneficial influence on medical care. In addition, one might envision improving critical care by having the same personal

3

physician involved with the total health care team in specialized units. Communicating the substance of the personal physician's knowledge and understanding of the patient to other specialists is an important function of the personal physician.

One might also anticipate that this role of continuity applies in general hospital care, in the home, and in the long-term care facility (4). Visits to the home and to the nursing home are absolutely indicated if we seek excellence in patient care of the elderly.

Many of our most serious problems in health care are related to failure in the continuity of care. With the population becoming increasingly older, with increasing specialization and emphasis on technology, and with the cost of care becoming very high, the greatest attention in the future must be given to the principle of continuity of care by a personal physician.

BOLSTERING FAMILY AND HOME

Every physician should enlist those means that would keep an elderly person either in the individual's own home or in an extended family setting. It should certainly be our goal as physicians to keep elderly persons functioning independently, preserving their lifestyles and self-respect as long as possible. The physician should use the prescription for a nursing home as specifically as a prescription for an antibiotic or an antihypertensive medication.

A number of forces have resulted in patients going to institutional settings when other alternatives might have been possible. Between 1960 and 1975, a massive push toward institutionalization took place, creating hundreds of thousands of nursing home beds. What forces contributed to excessive institutional care? Funding mechanisms have been directed solely toward reimbursement for institutional care rather than for other alternatives. With the increased mobility of families, there simply may not be family members available in the community to participate in the elderly person's care. Homes are architecturally based on a small, nuclear family and do not permit housing an elderly patient. Finally, the increasing movement of women into the work force has meant that fewer family members are available to remain home with the impaired or disabled elderly person.

What alternative can the physician recommend to these caregivers? A simple list includes homemakers, home health aides, other types of home care, day care, after care, specialized housing settings, visiting nurses, friendly visitors, foster home care, chore services, home renovation and repair services, congregate and home-delivered meal programs, transportation programs, and shopping services. Personal physicians should also understand and use legal and protective services for the elderly whenever indicated.

Who are the caregivers in American society? An examination of data from the 1982 National Long-Term Care Survey (5) revealed that caregivers to the disabled have the following characteristics: they are predominantly female; three-quarters of them live with the person for whom they provide care. One-third are themselves over 65 years old, poor or near-poor, and in fair-to-poor health. Some caregivers face conflicts between their caregiving duties and the needs of other family members and their jobs. Over 90% of the caregivers carry the burden without assistance from the formal health care system.

In the study by Stone et al. (5), 71.5% of caregivers to the functionally impaired elderly were female, daughters constituting 28.9%. Husbands accounted for 12.8% and sons for 8.5% of this population. In the case of sons, it is often the son's spouse, the daughter-in-law, who actually provides the care. The burden of caregiving is felt by many women today, sandwiched between the demands of their parents and of their children and grandchildren. It has been said that the empty nest syndrome has been replaced by a crowded nest syndrome. Many caregivers experience extreme burden and stress, and sometimes the question is, who is the real patient—the patient or the caregiver? The physician will often see the caregiver who is in more distress than the patient and in fact develops serious physical and emotional problems as a result of the burden and stress encountered.

The belief that old people are rejected by their families has been exploited as a social myth (6). Many families are struggling to cope with the needs of parents who are frail and debilitated. The family member, friend, or neighbor is often the crucial link in guaranteeing that the dependent elder will remain in the community. In repeated studies, the characteristics of the caregiver, more than those of the elderly patient, are essential considerations in predicting institutional placement.

Even when adult children and elderly parents are separated by distance, the quality of their relationship may be unaffected, with cohesion maintained despite limited face-to-face contact. At a certain distance, the telephone becomes an important means as a substitute for visits (7). Nevertheless, for many adult children, separation by distance causes increased tension and difficulty in their efforts to carry out the caregiver role. Family connectedness in the case of geographically distant older parents may be reduced to telephone communication, with visits for holidays, illness, or crisis (8).

Cost containment today, particularly in the prospective payment system, will require greater reliance on alternatives to institutional care. We can expect to see many new resources and support systems, including innovative experiments in housing and transportation, more home-delivered care, a cadre of respite workers, and perhaps tax credits for family-oriented care. Personal physicians can be significant advocates in their communities for the development of new resources and support systems to help keep elderly patients in their own homes or in the home of a family member. We can also expect to see increased educational media (television programs, brochures, books, and courses not only at local hospitals and long-term care facilities but also at the high school, community college, and university levels) that will provide information to the many families who are striving to keep an elderly member at home, either with spouse, with family, or alone.

COMMUNICATION SKILLS

Specific communication skills are critical in good management of the elderly patient. Most important in good communication is listening and allowing patients to express themselves. The physician should use an open-ended approach, interpreting what the patient is saying and reading between the lines. The physician can use intuition in deciding what the patient really means. Why did the patient really come to see the physician? The elderly patient complaining of headache or backache may be expressing depression or grief. We should not miss important verbal clues when the patient tells us, "Doctor, I really think these headaches started when I lost my husband."

It is helpful to leave the door open for other questions or comments by the patient, both at the conclusion of the visit and in the future. It is always helpful to say: "Are there other questions or concerns that you have at this time?" A physician anticipating a specific problem can make it easier for the patient to discuss this issue. For example, "You are doing well, but I know that you are concerned about your arthritis and whether or not you will be able to climb the stairs in your home. At some point, we may want to discuss the various alternatives that are open to you."

Just as the physician providing care to pediatric patients must deal with the children's parents, the physician providing care to the elderly patient must be able to deal with their adult children. These children play a vital role in decision making and providing support, and the physician must, therefore, possess skills in communicating with them and in dealing with their emotional reactions, such as guilt or grief. The physician taking care of an elderly patient with cancer must be prepared when the adult daughter tells him: "Whatever you do, please don't tell my father that he has cancer," especially when it is apparent that the parent is totally and fully aware of all aspects of his problem.

The physician should be careful when meeting with elderly patients who discuss an absent spouse or child or when dealing with adult children or grandchildren who are discussing the parent or grandparent who is not present. The physician should not necessarily accept the assumptions that are stated about the absent family member. Physicians must be able to listen carefully, ask questions, and collect information; our opinion of the situation might be entirely different if we had an opportunity to hear the view of the absent family member.

Peabody (9) in 1927 said: "The good physician knows his patients through and through, and his knowledge is bought dearly. Time, sympathy and understanding must be lavishly dispensed, but the reward is to be found in that personal bond which forms the greatest satisfaction of the practice of medicine." The physician who enters the patient's universe and understands the patient's perceptions, assumptions, values, and religious beliefs has a tremendous advantage. Frankl (10) in *Man's Search for Meaning*, demonstrated how physicians can help patients understand the meaning and value of their lives. Of course how elders find meaning in their lives is related to how they found meaning at other stages in their lives. It is therapeutic for patients to feel that the physician cares enough about them to understand their lives, particularly the meaning and purposes of their present existence. Frankl (11) stated in *The Doctor and the Soul* that human life can be fulfilled not only in creating and enjoying but also in suffering. He provides examples in which suffering becomes an opportunity for growth, an achievement, a means for ennoblement. Frankl's existential psychiatry, or logotherapy, is a useful psychological method that helps elderly patients appreciate the positive attributes, meanings, and purposes of their lives.

Yalom (12) defines existential psychotherapy as "a dynamic approach to therapy which focuses on concerns that are rooted in the individual's existence." Many individuals are tormented by a crisis of meaning (13). Many suffer an existential vacuum, experiencing a lack of meaning in life (10–14). The patient experiencing an existential vacuum may demonstrate many symptoms that will rush in to fill it in the form of somatization, depression, alcoholism, and hypochondriasis. The physician recognizing an existential vacuum can help the patient find meaning. Frankl's main theme is that meaning is essential for life. Engagement or involvement in life's activities is a therapeutic answer to a lack of meaning in life. The physician can help guide the patient toward engagement with life, life's activities, other people, and other satisfactions.

Frankl (10, 11) provides advice to all physicians in using hope as a therapeutic tool. The physician dealing with the elderly must focus on the significant role of hope in daily practice. As physicians, we must eventually understand the biologic basis of hope. We do not understand sufficiently the biochemical, neurophysiologic, and immunologic concomitants of different attitudes and emotions and how they are affected by what is communicated from the physician. Physicians have an opportunity to worsen panic and fear; physicians also have an opportunity to create a state of confidence, calm, relaxation, and hope.

In this day and age of increasing technology and subspecialization, the patient's recovery may still depend on the physician's ability to reduce panic and fear and to raise the prospect of hope. Cousins (15) describes the "quality beyond pure medical competence that patients need and look for in their physicians. They want reassurance. They want to be looked after and not just over. They want to be listened to. They want to feel that it makes a difference to the physician, a very big difference, whether they live or die. They want to feel that they are in the physician's thoughts." For example, in building the doctor–elderly patient relationship, nothing is more effective than the physician picking up the phone and calling the patient and saying: "I was thinking about your problem. How are you doing?" This expression of interest by telephone is a potent way to cement the relationship of doctor and patient.

Jules Pfeiffer's cartoon character the "modern Diogenes" carries on the following discourse upon meeting an inquisitive fellow traveler through the sands of time. "What are you doing with the lantern?" asks the traveler. "I'm searching," replies Diogenes. "For an honest man?" he asks. "I gave

that up long ago!" exclaims Diogenes. "For hope?" "Lots of luck." "For love?" "Forget it!" "For tranquility?" "No way." "For happiness?" "Fat chance." "For justice?" "Are you kidding?" "Then what are you looking for?" he implores of Diogenes. "Someone to talk to."

DOCTOR-PATIENT RELATIONSHIP

WHAT THE DOCTOR AND PATIENT BRING TO EACH ENCOUNTER

Physicians must understand what both they and the patient bring to each interaction, including both positive and negative feelings (16). The patient's views of old age may be negative and fearful, believing illness signifies misery, approaching death, loss of self-esteem, loneliness, and dependency. The physician's own fears about aging and death may color the interview as well. The doctor may simply not view helping the older, impaired patient as worthwhile. The physician may have low expectations for success of treatment, writing off the elderly patient as "senile," "mentally ill," or "hypochondriac." Doctors may have significant conflicts in their own relationships with parent figures or may feel threatened that the patient will die.

KNOWING THE PATIENT

Several steps recommended in building a sound doctor-patient relationship are particularly applicable to the elderly patient (9, 16). The first rule is that the physician should know the patient thoroughly; the second rule is that the physician should know the patient thoroughly; and the third rule is that the physician should know the patient thoroughly. The interested physician performs the first step in building a sound doctor-patient relationship by gathering a complete history, including the personal and social history, and doing a complete physical examination. Ideally, the physician should be a good listener, warm and sensitive, providing patients with ample opportunity to express multiple problems and reflect upon their life history and current life situation. Thus, the physician will be able to understand the meanings and purposes of the patient's present existence.

As stated above, family and friends represent the principal support system for the elderly and usually call for nursing home placement only as a last resort, after all alternatives have failed. However, the physician must be able to recognize the dysfunctional family. There are elderly who have been rejected by children. Like King Lear, these elderly may say: "How sharper than a serpent's tooth, it is to have a thankless child." There are elderly who have rejected a child for a variety of reasons. There are families with members estranged from each other for many years. The physician should understand what has happened over the years in the patient's marriage. Before the physician can hope to help families with such problems, it is important to recognize first that these problems exist.

CREATING A PARTNERSHIP WITH THE PATIENT

In all dealings with patients, physicians should be frank and honest and share information truthfully. Patients should feel a sense of partnership with the physician. In this partnership, the doctor first reviews his or her perception of the patient's problems. Then, for each problem, alternative choices are considered, and decision making is shared with the patient. Although there are situations in which frankness is counterproductive, with most patients, frankness is helpful. There are also situations in which elderly patients do not want to share in decision making, but simply want to surrender their autonomy to a relative such as spouse or adult child, or to the physician. Again, in most cases, the physician should attempt to enter a partnership with the patient and share as much decision making as possible.

Discussions with the patient or family members should be presented in a hopeful manner. As discussed above, it is important to offer a positive approach whenever possible. The physician's infusion of optimism and cheerfulness is therapeutic. The physician should help patients appreciate such positive attributes or purposes in their lives as religious beliefs, relationships with children and grandchildren, the enjoyment of friends, or the enjoyment of the relationship with doctors, nurses, and other health professionals in the immediate therapeutic environment.

The physician should be careful to hold discussions with family members with the patient's consent. If the patient is significantly mentally impaired, then it might be appropriate to deal with the closest relative. Complex ethical questions arise concerning confidentiality and decision making in regard to the elderly patient with partial mental impairment.

NEED FOR THOROUGH EVALUATION AND ASSESSMENT

The physician must avoid prejudging the patient. We must not allow preconceived notions of common patterns of illness to preclude the most careful individualized assessment of each patient. Conscientious history and physical examination are essential. Treatment choices should be considered only following a thorough evaluation. Judicious consideration of all factors may result in a decision to treat or not to treat certain problems in certain patients. Attention to lesser problems may be postponed according to the priorities of the moment, rather than complicate an already variegated therapeutic program.

Physicians must avoid "wastebasket" diagnoses. The past concept of "chronic brain syndrome" or "arteriosclerotic brain disease" is one such example. Not all mental disturbance in the elderly represents dementia; not all dementias in the elderly are arteriosclerotic. Neuropsychiatric disturbance in the elderly might be placed into a wastebasket and casually accepted as both expectable and untreatable when, in reality, a very treatable cause may be present. The physician must consider and seek out treatable disease.

The most common types of dementia include Alzheimer's disease and vascular dementia. There are other forms of dementia, some very treatable, including myxedema, chronic drug intoxication, pernicious anemia, folic acid deficiency, and chronic subdural hematoma. Neuropsychiatric disturbance may also include delirium or acute confusional state secondary to many types of medical illness or drug toxicity. Such delirious states can be helped if the primary disorder is recognized and treated.

It is often difficult to disentangle the physical from the emotional. For example, neuropsychiatric disturbance may be caused by severe depression that is a very treatable disorder. Emotional disorder may present in the elderly as a physical problem, such as musculoskeletal tension being the principal manifestation of depression. Conversely, physical disease in the elderly might present as a mental disorder with confusion, disorientation, or delirium often being the first sign of many common medical ailments including myocardial infarction, pulmonary embolism, occult carcinomatosis, pneumonia, urinary tract infection, or dehydration (Table 1.1).

Thus, it cannot be emphasized too many times that proper diagnosis is essential in making specific treatment plans, such as the treatment of urinary tract infection in the case of an acute delirious state, the treatment of folic acid deficiency in the case of a specific dementia, or the treatment of depression. Each of these is very specific. Treatment in each case would be irrational if a specific diagnosis were not known.

Table 1.1
Characteristics of Elderly Patients

1. Multiple organic, psychological, and social problems are present.
2. Functional or physiological capacities are diminished, e.g., creatinine clearance declines with age.
3. Adverse effects of drugs are more pronounced and more likely.
4. Physical disease might present as a mental disorder, with confusion, disorientation, or delirium often being the first sign of many common medical ailments.
5. Typical signs and symptoms of disease may be hidden or slight, e.g., pain may be absent in myocardial infarction, fever may be minimal in pneumonia.

It is often not sufficient to know the organic, anatomic or psychiatric diagnosis; rather we should seek a more total understanding of the elderly patient. At times, it is more important to assess the elderly patient's functional status, which might have greater significance than the diagnostic or anatomic label. For example, in the case of a cerebrovascular accident, knowledge of the exact anatomic location as determined by arteriography may not help the patient as much as understanding the patient's functional state. It may be more important to know whether the patient can walk or climb stairs; can handle bathing, eating, and dressing; can get out of bed and sit in a chair; can handle a wheelchair; or requires a cane or walker. All these functional concerns must be considered in evaluating an elderly patient.

Our diagnostic thinking in evaluating an elderly patient is affected by consideration of what is physiologic versus what is pathologic. Aging itself can be defined as the progressive deterioration or loss of functional capacity, which takes place in an organism after a period of reproductive maturity (Table 1.1). The Baltimore Longitudinal Study of Aging since 1958 has studied this decline in each of several specific functional capacities, such as glucose tolerance and creatinine clearance. There is a progressive deterioration of glucose tolerance with each decade of life. Indeed, hyperglycemia is so common in the elderly that to avoid labeling a disquietly high proportion of people as diabetics, Elahi, Clark, and Andres (17) formulated a percentile system that ranks a subject with age-matched cohorts. (Some individuals, however, show no evidence of deterioration of glucose tolerance or insulin tolerance to glucose with aging.) Although currently the accepted definitions allow the same diagnostic criteria to be applied at any age, it is often unclear who is truly diabetic. The rate of decline in creatinine clear-

ance also accelerates with advancing age (18). This phenomenon appears to represent true renal aging because it was seen in several hundred normal individuals who were free of specific diseases and not taking medications that might alter glomerular filtration rate. The physician must not be quick in treating a laboratory value that may simply represent an altered physiologic state and not a true disease or pathologic disorder.

Increased adverse effects of drugs are present in the elderly who often tolerate medications poorly (Table 1.1). Polypharmacy is a major problem in the care of the elderly patient. Not only do psychotropic medications cause an altered CNS response resulting in confusion and delirium, but also antibiotics or digitalis may cause these problems. Altered renal and hepatic functions may affect drug elimination. In general, the elderly demonstrate greater variability and idiosyncrasy in drug response than do younger individuals.

Prudence is, therefore, extremely important in prescribing drugs for the elderly individual. The physician must determine if the patient's complaint is justification for treatment. Is this medication absolutely necessary? The skill of the physician is required in weighing benefit versus risk. The benefit-risk balance is more crucial in the elderly patient than in younger individuals. The physician must attempt to keep the total number of medications down to as few as possible.

Also affecting our diagnostic ability in the elderly is that signs and symptoms of disease in the aged may be slight or hidden. Pain, white blood cell response, and fever and chills are examples of defense mechanisms that may be diminished in older persons (Table 1.1). The aged person may have pneumonia or renal infection without chills or a rise in temperature. Myocardial infarction, ruptured abdominal aorta, perforated appendix, or mesenteric infarction may be present without pain in the elderly (19).

Multiple clinical, psychological, and social problems (Table 1.1) are characteristic of the elderly (19). Clinically and pathologically, an elderly patient may have 10 or 15 problems (20). Geriatric patients should benefit from the use of a problem-oriented approach to medical records. Medical records should include not only the medical problem, but should demonstrate an understanding of functional, psychological, social, and family problems as well. The key feature of the problem-oriented record is the problem list, which serves as a table of contents of the patient's total medical history. It behooves us to use a problem list as a minimal or core component of a problem-oriented system in caring for the elderly patient. Without a problem list, we can easily lose track over time of the elderly patient's multiple problems; for example, that the patient was hospitalized in 1953 for a psychiatric problem or that in 1975, the patient suffered a compression fracture of the T10 vertebra secondary to slipping on ice. These problems may be lost to memory without some form of problem-oriented system. In addition, care is enhanced by maintaining a medication list that is kept current at each patient visit.

PREVENTION AND HEALTH MAINTENANCE

A tremendous revolution is taking place in the United States, with emphasis on prevention, health maintenance, and wellness. Unfortunately, not all the facts are in. For example, less is known about risk factors for heart disease and stroke for the elderly patient than for younger adults. However, enough is known about prevention that we are seeing a decline in the mortality rate from heart disease and cerebrovascular disease, which probably relates to increased preventive measures.

More and more physicians and nurses are emphasizing health maintenance and wellness in their practices and in their community educational programs. However, the drive for wellness is coming not only from the health professionals, but also from the public itself. Personal physicians have an opportunity in their practices to encourage preventive medicine and health maintenance at every age level and at each level of functional ability or disability.

A remarkable amount of new information is being discovered about the role of exercise and strength training in the prevention or reversibility of frailty and physiologic decline (21–23). It is expected that more will be learned and that the health of many elderly will be improved by exercise and physical activity.

How do physicians and health professionals determine the standard for health screening and health promotion? The *Guide to Clinical Preventive Services* (24) has represented a "gold standard" for health screening guidelines. But each practicing physician will have to follow the medical literature and evaluate the algorithms and guidelines that unfold in the decade ahead. How valuable are prostate screening antigen and ultrasound examinations in screening for carcinoma of the prostate in the elderly? What should the physician's response be to different levels of elevated total and LDL cholesterol and reduced HDL cholesterol in the elderly? How often should we be performing Papanicolau smears and mammogra-

phy on women 75 years and older who are residents in nursing homes? And in the office, what should our response be to the woman 75 years of age and older who refuses a gynecologic examination and mammography?

We can expect that it will require some time before we have algorithms or guidelines that are absolutely certain. We can expect that in each area of health screening and health promotion, our guidelines will not be written in stone, but will be reconsidered and reevaluated in the years ahead. Physicians and health professionals caring for the elderly will participate in the dynamic tension and debate that will continue in reaching a consensus on these questions. But at any time, with the state of knowledge that we do have in preventive medicine and health screening, there remains the differential between the physician's intellectual acceptance and awareness of these guidelines and the actual use of these guidelines on a regular, consistent basis.

A final note on measures to enhance health in the aging patient. Not only the community-based elder but (as stated above) even frail patients in nursing homes will benefit from strength training and exercise. The next decade will see more advances in nutrition, therapeutic measures to retard the aging process, and exercise, and we can expect that we can witness not only adding years to life but adding life to years.

INTELLIGENT TREATMENT WITH ATTENTION TO ETHICAL DECISION MAKING

The doctor should resist the temptation to treat a new problem that is poorly understood with still more medications. The question should be raised whether the present symptoms, such as confusion or depression, might be related to current drug use.

Therefore, the aphorism "First, do no harm." A similar concept was stated by Seegal (25) as the "principle of minimal interference" in the management of the elderly patient. "First, do no harm" and the "principle of minimal interference" should be remembered when one reviews the abundant examples of iatrogenic problems that the elderly experience (26, 27).

The principle of minimal interference can be applied not only to drug therapy, but to other decisions, including the use of diagnostic tests (the principle of diagnostic parsimony), surgical intervention, and decision making in regard to hospitalization or placement in a long-term care facility. The principle of minimal interference may result in decisions that are both humanistic and cost-effective; for example, a decision that the patient should remain at home, despite limited access to medical therapy, rather than reside in a long-term care facility; or the decision not to do a gastrointestinal workup in the evaluation of anemia when the patient is preterminal as a result of malignant brain tumor.

In the care of the elderly, there are times for minimal interference and there are times for maximal intervention. Again, certainly the patient with dementia caused by myxedema deserves every effort to replace thyroid hormone carefully. Elderly patients with severe congestive heart failure secondary to rheumatic or congenital heart disease deserve full consideration for definitive treatment, including surgery, for their cardiac problems. Elderly patients with depression deserve specific treatment for this very treatable disorder.

In the future, we will be faced with more and more difficult decisions of an ethical nature (see Section III, Ethical Issues in the Elderly Patient). For example, an 80-year-old man may present with a past history of resection of an abdominal aneurysm in 1980, multiple myocardial infarctions, and multiple strokes causing severe dementia. His main problem on the current hospitalization is pneumonia causing a worsening of his confused state. Because of periods of sinus arrest, a pacemaker is considered. Should a pacemaker be used in patients with significant dementia? Should pneumonia be treated in patients with severe dementia or terminal carcinoma? Difficult and ambiguous clinical problems such as these will face the personal physician with increasing frequency. The physician in the future will be called upon to make complex decisions according to the accepted traditions and values of the specific religion, nation, and society or culture, with major guidance from the patient's stated wishes, affirmed when the patient was fully competent. Section III of this text attempts to deal with the ethical dilemmas we face in daily practice in caring for the elderly.

In regard to all therapeutic decisions, personal physicians are at an advantage if their understanding of the patient is based on continuity of care. The physician then can consider the patient in totality including psychological, social, family, and environmental factors. To recommend intelligently any treatment plan, it is beneficial to know about the home or institutional environment, the family constellation, the availability of friends, access to transportation, and the economic situation of the patient. Also, as the physician grapples with complex decisions of an eth-

ical nature, specific knowledge of the patient's value systems and beliefs is critically important. Chapter 62 describes in detail the importance of eliciting a Values History from patients, not only when they are terminally ill, but during the entire doctor-elderly patient relationship.

INTERDISCIPLINARY COLLABORATION

The physician must understand when to call upon other health professionals. One must know when to call upon visiting home nurses, social workers, psychologists, or representatives of community agencies. One must know when to call for legal or financial counseling. All physicians would do well to work in closer harmony with the patient's or family's clergyman or pastor.

The physician should know when to recommend specific rehabilitative therapies. Specific use of physical, occupational, recreational, and speech therapies is vital for the proper care of certain problems. For example, the elderly patient with diabetic neuropathy and flapping gait might benefit from bilateral leg braces. Patients recovering from stroke might benefit from occupational therapy that reintroduces them to the activities of normal daily living and is not simply recreational or diversionary.

The improvement of health care of the chronically ill elderly requires that health professionals work together for the best interest of the patient. What is required is a genuine collaborative effort to act in a unified fashion to bring about a system that will best meet the needs of the frail elderly.

RESPECT FOR THE USEFULNESS AND VALUE OF THE AGED INDIVIDUAL

Much in our society works to reject or devalue the aged. We are certainly living in a youth-oriented era, and a physician must guard against viewing the elderly as useless, insignificant, or worthless. This lack of respect and devaluation occurs in society at large, in the work place, in the family, and in the entertainment media, but it should not occur in the doctor's office or other clinical settings. The anthropologist knows other cultures and societies where the elders of the community are most valued. An hour of watching American television reveals the youth orientation of our society. It is unfortunate that many elderly patients report that previous physicians treated them poorly because they were old.

An exceptional book, not actively directed to the elderly, but one that should be in the curriculum of medical students and residents, is *Respectful Treatment: A Practical Handbook of Pa-*

tient Care (28). The author, Martin Lipp, describes the therapeutic benefit of respect in the doctor-patient relationship, especially in dealing with those we consider problem patients: the angry patient; the dependent, passive patient; the complaining, demanding patient; the denying patient; the overly affectionate patient; the mentally ill patient; etc. Respect is therapeutic. Many patients feel weak and vulnerable, and they demonstrate low self-esteem by virtue of age, illness, and various psychological and personality factors. Respect is a message to the patient that quickly brings about a more sound doctor-patient relationship.

Discussions are held on the subject of calling patients, and elderly patients in particular, by their first names or by their last names preceded by Mr., Mrs., or Ms. An immediate demonstration of respect is calling elderly patients by their family names, with Mr., Mrs., or Ms. used appropriately.

We hope the next 20 years will bring considerable social change with redefinition of the age for retirement and many other social and economic changes that will allow the elderly to function as a continuing resource in our society. We can expect to see reduced restrictions on older workers, with particular reference to mandatory retirement. We can also expect to see more educational programs that will provide skilled training, job counseling, and placement for older men and women to initiate, enhance, and continue their voluntary participation in the work force. We should anticipate the breakdown of stereotypes and greater recognition of the value of the elderly as a human resource.

COMPASSIONATE CARE

In an increasingly technologic society, caring and compassion must be foremost in the practice of medicine. We must avoid the possible dehumanization that takes place when patients simply become subjects for study and treatment. Every year in the United States, we are seeing new accomplishments in medical technology and specialization. Computerized tomography, computerized nuclear medicine, magnetic resonance imaging, positron emission tomography (PET), organ transplants, achievements in cardiovascular surgery, achievements in hemodialysis, and achievement in intensive and critical care—all these are becoming part of our routine medical environment. In such a new medical world, it is imperative that compassionate care not be lost in daily encounters between health professionals and elderly patients.

In all the great religions, various forms of a Golden Rule are stated; many religions teach: "You must love your neighbor as you do yourself," and, "What you do not want done to yourself, do not do to others." Surpassing new technical achievements and new specialized knowledge is the need to express compassion (29). The physician's duty is "to cure sometimes . . . to comfort always."

Critically important is the attitude of the doctor toward the elderly patient. Is the physician willing to spend time with the patient? Is the physician willing to be involved in the chronic and long-term aspects of the patient as well as in the acute illness? Is the physician concerned with the social, psychological, and family aspects of the patient, in addition to clinical and organic aspects?

Care and compassion mean that physicians must dispense sufficient time in their encounters with elderly patients. There is actually evidence in one study (30) that physicians spend less time with elderly patients than with younger ones. Fifteen to 20 minutes may be minimal time to carry out a visit in the office, home, hospital, or long-term care facility. One and one-half hours, not necessarily in one sitting, may be required to complete an examination of a new patient, particularly one with multiple complex problems. More time will be required in each encounter if the various functions of counseling, psychological support, health maintenance, and prevention are to be carried out in addition to making decisions about treatment and possible rehabilitation.

Examples of failure in caring and compassion include the physician who waves at the door of the patient's room; the physician who quickly resorts to psychotropic drugs in the office, rather than taking the time to listen; and the physician on teaching rounds who never sees the patient and who limits the discussion to laboratory studies or some specific interesting aspect of the case in a nearby conference room.

The physician should be a good listener and read between the lines what the patient is saying. Often the physician can express warmth, understanding, or sympathy nonverbally. Staying close to the patient and maintaining eye contact is helpful. Sitting next to the patient's bed or on the edge of the bed in the hospital or long-term care facility brings the doctor right into the patient's small universe. The physician might put a hand on the patient's shoulder and pat, touch, or hold hands at appropriate points during the visit.

As the revered physician, Eugene Stead, Jr., would say: "What this patient needs is a doctor" (31). Our elderly patients, and in fact all of our patients, are yearning for a physician who will listen and understand. Again, we remember Peabody's words (9), "The good physician knows his patients through and through, and his knowledge is bought dearly. Time, sympathy and understanding must be lavishly dispensed, but the reward is to be found in that personal bond which forms the greatest satisfaction of the practice of medicine. One of the essential qualities of the clinician is interest in humanity, where the secret of the care of the patient is in caring for the patient."

CHANGING TIMES IN HEALTH CARE

In performing these essential aspects of care of the elderly patient, the physician may be distraught about the difficulties of these times in which a revolution in health care is taking place. The physician may feel discouraged during this period of increased competition, cost containment, alternative patterns of health care delivery, the malpractice threat, and other current forces in health care reform. The physician may be disheartened by a system that provides financial incentives for saving money and that puts the physician at risk for spending, that excessively scrutinizes and profiles the physician in the hospital, and that may often seem to emphasize the financial bottom line rather than excellence of patient care.

Despite this tug of war, the physician must simply have faith that excellence of patient care— care that is compassionate and humane, care that is characterized by continuity, care that is sensitive to psychosocial and family issues, and care that is characterized by all the other essential principles—will endure. Although the organization of health care delivery will undoubtedly change, we can expect that society will ultimately demand a quality of care that we would each want for ourselves.

OPPORTUNITIES FOR NEW DIRECTION AND CHANGE

As primary care or generalist physicians go about their daily professional duties, situations are noted in which precise or clear answers do not exist. This circumstance was mentioned above in prevention and health maintenance: the need for ongoing refinement of algorithms and guidelines for health promotion and health screening. But there are other areas that require reflection, research, and in some cases, societal response.

There is much mental illness that is poorly understood. There are elderly individuals who present with atypical features including paranoid ideation or eccentric behavior. We often lack the patient's full life history, and the emotional disorder does not fit into the DSM-IV classification. One elderly patient presented with fears of being watched by the CIA and the FBI and with concerns that people were saying he was masturbating and had bad body odor. Two attempts to arrange psychiatric consultation failed; the patient did not want to follow up with the psychotherapist. He appeared well in every other regard. After 6 months of office visits lasting 20 minutes each, his paranoid ideation improved, and he expressed gratitude that the treatment was helping tremendously. At 1 year, he was free of paranoid thoughts, although it was possible to ask about it, and he would reply that that was no longer a problem. Was his behavior somehow related to depression, isolation, or loneliness? At 3 years, he looks forward to his office visits and continues to express gratitude for the medical attention that cured him. There is much to learn about mental health disorders seen in the elderly who are living in the community. There is much that we do not yet understand.

We have discussed above the problem of the elderly in America who are geographically separated from their adult children. But the elderly are also often separated by emotional or other generational differences. This may not be an estrangement with hateful feelings (as expressed in King Lear's statement, "How sharper than a serpent's tooth it is to have a thankless child"). This is simply the fact that not all American families resemble the family gathered around the table for Thanksgiving as portrayed by Norman Rockwell.

Climo (7, 8) critically examines the consequences of geographic separation of elders and adult children. But American culture fosters disconnectedness. Although some American families do resemble the Norman Rockwell portrait, others do not. Many teenagers and young adults are thinking of the future and cannot identify with their parents or grandparents. Many middle-aged persons are still thinking of the future and still cannot identify with their elderly parents. Each is in a separate compartment and has difficulty with the cultural diversity that exists between generations. The members of each generation may have their own dress and hair code, music, values, religious beliefs, friends, and traditions. If they gather for Thanksgiving or a wedding, it may be an ordeal. The parents may not want the grandparents to know that a grandchild is having problems with drugs. The parents may have moved away from a faith community that had great meaning to the grandparents. Secrets may be commonplace between members or branches of a family.

In fulfillment of independent living with each generation determining its own existence, there is a disconnectedness, separation, isolation, and loneliness that each generation feels, particularly the elderly who are not busy with work or child-raising and are disappointed over their lack of connection with their children and grandchildren. Elders may feel dejected, wishing for more contact with their family members, their community, or other people, and the elders simply may not be able to make these connections. They may especially be separated from young people who have chosen a new direction for their lives. Perhaps the most striking evidence of disconnectedness in our society is the existence of large members of homeless elderly in many communities.

We have discussed above the work of Frankl (10, 11) and Yalom (12) and the presence of an existential vacuum. We have referred to existential psychotherapy and the use of hope as a therapeutic tool. The physician caring for 80- and 90-year-old patients must be prepared to hear the patient utter, "I don't know why I'm still here" or, "I don't know why God doesn't take me away. I have lived long enough." In such cases, the physician must be attuned to the possibility that these statements represent the subtle expression of suicidal ideation and should not be reluctant to discuss this with the patient.

Without entering too much into the world of theology, it might be appropriate for the physician to say such things as, "That's not for you to decide or ponder. There must be a reason you are still here. Apparently God must want you here for some reason. There is the friendship that you and I still enjoy, and the friendship that you enjoy with the visiting nurse (or home health aide). There's your nephew in New Hampshire and his family. You may see him only three or four times per year, but I know that you both care about each other. Again, your being here is not really for you or me to decide. All of us must make the best of each day while we are still here."

What about the extraordinarily independent patient who is feisty and maybe a bit eccentric? The patient will not accept what seems to be needed treatment or will refuse home health aides or day care. Others have divorced themselves from the medical system, at least for the present time, because of past experience that was burdensome, expensive, and seemingly unnecessary. Some will refuse supports such as having health aides because they do not want the burden of strangers in the home or the expense of this assistance (even though they can afford it). They do not want to divert their savings in case they need it in the future or in order not to reduce an inheritance to a loved one. They may recall bad experiences with a series of dentists whose bills ran into thousands of dollars. The patient may be wary of the medical system that kept her in the hospital emergency room for 12 to 36 hours and gave her repeated bone scans and other seemingly needless tests each time she suffered a fractured vertebra related to her osteoporosis. It would seem prudent to state the case for what is reasonable but to allow as much self-determination and autonomous action as possible. This respect for the patient's autonomy may enhance the doctor-patient relationship.

In fact, many elderly who exhibit extraordinary independence appear to do well despite their selective lack of participation in medical care or other support systems. Segerberg, in *Living To Be 100*, gives anecdotal descriptions of exceptional independence in 1200 centenarians (32). Extraordinary independence needs to be studied more as a positive factor in successful aging by at least some individuals.

As a society, we are beginning to realize that there are situations where it is burdensome and futile to combat death and lethal disease. More and more, there is the realization that at certain times, continued treatment may simply be too burdensome to the patient to be worth continuing, and there is now a rising interest throughout the country in living wills and other advance directives for health care. As physicians, we must learn to respect these directives if they were made with full informed consent by a competent patient (34). Many elderly have witnessed burdensome, expensive, and what appeared to be futile care provided to their friends and loved ones, and this has led to the importance of these health care directives, supported by the Cruzan Supreme Court decision and the Patient Self-Determination Act (34). The next decade will bring greater understanding and use of these advance directives, and thus the patient's preferences will be known and respected.

We can expect that more terminally ill patients will choose to go home to die with proper care from family, aides, caregivers, and volunteers, and as a profession, we should respect and support the terminally ill patient's wish to die at home (34). Home care, whether the patient is simply going home, staying home, or participating in a hospital or hospice home care program, will be a choice that our patients will make, and we can anticipate a marked increase in attention to home care in our health care system in the years ahead.

SUMMARY

In the care of the elderly patient, eleven essential principles should be considered: (a) the role of the physician as the integrator of the biopsychosocial model; (b) continuity of care; (c) bolstering the family and home; (d) good communication skills; (e) building a sound doctor-patient relationship; (f) the need for thorough evaluation and assessment; (g) prevention and health maintenance; (h) intelligent treatment with attention to ethical decision making; (i) interdisciplinary collaboration; (j) respect for the usefulness and value of the aged individual; and (k) compassionate care. The embodiment of these eleven principles represents a standard of excellence to which we can all aspire.

REFERENCES

1. Engel GL. The need for a new medical model: a challenge for biomedicine. Science 1977;196:129–136.
2. Engel GL. How much longer must medicine's science be bound by a seventeenth century world view? Psychother Psychosom 1992;57:3–16.
3. Wasson JH, Sauvigne AE, Mogielnicki RP, et al. Continuity of outpatient medical care in elderly men. A randomized trial. JAMA 1984;2532:2413–2417.
4. Reichel W. The continuity imperative. JAMA 1981;246:2065.
5. Stone R, Cafferata GL, Sangl J. Caregivers of the frail elderly: a national profile. Gerontologist 1987;27:616–626.
6. Shanas E. Social myth as hypothesis: the case of the family relations of old people. Gerontologist 1979;19:3–9.
7. Climo J. Visits of distant living adult children and elderly parents. J Aging Stud 1988;2:57–69.
8. Climo J. Distant parents. New Brunswick, NJ: Rutgers University Press, 1992.
9. Peabody FW. The care of the patient. JAMA 1927;88:877–882.
10. Frankl VE. Man's search for meaning. New York: Beacon Press, 1959.
11. Frankl VE. The doctor and the soul. New York: AA Knopf, 1955.
12. Yalom ID. Existential psychotherapy. New York: Basic Books, 1980.
13. Cassel EJ. The nature of suffering and the goals of medicine. N Engl J Med 1982;306:639–645.
14. Kushner H. When all you've ever wanted isn't enough. New York: Summit Books, 1986.
15. Cousins N. The physician as communicator. JAMA 1982;248:587–589.
16. Butler R. The doctor and the aged patient. In: Reichel W, ed. The geriatric patient. New York: Hospital Practice, 1978:199–206.
17. Elahi D, Clark B, Andres R. Glucose tolerance, insulin sensitivity and age. In: Armbracht HJ, Coe RM, Wongsurawat N, eds. Endocrine function and aging. New York: Springer-Verlag, 1990:48–63.
18. Rowe JW, Andres R, Tobin JR, Norris AH, Shock NW. The effect of age on creatinine clearance in men: a cross-sectional and longitudinal study. J Gerontol 1976;31:155–163.
19. Reichel W. Multiple problems in the elderly. In: Reichel W, ed. The geriatric patient. New York: Hospital Practice, 1978:17–22.
20. Howell TH. Causation of diagnostic errors in octogenarians. A clinicopathological study. J Am Geriatr Soc 1966;14:41–47.
21. Fiatarone MA, Evans WJ. The etiology and reversibility of muscle dysfunctions in the aged. J Gerontol 1993;48(special issue):77–83.
22. Frailty and injuries: cooperative studies of intervention techniques (FICSIT). J Am Geriatr Soc 1993;41:283–343.
23. Laws A, Reaven GM. Effect of physical activity on age-related glucose intolerance. Clin Geriatr Med 1990;6:849–863.
24. U.S. Preventive Services Task Force. Guide to clinical preventive services. Baltimore: Williams & Wilkins, 1989.
25. Seegal D. The principle of minimal interference in the management of the elderly patient. J Chron Dis 1964;17:299–300.
26. Reichel W. Complications in the care of 500 elderly hospitalized patients. J Am Geriatr Soc 1965;13:973–981.
27. Steel K, Gertman PM, Crescenzi C, Anderson J. Iatrogenic illness on a general medical service at a university hospital. N Engl J Med 1981;304:638–642.
28. Lipp MR. Respectful treatment: a practical handbook of patient care. 2nd ed. New York: Elsevier, 1986.
29. Glick S. Humanistic medicine in a modern age. N Engl J Med 1981;304:1036–1038.
30. Keeler EB, Solomon DH, Beck JC, Mendenhall RC, Kane RL. Effect of patient age on duration of medical encounters with physicians. Med Care 1982;20:1101–1108.
31. Wagner GS, Cebe B, Rozear MP, eds. E. A. Stead, Jr., What this patient needs is a doctor. Durham, NC: Carolina Academic Press, 1978.
32. Segerberg O. Living to be 100. New York: Charles Scribners Sons, 1982.
33. Doukas DJ, Reichel W. Planning for uncertainty: a guide to living wills and other advance directives for health care. Baltimore: Johns Hopkins University Press, 1993.
34. Sankar A. Dying at home: a family guide for caregiving. Baltimore: Johns Hopkins University Press, 1991.

2/ Multidimensional Assessment of the Older Patient

Joseph J. Gallo, Laura Stanley, Naomi E. Zack, William Reichel

AN OVERVIEW OF GERIATRIC ASSESSMENT

It is fitting to begin a text of geriatrics with a discussion of assessment, since a thorough assessment of the patient is the key to formulating a care plan and an appropriate schedule of health maintenance. While the traditional history and physical examination serves well for most patients with acute illness, additional considerations may influence the course of action in the face of chronic illness and age. This has always been so, but demographic trends, such as increased numbers of people surviving with controllable but not curable chronic illnesses, and societal attitudes, such as the emphasis on patient autonomy, demand that these "additional considerations" be explicitly and systematically addressed.

In this chapter we discuss multidimensional geriatric assessment and suggest a strategy to incorporate it into the varied settings in which older adults receive care. Comprehensive geriatric assessment comprises, in addition to a history and physical examination, an evaluation of functional status, mental status, social and economic factors, and the values of the patient and family, as well as preparation of an appropriate health maintenance plan. The geriatric assessment represents the "technology of geriatrics" (1, 2). There is increasing emphasis on providing geriatric assessment of this kind in the office, in the hospital, on consideration for nursing home placement, on admission to long-term care facilities, and at the time of major life changes, such as bereavement and retirement.

The consequences of medical diagnoses such as diabetes or hypertension on each of the dimensions of comprehensive assessment should be considered in every older patient. How might an additional medication for hypertension affect this patient's functional and mental status? Will nutritional status be further compromised by treatment of hyperlipidemia? Conversely, the multidimensional status of the older person must be considered in a larger context when addressing treatment options. What will be the implications of this patient's social and economic status on the treatment of disorders such as diabetes or cancer? Can this patient be cared for in sheltered housing? What value does this patient place on dying at home? Thus, geriatric assessment is complementary to, and in reciprocal relationship with, the standard medical evaluation.

The presenting symptom should also be considered for its relationship with functioning in each dimension; indeed, the presenting symptom itself may be a change in functional, mental, or social condition. Why the patient comes for care may have more to do with a strained or ailing caregiver than with deterioration in the patient's medical condition. Usually it is a family member, caregiver, or case manager, and not the patient, who requests geriatric assessment, often in the midst of a crisis.

We wish to emphasize at the outset that to be useful, the findings of an evaluation must be linked to treatment provided to the patient and caregiver. In some cases, information about the diagnosis and prognosis will be all that is required; in others, arrangements for formal support, changes in the medication regimen, further diagnostic testing to search for reversible causes of functional decline, and other modifications of the care plan may be necessary. Individual circumstances and values must be taken into account and preclude standard "rules" to follow in determining what to do with the information from assessment.

The dimensions of comprehensive geriatric assessment must be a focus for prevention of problems as well as for evaluation of established problems (3, 4). Anticipating effects of disorders on multiple dimensions and anticipating effects of status on treatment of disorders casts "geriatric assessment" in terms of "geriatric prevention." Thus, multidimensional geriatric assessment provides a flexible model for planning patient care and monitoring status.

The domains of multidimensional geriatric assessment are discussed in turn, although we realize that certain aspects of the evaluation wax and wane in importance depending on the particular situation. In Tables 2.1 through 2.7, several evaluative instruments are provided. In the text, we have indicated key questions that alert the clinician to areas that require further inquiry and special consideration in patient care.

FUNCTIONAL ASSESSMENT

ACTIVITIES OF DAILY LIVING

The ability to function in the world is predicated on the ability to perform certain daily activities or to compensate when the ability is impaired by disease or injury. The activities of daily living (ADLs) have been variously defined, but a standard listing, the Katz Index of ADLs (5), includes bathing, dressing, toileting, transfer, continence, and feeding (Table 2.1). While the term "functional assessment" is sometimes used to refer to multidimensional geriatric assessment, we prefer to reserve the term specifically for assessment of the patient's ADLs.

Approximately 5% of persons aged 65 to 69 years have difficulty with bathing; this percentage increases to about 30% for persons aged 85 years and older (6). The ADLs tend to be lost in a predictable sequence: bathing, dressing, transferring, using the toilet, grooming, and eating; for example, 12.0% of older adults in East Boston reported difficulty with bathing, while 2.6% reported difficulty with eating. With knowledge that a given ADL is lost, preservation of more basic ADLs in the sequence can be predicted, while abilities that were lost tend to be regained in the reverse sequence. Longitudinal studies have revealed that ADL performance predicts mortality (7).

Older adults who have trouble with ADLs need to compensate for the disability. Bathing, for example, may be avoided, done partially, or attempted without adequate safeguards such as handrails. Of course, involvement of another person is an important avenue for compensation when the older person has trouble with ADLs. The type and extent of the ADLs requiring compensation have implications for the caregiver.

The source of information on ADL status should be recorded when ADLs are assessed. Di-

Table 2.1
Katz Index of Activities of Daily Living[a,b]

1. Bathing (sponge, shower, or tub):
   - I: receives no assistance (gets in and out of tub if tub is the usual means of bathing)
   - A: receives assistance in bathing only one part of the body (such as the back or a leg)
   - D: receives assistance in bathing more than one part of the body (or not bathed)
2. Dressing:
   - I: gets clothes and gets completely dressed without assistance
   - A: gets clothes and gets dressed without assistance except in tying shoes
   - D: receives assistance in getting clothes or in getting dressed or stays partly or completely undressed
3. Toileting:
   - I: goes to "toilet room," cleans self, and arranges clothes without assistance (may use object for support such as cane, walker, or wheelchair and may manage night bedpan or commode, emptying it in the morning)
   - A: receives assistance in going to "toilet room" or in cleansing self or in arranging clothes after elimination or in use of night bedpan or commode
   - D: doesn't go to room termed "toilet" for the elimination process
4. Transfer:
   - I: moves in and out of bed as well as in and out of chair without assistance (may be using object for support such as cane or walker)
   - A: moves in and out of bed or chair with assistance
   - D: doesn't get out of bed
5. Continence:
   - I: controls urination and bowel movement completely by self
   - A: has occasional "accidents"
   - D: supervision helps keep urine or bowel control, catheter is used, or is incontinent
6. Feeding:
   - I: feeds self without assistance
   - A: feeds self except for getting assistance in cutting meat or buttering bread
   - D: receives assistance in feeding or is fed partly or completely by using tubes or intravenous fluids

[a]Adapted with permission from JAMA 1963;185:915, Copyright 1963, American Medical Association.
[b]Abbreviations: I, independent; A, assistance; D, dependent.

rect observation in the home or the nursing home is the most desirable method of evaluating performance but is cumbersome in most settings. Older persons may overstate their abilities and underestimate the amount of help they require, in reporting ADLs. Caregivers, on the other hand, may overestimate the help required. Ratings of "dependence" in an ADL involve some subjective judgment of many factors. How much help is required on a given day may vary depending on motivation, unforeseen situations, and fluctuation in medical conditions such as pain and stiffness from arthritis.

The assessment of mobility should include a description of bed mobility, the ability to transfer (as from bed to chair), and the ability to get to the toilet and bathtub. Evaluate the gait and functional performance by asking the patient to rise from a chair, walk a short distance, turn, walk back, and sit down (8). Find out if recommended ambulatory aids, such as canes and walkers, are actually used and considered to be helpful. For persons who use a wheelchair, consider how well the patient negotiates the environment. For older persons engaged in exercise on a regular basis or who seek advice about how to start, identify current activities, such as playing golf, walking, hiking, or swimming, and whether warmup and cooldown exercises accompany activity.

Nutrition is an important though frequently neglected domain of assessment. Evaluate the teeth and the ability to chew and swallow food safely, to gauge risk for malnutrition and associated problems. For many older persons, caloric intake is below the Recommended Daily Allowance, resulting in dietary deficiencies in vitamins and other nutrients (9). Older adults often do not consume sufficient amounts of fluids because thirst and food intake are diminished (10). In evaluating nutritional status, remember that age-related changes in the gastrointestinal tract are not as important as functional disability, poverty, poor general health, cultural beliefs about food, and the inability to obtain a fresh and varied diet.

The ability, time, and willingness of the older patient to carry out personal care, such as brushing the teeth, shaving, caring for dentures, bathing, and dressing, will be useful information in planning caregiver support. The older person's ability to get to the bathroom and to manage toileting and incontinence aids is an integral part of the assessment of bowel and bladder function and continence. Some activities require only sporadic help at certain times of the day (dressing and undressing) or week (bathing). The assistance required may be a device or mechanical aid (canes, walkers), modifications to the living environment (constructing a toilet on the first floor), or a person (family member, paid help). So, while it is useful to know that an individual requires assistance with an ADL, the source of the information, the consistency and timing of the help required, and the type of assistance needed rounds out the picture. This information serves as a benchmark for noting change in function, tailors the plan of care to the individual, and helps to organize caregiving.

INSTRUMENTAL ACTIVITIES OF DAILY LIVING

Additional daily activities are necessary for persons living in modern society: using the telephone, shopping for food and preparing meals, and managing money are "ADLs," but not in the same sense as the personal care tasks of such ADLs as bathing and dressing. The Lawton "instrumental" ADL scale (11) consists of items assessing the use of the telephone, traveling, shopping, preparing meals, doing housework, taking medication, and managing money (Table 2.2).

The tasks comprising the IADLs are laden with cultural and gender biases (12). For example, items on meal preparation may be biased against men, while for some traditional older couples, handling the money is the man's chore. Even so, a caregiver must assume these tasks if the older person is unable to do so.

IADLs include managing medications. In addition to obtaining a complete list of medications, assess the use of over-the-counter drugs, home remedies, vitamins, eye solutions, topical preparations, herbal remedies, and homeopathic substances. Some medications available over the counter have anticholinergic properties with the potential to cause mental status changes and urinary retention. If the older patient uses several sources of medical care, poor communication among clinicians may result in medications being discontinued or changed without proper regard to the total clinical picture. Ask about whether the patient and caregiver understand the purpose of each medication and who prescribed it.

Asking about IADLs may be a good way to detect problems, particularly cognitive impairment, in ambulatory older patients. For example, inability to use the telephone may be caused by a problem with processing information, sequencing steps of the task, or managing fine motor coordination. Difficulty with any of four IADLs (those that pertain to using the telephone, taking medications appropriately, handling money, and using transportation) were found to be important correlates of cognitive impairment in a French community sample of almost 3000 persons over the age of 65 years (13). The Fillenbaum five-item IADL screening questionnaire (14) includes getting to places out of walking distance, going shopping for groceries or clothes, preparing meals, doing housework, and handling money (Table 2.3). Poor performance on these IADLs signaled an in-

Table 2.2
Instrumental Activities of Daily Living[a,b]

1. Telephone:
    I: able to look up numbers, dial, receive and make calls without help
    A: able to answer phone or dial operator in an emergency but needs special phone or help in getting number or dialing
    D: unable to use the telephone
2. Traveling:
    I: able to drive own car or travel alone on bus or taxi
    A: able to travel but not alone
    D: unable to travel
3. Shopping:
    I: able to take care of all shopping with transportation provided
    A: able to shop but not alone
    D: unable to shop
4. Preparing meals:
    I: able to plan and cook full meals
    A: able to prepare light foods but unable to cook full meals alone
    D: unable to prepare any meals
5. Housework:
    I: able to do heavy housework (like scrub floors)
    A: able to do light housework, but needs help with heavy tasks
    D: unable to do any housework
6. Medication:
    I: able to take medications in the right dose at the right time
    A: able to take medications but needs reminding or someone to prepare it
    D: unable to take medications
7. Money:
    I: able to manage buying needs, writes checks, pays bills
    A: able to manage daily buying needs, but needs help managing checkbook, paying bills
    D: unable to manage money

[a]Adapted with permission from Multidimensional Functional Assessment Questionnaire. 2nd ed. Duke University Center for the Study of Aging and Human Development of Duke University 1978:169–170.
[b]Abbreviations: I, independent; A, assistance; D, dependent.

Table 2.3
The Five-Item Instrumental Activities of Daily Living Screening Questionnaire[a]

1. Can you *get to places* out of walking distance:
    1 Without help (can travel alone on bus, taxi, or drive your own car)?
    0 With some help (need someone to help you or go with you when traveling) or are you unable to travel unless emergency arrangements are made for a specialized vehicle such as an ambulance?
    — Not answered
2. Can you *go shopping* for groceries or clothes (assuming you have transportation):
    1 Without help (taking care of all your shopping needs yourself, assuming you have transportation)?
    0 With some help (need someone to go with you on all shopping trips), or are you completely unable to do any shopping?
    — Not answered
3. Can you *prepare your own meals*:
    1 Without help (plan and cook meals yourself)?
    0 With some help (can prepare some things but unable to cook full meals yourself), or are you completely unable to prepare any meals?
    — Not answered
4. Can you do your *housework*:
    1 Without help (can scrub floors, etc.)?
    0 With some help (can do light housework but need help with heavy work), or are you unable to do any housework?
    — Not answered
5. Can you *handle your own money*:
    1 Without help (writes checks, pays bills, etc.)?
    0 With some help (manage day-to-day buying but need help with managing your checkbook and paying your bills), or are you completely unable to handle money?
    — Not answered

[a]Reprinted with permission from Fillenbaum G. Screening the elderly: a brief instrumental activities of daily living measure. J Am Geriatr Soc 1985;33:698–706.

creased mortality at follow-up (14). Knowledge of IADL deficits can alert the clinician to concerns when the patient must be home alone. In certain circumstances, the patient may require 24-hour supervision or the installation of an emergency response system such as Lifeline.

A search for cognitive impairment, depression, and caregiver strain may be more fruitful if the patient is noted to have difficulty with any of the IADLs. While evaluation may be more detailed depending on the circumstances, at a minimum ask older ambulatory adults about functioning in the realms of transportation, shopping, and meal preparation: "Are you able to get around in your neighborhood?"; "Who shops for you?"; "Who prepares your meals?" In addition, ambulatory patients with difficulties in the IADLs should also be asked about ADLs; for example, "Do you have any difficulty dressing yourself?" Then consider further evaluation, including formal mental status assessment, depending on the clinical picture.

Inviting the patient or caregiver to describe a typical day can be an effective way of obtaining much of the information in the functional history and is potentially a less intrusive manner of interviewing, as it assumes participation and lends itself to open-ended questions. It also is an opportunity to observe how well activities and events are recalled and to discuss health issues as they arise in the course of daily activities.

SLEEP

Sleep disturbance is a common reason for seeking medical attention, resulting in the use of both physician- and self-prescribed medication. It is normal to find a marked increase in daytime naps after the age of 85 years (15). Sleep efficacy is impaired by age-related and pathological changes and is marked by increased nighttime awakening and prolongation of sleep latency (the time required to fall asleep). In the evaluation of the complaint of disturbed sleep, consider environmental factors (such as noise, moving to an institution, and hospitalization) and personal factors (such as dementia, depression, arthritis, angina, duodenal ulcer, chronic obstructive pulmonary disease, lower extremity cramping, periodic leg movements, and the adverse effects of medications).

A sleep diary that documents the routines and patterns of sleep may be useful in evaluating complaints of sleep disturbance. Early morning awakening may signal depression. Awakening during the night may indicate uncompensated congestive heart failure or excessive bronchial secretions resulting in daytime fatigue or sleepiness. Of particular significance are the use of alcohol, exercise, timing of meals, effective strategies such as relaxation, and nighttime rituals that have been effective in dealing with sleep disturbance in the past.

DRIVING

By the year 2020, the number of drivers over the age of 65 will increase to 50 million; of these, half will be over the age of 75 (16). Find out where and when the older person is driving as well as the length of travel. Both the number and type of medications are associated with the incidence of "near-miss accidents" (17). In the physical examination, assess the range of motion of the neck, upper extremities, and lower back. The clinical assessment should include an evaluation of visual acuity and visual fields, a hearing evaluation, and a review the individual's medication regimen and risk of functional impairment (18). The assessment of ADLs, IADLs, and cognitive status could be complemented by psychological testing such as the symbol-digit test, a test of category fluency, or the Motor-Free Visual Perception Test, all under active investigation for how performance on these tests relates to driving. The moral and legal obligations of health professionals to report to the Motor Vehicles Administration is now under scrutiny (19).

SEXUALITY

Older adults may want to continue sexual expression, closeness, and intimacy into the later years. It is unfortunate when ageism and personal discomfort in dealing with sexuality cause the sexual concerns of older adults to be overlooked. A safe, nonjudgmental, and sensitive environment allows potentially treatable or reversible problems such as impotence in men or diminished vaginal lubrication in women to be discussed, facilitating health education and counseling that may enhance quality of life. Education about sexually transmitted diseases and AIDS is important, yet is often neglected in this age group (20).

MENTAL STATUS

COGNITIVE FUNCTION

Evaluation of mental status begins with engagement of the older adult. Much can be learned from careful observation of the patient's dress, general appearance and grooming, posture, behavior, speech, and word choice (21). The history of the prior level of functioning, as evidenced by occupational and educational attainment, can also provide clues to the patient's current mental state. During the encounter, the examiner forms temporary hypotheses about the patient's mental status in the context of the concerns of the patient or family. This context and one's observations about the patient must not be lost in the application of standardized assessments of mental state.

Dementia is a pervasive acquired syndrome affecting language, memory, cognition, personality, and judgment, without clouding of consciousness (22). Clouding of consciousness, which may be manifested by inability to maintain attention, is the hallmark of delirium. Although many causes can underlie dementia, patients with superimposed delirium may show significant improvement if the underlying cause of the delirium can be treated. Brief methods of cognitive assessment cannot in themselves make a diagnosis of dementia. A diagnosis of dementia syndrome can only be made after a thorough history and physical examination that demonstrates that the impairment is global, including such dimensions as personality change, and preferably using standard criteria (22, 23).

Assessment of mental status remains one of the most important yet frequently neglected aspects of care. In the ambulatory setting, formal evaluation with standard instruments, such as the Mini-Mental State Examination (MMSE, 24) or the Short Portable Mental Status Questionnaire (SPMSQ, 25), may be particularly important for older adults who are having difficulty with IADLs. In other circumstances, such as on hospital or nursing home admission, evaluation with a standard mental status questionnaire provides a baseline for noting further change and can be an important piece of information in decision making. Older persons with poor cognitive performance on testing may be at increased risk for delirium following hospitalization, surgery, or medication use. Longstanding reversible causes of cognitive impairment may become irreversible, so that early detection in high-risk situations provides the best hope for prevention of disability. Discussion of the full mental status examination can be found in an excellent text (26).

The MMSE is one of the more widely known brief tests of mental status in clinical use (24). Literature on the performance of the MMSE is extensive and is reviewed by Tombaugh and McIntyre (27) and by Crum and her colleagues (28). Scores on the MMSE correspond to results of more elaborate psychological testing, to structural and functional brain abnormalities, and to the stage of Alzheimer's dementia. The MMSE has been translated and studied in many cultural settings.

The first part of the MMSE assesses orientation, memory, and attention (Table 2.4). The words *apple*, *table*, and *penny* have been used in the memory task in the Epidemiologic Catchment Area Program field survey and can be used to test registration (learning the word list) and recall (remembering the word list). Registration is scored on the first trial. The second part of the MMSE tests the ability to write a sentence, name objects, follow verbal and written commands, and copy a complex polygon design. A maximum score of 30 is possible.

As is true for all brief cognitive measures, the MMSE must be interpreted carefully, taking account of the patient's educational attainment and prior level of functioning and the clinical setting. Persons with less formal education may score more poorly than better educated persons despite no evidence of cognitive impairment. On the other hand, well-educated persons with early dementia may do very well on the MMSE. Norms for the interpretation of MMSE score in the light of the patient's age and educational level are available from the Epidemiologic Catchment Area study (28). Thresholds for assessing cognitive impairment from the MMSE were derived by examining the lowest quartile of MMSE scores within several educational levels. For persons with 0 to 4 years of education, using a threshold of 19 and below would identify persons scoring at a level less than 75% of persons in the same educational stratum. Corresponding thresholds are for persons with 5 to 8 years of schooling, 23 and below; for 9 to 12 years of schooling, 27 and below; for schooling at the college level and beyond, 29 and below (28).

Other brief mental status testing instruments have not been, to our knowledge, as thoroughly studied as the MMSE. The SPMSQ (Table 2.5) consists of 10 questions dealing with orientation, personal history, remote memory, and calculations. The test does not include any test of writing or constructional praxis as does the MMSE. Instructions for scoring the SPMSQ are included in Table 2.5.

PSYCHOLOGICAL ASSESSMENT

Although mental status testing usually emphasizes the cognitive aspects of mental life, it is important to consider the impact of psychological factors and life events on health and functioning. Life events in later life differ from life events in youth in the frequent association with loss, in the occurrence of several events in a short time period, in requiring more energy to cope, and in engendering feelings of powerlessness (9). Widowhood, chronic illness, retirement, and the deaths of friends and family all may result in altered lifestyle, residence, economic status, and functioning. Identify past coping styles in order to recognize and support healthy behaviors that may be used in times of crisis.

While epidemiologic studies using standard diagnostic criteria find decreasing rates of depression with age, studies using symptom checklists suggest that depressive symptoms increase with age (see Newmann (29) for a review). Depression may be more common in future cohorts of older adults. This and other evidence, including the high suicide rate in older adults, suggest that the form of depression may be different in older adults (29a). Depressive symptoms that do not meet criteria for major depression may still have significant functional and prognostic implications (30). It is especially important to consider depression, anxiety, and alcohol use in clinical situations characterized by newly diagnosed illness, by functional decline, and by bereavement and other losses.

Major depression is defined largely in terms of the vegetative symptoms of depression; for example, in addition to depressed mood and loss of

Table 2.4
Mini-Mental State Examination (MMS)

Maximum Score	Score	
		ORIENTATION
5	( )	1. What is the (year) (season) (date) (day) (month)?
5	( )	2. Where are we: (state) (country) (town) (hospital) (floor)?
		REGISTRATION
3	( )	3. Name 3 objects: 1 second to say each. Then ask the patient all 3 after you have said them.
		Give 1 point for each correct answer. Then repeat them until he learns all 3. Count trials and record.
		Trials
		ATTENTION AND CALCULATION
5	( )	4. Serial 7's. 1 point for each correct. Stop after 5 answers. Alternatively, spell "world" backwards, if cannot subtract.
		RECALL
3	( )	5. Ask for 3 objects repeated above. Give 1 point for each correct.
		LANGUAGE
9	( )	6. Name a pencil, and watch (2 points)
		7. Repeat the following "No ifs, ands or buts" (1 point)
		8. Follow a 3-stage command: "Take a paper in your right hand, fold it in half, and put it on the floor." (3 points)
		9. Read and obey the following: "Close your eyes" (1 point)
		10. Write a sentence. (1 point)
		11. Copy design. (1 point)

TOTAL SCORE

1. 1 point for each correct answer.
2. 1 point for each correct answer.
3. 1 point for each of the 3 object names that is correctly repeated the first time. Then repeat them until all 3 are repeated but give no further points.
4. 1 point for each correct subtraction. If the patient does not or cannot make any subtractions have him spell the word "world" backwards. If an attempted subtraction is made this is the preferred task.
5. 1 point for each object.
6. 1 point for each correctly named object. Give no points if an approximate but incorrect word is used.
7. 1 point if completely and correctly completed.
8. 1 point for each command followed.
9. 1 point only if the patient carries out the activity. No points if the sentence is read correctly but the act is not done.
10. Sentence should be grammatically correct and have subject, verb and predicate.
11. 1 point if each figure has 5 sides and the overlap is correct.

Reprinted with permission from Folstein MF, Folstein SE, McHugh PR. Mini-Mental State: A practical method for grading the cognitive state of patients for the clinician. J Psychiatr Res 12:189, 1975. Copyright 1975, Pergamon Journals, Ltd. Courtesy of Dr. Marshal Folstein.

Table 2.5
Short Portable Mental Status Questionnaire

SHORT PORTABLE MENTAL STATUS QUESTIONNAIRE (SPMSQ)
Eric Pfeiffer, M.D.

Instructions: Ask questions 1–10 in this list and record all answers. Ask question 4A only if patient does not have a telephone. Record total number of errors based on ten questions.

+	−	
		1. What is the date today?_____
		Month Day Year
		2. What day of the week is it?_____
		3. What is the name of this place?_____
		4. What is your telephone number?_____
		4A. What is your street address?_____
		(Ask only if patient does not have a telephone)
		5. How old are you?_____
		6. When were you born?_____
		7. Who is the President of the U.S. now?_____
		8. Who was President just before him?_____
		9. What was your mother's maiden name?_____
		10. Subtract 3 from 20 and keep subtracting 3 from each new number, all the way down.
		Total Number of Errors

To Be Completed by Interviewer

Patients Name: _____   Date: _____

Sex: 1. Male   Race: 1. White
2. Female   2. Black
3. Other

Years of Education: _____   1. Grade School
2. High School
3. Beyond High School

Interviewer's Name: _____

INSTRUCTIONS FOR COMPLETION OF
THE SHORT PORTABLE MENTAL STATUS QUESTIONNAIRE (SPMSQ)

Ask the subject questions 1 through 10 in this list and record all answers. All responses to be scored correct must be given by subject without reference to calendar, newspaper, birth certificate, or other aid to memory.

Question 1 is to be scored correctly only when the exact month, exact date, and the exact year are given correctly.

Question 2 is self-explanatory.

Table 2.5 *continued*

Question 3 should be scored correctly if any correct description of the location is given. "My home," correct name of the town or city of residence, or the name of hospital or institution if subject is institutionalized, are all acceptable.

Question 4 should be scored correctly when the correct telephone number can be verified, or when the subject can repeat the same number at another point in the questioning.

Question 5 is scored correct when stated age corresponds to date of birth.

Question 6 is to be scored correctly only when the month, exact date, and year are all given.

Question 7 requires only the last name of the President.

Question 8 requires only the last name of the previous President.

Question 9 does not need to be verified. It is scored correct if a female first name plus a last name other than subject's last is given.

Question 10 requires that the entire series must be performed correctly in order to be scored as correct. Any error in the series or unwillingness to attempt the series is scored as incorrect.

SCORING OF THE SHORT PORTABLE MENTAL STATUS QUESTIONNAIRE (SPMSQ)

The data suggest that both education and race influence performance on the Mental Status Questionnaire and they must accordingly be taken into account in evaluating the score attained by an individual.

For purposes of scoring, three educational levels have been established: a) persons who have had only a grade school education; b) persons who have had any high school education or who have completed high school; c) persons who have had any education beyond the high school level, including college, graduate school or business school.

For white subjects with at least some high school education, but not more than high school education, the following criteria have been established:

0–2	ERRORS	INTACT INTELLECTUAL FUNCTIONING
3–4	ERRORS	MILD INTELLECTUAL IMPAIRMENT
5–7	ERRORS	MODERATE INTELLECTUAL IMPAIRMENT
8–10	ERRORS	SEVERE INTELLECTUAL IMPAIRMENT

Allow one more error if subject has had only a grade school education.
Allow one less error if subject has had education beyond high school.
Allow one more error for black subjects, using identical education criteria.

interest in activities, the DSM-IV criteria include weight change, insomnia, fatigue, and inability to concentrate (22). The diagnosis of depression can be difficult in older persons because multiple physical symptoms and psychological complaints unrelated to depression are so common. Unexplained physical complaints may be ascribed by professionals and caregivers to hypochondriasis, fatigue may be misinterpreted as laziness, and sadness can be construed as grouchiness (31). Irritability in close personal relationships may be an overlooked symptom of depression (32). Although an isolated vegetative symptom is common among older adults, the constellation of symptoms in major depression is not and may represent a case of depression even in the face of proven medical illness.

It is imperative to exclude concomitant illnesses that can cause a secondary affective illness (such as a metabolic disorder) or which can complicate the treatment of depression (such as a cardiac dysrhythmia). Medications such as β-blockers can contribute to depression. Coexisting dementia must be considered in the evaluation

and treatment of depression in older persons as well (33, 34).

The Geriatric Depression Scale (Table 2.6) is one method of screening for depression and is a questionnaire consisting of 30 items to be answered simply "yes" or "no" (35–38). The GDS is scored by assigning one point for each answer that corresponds to the answers after the question in Table 2.6 so that higher scores are associated with greater levels of depression. Usually a threshold score of 10 or 11 is used to separate patients into depressed and nondepressed groups. The GDS attempts to be less reliant on somatic symptoms of depression than other depression instruments, such as the Zung Self-rated Depression Scale (39) or the Beck Depression Inventory (40); however, it is not clear that the GDS offers any practical advantage as a result.

Studies of the GDS suggest that the instrument may be useful in the detection of depression, at least in patients without cognitive impairment. Research suggests that caution must be exercised when the GDS is administered in the context of dementia (41–43). It is important to emphasize

Table 2.6
Geriatric Depression Scale

1 Are you basically satisfied with your life? (no)
2 Have you dropped many of your activities and interests? (yes)
3 Do you feel that your life is empty? (yes)
4 Do you often get bored? (yes)
5 Are you hopeful about the future? (no)
6 Are you bothered by thoughts you cannot get out of your head? (yes)
7 Are you in good spirits most of the time? (no)
8 Are you afraid that something bad is going to happen to you? (yes)
9 Do you feel happy most of the time? (no)
10 Do you often feel helpless? (yes)
11 Do you often get restless and fidgety? (yes)
12 Do you prefer to stay home at night, rather than do new things? (yes)
13 Do you frequently worry about the future? (yes)
14 Do you feel that you have more problems with memory than most? (yes)
15 Do you think it is wonderful to be alive now? (no)
16 Do you often feel downhearted and blue? (yes)
17 Do you feel pretty worthless the way you are now? (yes)
18 Do you worry a lot about the past? (yes)
19 Do you find life very exciting? (no)
20 Is it hard for you to get started on new projects? (yes)
21 Do you feel full of energy? (no)
22 Do you feel that your situation is hopeless? (yes)
23 Do you think that most people are better off than you are? (yes)
24 Do you frequently get upset over little things? (yes)
25 Do you frequently feel like crying? (yes)
26 Do you have trouble concentrating? (yes)
27 Do you enjoy getting up in the morning? (no)
28 Do you prefer to avoid social gatherings? (yes)
29 Is it easy for you to make decisions? (no)
30 Is your mind as clear as it used to be? (no)

Score one point for each response that matches the yes or no answer after the question.

aAdapted with permission from Yesavage JA, Brink TL. Development and validation of a geriatric depression screening scale: a preliminary report. J Psychiatr Res 1983;17:41. Copyright 1983, Pergamon Journals Ltd.

that many validity studies of the GDS exclude persons with cognitive impairment. A short version of the GDS may not have acceptable properties (44) and at best does not maintain validity in demented patients (41). The GDS is perhaps best used in combination with a short mental status instrument such as the MMSE.

Other psychiatric problems in late life have received less attention than depression, such as the anxiety disorders, alcohol use, and substance use, including the misuse of and addiction to prescription drugs by older people. Unexplained functional decline or behavioral problems may be traced to undetected cognitive impairment or psychiatric illness.

SOCIAL ASSESSMENT

Families provide most long-term care to older people. Practitioners who care for older persons face the question, "Who is the patient?" Support of family members in the caregiving role is critical to an older person's quality of life and to society's ability to cope with a burgeoning older population. Yet, behind the question, "Who is the patient?" lies an ethical question of patient autonomy.

In considering social assessment as a domain of multidimensional geriatric assessment, we recognize the potential conflicts between patient autonomy and caregiver beneficence, and between caregiver autonomy and patient care. The conflict between patient autonomy and caregiver beneficence arises when the patient's wishes, from the caregiver's point of view, do not seem like good judgment. The caregiver then attempts to enlist the physician or other health professional as an ally. The conflict between caregiver autonomy and patient care may arise when caregivers perceive questions about their health or ability to manage the tasks of caregiving as intrusive, or when the caregiver is impaired.

The status with regard to ADLs and IADLs is of paramount importance to caregivers. Caregivers may find themselves doing more and more for the older adult, starting with transportation and handling finances, walking a fine line between encouraging independence and providing necessary assistance. Functional "symptoms" may be the first clue to the caregiver that something is wrong. The timing and amount of help an older person requires is an important, though not the only, determinant of caregiver burden.

Dementia, especially when accompanied by disturbing behaviors such as hitting, increases caregiver stress (45). The perceptions of the caregiver regarding caregiving tasks and the amount of support available must be assessed (46). Physicians and other health professionals should not underestimate their role in supporting caregivers through referral to services such as respite care and also through therapeutic listening (47, 48).

Caregivers are often themselves over the age of 65 years. Functional limitations of even caregivers with the best of intentions may mean that caregiving tasks will be too demanding. Caregivers also succumb to depression, functional decline, cognitive impairment, and physical illness. The health of caregivers can deteriorate faster than the patient's, superseding the status of the older person in determining the level of caregiver burden (49). Clinicians need to be aware of the status of the caregiver and be prepared to ask the following questions (Table 2.7): Is there someone in whom they can confide? Are they satisfied with their relationships? Do they have opportunities for respite? Is there evidence of depression or substance abuse? Does the caregiver have medical illness, such as arthritis or heart disease, which will make certain tasks difficult or impossible?

Keep in mind situations that may portend increased risk for abuse or neglect of older adults. Mistreatment may be verbal, psychological, and financial as well as physical (50). Mistreatment of older persons may be unintentional, through ignorance of proper caregiving techniques. When caregivers have psychiatric illness, including alcohol or other substance abuse problems, the risk for abuse may be increased. Caregiver stress may be heightened by factors outside the caregiving relationship, such as job loss or marital problems. Open the door to discussion of emotions like anger by assessing the caregiver's ability and desire to continue in the role of caregiver. Ask the caregiver what tasks seem most burdensome and about frustration and anger they may experience with caregiving. A plan of care using available community resources for respite may prevent reliance on a single caregiver, which would otherwise increase susceptibility to unexpected lapses in care or even abuse from a tired, angry, and overburdened caregiver. Comments on caregivers apply to the staff in institutional settings where "burnout" and low morale can be a problem.

In addition to information about the primary caregiver, obtain information about other formal and informal supports the older person may use, including a visiting nurse, home health aide, homemaker, Meals on Wheels, a pharmacy that will make home deliveries, or privately hired aides or homemakers. Ascertain what is and what is not working and what assistance may need to be incorporated into the older person's formal and informal social network to maximize function.

Social workers and social service agencies often have established relationships with older persons and their families and are a valuable resource in an interdisciplinary, collaborative approach to geriatric care. Social workers are specifically trained in social assessment including the dynamics of family and patient-caregiver relationships, available benefits (such as Medicaid, Food Stamps, and Supplemental Social Security Insurance), and community resources (such as adult day care, support groups, and companion services). A social worker can provide counseling, psychotherapy, or resource information in the community and institution. An awareness of the social service agencies is essential; each state has an Office on Aging, with listings in the phone book, that can provide practitioners with information about local resources. Several excellent references for learning about caregiver support are available (47, 48, 51).

VALUES ASSESSMENT

Eliciting the patient's wishes in the event of terminal or irreversible illness, an important part of geriatric assessment, is discussed more fully in Section III. Suffice it to say here that an opportunity to express wishes with regard to life-sustaining technologies will usually be welcomed by the patient and family. Recommend that the patient designate a person to make health-care decisions in the event of incapacity. If the patient has impaired decision-making capacity, discuss treatment plans with the family in advance of a crisis situation whenever possible.

HISTORY AND PHYSICAL EXAMINATION

The examination of the older patient should consider the special approach mandated by sensory impairment, restricted mobility, and slower response time. Good communication skills are important when dealing with all patients, but particularly with older people. Remember that the presenting symptom may involve the most poorly compensated organ system, not the organ system expected, so that pneumonia or congestive heart failure presents as delirium. The history and physical examination should aim to uncover remedial problems, with a focus on geriatric problems such as falls, incontinence, and sensory deficits. Ask about driving habits as well.

Gait and overall functional performance should be evaluated (8). By observing the patient

Table 2.7
Caregiver Assessment[a]

1. Does the caregiver have a confidante?
2. Who visits the caregiver, how often, and is the caregiver happy with these relationships?
3. What aspects of caregiving are most disturbing?
4. Does the caregiver have symptoms of depression?
5. Does the caregiver have functional or physical limitations?

[a]Adapted with permission from Gallo JJ. The effect of social support on depression in caregivers of the elderly. J Fam Pract 1990;30:430–440.

undressing in the examination room, one can assess sequencing a task, manual dexterity, attention span, and distractibility. The physical examination can verify and contribute to the information gathered in the functional history and other aspects of the geriatric assessment.

Frequently neglected are examinations of the skin, breasts, prostate, and rectum. Breast and pelvic examinations are particularly important for the older woman who has had infrequent contact with health professionals. Specific aspects of the history and physical examination pertinent to the older adult can be found interspersed throughout this book.

HEALTH PROMOTION AND DISABILITY PREVENTION

We discuss health promotion and disability prevention last but certainly not because it is least in importance; indeed, from a public health point of view, the prevention of disability has implications for health care cost, quality of life, and postponement of the need for long-term care services (36). Since the focus is on functional capacity, not diagnostic category, we use the term "disability prevention," not "disease prevention." "Geriatric-oriented" prevention puts the multidimensional assessment on a "prevention" footing, such as the prevention of functional impairment.

Prevention can be categorized as standard disease prevention or geriatric-oriented prevention (3). Standard preventive medicine deals with cardiovascular disease, cerebrovascular disease, cancer, and immunization (influenza and pneumococcal vaccines). Geriatric-oriented prevention deals with preventing or minimizing the effects of difficulties in areas that may not fit into a disease model of illness. Detailed guidelines are available that evaluate the evidence for efficacy and inform clinical practice, as discussed in the next chapter (53–55). Recommendations for standard preventive procedures must be tailored to the individual patient, considering the total clinical picture and the multidimensional evaluation; for example, cancer screening in a debilitated patient does not seem warranted if an asymptomatic condition will not be treated.

INTEGRATION INTO THE SETTINGS OF GERIATRIC CARE

AMBULATORY CARE

The ambulatory care of the older person provides ample opportunity for anticipatory guidance and opportunistic case finding if the domains of geriatric assessment are considered within the context of the doctor-patient relationship (1–4). Carry out an assessment over several visits, if necessary. The future of health care will see a greater reliance on a continuing process of assessment that may be carried out over a prolonged period. Generalist physicians supported by nurses, social workers, nutritionists, and other health professionals will develop new patterns of office assessment as more is learned about this process. How the generalist physician and nurse incorporate the principles of multidomain assessment will evolve in the next decade. Right now the health care professional, with the patient, must prioritize the problems to be addressed in the visit. Better care means attending to all dimensions of patient care: physical, emotional, mental status, functional, social, economic, values, existential and spiritual, and health promotion and disability prevention factors.

The logistics and reimbursement patterns for geriatric assessment have not been worked out yet in everyday practice. In one office or clinic or community health center, the physician may perform a history and physical examination, evaluate mental status and mood, order appropriate tests, and communicate with other health care professionals. In some settings, the nurse may evaluate functional ability, nutrition, social activity, and social support by family and caregivers, and may make home visits when this is part of the assessment. Social workers may explore family dynamics, examine financial and living arrangements, perform the home visit, and act as the liaison for the team between the patient and various social agencies. Other professionals such as nutritionists, physical therapists, occupational therapists, and clergy may all work together or may be called upon in a consultative role.

How the generalist clinician will use the tools of geriatric assessment in daily practice will evolve, and we will witness changes in reimbursement with new fee codes that will be granted for clinical effort that exceeds what has been traditional office or clinic care. At this time, much effort is being given to enhance reimbursement for expanded service that exceeds the traditional comprehensive examination.

The generalist clinician may find it helpful to use a flow chart to keep track of cognitive, functional, social status, and health maintenance examinations, as well as medical conditions, over time (1). The use of computer technology to guide assessment and information management is a new field in geriatrics. Finally, close interdisciplinary working relationships with case managers, social service agencies, and others can be especially effective when caring for older adults with multisystem problems.

On an outpatient basis, the more complicated older patient with multiple problems may require referral to a specialized geriatric assessment program that exists in many hospitals and other settings. It is often a family member or caregiver who initiates this referral. Members of the multidisciplinary assessment team may consist of a physician and a nurse, or a physician and a social worker, or in some cases, a single professional—physician, nurse, or social worker, all of whom have the expertise in geriatric assessment.

Gerontological nurses practicing in the expanded role have skill in conducting a comprehensive assessment and managing acute and chronic health problems and wellness issues. Nurses often fulfill the role of "case manager" across the care continuum and provide leadership in assessment and management.

HOSPITALS

It is particularly challenging to maintain a comprehensive perspective in the hospital setting, yet the ultimate outcome may be less than optimum if treatment is approached without consideration of the dimensions of geriatric assessment. The cognitive, functional, emotional, and social status are all important to assess at the time of admission, so that planning for services required at discharge can begin immediately. Patients with cognitive impairment are at greater risk of delirium during hospitalization and after surgery. Also, preadmission functional status is a good predictor of posthospitalization status. "High-tech" care may loom over more mundane efforts such as assisting patients out of bed, implementing toileting schedules, or obtaining a much-needed hearing aid. The interruption of an established geriatric care plan by hospitalization may result in lost ground and iatrogenesis; for example, the benefits of superb intensive care may be undone by the development of decubiti.

As stated in Chapter 1, the first essential for the physician, nurse, and others who care for the older person is to act as an integrator of the biopsychosocial model. To accomplish this, the health professional must know the patient thoroughly. This is not to diminish the excellence of the medical specialties and subspecialties that have achieved much over the past 20 to 30 years. In the ideal model of health care described in Chapter 1, the patient is not seen from a single medical specialty point of view but with the full appreciation of other organ systems, emotional or psychosocial factors, information based on continuity over a period of time, knowledge of the patient's family and community, and an understanding of all the dimensions of geriatric assessment (56–60).

REHABILITATION SETTINGS

The principles of rehabilitation are particularly applicable to older adults with acute medical problems and functional deficits: (a) stabilization of the underlying or acute process, (b) prevention of secondary complications and functional deficits, and (c) facilitation of the individual's adaptation to the disability and to the environment (transportation, home modification, and the use of assistive devices and equipment) (61). Indeed, the emphasis on functional assessment in rehabilitation is central to the notion of geriatric assessment (62).

Geriatric assessment can be instrumental in identifying older patients who would benefit from rehabilitation programs. While rehabilitation programs are available at specialized rehabilitation hospitals, medically stable patients requiring a low-intensity program may be rehabilitated while in the nursing home or through arrangements with an outpatient clinic. Although functional deficits in older populations may be reversible, comprehensive rehabilitation programs for aged persons are not widely available (63).

LONG-TERM CARE

A comprehensive geriatric assessment is essential at the time of admission to a nursing home or other long-term care facility. Admission to long-term care often comes at a time of great stress and crisis for the older person and caregiver alike, after a hospitalization or a major disruption in the social support network. The importance of a comprehensive functional assessment is emphasized by the Omnibus Budget Reconciliation Act (OBRA) of 1987, which mandates that all persons admitted to Medicaid- and Medicare-eligible long-term care facilities be assessed in an organized way. OBRA directs facilities to "conduct comprehensive, accurate, standardized, and reproducible assessments of their residents' functional capacity." The Minimum Data Set (MDS) contains the components of the required assessment (64). Nurses, physical therapists, occupational therapists, recreational therapists, and social workers complete the mimimum data set within 15 days of the patient's admission to the long-term care facility and must review the data for accuracy at least quarterly thereafter.

The MDS includes assessment of medical conditions: alertness and coherence, memory, cognitive skills for daily decision making, and changes in cognitive status; communication and hearing problems; vision; modes of expression and the ability to understand others; and ADLs. Problems related to body movement are assessed in detail, including balance, contractures, gait, and the use of mobility appliances or devices such as canes, walkers, braces, prostheses, and wheelchairs. Psychosocial functioning and well-being is assessed through estimation of initiative and involvement, ability to relate to others, and the ability to express feelings. Mood and behavior patterns are noted, such as wandering, abusiveness, and refusing medicines or care. Preferred daily activity patterns are recorded as well as the setting for preferred activity, i.e., in the patient's own room, the community area, or outside the facility.

Although the MDS evaluation is time consuming, it has the advantage of encouraging the staff to engage the older person in establishing goals and a mutually agreed upon plan of care to reach the goals. Geriatric assessment in the long-term care setting is not a one-time event, but is ongoing, so that the goals and care plan reflect the changing needs of the resident.

HOME CARE

A home evaluation for every older adult as part of an initial assessment would be ideal. Home care programs with visiting physicians and nurse practitioners are available in many areas of the country. Usually the home assessment is done by a visiting nurse, and information from the assessment is relayed to the office- or hospital-based care provider.

A single home visit can often yield more information than many office visits, and some data are never fully appreciated in the office. In the home, the health care provider is on the older person's "turf," so that power is shifted to the older person. Good observational skills are required to fully assess the environment without being too intrusive; however, an experienced person can garner much information from even one home visit. An evaluation of environmental safety is crucial to understanding some of the issues affecting the older person's care and lifestyle, including the risk of falling. A bowl of candy positioned close to the diabetic's chair or bed, or boxes of crackers stacked on kitchen counters, may explain uncontrolled di-

abetes and clearly demonstrate the need for more diabetic teaching, closer monitoring, and possibly, support from a caregiver.

How medications are actually taken can be more easily checked at home than at the office or hospital. The use of home care equipment (such as oxygen), the layout of the home or apartment (such as the location of stairs), and ease of access to the bathroom and kitchen, are easier to appreciate when seen first-hand. Informal supports and an extended family network are more easily understood as people drop in or call during a home visit. The health care provider who makes regular home visits joins that group of supporters. Older persons come to rely upon caretakers, both formal and informal, who, by making home visits, enhance quality of life and help the older person remain at home.

CONCLUSION

The multidimensional geriatric assessment provides the foundation for the therapeutic plan in all the settings of geriatric care. The challenge of modern geriatrics is to consider the effects of medical disorders on each dimension of comprehensive assessment and to consider the multidimensional status of the older person when addressing treatment options, within the framework of a fragmented, "high-tech," and insurance-driven system. As health care reform beckons, mechanisms that foster appropriate geriatic care will need to be cultivated.

REFERENCES

1. Gallo JJ, Reichel W, Andersen L. Handbook of geriatric assessment. 2nd ed. Rockville: Aspen, 1995.
2. Epstein AM, Hall JA, Besdine R, et al. The emergence of geriatric assessment units: The "new technology of geriatrics." Ann Intern Med 1987;106:299–303.
3. Stults BM. Preventive health care for the elderly. West J Med 1984;141:832–845.
4. Lavizzo-Mourey R, Day SC, Diserens D, Grisso JA. Practicing prevention for the elderly. Philadelphia: Hanley & Belfus, 1989.
5. Katz S, Ford AB, Moskowitz RW, et al. Studies of illness in the aged: the index of ADL. JAMA 1963;185:914–919.
6. Coroni-Huntley J, Brock DB, Ostfeld AM, Taylor JO, Wallace RB, eds. Established populations for epidemiologic study of the elderly: resource data book. National Institute on Aging. Public Health Service. National Institutes of Health. NIH Publication No. 86–2443. Washington, DC, 1986.
7. Lichtenstein MJ, Federspiel CF, Schaffner W. Factors associated with early demise in nursing home residents: a case control study. J Am Geriatr Soc 1985;33:315–319.

8. Tinetti ME, Speechley M. Prevention of falls among the elderly. N Engl J Med 1989;320:1055–1059.

9. Miller CA. Nursing care of older adults. Glenview, IL: Scott, Foresman, Little, Brown Higher Education, 1990.

10. DeCastro JM. Age-related changes in natural spontaneous fluid ingestion and thirst in humans. J Gerontol 1992;47:321–330.

11. Lawton MP, Brody EM. Assessment of older people: self-maintaining and instrumental activities of daily living. Gerontologist 1969;9:179–186.

12. Teresi JA, Cross PS, Golden RR. Some applications of latent trait analysis to the measurement of ADL. J Gerontol 1989;44:S196–204.

13. Barberger-Gateau P, Commenges D, Gagnon M, Letenneur L, Sauvel C, Dartigues JF. Instrumental activities of daily living as a screening tool for cognitive impairment and dementia in elderly community dwellers. J Am Geriatr Soc 1992;40:1129–1134.

14. Fillenbaum G. Screening the elderly: a brief instrumental activities of daily living measure. J Am Geriatr Soc 1985;33:698–706.

15. Hayter J. To nap or not to nap? Geriatr Nurs 1985;6:104–106.

16. Malfetti JL. Older driver graduated licensing: summary of proceedings of the conference on driver competency assessment. In: State of California Department of Motor Vehicles, Program and Policy Administration, Research, and Development Section, 1990.

17. Lillie SM. Evaluation for driving. In: Yoshikawa TT, Cobbs EL, Brummel-Smith K, eds. Ambulatory geriatric care, St. Louis: Mosby, 1993:131–141.

18. Underwood M. The older driver: clinical assessment and injury prevention. Arch Intern Med 1992;152:735–740.

19. Canadian Medical Association. Physicians' guide to driver examination. 5th ed. Can Med Assoc J 1991;(suppl)Jul 15:1–64.

20. Catania JA. Older Americans and AIDS: transmission risks and primary prevention research needs. Gerontologist 1989;29:373–381.

21. Jones TV, Williams ME. Rethinking the approach to evaluating mental functioning of older persons: the value of careful observations. J Am Geriatr Soc 1988;36:1128–1134.

22. American Psychiatric Association. Diagnostic and statistical manual of mental disorders. 4th ed. Washington, DC: American Psychiatric Association, 1994.

23. McKhann G, Drachman D, Folstein M, et al. Clinical diagnosis of Alzheimer's disease. Neurology 1984;34:939–944.

24. Folstein MF, Folstein SE, and McHugh PR. "Mini-Mental State," a practical method for grading the cognitive state of patients for the clinician. J Psychiatr Res 1975;12:189–198.

25. Pfeiffer E. A short portable mental status questionnaire for the assessment of organic brain deficit in elderly patients. J Am Geriatr Soc 1975;23:433–441.

26. Strub RL, Black FW. The mental status examination in neurology. 2nd ed. Philadelphia, FA Davis, 1985.

27. Tombaugh TN, McIntyre NJ. The Mini-Mental State Examination: a comprehensive review. J Am Geriatr Soc 1992;40:922–935.

28. Crum RM, Anthony JC, Bassett SS, Folstein MF. Population-based norms for the Mini-Mental State Examination by age and educational level. JAMA 1993;269:2386–2391.

29. Newmann, J.P. Aging and depression. Psychol Aging 1989;4:150–165.

29a. Gallo JJ, Anthony JC, Muthen BO. Age differences in the symptoms of depression: a latent trait analysis. J Gerontol 1994;49:P251–264.

30. Blazer D. Clinical features of depression in old age: a case for minor depression. Curr Opinion Psychiatry 1991;4:596–599.

31. Chaisson-Stewart GM, ed. Depression in the elderly: an interdisciplinary approach. New York: J Wiley & Sons, 1985.

32. Rohrbaugh RM, Siegal AP, Giller EL. Irritability as a symptom of depression in the elderly. J Am Geriatr Soc 1988;36:736–738.

33. Depression Guideline Panel. Depression in primary care: clinical practice guideline, number 5. Rockville, MD: U.S. Department of Health and Human Services, Public Health Service, Agency for Health Care Policy and Research. AHCPR publication no. 93–0550 and 93–0551, April 1993.

34. Popkin MK, Tucker GJ. "Secondary" and drug-induced mood, anxiety, psychotic, catatonic, and personality disorders: a review of the literature. J Neuropsychiatr Clin Neurosci 1992;4:369–385.

35. Lachs MS, Feinstein AR, Cooney LM, et al. A simple procedure for general screening for functional disability in elderly patients. Ann Intern Med 1990;112:699–706.

36. Institute of Medicine. The second 50 years: promoting health and preventing disability. Washington, DC: National Academy Press, 1992.

37. Brink TL, Yesavage JA, Lum O. Screening tests for geriatric depression. Clin Gerontol 1982;1:37–43.

38. Yesavage JA, Brink TL, Rose TL, et al. Development and validation of a geriatric depression screening scale: a preliminary report. J Psychiatr Res 1983;17:37–49.

39. Zung WWK, Magill M, Moore JT, et al. Recognition and treatment of depression in a family medicine practice. J Clin Psychiatry 1983;44:3–6.

40. Beck AT, Beck RW. Screening depressed patients in family practice: a rapid technique. Postgrad Med 1972;52:81–85.

41. Burke WJ, Roccaforte WH, Wengel SP. The short form of the Geriatric Depression Scale: a comparison with the 30-item form. J Geriatr Psychiatry Neurol 1991;4:173–178.

42. Burke WJ, Houston MJ, Boust SJ, Roccaforte WH. Use of the Geriatric Depression Scale in dementia of the Alzheimer type. J Am Geriatr Soc 1989;37:856–860.

43. Kafonek S, Ettinger WH, Roca R, et al. Instruments for screening for depression and dementia in a long-term care facility. J Am Geriatr Soc 1989;37:29–34.

44. Alden D, Austin C, Sturgeon R. A correlation between the Geriatric Depression Scale long and short forms. J Gerontol 1989;44:P124–125.

45. Rabins P, Mace NL, Lucas MJ. The impact of dementia on the family. JAMA 1982;248:333–335.

46. Gallo JJ. The effect of social support on depression in caregivers of the elderly. J Fam Pract 1990;30:430–440.

47. Huttman ED. Social services for the elderly. New York: The Free Press, 1985.

48. Hooyman NR, Lustbader W. Taking care: supporting older people and their families. New York: The Free Press, 1986.

49. Brown LJ, Potter JF, Foster BG. Caregiver burden should be evaluated during geriatric assessment. J Am Geriatr Soc 1990;38:455–460.

50. Aravanis SC, Adelman RD, Breckman R, Fulmer TT, Holder E, Lachs M, O'Brien JG, Sanders AB. Diagnostic and treatment guidelines on elder abuse and neglect. Arch Fam Med 1993;2:371–388.

51. Mace NL, Rabins PV. The 36-hour day. Rev ed. Baltimore: Johns Hopkins University Press, 1991.

52. Keeler EB, Kane RL, Solomon DH. Short- and long-term residents of nursing homes. Med Care 1981;19:363–369.

53. U.S. Preventive Services Task Force. Guide to clinical preventive services. Baltimore, Williams & Wilkins, 1989.

54. Woolf SH, Kamerow DB, Lawrence RS, et al. The periodic health examination of older adults: the recommendations of the U.S. Preventive Services Task Force, Part I. J Am Geriatr Soc 1990;38:817–823.

55. Woolf SH, Kamerow DB, Lawrence RS, et al. The periodic health examination of older adults: the recommendations of the U.S. Preventive Services Task Force, Part II. J Am Geriatr Soc 1991;39:316–317.

56. Extending life, enhancing life: a National Research Agenda on aging. Washington, DC: National Academy of Sciences, 1991.

57. Reichel W. The continuity imperative. JAMA 1981;246:2065.

58. Engel GL. How much longer must medicine's science be bound by a seventeeth century world view? Psychother Psychosom 1992;57:3–16.

59. Fulmer TT, Walker MK. Critical care nursing of the elderly. New York: Springer Series on Geriatric Nursing, 1992.

60. Brody SJ, Morrison MH. Aging and rehabilitation beyond the medical model. Generations 1992;25:23–26.

61. Brummel-Smith K. Geriatric rehabilitation. Generations 1992;25:27–30.

62. Williams TF. Rehabilitation in the aging. New York: Raven, 1984:xiii.

63. Wray LA, Torres-Gil FM. Availability of rehabilitation services for elders. Generations 1992;25:31–36.

64. Levenson SA, ed. Medical direction in long-term care: a guidebook for the future. Durham, NC: Carolina Academic Press, 1993.

3/ Health Maintenance and Prevention for Older Persons

John B. Murphy, Elise M. Coletta

The goal of preventive health efforts should be to improve (or maintain) the quality of life while maximizing length of life. There are good data to demonstrate the efficacy of some preventive health activities, even for persons of advanced age. A nihilistic approach to preventive health care of elderly persons is not justifiable. Nonetheless, a cautious or skeptical approach is warranted. Far too often, preventive health interventions of demonstrated efficacy in younger populations are presumed to be equally effective when applied to older persons. Such presumptions disregard the unique qualities of older persons and can expose them to ineffective and, in some cases, harmful interventions.

Prevention has been characterized as primary, secondary, and tertiary. Primary prevention refers to efforts designed to prevent disease before it ever occurs. Counseling, immunizations, and chemoprophylaxis are forms of primary prevention. Secondary prevention refers to identifying diseases or conditions in their asymptomatic phase (also known as screening), and tertiary prevention refers to preventing progression of disease once it becomes symptomatic. This chapter focuses on primary and secondary prevention.

The distinction between preventive health interventions in asymptomatic individuals, and diagnosis in symptomatic individuals with the index disease or condition cannot be overemphasized. In this chapter we focus on asymptomatic individuals without specific risk factors for the disease discussed.

The research database that supports clinical decision making as it relates to prevention for elderly persons has numerous gaps and omissions. Given the difficulty and cost of conducting large-scale trials to validate primary and secondary preventive health efforts for older persons, it is likely that many of the shortcomings of our existing database will persist for some time. This places physicians in the position of using their judgment in making decisions about preventive health interventions. As is the case when dealing with other age groups, astute clinicians will routinely incorporate known risk factors for a given disease and the risks of the intervention into their decision-making process.

For the older patient, additional variables need to be considered. Although the average life expectancy for a given individual is an important variable, a more important concept is active life expectancy (ALE). ALE was operationally defined by Katz et al. and refers to that period of life free of disability in activities of daily living (ADLs)(1). A fundamental tenet of ALE as a measure of health status is that avoiding death and disease is not the only criterion for assessing the health of people in old age; functional status and independence play an important role in defining both health and quality of life. Furthermore, functional status is a powerful predictor of mortality and other health outcomes. As such, ALE (Table 3.1) and a patient's functional status should be considered by clinicians who must exercise their judgment in deciding which preventive measures to offer a given patient.

Primary and secondary prevention recommendations vary greatly depending upon the organization that is making the recommendations. There are understandable reasons for the differences, particularly when "gold standard" randomized trials are not available to support the recommendations. It is not surprising that subspecialty societies and organizations, such as the American Cancer Society, have more extensive and/or "aggressive" recommendations for the diseases or conditions on which they focus. This undoubtedly stems, in part, from an honest zeal to do the most possible to minimize the impact of these diseases, but it also stems from selection bias. The patient population walking into the primary care physician's office clearly differs from that seen in a university hospital subspecialty clinic. There is no question that the prevalence of disease in the subspecialist's office is higher, and as such, it will be the subspecialist's impression that yet unproven interventions have greater efficacy. It necessarily follows, however, that such potential for selection bias must be incorporated into general screening recommendations. For this reason, the recommendations of more broadly based groups, such as the USPSTF or the Canadian Task Force on the Periodic Health Examination, probably hold greater validity for the clinician in practice.

At least as important as issues related to which preventive health interventions are important, are issues related to how to conduct preventive health interventions. In short, what to do is much simpler than how to go about doing it. However, a discussion of the process of practicing prevention is beyond the scope of this chapter.

PRIMARY PREVENTION
COUNSELING

Tobacco

Nineteen percent of Americans age 65 to 74 smoke, as do 9% of those 75 or older (2). Even minimal counseling by health care providers has been shown to be effective in smoking cessation, and the health benefits of smoking cessation clearly extend to quitting at older ages (3). These benefits include improved pulmonary function; decreased risk of coronary artery disease, peripheral vascular disease, stroke, and lung cancer; and decreased risk of hip fracture for women using estrogen replacement therapy (ERT) (4–7).

Exercise

More than 40% of persons age 65 and older report no leisure-time physical activity, and less than 10% participate in regular aerobic exercise (8). Increasing physical activity not only reduces coronary heart disease risk, but also can improve musculoskeletal conditions and bone density and enhance a sense of well-being for older persons (7–10). Fall risk may be reduced as well. All older persons should be encouraged to engage in a regular program of physical activity tailored to their personal condition.

Diet

The ideal low-fat, high-fiber diet with lots of fresh fruits and vegetables, lean meats, and non-fat dairy products does not match well with the characteristics of the current cohort of older Americans. This group tends to be marginally well off financially and to have poor dentition, a high prevalence of heart disease, lung disease, and joint conditions, and difficulty with transportation. Many of the optimum foods (lean meats, fresh fruits and vegetables) cannot be procured at the corner convenience store and thus, for the individual who has difficulty with transportation, may be obtainable only when a family member or friend can drive him or her to a larger grocery store. The perishability of these foods may also be a problem. Furthermore, many of the advantageous foods, particularly fruits, low-fat dairy products, and lean meats, are heavy and may be difficult to carry for the older individual with coronary artery disease, chronic lung disease, or arthritis. Most of these foods are relatively expensive, which creates a further impediment to procurement by an older population that is relatively poor. For these reasons, dietary recommendations, although very important, must be tempered, to avoid precipitating malnutrition in an often marginally nourished group of individuals.

A large proportion of community-dwelling elders consume diets that fail to meet the minimum recommended dietary allowances (RDA) (11). Preliminary data suggest that daily supplementation with a multivitamin (approximating the U.S. RDA) may improve immune function and result in fewer infection-related sick days for older persons (12).

The effect of calcium intake on the rate of fracture in older women has not been evaluated in a controlled clinical trial (13). However, in postmenopausal women, calcium supplementation in the range of 1 to 2 grams has been demonstrated to significantly decrease the rate of bone loss (14–15). For this reason, most authorities recommend a calcium intake of 800 to 1500 mg daily for postmenopausal women, unless contraindicated by

Table 3.1
Total and Active Life Expectancies[a]

Age	Total Life Expectancy (yr)		Active Life Expectancy (yr)	
	Men	Women	Men	Women
65	15–17	19–21	11–13	15–17
75	8–11	11–13	6–7	8–9
85	4–6	6	2–3	2–4
90+	1–2	<1	<1	

[a]Adapted from Branch LG, Guralnik JM, Foley DJ, et al. Active expectancy for 10,000 Caucasian men and women in three communities. J Gerontol 1991;46:M145–150.

concurrent medical illnesses (13, 16). Table 3.2 lists the calcium content of selected foods. Vitamin D deficiency is a common, but often unrecognized, contributing factor to the development of fractures in elders. Thus, dietary supplementation of vitamin D to 600–800 international units/day is recommended (13, 16, 17).

Alcohol

Data from controlled trials suggesting that counseling about alcohol consumption prevents alcohol abuse are lacking. However, the proportion of older persons who drink is increasing and is estimated to be between 2 and 15% of the general population (19). Furthermore, elders are felt to be at greater risk for alcohol abuse because of physiological changes in alcohol distribution and metabolism, the concurrent use of prescription and nonprescription medications, the presence of comorbid illness, and an increased risk for falls and accidents. Thus, as recommended by the USPSTF, it seems reasonable to inquire about a patient's alcohol intake (although no specific screening questionnaire or laboratory test can be currently recommended) and to intervene when a concern is identified (20).

Accidental Injury

There are few data from controlled trials to suggest that counseling prevents accidents and injuries; however, accidents are the seventh leading cause of death for persons age 65 and older. Thus, it seems prudent, as recommended by the USPSTF, to advise patients to use automobile safety belts and helmets when riding bicycles and to counsel patients on abstinence from alcohol when driving and on home safety (21). Sample home safety recommendations include advice on adequate lighting, removing or repairing floor structures that predispose to tripping (e.g., loose rugs, electric cords), and installation of handrails and traction strips in bathrooms and stairways.

Advance Directives

Advance directives are covered extensively elsewhere in this text. However, it is important to incorporate discussions related to advance directives into routine health maintenance to prevent unwanted medical interventions.

Medications

Some 60 to 80% of community-dwelling elders regularly use prescription medications, 50 to 76% routinely use nonprescription drugs, and up to 14% are taking five or more prescription medications (22). The potential for adverse drug reactions and drug interactions probably increases with age (in part related to the number of medications and comorbid illness), and thus, counseling to avoid all unnecessary medications may be beneficial.

IMMUNIZATIONS

Pneumococcal

Pneumococcal polysaccharide vaccine is currently recommended for all persons age 65 and older (23). However, only 14% of persons 65 and older have received pneumococcal vaccine. The reasons for this are multifactorial but include conflicting evidence about vaccine efficacy. It appears that efficacy is good to excellent in younger immunocompetent recipients, but protective efficacy appears to wane with age and in immunocompromised individuals. Thus, it is likely that in the near future, the age recommendation for consideration of pneumococcal vaccine will shift to an earlier age (less than 55 years). It is also currently recommended that individuals at high risk of pneumococcal disease (asplenic patients, transplant recipients, those with chronic renal failure or nephrotic syndrome) be revaccinated every 6 years. If universal immunization at the age of 55 becomes the recommended practice or if longitudinal studies show waning antibody levels, booster immunization may become routine for all patients.

Influenza

Influenza vaccine has been available since the 1950s. However, 19 of the postvaccine annual influenza epidemics in the United States have been associated with more than 10,000 excess deaths, and two of these epidemics were associated with

Table 3.2
Calcium Content of Selected Foods[a]

Food	Serving Size	Calcium Content (mg)
Parmesan cheese	1 ounce (oz)	390
Sardines	8 medium	354
Yogurt	8 oz	345
Milk (skim)	8 oz	303
Cheddar cheese	1 oz	211
Broccoli	1 spear	205
American cheese	1 oz	195

[a]Adapted from Anonymous. Calcium supplements. Med Lett 1989;31:101–102.

40,000 excess deaths (23). Approximately 88 to 90% of the excess deaths occurred in persons 65 years of age or older. For this reason, the influenza vaccine is recommended for all persons age 65 and older. Although influenza immunization provides 65 to 80% protection in young individuals, the vaccine may be only 30 to 40% effective in preventing clinical illness in older persons (23). However, it can still benefit older individuals who develop the illness by lessening the severity of the disease, the likelihood of hospitalization, and the risk of death.

Additionally, compliance with influenza vaccine recommendations is affected by concern about the perceived frequency of adverse reactions. This concern is not justified because there is no difference in the frequency of adverse reactions in individuals receiving influenza vaccine and those receiving placebo (24). Antigenic variation among influenza viruses (shift and drift) as well as the short duration of vaccine-induced immunity require that individuals receive influenza vaccine each fall, and no opportunity should be bypassed in an effort to immunize patients. This includes routine office visits, hospitalizations for acute illnesses, and office- or community-based immunization programs. Amantadine hydrochloride, an antiviral drug, can prevent influenza A or be used therapeutically to reduce symptoms of influenza A infections (if given within the first 24 hours of symptoms). However, it is not a substitute for vaccination.

Tetanus

The occurrence of tetanus has decreased dramatically because of the use of tetanus toxoid (23). However, of all reported cases of tetanus between 1982 and 1989, 60% occurred in individuals age 60 and older, and most persons who die from tetanus are older. Serosurveys done since the late 1970s indicate that while less than 10% of young adults lack protective levels of circulating antitoxin against tetanus, 50 to 70% of older persons lack protective levels of circulating antitoxin (25). For these reasons it is currently recommended that older individuals continue to receive booster vaccinations middecade every 10 years (i.e., age 65, 75, 85, etc.). For individuals who have no history of previously receiving tetanus vaccination a primary series of three doses is recommended. The first two doses should be given at least 4 weeks apart, and the third dose should be given 6 to 12 months after the second.

No other vaccinations are currently recommended for asymptomatic low-risk elderly individuals. However, it is becoming increasingly clear that adults are the primary vector for pertussis illness in unimmunized or partially immunized children (26). Furthermore, pertussis is not exclusively a disease of childhood. It is an important respiratory disease in adults as well (26). Nonetheless, the currently licensed whole-cell pertussis vaccines are not recommended for routine use in adults because the incidence of side effects is too high for use in nonemergency situations. Trials of acellular pertussis vaccine in adults do demonstrate safety, and in the future it is possible that some form of pertussis vaccination will also be recommended throughout early and late adult life.

CHEMOPROPHYLAXIS

Aspirin

The Physicians' Health Study (a randomized, double-blind, placebo-controlled trial) demonstrated a conclusive reduction in the risk of myocardial infarction in men who took low-dose aspirin (325 mg of aspirin every other day) (27). Subgroup analysis illustrated that men age 60–69 and 70–84 received the most benefit. There was a nonsignificant increase in stroke rate in men taking aspirin, which did not change across age groups. The British doctors' trial illustrated no significant reduction in cardiovascular disease in men taking aspirin (28). However, an overview of both the British and U.S. physicians' studies demonstrated a significant 33% reduction in the risk of first myocardial infarction (29). For these reasons, many authorities cautiously recommend low-dose aspirin for men over age 50 for the primary prevention of heart disease (30).

Currently no randomized trial using aspirin in women has been completed. The Nurses' Health Study (a prospective cohort study) has demonstrated a reduced risk of myocardial infarction in women using low-dose aspirin (one to six 325-mg aspirin per week) who were 50 years or older (31). In this group there was no increase in stroke risk. Lacking evidence from randomized trials, many authorities have been cautious and fall short of recommending aspirin for primary prevention of heart disease in women (32).

Estrogen

In postmenopausal women, the most effective agent for prevention of bone loss and fracture is estrogen (13). One-third to one-half of the total bone loss a women sustains in her lifetime is estrogen related. Most of the bone loss caused by estrogen lack occurs within 6 years of menopause, but estrogen-mediated bone loss can continue for up to 20 years after menopause. Estrogen has been shown to be of benefit if started in women with early osteoporosis (13), but there are insufficient data to determine the latest age at which newly prescribed estrogen still has a substantial effect on bone mass and fracture rate. At present, there is no evidence that continuing estrogen after age 70 is effective in the prevention of osteoporosis (17).

Epidemiologic evidence of a cardioprotective effect of unopposed estrogen therapy may provide an additional reason for considering hormonal replacement (33). This cardioprotective effect is due, in part, to a favorable change in the lipid profile by estrogen (34). However, there is no information on cardioprotection when estrogen is started at or after age 65. The cardioprotective effect of estrogen may warrant longer use if proposed additional nonatherosclerotic, non-lipid-related mechanisms of action are verified. These mechanisms may imply that current use of estrogen is required for the cardioprotective effect (34). To eliminate the increased risk of endometrial cancer, progestin therapy must be added to estrogen for non-hysterectomized women. The potential mediating effect on cardioprotection by the addition of progestin and the conflicting data on promotion of breast cancer by estrogen prohibit any present unequivocal recommendation for general use in older woman at average risk for osteoporosis or heart disease (35, 36).

SECONDARY PREVENTION

Coronary Heart Disease

Coronary heart disease (CHD) accounts for nearly half of the total mortality in the U.S. population older than 65 years. The primary emphasis on screening for CHD risk factors in the U.S. has been focused on assessment of serum lipids, and, in particular, total serum cholesterol. The Framingham Study found that cardiovascular disease mortality is related to total cholesterol in subjects under 50 years, but not in those over 50 years (37). However, the level of HDL cholesterol may have some predictive importance in subjects over 60 years of age (38). In the Honolulu (Hawaii) Heart Program, serum cholesterol was an independent predictor of CHD even among men older than 65 years (39).

The picture is further complicated by individuals with low serum cholesterol, who appear, in the Framingham data, to have increased mortal-

ity. It is felt that this group of individuals may well be suffering from protein-calorie malnutrition secondary to other conditions (40). These conflicting data have led most authorities to agree that a significantly elevated serum cholesterol continues to be a risk factor for CHD in older persons, but because of the increasing prevalence of competing risk factors (e.g., hypertension and diabetes mellitus), the predictive power of plasma cholesterol concentrations for CHD events in older persons is somewhat diminished (41).

It is clear that cholesterol-lowering drugs can effectively lower elevated serum cholesterol levels in persons age 65–75 years (42). However, to date no study has demonstrated long-term safety of these drugs nor is there evidence of drug efficacy in an older population, in terms of decreasing CHD morbidity and mortality or total mortality (43). An ongoing trial, Cholesterol Reduction In Seniors Program (CRISP), is designed to ascertain whether lowering total cholesterol in individuals with total cholesterol values between 240 and 300 mg/dL will reduce cardiovascular morbidity and mortality and overall mortality. Until the results of this study are available (and this may be some time because CRISP has been modified), clinicians must rely on clinical judgment and modeling studies that predict the potential benefit of cholesterol lowering in older persons.

Two well-conducted modeling studies predict very modest increases in life expectancy for persons over 65 years of age who make significant reductions in their serum cholesterol levels (44, 45). Grover et al. estimated a 35- to 50-day increase in life expectancy for a 65-year-old man who lowered his cholesterol from 240 to 200 mg/dL, and a 3- to 4-month increase in average life expectancy if the cholesterol was lowered from 300 to 200 mg/dL (44). Similarly, Taylor et al. estimated a 2- to 5-month increase in life expectancy for hypertensive smokers with a total cholesterol of 300 mg/dL if they were to reduce their cholesterol by up to 20% (45). Such modest potential gains in total life expectancy (not ALE), balanced against the costs and potential risks of long-term drug therapy, do not support a recommendation to screen for elevated cholesterol in persons beyond age 65.

Secondary screening for asymptomatic CHD with electrocardiograms (ECGs), either resting or exercise, is not currently recommended by the USPSTF or Canadian Task Force on the Periodic Health Examination (CTF). The poor specificity and sensitivity of such tests make them suboptimal tools for screening (46). Furthermore, the availability of a prior ECG has not been shown to have significant effect on the evaluation of patients with acute chest pain (47). Nonetheless, the American College of Cardiology recommends an ECG every 5 years, and the American Heart Association (AHA) recommends a baseline ECG at ages 40 and 60.

Both groups suggest exercise testing for sedentary persons embarking on vigorous exercise programs and for asymptomatic patients over age 40 with more than two risk factors for CHD (cholesterol level above 240 mg/dL, blood pressure above 160/90, tobacco use, diabetes, or a positive family history). We see no compelling evidence for, and thus recommend against, the use of screening ECGs. Although data are lacking, we agree with the suggestion to screen high-risk older patients before endorsing a vigorous exercise program, but see no reason to screen low-risk individuals embarking on a moderate exercise program in which activity is gradually increased in intensity and duration.

Hypertension affects 58 million Americans, contributing to over 20% of ischemic heart disease. The efficacy of reducing blood pressure has been well documented in studies on older persons (48). This includes persons with diastolic hypertension as well as those with isolated systolic hypertension. Thus routine blood pressure screening with each visit is supportable.

STROKE

Cerebrovascular disease is the third leading cause of death for older persons. Seventy-five percent of strokes occur after age 65, and the incidence of stroke rises steeply with age. Listening for carotid bruits is neither specific nor sensitive enough to warrant routine performance. While carotid endarterectomy (CEA) is of documented benefit in patients with a significant symptomatic stenosis of the carotid artery, currently few data support the benefit of CEA in asymptomatic patients (49, 50). Therefore, to date there is no role for screening asymptomatic patients with Doppler studies of the carotid arteries or carotid auscultation. Given the efficacy of CEA in patients with a transient ischemic attack, it is important to ask about TIAs.

Hypertension has been estimated to contribute to up to 90% of strokes, and screening for hypertension is warranted for the prevention of stroke, particularly for elders (48). The treatment of atrial fibrillation (AF) with warfarin (for those with valvular and nonvalvular atrial fibrillation) has been conclusively shown to decrease risk of stroke in younger and older individuals (51).

Thus, routinely checking the pulse for AF is also warranted.

CANCER

Cervical Cancer

Approximately 13,000 new cases of invasive cervical cancer are diagnosed each year, and about 6000 women die from this disease annually. Forty percent of deaths occur in women age 65 and older (52). Nonetheless, elderly women do not appear to benefit from Papanicolaou (PAP) testing if repeated cervical smears have been adequate and normal before age 65 (53). However, many older women have not previously been adequately screened. It is estimated that as many as 25% of women over the age of 65 in the U.S. have never had a PAP smear and up to 75% have not had regular screening (54).

In addition to low levels of screening, there are also questions related to the adequacy of sampling in older women. It is generally felt that the squamocolumnar junction is the site of optimum sampling for the detection of cervical cancer. The squamocolumnar junction migrates rostrally with age and thus may be more difficult to sample in an older woman. The presence of endocervical cells is generally felt to be consistent with an adequate sample. Thus, screening for cervical cancer with PAP smears can be safely stopped in women 65 and older in the absence of recent risk factors and previous cervical disease, if the woman has had a minimum of three recent adequate (endocervical cells present) normal cervical smears.

Breast Cancer

The incidence of breast cancer rises with age and does not level off until age 85 or above. The effectiveness of screening for breast cancer using mammography and the clinician breast examination effectiveness have been unequivocally demonstrated for women in the age range 50 to 74, and many studies have also shown clear benefit for women age 40 to 49. What is unclear (because of a lack of data) is whether there is additional benefit in screening women beyond the age of 74. The USPSTF recommends concluding screening at approximately age 75 unless pathology has been previously detected. The American Geriatrics Society has recommended screening until age 85. Data to support a specific cutoff are currently lacking, and in the absence of such data, we recommend routinely screening until age 75. For those functionally independent individuals with no major comorbid illnesses, screening can be continued through age 85. Beyond age 85, for individuals who have no previously identified breast disease, screening may be of limited value because the ALE at 85 is only 2 to 4 years.

Colon Cancer

Colorectal cancer increases in incidence throughout old age and unlike breast cancer continues to rise beyond age 85. To date, a single randomized controlled trial has examined the efficacy of fecal occult blood (FOB) testing as a screening test for colon cancer (55). There are no randomized trials that have evaluated the efficacy of sigmoidoscopy or digital rectal examination (DRE). Currently, a number of additional randomized trials are assessing the efficacy of FOB testing. The single completed FOB study is a well-designed, large, randomized trial that at the end of 13 years showed reduced colon cancer mortality in the experimental group compared with controls. Prior to 13 years there was no significant benefit.

This study provides significant justification for FOB screening. However, the long time period from trial initiation until demonstrated benefit, in spite of a large sample size, diminishes the importance of FOB testing in older populations. Competing risks make it unlikely that the older person will benefit from FOB testing. Furthermore, 50% of FOB studies are negative even in the face of colon cancer (56). For individuals with an ALE of 13 years or more, FOB testing may be beneficial. This corresponds to an age of roughly 70 years. Ongoing studies and subgroup analysis of the older population in the existing randomized trial may provide additional data regarding screening recommendations for colon cancer with FOB.

There are also additional parameters regarding older persons that may make it less advantageous to screen for colon cancer. Although the adenoma-carcinoma sequence has been well documented, it is estimated that at least 10 years are required for the progression from a small adenoma to malignancy. It is further estimated that 95% of all adenomas (and perhaps more) will never reach a malignant stage in a given individual's lifetime. Furthermore, the prevalence of adenomas in autopsy studies of individuals who did not die from colon cancer increases dramatically with age. In one autopsy series, 40 to 70% of individuals over the age of 65 had one or more adenomas at autopsy (57). Extrapolating from these findings to the population at large, assuming that 50% of these adenomas were within the reach of the flexible sigmoidoscope, suggests that one in four older persons

(50% of individuals with adenomas) would have adenomas identified on screening sigmoidoscopy. Standard practice would then dictate at least an air-contrast barium enema and preferably colonoscopy in follow-up. This would expose one quarter of our older population to colonoscopy and polypectomy, when it is estimated that a very small minority of these individuals are likely to have adenomas that progress to carcinoma. This would have tremendous cost implications and produce significant morbidity when there are no clear data to support the screening sigmoidoscopy. Additionally, DREs cannot reach most cancers and have never been proven to be efficacious. For these reasons, routine sigmoidoscopy and DRE are not recommended for colon cancer screening.

Prostate Cancer

The USPHSTF recommended against screening for prostate cancer with prostatic specific antigen, acid phosphatase, or transrectal ultrasound and made no recommendation regarding DRE. Recent data supports the use of prostatic specific antigen as a screening test in combination with DRE and transrectal ultrasound measurements (58).

However, these studies were conducted in referral and/or volunteer populations and do not distinguish between individuals with prostate cancer that will have a significant effect on the quality or quantity of their remaining lives and those with incidental prostatic cancer. To date, screening for prostate cancer is a clinical dilemma, with no clear evidence to suggest decreased mortality as the result of any screening test (58). No controlled trials have demonstrated that detecting more or earlier prostate cancer can improve quantity or quality of life (59).

In the absence of clear data, Mold et al. recently published a decision analysis to further investigate this issue (60). They concluded that the evaluation and treatment of prostatic nodules found by DRE in asymptomatic men in the primary care setting does not lead to significant improvement in life expectancy and adversely affects quality of life. Since most older men will die with and not from prostate cancer and since there are no data to support prostate cancer screening, we recommend against screening for prostate cancer until clear evidence demonstrating decreased morbidity or mortality becomes available.

Skin Cancer

Nonmelanoma skin cancers are the most common malignancies found in older individuals. The incidence of both basal and squamous cell carcinomas increases with age. When identified at an early stage, both types of skin cancer are very treatable. We know of no randomized trials on the efficacy of clinician skin examination. Nonetheless, given the high prevalence of these conditions, the low risk of false-positive screening skin examinations and the availability of acceptable low-cost, effective treatment options, we recommend routine examination of the skin as part of an annual examination for older individuals.

Other Cancers

We know of no data to support screening for lung cancer, ovarian cancer, uterine cancer (aside from asking about postmenopausal bleeding), or other malignancies in older individuals who are asymptomatic and have no risk factors for these conditions.

OTHER SCREENING MANEUVERS

Hearing

Hearing problems are one of the most prevalent conditions found in older Americans, with at least 36% of those age 75 and over affected. Mulrow et al., in a randomized trial, demonstrated the efficacy of screening for hearing deficits in an older population by using a hand-held otoscope with a built-in audiometer that delivered a 40-decibel tone at frequencies of 500, 1000, 2000, and 4000 Hz (61). Efficacy was assessed on the basis of improvement in (a) communication, (b) social, emotional, and cognitive function, and (c) mood in the group provided with hearing aids. Based on these findings and the high prevalence of hearing problems in older populations, a recommendation for routine screening for hearing deficits with a desktop audiometer or a hand-held audiometer is supportable. A recommended frequency of screening is open to question.

Visual Acuity

The incidences of glaucoma, cataracts, and macular degeneration all increase with age. Unfortunately, office glaucoma screening by primary care physicians using Schiotz tonometry and/or ophthalmoscopy has not been effective (62). Given

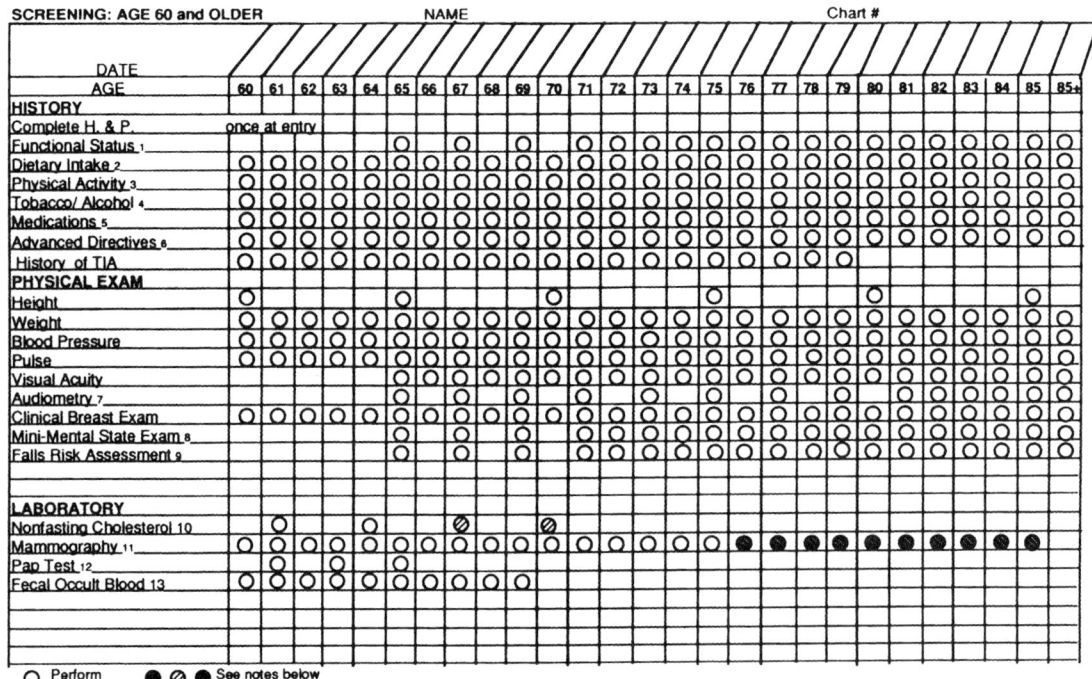

Figure 3.1 Screening age 60 and older.

that refractive problems are also common in older populations, it is recommended that regular annual screening be conducted by an eye specialist for all persons age 65 and older.

Osteoporosis and Fall-related Fractures

The importance of bone density in the development of osteoporosis-related fracture has led some to suggest limited use of densitometry to predict fracture risk in postmenopausal women. Given that most women over age 75 have bone densities below "fracture threshold," it is doubtful that densitometry will become a useful screening test in this population (9, 17). Although there are few data, a screening maneuver such as the "get-up and go" test (patients are observed as they rise from a chair, walk 3 meters, and return to the chair) may identify individuals at risk for falls.

Functional Assessment

Screening functional assessment is a hotly debated issue (63, 64). It is our opinion that a screening functional assessment that includes the domains of physical function (ADLs, IADLs, and mobility) and cognition (e.g., Mini-Mental State Examination) is worthwhile. We support physical function screening because functional impairments (the result of unidentified disease) and disease progression that often go undetected can be identified by a screening functional assessment. As for cognition testing, many persons with cognitive deficits will have irreversible dementias. Nonetheless, even when this is the case, the primary care physician can substantially improve the quality of a patient's life by early identification.

Summary

Our screening recommendations for older individuals are outlined in Figure 3.1. Our recommendations are parsimonious for two reasons. First, we are concerned about the potential harm of using unproven screening strategies. Second, even when there are effective screening strategies, many persons who should be screened have not received adequate screening. We agree with Clayman when he suggests that it is much wiser to invest our scarce resources in improving the screening rates for clearly efficacious interventions before investing in strategies whose efficacy is in question (65).

REFERENCES

1. Katz S, Branch LG, Branson MH, et al. Active life expectancy. N Engl J Med 1983;309:1218–1224.
2. Tobacco use by adults. MMWR 1989;38:685.
3. Hermanson B, Omen GS, Kromal RA, et al. Beneficial six-year outcome of smoking cessation in older men and women with coronary artery disease: results from the Cass registry. N Engl J Med 1988;319:1365–1369.
4. Kiel D, Baron JA, Anderson JJ, et al. Smoking eliminates the protective effect of oral estrogen on the risk of hip fracture among women. Ann Intern Med 1992;116:716–721.
5. Kawachi I, Graham HC, Stampfer MJ, et al. Smoking cessation and decreased risk of stroke in women. JAMA 1993;269:232–236.
6. Higgins MW, Enright PL, Kronmal RA, et al. Smoking and lung function in elderly men and women: the cardiovascular health study. JAMA 1993;269:2741–2748.
7. Paffenbarger RS, Hyde RT, Wing HL. The association of changes in physical activity level and other lifestyle characteristics with mortality among men. N Engl J Med 1993;328:538–545.
8. Healthy People 2000: National Health Promotion and Disease Prevention Objectives, U.S. Department of Health and Human Service. DHHS Publ no. (PHS) 91–50213, 1991:24.
9. Riggs BL, Melton LJ III. Involutional osteoporosis. N Engl J Med 1986;314:1676–1686.
10. Morley MC, Cowper PA, Feussner JR, et al. Two-year trends in physical performance following supervised exercise among community-dwelling older veterans. J Am Geriatr Soc 1991;39:549–554.
11. Ryan AS, Craig LD, Finn SC. Nutrient intakes and dietary patterns of older Americans: a national study. J Gerontol Med Sci 1992;47:M145–M150.
12. Chandra RK. Effect of vitamin and trace element supplementation on immune response and infection in elderly subjects. Lancet 1992;340:1124–1127.
13. Riggs BL, Melton LJ. The prevention and treatment of osteoporosis. N Engl J Med 1992;327:620–627.
14. Prince RL, Smith M, Dick IM, et al. Prevention of postmenopausal osteoporosis: a comparative study of exercise, calcium supplementation, and hormone replacement therapy. N Engl J Med 1991;325:1189–1195.
15. Reid IR, Ames RW, Evans MC, et al. Effect of calcium supplementation on bone loss in postmenopausal women. N Engl J Med 1993;328:460–464.
16. Heaney RP. Thinking straight about calcium. N Engl J Med 1993;328:503–505.
17. Resnick NM, Greenspan SL. "Senile" osteoporosis reconsidered. JAMA 1989;261(7):1025–1029.
18. Chapuy MC, Arlot ME, Duboeuf F, et al. Vitamin D3 and calcium to prevent hip fractures in elderly women. N Engl J Med 1992;327(23):1637–1642.
19. Laforge RG, Mignon SI. Alcohol use and alcohol problems among the elderly. RI Med 1993;76:21–26.
20. U.S. Preventive Services Task Force. Guide to clinical preventive services: an assessment of the effectiveness of 169 Interventions. Baltimore: William & Wilkins, 1989:277–286.
21. U.S. Preventive Services Task Force. Guide to clinical preventive services: an assessment of the effectiveness of 169 interventions. Baltimore, William and Wilkins, 1989:315–329.
22. Chrischilles EA, Foley DJ, Wallace RB, et al. Use of medications by persons 65 and over: data from the Established Populations for Epidemiologic Studies

of the Elderly. J Gerontol: Med Sci 1992;47:M137–M144.

23. Gardner P, Shaffner W. Immunization of adults. N Engl J Med 1993;328:1252–1257.

24. Margolis KL, Nichol KL, Poland GA, Pluhar RE. Frequency of adverse reactions to influenza vaccine in the elderly: a randomized, placebo-controlled trial. JAMA 1990;264:1139–1141.

25. Weiss BP, Strassburg MA, Feeley JC. Tetanus and diphtheria immunity in an elderly population in Los Angeles County. Am J Public Health 1983;73:802–804.

26. Herwaldt LA. Pertussis and pertussis vaccines in adults. JAMA 1993;269:93–94.

27. Steering Committee of the Physician's Health Study Research Group. Final report of the aspirin component of the ongoing physician's health study. N Engl J Med 1989;321:129–135.

28. Peto R, Gray R, Collins R, et al. Randomized trial of prophylactic daily aspirin in British male doctors. Br Med J 1988;296:313–316.

29. Hennekens CH, Peto R, Hutchinson GB, Doll R. An overview of the British and American aspirin studies. N Engl J Med 1988;318:923–924.

30. Manson JE, Tosteson H, Ridker P, et al. The primary prevention of myocardial infarction. N Engl J Med 1992;326:1406–1416.

31. Manson JE, Stampfer MJ, Colditz GA, et al. A prospective study of aspirin use and primary prevention of cardiovascular disease in women. JAMA 1991;266:521–527.

32. Appel LJ. Preventing heart disease in women: another role for aspirin? JAMA 1991;266:565–566.

33. Stampfer MJ, Colditz GA, Willett WC, et al. Postmenopausal estrogen therapy and cardiovascular disease. Ten-year follow-up from the Nurses' Health Study. N Engl J Med 1991;325(11):756–762.

34. Barrett-Connor E. Risks and benefits of replacement estrogen. Annu Rev Med 1992;43:239–251.

35. Heinrich JB. The postmenopausal estrogen/breast cancer controversy. JAMA 1992;268(14):1900–1902.

36. Steinberg KK, Thacker SB, Smith J, et al. A meta-analysis of the effect of estrogen replacement therapy on the risk of breast cancer. JAMA 1991;265(15):1985–1990.

37. Anderson KM, Castelli WP, Levy D. Cholesterol and mortality: 30 years of follow-up from the Framingham Study. JAMA 1987;257:2176–2180.

38. Castelli WP, Garrison RJ, Wilson PW, et al. Incidence of coronary heart disease and lipoprotein cholesterol levels: the Framingham Study. JAMA 1986;256:2835–2838.

39. Benfante R, Reed D. Is elevated serum cholesterol level a risk factor for coronary heart disease in the elderly? JAMA 1990;263:393–396.

40. Morley JE. Nutritional status in the elderly. Am J Med 1986;81:679–695.

41. Kaffonek SD, Kwiterovich PO. Treatment of hypercholesterolemia in the elderly. Ann Intern Med 1990;112:723–725.

42. Bach LA, Cooper ME, O'Brien RC, Gerums G. The use of simvastatin, HMG CoA reductase inhibitor, in older patients with hypercholesterolemia and atherosclerosis. J Am Geriatr Soc 1990;38:10–14.

43. Pacala JT. The relation of serum cholesterol to risk of coronary heart disease: implications for the elderly. J Am Board Fam Pract 1990;3:271–282.

44. Grover S, Abrahamowicz M, Joseph L, et al. The benefits of treating hyperlipidemia to prevent coronary heart disease: estimating change in life expectancy and morbidity. JAMA 1992;267:816–822.

45. Taylor WC, Pass TM, Shepard D, Komaroff AL. Cholesterol reduction and life expectancy: A model incorporating multiple risk factors. Ann Intern Med 1987;106:605–614.

46. Sox HC, Garber AM, Uttenberg B. The resting electrocardiogram as a screening test. Ann Intern Med 1989;111:489–502.

47. Lee TH, Cook EF, Weisberg MC, et al. Impact of the availability of a prior electrocardiogram on the triage of the patient with acute chest pain. J Gen Intern Med 1990;5:381–388.

48. SHEP Cooperative Research Group. Prevention of stroke by antihypertensive drug treatment in older persons with isolated systolic hypertension. JAMA 1991;265:3255–3264.

49. North America Symptomatic Carotid Endarterectomy Trial Collaborators. Beneficial effect of carotid endarterectomy in symptomatic patients with high-grade carotid stenosis. N Engl J Med 1991;325:445–453.

50. The CASANOVA Study Group. Carotid surgery versus medical therapy in asymptomatic carotid stenosis. Stroke 1991;22:1229–1235.

51. Special Report, Preliminary report of the stroke prevention in atrial fibrillation study. N Engl J Med 1990;322:863–867.

52. American Cancer Society. Cancer Statistics, 1989. CA 1989;30:3–20.

53. Canadian Task Force on Cervical Cancer Screening. Cervical cancer screening programs: summary of the 1982 Canadian Task Force report. Can Med Assoc J 1982;127:581–589.

54. Mandelblatt JS, Fahs MC. The cost-effectiveness of cervical cancer screening for low income elderly women. JAMA 1988;259:2409–2413.

55. Mandel JS, Bond JH, Church TR, et al. Reducing mortality from colorectal cancer by screening for fecal occult blood. N Engl J Med 1993;328:1365–1371.

56. Ahlquist DA, Wieand HS, Maertel CG, et al. Accuracy of fecal occult blood screening for colorectal neoplasia. JAMA 1993;269:1262–1267.

57. Rickert RR, Averbach O, Garfinkle L, Hammond C, Frasca J. Adenomatous lesions of the large bowel, an autopsy survey. Cancer 1979;43:1847–1857.

58. Littrup P, Lee F, Mettlin C. Prostate cancer screening: current trends and future implications. CA 1992;42:198–209.

59. Lange PH. The next era for prostate cancer: controlled clinical trials. JAMA 1993;269:95–96.

60. Mold J, Holtgrave D, Bisonni R. The evaluation and treatment of men with asymptomatic prostatic nodules in primary care: a decision analysis. J Fam Pract 1992;34:561–568.

61. Mulrow CD, Aguilar C, Endicott J, et al. Quality of life changes and hearing impairments: a randomized trial. Ann Intern Med 1990;113:188–194.

62. Tucker JB. Screening for open-angle glaucoma. Am Fam Physician 1993;48:75–80.

63. Warshaw G. Are environmental questionnaires of clinical value in everyday office practice? An affirmative view. J Fam Pract 1990;30:194–200.

64. Jones T, Williams M. An opposing view. J Fam Pract 1990;30:197–200.

65. Clayman CB. Mass screening for colorectal cancer: are we ready? JAMA 1989;261:609.

4/ Drugs and the Elderly

Anne L. Hume, Norma J. Owens

At present, individuals over the age of 65 comprise approximately 12.5% of the population and receive almost 32% of all prescribed medications (1). Data indicate that two-thirds of the elderly take between 5 and 12 medications each day. Cardiovascular, analgesic, and psychotropic drugs are the most commonly prescribed medications for this age group (1).

While drug therapy may be beneficial, adverse drug reactions are common among the elderly, and only recently have their long-term societal effects been recognized. For example, many psychotropic agents have been associated with falling and hip fractures (2, 3). The consequences to the older individual are readily apparent, as are the potential negative effects on the family. However the public health impact of accelerated functional decline, perhaps caused by the use of an inappropriate medication, and the economic costs of increased hospital and nursing home care have only recently been recognized (4).

This chapter reviews major issues associated with the use of medications by the elderly. The chapter is divided into four sections: Pharmacology and Aging, Adverse Drug Reactions in the Elderly, Principles of Safe and Effective Drug Use in the Elderly, and an overview, Selected Pharmacologic Groups.

PHARMACOLOGY AND AGING

The physiologic changes associated with aging may both influence and interact with many pharmacokinetic and pharmacodynamic processes, as shown in Table 4.1. In this overview, age-related changes on the major components of pharmacokinetics and pharmacodynamics are considered in isolation from one another. One point with this simplistic approach deserves specific emphasis: many changes believed to be age related physiologic changes are not age related at all, but rather reflect the effects of coexisting diseases, drugs, nutrition, and environmental factors.

LIMITATIONS OF CURRENT STUDIES

Many studies of age-related physiologic changes and pharmacokinetic and pharmacodynamic variables have major methodologic problems in their design. These problems, in turn, limit their clinical applicability (5). Study designs typically have utilized a cross-sectional, rather than a longitudinal, approach. In addition, periods of observation in prospective studies have been brief for physiologic processes and diseases occurring over years (5).

The major concerns, however, focus on the actual study population of "elderly." Because of the absence of a useful marker of biologic age, arbitrary definitions of "elderly" rely solely on chronologic age (5). In the few available studies of investigational drugs in older persons, the participants are representative only of the "fit" elderly who are free of concurrent disease and drug therapy. The frail elderly who actually receive the new drug may not respond as favorably as did the original study population. For example, they may frequently be at risk of serious toxicity because of a lack of information about the appropriate dosage. The frail elderly have been defined in terms of their poor outcomes associated with hospitalization (e.g., death, discharge to a nursing home, generation of large institutional costs), increased use of outpatient services, or impaired functional status (6). Finally, study participants rarely have concomitant nutritional deficiencies and alcohol use. All of these factors, as well as inherent genetic variation, may have significant effects on the pharmacokinetic and pharmacodynamic variables of a given drug in older persons (7).

PHARMACOKINETICS

Absorption

Oral Absorption. Drug absorption from the gastrointestinal tract is influenced by coexisting diseases, concomitant medications, specific physiochemical properties of the drug, and possibly

Table 4.1
Possible Physiologic Changes and Pharmacologic Outcomes Associated with Aging

Physiologic Change	Pharmacologic Outcome
Increased gastric pH Decreased gastrointestinal motility Decreased splanchnic blood flow	Altered rate or extent of drug absorption (?)
Decreased lean muscle mass Decreased total body water Increased adipose tissue Changes in albumin and other protein concentrations	Altered volume of distribution (?)
Decreased hepatic blood flow Decreased total liver mass Changes in hepatic microsomal enzyme systems (?)	Decreased hepatic drug metabolism (?)
Decreased glomerular filtration rate Decreased renal plasma flow Decreased renal tubular secretion	Decreased renal elimination of drugs and metabolites (?)

age-related physiologic changes (7, 8). Common coexisting diseases such as congestive heart failure may slow or reduce drug absorption. Concomitant drugs, including bile acid sequestrants, laxatives, and anticholinergic agents, may alter the rate or extent of absorption. The result may be an inadequate response or an unexpected failure, as in the case of cholestyramine and warfarin. Specific physiochemical properties of a drug such as the need for an acidic environment may also be important (8). Possible age-related physiologic changes include increased gastric pH, decreased gastric emptying and intestinal motility, and reduced splanchnic blood flow (7, 8).

The available literature indicates that the rate of drug absorption in the healthy older person is either unchanged or reduced, while the total amount absorbed is comparable to that absorbed by younger individuals. However, broad statements about drug absorption in the elderly have been based on studies with serious methodological flaws and may not be correct in the presence of concomitant diseases and drugs (8).

Presystemic Clearance. Some drugs administered orally are well absorbed from the gastrointestinal tract but are extracted by the liver at a very rapid rate ("first-pass" effect, or presystemic clearance). The net result is that systemic concentrations are low. Age-related decreases in portal blood flow may increase the systemic bioavailability (and subsequent concentrations) of these drugs (7). Along with potential age-related declines, medications such as histamine-2 (H2) blockers may reduce hepatic blood flow, further

decreasing presystemic clearance and potentially increasing systemic concentrations (9).

Transdermal Absorption. Transdermal drug administration has many advantages over other routes. The first-pass effect is avoided, and the duration of activity may be prolonged. Patient compliance may also be improved.

The stratum corneum of older skin is drier, and because of the reduced sebaceous gland functioning, the lipid content of the skin may be reduced (10). In one of the few studies available, the percutaneous absorption of testosterone and estradiol did not differ between young and older individuals, but absorption of hydrophilic compounds including hydrocortisone was reduced in the older age group (11).

Distribution

Body Composition. Age-related physiologic changes involve body composition, plasma protein binding, and organ blood flow and may influence the distribution of drugs in older persons. Declines in total body water and lean muscle mass have been reported in older individuals, while the percentage of adipose tissue is increased. When the latter change occurs is unknown, although a recent report indicated that the percentage of body fat does not increase significantly after the age of 40 (12). The findings suggested that the change in body fat was due to weight gain alone, rather than being a true age-associated effect, and that previous studies failed to correct for the increased body mass index occurring at middle age (12).

The importance of changes in body composition depends on the physiochemical properties of the drug. Water-soluble drugs such as digoxin may have a reduced volume of distribution in older persons, resulting in an increased initial plasma concentrations. Lipophilic medications such as the benzodiazepines may have an increased volume of distribution (7).

Protein Binding. Many drugs are bound to plasma proteins. The factors influencing protein binding include protein concentrations, concurrent diseases and drugs, and nutritional status, all of which may be important in older persons. Basic drugs such as lidocaine and propranolol have a higher binding affinity for α-1-acid glycoprotein, which increases in response to many diseases. Potentially the protein binding of these drugs may increase as well. Whether or not the concentration of this protein increases with age is controversial (7, 8), although one recent study has reported no relationship between advancing age and α-1-acid glycoprotein concentrations (13).

Acidic drugs such as phenytoin bind primarily to albumin, which decreases slightly in healthy older individuals and probably is of little significance. However, in the frail elderly with multiple chronic diseases and marginal nutritional status, the larger declines in albumin concentrations might result in clinically important increases in unbound drug concentrations. For example, chronic renal failure is associated with qualitative and quantitative changes in the binding affinity of albumin. For drugs such as phenytoin, the free pharmacologically active concentration of the drug may be increased. Concomitant medications may also displace highly protein-bound drugs from albumin (7, 8).

Metabolism

The clearance of drugs metabolized by the liver depends on both the activity of the different enzyme systems and hepatic blood flow (7). Total liver mass and hepatic blood flow may decrease with advancing age such that a 65-year-old person may have 40 to 45% lower blood flow than a young adult (8). Hepatic drug metabolism is also influenced by concomitant diseases, drugs, nutritional status, gender, genetics, and environmental factors such as smoking and vitamin supplementation. These factors may have a more pronounced effect on drug metabolism than those associated with aging alone (7, 8).

Drugs having a slower rate of metabolism (low intrinsic clearance) might be expected to have a reduced clearance rate in older persons. Studies using antipyrine, a model for intrinsic metabolic clearance, have demonstrated reduced clearance among older age groups (14). Drugs that have a rapid rate of metabolism, including propranolol and certain antidepressants, have a high extraction rate by the liver. For these drugs, the primary rate-limiting step in metabolism is hepatic blood flow. As discussed previously, age-related decreases in hepatic blood flow may result in increased systemic concentrations of these drugs.

Biotransformation of drugs in the liver has been classified into either phase I reactions of oxidation, reduction, and hydrolysis or phase II conjugation reactions of glucuronidation, acetylation, or sulfation. Phase I pathways are slowed or unchanged in older persons, while phase II reactions generally are unaffected by aging (7, 8).

In a study of 26 healthy young individuals (mean age, 30) and 21 healthy older persons (mean age, 69), the clearance of triazolam was reduced by 50% in the older group (15). Performance on psychomotor tests reflected the pharmacokinetic differences between the two groups. This study is important because the "older" group were very healthy young-old and not the frail elderly whose concomitant diseases and drug therapy further decrease the clearance of triazolam.

Several other considerations are important in the hepatic metabolism of drugs. Genetics can influence the metabolism of many drugs such as antidepressants, possibly resulting in variable therapeutic and toxic effects. Whether phenotype status for drug metabolism changes with age is uncertain (7). Many drugs such as warfarin are available as racemic mixtures of different enantiomers or optical isomers. These compounds differ in their metabolism as well as their therapeutic effects. No one laboratory test is a reliable quantitative measure of hepatic function for guiding appropriate dosage adjustments in hepatic disease.

Renal Elimination

The renal clearance of many drugs may be reduced in older persons. Declines in glomerular filtration rate, renal plasma flow, and tubular secretion have been associated with advancing age. However, recent evidence from the Baltimore Longitudinal Study of Aging indicates that a decline in renal function is not an inevitable outcome of aging. In this study, one-third of individuals followed over a 23-year period had no change in their renal function (16). Once again, the purported changes in renal function may, in fact, represent the effects of subclinical disease and not simply age per se (17).

Serum creatinine concentrations frequently are within the normal range in older persons. This finding may be expected because of concomitant decreases in muscle mass and resulting creatinine production. Creatinine clearance (Cl) (18) can be estimated by the formula:

$$Cl = (140 - age) \times weight\ (kg)/72$$
$$\times serum\ creatinine$$

For women, the resulting value should be multiplied by 0.85. While this formula (as well as others) has been validated in prospective studies of general medical patients, a recent report suggests that it may not be accurate in frail nursing home residents. Among 19 frail older women, this formula gave estimates that exceeded by 20% or more the actual measured creatinine clearance (19). This may be important for drugs such as the aminoglycosides, which are renally eliminated.

Drugs that are excreted by the kidney may accumulate in the presence of renal insufficiency. Their dosages should always be reduced to prevent toxicity. These drugs include digoxin, cimetidine, and atenolol among many others. Drugs that have active metabolites, such as procainamide, should also be used with great caution. In the case of procainamide, its primary metabolite, *N*-acetylprocainamide, is a long-acting active antiarrhythmic agent that can accumulate in the presence of severe renal impairment.

PHARMACODYNAMICS

Pharmacodynamics is the study of the effects of drugs at the receptor level. Unlike pharmacokinetics and aging, limited pharmacodynamic data currently exist. Contradictory findings may reflect the methodological problems associated with this type of research (8).

Recently the pharmacodynamic effects of verapamil have been studied in three groups of men with hypertension: 7 between the ages of 23 and 36, 10 between 61 and 74, and 7 between 75 and 102 (20). The investigators demonstrated greater decreases in blood pressure and heart rate in the two older groups. They emphasize that the clinical outcomes with calcium channel blockers are the sum of direct pharmacodynamic effects and indirect reflex effects, the latter influenced by both aging and concomitant disease (20).

The effect of aging on the pharmacodynamic response to warfarin remains controversial (21, 22). Older patients have been reported to exhibit a greater response to equivalent warfarin concentrations than do younger individuals (23). While

some investigators (24) have not demonstrated a difference in the risk of either major or minor bleeding in older age groups, data from a large cohort (25) indicated that the relative risk of major bleeding with warfarin was 3.2 for patients 65 years of age or older. The differences in the findings of many studies may be related to definitions of major or minor bleeding as well as other methodological issues (21).

ADVERSE DRUG REACTIONS IN THE ELDERLY

In a now classic article, Steele and colleagues (26) determined that older persons experienced an increased incidence of iatrogenic complications with medication use in the hospital setting. In the 815 patients studied, over half of the complications experienced were directly related to medication exposure. Patients with complications were older, used more medications, and had a longer length of hospital stay.

The results of the Harvard Medical Practice Study provide further support for drugs as a major cause of adverse events among hospitalized patients (27). Of the 1133 adverse events identified, complications from drug therapy were the most common type of adverse event, comprising 19.4% of all adverse events in the sample. The rates of drug-related adverse events varied with age, ranging from 2.36 adverse events per 1000 discharges in patients up to 15 years of age to 11.46 in individuals over the age of 65. Subtle effects from drug therapy may also have contributed to falls and hip fractures, which were considered a separate category.

While adverse drug reactions may be common in older persons, the traditional belief that age is an independent risk factor for their development has been questioned. In a review of age as a risk factor for adverse drug reactions, patient-specific physiologic parameters, burden of disease, and functional abilities have emerged as more important predictive factors than simple chronologic definitions of elderly (21).

DRUGS AND FUNCTIONAL STATUS

Traditionally the adverse effects of drugs have been defined in terms of readily observable outcomes such as rash. This approach disregards the fact that a medication that causes drowsiness may be the major precipitating factor in a sequence of events resulting in a hip fracture in an otherwise healthy 80-year-old individual. Increasingly, the detrimental effects of medications on functional status must be considered as preventable adverse drug reactions in the elderly. Drugs can influence the functional status in three major areas: mobility, continence, and mental functioning (28).

Mobility

Drug-induced causes of immobility have received more attention since the publication of convincing evidence of the association between hip fracture and psychotropic drug use. Using a retrospective case-control design in over 1000 older patients with hip fracture, Ray and colleagues (2) showed that the frequency of psychotropic drug use was higher among persons who suffered a fall with a subsequent hip fracture. The classes of psychotropic drugs included anxiolytic/benzodiazepines, antidepressants, and antipsychotics. The investigators controlled for the time of drug use, showing that only current users of these medications were at increased risk, in contrast to previous users, differentiating between drug and disease effects. Another strength of the study was the presence of a dose-response. Individuals using higher standardized doses of these medications had the highest rate of hip fracture. While a cause-and-effect relationship cannot be proved, the data have been confirmed by subsequent studies, particularly for long-acting benzodiazepines and hip fracture (3). The mechanism of falls caused by drugs from different pharmacologic groups is unknown. While postural hypotension could be postulated as a mechanism for the antidepressants and antipsychotics, it is unlikely for benzodiazepines. Nonspecific sedative effects inherent with many drugs acting within the central nervous system (or what is sometimes referred to as psychomotor retardation) may be a common factor. For the frail older person, extreme caution must be recommended in prescribing these drugs.

Continence

Drugs may also impair a person's ability to control urination. Urinary retention may be caused by many medications including anticholinergic agents, drugs with anticholinergic side effects, and smooth muscle relaxants such as nifedipine (29). Inhibiting the cholinergic pathway prevents the bladder from contracting, which may lead to overflow incontinence. This is especially troublesome in older men with prostatic hypertrophy. Additionally, the α-agonists such as phenylpropanolamine tighten the urinary sphincter, which can contribute to urinary retention in men. In women, however, who are more likely to experience stress incontinence secondary to pelvic floor

atrophy, α-agonists may improve sphincter tone. This paradox is true for α-blockers such as prazosin. By relaxing the urinary sphincter, prazosin may alleviate urinary incontinence in men suffering from prostatic hypertrophy; in women it may worsen stress incontinence (28). Thus, patients must be informed and questioned about changes in their ability to remain continent when medications are added to their regimens.

Mental Functioning

Drug-induced changes in cognition are common adverse drug reactions in older persons (28). The identification of cognitive changes may be difficult in clinical practice when treating patients with multiple underlying risk factors and limited therapeutic choices. Regardless, cognitive abilities must be maintained and are essential for optimal patient functioning and independence. This must be a defined goal or outcome of any drug therapy in the elderly.

Any medication altering a patient's electrolyte profile may contribute to a change in mentation. This is especially true for patients with multiple risk factors for delirium. The risk factors for delirium in hospitalized older persons were evaluated in 325 persons who were 65 years of age or older and admitted to a medical or surgical ward of a tertiary-care hospital (30). One-third of the patients developed delirium during hospitalization. Patient factors on admission associated with the subsequent development of delirium included age greater than 80, prior cognitive impairment, or a fracture as a cause of admission. In the final multivariate model, which controlled for prior cognitive impairment, age, and other confounders, the use of neuroleptics was an independent predictor of delirium (OR, 4.48; 95% CI, 1.8–10.5). Narcotic use was also predictive of delirium in the final model (OR, 2.5; 95% CI, 1.24–5.2). Anticholinergic agents, H2-blockers, digoxin, benzodiazepines, corticosteroids, and nonsteroidal antiinflammatory agents (NSAIA) were not associated with the development of delirium. Evaluation of medication exposure was problematic in this study, as a more detailed analysis was not done to assess the effect of dose, duration, or type of administration (such as around-the-clock or only as needed), except for the anticholinergic agents (30).

Excessive medication use was associated with a worsening of preexisting cognitive impairment in ambulatory older persons who were referred for dementia. Of 300 patients evaluated, 35 were determined to be experiencing a drug-induced worsening of cognition. Upon discontinuation of the offending medication, all patients improved in their cognitive skills, with 10 returning to a normal baseline. Offending drugs included benzodiazepines, antihypertensive agents, neuroleptics, cimetidine, and analgesics (31).

Another important cause of drug-induced cognitive impairment are the anticonvulsants (32). The barbiturates, phenytoin, and benzodiazepines have been implicated in causing impairments in concentration, mental energy, mood, and memory. These effects have been most often studied in children and occur more frequently with regimens containing multiple anticonvulsants. Recent reports continue to document this adverse effect on intelligence in children (33). When prescribed for older persons, especially those with underlying cognitive problems, adherence to the recommendation for single-agent therapy in conditions warranting treatment should be followed.

Benzodiazpines have been recognized to cause anterograde amnesia. These effects may be worsened in older persons because of pharmacokinetic changes. Generally, if a benzodiazepine is necessary, a drug should be chosen with a short half-life to minimize accumulation. Individuals in the 65-to-75 age group should receive half the recommended adult dose. Specific data on appropriate doses for individuals over the age of 75 are not available, and one-quarter of the recommended adult dosage is a conservative starting dose.

Soon after cimetidine was first used in the treatment of peptic ulcer disease, reports of a drug-induced delirium and confusion were published. Research has since shown that cognitive changes occur when the drug is used in high dosages (i.e., 300 mg i.v. every 6 hr) and in individuals with hepatic and/or renal impairment (34). Controversy continues as to whether or not this adverse effect occurs with all H2-blockers or just with cimetidine (35). Regardless, the data indicate a dose effect, prompting advice for dosage reduction in older patients. Recent guidelines suggest, for instance, that in persons over the age of 85 years no more than 200 mg per day of cimetidine should be given. Less specific information exists for the newer H2-blockers.

Drug-induced depression in older individuals is often reported as convincing case reports in the literature. However, the reports provide little information on the frequency of occurrence or specific patient risk factors. The presentation of drug-induced depression is usually atypical in an older person in that vegetative symptoms of sleeplessness, appetite suppression, and constipation, as well as lability of mood, predominate. The onset of symptoms is usually insidious occurring over months rather than abruptly after a medication is started (36). Reserpine is often cited as a cause of depression, but more recent studies suggest that dosages of 0.25 mg per day of reserpine or less are no more likely to cause depression than are diuretics or other antihypertensive agents (37).

PRINCIPLES OF SAFE AND EFFECTIVE DRUG USE IN THE ELDERLY

BASIC ELEMENTS OF APPROPRIATE PRESCRIBING PRACTICES

The Healthy People 2000 Report (38) has identified the reduction of polypharmacy as a priority for health promotion and disease prevention among older populations. This goal may be achieved through the development of a coordinated medication plan. Prescribers must assure that new medicines do not adversely interact with current drugs, pharmacists prospectively monitor for potential medication-related problems and intervene to prevent their occurrence, and older persons and their families actively participate and agree with the intended outcomes of drug therapy (38). A basic tenet of safe and effective drug use is that nonpharmacologic therapy is always initiated first whenever appropriate. Drug therapy should never overshadow lifestyle and dietary interventions.

Comprehensive Medication Database

The first step in planning for safe and effective drug use is to develop a comprehensive medication database. The need for a listing of all drugs that an older individual may be taking is obvious and is valuable in solving a potential drug-induced disease or a drug-drug interaction. However, data on the precise dose, dosage form, and schedule of administration frequently are lacking in many drug histories.

The lack of detailed information on precise dosage forms has become an important prescribing issue since the introduction of multiple sustained-release products for drugs, including theophylline and diltiazem. Sustained-release products may improve patient compliance and reduce dose-to-dose variability in drug concentrations. However, different dosage forms of the same drug rarely are bioequivalent and may result either in inadequate therapeutic response or in toxicity if switched indiscriminantly. Newer dosage forms usually have had a simple suffix such as XL, SR, CD, or LA added to an existing brand name. The omission or addition of a suffix may result in serious consequences if, for example, a new prescription is written for Procardia 90 mg every morning, instead of Procardia XL and subsequently is filled with the regular-release product by the pharmacist. In addition, without a detailed knowledge of the dosage form that a patient takes, it is easy to change release characteristics of many products. For example, if an order is written for theophylline 200 mg every 12 hours through a nasogastric tube and the patient receives Theo-Dur, the tablets would have to be crushed, thereby destroying its sustained-release properties (39).

Data must also be collected on the routine use of nonprescription or over-the-counter (OTC) drugs. Frequently OTC drugs are not perceived by patients to be medications, and thus physicians may not be informed about their use. Practitioners may assume OTC drugs to be free of drug-drug interactions or side effects. For example, a recent study with OTC ibuprofen would at first appear to support this belief. In a study of 25 controlled hypertensive subjects between the ages of 60 and 80, ibuprofen in a dosage of 400 mg three times daily for 10 days was demonstrated to be as safe as aspirin or acetaminophen on blood pressure and renal function (40). However, the participants lacked the major risk factors such as congestive heart failure for developing NSAIA-induced acute functional nephrotoxicity and were using the product exactly as indicated. Whether OTC ibuprofen is as benign in the frail elderly woman with mild congestive heart failure and impaired cognition is unknown. On a very basic level, the safe use of OTC drugs requires adequate eyesight and intact cognition to read and interpret the tiny directions currently on many products. Thus OTC drugs might represent a potential source of drug-induced disease and drug interactions and should be included in a comprehensive medication database.

Finally, information about "borrowed" medications and prescriptions saved from prior illnesses should also be documented. Knowledge of natural food products that a patient may be taking is also essential, as they may contain substances with active pharmacologic properties.

Appropriateness of Drug Therapy

The second step in developing a coordinated plan for safe and effective drug use is to evaluate the appropriateness of all drug therapy. A Medication Appropriateness Index has been developed and has identified practical questions to be considered in evaluating drug therapy (41). The following discussion focuses on some of those questions as shown in Table 4.2.

Is there an indication for the drug and is it effective for the condition? Every drug should be paired with a well-documented diagnosis. In the Senior Care Study, the frequency of medication use without a linked patient diagnosis ("unpaired drugs") and the use of inappropriate medication choices in frail older patients was recently reported (42). During hospitalization, 37% of patients were prescribed one or more unpaired drugs, and 26% received inappropriate medication choices. Cardiac drugs including digoxin accounted for over one-third of the unpaired drugs. "Unmatched" medications should be discontinued or at least reevaluated whenever possible. The prescription of multiple medications for older persons occurs because of a high burden of illness and associated symptoms. However the literature clearly has shown an association between multiple drug use and poor patient outcomes (6).

Is the dosage correct given the patient's renal and/or hepatic function? Aging is a dynamic process. The presence of concomitant diseases and the use of drugs that reduce renal or hepatic function mandate periodic reevaluation of all drug dosages. The available literature reporting the effect of age on drug dosage has been based on the "young-old" and may not be applicable to individuals over the age of 75 years. Thus, the present guidelines that suggest a 50% reduction in the dosage of benzodiazepines, for example, apply only to persons between the ages of 65 and 75 years. Extreme caution must be used in determining the appropriate dosage of drugs for individuals over the age of 75 (6).

Is the duration of therapy acceptable? Before prescribing any drug, an appropriate indication and well-defined outcomes are essential. The expected or intended duration of therapy should also

Table 4.2
Possible Considerations in Evaluating the Appropriateness of Drug Therapy

1. Is there a specific indication for the drug? Is the drug effective?
2. Is the dosage correct given hepatic or renal function?
3. Is the duration of therapy well defined with specific outcomes?
4. Are the directions for use practical?
5. Have important drug-drug and drug-disease interactions been avoided?
6. Is duplication minimized? Are medications being used to treat the side effects of other drugs?
7. Are the least expensive drugs being used?

be clearly defined. The use of benzodiazepines in older individuals for a grief reaction following the loss of a spouse or friends may be appropriate with readily identifiable outcomes, including relief of insomnia. However, their misuse usually has occurred when the duration of therapy was not adequately discussed and the initial short-term prescription became a long-term problem.

Are the directions correct and, at the same time, practical? The impractical nature of some drug regimens is easily overlooked. Complicated dosing regimens for drugs such as warfarin or diuretics are common in the hospital setting and permit careful titration of therapy. At home, however, they present many potential problems for the older individual who is cognitively impaired. Dosing regimens should be as simple as possible and where possible linked to specific events such as "at bedtime."

Are there clinically significant drug-drug or drug-disease interactions present? The use of ophthalmic β-blockers in patients with pulmonary or cardiovascular disease is a classic example of drug-disease interaction. While oral and intravenous β-blockers are well recognized to produce pulmonary and cardiovascular side effects, these outcomes have been associated with ophthalmic use only recently (43). Respiratory distress, including fatal bronchospasm, and cardiovascular effects, including conduction defects and heart failure, have been reported with the use of ophthalmic β-blockers in patients with preexisting cardiovascular disease. Because the drugs are topical, their systemic effects are easily overlooked and a drug-disease interaction missed in susceptible patients. However, the cul-de-sac of the eye is an important site for systemic drug absorption because of subsequent drainage into the lacrimal duct and ultimately into the ophthalmic and facial veins.

Is there unnecessary duplication? The patient who already has a benzodiazepine prescription for daytime anxiety does not need a second for hypnotic effects. Relatedly, are medications being used to treat the side effects of other drugs? This practice should be discouraged whenever possible. For example, the relationship between the use of anticholinergic drugs and laxatives in a population of 800 nursing home residents from 12 intermediate care facilities was recently measured (44). Patients ranged in age from 65 to 105 years, with a mean of 84.7 years. After controlling for potential confounders, the use of laxatives was significantly higher among residents receiving anticholinergic antidepressants (OR, 3.12; 95% CI, 1.21, 8.03) and neuroleptics (OR, 2.01; 95% CI,

1.09, 3.71) and diphenhydramine (OR, 2.18; 95% CI, 1.01, 4.71). The relationship disappeared when the less anticholinergic antidepressants were included in the model. For most drugs prescribed to older patients, alternatives lacking specific characteristics such as anticholinergic properties exist and are a more rational approach.

Is this drug the least expensive alternative, compared with others of equal utility? Most new medications do not represent an important therapeutic advance, but they usually are more expensive than older products. Many clinicians are reluctant to ask patients how they pay for their prescriptions. This is a critical step in reducing drug costs for older patients. The use of generic drugs when available and appropriate may save money for patients. The use of drugs that have a flat cost regardless of the dose will also reduce costs; this has been the case with several of the newer angiotensin converting enzyme (ACE) inhibitors, for which the cost for 100 tablets of the lowest strength is almost identical to that of the highest. In addition, the use of the lowest dose for the appropriate duration, as in the case of H2-blockers, will also reduce medication costs.

After initially reviewing the appropriateness of a given drug regimen, this process should be repeated periodically. In primary care, the older patient who has had multiple hospitalizations or who is receiving prescriptions from many providers is at particular risk of accumulating drugs.

Medication Counseling

Talking with older patients about their medications is "low-tech" and frequently overlooked as an intervention. Inadequate communication remains a major cause of noncompliance with prescribed regimens, treatment failures, medication misuse, and adverse reactions. Medication counseling usually is at the end of an office visit, when many older patients may not remember the precise details of what was discussed (45).

Medication counseling should always begin with a discussion about whether or not a drug is even needed. Nonpharmacologic interventions should be used whenever feasible. A single strategy for medication counseling, such as the use of pamphlets, will not work for every elderly patient in every practice setting.

Patient counseling must be conducted in an atmosphere that is sensitive to individual's cultural or ethnic background, concomitant diseases, and age-related declines. The concept of chronic medication use may be new to certain cultural or ethnic groups. If the chronic nature of a disease such as hypertension has not been discussed, an individual may assume that the blood pressure treatment is completed and the disease cured, when the last refill is obtained.

Counseling the older patient must also recognize the possible presence of visual, auditory, or cognitive impairments. Meyer and Schuna (46) have reported that impaired cognition results in few problems with the mechanical processes involved in opening prescription bottles and removing tablets. However, reading the prescription label, interpreting directions, and recognizing tablet colors were influenced significantly by the presence of impaired cognition. While a spouse or other family member should be present when discussing medications, the potential for subtle cognitive impairment even in these individuals should be appreciated. The individual responsible for medication use in the home must be well informed, involved, and cognitively intact to prevent drug-related problems.

Patient medication counseling is one component of the Omnibus Budget Reconciliation Act (OBRA) of 1990, which became effective in January 1993 (47). Pharmacists are now mandated to provide patient counseling to individuals receiving Medicaid benefits. Information that must be discussed includes name and description of the drug, dosage, route, frequency, duration of therapy, special directions including those for a missed dose, side effects, food and drug interactions, disease state effects, storage and stability, refills, and self-monitoring techniques. Although logistic and legal concerns have been raised about OBRA '90, the intent is to enhance compliance while reducing medication-related problems.

Promoting Adherence

While noncompliance with medications has been perceived as a major problem among all older persons, little evidence supports this belief. The number of prescribed medications is a more important determinant of compliance than any age-related effect (48). Basic considerations in promoting adherence center on reducing the number of prescribed drugs, simplifying dosage regimens, and evaluating the patient's functional ability to take medication.

Compliance can be measured using either direct or indirect methods, which vary in their sensitivity and specificity (49). The determination of drug or metabolite concentrations in blood, urine, or saliva is the most common direct method. Indirect measures include therapeutic response, self-report, pill counts, and pharmacy records.

Electronic monitoring of compliance is possible with the Medication Event Monitoring System (MEMS), which uses a microprocessor in a prescription cap to record the date and time the bottle is opened. McKenney and colleagues (50) reported the value of using MEMS for ambulatory older persons with hypertension. Individuals using MEMS had an average compliance rate of 95.1%, with average reductions in their systolic and diastolic blood pressures of 7.6 mm Hg and 8.8 mm Hg, respectively, over a 6-month period. Control subjects averaged a compliance rate of 78% and decreases of 2.8 mm Hg and 0.2 mm Hg in systolic and diastolic blood pressures, respectively.

Problem Areas in Prescribing

Inappropriate prescribing practices continue to be a problem in long-term care facilities. This is despite increased attention to the potential adverse outcomes associated with inappropriate prescribing practices, as well as new Federal regulations (51). A prospective study (52) recently quantified the appropriateness of medications received by 1106 residents between the ages of 65 and 107 from 12 nursing homes. Using explicit criteria, 19 drugs to be avoided and 11 dose or duration limits were identified. Of the nursing home residents, 40% received at least one inappropriate drug, and inappropriate medications were 7% of all prescriptions. Among the inappropriate medications, long-acting benzodiazepines, dipyridamole, and propoxyphene accounted for almost 75% of the drugs that should be avoided in the elderly. The most common drugs with duration limits included H2-blockers (69.8%), short-acting benzodiazepines (16.3%), and oral antibiotics (14.0%). Iron supplements (72.3%), H2-blockers (18.5%), and antipsychotic agents (9.2%) were identified as drugs that had their dosage limits exceeded among the medication orders. Women received more drugs than men (7.3 vs. 6.6). Women also had a greater number of inappropriate medication orders, although the difference was not statistically significant (52). Other studies have also identified differential prescribing practices based on gender (53).

While the prevalence of inappropriate prescribing patterns has been identified in many studies, newer research must focus on specific, well-defined patient outcomes and on effective intervention strategies. Many traditional interventions to improve prescribing are ineffective (54). As part of OBRA '90, prospective drug use review of Medicaid prescriptions is also now required of pharmacists. States are also responsible for establishing a retrospective drug use review and educational outreach program for pharmacists and physicians (47). The efficacy of these programs has yet to be demonstrated.

SELECTED PHARMACOLOGIC GROUPS

Diuretics

Diuretics can be divided into three general groups: thiazides and related drugs, loop diuretics, and potassium-sparing agents. Thiazides include hydrochlorothiazide, chlorthalidone, metolazone, and indapamide among many others. Alone or in combination with potassium-sparing diuretics, hydrochlorothiazide remains the most commonly prescribed thiazide diuretic. Chlorthalidone has a half-life in excess of 40 hours and can result in significant hypokalemia. Metolazone differs from other thiazides in that its antihypertensive activity persists even as the creatinine clearance drops below 30 mL/min, while indapamide is lipid neutral (55).

Loop diuretics include furosemide and bumetanide. In general, loop diuretics are less effective than thiazides as antihypertensive agents. The use of loop diuretics as antihypertensive agents is limited primarily to those patients who have a creatinine clearance below 30 mL/min or who have concomitant edema. Potassium-sparing diuretics include triamterene, amiloride, and spironolactone. They are used to minimize or correct the hypokalemia associated with thiazide diuretics, as amiloride and triamterene lack significant antihypertensive properties. Hyperkalemia secondary to potassium-sparing diuretics has occurred in the presence of concomitant renal insufficiency, diabetes mellitus, ACE inhibitors, and potassium supplementation. Although uncommon, older patients receiving triamterene may develop nephrolithiasis (55).

The use of thiazide diuretics in newly diagnosed elderly hypertensives has declined, even among otherwise healthy individuals (56). The reasons for this decline may include concerns about their potential adverse effects on concomitant risk factors for coronary heart disease. Diuretics and β-blockers, however, are the only antihypertensive classes that have been shown to reduce the morbidity (especially that caused by stroke) and mortality in hypertension (57).

Three recent studies (58–60) have demonstrated the benefits of diuretics in older patients with hypertension. In the Systolic Hypertension in Elderly Program (SHEP), a placebo-controlled trial of 4736 participants with isolated systolic hypertension, chlorthalidone was used in doses of 12.5 to 25 mg daily, with atenolol or reserpine added if blood pressure was not controlled. Serum potassium concentrations were monitored closely, and potassium supplements were given if the level was below 3.5 mEq/L. Overall, the regimen resulted in a 36% reduction in the number of fatal and nonfatal strokes and a 27% decrease in the number of fatal and nonfatal myocardial infarctions. The reduction in stroke occurred in all age groups (58). While the individuals studied in SHEP were very healthy and may not be representative of all older patients who have multiple diseases, thiazides clearly have a major role in the management of mild-to-moderate hypertension.

Recent research has suggested that thiazide diuretics may reduce the risk of hip fractures in older men and women. The biologic basis may be that thiazides reduce urinary calcium excretion, thereby improving calcium balance and decreasing bone resorption (61). A 32% reduction in the adjusted risk of hip fractures among thiazide users was reported in a 4-year cohort study of 9518 men and women 65 years of age or older (62). In a nested case-control study, the risk of hip fractures was reduced among individuals who had used thiazides for at least 2 years (63), although other epidemiologic studies have not demonstrated similar benefits (64). While promising, the use of thiazides has not yet been determined to reduce calcium loss from the proximal femur and to decrease the fracture rate in prospective clinical trials.

In low doses, thiazide diuretics are safe, effective, and inexpensive first-line antihypertensive agents for many older individuals when carefully monitored (57, 65). Doses should be limited to 12.5 to 25 mg of hydrochlorothiazide (or an equivalent thiazide) per day, as higher doses may worsen serum electrolyte, glucose, and lipoprotein concentrations. Serum potassium concentrations should be monitored routinely, and supplementation should be initiated when levels approach 3.5 mEq/L. The presence of persistent hypokalemia, despite appropriate supplementation, may suggest concomitant hypomagnesemia, which must be corrected first. Hyponatremia associated with fatigue and mental status changes has also occurred with thiazide use in the elderly. Contributing factors may include erratic salt and water intake, presence of concomitant diseases that influence water regulation, and the presence of a distal tubule defect (66).

β-BLOCKERS

β-Blockers can be differentiated on the basis of cardioselectivity, lipid solubility, intrinsic sympathomimetic activity, and presence of concomitant α-blocking activity. Cardioselective β-blockers such as atenolol exert most of their effects on cardiac β-1 receptors and less on β-2 receptors. Cardioselectivity is relative and disappears with increasing doses of a β-blocker. β-Blockers also differ in their lipid solubilities. Previously, only the highly lipid-soluble agents such as propranolol and metoprolol were believed to penetrate the central nervous system to a significant degree. Drowsiness and other central nervous system side effects could be minimized by choosing a hydrophilic drug such as nadolol. However, it is now recognized that all β-blockers cross the blood-brain barrier.

The third property is intrinsic sympathomimetic activity (ISA). At low levels of sympathetic nervous system activity, β-blockers with ISA, such as pindolol, may have slight agonist properties and produce less resting bradycardia. ISA is also associated with fewer adverse effects on lipid and lipoprotein concentrations. However, with the possible exception of acebutolol, β-blockers with significant ISA do not provide protection against recurrent myocardial infarction ("cardioprotection").

Many beliefs surround the use of β-blockers in the elderly. A long-standing belief is that older hypertensives do not respond to β-blockers. While β-blockers may be less effective than calcium channel blockers, atenolol and other drugs in this class may be effective in over 50% of older hypertensive patients (57, 67).

Another common belief is that β-blockers always impair psychological functioning, including cognitive ability. This has been challenged in several recent studies of older hypertensives (68, 69). Drowsiness was no more common with atenolol or metoprolol than with placebo in 27 older patients with hypertension. Mental performance using Trails-A maze testing was improved with metoprolol, although the treatment periods were only 2 weeks for each β-blocker and the patients were relatively young, with mean age of 63 ± 3 years (68). The effects of atenolol and nifedipine on cognitive functioning and mood have been compared in 31 hypertensive patients between the ages of 60 and 81. While neither atenolol or nifedipine produced major effects on cognition during the 4 weeks of drug treatment, nifedipine was associated with subtle impairments in learning and memory in several patients (69). These studies have included healthy young-old who may not be representative of the frail elderly with multiple coexisting diseases.

The other side effects of β-blockers are well known and an extension of their pharmacologic properties. The withdrawal syndrome following abrupt discontinuation is a final important consideration in using β-blockers in the elderly. Given the prevalence of silent coronary artery disease in older individuals, β-blockers should be carefully tapered whenever possible in this population.

CALCIUM CHANNEL BLOCKERS

Calcium channel blockers include at least three distinct pharmacologic groups including nifedipine (or dihydropyridines), diltiazem, and verapamil. Calcium channel blockers have good oral absorption from the gastrointestinal tract. Bioavailability is low, however, because of presystemic clearance. With chronic dosing, bioavailability increases because of saturation of the first-pass effect.

Vasodilation, negative inotropic effects, and cardiac conduction effects are three major properties of calcium channel blockers. Vasodilation is greatest with nifedipine, while negative inotropic properties predominant with verapamil. Cardiac conduction disturbances are associated most frequently with verapamil, to a lesser extent with diltiazem, and rarely with the dihydropyridine calcium channel blockers. The hemodynamic effects of calcium channel blockers portrayed in comparison charts have been derived from studies in normal healthy individuals. Actual clinical responses among the elderly are the result of direct and indirect hemodynamic effects including age-related decreases in baroreceptor responsiveness and the presence of concomitant cardiovascular diseases.

Calcium channel blockers may be unique in their ability to slow the progression of atherosclerosis, as many cellular processes may be influenced by calcium. The International Nifedipine Trial on Anti-atherosclerosis Therapy (INTACT) reported a significant reduction in the number of new atherosclerotic lesions per patient among individuals receiving nifedipine 80 mg per day, compared with placebo. However, for preexisting coronary artery lesions, regression and progression did not differ between the two treatment groups (70).

Unlike β-blockers, secondary prevention trials with calcium channel blockers have been disappointing. The Multicenter Diltiazem Postinfarction Trial of 2466 patients between the ages of 25 and 75 who had an acute myocardial infarction failed to demonstrate a significant difference between diltiazem and placebo after a mean of 25 months. Subgroup analyses subsequently showed a significant increase in the risk of reinfarction or death among individuals taking diltiazem who had an ejection fraction below 40% (71).

Calcium channel blockers are effective antihypertensive agents in older persons, although their actual effects on morbidity and mortality are unknown. They do not adversely affect coexisting diseases such as chronic obstructive lung disease and gout. Adverse effects of calcium channel blockers usually are an extension of their pharmacologic properties. Constipation is also common with verapamil and can be minimized by the concomitant use of stool softeners. Pedal edema typically is associated with nifedipine and related calcium channel blockers.

Many different dosage forms of calcium channel blockers have recently become available. The value of sustained-release verapamil is questionable, as the parent drug has a half-life of at least 4 hours, while its active metabolite is even longer acting. Nifedipine, however, is absorbed rapidly, resulting in hypotension and reflex tachycardia, and because of a half-life of 2.5 hours, it must be dosed every 6 to 8 hours (55). The sustained-release preparation of nifedipine has alleviated these problems and the dose-to-dose variability.

ACE INHIBITORS

ACE inhibitors differ in their structure, pharmacokinetics, duration, and potency. ACE inhibitors may also differ in their ability to inhibit ACE in different target tissues. Captopril is the only ACE inhibitor that contains a sulfhydryl moiety. Enalapril, fosinopril, and ramipril are hydrolyzed into active compounds resulting in a prolonged onset and duration of activity. With the exception of fosinopril, ACE inhibitors are eliminated renally, and doses should be reduced by approximately 50% when the creatinine clearance is less than 30 mL/min.

Recent studies have demonstrated the efficacy of ACE inhibitors in older persons with hypertension, although they are less effective than calcium channel blockers (57, 72). Their beneficial effects on some quality-of-life parameters (73) are well recognized. Recently ACE inhibitors have been reported to differ in their effects on quality-of-life variables. In a study of 379 hypertensive men between the ages of 55 and 79 (mean age 64), the effects of captopril and enalapril were compared in terms of blood pressure control, major side effects, patient withdrawals, and quality-of-life parameters. The use of captopril was associated

with more positive changes in overall quality of life, sleep, vitality, and emotional control (74). The observed changes with captopril and enalapril varied according to baseline health status. While low quality-of-life scores at baseline were either stable or improved with both drugs, individuals with higher initial scores were generally stable with captopril and worsened with enalapril. The reasons for these findings are unknown and not entirely consistent with the literature. While they may reflect differences in the central nervous system penetration of the two drugs, other investigators have cited important methodological problems (75, 76).

While safe in the elderly, significant hypotension may occur if the patient is sodium or volume depleted. The hypotension can be minimized by decreasing or discontinuing the diuretic for several days before initiation of the ACE inhibitor. In addition, careful titration with very low doses of a short-acting ACE inhibitor such as captopril may minimize hypotension.

Dermatologic reactions and cough are also common. The dry nonproductive cough occurs in as many as 20% of patients taking ACE inhibitors. While discontinuing the drug is always preferred, a reduction in the dose may lessen the coughing in some patients. Case reports have suggested that nifedipine or a NSAIA may be effective in lessening the cough while continuing the ACE inhibitor (77, 78). However, NSAIA may blunt the antihypertensive activity of ACE inhibitors and, in the setting of congestive heart failure, may produce acute renal failure.

Hyperkalemia can develop with all ACE inhibitors, usually in the presence of diabetes mellitus, severe renal insufficiency, sodium-restricted diets, concomitant use of potassium-sparing diuretics, potassium supplements including salt substitutes, and NSAIAs. Angioedema of the face, lips, tongue, glottis, larynx, and mucous membranes has been reported with the first dose of all ACE inhibitors and can be life-threatening. Finally, the possibility of renal artery stenosis should always be considered in any older person who has recently developed severe hypertension and develops acute renal failure from an ACE inhibitor.

CHOLESTEROL-LOWERING DRUGS

Four major groups of cholesterol-lowering medications are currently available. The bile acid sequestrants include colestipol and cholestyramine; the fibric acid derivatives are gemfibrozil and clofibrate; the statins include lovastatin, simvastatin, fluvastatin, and pravastatin; and a miscellaneous category consists of niacin, probucol, and dextrothyroxine.

In one study, the use of cholesterol-lowering drugs increased fivefold between 1983 and 1988, primarily as a result of the availability of gemfibrozil and lovastatin (79). Individuals over the age of 60 accounted for 59% of the reported prescriptions for cholesterol-lowering agents, and their use was more common among women. Their long-term benefit in reducing morbidity and mortality has not yet been demonstrated in the elderly, and elevated cholesterol concentrations may not be an important risk factor among elderly women (80). Extrapolating the findings from major lipid studies to the frail elderly and to women should be avoided. Only a large-scale clinical trial will demonstrate the value, if any, of lowering cholesterol in otherwise healthy older persons.

NITRATES

Nitrates include nitroglycerin, isosorbide dinitrate, isosorbide-5-mononitrate, erythrityl tetranitrate, and pentaerythritol tetranitrate. Isosorbide mononitrate is the primary active metabolite of isosorbide dinitrate and differs from its parent compound and nitroglycerin in that it does not undergo significant first-pass metabolism.

Information comparing the pharmacokinetics and pharmacodynamics of nitrates in older and young individuals is limited. Greater systemic bioavailability might be expected with the use of nitroglycerin or isosorbide dinitrate in elderly patients, as both drugs have a high degree of first-pass metabolism. In addition, it is unknown if age-related differences occur in the percutaneous absorption of nitrates from transdermal preparations. In one study (81), anginal symptoms among elderly were relieved more rapidly with the use of an oral nitroglycerin spray than with sublingual tablets, possibly the result of dryness in the mouth which might slow the dissolution of sublingual tablets. Whether this is a clinically significant age-related change in older individuals is unknown, as a middle-aged comparison group was not included.

Hemodynamic sensitivity to nitrates does not appear to be altered with increasing age. However, baroreceptor activity can decline, and the elderly may not be able to increase their heart rate adequately in response to nitrate-induced vasodilation. Therefore, postural symptoms from nitrate administration may be greater in older patients.

A critical issue in the use of all nitrates is the development of tolerance. Nitrate tolerance is prevented by having a daily 10-hour nitrate-free interval, which can be during sleep when sympathetic tone and myocardial oxygen demand is low, unless the patient is having anginal symptoms during REM sleep (82). With a nitroglycerin patch, applying the product early in the morning and then removing it in the early evening should be adequate. Recent claims about new nitrate dosage forms and their purported lack of tolerance simply indicate that the drug-free interval has already been incorporated into the labeled prescribing directions and not an intrinsic advantage of the product.

THROMBOLYTIC AGENTS

Thrombolytic agents are an important advance in cardiovascular therapeutics and currently include streptokinase, urokinase, alteplase, and anistreplase. When administered within 4 hours of the onset of symptoms, thrombolytics can restore the patency of the infarct-related vessel and maintain ventricular function, as well as reduce mortality (83). However, these benefits can be accompanied by life-threatening bleeding including intracranial hemorrhage, which varies according to age (84). Data from the Thrombolysis in Myocardial Infarction (TIMI) trials also indicated an increasing incidence of major hemorrhage with advancing age: 8.7% in individuals less than 65 years of age, 14.5% among patients between 65 and 69 years old, and 24.7% for patients between 70 and 74 years old (85).

Most studies of thrombolytic therapy have excluded individuals over the age of 75, despite their high risk of morbidity and mortality from acute myocardial infarction, because of concern about hemorrhagic complications. Recent findings from the Global Utilization of Streptokinase and Tissue Plasminogen Activator for Occluded Coronary Arteries (GUSTO) study, which included some patients over 75 years of age, have reinforced concerns about the risk of hemorrhagic stroke in older patients who receive thrombolytic agents (86).

While considering the risks and benefits in using thrombolytic agents, several practical limitations to their use in the elderly may exist. The time between the onset of chest pain and presentation in the emergency room may vary with age (87). Individuals less than 55 years of age presented within an average of 4.1 hours, those between 55 and 64 years at 5.2 hours, those between 65 and 74 at 5.1 hours, and those over 75 years at 6.1 hours. The authors reported that 24% of individuals over the age of 75 presented more than

6 hours after the onset of symptoms, which would significantly limit the expected benefit from thrombolytic therapy. In addition, many elderly patients presented with atypical symptoms and electrocardiogram findings, which might further delay the appropriate initiation of thrombolytic therapy.

NONSTEROIDAL ANTIINFLAMMATORY AGENTS

NSAIAs can be divided into broad groups as shown in Table 4.3. The drugs vary in their duration of action, dosing, potency, tissue penetration, and cost (88). Although effective in older populations, the use of NSAIAs has been associated with many side effects, including gastropathy and nephrotoxicity, in the elderly. Proposed risk factors for NSAIA-induced gastropathy have included a history of peptic ulcer disease or gastrointestinal bleeding, advanced age, large doses, cigarette smoking, and concomitant ethanol and other ulcerogenic drug exposure.

Once a NSAIA-induced ulcer has been identified, the need for continued therapy should be reevaluated. If the NSAIA can be discontinued, ulcers heal rapidly with any standard therapy for peptic ulcer disease. When continued therapy is warranted, the choice of an ulcer treatment is more problematic. Studies with H2-antagonists and sucralfate have been conflicting, but ulcers less than 5 mm in diameter often heal spontaneously despite continued NSAIA therapy (88). Omeprazole in a dose of 40 mg per day was more effective than ranitidine 150 mg twice daily in healing large gastric ulcers, despite continued NSAIA therapy (89).

Prevention of NSAIA-induced gastropathy must begin with a reevaluation of the actual need for the drug. Acetaminophen or a nonacetylated salicylate may be as effective as a NSAIA for osteoarthritis (90). While food or H2-blockers may decrease dyspeptic symptoms, the risk of developing a gastric ulceration and clinically significant gastrointestinal bleeding is not reduced.

The only drug approved for the prevention of NSAIA-induced gastric ulceration is misoprostol, which has both antisecretory and mucosal protective poperties (91). The recommended dose is 200 μg four times daily, with meals and at bedtime. Diarrhea and abdominal pain are common, with the diarrhea dose-related and generally transient.

Table 4.3
Selected Pharmacologic Characteristics of Nonsteroidal Antiinflammatory Agents

Drug	Half-Life[a] (hr)	Protein Binding (%)	Elimination (Hepatic/Renal)	Interaction with Oral Anticoagulants
Acetic acids				
Diclofenac (Voltaren)	1.5	99	Hepatic	Uncommon
Indomethacin (Indocin)	4	90	Hepatic	Possible
Tolmetin (Tolectin)	1	99	Hepatic	Uncommon
Nabumetone (Relafen)	25	99	Hepatic	Possible
Etodolac (Lodine)	8	95	Hepatic	Uncommon
Ketorolac (Toradol)	5	99	Hepatic	Uncommon
Sulindac (Clinoril)	18[b]	93 (sulfide metabolite)	Hepatic	Uncommon
Propionic acids				
Fenoprofen (Nalfon)	3	99	Hepatic	Possible
Flurbiprofen (Ansaid)	6	99	Hepatic	Possible
Ibuprofen (Motrin)	1.9	99	Hepatic	Uncommon
Ketoprofen (Orudis)	2	99	Hepatic/renal	Uncommon
Naproxen (Naprosyn)	14	99	Hepatic	Uncommon
Oxaprozin (Daypro)	50	99	Hepatic	Uncommon
Oxicams				
Piroxicam (Feldene)	50	99	Hepatic	Possible
Salicylates				
Aspirin	2–25[c]	95 (salicylate)	Hepatic/renal	Common[c]
Diflunisal (Dolobid)	10	99	Hepatic	Possible

[a]Derived from healthy young adults.
[b]Active metabolite.
[c]Dose-dependent.

The diarrhea may be lessened by starting at 100 μg two to three times daily and gradually increasing the dose as tolerated. In one study, patients receiving 100 μg four times daily experienced diarrhea less frequently than individuals taking 200 μg four times daily, while maintaining a similar rate of efficacy in preventing NSAIA-induced gastric ulcers (92). While risk factors for NSAIA-induced gastropathy have been proposed, identifying actual candidates for whom long-term prophylaxis with misoprostol would be cost-effective remains problematic. Studies of the cost-effectiveness of misoprostol have been conflicting as a result in major differences in the assumed risks associated with the use of NSAIA (91).

ORAL HYPOGLYCEMIC AGENTS

First-generation sulfonylureas include tolbutamide, tolazamide, acetohexamide, and chlorpropamide. Their use has declined since the introduction of glyburide and glipizide, which offer potential advantages in terms of fewer drug interactions and side effects. Chlorpropamide should specifically be avoided in elderly diabetics because of its prolonged half-life, which approaches 72 hours, and the accompanying risk of hypoglycemia. In addition, the use of chlorpropamide has been associated with the development of hyponatremia in older patients (93).

Although sulfonylureas are similar in their efficacy, a recent study (94) reported that glyburide reduces basal hepatic glucose production and fasting glucose concentrations better than glipizide. Glipizide decreases postprandial glucose concentrations more than does glyburide, which may be due to the more rapid absorption of glipizide. The actual clinical importance of these findings remains to be established.

Both glipizide and glyburide can be administered once daily. Glipizide should not be taken with food; the absorption of the drug may be reduced. The presence of food does not affect the absorption of glyburide.

Questions remain about the dosing of these agents and their use with insulin. In one study (95), daily dosages above 10 mg provided only minimal additional benefit in terms of blood glucose or hemoglobin A1C concentrations. Combination therapy with a sulfonylurea and NPH insulin at bedtime have been advocated for some diabetics. This practice, however, remains controversial. A recent study of four insulin regimens, including one combination therapy, did not demonstrated differences in glycemic control. Weight gain was slightly less and hyperinsulinemia was decreased with combination therapy (96).

PSYCHOTROPIC AGENTS

Psychotropic agents are commonly used in the elderly. As discussed above, they are frequently used in the absence of a definitive psychiatric diagnosis and represent an "unpaired" drug. Even when used cautiously for appropriate indications, psychotropic drugs may result in adverse effects on the functional status of many older individuals.

Antipsychotic Agents

Antipsychotic agents are effective for the treatment of psychiatric conditions, including schizophrenia and other diseases in which delusions or psychosis are present. Their use in the elderly, especially in the nursing home setting, has been much higher than necessary for the treatment of patients with a psychiatric diagnosis. Their increased use is primarily due to attempts to control behavioral problems in demented patients. However, few data exist to document their efficacy for this purpose. In a meta-analysis of 33 studies of patients with primary dementia, the effectiveness of antipsychotic agents prescribed for agitation was recently evaluated (97). A statistically significant mean effect size of 0.18 was shown for the use of an antipsychotic vs. placebo. No antipsychotic was more effective than another. Only 18 out of 100 patients would be expected to respond on the basis of their effect size.

Antipsychotic agents are also misused frequently when prescribed on an "as needed," or "prn," dosing regimen. They are not effective when used in this manner, and it is likely that the patient will only experience the acute sedative properties of these drugs (98).

Because of misuse of these drugs, regulations have been developed that define appropriate and inappropriate indications for antipsychotic use. One reason for tighter regulatory control has been their potential toxicity, including hypotension, a lowering of the seizure threshold, alterations in water homeostasis, anticholinergic effects, and the development of extrapyramidal symptoms. Many of these side effects promote the use of additional medications such as anticholinergic agents for the treatment of antipsychotropic agent–induced extrapyramidal symptoms. All movement disorders further impair an individual's ability to ambulate, and some are potentially irreversible. Tardive dyskinesias have been consistently shown to occur more often in older persons (99). Further complicating the development of movement disorders from antipsychotic agents in dementia is the underlying pathophysiology of

Alzheimer's disease; patients are more likely to develop movement disorders of the dopaminergic pathway as a long-term complication of the disease. Another serious complication of antipsychotic agents is the development of neuroleptic malignant syndrome, a hyperpyrexic condition associated with hypertonicity of the skeletal muscles and an instability of the autonomic nervous system (100).

Benzodiazepines

As shown in Table 4.4, many benzodiazepines are available to treat anxiety and short-term insomnia in older individuals. Benzodiazepines are generally safe and effective. Problems with their use usually develop when predictable pharmacokinetic and pharmacodynamic changes are overlooked, and for example, "normal" doses of long-acting agents are prescribed for an indeterminant course of therapy.

Benzodiazepines commonly cause sedation, ataxia, and impaired psychomotor performance. They also may produce anterograde amnesia in which patients report the inability to acquire or store information. While these effects are temporary, they may precipitate falls or delirium in susceptible individuals. Benzodiazepines also produce paradoxical effects of anger, hostility, and other self-destructive acts. Shader and Greenblatt (101) have suggested that these reactions may occur in persons with underlying anger that is expressed through the disinhibiting anxiolytic effects of these drugs.

The relative safety or toxicity of one benzodiazepine versus another has frequently been debated in the literature. Using data reported to the FDA, triazolam had been shown to have a higher rate of behavioral toxicity than temazepam. However, after controlling for age and the appropriateness of dose, this difference disappeared (102). Most of the reported reactions with triazolam have been associated with higher doses, such as 0.25 mg in persons over the age of 65 years.

Antidepressants

Depression commonly occurs in older individuals. It may present in an atypical manner with significant cognitive impairment. Medications can be an important contributing factor in the development of depression in older patients at risk.

Unlike other psychotropic agents, antidepressants are probably underused in the elderly. The antidepressants currently available are shown in Table 4.5. As the number of drugs continues to increase, a comprehensive strategy for choosing among the various agents is essential. In general, if all antidepressants are equally effective, the goal should be to either avoid or to promote certain side effects for individual geriatric patients.

One strategy might be to focus only on those antidepressants that lack major anticholinergic effects. Agents such as amitriptyline, imipramine, doxepin, and protriptyline all possess significant anticholinergic properties. While these drugs have been used in older individuals for many years, newer antidepressants may offer impor-

Table 4.4
Selected Pharmacologic Characteristics of Benzodiazepines

	Peak Levels (hr)	Half-Life (hr)	Major Active Metabolites	Half-Life of Active Metabolites (hr)
Alprazolam (Xanax)	0.5–1.5	12–19	Hydroxyalprazolam	
Chlordiazepoxide (Librium)	2–4	5–30	Desmethylchlordiazepoxide	30–60
			DMD	
			Demoxepam	
Clorazepate (Tranxene)		30–60	Desmethyldiazepam (DMD)	30–60
Diazepam (Valium)	1–2	20–50	DMD	30–60
Flurazepam (Dalmane)	—[a]	—[a]	Desalkylflurazepam	50–100
Halazepam (Paxipam)	1–3	7	DMD	30–60
Lorazepam (Ativan)	2	10–20	None	
Oxazepam (Serax)	1–2	5–10	None	
Prazepam (Centrax)	6	78	DMD	30–60
			Hydroxyprazepam	
Quazepam (Doral)	1.5	40	Oxoquazepam	40–80
Temazepam (Restoril)	2–3	9–12	None	
Triazolam (Halcion)	0.5–1.5	2–3	Hydroxytriazolam	

[a]Rapidly and completely metabolized to desalkylflurazepam.

Table 4.5
Selected Pharmacologic Characteristics of Available Antidepressants

Drug	Sedation	Insomnia	Anticholinergic Effects	Orthostatic Hypotension	Delay in Cardiac Conduction	Nausea
Amitriptyline	+ + +	0	+ + +	+ + +	Yes	0
Desipramine	+	+	+	+	Yes	0
Doxepin	+ + +	0	+ +	+ + +	Yes	0
Imipramine	+ +	0	+ +	+ +	Yes	0
Nortriptyline	+ +	0	+	+	Yes	0
Protriptyline	+	+ +	+ +	+	Yes	0
Trazodone	+ + +	0	0	+ +	Low	+
Fluoxetine	0	+ +	0	0	Low	+ +
Sertraline	0	+	0	0	Low	+
Paroxetine	0	+	0	0	Low	+

tant advantages. The anticholinergic properties of antidepressants are well recognized to cause dry mouth, constipation, and urinary retention, which may already be present in an older individual. Confusion and delirium have also been associated with the use of highly anticholinergic antidepressants in older patients with a preexisting cognitive impairment. However, the anticholinergic effect of blurring vision is easily overlooked. In the presence of age-related declines in vision or decreases in proprioception caused by disease, the potential for blurred vision to place an individual at even greater risk of falling must be considered and specifically avoided.

The ability of antidepressants to produce orthostatic hypotension by α-adrenergic blockade should also be minimized, especially to lessen the risk of falls in older individuals. Antidepressants that slow cardiac conduction or are associated with a high risk of seizures should also be specifically avoided in the elderly.

After considering these major factors, the preferred agents might be limited to desipramine, nortriptyline, trazadone, and the selective serotonin-reuptake inhibitors (SSRIs) such as fluoxetine. From here, the selection of an antidepressant might be based on individual patient characteristics. For instance, in an anxious patient unable to sleep the use of trazadone could be advised as it is very sedating. In the patient with psychomotor impairment who is withdrawn, the choice might be desipramine, which is not very sedating, or one of the SSRI such as fluoxetine.

Trazadone has been used extensively in the elderly, especially before the availability of SSRIs. Although generally safe, priapism has been associated with the use of trazodone, and on rare occasions surgical intervention has been required.

Fluoxetine and the new SSRIs are also an important advance in the treatment of depression. Although as effective as the older drugs, their side-effect profile is very different from traditional antidepressant agents. Anxiety, nervousness, insomnia, and tremor may occur with this class. Although the drug interactions with SSRIs have been limited primarily to other psychotropic drugs, this may become an important issue with their use in the elderly as more experience with this class emerges.

Appetite stimulation is usually a desired effect in older depressed patients and is more likely to occur with the older sedating antidepressants, as appetite stimulation mirrors the anticholinergic profile of these drugs. The relative lack of appetite stimulation, or in fact anorexia, has been a concern with fluoxetine. A recent report indicated that the use of fluoxetine may be associated with nausea and anorexia, as well as a weight loss on average of 4.6 kg, among a small group of medically ill patients over the age of 75 years (103).

Hyponatremia is a common electrolyte disorder in the elderly. Although rare, hyponatremia has been associated with the use of all antidepressants, especially in older individuals and among persons taking diuretics. The precise etiology of antidepressant-induced hyponatremia is unknown, but it frequently has occurred in patients who had multiple risk factors for developing hyponatremia. Whether one antidepressant causes hyponatremia more than another cannot be determined on the basis of isolated case reports. More importantly, if hyponatremia develops and an antidepressant is still needed, data are lacking as to the best alternative agent or class to select.

After selecting an antidepressant, careful attention to the proper dose is essential to the successful use of these drugs in older persons. Most antidepressants have prolonged half-lives, and some have long-acting active metabolites. Recommended beginning doses for desipramine and nortriptyline, for example, are 10 mg at night, increasing to usually no more than 50 to 75 mg per day.

COGNITION-ENHANCING MEDICATIONS

Alzheimer's disease is the most common dementing illness, affecting approximately 1.4 million Americans. While a cure is not available, the Food and Drug Administration recently approved tacrine, the first medication indicated for the treatment of Alzheimer's disease. Many other drugs are under study in an effort to develop an effective treatment to improve cognition. Cholinergic enhancers have included lecithin, choline, physostigmine, and tacrine (which will be reviewed in detail later in this chapter). Drugs such as nimodipine may attenuate the negative effects of excitatory amino acids such as glutamate, which interact with the N-methyl-D-aspartate (NMDA) receptor. Miscellaneous agents including captopril, l-deprenyl, nerve growth factor, and ergoloid mesylates among others are also under investigation (104).

Methodological Issues

Before discussing tacrine, careful attention must be focused on methodological considerations in studies of drug treatments for Alzheimer's disease. One of the most important criteria that all clinical trials in this area must meet is the use of a uniform definition for the diagnosis of Alzheimer's disease. Usually a diagnosis of "probable" Alzheimer's disease is made because "definite" Alzheimer's disease can only be determined from a biopsy specimen from the brain of an affected patient. The National Institute of Neurological and Communicative Disorders and Stroke has established criteria for the diagnosis of Alzheimer's disease for use in research protocols (105).

Second, many standard pharmaceutical issues such as dose and duration of therapy vary among the reported studies. For instance, in the reports of the most extensively studied compound, tacrine hydrochloride, the prescribed doses range widely, with some investigators using doses of 250 mg per day, while others use doses between 40 and 80 mg per day. The use of concomitant lecithin also differs between studies. By itself, lecithin has never been shown to be of benefit (104). Controversy also exists as to the necessary duration of an experimental therapy for Alzheimer's disease. Is a 6-week trial adequate to evaluate the efficacy of a treatment in a disease with a long and insidious course?

The most heated controversy surrounds the type of measure used to assess outcomes of drug therapy. Most studies use some type of mental status examination such as the Folstein Mini-Mental Status Examination to evaluate changes in cognitive status from baseline. This test is an efficient screening tool for moderately impaired individuals, but it lacks sensitivity and exhibits a threshold effect. Statistically significant, but perhaps clinically irrelevant, results may occur if caution is not used when interpreting the results of outcome measurements. Guidelines have been proposed for determining the clinical relevance of studies evaluating cognitive improvement in demented patients (106). A statistically significant drug effect should be greater than half of the standard deviation of the outcome measure to also be clinically relevant (106).

Cholinergic Medications

The most extensive research for a drug treatment of Alzheimer's disease has focused on agents that increase the concentrations of acetylcholine in the brain. Upon autopsy, the brains of patients who have died of Alzheimer's disease show profound deficiencies of acetylcholinesterase and muscarinic and nicotinic receptors. This information, combined with evidence that young subjects given histamine-1 receptor antagonists such as scopolamine develop memory impairments similar to those of patients with Alzheimer's disease, led to the development of the "cholinergic hypothesis." This hypothesis simply states that a lack of acetylcholine is at least in part the cause of the cognitive dysfunction in individuals suffering from Alzheimer's disease (107). To further support the cholinergic hypothesis, investigators recently have characterized the increased sensitivity of older individuals without central nervous system disease to the anticholinergic effects of scopolamine (108). As a result, many clinical trials have reported on the value of improving cholinergic transmission. The three methods available for improving cholinergic transmission include increasing acetylcholine synthesis and release with presynaptic compounds, preventing the breakdown of acetylcholine, and using postsynaptic compounds to stimulate acetylcholine receptors directly.

Administration of acetylcholine precursors such as choline or lecithin has failed to show a cognitive benefit in patients with Alzheimer's disease (104). The direct stimulation of cholinergic postsynaptic receptor sites has also failed to show substantial improvement in most clinical trials.

One recent study suggests, however, that long-term administration of acetyl-L-carnitine may prevent deterioration (compared with placebo) in patients with Alzheimer's disease. Acetyl-L-carnitine is a naturally occurring substance that is structurally similar to acetylcholine and acts to improve both cholinergic activity and oxidative brain metabolism (109).

Tacrine Hydrochloride

Ten randomized, controlled clinical trials have compared tacrine hydrochloride with placebo in patients with Alzheimer's disease. Summers and colleagues were the first to publish a positive study with tacrine (110). However, because of methodological problems, more rigorous studies have been undertaken. Six published trials were prospective, randomized, double-blind crossover studies involving modest numbers of patients who were receiving tacrine in doses ranging from 100 mg per day to 250 mg per day (111–116). Of the two studies demonstrating positive results, statistically significant improvements on two measures of cognition were reported, without any change in the activities of daily living (113, 114).

More recently, Farlow and colleagues (117) conducted a large-scale, parallel, placebo-controlled trial using doses up to 80 mg per day. At the end of treatment with tacrine, both clinician-rated global assessment and caregiver-rated global assessment showed significant improvement. At the highest dose studied, 51% of patients achieved significant cognitive improvement, roughly equivalent to a 6-month gain in performance. A 30-week, placebo-controlled, parallel study was also recently completed, and the preliminary data showed that some patients can tolerate as much as 160 mg of tacrine per day. The positive benefits demonstrated by Farlow (117) were confirmed in that both clinician global ratings and cognition on a functional performance assessment scale improved significantly (118).

Tacrine has been associated with significant side effects resulting in a high rate of withdrawals from the previously cited studies. Common but minor side effects included an 8 to 14% rate of nausea and vomiting, 11 to 13% headaches, 5 to 8% diarrhea, and 3 to 8% of patients reporting abdominal pain (116). Other effects have included excessive micturition, dizziness, and diaphoresis.

The most significant adverse effect associated with tacrine treatment are elevations of hepatic transaminases. The liver enzymes return to baseline after discontinuation of the drug. The proportion of patients with elevated liver enzymes from clinical trials with tacrine has ranged from 40 to 46%, with about half of the patients experiencing elevations that were greater than three times the normal values. In a more thorough review of 30 patients who had Alzheimer's disease and were treated with tacrine, half of the patients showed elevations in liver enzymes at some time during the study (119). Patients experienced this toxicity from 17 to 38 days after the initiation of tacrine, and the liver enzymes returned to normal within 14 to 28 days after discontinuing the drug. Hepatotoxicity was dose-dependent, with some patients able to continue treatment at a reduced dosage, while others were restarted at a lower dosage after temporarily discontinuing tacrine.

Twenty-seven percent of patients demonstrated more severe liver toxicity. One patient developed a rise in bilirubin to 107 mmol/L with clinical jaundice. Eight patients had symptoms suggestive of hepatitis, including malaise, anorexia, nausea, and vomiting, although these may also occur secondary to the expected cholinergic effects of tacrine. Nine of 12 women developed hepatotoxicity, compared with 6 of 18 men, which may suggest a gender difference in the occurrence of this side effect (119). The predisposition for liver toxicity to occur in women has been confirmed in another large trial (116).

In summary, tacrine is the first new agent to be approved for the primary treatment of Alzheimer's disease. However, the cognition-enhancing effects of tacrine are modest, and the drug is associated with a significant risk for hepatotoxicity. While few other drugs are available to treat Alzheimer's disease, many compounds are under investigation. It is likely that within the next 10 years, clinicians may be able to choose from many medications and that drug regimens will be multidimensional, with agents to enhance cholinergic transmission as only one treatment approach.

REFERENCES

1. Baum C, Kennedy DL, Knapp DE, et al. Drug utilization in the U.S.—1986. Rockville, MD: Department of Health and Human Services, Food and Drug Administration, 1987.
2. Ray WA, Griffin MR, Schaffner W, Baugh DK, Melton LJ. Psychotropic drug use and the risk of hip fracture. N Engl J Med 1987;316:363–369.
3. Ray WA, Griffin MR, Downey W. Benzodiazepines of long and short elimination half-life and the risk of hip fracture. JAMA 1989;262:3303–3307.
4. Siu AL, Beers MH, Morgenstern H. The geriatric "medical and public health" imperative revisited. J Am Geriatr Soc 1993;41:78–84.
5. Kitler ME. Clinical trials in the elderly. Pivotal points. Clin Geriatr Med 1990;6:235–255.
6. Owens NJ, Fretwell MD, Willey C, Murphy SS. Distinguishing between the fit and frail elderly

and optimising pharmacotherapy. Drugs Aging 1993;3:101–105.

7. Montamat SC, Cusack BJ, Vestal RE. Management of drug therapy in the elderly. N Engl J Med 1989;321:303–309.

8. Mayersohn MB. Special pharmacokinetic considerations in the elderly. In: Evans WE, Schentag JJ, Jusko WJ, eds. Applied pharmacokinetics. Vancouver: Applied Therapeutics, 1992:1–43.

9. Feely J, Wilkinson GR, Wood AJJ. Reduction of liver blood flow and propranolol metabolism by cimetidine. N Engl J Med 1981;304:692–695.

10. Roskos KV, Maibach HI. Percutaneous absorption and age. Implications for therapy. Drugs Aging 1992;2:432–439.

11. Roskos KV, Maibach HI, Guy RH. The effect of aging on percutaneous absorption in man. J Pharmacokinet Biopharm 1989;17:617–623.

12. Silver AJ, Guillen CP, Kahl MJ, Morley JE. Effect of aging on body fat. J Am Geriatr Soc 1993; 41:211–213.

13. Veering BT, Burm AG, Souverijn JH, Serree JM, Spierdijk J. The effect of age on serum concentrations of albumin and alpha-1-acid glycoprotein. Br J Clin Pharmacol 1990;29:201–206.

14. Vestal RE, Norris AH, Tobin JD, et al. Antipyrine metabolism in man: influence of age, alcohol, caffeine, and smoking. Clin Pharmacol Ther 1975; 18:425–432.

15. Greenblatt DJ, Harmatz JS, Shapiro L, Engelhardt N, Gouthro TA, Shader RI. Sensitivity to triazolam in the elderly. N Engl J Med 1991; 324:1691–1698.

16. Lindeman RD, Tobin J, Shock NW. Longitudinal studies on the rate of decline in renal function with age. J Am Geriatr Soc 1985;33:278–285.

17. Lindeman RD. Changes in renal function with aging. Implications for treatment. Drugs Aging 1992; 2:423–428.

18. Cockcroft DW, Gault MH. Prediction of creatinine clearance from serum creatinine. Nephron 1976; 16:31–41.

19. Drusano GL, Muncie HL, Hoopes JM, Damron DJ, Warren JW. Commonly used methods of estimating creatinine clearance are inadequate for elderly debilitated nursing home patients. J Am Geriatr Soc 1988;36:437–441.

20. Abernethy DR, Schwartz JB, Todd EL, Luchi R, Snow E. Verapamil pharmacokinetics and disposition in young and elderly hypertensive patients. Ann Intern Med 1986;105:329–339.

21. Gurwitz JH, Avorn J. The ambiguous relation between aging and adverse drug reactions. Ann Intern Med 1991;114:956–66.

22. Levine MN, Hirsh J, Landefeld S, Raskob G. Hemorrhagic complications of anticoagulant treatment. Chest 1992;102:352–359.

23. Shepherd AM, Hewick DS, Moreland TA, et al. Age as a determinant of sensitivity to warfarin. Br J Clin Pharmacol 1977;4:315–320.

24. Gurwitz JH, Goldberg RJ, Holden A, Knapic N, Ansell J. Age-related risks of long-term oral anticoagulant therapy. Arch Intern Med 1988; 148:1733–1736.

25. Landefeld CS, Goldman L. Major bleeding in outpatients treated with warfarin: incidence and prediction by factors known at the start of outpatient therapy. Am J Med 1989;87:144–152.

26. Steele K, Gertman PM, Crescenzi C, Anderson J. Iatrogenic illness on a general medical service at a university hospital. N Engl J Med 1981;304:638–642.

27. Leape LL, Brennan TA, Laird N, et al. The nature of adverse events in hospitalized patients. Results of the Harvard Medical Practice Study II. N Engl J Med 1991;324:377–384.

28. Owens NJ, Silliman RA, Fretwell MD. The relationship between comprehensive functional assessment and optimal pharmacotherapy in the older patient. Drug Intell Clin Pharm 1989; 23:847–854.

29. Resnick NM, Yalla SV. Management of urinary incontinence in the elderly. N Engl J Med 1985; 313:800–805.

30. Schor JD, Levkoff SE, Lipsitz LA, et al. Risk factors for delirium in hospitalized elderly. JAMA 1992;267:827–831.

31. Larson EB, Kukull WA, Buchner D, Reifler BV. Adverse drug reactions associated with global cognitive impairment in elderly patients. Ann Intern Med 1987;107:169–173.

32. Reynolds EH, Trimble MR. Adverse neuropsychiatric effects of anticonvulsant drugs. Drugs 1985; 29:570–581.

33. Farwell JR, Lee YJ, Hirtz DG, Sulzbacher SI, Ellenberg JH, Nelson KB. Phenobarbital for febrile seizures. N Engl J Med 1990;322:364–369.

34. Schentag JJ, Cerra FB, Calleri G, DeGlopper E, Rose JQ, Bernhard H. Pharmacokinetic and clinical studies in patients with cimetidine-associated mental confusion. Lancet 1979;i:177–181.

35. Cantu TG, Korek JS. Central nervous system reactions to histamine-2 receptor blockers. Ann Intern Med 1991;114:1027–1034.

36. Ganzini L, Walsh JR, Millar SB. Drug-induced depression in the aged. Drugs Aging 1993;3:147–158.

37. Goldstein G, Barry MJ, Cushman WC, et al. Treatment of hypertension in the elderly: II. Cognitive and behavioral function. Hypertension 1990; 15:361–369.

38. Healthy People 2000. Washington, DC: Department of Health and Human Services; 1991. DHHS publication no. [PHS] 91–50212.

39. Lesar TS. Common prescribing errors. Ann Intern Med 1992;117:537–538.

40. Furey SA, Vargas R, McMahon FG. Renovascular effects of nonprescription ibuprofen in elderly hypertensive patients with mild renal impairment. Pharmacotherapy 1993;13:143–146.

41. Hanlon JT, Schmader KE, Samsa GP, et al. A method for assessing drug therapy appropriateness. J Clin Epidemiol 1992;45:1045–1051.

42. Owens NJ, Sherburne NJ, Silliman RA, Fretwell MD. The Senior Care Study. The optimal use of medications in acutely ill older patients. J Am Geriatr Soc 1990;38:1082–1087.

43. Everitt DE, Avorn J. Systemic effects of medications used to treat glaucoma. Ann Intern Med 1990;112:120–125.

44. Monane M, Avorn J, Beers MH, Everitt DE. Anticholinergic drug use and bowel function in nursing home patients. Arch Intern Med 1993;153:633–638.

45. Kessler DA. Communicating with patients about their medications. N Engl J Med 1991;325:1650–1652.

46. Meyer ME, Schuna AA. Assessment of geriatric patients' functional ability to take medication. Drug Intell Clin Pharm 1989;23:171–174.

47. Omnibus Budget Reconciliation Act of 1990. Department of Health and Human Services. Health Care Financing Administration. 42 CFR Part 456. Federal Register 1992;57:212.

48. Spagnoli A, Ostino G, Borga AD, et al. Drug compliance and unreported drugs in the elderly. J Am Geriatr Soc 1989;37:619–624.

49. Stephenson BJ, Rowe BH, Haynes RB, Macharia WM, Leon G. Is this patient taking the treatment as prescribed? JAMA 1993;269:2779–2785.

50. McKenney JM, Munroe WP, Wright JT. Impact of an electronic medication compliance aid on long-term blood pressure control. J Clin Pharmacol 1992;32:277–279.

51. Burke WJ. Neuroleptic drug use in the nursing home: the impact of OBRA. Am Fam Physician 1991;43:2125–2130.

52. Beers MH, Ouslander JG, Fingold SF, et al. Inappropriate medication prescribing in skilled nursing facilities. Ann Intern Med 1992;117:684–689.

53. Hohmann AA. Gender bias in psychotropic drug prescribing in primary care. Med Care 1989; 27:478–490.

54. Soumerai SB, McLaughlin T, Avorn J. Improving drug prescribing in primary care: a critical analysis of the experimental literature. Milbank Q 1989; 67:268–317.

55. Gilman AG, Goodman LS, Rall TW, Murad F, eds. Goodman and Gilman's the pharmacological basis of therapeutics. 8th ed. New York: Macmillan, 1990.

56. Psaty BM, Savage PJ, Tell GS, et al. Temporal patterns of antihypertensive medication use among elderly patients. The Cardiovascular Health Study. JAMA 1993;270:1837–1841.

57. Joint National Committee on Detection, Evaluation, and Treatment of High Blood Pressure. The fifth report of the Joint National Committee on Detection, Evaluation and Treatment of High Blood Pressure (JNC V). Arch Intern Med 1993;153: 1023–1038.

58. The SHEP Cooperative Research Group. Prevention of stroke by antihypertensive drug treatment in older persons with isolated systolic hypertension: final results of the Systolic Hypertension in the Elderly Program (SHEP). JAMA 1991;265: 3255–3264.

59. MRC Working Party. Medical Research Council trial of treatment of hypertension in older adults: principal results. Br Med J 1992;304:405–412.

60. Dahlof B, Lindholm LH, Hansson L, Schersten B, Ekbom T, Wester PO. Morbidity and mortality in the Swedish Trial in Old Patients with Hypertension (STOP-Hypertension). Lancet 1991;338: 1281–1285.

61. Sutton RA. Diuretics and calcium metabolism. Am J Kidney Dis 1985;1:4–9.

62. LaCroix AZ, Wienpahl J, White LR, et al. Thiazide diuretic agents and the incidence of hip fracture. N Engl J Med 1990;322:286–290.

63. Ray WA, Griffin MR, Downey W, Melton LJ. Long-term use of thiazide diuretics and risk of hip fracture. Lancet 1989;1:687–690.

64. Heidrich FE, Stergachis A, Gross KM. Diuretic drug use and the risk for hip fracture. Ann Intern Med 1991;115:1–6.

65. Applegate WB, Rutan GH. Advances in management of hypertension in older persons. J Am Geriatr Soc 1992;40:1164–1174.

66. Ashouri OS. Severe diuretic-induced hyponatremia in the elderly. A series of eight patients. Arch Intern Med 1986;146:1355–1357.

67. Massie BM, Cushman WC, Reda DJ, Materson BJ. Monotherapy of hypertension: results of major subgroup analyses at one year. Circulation 1991; 84:II-137.

68. Gengo FM, Fagan SC, de Padova A, Miller JK, Kinkel PR. The effect of beta-blockers on mental performance in older hypertensive patients. Arch Intern Med 1988;148:779–784.

69. Skinner MH, Futterman A, Morrissette D, Thompson LW, Hoffman BB, Blaschke TF. Atenolol compared with nifedipine: effect on cognitive function and mood in elderly hypertensive patients. Ann Intern Med 1992;116:615–623.

70. Lichtlen PR, Hugenholtz PG, Rafflenbeul W, Hecker H, Jost S, Deckers JW. Retardation of angiographic progression of coronary artery disease by nifedipine. Results of the International Nifedipine Trial on Antiatherosclerotic Therapy (INTACT). Lancet 1990;335:1109–1113.

71. The Multicenter Diltiazem Postinfarction Trial Research Group. The effect of diltiazem on mortality and reinfarction after myocardial infarction. N Engl J Med 1988;319:385–392.

72. Applegate WB, Phillips HL, Schnaper H, et al. A randomized, controlled trial of the effects of three antihypertensive agents on blood pressure control and quality of life in older women. Arch Intern Med 1991;151:1817–1823.

73. Croog SH, Levine S, Testa MA, et al. The effects of antihypertensive therapy on the quality of life. N Engl J Med 1986;314:1657–1664.

74. Testa MA, Anderson RB, Nackley JF, Hollenberg NK and the Quality-of-Life Hypertension Study Group. Quality of life and antihypertensive therapy in men: a comparison of captopril with enalapril. N Engl J Med 1993;328:907–913.

75. Santanelb NC, Guess H, Heyse JF. Captopril, enalapril, and quality of life. (Letter) N Engl J Med 1993;329:505.

76. Ware JE. Captopril, enalapril, and quality of life. (Letter) N Engl J Med 1993;329:506.

77. Israili ZH, Hall WD. Cough and angioneurotic edema associated with angiotensin-converting enzyme inhibitor therapy. A review of the literature and pathophysiology. Ann Intern Med 1992; 117:234–242.

78. Fogari R, Zoppi A, Tettamanti F, et al. Indomethacin or nifedipine for cough induced by captopril therapy. J Cardiovasc Pharmacol 1992;19:670–675.

79. Wysowski DK, Kennedy DL, Gross TP. Prescribed use of cholesterol-lowering drugs in the United States, 1978 through 1988. JAMA 1990;263:2185–2188.

80. Forette B, Tortrat D, Wolmark Y. Cholesterol as a risk factor for mortality in elderly women. Lancet 1989;1:868–870.

81. Reisin LH, Landau E, Darawshi A. More rapid relief of pain with isosorbide dinitrate oral spray

than with sublingual tablets in elderly patients with angina pectoris. Am J Cardiol 1988;61:2E.

82. Parker JO, Farrell B, Lahey KA, Moe G. Effect of intervals between doses on the development of tolerance to isosorbide dinitrate. N Engl J Med 1987; 316:1440–1444.

83. Williamson BD, Muller DWM, Topol EJ. Should older patients with acute myocardial infarction receive thrombolytic therapy? Drugs Aging 1992; 2:461–468.

84. Lew AS, Hod H, Cercek B, Shah PK, Ganz W. Mortality and morbidity rates of patients older and younger than 75 years with acute myocardial infarction treated with intravenous streptokinase. Am J Cardiol 1987;59:1–5.

85. Chaitman BR, Thompson B, Wittry MD, et al. The use of tissue-type plasminogen activator for acute myocardial infarction in the elderly: results from the Thrombolysis in Myocardial Infarction Phase I, Open Label Studies and the Thrombolysis in Myocardial Infarction Phase II Pilot Study. J Am Coll Cardiol 1989;14:1159–1165.

86. The GUSTO Investigators. An international randomized trial comparing four thrombolytic strategies for acute myocardial infarction. N Engl J Med 1993;329:673–682.

87. Weaver WD, Litwin PE, Martin JS, et al. Effect of age on use of thrombolytic therapy and mortality in acute myocardial infarction. J Am Coll Cardiol 1991;18:657–662.

88. Brooks PM, Day RO. Nonsteroidal antiinflammatory drugs—differences and similarities. N Engl J Med 1991;324:1716–1725.

89. Walan A, Bader JP, Classen M, et al. Effect of omeprazole and ranitidine on ulcer healing and relapse rates in patients with benign gastric ulcer. N Engl J Med 1989;320:69–75.

90. Bradley JD, Brandt KD, Katz BP, et al. Comparison of an antiinflammatory dose of ibuprofen, an analgesic dose of ibuprofen, and acetaminophen in the treatment of patients with osteoarthritis of the knee. N Engl J Med 1991;325:87–91.

91. Walt RP. Misoprostol for the treatment of peptic ulcer and antiinflammatory-drug-induced gastroduodenal ulceration. N Engl J Med 1992; 327:1575–1580.

92. Graham DY, Agrawal NM, Roth SH. Prevention of NSAID-induced gastric ulcer with misoprostol: multicentre, double-blind, placebo-controlled trial. Lancet 1988;2:1277–1280.

93. Ruoff G. The management of non-insulin-dependent diabetes mellitus in the elderly. J Fam Pract 1993;36:329–335.

94. Groop L, Luzi L, Melander A, et al. Different effects of glyburide and glipizide on insulin secretion and hepatic glucose production in normal and NIDDM subjects. Diabetes 1987;36:1320–1328.

95. Stenman S, Melander A, Groop PH, Groop LC. What is the benefit of increasing the sulfonylurea dose? Ann Intern Med 1993;118:169–174.

96. Yki-Jarvinen H, Kauppila M, Kujansuu E, et al. Comparison of insulin regimens in patients with non-insulin-dependent diabetes mellitus. N Engl J Med 1992;327:1426–1433.

97. Schneider LS, Pollock VE, Lyness SA. A meta-analysis of controlled trials of neuroleptic treatment in dementia. J Am Geriatr Soc 1990;38:553–563.

98. Druckenbrod RW, Rosen J, Cluxton RJ. As-needed dosing of antipsychotic drugs: Limitations and guidelines for use in the elderly agitated patient. Ann Pharmacother 1993;27:645–648.

99. Kane JM, Smith JM. Tardive dyskinesia: prevalence and risk factors, 1959 to 1979. Arch Gen Psychiatry 1982;39:473–481.

100. Guze BH, Baxter LR. Neuroleptic malignant syndrome. N Engl J Med 1985;313:163–166.

101. Shader RJ, Greenblatt DJ. Use of benzodiazepines in anxiety disorders. N Engl J Med 1993;328:1398–1404.

102. Wysowski DK, Barash D. Adverse behavioral reactions attributed to triazolam in the Food and Drug Administration Spontaneous Reporting System. Arch Intern Med 1991;151:2003–2007.

103. Brymer C, Winograd CH. Fluoxetine in elderly patients: is there cause for concern? J Am Geriatr Soc 1992;40:902–905.

104. Miller SW, Mahoney JM, Jann MW. Therapeutic frontiers in Alzheimer's disease. Pharmacotherapy 1992;12:217–222.

105. McKhann G, Drachman D, Folstein M, Katzman R, Price D, Stadlan EM. Clinical diagnosis of Alzheimer's disease: report of the NINCDS-ADRDA work group under the auspices of the Department of Health and Human Services Task Force on Alzheimer's Disease. Neurology 1984;34:939–944.

106. Engel RR, Satzger W. Methodological problems in assessing therapeutic efficacy in patients with dementia. Drugs Aging 1992;2:79–85.

107. Bartus RT, Dean RL, Beer B, Lippa AS. The cholinergic hypothesis of geriatric memory dysfunction. Science 1982;217:408–417.

108. Molchan SE, Martinez RA, Weingartner HJ, et al. Increased cognitive sensitivity to scopolamine with age and a perspective on the scopolamine model. Brain Res Rev 1992;17:215–226.

109. Spagnoli A, Lucca U, Menasce G, et al. Long-term acetyl-L-carnitine treatment in Alzheimer's disease. Neurology 1991;41:1726–17.

110. Summers WK, Majovski LV, Marsh GM, Tachiki K, Kling A. Oral tetrahydroaminoacridine in long-term treatment of senile dementia, Alzheimer's type. N Engl J Med 1986;315:1241–1245.

111. Chatellier G, Lacomblex L. Tacrine and lecithin in senile dementia of the Alzheimer type: a multicentre trial. Br Med J 1990;300:495–499.

112. Fitten LJ, Perryman KM, Gross PL, Fine H, Cummins J, Marshall C. Treatment of Alzheimer's disease with short and long-term oral THA and lecithin: a double blind study. Am J Psychiatry 1990; 147:239–242.

113. Gauthier S, Bouchard R, Lamontagne A, et al. Tetrahydroaminoacridine-lecithin combination treatment in patients with intermediate-stage Alzheimer's disease. Results of a Canadian double-blind, crossover, multicenter study. N Engl J Med 1990;322:1272–1276.

114. Eagger SA, Levy R, Sahakian BJ. Tacrine in Alzheimer's disease. Lancet 1991;337:989–992.

115. Molloy DW, Guyatt GH, Wilson DB, Duke R, Rees L, Singer J. Effect of tetrahydroaminoacridine on cognition, function and behaviour in Alzheimer's disease. Can Med Assoc J 1991;144:29–34.

116. Davis KL, Thal LJ, Gamzu ER, et al. A double-blind, placebo-controlled multicenter study of tac-

rine for Alzheimer's disease. N Engl J Med 1992;
327:1253–1259.

117. Farlow M, Gracon SI, Hershey LA, Lewis K, Sadowsky C, DolanUreno J. A controlled trial of tacrine in Alzheimer's disease. JAMA 1992;268:2523–
2529.

118. FDC Reports—"The Pink Sheet" 1993;55:7–
9.

119. O'Brien JT, Eagger S, Levy R. Effects of tetrahydroaminoacridine on liver function in patients
with Alzheimer's disease. Age Aging 1991;20:129–
131.

5/ Common Complaints of the Elderly

Thomas D. McRae

The physician can approach common complaints in the elderly from two different perspectives: the traditional medical view of what diseases occur most often or the patients' view of what bothers them most, which they may or may not report to physicians. To deliver optimal health care to the elderly, the physician must realize that these two views are often quite different and must be prepared to explore both. Neglecting either may result in missed opportunities to improve significantly the patient's quality of life, or worse, such neglect may lead to significant iatrogenic disease. The goal of this chapter is to familiarize the reader with both perspectives and to encourage both lines of thinking when treating older patients.

Numerous surveys have documented the diseases most common to the elderly. Not surprisingly, the results vary significantly with the population studied and with the perspective from which it is studied. Thus, community-residing elders present one set of problems, while those in nursing homes present another. Likewise, all-cause mortality presents one set of diseases, while hospital discharges or physicians' office visits present still others. Furthermore, studies focusing on a single problem such as falls or incontinence yield other varying data. In reality, no single approach to this traditional epidemiologic question is best. What is probably most useful is to form a gestalt based on the varying samples, keeping in mind the variability involved, when looking at any given individual.

With all-cause mortality, data from the National Center for Health Statistics (1) show that although the numbers have been declining in recent years, cardiovascular disease remains the leading cause of death in both elderly men and women, accounting for 600,000 deaths in 1990— a rate of approximately 1,900/100,000 U.S. residents older than 65. Neoplasms are the second most common cause of death, and their numbers are rising, so that in the not too distant future,

they will likely surpass cardiovascular disease in the young elderly (ages 65 to 74), though cardiovascular disease will probably remain the leading cause in persons 75 and older. For men, the most common sites of occurrence are prostate, lung, and colon and rectum; while the leading causes of mortality are lung, prostate, and colon and rectum. For women, the most common sites of occurrence are breast, colon and rectum, and lung; while their leading causes of mortality are lung, breast, and colon and rectum (2). Cerebrovascular disease remains the third leading cause of death in the elderly. It dropped there in about 1980, and the numbers continue to decline, apparently because of improved control of hypertension and other risk factor reductions. Pneumonia and influenza hold fourth place overall as a leading cause of death in people over 65, and chronic obstructive lung diseases are fifth. If the data are broken down by sex, this overall pattern holds for women, but in men, chronic obstructive lung diseases are fourth, and pneumonia and influenza are fifth.

Besides mortality, data from the National Center for Health Statistics (3) also show the leading causes of hospitalization for persons over the age of 65 in the United States. The top five primary discharge diagnoses for men in 1990 were heart disease, neoplasms, pneumonia, cerebrovascular disease, and hyperplasia of the prostate. For women, they were heart disease, neoplasms, cerebrovascular disease, fractures, and pneumonia. The five most common inpatient operations performed on men in 1990 were prostatectomy, cardiac catheterization, coronary artery bypass, pacemaker insertion or placement, and inguinal hernia repair. Elderly women's most common inpatient invasive procedures were cardiac catheterization, fracture reduction, pacemaker insertion or replacement, biopsies on the digestive system, and cholecystectomy. Of particular note regarding these latter data is the apparent dramatic increase in the numbers of invasive cardiac procedures performed on the elderly since 1980.

As noted above, deaths from cardiovascular disease are declining in this age group. At the same time, health care costs continue to skyrocket and seem to defy control. A study of the actual benefits of these procedures to patients versus their cost to the patient and to society is long overdue.

The National Center for Health Statistics also tracks the leading causes of psychiatric hospitalization (4). In 1986, affective disorders were far and away the most common cause of psychiatric admission of the elderly, accounting for 52% of admissions to all types of nonfederal hospitals. Organic disorders accounted for 20%. Schizophrenia was the primary diagnosis in 8%, and alcohol-related disease was diagnosed in 5%. The high rate of admission for affective disorders serves a reminder that in elderly males, especially white males, suicide is a major concern. In 1989, the number of deaths due to suicide was 12.2/100,000 in the U.S. population as a whole (5). For white men of all ages, it was 21.4/100,000. For elderly white men, it ranged from 35.1/100,000 for 65- to 74-year-olds to 71.9/100,000 for those 85 and older—nearly three times that of any other age cohort!

Perhaps having more impact on the daily practices of primary care providers, the National Ambulatory Care Survey (6) provides data on the most common causes of visits to physicians' offices. In this 1975 survey, nearly two-thirds of the visits were to general or family practitioners and internists, and fully two-thirds of the visits were accounted for by six groups of diagnoses: diseases of the circulatory system (25.9%), diseases of the nervous system and sense organs (9.4%), diseases of the musculoskeletal system and connective tissue (9.3%), diseases of the respiratory system (8.4%), special conditions and examinations without illness (6.9%), and endocrine, nutritional, and metabolic diseases (6.3%). The 10 most commonly recorded individual diagnoses, however, do not completely reflect this distribution. While essential hypertension and chronic ischemic heart disease are first and second, diabetes mellitus is third, and medical and surgical aftercare and osteoarthritis are fourth and fifth. Symptomatic heart disease, arthritis (unspecified), cataracts, medical or special examination, and neuroses round out the top 10, which cumulatively account for 36.1% of all visits.

A more recent study, the 1988 National Health Interview Survey (7), provides the patients' perspective on acute and chronic conditions in the ambulatory elderly. Respondents to this survey reported conditions that required medical attention or resulted in restriction of activity. For the acute conditions, the numbers reported are incidence estimates of conditions per 100 persons per year. Respiratory conditions (43.9/100 persons/year) were more than twice as common as any others. Of these, influenza (20.0) and the common cold (15.8) were the most frequent, while the incidence of pneumonia was only 1.4. Injuries were also very common (20.6). Other common acute conditions were digestive system disorders (6.4); infective and parasitic diseases, mostly unspecified viral illnesses (5.6); acute musculoskeletal conditions (4.7); acute urinary conditions (4.4); and skin conditions (2.4). Notable for its absence was unspecified fever. For the chronic conditions, the numbers given are prevalence estimates of conditions per 1000 of the population 65 and over. In general, for the most common diagnoses, the prevalence figures all increase for persons over the age of 75. The 10 most prevalent conditions reported in this survey were the following: arthritis (485.7), hypertension (373.0), hearing impairment (315.2), heart disease (295.8), chronic sinusitis (173.0), cataracts (167.7), deformity or orthopedic impairment (161.1), diabetes mellitus (92.4), visual impairment (90.7), and tinnitus (83.9). To put these numbers in context, a prevalence of 485.7 represents nearly 14 million persons 65 and over with arthritis, while slightly more than 2.4 million have tinnitus. Despite these figures, more than 70% of the respondents reported themselves to be in good-to-excellent health. However for the subset of black respondents, this number drops significantly to about 52%.

Another example of the patients' perspective on the most common diagnoses in a community-residing elderly population is provided by the Dunedin Program. Based on a series of questionnaires administered to people over the age of 65 living in this Florida community, Hale and colleagues (8) report a surprisingly high prevalence of certain symptoms. Their four most common symptoms reported by women responding to a list of 28 symptoms put in lay language were nocturia (80.4%), pedal edema (30.5%), cold feet and legs (28.6%), and constipation (23.7%). The average age of these women was 75.0, and their mean number of reported symptoms was 3.99, which was significantly greater than the 3.22 mean reported by the men in the study, whose average age was 75.6. The four most common symptoms for these men were nocturia (79.8%), irregular heartbeat (24.8%), cold feet and legs (23.6%), and tinnitus (23.1%).

Even though they cover diagnoses reported by physicians and diagnoses and symptoms reported by patients, the data sets just discussed do not tell the whole story about the most common diagnoses in the noninstitutionalized elderly. In a landmark study done in Edinburgh in 1964, Williamson and colleagues (9) documented the phenomenon of the "iceberg of unreported illness." They examined patients in the community and found an average of 3.26 diagnoses for men, of which an average of 1.87 were unknown to their family doctors; women averaged 3.42 diagnoses, with an average of 2.03 diagnoses that their family doctors did not recognize. The four most common diagnoses found were the same for both men and women: defects of vision and hearing, musculoskeletal and foot disorders, atherosclerotic peripheral vascular disease, and psychiatric disorders (dementia, depression, and neuroses).

Despite the intervening years of increasing physician awareness of the problems of the elderly, this phenomenon does not seem to have gone away. Several studies of comprehensive geriatric assessment in recent years have found significant problems of which patients' physicians were not aware. For example, Rubenstein and colleagues (10), in reviewing 6 years of data on their acute inpatient geriatric evaluation unit at the Sepulveda Veteran's Administration Medical Center, reported an average of 3.14 new diagnoses found per patient. Of these, 0.71 were "major" and 2.43 were "minor." The most common major diagnoses were depression, malnutrition, reversible incontinence, gastrointestinal disorders (including bleeding, obstruction, and multiple polyps), hypothyroidism, and reversible dementia. Their most common minor disorders were low-grade anemia, minor psychiatric conditions, hearing impairment, minor gastrointestinal disorders (including constipation, peptic ulcer, and diverticulosis), bone and joint disorders, minor infections, and gait disorders and falls. Similarly, Winograd (11) reported finding 50 new diagnoses in 71 patients referred for geriatric consultation in a non-VAMC setting. The most common of these were cardiovascular disorders, adverse medication effects, malnutrition, misdiagnosis of dementia, and gait disorders. In community assessment, Williams and colleagues (12) found substantial percentages of new diagnoses in their population, including psychiatric disorders (45%), rheumatic disease (36.6%), dementing illness (32.1%), cardiovascular disease (31.3%), gastrointestinal disease (24.4%), and hypertension (21.4%).

One explanation for the lack of agreement between these common complaints of the elderly and the diagnoses most often reported by physicians may lie with the elderly themselves. Older persons may not bring complaints to the physician for a variety of reasons. They may attribute the symptom to the aging process and not think it worth mentioning, i.e., they do not want to "bother" the doctor. Other possibilities include simple embarrassment or fear that reporting the symptom may lead to hospitalization or institutionalization. Interview data gathered by Brody and Kleban support this hypothesis (13).

Another explanation is put forward by Fried and colleagues (14), namely that the traditional medical model of one symptom or set of symptoms yielding one diagnosis may not be adequate when dealing with the elderly. These authors tested this hypothesis both by retrospective chart review and by prospective evaluation of patients attending a geriatric assessment clinic. They found that barely 40% of the cases studied corresponded to the traditional model. For the remaining cases they developed four additional models: the synergistic morbidity model, the attribution model, the causal chain model, and the unmasking event model.

The synergistic morbidity model proposes the existence of a number of generally chronic diseases that add together to produce disability until a functional threshold is passed which causes the patient to seek medical attention. The example given by the authors is that of a 79-year-old woman who presents with the complaint of decreased social functioning secondary to urinary incontinence. This turns out to be due to her increased need to urinate secondary to diuretic therapy for worsening congestive heart failure and her decreased ability to get to the bathroom in time, secondary to worsening osteoarthritis.

In the attribution model, patients sense worsening health status and attribute it to worsening of a previously diagnosed problem, often causing them to delay further evaluation. When evaluation is performed, it leads to the diagnosis of a new, unrecognized condition as the cause of the decline in well-being. One example given by the authors is that of a 74-year-old man who presented with the complaint of feeling unwell, which he attributed to worsening of his longstanding constipation. Careful investigation, however, revealed that his bowel habits had not changed but that he had developed a new paranoid disorder, characterized by feelings of persecution by his neighbors and leading him to feel unwell. He rapidly improved with treatment with an antipsychotic medication. If treatment had focused solely on his gut, this improvement would not have been likely.

A variant of this model is the facilitating complaint. In this variant, patients attribute their presentation for care to the worsening of a previously known condition but recognize that their real concern is another problem that they may not perceive as a legitimate reason for seeking care. The authors describe a 68-year-old woman with known asthma and arthritis. The real concern of both the patient and her daughter was mild memory impairment. When confronted with this, both admitted that the presenting complaints were secondary.

The causal chain model postulates that the presenting complaint represents the "last straw" in a series of symptoms or diseases that all began with a single initial event and which have multiple points of interaction or feedback loops along the chain. Often this represents the interaction of medical and psychiatric illnesses. To illustrate this model, Fried and colleagues relate the case of a 76-year-old woman who presented with a 6-month history of weight loss and epigastric pain brought on by eating. Full evaluation revealed that her problems actually had begun 2 years previously with cataract surgery on her right eye. This led to a retinal detachment in that eye, which resulted in near blindness. The patient's poor vision caused her to be less active in community organizations in which she had been a leader. This led to dysphoria, social isolation, sleep disturbance, anorexia, and weight loss. Several months after this, epigastric pain precipitated by food intake began. Careful assessment revealed diagnoses of major depression and gastritis, both of which responded to therapy. Focusing solely on this patient's GI complaints would likely have missed her more significant problem of depression; and not recognizing the causal chain in this case would have given her no assistance in coping with her low vision.

The final model proposed by Fried et al. is the unmasking event model. This model proposes that a major stressful event, usually external to the patient, reveals a condition that had previously been stable, well compensated, and unrecognized. This unmasking may be dramatic enough to make the problem appear acute. The classic example presented by the authors is that of an 80-year-old woman who comes to live with her daughter after the death of her husband. The daughter brings her in for evaluation of new memory problems. Evaluation of the patient finds Alzheimer's disease, which has likely been present for a number of years but was not recognized and perhaps even denied while the husband was alive.

As suggested earlier, these models led to appropriate diagnosis and treatment in nearly 60% of cases, whether studied retrospectively or prospectively. Of the four models, the most frequently used was the attribution model. The authors note that a variety of forces are likely at work to limit the usefulness of the medical model, thus making these other models necessary.

Truisms and rules of thumb abound in every field of medicine, and geriatrics is no exception. One popular mnemonic for remembering the most common diseases in the elderly is to think of the "i's"—immobility, instability, incontinence, intellectual impairment, impaired homeostasis, impaired vision and hearing, insomnia, and iatrogenic disease. One approach to this chapter might have been to discuss briefly each of these. They are, however, all covered in depth in later chapters, because they are all important. And, while in many ways they are the essence of what makes geriatric medicine unique, limiting one's view to them exclusively narrows the breadth of vision necessary to provide optimal care to the elderly, in the same way that ignoring them does. This chapter seeks instead to encourage the dual vision of traditional epidemiology and the elderly person's perspective. Remember the common killers and the acute diseases, but also remember the chronic diseases and the missed diagnoses. Most of all, remember to think creatively, because as Fried and her colleagues showed, more often than not, Occam's razor just doesn't cut it.

REFERENCES

1. National Center for Health Statistics. Health, United States, 1991. Hyattsville, MD: Public Health Service, 1992.
2. Boring CC, Squires TS, Tong T. Cancer statistics, 1993. CA 1993;43:7–26.
3. National Center for Health Statistics. Health, United States, 1991. Hyattsville, MD: Public Health Service, 1992:229–232.
4. National Center for Health Statistics. Health, United States, 1991. Hyattsville, MD: Public Health Service, 1992:241.
5. National Center for Health Statistics. Health, United States, 1991. Hyattsville, MD: Public Health Service, 1992:177–178.
6. National Center for Health Statistics. Advance data from vital and health statistics: nos 21–30. National Center for Health Statistics. Vital Health Stat 1990;16(3):1–11.
7. National Center for Health Statistics. Current estimates from the National Health Interview Survey, 1988. National Center for Health Statistics. Vital Health Stat 1989;10(173):15,84–85,96–97,114.
8. Hale WE, Perkins LL, May FE, Marks RG, Stewart RB. Symptom prevalence in the elderly: an evaluation of age, sex, disease and medication use. J Am Geriatr Soc 1986;34:333–340.

9. Williamson J, Stokoe IH, Gray S, et al. Old people at home: their unreported needs. Lancet 1964;May 23:1117–1120.

10. Rubenstein LZ, Josephson K, Wieland GD, et al. Geriatric assessment on a subacute hospital ward. Clin Geriatr Med 1987;3(1):131–143.

11. Winograd CH. Inpatient geriatric consultation. Clin Geriatr Med 1987;3(1):193–202.

12. Williams ME. Outpatient geriatric evaluation. Clin Geriatr Med 1987;3(1):175–183.

13. Brody EM, Kleban MH. Physical and mental health symptoms of older people: who do they tell? J Am Geriatr Soc 1981;29:442–448.

14. Fried LP, Storer DJ, King DE, Lodder F. Diagnosis of illness presentation in the elderly. J Am Geriatr Soc 1991;39:117–123.

6/ Diagnosis and Management of Heart Disease

Arthur J. Moss

Cardiovascular performance declines progressively with age, and at the same time the older individual is at a progressively increased risk of having one or more of the numerous cardiac diseases that afflict mankind. Elderly patients, in contrast to their younger brethren, have to contend with both an aging heart and superimposed cardiac disease—a combination that markedly increases the likelihood of disability and death. The physician must differentiate between the physiologic decline in cardiac performance that ensues with age and problems resulting from specific cardiovascular diseases.

What is the potential functional state of an elderly individual without cardiac disease? The physiologic characteristics of a world champion distance runner, age 77, were reported by Webb et al. in 1977 (1). The subject held 14 recognized world records in track for competitors in the 74- to 76-year-old category. At age 77, the individual ran record races of 1 mile at 6:53.6 (min: sec.tenths) and 10,000 meters in 47:30.0. Physiologic studies of this subject revealed that he was slim and trim (height, 5′ 9 1/2″; weight, 151 lb), with resting blood pressure, 120/70 mm Hg; resting heart rate, 55 beats/min; maximum heart rate, 160 beats/min; and maximum minute ventilation of 83 L/min (normal range: 45 to 80 L/min for men of equivalent age). This single-patient study provides some insight into the optimal performance that can be achieved in a trained elderly individual without complicating cardiopulmonary disease—an image that we should keep in mind as we care for patients in the older age group.

CARDIOVASCULAR PATHOPHYSIOLOGY AND AGING

An enormous amount of valuable data has been accumulated about the cardiac aging process from in vitro biologic studies of senescent animal hearts. In addition, investigations of intact hearts from senescent animals and evaluation of cardiovascular performance in aging human beings provide important background information for understanding the setting of cardiac disease in the elderly (2). Comprehensive reviews of this subject are provided in a monograph edited by Weisfeldt, entitled The Aging Heart, (3) and in the book The Biology of Aging (4).

ANATOMIC AND BIOCHEMICAL CHANGES

Anatomic Changes

Age-related anatomic changes occur in the myocardial collagen and in the conduction system. Collagen becomes more plentiful, and it increases the stiffness of the heart. These changes reduce ventricular diastolic compliance more than systolic contractility, and they may affect impulse transmission. Myocardial deposition of lipid substances is also common. Sclerodegenerative changes develop in the conduction system with patchy fibrosis, a loss of myofibers, and an increase in the elastic tissue in the His-Purkinje network. The number of pacemaker cells in the sinoatrial node decreases with age. It has been estimated that after age 75 years, the sinus node contains less than 10% of the pacemaker cells present in younger patients (5). These anatomic findings explain, in part, the increased prevalence of high ventricular filling pressures, fascicular block conduction disturbances, and sinus node dysfunction in the elderly.

Energy Production

Various myocellular mitochondrial enzyme activities (fatty acid oxidation, the tricarboxylate cycle, and oxidative phosphorylation) progressively decrease with age. This diminution is explained in part by a reduction in the number of mitochondria per unit volume or weight and also by a shift of specific enzyme activity away from active fatty acid oxidation. It is reasonable to speculate that a reduction in this enzymatic machinery in the older heart contributes to diminished work performance in the intact organ.

Electrophysiologic Properties

Various characteristics of the excitation-contraction process change with age (6). In an isometric contraction, the transmembrane action potential, the myoplasmic calcium transient that initiates contraction, and the contraction itself are longer in senescent than in young adult rat hearts. In isotonic preparations, the rate and magnitude of myofiber shortening are decreased in the senescent animal. The myosin isoenzyme composition shifts from predominantly rapid ATP hydrolytic isoenzymes in the young heart to slower hydrolytic isoenzymes in the older heart. The time required for restitution of the excitation-contraction coupling cycle (reuptake of calcium by the sarcoplasmic reticulum) is prolonged in older myocardium. These time-dependent processes that are prolonged with age result in increased dynamic muscle stiffness during contraction and decreased relaxation (reduced diastolic compliance) in the senescent heart.

Spontaneous automaticity in the pacemaker cells of the sinus node and in the Purkinje network of the ventricles declines with age. This effect results primarily from a reduction in the rate of phase 4 depolarization in pacemaker cells—an alteration that may contribute to enhanced arrhythmogenesis and bradycardia in the elderly and an increased susceptibility to the bradycardic effects of antiarrhythmic agents. The conduction velocity of the electrical impulse is minimally altered in Purkinje fibers of senescent animals, but conduction is slowed through nodal tissue, such as the atrioventricular node, possibly from the disordered pacemaker cells in the junctional regions.

Cardiac Receptors

One of the most striking changes that occurs in the aged heart is a decline in the response to stress. Studies involving adrenergic-mediated stress in the aged heart by Lakatta (7) and Vestal et al. (8) reveal a decline in postsynaptic response to β-adrenergic stimulation, suggesting a reduction in either the number or the function of the receptors. Other investigators have shown that isolated muscle from old animals has fewer adrenergic receptors than muscle from young animals. In addition, current evidence indicates that the number of cardiac receptors for digitalis de-

clines with age, a finding that may explain why digitalis is less effective as an inotropic agent in older people than in younger people. These findings with regard to adrenergic and digitalis receptors may be part of a universal characteristic of aging—a reduction in the number of all hormonal receptors with age. The net result would be a diminished effectiveness for agonists (catecholamines) and an enhanced sensitivity to antagonists (β-blockers, calcium entry blockers) in the elderly patient.

Molecular Genetic Considerations

Studies on the genetic control of the cardiac aging process are in their infancy. One hypothesis is that increased cardiac loading that develops with age could be the stimulus that signals one or more genes to alter their protein expression, resulting in changes in membrane (ionic channels), regulatory (G protein/kinase), or contractile (actin, myosin, troponin) protein structure and function. However, genetics alone will never provide the entire answer to aging. Of note, there is a large mean difference in the age of death for monozygotic twins—a finding suggesting the importance of environmental factors in aging and/or disease.

ALTERED CARDIOVASCULAR FUNCTION

Rhythm Disorders

Sinus node dysfunction may manifest itself in terms of sustained sinus bradycardia at rates below 50 beats/min, intermittent sinus arrest with varying durations of asystole, or the atrial brady-tachy syndrome with alternating episodes of atrial tachycardia followed abruptly by profound sinus arrest. Patients with sinus node dysfunction may present clinically with fatigue or tiredness due to the bradycardia with reduced cardiac output, syncope from the asystolic sinus arrest, or troublesome palpitations or angina from the tachycardia. Sinus node dysfunction is quite prevalent in patients over 70 years of age and is responsible for considerable morbidity.

Atrioventricular block unrelated to acute myocardial infarction is a disorder primarily of older individuals. It may present as abrupt syncope, the so-called Morgagni-Adams-Stokes attack, or simply with fatigue and palpitations from varying degrees of heart block. Two common causes of heart block in the geriatric patient are Lenegre's disease and Lev's disease. The former is an idiopathic sclerodegenerative process involving the Purkinje conducting system. Lenegre's disease is one of the most common causes of right bundle branch block and left anterior hemiblock in older patients, and there is usually a slow progression to complete heart block over several years. Lev's disease is a degeneration of the fibrous supporting tissues of the heart, with invasion of the adjacent conducting system by fibrosis and calcification. Calcification may begin either in the aortic or mitral valve annulus and extend into the bundle of His or the proximal bundle branches to produce bundle branch block, hemiblock, or complete heart block.

Ventricular arrhythmias occur more frequently in the older group than the younger age group, even in the absence of demonstrable organic heart disease. Several studies have used 24-hour Holter recordings to evaluate the frequency and complexity of ventricular premature beats (VPBs) in different age groups. VPBs are common in overtly healthy elderly individuals, and 50% have complex VPBs (multiform, paired, or ventricular tachycardia) on Holter or exercise recordings (9). These findings argue for restraint in the treatment of asymptomatic ventricular irritability in older patients, especially those without evident heart disease.

Left Ventricular Dysfunction

Longitudinal studies of aging and studies comparing cardiovascular function in younger and older healthy subjects have demonstrated decreases in maximum stroke volume, cardiac output, and oxygen uptake in the older individuals in response to exercise. A study by Rodeheffer et al. (10) assessed the effects of age on left ventricular function at rest and during upright bicycle exercises. Age did not influence left ventricular dynamics at rest, but the ejection fraction was significantly reduced during exercise in subjects over age 60 years. Furthermore, wall motion abnormalities during exercise occurred with increasing frequency in older subjects, and these changes were not associated with abnormalities in end-diastolic volume or blood pressure. Recent studies indicate that left ventricular relaxation is progressively impaired in late middle age and old age, presumably a marker of cardiac aging (11).

The age-related decrease in left ventricular function may be due to one of four mechanisms: a reduction in the Frank-Starling heterometric regulation, increased afterload, decreased contractility due to disease, or decreased contractility due to aging. The available evidence favors the last explanation, and this would be consistent with the impaired release and uptake of calcium by the sarcoplasmic reticulum and the diminished number of myocardial adrenergic receptors reported in senescent animals.

Disordered Regulation of Blood Pressure

Many factors influence the regulation of blood pressure, including cardiac output (determined by heart rate, blood volume, venous return, and cardiac contractility), peripheral arteriolar resistance, the status of the renin-angiotensin-aldosterone system, the functional state of the baroreceptor reflexes, and the autonomic nervous system. The mean blood pressure increases progressively with age as a result of increased peripheral resistance. Wide fluctuations in blood pressure are commonly observed in elderly subjects as a result of increased aortic rigidity, autonomic neuropathy, and decreased baroreceptor function. Hypertension and orthostatic hypotension may coexist in the same patient, and therapy for one condition often exacerbates the associated condition.

CARDIAC DISEASES IN THE ELDERLY

Various pathologic studies of hearts of aged patients reveal the usual cardiac lesions observed in younger age groups as well as less commonly recognized disorders somewhat specific to the elderly. These cardiac diseases in the geriatric patient are usually manifest by alterations in cardiac rhythm, by congestive heart failure, or with ischemic chest pain.

COMMONLY OCCURRING CARDIAC DISEASES

Coronary Heart Disease

Ischemic heart disease, both acute myocardial infarction and chronic coronary disease, is the most common pathologic finding in elderly patients with congestive heart failure, but it also is frequently found in patients not in failure. With an acute myocardial infarction, elderly patients have a fourfold increased mortality rate compared with younger patients. Advanced age is associated with disproportionately high in-hospital mortality rates, even in the so-called good-risk myocardial infarction patient and in those given thrombolytic therapy. The major causes of death in hospitalized patients aged 70 and older with acute myocardial infarction are shock and cardiac rupture (12). This high incidence of myocardial rupture in the elderly may be due to impairment of reparative processes that affect the aged myocardium or possibly be secondary to an increased occurrence of hypertension in the elderly. The symptom presentation of coronary heart disease in the elderly may be quite atypical, and classic anginal chest pain is less frequent in older than in younger patients. Non–Q wave myocardial infarction is more prevalent in the elderly.

Hypertensive Heart Disease

It is now recognized that hypertension is one of the leading causes of congestive heart failure in all age groups, especially in the elderly. Hypertension may remain silent for many years, and the ravages of this disorder may not be evident until the individual passes retirement age. Concentric left ventricular hypertrophy with or without chamber dilation, elevated left ventricular filling pressures, and ECG evidence of either hypertrophy or a bundle branch block pattern are the usual findings.

Aortic Stenosis

Aortic stenosis, in which the aortic leaflets are sclerosed and calcified with reduced cusp motion, may be due to rheumatic heart disease with commissural fusion, a congenitally deformed bicuspid aortic valve, or degenerative calcification of a normal valve. With the decline in acute rheumatic fever, the elderly patients are the remaining reservoir for rheumatic aortic stenosis. Within a generation, rheumatic aortic stenosis will be a rare cause of this disorder. In contrast, bicuspid and degenerative aortic valve disease will make up the major proportion of elderly patients with aortic stenosis. As with younger patients with aortic stenosis, the occurrence of syncope, angina, or congestive heart failure has ominous implications.

Aortic Insufficiency

Aortic incompetence is the most common valve lesion found in the elderly. It may occur as an isolated lesion or in association with aortic stenosis or rheumatic mitral valve disease. Syphilitic aortic insufficiency is now a rare disease that is found almost exclusively in the older age groups. Dilation of the aortic root in association with longstanding hypertension is a frequent cause of an aortic insufficiency murmur, but it rarely causes significant regurgitation. Significant aortic regurgitation with left ventricular volume overload often produces some of the largest hearts observed in clinical medicine. The patients may do surprisingly well for many years despite an enormous heart and chronic congestive heart failure. The development of angina pectoris and atrial fibrillation are often associated with a rapidly deteriorating clinical course.

Mitral Valve Disease

Most patients with significant rheumatic mitral stenosis, insufficiency, or a combination of both usually develop progressive cardiac dysfunction before entering the geriatric age group. Those who make it into the older ages have usually been spared the complication of reactive pulmonary hypertension. Papillary muscle dysfunction in association with chronic coronary disease and a prior diaphragmatic myocardial infarction is a frequent cause of mitral insufficiency in this age group.

Bacterial Endocarditis

Bacterial endocarditis, often presenting with protean manifestations, is occurring with increasing frequency in the elderly. Preexisting mitral or aortic valve disease is not a prerequisite. Since many of the elderly are edentulous, *Streptococcus viridans* is less frequently the offending organism in this age group than in younger patients. Because of the high frequency of urologic disorders in older patients, enterococcal infection of the valves has become more prevalent. The mitral valve is more frequently involved than the aortic, usually with vegetations on the line of valvular apposition. Fever, anemia, and a heart murmur are the triad that should raise suspicion of possible bacterial endocarditis. However, these findings coexist in many elderly hospitalized patients without endocarditis. By the same token, elderly patients with endocarditis may be afebrile. Thus, if a patient with recent clinical deterioration has an unexplained anemia and a heart murmur, then blood should be drawn for aerobic and anaerobic cultures. Prolonged incubation (3 to 4 weeks) and specialized media are often needed to isolate organisms in the HACEK (*Haemophilus-Actinobacillus - Cardiobacterium - Eikenella - Kingella*) group. Fungal endocarditis should be considered in patients with suspected endocarditis and negative blood cultures.

Cor Pulmonale

Pulmonary hypertension with right ventricular hypertrophy and congestive heart failure is a troublesome problem in all age groups, and especially in the elderly. The hypoxia often results in secondary polycythemia. Complicating atrial arrhythmias are common and often compound the management problem. Chronic cor pulmonale is usually secondary to hypoxic chronic lung disease (chronic bronchitis-emphysema). Special factors in the older age group include the late secondary effects from kyphoscoliosis and other thoracic deformities, as well as the hypoxic diffusion problems associated with diffuse pulmonary parenchymal disease, for example, pulmonary fibrosis or late-stage sarcoidosis. Multiple pulmonary emboli are an infrequent cause of pulmonary hypertension in the elderly.

Cardiomyopathy

This disorder of cardiac muscle is often categorized by etiology as well as by the type of functional derangement. For the vast majority of elderly patients with cardiomyopathy but without overt systemic disease, the etiology is not uncovered and the patient is categorized as having idiopathic cardiomyopathy. Alcoholic cardiomyopathy and hemochromatosis with cardiomyopathy should be considered, since both disorders are treatable. Functionally, cardiomyopathy may be subdivided into congestive, restrictive, and obstructive types. The latter is of particular interest because hypertrophic obstructive cardiomyopathy (HOCM) is being diagnosed more frequently in the elderly with the increasing use of echocardiography. Patients with HOCM may present with angina or syncope, and therapy with β-blockers (diametrically opposite that given for most other cardiomyopathies) may be associated with dramatic symptomatic improvement. The anatomic substrate for HOCM is asymmetric septal hypertrophy with narrowing of the aortic outflow tract, disordered muscle bundles in the septum with fiber disarray, and abnormalities in the mitral valve support apparatus.

Pericarditis

Acute pericarditis occurs infrequently in the elderly, but effusive pericarditis secondary to neoplasm or tuberculosis, constrictive pericarditis from prior pericardial disease, and uremic pericarditis have a higher incidence in the older population than is generally appreciated. Diagnosis has been facilitated by echocardiography, especially the presence of pericardial effusion. Pericardial tamponade with the classic diagnostic triad of pulsus paradoxus, Kussmaul's sign, and pulsating neck veins may occur in association with both benign and malignant conditions; aggressive and prompt therapy (needle aspiration and/or surgical drainage) is indicated.

Dissecting Aneurysm

Aortic dissection is the most common fatal condition that involves the aorta. A review of the clinical experience from the Mayo Clinic involving 235 patients with acute or chronic dissection indicates that hypertension was the most common predisposing factor (13). The peak incidence is in the sixth and seventh decades of life, and men are more commonly affected than women. The acute onset of severe chest pain was the most common initial complaint (75%). Less common manifestations included congestive heart failure, syncope, cerebrovascular accident, shock, paraplegia, and lower extremity edema. Because of the diverse initial features and protean manifestations of this disorder, dissecting aneurysm should always be included in the differential diagnosis of unexplained symptoms of cardiovascular origin.

CARDIAC DISORDERS SOMEWHAT SPECIFIC TO THE ELDERLY

Calcific Degenerative Diseases

Calcification of the fibrous skeleton of the heart with involvement of the mitral annulus is often associated with a murmur of mitral insufficiency and atrioventricular conduction abnormalities. This degenerative condition is more frequent in females than in males and is especially common in patients with diabetes mellitus and a history of prior hypertension. The diagnosis may be substantiated by the presence of a J-shaped calcification on lateral chest x-ray of the heart or by echocardiography with prominent reflectivity in the mitral annular region. A second degenerative condition commonly encountered in the elderly is calcification and sclerosis of the fibrosa portion of the aortic cusps with reduced cusp mobility. An aortic systolic murmur of moderate intensity is usually present. Progression from sclerosis to stenosis is infrequent, since there is minimal if any fusion of the commissures. Innocuous aortic valve sclerosis must be differentiated from calcific aortic valve stenosis, in which the orifice area of the aortic valve is significantly reduced, with secondary hemodynamic effects.

Myxomatous Degeneration of the Cardiac Valves

Primary myxomatous degeneration of the cardiac valves, but principally of the mitral and aortic valves, may produce varying degrees of valvular insufficiency. The etiology of this condition is not known, but the normal aging process is a contributing factor. The histologic pattern in the myxomatous degeneration of the mitral valve is similar to that seen in patients with mitral valve prolapse. Although this disorder may occur at any age, it is generally more severe in the elderly. Frequently, there is disruption of the support apparatus, with chordal rupture (mitral valve), enlargement of the mitral annulus, or aortic root dilation. The echocardiogram provides precise diagnostic information.

Senile Cardiac Amyloidosis

Senile cardiac amyloidosis is clinically distinct from primary systemic amyloidosis because the deposits of amyloid material are localized to the myocardium, and the condition occurs almost exclusively in individuals of advanced age. Senile cardiac amyloid has been found at autopsy in 10% of patients over 80 years and in 50% of those over 90 years of age. The patients usually present with congestive heart failure, ventricular conduction disturbances, and cardiac arrhythmias in the absence of angina or hypertensive disease. Congestive heart failure ensues from diminished contractility and a reduction in the diastolic compliance characteristics of both ventricular chambers. Recent clinical studies indicate unique echocardiographic findings in this condition with a thickened ventricular wall, reduced wall motion, and a generalized increased reflectivity from the entire myocardium. Patients with senile cardiac amyloidosis may have an increased sensitivity to digitalis preparations.

Thrombotic Endocarditis

Nonbacterial thrombotic (marantic) endocarditis is frequently observed at autopsy in elderly, debilitated patients, especially those with underlying malignant disease. Thrombotic endocarditis is most frequently associated with adenocarcinomas of the lung, colon, or pancreas. The mitral and aortic valves are most commonly involved, frequently both valves are affected, and this type of endocarditis is not associated with significant valvular dysfunction. The disorder is usually manifested clinically by unexplained systemic emboli and negative blood cultures.

Senile Cardiomyopathy

This unexplained pathologic finding has been found at autopsy examination in patients with and without congestive heart failure. The heart is generally decreased in size and is distinctly brown (brown atrophy). It occurs in severe inanition and chronic wasting diseases such as pulmonary tuberculosis, cancer, and chronic sepsis. Although this disorder may be found in young adults, it primarily affects elderly persons.

DIAGNOSTIC CONSIDERATIONS

ROUTINE CLINICAL EVALUATION

In the elderly patient, the usual clinical evaluation may be less precise than can be achieved in younger patients. The clinical history that is central to all medical workups may be incomplete because of the frequent occurrences of confusion and memory deficits in older individuals. Therefore, it is essential to obtain supplementary information from knowledgeable family members or health service personnel where appropriate. Even when elderly patients are mentally alert with intact cognitive function, the history may be misleading, since many cardiac disorders have vague symptom presentations in the older age group. For example, in those over 70 years of age, acute myocardial infarction does not usually present with severe precordial chest pain. Dyspnea, syncope, stroke, and gastrointestinal symptoms are often the presenting complaint in elderly patients with an acute coronary event.

Laboratory tests and procedures in the older patients also leave something to be desired. Many times the patients may not be strong enough to complete a vigorous test, and often the standards of "normality" have not been defined for this age group. A common error is to apply the criteria of normality obtained from younger patients to this unique older population and thus inadvertently overdiagnose and assign disease entities to these patients when in fact none exist.

ECHOCARDIOGRAM AND DOPPLER ULTRASOUND

The echocardiogram provides dynamic visualization of cardiac structures with particular evaluation of the pericardium and pericardial space, ventricular walls, ventricular septum, valves, the atrial and ventricular chamber sizes, and the presence of mass lesions such as thrombus or myxoma. Two echocardiographic techniques are currently available: (*a*) routine noninvasive transthoracic echocardiography (TTE) and (*b*) semiinvasive transesophageal echocardiography (TEE). Doppler ultrasound studies are usually performed in association with both techniques and provide information about blood flow in the evaluation of dysfunctional valves and intracardiac shunts.

Echocardiography has been particularly helpful in the diagnosis of pericardial effusion, asymmetric septal hypertrophy, mitral valve prolapse, flail mitral valve, mitral stenosis, aortic stenosis, ventricular aneurysm, ventricular thrombus, atrial myxoma, and infective endocarditis. Echocardiography provides invaluable information about cardiac performance, including the ejection fraction and regional wall motion abnormalities. Stress echocardiography involving pharmacologic (dopamine) and exercise protocols is being used to evaluate dynamic and regional myocardial dysfunction secondary to coronary disease.

Many elderly patients have chest deformities such as senile emphysema or rib cage distortion that contribute to technical difficulties in TTE. The success rate for technically satisfactory TTE is very high in young patients, but the studies are frequently of limited quality in the elderly. TEE has overcome this problem. The TEE requires adequate sedation of the patient and local anesthesia of the pharynx, to position the probe in the esophagus in close proximity to the heart. TEE has proven to be safe in the elderly (14). The TEE images are usually of very high quality, but their interpretation requires considerable experience and expertise by the ultrasonographer. TEE is a highly accurate method for detecting atrial thrombi, particularly those involving the atrial appendage, valvular vegetations, and aortic dissection.

HOLTER MONITORING

Twenty-four-hour Holter ECG monitoring has become a valuable diagnostic technique in the evaluation of cardiac rhythm disturbances. Many elderly patients experience transient syncope, dizziness, and palpitations, and Holter monitoring may uncover a potentially life-threatening arrhythmia for which effective therapy is available. Holter monitoring has been used in the routine evaluation of postinfarction patients prior to hospital discharge. The frequency of transient yet asymptomatic ventricular tachycardia, heart block, and sinus node dysfunction is considerably higher in the older group than in younger patients. Similarly, 24-hour Holter recordings are indicated in all patients after pacemaker implantation, to assess the sensing and pacing function of the newly implanted units. Finally, follow-up Holter monitoring has provided valuable insight into the efficacy of antiarrhythmic drug therapy, especially as it relates to the suppression of ventricular premature beats and the control of the ventricular response rate to atrial fibrillation. In this regard, recent studies have shown that for individual patients, a 70 to 80% reduction in the

frequency of ventricular premature beats from baseline is required before ascribing the effect to the administered antiarrhythmic agent.

Holter ECG monitoring has also been used to evaluate patients for "silent myocardial ischemia" as defined by asymptomatic ST-segment depression during ambulatory activity. To date, this technique has not proven to be as useful as originally proposed. In a recent prospective study of stable patients with established coronary disease, Holter-recorded, ischemic-type ST-segment depression was not associated with an increased rate of subsequent cardiac events during 2-year follow-up, compared with those without ST-segment depression (15). Holter monitoring should not be used to screen stable elderly patients for evidence of silent myocardial ischemia.

EXERCISE TOLERANCE TEST

A variety of activity protocols exist, but common to all is the adjustment of the work load to the patient's capacity, continuous ECG monitoring, intermittent recording of blood pressures, and attention to the patient's symptomatic state during the activity test, with emphasis on safety. The exercise protocol used depends on the indications for the test. The indications may include functional evaluation after myocardial infarction, evaluation of patients with chest pain, determination of the severity of underlying cardiac disease, or the determination of activity-related arrhythmias.

The treadmill is the most widely used technique for activity testing, and its major advantage is the adjustment of the grade and speed of walking to the agility of the patient. The submaximal Bruce protocol, which is targeted to 75 to 90% of the maximum age-predicted heart rate, may be too difficult for elderly patients. The initial walking rate begins at 1.7 miles/hr at a 10% grade, and the speed and grade are progressively increased at 3-min intervals. Most elderly patients cannot follow this protocol, and frequently the activity test is terminated prematurely because of leg and joint problems rather than cardiac symptoms or signs.

Elderly patients seem to perform better when the speed is kept constant and the grade gradually increased. The modified Naughton protocol (Table 6.1) is particularly useful in the older patient; the speed is kept constant at 2.0 miles/hr, the initial grade is flat at 0 , and the grade is increased by 3.5% every 2 min. For low-level activity testing, the protocol is terminated after 8 min, with peak level of activity equivalent to stage 1 of

Table 6.1
Modified Naughton Protocol for Activity Testing in the Elderly Patient

Stage	Time (min)	Speed (mph)	Grade (%)	METs[a]
1	0–2	0	0	1
2	2–4	2	0	2
3	4–6	2	3.5	3
4	6–8	2	7.0	4
5	8–10	2	10.5	5
6	10–12	2	14.0	6
7	12–14	2	17.5	7

[a]Metabolic equivalents.

the standard Bruce protocol. For higher-level testing, the protocol can be continued for additional time at steeper grades.

This low-level exercise test can be performed in postinfarction patients prior to hospital discharge without major problems. This predischarge activity evaluation has proved useful for recommending safe activity levels at home and in uncovering serious ischemic and arrhythmic disorders. A higher-level exercise test such as the standard Bruce protocol may be used in the diagnostic and functional evaluation of ambulatory outpatients. Regardless of the test used, a maximum target heart rate should be chosen either on the basis of clinical judgment or by established norms according to the age of the patient, and the test should be terminated when adverse symptoms or signs appear. Elderly patients, especially elderly women, have a higher percentage of false-positive ischemic ST-segment changes with activity testing, and stringent criteria of > 2.0 mm ST-segment shifts should be used for defining abnormality.

RADIONUCLIDE IMAGING

Radionuclide techniques are widely applied for the evaluation of cardiac function (ejection fraction) and myocardial perfusion (thallium imaging). The tests are essentially noninvasive and require the intravenous administration of a small amount of radioactive tracer and precordial counting with a gamma scintillation camera. The function and perfusion studies can be done at rest and after exercise.

The radionuclide ejection fraction (RNEF) can be obtained either by first-pass or gated techniques. The former method involves recording the time-activity curves of the passage of a bolus of radioactive substance through the heart, usually for 5 to 10 heart beats. Peaks and valleys of the time-activity curve correspond to end-diastole and end-systole, and the ejection fraction is computed from these measurements. The most commonly used gated equilibrium method requires in vitro labeling of the red blood cells with the radiopharmaceutical agent and imaging of the cardiac blood pool at least 5 minutes after intravenous administration of the labeled blood. End-systolic and end-diastolic volumes are determined by synchronization with the R wave of the patient's ECG, and the data from many cardiac cycles are added in phase to one another. Information on regional wall motion can be obtained with both techniques.

Recent studies on healthy volunteers indicate that the resting RNEF does not deteriorate with age. Port et al. (16) reported that the resting RNEF was above the normal value of 0.60 in most healthy subjects over age 60. However, during exercise, the RNEF declined abnormally in most elderly subjects, indicating underlying subclinical myocardial dysfunction and a reduction in reserve capacity. These RNEF techniques provide valuable quantitative information on cardiac performance in patients with coronary heart disease, congestive heart failure, ventricular aneurysm, hypertensive heart disease, and cardiomyopathy. An RNEF below 0.35 reflects significant underlying heart disease, and an RNEF below 0.20 is associated with an ominous prognosis. Serial RNEF measurements can be helpful in evaluating the efficacy of therapeutic interventions such as afterload reduction, digitalization, and diuresis. The RNEF technique is particularly useful in the elderly patient, since precise information can be obtained with minimal effort on the part of patient.

Two thallium-201 scintigraphic techniques are available for detecting reversible myocardial perfusion defects (ischemia and/or scar) in patients with coronary disease. In the exercise protocol, thallium-201 is injected intravenously at peak exercise (treadmill or bicycle), and the heart is imaged with a gamma scintillation camera in three projections immediately after exercise and then again 3 to 4 hours later. In the pharmacologic protocol, thallium-201 is injected in the supine patient 3 minutes after infusion of intravenous dipyridamole, and images are collected a few minutes after the thallium-201 injection and again 3 hours later. Perfusion defects that are present early and late after the thallium-201 injection indicate myocardial scar. Defects that fill in during the recovery phase indicate an area of reversible ischemia, usually due to a culprit coronary stenotic lesion. These two techniques are equally effective in detecting reversible myocardial ischemia and/or scar. The dipyridamole study is particularly useful in elderly patients who can not exercise maximally because of musculoskeletal problems.

HEMODYNAMIC MONITORING IN THE ICU

Critically ill patients with myocardial, circulatory, or respiratory problems require hemodynamic monitoring to provide appropriate and optimal therapy. The elderly patient is especially vulnerable to volume fluctuations, and measurements of the left ventricular filling pressure, cardiac output, and the calculated peripheral vascular resistance provide invaluable insight for therapeutic intervention with inotropic agents, afterload reduction, volume addition, and diuresis. In 1970, Swan, Ganz, and colleagues introduced the flow-directed, balloon-tipped, pulmonary artery catheter. With either a venous cutdown or a percutaneous venous puncture, the catheter is advanced from a peripheral vein into the pulmonary artery without the absolute requirement for fluoroscopy, although the latter may aid in its placement. The pulmonary arterial systolic and diastolic pressures are recorded, and when the balloon is inflated, the catheter becomes "wedged," with pressure measurements reflecting left atrial pressure. The presently designed catheter also records right atrial pressure and has a thermistor probe for measurement of cardiac output by the thermodilution technique. Since a considerable discrepancy may exist between the functions of the right and left ventricles in critically ill patients with hemodynamic embarrassment, the balloon-tipped pulmonary artery catheter provides essential information for the proper management of these individuals. An intraarterial line also should be placed to record systemic pressure directly. In patients with the low output state, a cuff blood pressure is not an accurate measure of the systemic arterial pressure.

CARDIAC CATHETERIZATION AND CORONARY ANGIOGRAPHY

These diagnostic procedures are reserved for patients with significant valvular or coronary heart disease who may require invasive interventions for treatment of life-threatening or disabling cardiac disease. In experienced hands, these procedures are associated with only a minimally increased risk in older patients, compared with those who are younger. Quantitation of the severity of valvular stenotic or insufficient lesions and direct visualization of the coronary arterial tree and the left ventricular contraction pattern are essential for proper decision making in these patients. Significant valvular and coronary disease is eminently correctable, even in patients in the 70- and 80-year age groups.

MANAGEMENT OF SELECTED CARDIAC DISORDERS

During the past decade there have been significant advances in the management of the entire spectrum of cardiac disorders. Better understanding of the pathophysiologic mechanisms of disease and the introduction of new pharmacologic agents and invasive interventions have brought a significant improvement in the quality and longevity of life. This section focuses on the current management of nine common cardiac disorders, with emphasis on the use of validated therapies. As has been pointed out in other chapters in this book, drug absorption, distribution, metabolism, excretion, and organ responsiveness may be different in the geriatric age group from those of younger patients. Invasive interventions are associated with an increased complication rate in the geriatric population. A conservative therapeutic approach together with careful follow-up are essential for optimal efficacy and safety in this age group. For a comprehensive presentation of the management of the following selected cardiac disorders, the reader is referred to standard cardiology texts.

CONGESTIVE HEART FAILURE

Congestive heart failure (CHF), a major problem in the elderly, has many diverse causes, but long-standing hypertension and chronic coronary heart disease (ischemic cardiomyopathy) account for most cases. The severity of the CHF depends largely on the extent of myocardial involvement and the degree of global cardiac dysfunction. Significant compromise of coexisting organ system function, such as that of the kidneys and liver, exacerbate the CHF and reduce the effectiveness of therapeutic measures. Reduction in physical activity, restriction of dietary salt, digitalis, and diuretics are the mainstays of therapy. More potent diuretics, angiotensin converting enzyme (ACE) inhibitors, and new inotropic agents have expanded the therapeutic armamentarium available to the physician.

Diuretics

The available diuretics may be categorized into three groups depending on their site and mechanism of action: (a) loop diuretics, (b) distal convoluted tubule diuretics, and (c) potassium-sparing diuretics. The loop diuretics (furosemide, bumetanide, and ethacrynic acid) are the most potent agents available. Furosemide has an excellent dose-response relationship over a wide range of doses. In refractory cases of CHF and in patients with significant underlying renal disease, large oral doses of the loop diuretics may be ineffective; much smaller intravenous doses may produce a profound diuresis. When using intravenous loop diuretics in older patients, it is best to start with small doses, in the range of half of the usual starting dose, and gradually increase the dose as determined by the response.

Thiazide diuretics, which act in the distal convoluted tubule, are categorized as moderately potent agents. These drugs are poorly effective in patients with reduced glomerular filtration rates (<30 mL/min) and thus are of limited potency when administered alone to older patents with severe CHF. However, these agents may induce a profound diuresis when used in combination with the more potent loop diuretics.

The potassium-sparing diuretics (spironolactone, triamterene, and amiloride) are the weakest of the diuretics and should be used with caution in elderly patients. The antikaluretic action of these agents may produce unexpected hyperkalemia with secondary cardiac conduction disturbances, especially in patients with preexisting renal disease and in patients receiving ACE inhibitors.

Angiotensin Converting Enzyme (ACE) Inhibitors

The treatment of CHF has improved in recent years, most importantly with the addition of ACE inhibitors to the traditional regimen of cardiac glycosides and diuretics. ACE inhibitors counteract the vasoconstrictive mechanisms that secondarily develop in the setting of left ventricular dysfunction and low cardiac output. Activation of the renin-angiotensin-aldosterone and sympathetic nervous systems augments left ventricular impedance (afterload), further exacerbating left ventricular failure. Two recent large-scale clinical trials have demonstrated that ACE-inhibitor therapy reduces mortality and morbidity in patients with overt heart failure, inhibits progression of mild heart failure, and reduces pathologic ventricular remodeling and mortality in patients with acute myocardial infarction and reduced ejection fraction (17, 18).

Several ACE inhibitors are now available, including captopril, enalapril, lisinopril, ramipril,

benazepril, fosinopril, and quinapril. ACE inhibitors have become the cornerstone in the treatment of CHF. It is recommended that these agents should initially be administered in small doses, and the dose progressively increased to full dosage to achieve maximal hemodynamic effect. Although this strategy works in the younger patients, a multiplicity of potentially serious adverse effects limits their use and full dosage in older patients. The major adverse effects of ACE inhibitors include orthostatic hypotension and azotemia, especially in patients with preexisting renal disease. Minor effects include an irritative, nonproductive cough, alteration in taste, and allergic dermatitis.

Most ACE inhibitors are primarily excreted by the kidney, and kidney function declines with age. Pharmacokinetic studies have demonstrated increased serum concentrations of ACE inhibitors in patients with renal insufficiency. Thus, particular attention to dosage is necessary in the older patient. Patients with one nonfunctioning kidney and renovascular compromise of the other kidney are at very high risk of developing progressive renal failure with ACE inhibitors. Routine blood urea nitrogen and creatinine determinations should be obtained periodically after initiating therapy with these agents.

Other Agents

For patients with CHF who cannot tolerate ACE inhibitors, therapy with hydralazine plus topical (nitroglycerin ointment) or oral (isosorbide dinitrate) nitrates provides good afterload and preload reduction. An α-adrenergic blocker such as prazosin produces arteriolar and venous vasodilation and may be used in place of the hydralazine-nitrate combination. Prazosin and other α-adrenergic blockers are frequently associated with orthostatic hypotension with initial dosing and tachyphylaxis during chronic administration, and these effects limit the usefulness of these agents in the older age group.

In patients who develop intractable CHF despite a maximal regimen of digoxin, diuretics, and ACE inhibitors, hospitalization with bed rest, low-salt diet (2 g sodium), oxygen, and intravenous diuretics is required. The addition of a short course of intravenous renal dose dopamine (<5 μg/kg/min) or dobutamine (<10 μg/kg/min) for 72 hours is frequently associated with improved left ventricular function and augmented diuresis. Phosphodiesterase inhibitors (amrinone or milrinone) have not been very effective in my experience.

Patients with CHF have augmented adrenergic tone, and the excess catecholamines contribute to tachycardia and myocellular dysfunction and injury. Low-dose beta blockade has proven beneficial in certain subgroups with CHF, and cautious therapy with these agents is appropriate, especially in patients with dilated cardiomyopathy.

ANGINA PECTORIS

Angina pectoris in the elderly may have atypical presentations, and age-related neurologic and cognitive deficits may complicate the history. The pattern of the discomfort or weakness, which comes on with physical or emotional activity or else awakens the patient at night, is more important in establishing the diagnosis than the character or location of the pain. A therapeutic trial with sublingual nitroglycerin may provide the most sensitive and specific diagnostic information. The ECG may reveal nonspecific ST and T wave changes, a left bundle branch block pattern, or Q waves of an old myocardial infarction, but these findings are not sufficient to establish an unequivocal diagnosis of angina. Exercise testing is often indicated to establish the diagnosis and to determine the relative severity of the coronary disease process. Precipitation of the patient's characteristic discomfort within the first few minutes of activity testing, usually with significant ST and T wave changes that regress after activity termination, indicates major double- or triple-vessel coronary artery disease or left main coronary artery stenosis. In equivocal situations, a stress thallium study should be obtained. Coronary angiography should be used for more precise diagnosis, depending on the age of the patient, the intractability of the angina, and the potential for intervention with coronary artery bypass surgery or angioplasty.

Although anginal pains are usually due to coronary disease, two noncoronary conditions that may present with angina in the elderly are hypertropic obstructive cardiomyopathy and aortic valvular stenosis. The heart murmurs in both of these conditions may be minimal, and the echocardiogram should be used to diagnose or rule out these obstructive outflow tract conditions.

The more troublesome forms of angina in the elderly include decubitus (rest) angina, nocturnal angina, and postprandial angina. Common to all three patterns of angina is extensive triple-vessel coronary disease or left main coronary artery stenosis. General management involves aspirin, normalization of blood pressure, decongestive therapy, correction of brady-tachy rhythm disturbances, and treatment of coexisting medical problems such as thyroid abnormalities.

Medical Management

β-Adrenergic blocking agents, first- and second-generation calcium antagonists, and nitrates are the mainstays of anginal treatment. There is considerable variability in the elderly patient's tolerance of currently available β-blocking drugs. These drugs have unquestioned efficacy, but because of variable absorption and the potential for serious adverse side effects such as bradycardia, CHF, bronchial asthma, and depression, caution must be exercised in patient selection and drug dosage. In the over-70 age group, metoprolol is a good choice, starting at 25 mg twice daily, with doubling of the dose if well tolerated. Dosage of metoprolol must be individualized.

Calcium antagonists include the first-generation diltiazem, nifedipine, and verapamil agents and the second-generation dihydropyridine groups—amlodipine, felodipine, nicardipine, nimodipine, nisoldipine, and nitrendipine. In the absence of left ventricular dysfunction, each of the aforementioned agents is effective in reducing the frequency of angina, although a much larger clinical experience exists with the first-generation drugs. The long-acting preparations are preferable for once- or twice-a-day administration. Sustained-release diltiazem (120 mg) or nifedipine (30 mg) once or twice daily is usually well tolerated. Verapamil is generally best avoided in the elderly patient because of its cardiodepressant, atrioventricular blocking, and constipating effects. Diltiazem should not be used in patients with left ventricular dysfunction or sinus node dysfunction. Nifedipine frequently causes ankle edema from its vasodilatory effects, especially in elderly patients with chronic venous disease. The impact of the cardiovascular effects of calcium antagonists must be considered when selecting one of these agents for antianginal therapy.

Oral nitrates such as isosorbide dinitrate and transdermal nitrate preparations have excellent efficacy in controlling angina. The limiting effects of these agents are headache, hypotension, and tachyphylaxis. Transdermal nitrates are especially effective in the management of nocturnal angina, with application of the patch at bedtime and removal in the morning to avoid tolerance. Prophylactic sublingual nitroglycerin is extremely useful in patients with advanced coronary disease who develop angina with specific activities.

Invasive Therapies

During the past 5 years there has been a dramatic increase in the use of diagnostic coronary angiography for the evaluation of coronary disease in the older population. The reason for this is the increased symptomatic efficacy and possible increased survival with percutaneous transluminal coronary angioplasty (PTCA) and coronary artery bypass graft (CABG) surgery in this age group. The technical success rate for PTCA in the elderly is very high (80 to 85%), but age is associated with increased procedure-related death (<1%), nonfatal infarction, stroke, renal insufficiency, and femoral arterial problems. Symptomatic restenosis within 6 months after initial PTCA is in the range of 30 to 35%. Most elderly patients with angina have multivessel disease, and PTCA should be selectively used to dilate only the primary or culprit lesion to minimize complications. Directional atherectomy has had only limited success in this age group, probably because of the high frequency of calcified lesions.

CABG surgery in the geriatric population is usually reserved for patients with left main coronary disease or multivessel coronary disease and left ventricular dysfunction. Complete revascularization is usually performed, and observational data indicate that these patients do remarkably well after successful surgery. Relative contraindications for CABG surgery include left ventricular ejection fraction below 0.20, major comorbidity, significant renal, hepatic, or pulmonary dysfunction, and poor motivation on the part of the elderly patient for a major operation. The total operative mortality and morbidity rate is between 5 and 15%. Convalescence is usually prolonged, in the range of 3 to 6 months. Short- and long-term graft patency is lower in the older age group because of the frequent presence of venous varicosities in the graft vessel and sclerosis of the coronary arteries, which complicates vein-artery anastomosis. Internal mammary arteries are being preferentially used in all age groups because of the increased graft patency rate associated with this approach. There are now many older patients who have had a prior CABG operation, have recurrent, refractory angina, and are undergoing CABG redos with proportionately increased complication rates. CABG surgery in the elderly is a major undertaking, and risk-benefit considerations must be carefully weighed.

UNSTABLE ANGINA

Unstable angina warrants special consideration, since these patients require prompt hospitalization and aggressive management because of the high likelihood of developing acute coronary occlusion and myocardial infarction. The usual definition of unstable angina includes new-onset angina, progressive or crescendo angina, or prolonged angina without prompt relief by nitroglycerin. The unstable angina is usually associated with transient electrocardiographic ST and T wave changes, but without myocardial enzyme elevation. The patient should be hospitalized because of the risk of an unfavorable outcome.

Aggressive therapy includes aspirin and intravenous heparin, intravenous nitroglycerin with intraarterial blood pressure monitoring, and maximization of β-blockers and calcium antagonists. Usually, this multipronged therapy provides clinical stabilization. Prompt diagnostic coronary angiography is indicated to evaluate the extent and severity of the coronary disease. PTCA or CABG surgery is indicated if one or more amenable, life-threatening lesions are found. Not infrequently, the extensive nature of the coronary disease progress does not permit invasive therapy. In such situations, augmented dosage of the conventional antianginal therapy, combination of calcium antagonists with different mechanisms of action, and warfarin anticoagulation in combination with aspirin have provided improved control of the angina. Many of the elderly patients have underlying sinus node dysfunction, with sinus bradycardia that limits full dosage of β-blockers and calcium antagonists. The elimination of profound bradycardia with dual-chamber atrioventricular sequential pacing frequently permits optimization of the antianginal therapy with remarkable clinical improvement. Combined therapy maximized to the individual patient is essential in unstable angina.

ACUTE MYOCARDIAL INFARCTION

Thrombolytic Therapy

Thrombolytic therapy is now being used to open acute thrombotic occlusions of coronary vessels in patients of all age groups seen within 4 to 6 hours of onset of acute myocardial infarction. The currently available thrombolytic agents include streptokinase, recombinant tissue plasminogen activator (rt-PA), and anisolated streptokinase plasminogen activator complex (APSAC). Review of several large comparative trials indicates that the currently available thrombolytic agents have similar efficacy and safety profiles in the very early treatment of acute myocardial infarction. However, a vigorous debate continues over which thrombolytic agent is the "best."

In 1993, Forman et al. (19) pooled the data from major thrombolytic trials involving nearly 10,000 elderly patients. Thrombolytic therapy reduces mortality by 17% in the higher age groups and by almost 20% in the very old patients. However, the risk of hemorrhage, particularly intracerebral hemorrhage, also increases with age, possibly to a greater degree with rt-PA than with streptokinase. Overall, thrombolytic therapy has been found to be beneficial and cost-effective for suspected acute myocardial infarction in elderly patients in a wide variety of clinical circumstances (20).

A reasonable regimen includes streptokinase, heparin, and aspirin to treat patients within the first 6 hours of infarction. Exceptions are patients who have recently received streptokinase and those who are hypotensive, since allergic reactions to a second dose of streptokinase have been reported, and streptokinase may aggravate hypotension in the latter subgroup. Recently, there has been increasing interest in the use of immediate PTCA as an alternative to thrombolytic therapy to achieve a higher coronary patency rate and a lower hemorrhagic stroke rate. The available data do not support the routine use of this procedure in the elderly. It may have special use in patients with shock complicating a large evolving infarction.

β-Blocker Therapy

In pooled data from three large β-blocker trials involving over 8500 older patients, early β-blocker therapy with metoprolol or propranolol administered within the first 24 hours of the acute event was associated with a 23% reduction in mortality. Although there are some obvious contraindications to the early use of β-blockers in the elderly (CHF, sinus bradycardia less than 50 bpm, heart block, hypotension, asthma, and depression), those without contraindications may well benefit from this intervention.

Other Agents

Lidocaine is no longer recommended for routine antiarrhythmic prophylaxis in acute infarction, but it should be administered in conservative dosage to those with frequent or repetitive ventricular ectopic beats. ACE inhibitor therapy has been recommended in patients with large anterior myocardial infarctions, to reduce dysfunctional left ventricular remodeling. Heparin anticoagulation may prevent mural thrombi in acute infarctions complicated by low cardiac output, especially those with anterior-apical wall motion

abnormalities. Chronic warfarin anticoagulation is indicated if thrombi are detected by echocardiography during the acute process. Calcium antagonists have no prophylactic benefit in patients with acute infarction and may exacerbate CHF in patients with left ventricular dysfunction (21). Controversy exists regarding the benefit of diltiazem in patients with non–Q wave infarction. Finally, aspirin should be routinely administered to all infarct patients unless there is a contraindication. The short- and long-term benefits from aspirin are quite impressive.

ATRIAL FIBRILLATION

Atrial fibrillation commonly occurs in the elderly, frequently complicates CHF, and may develop in the absence of demonstrable heart disease. The loss of the atrial "kick" with reduction in cardiac output and the variable and erratic rate may exacerbate left ventricular dysfunction. Acute onset of temporary atrial fibrillation may be caused by fever, electrolyte imbalance, myocardial infarction, pericarditis, or a pulmonary embolus, and the arrhythmia usually resolves with treatment of the underlying condition and acute digitalization. Paroxysmal recurrent atrial fibrillation often accompanies sinus node dysfunction, and the associated brady-tachy rhythm disorders may require pacemaker therapy in addition to pharmacologic measures. Chronic atrial fibrillation is usually secondary to ischemic or hypertensive heart disease, but apathetic thyrotoxicosis, rheumatic heart disease, and the usual spectrum of cardiac disorders also occur in the elderly and may contribute to this rhythm disorder (22).

Management of atrial fibrillation involves (a) rate control; (b) conversion, either pharmacologically or electrically; and (c) reduction of systemic embolization. Rate control can usually be achieved with digitalization, and the parenteral or oral route of therapy is usually dictated by the urgency of the situation and the clinical state of the patient.

Digoxin is the digitalis drug of choice, and a loading dose is indicated for prompt control of a rapid ventricular response to atrial fibrillation. A loading dose of 0.75 mg or 0.5 mg of digoxin with 0.25 mg maintenance dose daily should produce digoxin levels within the therapeutic range (1 to 2 ng/mL) within 48 hours when renal function is normal. With impaired renal function or in the octogenarian age group, a reduced maintenance dose of 0.125 mg should be used. Propranolol in small doses (1.0 mg intravenously or 10 mg orally every 6 hours) or diltiazem 120 to 180 mg per day in divided doses or in the sustained-release formulation is useful in combination with digoxin to slow rapid atrial fibrillation and to prevent accelerated rates during activity in patients receiving chronic digitalis therapy.

Cardioversion from atrial fibrillation to sinus rhythm should be considered in acute-onset rapid atrial fibrillation that is poorly tolerated hemodynamically. Synchronized, direct current electrical cardioversion is the procedure of choice in such a situation, and quinidine conversion should be avoided. Elective cardioversion of chronic atrial fibrillation carries a significant risk in the older population because of the high frequency of underlying sinus node dysfunction. This disorder is often associated with asystolic atrial arrest or systemic embolization from mural atrial thrombi, and cardioversion is contraindicated in the very elderly with chronic atrial fibrillation except in unusual situations. Furthermore, atrial fibrillation frequently recurs after cardioversion in these patients.

If cardioversion is carried out, prophylactic anticoagulation for a month or more with warfarin before cardioversion is indicated. A recent study suggests that if transesophageal echocardiography excludes atrial thrombi, electrical cardioversion can be carried out without prolonged anticoagulation (23). Maintenance of sinus rhythm after pharmacologic or electrical cardioversion is a challenge, and a variety of antiarrhythmic agents have been tried. Recent experience with low-dose amiodarone (600 mg a day for 4 days, then 100 mg or 200 mg daily thereafter) has been most favorable, with very few adverse side effects.

It has recently been appreciated that chronic atrial fibrillation is often associated with subclinical systemic emboli, frequently involving the brain, with secondary neurologic abnormalities including progressive dementia. Anticoagulants are recommended in patients with recurrent or chronic atrial fibrillation. Oral warfarin is the drug of choice. Many elderly patients cannot be safely anticoagulated with the warfarin, and in such situations anti–platelet aggregating therapy with aspirin should be used.

Warfarin anticoagulation is not without risk. The incidence of warfarin-associated bleeding may be reduced by attending to modifiable risk factors (accuracy and reliability of the prothrombin time determination), frequent monitoring early in treatment, and careful patient selection. Older age, in and of itself, is not a risk factor. Nonstandardized reporting of the prothrombin time (PT) and the PT ratio (PT/normal mean PT) has

been a problem in the past because the thromboplastins used to measure the PT can vary markedly in sensitivity; the PT ratio does not reflect this. Problems of unreliable reporting of PT can carry special risk in the elderly, since small changes in warfarin dosage could result in substantial swings in actual anticoagulant effect. To correct this problem, the World Health Organization developed the international normalized ratio (INR), a calculated value referenced to a standard preparation of thromboplastin, i.e., INR = (PT ratio)x, where x is the international sensitivity index for thromboplastin (referenced value = 1.0). For the prevention of systemic embolism in patients with atrial fibrillation, the recommended INR value is 2.0 to 3.0.

VENTRICULAR ARRHYTHMIAS

Ventricular premature beats are common in the elderly, and standard antiarrhythmic agents such as lidocaine, quinidine, procainamide, and disopyramide are poorly tolerated. Thus, the indications for treating simple or complex patterns of ventricular arrhythmias are quite stringent, and only ventricular arrhythmias of truly life-threatening potential should be treated. In the over-70 age group, repetitive ventricular premature beats (nonsustained or sustained ventricular tachycardia) complicating acute myocardial infarction should be treated with intravenous lidocaine. However, the loading and maintenance doses of lidocaine should be reduced to one-half the usually recommended values, and the duration of therapy should be attenuated to 12 hours unless a life-threatening arrhythmia persists. Lidocaine toxicity with respiratory depression, confusion, hypotension, and seizures is common in the elderly, and lidocaine administration requires careful monitoring for adverse side effects.

In the absence of acute cardiac disease, asymptomatic short runs of nonsustained ventricular tachycardia at rates less than 150 beats/min or lesser degrees of ventricular irritability do not require prophylactic antiarrhythmic therapy. Patients with recurrent life-threatening ventricular tachyarrhythmias, often with associated symptoms of lightheadedness or near syncope, should be seen by a cardiac consultant, since specialized testing and complex therapy are usually required to control the potentially malignant arrhythmias.

Electrophysiologic stimulation (EPS) is usually performed in such high-risk patients to evaluate inducibility of ventricular tachycardia or fibrillation with double or triple stimuli delivered to the right ventricle via transvenous electrode catheters. If ventricular inducibility is achieved, EPS is again carried out to determine if induced ventricular tachyarrhythmia can be suppressed by intravenous procainamide. Inducible ventricular arrhythmias that are not suppressed by procainamide are associated with a poor prognosis, especially in coronary patients with left ventricular dysfunction. Identified high-risk patients are usually treated either with amiodarone or an implantable cardioverter defibrillator (ICD). Presently, the only approved procedures for ICD implantation are the transthoracic approach requiring a thoracotomy for placement of patch electrodes on the epicardium and the transvenous approach. This latter approach will surely increase the number of patients who can be treated with an ICD, especially high-risk patients in the geriatric age group. Patients who have sustained an out-of-hospital aborted cardiac arrest unrelated to acute myocardial infarction should have an ICD implanted.

BRADYARRHYTHMIAS AND THE ATRIAL BRADY-TACHY SYNDROME

Elderly patients are at high risk for developing sinus node and atrioventricular conduction disturbances with sinus bradycardia, intermittent sinus arrest, intermittent atrial bradycardia alternating with paroxysmal atrial tachycardia/fibrillation, and atrioventricular block. These patients often present with recurrent lightheadedness, syncope, and troublesome palpitations poorly responsive to medication. Pacemaker therapy has proved to be particularly efficacious for these troublesome arrhythmias because the episodes of tachycardia are usually precipitated and preceded by bradycardia.

Dual chamber atrioventricular pacing (DDD) is the preferred treatment for these disorders so long as chronic atrial fibrillation is not present. Atrioventricular synchrony is maintained, thereby maximizing the atrial contribution to ventricular performance. Rate-responsive dual-chamber pacemakers (DDDR) are now available and provide appropriate physiologic increase in pacing rate with physical activity. Such therapy has significantly improved the quality of life of the elderly patient with bradyarrhythmia syndromes. Atrial fibrillation with slow ventricular response and long pauses requires single-chamber ventricular pacing. Rate-responsive ventricular demand pacing (VVIR) is indicated in these patents.

The induction of pacemaker malfunction by the electric fields from microwave ovens, electric blankets, and electric beds is vastly overrated, and these problems are essentially nonexistent with the current generation of pacemakers. Follow-up of patients with implanted pacemakers is imperative, since the pacemaker generators have a limited life expectancy (varying from 4 to 8 years, depending on the characteristics of the generator), and the generators must be replaced before battery failure. Regular transtelephone monitoring of pacemaker function (rate, pulse width, sensing, magnet characteristics) at monthly intervals is essential if one is to identify potential pacemaker problems before they assume life-threatening consequences. Numerous commercial monitoring systems are available, as well as programs run by major pacemaker clinics. The cost for such monitoring is covered by Medicare, provided the guidelines outlined by the federal government are followed. Periodic monitoring is extremely useful in picking up sensing and pacing problems whether related to the generator or the electrode.

In addition to regular telephone monitoring, each pacemaker patient should be followed at less frequent intervals by a cardiologist who is knowledgeable in the field of pacemakers. Generally, the cardiologist should see the patient 1 month after pacemaker implantation to check the function of the implanted unit and to reprogram the parameters of the generator (rate, output, sensitivity, hysteresis) if so indicated. Thereafter, the frequency of cardiologic follow-up may be reduced to 9- to 12-month intervals, providing a monthly or every other month telephone monitoring schedule has been established.

SYNCOPE

Syncope is a frequent and troublesome disorder in the elderly that contributes to significant disability from secondary trauma related to the falls. A detailed clinical history is essential for identifying the cause of the syncope. Slow onset–slow offset syncope is usually due to metabolic disorders such as hyperventilation or hypoglycemia. Abrupt onset–slow offset syncope suggest a neurologic seizure disorder. Abrupt onset–abrupt offset syncope almost always has a cardiovascular etiology. Clinical examination permits identification of orthostatic hypotension and systolic murmurs of aortic stenosis or hypertrophic obstructive cardiomyopathy. The severity of the latter conditions are easily evaluated by echo/Doppler studies.

Vasodepressor syncope with vasovagal reaction is characterized by severe hypotension and paradoxical bradycardia, usually precipitated by sympathetic excitation. The diagnosis of this neurocardiogenic syncope can now be established with upright-tilt testing. If upright-tilt testing without the infusion of isoproterenol reproduces hypotension and bradycardia in less than 15 minutes and causes presyncope or syncope, the diagnosis of neurocardiogenic syncope can be made, and treatment with metoprolol or disopyramide is appropriate. Implantation of a pacemaker is not indicated.

Intermittent sinus arrest or atrioventricular heart block may be suggested by the response to carotid sinus stimulation or by 24-hour Holter monitoring or event recordings. These patients usually have evidence of sinus node dysfunction or conduction abnormalities such as right bundle branch block with left axis deviation (bifascicular block) or left bundle branch block.

Transient hypotensive ventricular tachyarrhythmias are usually associated with significant left ventricular dysfunction and manifest ventricular irritability (frequent VPBs during clinical evaluation). Holter monitoring and EPS testing are required to substantiate the fact that these intermittent arrhythmias are the cause of the syncope.

Rare causes of syncope include atrial myxoma, superior vena cava obstruction from tumor, bilateral severe carotid stenosis/obstruction, subclavian steal syndrome, and bilateral vertebral stenosis/obstruction with drop attacks from compromise of the posterior circulation to the brainstem.

Virtually all of these conditions are suggested by the history and physical examination or by selected noninvasive tests. Only rarely are invasive tests such as EPS and angiographic studies required to diagnose the cause of the syncope.

VALVULAR HEART DISEASE

Although all types of significant valvular disease may occur in the elderly, the most common hemodynamically significant lesions requiring operative intervention are aortic stenosis (rheumatic or congenital bicuspid valvular stenosis) and mitral insufficiency (rheumatic, myxomatous valvular degeneration, or ruptured chordae or papillary muscles). The proper timing of surgical intervention is usually based on clinical and laboratory evidence of hemodynamic deterioration during follow-up. Serial, semiquantitative evaluation of the progression and severity of the valvular disease is best performed by echocardiography and Doppler ultrasound. Cardiac catheterization is indicated when more precise information is needed to make the decision regarding

operative intervention. Furthermore, the status of the coronary arteries must be investigated before surgery. Critical factors that profoundly influence operative mortality include (a) the extent of valvular and aortic calcification; (b) the degree of myocardial and cardiac dysfunction; (c) the severity of coexisting pulmonary hypertension from active or passive pulmonary vascular disease; (d) the location and extent of coexisting coronary disease; and (e) the type and extent of diseases of other organ systems. Valvular replacement surgery produces a greater insult to the circulatory system than CABG surgery, and the net result is a more complicated perioperative course and a delayed functional recovery. If the porcine bioprosthesis is used in the aortic position, long-term anticoagulation is not required. Otherwise, warfarin anticoagulation is indicated despite the increased hemorrhagic risk. Once again, risk-benefit considerations dictate an operative recommendation only for those patients with a life-threatening valvular lesion as manifest by progressive cardiac-related symptomatology and appropriate objective findings.

Operative mortality for valve surgery in the octogenarian is about 15%, with lower mortality rates in those with valve replacement alone and higher rates when combined with CABG surgery (24, 25). Perioperative complications are common in the very elderly, with serious cerebral vascular insults in many of the patients. Among those who survive the surgery unscathed, actuarial survival is remarkably good, with 80% doing well at 1 year.

Balloon valvulotomy for aortic and mitral valvular stenosis has not been very successful in the older patient, and it has been associated with considerable complications. This technique has very limited value in the older patient.

GENDER-RELATED ISSUES

In the post-65-year age group, women make up a significantly larger percentage of the population and account for a predominantly larger number of cardiovascular events than do men. Women have smaller hearts and blood vessels, more delayed onset of atherosclerosis, a higher frequency of glucose intolerance and diabetes mellitus, and more marked osteoporosis than men. Data from many sources suggest that unconscious gender bias exists in the diagnosis and treatment of women with cardiovascular disease (26, 27), with overall poorer outcomes for women after adjustment for various confounding medical and social factors.

Over the years, women have been improperly excluded from most of the major cardiovascular clinical studies and trials, frequently because of reproductive concerns in the younger age group and age-related comorbidity concerns in the older age group. The net result is a more incomplete scientific database for women than for men. Thus, the cardiovascular diagnostic and therapeutic strategies that are applied to women are predominantly based on data derived from men, even though the pathophysiology of the disease process and therapeutic responsiveness may be quite different in the two sexes.

A few points warrant special comment. Patients seek medical care on the basis of symptoms. Women seem to have more symptoms suggesting cardiovascular disease than do men, yet the specificity of the symptoms being associated with demonstrable cardiovascular disease is lower in women. Exercise testing, the cornerstone of the diagnostic algorithm, is a less reliable predictor of coronary disease in women. Women have been referred for coronary angiography at a lower rate than men. Whether related or not, women undergoing CABG surgery have a higher operative mortality than men after adjustment for relevant confounding variables including age. Similar findings have been noted after acute myocardial infarction. Chest pain with evidence of myocardial ischemia and normal coronary arteries (syndrome X) is more common in women. CHF and left ventricular diastolic dysfunction has a greater prevalence in women than in men, possibly related to the increased prevalence of hypertension and diabetes in women. Physicians refer fewer women for exercise rehabilitation after a coronary event despite equivalent functional benefit from such programs in men and women.

Women have certain sex-related conditions that predispose them to specific cardiovascular problems and therapy. Elderly women have more orthostatic hypotension than men of equivalent age and thus are at increased risk of falling and fracturing a hip. Postmenopausal hormonal replacement is now recommended in women because of its favorable effect on serum lipids, and it is estimated that such therapy would result in a 42% reduction in the risk of coronary disease in users compared with nonusers. Finally, taxol, a very potent drug for the treatment of advanced ovarian carcinoma, is associated with sinus bradycardia and heart block.

Concerns about women's cardiovascular health are now being actively addressed. The multimillion-dollar National Institutes of Health–sponsored Women's Health Initiative has been launched, and during the next decade there should develop a better scientific foundation for understanding, diagnosing, and treating cardiovascular disease in women.

PROPHYLACTIC CARDIOLOGY

The practice of "preventive" cardiology in the aging population is similar to that in the general population. Although the potential for long-term benefit is attenuated by the age of the older population, risk-benefit considerations and the importance of optimizing the quality of life of our older citizens during their remaining advanced years support the concept of prophylaxis, a strategy to reduce the rate of progression of cardiovascular diseases.

For the older patient, one approach places emphasis on a few important measures that enhance the likelihood of reducing morbidity, and possibly mortality, from cardiovascular disease. It is reasonable to tolerate mildly or even moderately elevated cholesterol levels in this age group. Dietary recommendations alone are prudent for cholesterol levels above 250 mg/dL in association with increased LDL-cholesterol. A reasonable and well-tolerated approach for cholesterol levels above 300 mg/dL is drug therapy with an HMG–coenzyme A reductase inhibitor. The central features of a general prophylactic strategy include (a) low dose aspirin (80 mg daily) in those without a contraindication; (b) cessation of tobacco use in smokers; (c) therapy with estrogen and/or progestin in postmenopausal women if they accept the risk/benefit recommendation; (d) reduced salt intake when appropriate; and (e) control of hypertension and hyperglycemia. Exercise and dietary weight reduction programs should be individualized. Cardiac rehabilitation programs are appropriate for most patients who have had a coronary event or heart surgery.

REFERENCES

1. Webb JL, Urner SC, McDaniels J. Physiologic characteristics of a champion runner age 77. J Gerontol 1977;32:286–290.
2. Higginbotham MB, Morris KG, Williams RS, et al. Physiologic basis for the age-related declilne in aerobic work capacity. Am J Cardiol 1986;57:1374–1379.
3. Weisfeldt ML, ed. The aging heart. Its function and response to stress. Vol 12. New York: Raven Press, 1980.
4. Scheider EL, Rowe JW, eds. Handbook of the biology of aging. 3rd ed. San Diego: Academic Press, 1990.
5. Davies MJ. Pathology of the conduction system. In: Caird FI, Dall JLC, Kennedy RD, eds. Cardiology in old age. New York: Plenum, 1976:57–80.
6. Lakatta E. Heart and circulation. In: Schneider EL, Rowe JW, eds. Handbook of the biology of aging. San Diego: Academic Press, 1990:181–216.

7. Lakatta EG. Age-related alternations in cardiovascular response to adrenergic mediated stress. Fed Proc 1980;39:3173–3177.

8. Vestal RE, Wood AJJ, Shand DG. Reduced beta-adrenoreceptors sensitivity in the elderly. Clin Pharmacol Ther 1979;26:181–186.

9. Fleg JL. Ventricular arrhythmias in the elderly: prevalence, mechanisms, and therapeutic implications. Geriatrics 1988;43:23–29.

10. Rodeheffer RJ, Gerstenblith G, Becker L, Fleg JL, Weisfeldt ML, Lakatta EG. Exercise cardiac output is maintained with advancing age in healthy human subjects: cardiac dilatation and increased stroke volume compensate for diminished heart rate. Circulation 1984;69:203–213.

11. Cacciapouti F, D'Avino M, Lama D, Bianchi U, Perrone N, Varricchio M. Progressive impairment of left ventricular diastolic filling with advancing age: a Doppler echocardiographic study. J Am Geriatr Soc 1992;40:245–250.

12. Latting CA, Silverman ME. Acute myocardial infarction in hospitalized patients over age 70. Am Heart J 1980;100:311–318.

13. Spittell PC, Spittell JA, Joyce JW, et al. Clinical features and differential diagnosis of aortic dissection: experience with 236 cases (1980 through 1990). Mayo Clin Proc 1993;68:642–651.

14. Zabalgoitia M, Gandhi DK, Evans J, Mehlman DJ, MrPherson DD, Talano JV. Transesophageal echocardiography in the awake elderly patient: its role in the clinical decision-making process. Am Heart J 1990;120:1147–1153.

15. Moss AJ, Goldstein RE, Hall WJ, et al. Detection and significance of myocardial ischemia in stable patients after recovery from an acute coronary event. JAMA 1993;269:2379–2385.

16. Port S, Cobb FR, Coleman RE, et al. Effect of age on the response of the left ventricular ejection fraction to exercise. N Engl J Med 1980;303:1133–1137.

17. The SOLVD Investigators. Effect of enalapril on survival in patients with reduced left ventricular ejection fractions and congestive heart failure. N Engl J Med 1991;325:293–302.

18. Pfeffer MA, Braunwald E, Moye LA, et al. Effect of captopril on mortality and morbidity in patients with left ventricular dysfunction after myocardial infarction—results of the Survival and Ventricular Enlargement Trial. N Engl J Med 1992;327:669–677.

19. Foreman DE, Wei JY. MI: Making therapeutic choices when the options are unclear. Geriatrics 1993;7:32–45.

20. Krumholz HM, Pasternak RC, Weinstein MC, et al. Cost effectiveness of thrombolytic therapy with streptokinase in elderly patients with suspected acute myocardial infarction. N Engl J Med 1992;327:7–13.

21. The Multicenter Diltiazem Post Infarction Trial Research Group. The effect of diltiazem on mortality and reinfarction after myocardial infarction. N Engl J Med 1988;319:385–392.

22. Kannel WB, Abbott RD, Savage DD, McNamara PM. Epidemiologic features of chronic atrial fibrillation. N Engl J Med 1982;306:1018–1022.

23. Manning WJ, Silverman DI, Gordon SPF, Krumholz HM, Douglas PS. Cardioversion from atrial fibrillation without prolonged anticoagulation with use of transesophageal echocardiography to exclude the presence of atrial thrombi. N Engl J Med 1993;328:750–755.

24. Pasic M, Carrel T, Laske A, et al. Valve replacement in octogenarians: increased early mortality but good long-term result. Eur Heart J 1992;13:508–510.

25. Culliford AT, Galloway AC, Colvin SB, et al. Aortic valve replacement for aortic stenosis in persons aged 80 years and over. Am J Cardiol 1991;67:1256–1260.

26. Laskey WK. Gender differences in the management of coronary artery disease: bias or good clinical judgment? Ann Intern Med 1992;116:869–871.

27. Wenger NK, Speroff L, Packard B. Cardiovascular health and disease in women. N Engl J Med 1993;329:247–256.

7/ Hypertension in the Elderly

Rex L. Mahnensmith

Data from four National Health Surveys conducted between 1960 and 1990 indicate that over half of persons aged 60 years or over in the United States are hypertensive (1–4). The most recent survey, completed in 1990, documented a 60% prevalence of hypertension among elderly whites, a 71% prevalence among elderly blacks, and a 61% prevalence among elderly Hispanic Americans (4). Additionally, the screening program for the Systolic Hypertension in the Elderly Program documented a 75% prevalence of hypertension among a population of 5566 persons aged 75 or older (5). Similar prevalence data have been recorded for elderly populations outside the United States (6).

In times past, practitioners were advised that progressive elevations in systemic BP were normal to the aging process, were well tolerated by the aging patient, were necessary to sustain organ perfusion, and should not be lowered with pharmaceutical interventions, lest annoying and threatening hypoperfusion syndromes be precipitated (7, 8). However, it is now clear that a steady rise in BP with age, particularly systolic BP, is not biologically normal. People from agrarian cultures who are accustomed to daily physical labor and gain nourishment largely from plant sources do not exhibit an age-related rise in systolic BP (6, 9). In highly industrialized populations, groups with similar lifestyles and customs can be found who also do not exhibit an age-related rise in systolic BP. Where it is seen in industrialized cultures, this age-related rise in BP seems to correlate with high dietary salt intake and progressive increases in body weight over time (9). Furthermore, migration of adults from a rural to urban context is associated with higher BP over time, suggesting an important contribution from lifestyle, customs, and habits (6, 9).

It is additionally clear that elevated BP in persons aged 60 years or older constitutes a definite threat to life and well-being. Long-term observations from the Framingham Heart Studies have revealed that risk of a fatal cardiovascular event for men aged 65 to 75 years is increased 2.4 times when BP exceeds 160/95 mm Hg, compared with normotensive men (BP < 140/90 mm Hg) of the same age, and increased 2.1 times when arterial pressures range between 140/90 and 160/95 mm Hg. In women, the risk is even greater. Among women aged 65 to 74 years, fatal cardiovascular events are nearly 8 times more frequent when arterial BP exceeds 160/95 mm Hg and 4.3 times more frequent when BPs range 140/90 to 160/95 mm Hg, compared with normotensive women (10). The Framingham studies along with others have also established that isolated systolic BP elevations are progressive and confer greater cardiovascular risk than diastolic elevations among the elderly and thus stand as an independent risk factor for cardiac disease, stroke, and death (11–13).

Despite the strength of these data, practitioners continue to exhibit uncertainty when deciding whether to treat a given elderly hypertensive patient. Recommendations regarding treatment abound, but so do cautions and admonitions (4, 7, 8, 14, 15). One result is that many hypertensive patients do not receive treatment (16). Practitioners should have ears for both voices, for there is clear and well-documented benefit to BP lowering in the hypertensive elderly, yet the elderly individual is more likely than any other to experience adverse effects not only from the medications themselves but from excessive BP lowering, too. The explanation for this vulnerability probably resides with the relatively advanced vascular disease that accompanies the aged hypertensive state. Both large and small arteries are stiff, and peripheral arteriolar lumens are markedly narrowed, and some completely occluded (12, 17). These structural alterations are both cause and consequence of elevated arterial pressures and present a physiologic paradox unique to the elderly hypertensive patient—while contributing in a principal way to the pathogenesis of hypertension and high-pressure damage to vital end-organs in the elderly, these vascular changes are also responsible for generalized reductions of vascularity and blood flow to these organs and thus threaten them with ischemia and hypoperfusion syndromes. It is this paradox that confounds our attempts at BP lowering in this patient population and gives the practitioner pause.

Notwithstanding, thoughtful pause in therapeutic decision making should not become indecisive paralysis. Hypertensive elderly patients benefit from cautious BP lowering and should be treated. The pathogenesis and hemodynamic character of hypertension in the elderly is increasingly understood, and a full understanding of these pathophysiologic issues can yield a logical strategy for therapeutic intervention that addresses the threat of high-pressure injury as well as that of low organ blood flows. We are also greatly benefited by a growing number of prospective, placebo-controlled interventional trials focusing exclusively on hypertension in elderly persons, which provide guidance for therapy and reassurance that therapy can indeed be undertaken safely and with benefit to a large number of patients.

PATHOPHYSIOLOGIC ISSUES IN THE ELDERLY HYPERTENSIVE PATIENT

Mean arterial pressure (MAP) in a person of any age is a function of cardiac output (CO) and systemic vascular resistance (SVR), where MAP = CO × SVR. An increase in either of these variables can raise arterial BP. Young and middle-aged hypertensives typically exhibit a high-normal or normal cardiac output with either a normal or mildly elevated systemic vascular resistance, while the elderly hypertensive is characterized by a subnormal cardiac output coupled to a very high systemic vascular resistance (12, 17, 18). How this physiologic condition evolves is relevant.

In all age groups, the central factor in the genesis of essential hypertension involves an increase in vascular smooth muscle tone, particularly that of small arteries and arterioles (9). Mechanisms for this are multiple, and relative contributions in individual patients vary. Operative factors include a genetic predisposition, sympathetic overactivity, renin-angiotensin overactivity, and cell membrane sodium and calcium transport abnormalities, all of which conspire to create sustained vascular smooth muscle constriction (9). In hypertensive elderly, it is well-documented that plasma norepinephrine levels are slightly elevated with little circadian variation and calcium

channel blockers produce consistent vasorelaxation, while plasma renin levels are relatively low, which has led to a conclusion that active vasoconstriction in this age group is due largely to calcium currents and sympathetically driven constriction (9, 19).

However, more important than active vasoconstriction in the production of heightened vascular resistance is a progressive architectural alteration of both central and peripheral arteries, which results in fixed vascular narrowing. A number of processes are involved in this change, including progressive vascular smooth muscle hypertrophy and replication and accumulation of collagen matrix and calcium in vessel walls (9, 17). Histologically, one sees concentric replication of hypertrophied smooth muscle cells layered in a thick fibrous matrix, elastic lamina disruption, migration of smooth muscle cells from media to intima, endothelial disorganization, and marked thickening of vascular walls. Such thickening of the walls of resistance arterioles severely encroaches lumen patency. It also renders larger artery walls noncompliant. Aging contributes importantly to these changes as does prolonged exposure to the dynamic stresses of arterial hypertension.

These structural changes directly heighten vascular resistance and magnify active constricting influences (9). They also create marked alterations in the dynamics of arterial blood flow (12, 20). In particular, owing to the noncompliant nature of an aged hypertensive aorta, systolic pulse pressure waves are not dampened as they travel through the arterial network. Thus, the rate of rise in intraarterial pressure with cardiac ejection is steeper than normal, the peak that this pressure wave reaches is higher than normal, and the forward velocity of the pulse wave is faster than normal (Fig. 7.1) (20). Additionally, the high resistance of the peripheral arteriolar network sustains the high pressure and creates brisk retrograde wave reflections that rebound back upstream with sufficient velocity to meet the next forward pulse wave in midsystole, which further augments systolic pressures and creates intraluminal turbulence (17, 20).

As might be predicted, stresses within this aged vascular network are dynamic and great. Throughout the arterial network the pulsatile energy of systolic waves creates fatigue and fracture of arterial wall elastin and accelerates its breakdown, while repeated high-pressure impacts in precapillary arterioles cause endothelial breakdown and frank tissue injury. These dynamic stresses underlie the familiar pressure-related complications of hypertension—lacunar infarcts,

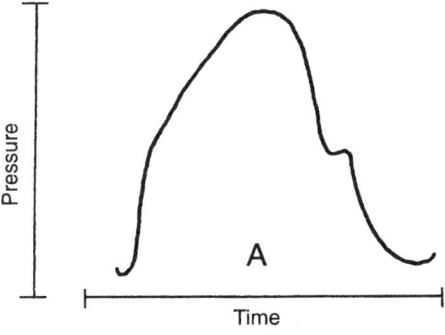
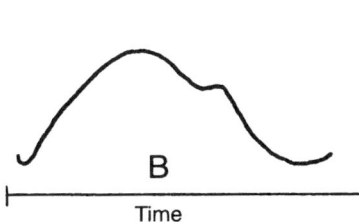

Figure 7.1. Hypertensive pulse wave (*A*) compared with normotensive pulse wave (*B*). The pulse wave in a hypertensive elderly person features more rapid rise in pressure plus a higher and more sustained peak. Arterial noncompliance creates the rapid rise and higher peak of pressure; accelerated retrograde pulse waves rebounding from tight peripheral arterioles contribute to the sustained peak and create turbulence (19).

hemorrhagic strokes, retinal damage, aortic aneurysm formation, and progressive renal insufficiency. The heart is also victim to these stresses, for it can continue to sustain adequate forward output in the face of high outflow resistance only by undergoing hypertrophy itself. Yet this hypertrophy eventually compromises cardiac performance, for with hypertrophy the myocardium stiffens, which reduces end-diastolic volume and, in turn, forward stroke volume. Myocardial "adaptation" to sustained afterload stresses thus becomes maladaptive, and this sequence of change underlies the evolution of congestive heart failure in this patient population (21).

High-pressure stresses, however, are only one category of threat to the elderly hypertensive individual. Ischemia is the other. As elastin breaks down and endothelium is rent, collagen formation is stimulated and an expanding disorganized matrix is laid down. Generalized arteriosclerosis thus evolves and becomes advanced over years. Atheroma formation is similarly stimulated in larger vessels. Coronary atherosclerosis, high afterload stress, high myocardial tension, and progressive myocardial hypertrophy all underlie the high prevalence of ischemic cardiac disease in these patients. Both large and small vessel atherosclerosis underlie the high incidence of stroke and renal insufficiency. It is essential to realize that the same vascular pathology that perpetrates high-pressure complications also creates hypoperfusion-ischemic problems, for ischemic injury and resulting functional compromise are as common in the older hypertensive as high-pressure complications (17). This has practical import in therapeutic decision making.

A mild plasma volume contraction and an unusual propensity to orthostasis are other practical pathophysiologic characteristics of hypertension in the elderly (18, 19). High-pressure natriuresis coupled to a smaller capacitance of the narrowed arterial network perpetuate a relative plasma volume contraction. Aged kidneys also exhibit a urinary concentrating defect. Orthostasis derives from the rigid vascular network coupled to impaired baroreceptor activity, a decline in parasympathetic responsiveness, and the mild decrease in effective circulating blood volume (15, 19). These physiologic changes enlarge the threat of organ hypoperfusion that exists from precapillary arteriolosclerosis. Furthermore, data exist that demonstrate that organ blood flow autoregulation is impaired in hypertensive elderly, particularly blood flow into and through the cerebral and renal vascular trees (15, 21). The convergence of these problems renders the hypertensive elderly person particularly vulnerable to critical reductions in tissue blood delivery from relatively modest short-term declines in mean arterial pressure (8, 21).

A final feature of elderly hypertension is salt sensitivity. Salt sensitivity denotes an unusual propensity to BP elevation from salt ingestion and derives primarily from a reduced capacity for renal salt excretion. Renal arteriolosclerosis and glomerulosclerosis are the principal constraints to efficient sodium homeostasis, but an age-related decline in renal prostaglandins may also contribute, for these are important sodium homeostatic agents (19, 21). In practical terms, salt balance is maintained, but with retarded efficiency and at the expense of a higher mean arterial pressure.

EVALUATION OF THE PATIENT WITH HYPERTENSION

Documentation that hypertension is real and sustained is the first priority for the practitioner, as variability of ambient BPs increases with age (12, 13, 15). BPs should be measured on at least three separate occasions in both arms over a period of 2 to several weeks before initiating therapy, although initial BP readings that exceed 210 mm Hg systolic or 120 mm Hg diastolic or are associated with end-organ damage may require immediate therapy (4). BP measurements should be made with a cuff of appropriate size and include orthostatic measurements, as orthostatic tendencies grow as vascular rigidity and systolic elevations become more pronounced in the elderly.

Attention should also be given to the possibility of "pseudohypertension" in this patient population (12). Pseudohypertension denotes a false indication of severity of hypertension from sphygmomanometer measurements. This phenomenon is apparent when rigidly sclerotic brachial arteries cannot be occluded by the cuff. Systolic Korotkoff sounds remain audible at very high systolic cuff pressures, but true intraarterial pressures are actually much lower. Pseudohypertension should be suspected when measured systolic pressures are very high by cuff but minimal hypertensive changes are apparent in the heart or retina. Suspicion is heightened when a brachial or radial artery remains palpable after its pulse has been eliminated by raising cuff pressures above the apparent systolic cutoff. Another clue is when cautious therapy produces significant orthostatic hypotension and symptoms. Pseudohypertension can be confirmed only by direct intraarterial pressure measurements and correlation with cuff readings.

Assessment for end-organ injury is the next priority. This requires a comprehensive history and physical examination, urinalysis, blood chemistry panel, complete blood count, and a 12-lead electrocardiogram. Attention is focused on the possible existence of coronary or myocardial disease, cerebral and peripheral vascular insufficiency, aortic aneurysm development, and renal insufficiency. Echocardiography is not warranted in everyone, but if congestive heart failure is a clinical problem or if left ventricular hypertrophy is apparent on the electrocardiogram, then echocardiography should be done. Knowledge of ventricular performance and size can guide medication selection. Chest radiography is an insensitive way to screen for hypertensive cardiac disease but may reveal thoracic aortic disease. The examination should include a search for other cardiovascular risk factors, such as smoking, dyslipidemias, and obesity. These factors, if present, should be targets of management and may influence choice of drug therapy.

Of equal importance is an assessment of comorbid illnesses or functional limitations that may also influence choice of therapy. Important conditions in this regard are diabetes mellitus, clinical coronary insufficiency, congestive heart failure, peripheral or cerebral vascular insufficiency, renal insufficiency, cognitive or neurologic impairments, depression, sexual dysfunction, and obstructive airways disease (Table 7.1).

Screening for secondary causes of hypertension is not routinely recommended. However, if hypertension evolves as a new clinical problem in an elderly person or is particularly refractory to a two- or three-drug medication program, then one should screen for renovascular stenosis. Hypertension with renal insufficiency and/or an abdominal bruit are other reasons to screen for this diagnosis. Screening is best accomplished with captopril renography (22). This test requires that patients not take an angiotensin converting enzyme (ACE) inhibitor for at least 1 week. Then, on a selected day, a conventional isotope renogram is performed. Renal isotope uptake and excretion over time is plotted, and the plot of one kidney is compared with that of the other. A delay in uptake or time to peak is taken as an indication that one kidney may have renal artery stenosis. After a 1-hour washout period, a 25-mg dose of captopril is crushed, dissolved in water, and administered to the patient. The stomach must be empty. Then, 1 hour later, isotope renography is repeated. A kidney possessing a clinically renal artery stenosis will exhibit reduced isotope uptake and excretion over time compared with the precaptopril scan. This test has approximately 90% sensitivity and specificity (22).

Other types of secondary hypertension such as primary hyperaldosteronism or pheochromocytoma are much rarer in this patient group. If unprovoked hypokalemia is documented, then screening for primary hyperaldosteronism is justifiable. This is best done with a random plasma renin and aldosterone level. Primary aldosteronism will invariably be associated with suppressed plasma renin yet elevated aldosterone levels. If paroxysms of hypertension with palpitations and flushing are clearly present or if hypertension is particularly refractory, then screening for pheochromocytoma should be undertaken. This is accomplished with a 24-hour urine sample for catecholamine and metanephrine levels.

STRATEGIES FOR THERAPY

That treatment of hypertension in the elderly is beneficial is beyond refute. The original Veter-

Table 7.1
Comorbid Medical Problems and Choice of Antihypertensive Therapy[a]

Medical Problem	Drugs That May Improve the Condition	Drugs That May Worsen the Condition
Cerebrovascular insufficiency	Calcium antagonist ACE inhibitor	Diuretic Reserpine
Coronary insufficiency	Calcium antagonist β-Blocker	Hydralazine
Dementia	Calcium antagonist ACE inhibitor	Reserpine α-Blocker
Depression	. . . . .	Reserpine β-Blocker
Diabetes mellitus	ACE inhibitor	Thiazide diuretic β-Blocker
Heart block	. . . . .	β-Blocker Calcium antagonist
Heart failure: diastolic dysfunction	Calcium antagonist β-Blocker	Hydralazine
Heart failure: systolic dysfunction	Diuretic ACE inhibitor	Calcium antagonist β-Blocker
Obstructive airways disease	Calcium antagonist	β-Blocker Reserpine
Orthostasis	. . . . .	Diuretic Alpha blocker β-Blocker Reserpine
Peripheral vascular insufficiency	Calcium antagonist ACE inhibitor	β-Blocker Diuretic
Renal insufficiency	Calcium antagonist	β-Blocker
Sexual dysfunction	Calcium antagonist ACE inhibitor	β-Blocker Diuretic Reserpine

[a]Adapted from the fifth report of the Joint National Committee on Detection, Evaluation, and Treatment of High Blood Pressure (JNC V). Arch Intern Med 1993;153:154–183 and Houston MC. New insights and new approaches for the treatment of essential hypertension: selection of therapy based on coronary heart disease risk factor analysis, hemodynamic profiles, quality of life, and subsets of hypertension. Am Heart J 1989;117:911–951.

ans' Administration trial from the 1960s, the Australian Trial of Mild Hypertension which was conducted through the 1970s, and the more recent Hypertension Detection and Follow-Up Program (HDFP) each reported subgroup analyses of their data which concluded that antihypertensive therapy in the elderly was safe and effective (23–25). In fact, data from the HDFP indicated that intervention was even more beneficial in elderly than in younger cohorts, observations attributed to the higher likelihood and prevalence of complications from hypertension in the elderly. But these trials were not designed nor did they intend to examine risks and treatment of hypertension in the elderly. They were more general in scope and were not powerful enough to make conclusive statements about intervention in the elderly specifically. Hence, several prospective, placebo-controlled trials focusing exclusively on the elderly

were commenced and have now been completed. These trials provide practical guidance for implementing therapy for the elderly.

RECENT TRIALS FOCUSING EXCLUSIVELY ON THE ELDERLY

European Working Party on Hypertension in the Elderly Trial (EWPHE). This trial was a double-blind, placebo-controlled trial conducted from several hypertension centers across Europe (26, 27). It enrolled 840 patients aged 60 to 97 years with BPs ranging from 160 to 239 mm Hg systolic *and* 90 to 119 mm Hg diastolic and examined impact of BP reduction on stroke, incidence of cardiac events, and overall mortality. Hydrochlorothiazide plus triamterene were used as initial therapy, and methyldopa was added if necessary. Over a mean treatment period of 4.6 years, statistically significant reductions in stroke events (36%) and all cardiovascular events (34%) were documented. There was also a 47% reduction of fatal coronary events, but nonfatal myocardial infarctions and new evolution of angina occurred with nearly identical frequency in both placebo and treatment groups. The greatest cardiac benefit was a 63% reduction in occurrence of severe congestive heart failure in the treatment group. Treatment benefit was seen whether the patient had preexisting cardiac problems or mild, moderate, or severely elevated BP at entry. While treatment was well tolerated, mild hypokalemia and an increased incidence of glucose intolerance were noted with active treatment. Treatment benefit was not documented for patients above 80 years of age.

Elderly Patients in Primary Care Trial. This trial was conducted in England and Wales concurrently with the broader-scoped EWPHE Trial (28). Like the EWPHE Trial, the intent was to examine the impact of antihypertensive treatment (compared with placebo) on stroke and cardiac events in hypertensive elderly patients; but unlike the EWPHE Trial, this trial initiated therapy with a β-blocker, then added a diuretic if necessary, continued therapy for 8 years, and cared for the patients in a primary care setting. Patients were enrolled if their BPs were 170 to 280 mm Hg systolic *or* 105 to 120 mm Hg diastolic on successive measurements. With 884 patients aged 60 to 79 years completing the trial, there was no significant effect of therapy on incidence of fatal or nonfatal myocardial infarction, but there was a 42% reduction in stroke incidence and a 22% reduction in overall cardiovascular mortality. Benefit was similar whether patients were 60 to 69 years old or 70 to 79 years old.

Systolic Hypertension in the Elderly Program. This U.S. trial was organized specifically to evaluate whether antihypertensive drug therapy would reduce incidence of stroke and cardiac events in elderly persons with isolated systolic hypertension (29). From a mass screening program, 4736 persons with systolic BPs ranging from 160 to 219 mm Hg *and* diastolic BP *less than* 90 mm Hg were enrolled and randomized to placebo or active treatment, which was a step-care protocol using chlorthalidone as initial and a β-blocker as second-line therapy. Over a mean treatment period of 4.5 years, 72% of the patients receiving active treatment reached target BP (systolic BP < 160 mm Hg). A statistically significant 36% reduction in stroke events and 27% reduction in cardiac events was documented. Therapy was well tolerated, although mild hypokalemia and glucose intolerance were again noted in the active treat-

ment group. In contrast to the EWPHE Trial, treatment benefit was apparent for patients over the age of 80 years. This study was important because isolated systolic hypertension is unique among the elderly and convincing benefit from antihypertensive treatment in the elderly had heretofore been documented only for diastolic hypertension. This study made a clear statement that isolated systolic hypertension carries significant morbidity and treatment diminishes its associated morbidity.

Swedish Trial in Old Patients with Hypertension. Unique from other trials, this trial specifically recruited "older elderly" hypertensive patients (i.e., patients aged 70 to 84 years) to assess whether antihypertensive therapy would reduce incidence of stroke and cardiac disease (30). Patients had to have systolic BP 180 to 230 mm Hg *and* diastolic BP 90 mm Hg to be enrolled. Patients were randomized to receive placebo, a β-blocker, or hydrochlorothiazide plus amiloride as initial therapy and either diuretic or β-blocker as second-line therapy. With 4 years of therapy in 1627 patients, stroke occurrence was reduced by 47% and primary cardiac death by 50%. Significant reductions in occurrence of congestive heart failure, acceleration of hypertension, and transient cerebral ischemic attacks were also observed. Treatment benefit was clear for patients up to 80 years, but it was less clear for patients between 80 and 84 years of age.

Medical Research Council (of Great Britain) Trial. This trial aimed at evaluating benefit of therapy of "mild" hypertension in a large elderly population (31). Toward this end, 4396 patients aged 65 to 74 years with systolic BP 160 to 209 mm Hg *and* diastolic BP up to 115 mm Hg were randomized to receive either hydrochlorothiazide plus amiloride, atenolol, or placebo as initial therapy. If a second drug was needed to achieve target BP (150 to 160 mm Hg systolic), then the other agent was used. Compared with placebo, active treatment lowered occurrence of stroke by 25% and coronary events by 19% over the 7-year observation period. When the data were analyzed according to β-blocker versus diuretic, benefit compared with placebo was seen only among those patients treated with the diuretic, not with the β-blocker. A large drop-out rate from the β-blocker group because of untoward effects and failure to control BP may explain this difference. This study confirmed that therapy of mild hypertension in the elderly is beneficial, though the benefits were not as dramatic as those for more severe hypertension, and pointed out that low-dose diuretic therapy is better tolerated and more effective than β-blocker therapy in the elderly for mild hypertension.

Veterans Affairs Cooperative Study of Treatment of Hypertension in the Elderly. This study was designed to compare efficacy of various antihypertensive regimens on BP control and assess for drug-related cognitive or behavioral alterations in elderly hypertensive men (32, 33). Endpoints such as stroke, heart attack, or angina were not measured. Low- or high-dose hydrochlorothiazide was given as initial therapy, and then nonresponders were randomly assigned to receive hydralazine, methyldopa, reserpine, or metoprolol. Only 50% of the men reached target BP with low-dose hydrochlorothiazide (25 to 50 mg), but only 58% reached target BP with higher doses (50 to 100 mg), and these manifested greater incidence of adverse metabolic effect. Each of the other medications improved BP control, with no difference in efficacy among them (32). No deterioration in cognitive or behavioral function with BP control was observed regardless of therapeutic agent (33). While limited to men and of short duration, this study has practical value in pointing out that higher-dose diuretic therapy offers no advantage over lower doses, and cognitive functions are not necessarily impaired by successful BP lowering.

DEVELOPING A PRACTICAL STRATEGY FOR THERAPY

These trials clearly document that isolated diastolic, isolated systolic, and combined systolic-diastolic hypertension confer morbidity and mortality in the elderly that can be significantly mitigated with successful BP lowering by carefully applied pharmacotherapy. Current standard of care holds that BP elevations exceeding 160 mm Hg systolic or 90 mm Hg diastolic should be treated with pharmacotherapy (4, 35). Nonpharmacologic means should be used in any patient with BP ranging between 140 to 159 mm Hg systolic or 85 to 90 mm Hg diastolic (see below). However, if such a patient has evidence of end-organ damage or concurrent cardiovascular disease, then pharmacotherapy is indicated (4, 34, 35). Hence, the decision to initiate treatment of hypertension in individual patients should be based on severity of BP elevation and evidence of end-organ or vascular damage (4). Treatment should be initiated with a single drug and titrated to reduce systolic BP to less than 160 mm Hg *and* diastolic BP less than 90 mm Hg (4). For those patients with systolic BP between 140 and 159 mm Hg, or 85 and 90 mm Hg with end-organ damage

or coexisting cardiovascular disease, degree of BP lowering becomes an individualized judgment. Lowering BP too far may produce ischemic symptoms (4). Because only diuretics and β-blockers have been used in trials that demonstrate reduction in cardiovascular morbidity and mortality, the Joint National Committee on Detection, Evaluation, and Treatment of High Blood Pressure recommends these drugs as preferred initial agents (4). However, this committee acknowledges that calcium antagonists and ACE inhibitors are equally effective in lowering BP in this age group and may have special benefits for patients with comorbid conditions such as diabetes mellitus, coronary or cerebral vascular insufficiency, congestive heart failure, or renal insufficiency (4, 34, 35). The above trials excluded patients with these conditions, which are prevalent among the elderly. Thus, patient factors such as concurrent disease and cardiovascular condition must be considered in the practical decision of which therapy for which patient.

PATIENT FACTORS IN PLANNING THERAPY

While BP lowering can be effectively accomplished in the elderly with medications from any of the drug families, certain antihypertensive drugs may worsen some medical problems while improving others (4, 34). For example, angina with hypertension may be best treated with a calcium antagonist as initial therapy, while hypertension with congestive heart failure due to systolic dysfunction may be best treated with an ACE inhibitor but aggravated by verapamil. Yet, verapamil may be the ideal drug for a hypertensive patient with stiff left ventricular hypertrophy and heart failure due to diastolic dysfunction. Diabetes mellitus due to insulin resistance may be worsened by a β-blocker or diuretic but improved by an ACE inhibitor. Dyslipidemia similarly may be worsened by a diuretic or β-blocker. Depression or cognitive impairments may be worsened by reserpine, a β-blocker, or by central α-agonist therapy. Diuretics may aggravate gouty arthritis through hyperuricemia and potentiate arrhythmic tendencies or digitalis toxicity by lowering serum potassium. Hence, one's evaluation for end-organ damage and coexisting illnesses should lead to consideration of the impact of a given medication on the function of the end-organ and whether that medication will aggravate or ameliorate a given comorbid problem. Medications that will aggravate a condition should not be used. Selection of a single medication that effectively treats a coexisting problem will simplify therapy, amplify benefit, probably improve compliance, and reduce costs (4, 34) (Table 7.1).

CONSIDERATIONS OF SPECIFIC MEDICATIONS

Thiazide Diuretics. Diuretics lower BP by first inducing plasma volume contraction, then reducing sodium and water content of vascular walls, which achieves a minor but measurable degree of vasorelaxation. Benefit seen with diuretics in the several antihypertensive trials is largely a protection from pressure-related injury and probably derives from these combined actions. Even though diuretic effectiveness and benefit are beyond refute, diuretics control BP in only 50% of patients and have hazards and even some actions that could be considered unphysiologic in the elderly. Hypokalemia is probably the leading hazard, an effect frequently noted in the reported trials. Potassium-sparing diuretic combinations mitigate this effect, but not totally. Hypokalemia potentiates arrhythmic occurrences in patients with left ventricular hypertrophy or ischemic heart disease, which are relatively common in hypertensive elderly (4, 34). Glucose intolerance is also a concern, and for this reason, diuretics should be used as adjunctive therapy, not first-line therapy, in the diabetic patient who is diet-controlled or requires oral hypoglycemic therapy. Thiazide diuretics can elevate plasma lipids (though there is no proof that this contributes to morbidity) and precipitate gout. Furthermore, diuretics do reduce plasma volume, which may aggravate orthostasis or reduce organ perfusion in the many elderly hypertensive patients who are already relatively plasma volume contracted. While it is said that elderly patients tend to be "salt-sensitive," this does not necessarily imply that these patients are chronically salt and water overloaded and require daily diuresis. On the contrary, this designation implies that the patient is particularly sensitive to excessive salt intake, which would inordinately raise BP, and at the same time is particularly sensitive to salt depletion, which can precipitously drop BP. Given the stiffness of the vasculature and already reduced organ blood flows, further reductions in intravascular volume can easily result in organ hypoperfusion and magnification of orthostasis. Finally, thiazide diuretics have been associated with morbid hyponatremia in the elderly, particularly those who practice stringent salt restriction or take other medications that potentiate vasopressin release, such as oral hypoglycemics.

With these caveats in mind, thiazide diuretics nevertheless stand as the drug of choice to commence antihypertensive therapy in the uncomplicated patient who does not exhibit overt end-organ damage or have coexisting illnesses that would improve with another type of antihypertensive medication (4). Since recent studies have documented that the natriuretic and antihypertensive dose-response curve for hydrochlorothiazide plateaus between 25 and 50 mg per day while metabolic or toxic side-effects continue to accrue at higher doses, the formal recommendation is to begin therapy with 12.5 or 25 mg of hydrochlorothiazide or its equivalent per day in a potassium-sparing combination and add a second medication if the low-dose diuretic is insufficient in lowering BP to target (4, 32). Loop diuretics such as furosemide should not be used as primary antihypertensive agents in the uncomplicated patient since they are short acting and unnecessarily potent. A patient with renal insufficiency may require a loop diuretic, however, to achieve daily salt homeostasis. Continued surveillance for diuretic-related complications is essential.

Calcium Antagonists. By impeding calcium movement into cells, calcium antagonists reduce the contraction and tone of cardiac and vascular smooth muscle. Accordingly, arteriolar resistances and central arterial compliance improve, and arterial pressures fall. Yet, as arterial pressures decline, organ blood flows increase, so there is little reflex stimulation of catecholamine or renin-angiotensin production, and sodium excretion is sustained (21, 34). Calcium antagonists have particular cardiac benefits by promoting regression of cardiac hypertrophy and coronary dilation, although their cardiac depressant action is a potential drawback for the patient with systolic dysfunction or cardiac conduction disease. Calcium antagonists do not elevate lipid levels and in fact improve HDL and LDL cholesterol profiles and have been shown to improve insulin resistance and be directly antiatherogenic in both animals and humans (34). Because of these actions, these agents are particularly well suited for the hypertensive elderly, and their effectiveness in these patients is widely documented (34). Their higher cost notwithstanding, calcium antagonists seem ideal first-choice agents for the elderly hypertensive patient with diabetes mellitus, overt coronary disease, peripheral or cerebrovascular disease, renal insufficiency, or left ventricular hypertrophy (4, 21, 34, 35). And, if low-dose diuretic therapy proves inadequate in lowering BP for the uncomplicated patient or provokes untoward side effects, then calcium antagonists seem most appropriate as the logical alternate choice. Side effects that may complicate therapy with a calcium antagonist include heart block, a reduction in cardiac systolic ejection fraction, orthostasis, and constipation.

Angiotensin Converting Enzyme Inhibitors. ACE inhibitors are effective in the elderly despite the fact that renal renin output is generally reduced in this patient population (12). They lower BP by inhibiting production of angiotensin II and aldosterone and promoting vasoactive kinin production. Accordingly, ACE inhibitors reduce peripheral resistance principally through vasorelaxation, although over time regression of vascular smooth muscle hypertrophy is observed (34). Because of these actions, cerebral and renal blood flows are sustained or improved as intraarterial pressures decline and reflex activation of the sympathetic nervous system does not occur (34). For similar reasons, sodium retention is averted. Special benefit is apparent for the patient with congestive heart failure, particularly if systolic ejection function is compromised, as reduction in cardiac afterload with ACE inhibitors substantially improves forward cardiac output (4, 34). Benefit is apparent also for the patient with renal insufficiency, as these agents reduce intraglomerular pressures and retard progression of glomerulosclerosis. On the other hand, ACE inhibitors can abruptly reduce glomerular filtration rate in the patient with bilateral renal artery stenoses or advanced nephrosclerosis by lowering intraglomerular filtration pressures, which are critically dependent on postglomerular angiotensin-mediated vasoconstriction, and may promote hyperkalemia in the patient with renal insufficiency by reducing aldosterone synthesis, which is also partly angiotensin-dependent. Aside from these concerns and a not uncommon cough which these agents can produce, ACE inhibitors should be considered a first-choice medication for the patient with heart failure and an excellent synergistic medication to diuretics and/or calcium antagonists when a multidrug regimen is required to achieve BP control (21, 34). If an ACE inhibitor and diuretic are used together, the physician must avoid potassium-sparing diuretics and monitor closely for azotemia and hypotension, which may be potentiated by this combination (4).

β-Blockers. β-Blockers reduce BP chiefly by reducing cardiac ejection force and limiting production of renin and angiotensin. Although β-blockers were used widely in the antihypertensive trials involving the elderly, β-blockers are probably best regarded as third-line therapy in the elderly (34). First, reduction of cardiac output is not a physiologically appropriate goal for the elderly hypertensive person, who will typically possess an already reduced cardiac output. Second, tolerance for this class of drugs is relatively poor among the elderly, with fatigue and mental slowing being chief concerns (12, 31). Third, since peripheral β-blockade leaves α-constrictive action unopposed, β-blockers do not reduce vascular resistance nor raise organ blood flows when BP lowering is achieved. In fact, when studied, β-blockers have been shown most consistently to lower cerebral and renal blood flows as they lower BP, actions that would be considered undesirable for the elderly patient (34). For these reasons, use of β-blockers should be reserved for patients with coronary insufficiency, recent myocardial infarction, an expanding aortic aneurysm, or asymmetric ventricular hypertrophy where reduction of ejection force, heart rate, or cardiac work would produce direct benefit. Even in these patients, a calcium antagonist with negative inotropic and chronotropic properties may be a better first-choice agent because of the preservation of organ perfusion that calcium antagonists achieve as BP is lowered. Side effects that may complicate β-blocker therapy in the elderly include bradycardia or heart block, congestive heart failure, mental slowing, fatigue, depression, a worsening of glucose intolerance, reduced sympathetic response to hypoglycemia, bronchospasm, or impotence. β-Blockers also block the appropriate sympathetic response to postural changes, which may aggravate orthostasis.

α-Adrenergic Blockers or Central α-Agonists. α-Adrenergic blockers achieve vasorelaxation and reduction in BP through peripheral blockade of norepinephrine-mediated vasoconstrictive action on vascular smooth muscle cells. Central α-agonists lower BP by reducing central catecholamine output. Owing to these actions, cerebral and renal blood flows increase while cardiac output is generally preserved as BP is lowered (34). Though effective in the elderly, their side-effect profile limits their usefulness in the elderly. Mental slowing, orthostasis, and depression are common. Combining them with diuretics can make orthostasis even more likely, so this is unwise. There is a small resurgence of interest in peripheral α-blockade for the man with prostatic hypertrophy, in which α-blockade can relax the urethral sphincter while lowering BP concurrently. Despite this benefit and favorable actions on serum lipids and insulin sensitivity, both central and peripheral α-blockers will probably remain in an adjunctive position, since aggravation of orthostasis, sexual dysfunction, depression, and somnolence remain concerns, and there are better nondiuretic alternatives.

Direct Vasodilators. Direct vasodilators such as hydralazine or minoxidil aggravate orthostasis, promote sodium retention, and stimulate tachycardia. They are inappropriate as first-line agents and are superseded in effectiveness by calcium antagonists.

Ganglionic Blockers. Ganglionic blockers such as guanethidine and guanadrel aggravate orthostasis, create bowel dysfunction and impotence, and result in mental slowing. Their side-effect profile is therefore unacceptable for the elderly, and their effectiveness is superseded by other drug classes.

SPECIAL CHALLENGES IN PHARMACOLOGIC THERAPY

Pharmacologic therapy in the elderly hypertensive is fraught with more potential side effects than in younger patients (4). Tendency to orthostasis, reduced baroreceptor sensitivities, diffuse arteriosclerosis, reduced cardiac output, and salt sensitivity predispose elderly patients to symptomatic hypotension with doses of drugs that otherwise would not produce problems in younger hypertensives. Altered volume of distribution and reduced renal clearance of drugs are characteristic of elderly patients, because fat stores are generally increased and total body water, lean body mass, and GFR generally decreased. For these reasons, it is recommended that therapy in the elderly be initiated with a 50% lower dose than is recommended for younger adults and dose intervals be appropriately spaced to account for reduced GFR (4). Doses should be raised cautiously.

The physician must also practice vigilance for drug-drug interactions. Not only can drug-drug interactions create toxicity, such as possible digitalis toxicity with calcium antagonist use in a patient already on digoxin, but prescribed drugs may also subvert antihypertensive efficacy. For example, nonsteroidal antiinflammatory agents promote renal sodium retention and thereby countervail diuretic efficacy, and many sympathomimetic agents directly raise BP through vasoconstriction. Important interactions between antihypertensive medications and other drugs are reviewed in the Fifth Report from the Joint National Committee (4).

As with any other age group, periodic review of the antihypertensive program with consideration of stepdown or change of therapy should be done (4). At times, nonpharmacologic methods may succeed, and once-necessary medication can be discontinued or reduced in dosage. If a patient loses weight or becomes frail for other reasons, dose requirements may change. If a new medical problem supervenes, a different program may serve the patient better. And, it is always proper to question one's initial judgment about the diagnosis of hypertension in the first place. Most antihypertensive trials have demonstrated a reduction in average BP for untreated patients over time (4, 6, 17). Attempts at dose reductions after 6 to 8 months of control thus have some justification, particularly with the patient who has been successful with nonpharmacologic interventions and lifestyle modifications.

NONPHARMACOLOGIC THERAPY

Lifestyle modifications are just as appropriate for the elderly hypertensive person as for the younger hypertensive, though probably somewhat more difficult to achieve. Weight reduction, increased physical activity, dietary sodium moderation, cessation of smoking, and alcohol moderation are all recommended as beneficial (4). Additionally, patients should be counseled regarding other medications, such as decongestants, ophthalmic medications, and nonsteroidal antiinflammatory medications, which may raise BP or promote salt retention through their independent actions. Some elderly patients with mild or stage 1 hypertension may be managed by nonpharmacologic methods alone, but if target organ damage is apparent or if cardiovascular risk factors are present, then pharmacologic intervention is indicated without delay (4). Lifestyle and diet modification is appropriate for all patients requiring medication.

SUMMARY AND RECOMMENDATIONS

Hypertension is a disorder of arterial BP regulation that is expressed differently among patients of varying age. Among the young, high BP is characterized by high cardiac output and normal vascular resistance, and dynamic high-pressure problems constitute the greatest and most immediate threat. Accordingly, the goal of therapy with the younger patient is to reduce arterial pressure promptly and physiologically with drugs that have the fewest and least harmful side effects. Among the elderly, however, cardiac output is typically subnormal, and systemic vascular resistance is very high. Progressive arteriolar narrowing and central arterial stiffening are the major pathogenic issues for the elderly, for they cause even higher arterial pressures, create progressively greater workloads for the heart, and generate damaging pulse-flow systolic stresses that persistently threaten organs with pressure-related injury. Yet, the same vascular disease that participates in the genesis of hypertension among the elderly presents a hypoperfusion compromise to vital organs, impairing their function in the short term, and producing progressive ischemic injury over the long term. Thus, ischemic and high-pressure threats frequently coexist in the elderly hypertensive patient. Impaired baroreceptor functions, a propensity to orthostasis, altered autoregulation of organ blood flows, and salt sensitivity are other typical features of elderly hypertension. Mitigating high-pressure threats with antihypertensive therapy that reduces cardiac output further, significantly contracts intravascular volume, or lowers BP too rapidly or too far can magnify the ischemic threat and diminish or cancel overall benefit.

Accordingly, our broad therapeutic intent for the elderly hypertensive person must include protection of organs from both pressure-related and ischemic-related injury with preservation of organ blood flow and function as we lower arterial pressures. Present consensus recommends that systolic BP be lowered to less than 160 mm Hg if starting BP is greater than 180 mm Hg. If initial systolic BP is 160 to 179 mm Hg, the target is to reduce BP by 20 mm Hg. Diastolic BP should be lowered below 90 mm Hg, or 85 mm Hg if therapy is well tolerated (4, 12). However, simply lowering BP below a selected threshold is *not* a sufficient goal. Therapeutic logic dictates that we tailor our antihypertensive therapy to the pathophysiology and clinical condition of the patient and aim to directly mitigate active associated problems, such as heart failure or angina or peripheral vascular insufficiency.

Based on large-scale patient trials, diuretic therapy is clearly beneficial in the uncomplicated patient but has certain physiologic tradeoffs. Diuretics should not be used by rote or by recipe. They should be used circumspectly in low doses and coupled to calcium antagonists or ACE inhibitors when cardiac, renal, or metabolic concerns are present or when low-dose diuretic therapy alone does not bring BP into target range. Physiologically, calcium antagonists probably have the best profile for the elderly hypertensive. However, they suffer from their relatively high cost and from the fact that they have not yet been studied as rigorously as diuretics in large population trials. Yet, when coexisting medical problems warrant, the elderly hypertensive patient may be best served when calcium antagonists or ACE inhibitors are offered as principal therapy.

REFERENCES

1. Roberts J. Blood pressure of persons 18–74 years: United States 1971–1972. DHEW Publ no. 75–1632;1975.
2. Roberts J, Maurer K: Blood pressure levels of persons 6–74 years. DHEW Publ no. 78–1648;1977.
3. Rowland M, Roberts J. Blood pressure levels and hypertension in persons ages 6–74 years: United States 1976–1980. DHHS Publ no. 82–1250;1982.
4. The fifth report of the Joint National Committee on Detection, Evaluation, and Treatment of High Blood Pressure (JNC V). Arch Intern Med 1993;153:154–183.
5. Hulley SB, Furberg CD, Gurland B, et al. Systolic Hypertension in the Elderly Program (SHEP): antihypertensive efficacy of chlorthalidone. Am J Cardiol 1985;56:913–920.
6. Kaplan N. Hypertension in the population at large. In: Kaplan N, ed. Clinical hypertension. 5th ed. Baltimore: Williams & Wilkins, 1990:1–25.
7. Jackson G, Mahon W, Pierscianowski T, Condon J. Inappropriate anti-hypertensive therapy in the elderly. Lancet 1976;1:1317–1318.
8. Jones J, Graham D. Hypertension and the cerebral circulation—its relevance to the elderly. Am Heart J 1978;96:270–271.
9. Kaplan N. Primary hypertension: pathogenesis. In: Clinical hypertension. 5th ed. Baltimore: Williams & Wilkins, 1990:54–111.
10. Kannel WB, Gordon T. Evaluation of cardiovascular risk in the elderly: The Framingham Study. Bull NY Acad Med 1978;54:573–591.
11. Kannel WB, Wolf PA, McGee OL, Bawber TR, McNamara P, Castelli WP. Systolic blood pressure, arterial rigidity, and risk of stroke: The Framingham Study. JAMA 1981;245:1225–1229.
12. Mann SJ. Systolic hypertension in the elderly. Arch Intern Med 1992;152:1977–1984.
13. Sagie A, Larson MG, Levy D. The natural history of borderline isolated systolic hypertension. N Engl J Med 1993;329:1912–1917.
14. Davidson RA, Caranasos GJ. Should the elderly hypertensive be treated? Arch Intern Med 1987;147:1933–1937.
15. Lipsitz LA. Orthostatic hypotension in the elderly. N Engl J Med 1989;321:950–957.
16. Ray WA, Schaffner W, Oates JA. Therapeutic choice in the treatment of hypertension. Am J Med 1986;81(suppl 6C):9–16.
17. Kaplan N. Primary hypertension: natural history. Chapter 4. In: Kaplan N, ed. Clinical hypertension. 5th ed. Baltimore: Williams & Wilkins, 1990:112–135.
18. Kirkendall W, Hammond J. Hypertension in the elderly. Arch Intern Med 1980;140:1155–1161.
19. Weber M, Neutel J, Cheung D. Hypertension in the aged: a pathophysiologic basis for treatment. Am J Cardiol 1989;63:25H–32H.
20. O'Rourke M. Arterial stiffness, systolic blood pressure, and logical treatment of arterial hypertension. Hypertension 1990;15:339–347.
21. Weir M, Sowers J. Physiologic and hemodynamic considerations in blood pressure control while maintaining organ perfusion. Am J Cardiol 1988;61:60H–66H.
22. Mann SJ, Pickering TG. Detection of renovascular hypertension. Ann Intern Med 1992;117:845–853.

23. Veterans Administration Cooperative Study Group on Antihypertensive Agents. Effects of treatment on mortality in hypertension. III. Influence of age, diastolic blood pressure, and prior cardiovascular disease; further analysis of side effects. Circulation 1972;45:991–1004.
24. Managment Committee. Treatment of mild hypertension in the elderly. Med J Aust 1981;2:398–402.
25. Hypertension Detection and Follow-up Program Cooperative Group. Five-year findings of the HDFP. II. Mortality by race, sex, and age. JAMA 1979; 242:2572–2577.
26. Amery A, Brixho P, Clement D, et al. Mortality and morbidity results from the European Working Party on High Blood Pressure in the Elderly Trial. Lancet 1985;1:1349–1354.
27. Amery A, Brixho P, Clement D, et al. Efficacy of antihypertensive drug treatment according to age, sex, blood pressure, and previous cardiovascular disease in patients over the age of 60. Lancet 1986;2:589–592.
28. Coope J, Warrender TS. Randomised trial of treatment of hypertension in elderly patients in primary care. Br Med J 1986;293:1145–1151.
29. SHEP Cooperative Research Group. Prevention of stroke by anti-hypertensive drug treatment in older persons with isolated systolic hypertension. JAMA 1991;265:3255–3264.
30. Dahlof B, Lindholm L, Hansson L, et al. Morbidity and mortality in the Swedish Trial in Old Patients with Hypertension (STOP-Hypertension). Lancet 1991;338:1281–1285.
31. MRC Working Party. Medical Research Council trial of treatment of hypertension in older adults: principal results. Br Med J 1992;304:405–412.
32. Materson BJ, Cushman, WC, Goldstein G, et al. Treatment of hypertension in the elderly: I. Blood pressure and clinical changes. Results of a Department of Veterans Affairs Cooperative Study. Hypertension 1990;15:348–360.
33. Goldstein G, Materson BJ, Cushman WC, et al. Treatment of hypertension in the elderly. II. Cognitive and behavioral function. Results of a Department of Veterans Affairs Cooperative Study. Hypertension 1990;15:361–369.
34. Houston MC. New insights and new approaches for the treatment of essential hypertension: selection of therapy based on coronary heart disease risk factor analysis, hemodynamic profiles, quality of life, and subsets of hypertension. Am Heart J 1989;117:911–951.
35. Kaplan NM. Maximally reducing cardiovascular risk in the treatment of hypertension. Ann Intern Med 1988;109:36–40.

SYNDROME X

"Syndrome X" is a designation applied to a cluster of metabolic abnormalities, including insulin resistance, hyperinsulinemia, abnormal glucose tolerance, elevated blood VLDL triglyceride concentrations, and decreased blood HDL cholesterol concentrations, which occurs in association with systemic arterial hypertension (1). A high incidence of progressive coronary and peripheral vascular disease is present among patients who exhibit this cluster of problems. Hyperinsulinemia and insulin resistance are proposed as causal to this syndrome and its clinical expression, including the initiation and perpetuation of hypertension (1–4). However, the evidence in this regard is largely epidemiologic and correlational. Direct causality has been difficult to prove (5).

The strongest correlation between insulin resistance, hyperinsulinemia, abnormal glucose tolerance, dyslipidemia, and hypertension is found among obese individuals who exhibit overt non-insulin-dependent diabetes mellitus and obesity (4, 5). Coronary and peripheral vascular disease is highly prevalent among these patients, and simple control of their hypertension does not seem to impact greatly on the evolution of cardiovascular complications (1). However, a strong positive correlation between hyperinsulinemia and elevated blood pressures (BPs) independent of obesity has been documented in several studies (3, 6–8). This observation lends support to the postulate that hyperinsulinemia and/or insulin resistance may be an important pathogenetic factor in the evolution of hypertension in certain patients, including many who are elderly.

Insulin may contribute to elevated BPs through several mechanisms. Insulin exerts an antinatriuretic action on the kidney, which in the steady state would be overcome only through sustained elevations in BP and a shift in the pressure-natriuresis relationship of the kidney (2, 5). Insulin also stimulates the sympathetic nervous system (3, 5, 8). A chronically stimulated sympathetic nervous system could raise BP by increasing peripheral vascular resistance, inducing sodium retention by a direct tubular action, and through vasoconstriction of preglomerular arterioles, which will raise renin levels and induce further vasoconstriction and sodium retention through angiotensin and aldosterone. Insulin also can exert a mitogenic effect on vascular smooth muscle and thereby contribute to fixed vascular narrowing and growth of atheromata (3, 9). Angiotensin and catecholamines have similar properties (3, 9).

Hyperinsulinemia and/or insulin resistance may be a fundamental factor in the genesis of the heightened vascular resistance and salt-sensitive state that is central to hypertension among the elderly. In industrialized cultures, advancing age is associated with a decrease in lean body mass and an increase in adipose tissue (10). Increased adiposity is strongly correlated with insulin resistance and hyperinsulinemia and is reported to be a major contributing factor for age-associated increases in BPs. Salt sensitivity derives from various mechanisms, including reduced glomerular filtration rate and a relatively noncompliant vasculature, but is also strongly associated with adiposity (4, 5, 10). As discussed in the previous sections, salt sensitivity denotes an unusual increase in BP following a salty meal and a relative delay in excretion of the ingested sodium. Through its effects on both the kidney and the sympathetic nervous system, relative hyperinsulinemia following a meal may be operative in this phenomenon. As hyperinsulinemia resolves with weight loss, salt sensitivity similarly declines (2, 3, 10).

This concept of a hypertensive-metabolic-cardiovascular risk factor complex has important therapeutic implications. One significant realization is that these factors aggravate and magnify each other. Hypertension aggravates the vascular pathology, and vascular pathology magnifies the hypertension. Insulin resistance certainly contributes to dyslipidemia, and hyperinsulinemia and dyslipidemia certainly contribute to atherosclerosis. Thus, cardiovascular risk factor modification in these hypertensive patients requires a comprehensive and concerted approach that aims fundamentally at all the factors that are pathogenetically operative (8, 11). As central pathogenetic factors in this process, hyperinsulinemia and dyslipidemia must be considered no less important than high BP itself as a contributor to morbidity and mortality. As noted, successful lowering of BP does not appear to be as beneficial in this patient group as in another without the features of "syndrome X" (1). Ideally, then, our therapeutic interventions must aim to mitigate all associated risk factors and aggravate none (11, 12).

Weight reduction, increased physical activity, and a change in diet from simple carbohydrate and saturated fat to complex carbohydrates and lean high-biologic-quality protein sources are proven means toward subverting these metabolic risk factors (3, 10). Thiazide diuretics and β-blockers are concerns in the pharmacologic treatment of these patients, for both have been shown to raise insulin resistance and promote dyslipidemia while lowering systemic BPs (3, 9). Theoretically, these agents could promote untoward vascular change while mitigating the hypertensive threat. This eventuality has not been clearly proven, although the issue is a continuing debate (9, 11–14). If duretics must be used, their doses should be kept low (e.g., 12.5 to 25 mg hydrochlorothiazide per day) and hypokalemia avoided. Insulin resis-

tance and the dyslipidemic effects of thiazides appear to bear a positive relationship to dose and the occurrence of hypokalemia. Agents such as angiotensin converting enzyme inhibitors and calcium antagonists, which improve insulin sensitivity and attenuate atherogenesis, have theoretic advantage in the hyperinsulinemic patient (9). Both of these families improve renal natriuresis as well (9).

Recognition of the patients likely to exhibit the features of "syndrome X" is thus important. Most commonly, this will be the obese individual with either overt diabetes mellitus or subclinical glucose intolerance. However, even the elderly nonobese individual may exhibit relative hyperinsulinemia and insulin resistance that underpins a dyslipidemic state and progressive vascular disease, so it is appropriate to consider the existence of "syndrome X" in most if not all elderly hypertensive individuals (9, 10). It would not be practical to assay insulin levels or perform formal glucose tolerance tests in all hypertensive elderly patients, but measurement of serum lipid profiles with fasting and postprandial blood glucose concentrations is recommended along with a searching history and physical examination for evidence of vascular insufficiency in any aspect of the arterial tree (13).

REFERENCES

1. Reaven GM. Role of insulin resistance in human disease. Diabetes 1988;37:1595–1607.
2. Aviv A. The roles of cell Ca^{++}, protein kinase C and the Na$^+$-H$^+$ antiporter in the development of hypertension and insulin resistance. J Am Soc Nephrol 1992;3:1049–1063.
3. Bain SC, Dodson PM. The chronic cardiovascular risk factor syndrome (syndrome X): mechanisms and implications for atherogenesis. Postgrad Med J 1991;67:922–927.
4. Sowers JR, Standley PR, Ram JL, Zemel MB, Resnick LM. Insulin resistance, carbohydrate metabolism, and hypertension. Am J Hypertens 1991;4:466s–472s.
5. Brands MW, Hall JE. Insulin resistance, hyperinsulinemia, and obesity-associated hypertension. J Am Soc Nephrol 1992;3:1064–1077.
6. Swislocki ALM, Hoffman BB, Reaven GM. Insulin resistance, glucose intolerance, and hyperinsulinemia in patients with hypertension. Am J Hypertens 1989;2:419–423.
7. Ferrannini E, Buzzigoli G, Bonadonna R, et al. Insulin resistance in essential hypertension. N Engl J Med 1987;317:350–357.
8. Ferrannini E, Natali A. Essential hypertension, metabolic disorders, and insulin resistance. Am Heart J 1991;121:1274–1282.
9. Houston MC. New insights and new approaches for the treatment of essential hypertension: selection of

therapy based on coronary heart disease risk factor analysis, hemodynamic profiles, quality of life, and subsets of hypertension. Am Heart J 1989;117:911–951.

10. Sowers JR, Khoury S, Imam K, Byyny R. Therapeutic approach to hypertension in the elderly. Prim Care 1991;3:593–605.

11. Kaplan NM. Maximally reducing cardiovascular risk in the treatment of hypertension. Ann Intern Med 1988;109:36–40.

12. Kaplan NM. The appropriate goals of antihypertensive therapy: neither too much nor too little. Ann Intern Med 1992;116:686–690.

13. Joint National Committee on Detection, Evaluation, and Treatment of High Blood Pressure. The fifth report of the Joint National Committee on Detection, Evaluation, and Treatment of High Blood Pressure. Arch Intern Med 1993;153:154–183.

14. Alderman MH. Which antihypertensive drugs first—and why! JAMA 1992;267:2786–2787.

8/ Exercise in the Elderly

Jan Busby-Whitehead

The hallmark of aging is a structural and functional decline in the cells and tissues of all organs. The resulting physiologic changes include decreased muscle mass and strength; decreased maximal heart rate, exercise tolerance, and aerobic capacity; and increased body fat. Functional status is quite heterogeneous among older individuals of similar chronological age; therefore, other factors in addition to genetic processes must contribute to this variation. The development of subclinical and overt disease processes such as atherosclerotic coronary artery disease may adversely affect cardiac and physical function and promote sedentary behavior. Lifestyle behaviors such as cigarette smoking, imprudent diet, and physical inactivity may also contribute directly to the age-related decline in functional status (1–3).

Exercise may help prevent or slow the progression of functional loss. Numerous scientific studies provide evidence that physical activity leads to better mental and physical health (4). Exercise may have an important role as a therapeutic agent for the prevention and treatment of various diseases such as hypertension, obesity, non-insulin-dependent diabetes mellitus, osteoporosis, and depression (5). Current evidence also suggests that regular physical activity may improve morbidity and mortality from cardiovascular disease (6).

This chapter briefly reviews the relationship of physical activity to disease, possible mechanisms by which exercise promotes beneficial changes, the benefits and risks of exercise, the evaluation of older people for exercise programs, and guidelines for exercise prescriptions.

PHYSICAL ACTIVITY AND DISEASE

Coronary Artery Disease. Many epidemiologic studies have shown that lower levels of cardiorespiratory fitness and physical activity are independent risk factors for coronary artery disease (CAD) in men. In the British Civil Servant Study, only strenuous physical activity was associated with a decreased risk of CAD (7). However, in the Multiple Risk Factor Intervention Trial, U.S. Railroad Study, and the Kuopio Ischemic Heart Disease Risk Factor Study, activity of low-to-moderate intensity was associated with reduced mortality from CAD (8–10). In the Kuopio study, 2 hours of conditioning exercise weekly was sufficient to reduce the risk of acute myocardial infarction. Mechanisms by which aerobic exercise may reduce risk for cardiovascular disease include improvement of balance between myocardial oxygen demand and supply, reduced risk for lethal ventricular arrhythmias, development of eccentric ventricular hypertrophy, decreased blood coagulability by reducing adhesiveness of platelets and increased fibrinolysis, and improved plasma lipid and lipoprotein profile (4).

In Paffenbarger's study of leisure-time activity in Harvard alumni, the relative risk for all-cause mortality was related to physical activity in a dose-dependent way (6). The greatest risk was found for those who expended fewer than 500 kcal/week, intermediate risk for those expending between 500 and 1999 kcal and the least risk for those expending more than 2000 kcal per week. A caloric expenditure of 2000 kcal weekly represents the energy expended in walking 3 miles daily for 7 days. In this study, the most active participants also had the lowest risk of cardiac events.

Hypertension. Population studies have also found an inverse correlation between physical activity and blood pressure. Chronic aerobic training has been shown to lower blood pressure modestly independent of weight loss or reduced body fat (11). A recent meta-analysis of 25 longitudinal studies reported average reductions in systolic pressure of 10.8 mm Hg and reduction in diastolic pressure of 8.2 mm Hg (12). Moderate-intensity exercise was as effective as higher-intensity exercise in achieving lower pressures. Possible mechanisms by which repeated physical activity affects blood pressure include a decline in resting cardiac output, a decline in sympathetic nervous system activity, and a decline in total peripheral resistance. Concomitant weight loss and dietary changes such as decreased sodium or alcohol intake may be contributing factors (13).

Diabetes Mellitus.   Cross-sectional and longitudinal studies have shown an inverse relationship between physical activity and the prevalence of non-insulin-dependent diabetes mellitus (NIDDM) (14). Regular aerobic exercise combined with proper diet may prevent the development of NIDDM and improve glycemic control in patients who have the disease. Insulin sensitivity is improved in skeletal muscle and other tissues with a single session of aerobic exercise, resulting in decreased blood glucose levels in diabetic patients. This effect is thought to occur because of an increase in cell membrane glucose transporter number and activity (15).

Obesity.   People who are obese tend to be less physically active. Regular exercise contributes to maintenance of ideal body weight through caloric expenditure. In addition, exercise may improve body fat distribution, as some training studies suggest that upper abdominal subcutaneous fat is mobilized in preference to peripheral subcutaneous fat (16).

Osteoporosis.   Peak bone mass occurs by the third decade and declines gradually throughout middle and old age, with an accelerated loss occurring in postmenopausal women. Although bone clearly responds to the physical stress of weight-bearing exercise, the amount and type necessary to attenuate bone loss is unclear (17).

Psychological.   Most older persons who exercise regularly enjoy an improved sense of well-being and self-efficacy. However, a significant relationship between levels of physical activity and the incidence of depression has not been proven (18).

EVALUATION OF OLDER PATIENTS PRIOR TO CONDITIONING

An older individual should undergo a complete medical evaluation prior to beginning an exercise program. The history and physical examination should be targeted to the cardiovascular, pulmonary, musculoskeletal, and neurologic systems, as the presence of comorbid disease is common in this population. Laboratory tests should be performed to rule out impaired renal or liver function, anemia, and diabetes mellitus. In addition, a resting 12-lead electrocardiogram should be performed. Many authorities believe that a physician-monitored exercise treadmill test should be done in older persons to screen for cardiac ischemia, exercise-induced arrhythmias or asthma, exaggerated hypertensive response, or other abnormalities that would preclude participation in an exercise training program (19). Others believe that asymptomatic, healthy older persons without major risk factors for CAD, diabetes mellitus, or hypertension and no previous history of these conditions are at low risk for CAD and therefore do not require testing (20).

Exercise tolerance testing also permits assessment of maximal aerobic capacity, which can be used for determining exercise goals and monitoring progress. The test is performed with a bicycle or treadmill, according to a standardized multistage protocol (21). Disadvantages include availability of equipment and trained personnel and cost. Contraindications to exercise stress testing include unstable angina, recent myocardial infarction, uncontrolled arrhythmias, severe aortic stenosis, third-degree heart block, dissecting aneurysm, myocarditis or pericarditis, recent pulmonary embolism or other thromboembolic disease, congestive heart failure, significant emotional disturbance, or neurologic or musculoskeletal limitations. Physicians performing the test should also be familiar with the indications for stopping a test and the criteria for an abnormal test. Persons with abnormal tests should be referred to the appropriate specialist for further evaluation.

THE EXERCISE PRESCRIPTION

The exercise prescription, tailored individually for each patient, describes the type, frequency, duration, and intensity of the proposed activity. It should include information on the warmup, conditioning, and cool-down components of each exercise session. Various activities may be prescribed for improving aerobic fitness. Activities that involve a large proportion of the total muscle mass, maximize the use of large muscles and dynamic muscle contraction, and minimize the work of the heart per unit training effect will be most effective. Walking may be the most beneficial exercise for the older person in terms of safety, effectiveness, and simplicity. Cardiac patients generally require a supervised exercise program and those at highest risk will also require ECG monitoring (22).

For all individuals, the exercise session should begin with 5 minutes of slow jogging followed by stretching exercises. This warmup, designed to bring about gradual increases in blood flow as well as increases in tissue and general body temperatures may prevent muscle aches, pains, and injuries and possibly reduce the incidence of cardiac rhythm abnormalities during the conditioning period. A general rule of thumb is that mild perspiration should appear before the person begins vigorous activity.

Frequency is an important component of the exercise prescription. Most studies have reported little change in physical fitness if exercises are done fewer than three times a week and no added benefit if training is done more than 5 days weekly (23). The duration of the exercise sessions is usually set at 20 minutes initially and advanced to 30 to 60 minutes as the individual progresses with training. Early studies reported that 20 to 30 minutes of continuous aerobic exercise were necessary to achieve a cardiovascular training effect. A recent study, however, has shown that three 10-minute walks during the same day have the same fitness impact as one 30-minute walk (24). This new finding may have important implications for compliance.

A minimum exercise intensity is thought to be required for a person with a low fitness level to achieve a cardiovascular training effect. This level, as determined by the American College of Sports Medicine (ACSM), has decreased from 70% of maximal aerobic capacity in 1975 to 50% in 1986 and 40 to 50% in 1990. Low intensity is generally defined as <50%, moderate intensity as 50 to 70%, and high intensity as >70% of maximal aerobic capacity. The intensity may be determined in one of two ways. If maximal aerobic capacity was measured during an exercise stress test, exercise intensity can be related to the maximal heart rate.

Alternatively, the maximal heart rate predicted by age can be determined by a formula (220 − age = maximal predicted heart rate). The target heart rate is calculated as percentage of maximal exercise capacity; e.g., 40% × (maximal heart rate − resting heart rate) plus the resting heart rate. For example, for a 70-year-old patient with a resting heart rate of 72 and predicted maximal heart rate of 150 (220 − 70) who will be exercising at 40% of maximal exercise capacity, the target heart rate would be 40% × (150 − 72) + 72 = 103 beats per minute.

Because a linear relationship exists between oxygen consumption and heart rate during submaximal work loads, the target heart rate can be monitored during exercise as a representation of training intensity. Exercise may also be prescribed in terms of metabolic equivalents (METS), which is the oxygen consumption during rest, or 3.5 mL O_2/kg/min. METS have been determined

for most activities. The usual safe range of exercise intensity is 4 to 7 METS for older persons with normal exercise stress tests (25).

Many older persons will benefit from supervision of the initial physical activity to confirm that exercise capacity is not exceeded. If the program is unsupervised, individuals should be carefully instructed on how and when to take their pulse to ensure that they are exercising at an appropriate level. Training duration and intensity should progress slowly, in a stepwise fashion, usually over 6 months or longer as needed. Depending on the initial exercise capacity, persons should begin at 40 to 50% of their maximal aerobic capacity for 10 to 20 minutes of continuous exercise. The duration of the session should be gradually increased to 30 to 45 minutes. Intensity may then be increased, usually not more than 10% per month.

A 10-minute cool-down session of slow walking and stretching exercises should conclude each exercise session. Older persons should be counseled to wear appropriate supportive footwear and loose clothing and to consult a physician if they develop pain in the chest, arm, neck, or jaw; severe shortness of breath; fainting or dizziness; irregular heartbeat during or after exercise; and injury or joint swelling.

RISKS OF EXERCISE

The possible adverse effects of exercise that are of most concern are sudden death, injury, and osteoarthritis. The most serious, yet most uncommon, of these is sudden death, defined as death occurring either during the actual activity or within 1 hour of its completion. Although reported rates of sudden death vary from 4 to 56 times greater than chance, the absolute risk is low: one cardiac death per 396,000 hours of jogging or one death per 15,000 to 18,000 exercisers per year (26). In most documented cases of sudden death, autopsies have revealed preexisting CAD, coronary vessel anomalies, or hypertrophic cardiomyopathy (27).

Few data exist on the risks of injury associated with the physical activities performed by older people, such as walking or gardening. Injuries sustained by participants in organized exercise programs are primarily due to overuse and are relatively common. The ankle is the joint most likely to be injured. Most nontraumatic musculoskeletal injuries in runners are directly related to distance run and increasing mileage. Age and obesity do not appear to be contributing factors in current studies. There are no good studies of nontraumatic musculoskeletal injuries related to walking or cycling or gardening (25).

Preexistent musculoskeletal problems may be a deterrent to beginning an exercise regimen. One study reported that over 50% of older individuals involved in a variety of new activities developed injuries that represented exacerbations of prior conditions (29). For previously healthy individuals, injury rates ranging from 10% to 50% for both novice and experienced exercisers have been reported. Significantly lower rates of injury are associated with low-impact exercise such as walking) than with higher-impact activities such as aerobic dance and jogging. Almost all organized walk/jog exercise programs reporting injuries cite the primary involvement of the lower extremities. Because most participants recover from the injury and maintain training intensity by substituting an uphill treadmill walk for jogging, high impact rather than intensity has been implicated as the cause of injury. Older women seem to be more susceptible than men to lower extremity injury during jogging (26).

The fear that physical activity may stimulate the development of osteoarthritis or exacerbate a preexisting condition has kept some patients from participating in an exercise program and may prevent physicians from recommending that they do so. Because osteoarthritis affects 85% of all persons 70 years or older, it is important to know whether activities should be limited in this population. Cross-sectional studies found no difference in the prevalence of musculoskeletal complaints, symptomatic osteoarthritis, or radiographic evidence of osteoarthritis in long-distance runners compared with nonrunners (28). A recent 2-year longitudinal study also showed no difference in the progression of osteoarthritis between runners and controls (29). Studies have been limited by problems in identifying osteoarthritis in its earliest developmental stage.

Physical inactivity may in fact promote the development of osteoarthritis through repetitive stress placed on joints supported by weak muscles and stiff tendons. Regular weight-bearing exercise may help prevent osteoarthritis by improving muscle strength, increasing bone density, and reducing obesity. For patients with early arthritis, regular weight-bearing exercise may halt disuse atrophy and stimulate cartilage growth.

STRENGTH TRAINING

A decrease in functional mobility and recurrent falls are associated with the well-documented decline in muscle strength in older people. This age-related muscle weakness may be related to physical inactivity (disuse syndrome), nutri-

tionally inadequate diet, comorbid disease, and the biologic aging process. Several clinical trials of healthy, community-dwelling men and women under 80 years of age have reported increases of 17 to 72% over baseline maximum isometric strength after 6 weeks of static exercise (30). Recently, significant gains in muscle strength and mass were noted in a group of frail institutionalized nonagenarians (31). However, a long-term program of strength training appears to be necessary to sustain improvements in muscle function. Strength training appears to be well accepted by both men and women and to date has proven to be a safe intervention with appropriate supervision.

COMPLIANCE

Patient dropout rates as high as 50% from recommended exercise programs have been documented (32). Studies have shown that patients are more likely to participate in such a program if advised to do so by their physicians. Defining clearly the expected health benefits of exercise, such as lowering blood pressure or improving strength, will improve compliance. Older individuals are also more likely to participate in activities that easily fit into their daily schedule. Any proposed activity that requires transportation, someone to exercise with, special equipment, or high cost will limit participation. Regular, stepwise, low-level exercise is preferable to infrequent bouts of strenuous physical activity. Encouragement by the physician or staff members by telephone contact at biweekly or monthly intervals may be useful. A 6-month and 1-year visit to assess improvement in fitness is encouraged.

SUMMARY

Regular physical exercise has beneficial effects on many of the chronic diseases that burden the elderly. In addition, aerobic exercise reduces morbidity and mortality from cardiovascular disease, the primary cause of death for older men and women in the United States. A combined program of aerobic and strength training has great potential for preventing the functional decline associated with aging and preserving an active, independent lifestyle for older people.

REFERENCES

1. Schoenborn CA. Health habits of U.S. adults: the "Alamed 7" revisited. Public Health Rep 1986; 101:571–580.
2. Stephens T, Jacobs DR, White CC. A descriptive epidemiology of leisure-time physical activity. Public Health Rep 1985;100:147–158.

3. King AC, Blair SN, Bild DE, et al. Determinants of physical activity and interventions in adults. Med Sci Sports Exerc 1992;24:5221–5236.

4. Blair SN, Kohn LW III, Gordon NF. How much physical activity is good for health? Annu Rev Publ Health 1992;13:99–126.

5. Harris SS, Caspersen CJ, DeFriese GH, Estes H. Physical activity counseling for healthy adults as a primary preventive intervention in the clinical setting. JAMA 1989;261:3590–3598.

6. Paffenbarger RS Jr, Hyde RT, Wing AL, Hsieh CC. Physical activity, all-cause mortality and longevity of college alumni. N Engl J Med 1986;314:605–613.

7. Morris JN, Everitt MG, Pollard R, Chave SPW, Semmence AM. Vigorous exercise in leisure-time: protection against coronary heart disease. Lancet 1980;2:1207–1210.

8. Leon AS, Connett J, Jacobs DR Jr, Rauramaa R. Leisure-time physical activity levels and risk of coronary heart disease and death: the Multiple Risk Factor Intervention Trial. JAMA 1987;258:2388–2395.

9. Slattery ML, Jacobs DR Jr, Nichaman MZ. Leisure-time physical activity and coronary heart disease death: the U.S. Railroad Study. Circulation 1989; 79:304–311.

10. Lakka TA, Venalainen JM, Rauramaa R, Salonen R, Tuomilehto J, Salonen JT. Relation of leisure-time physical activity and cardiorespiratory fitness to the risk of acute myocardial infarction in men. N Engl J Med 1994;330:1549–1554.

11. Gordon NF, Scott CB, Wilkinson WJ, Duncan JJ, Blair SN. Exercise and mild essential hypertension. Recommendations for adults. Sports Med 1990; 10:390–404.

12. Hagberg JM. Exercise, fitness, and hypertension. In: Bouchard C, Shephard RJ, Stephens T, Sutton J, McPherson B, eds. Exercise, fitness, and health. A consensus of current knowledge. Champaign, IL: Human Kinetics 1990:445–466.

13. Duncan, JJ, Farr JE, Upton J, Hagan RD, Oglesby ME, Blair SN. The effects of aerobic exercise on plasma catecholamines and blood pressure in patients with mild essential hypertension. JAMA 1985;254:2609–2613.

14. Helmrich SP, Ragland DR, Leung RW, Paffenbarger RS. Physical activity and reduced occurrence of non-insulin dependent diabetes mellitus. N Engl J Med 1991;325:147–152.

15. King P, Hirshman M, Horton Ed, Horton ES. Glucose transport in skeletal muscle membrane vesicles from control and exercised rats. Am J Physiol 1989;257:C1128–1138.

16. Despres J-P, Tremblay A, Nadeau A, Bouchard C. Physical training and changes in regional adipose tissue distribution. Acta Med Scand 1988; 723(suppl):205–212.

17. Snow-Harter C, Marcus R. Exercise, bone mineral density and osteoporosis. In: Holloszy JO, ed. Exercise and sport sciences reviews. Baltimore: Williams & Wilkins, 1991;19:351–388.

18. Hughes JR. Psychological effects of habitual aerobic exercise: a critical review. Prev Med 1984;13:66–78.

19. Fleg JL, Goldberg AP. Exercise in older people: cardiovascular and metabolic adaptations. In: Hazzard WR, Andres R, Bierman EL, Blass JP, eds. Principles of geriatric medicine and gerontology. 2nd ed. New York: McGraw-Hill, 1989:85–100.

20. Kligman EW, Pepin E. Prescribing physical activity for older patients. Geriatrics 1991;47(8):33–47.

21. Bruce RA. Exercise testing of patients with coronary artery disease. Principles and normal standards for evaluation. Ann Clin Res 1971;3:323–332.

22. American College of Sports Medicine. Guidelines for exercise testing and prescription. 4th ed. Philadelphia: Lea & Febiger, 1991:314.

23. DeBusk RF, Stenestrand U, Sheehan M, Haskell WL. Training effects of long versus short bouts of exercise in healthy subjects. Am J Cardiol 1990; 65:101–113.

24. Johnson RJ. Sudden death during exercise. Postgrad Med 1992;92:195–206.

25. Pollack ML, Carroll JF, Graves JE, et al. Injuries and adherence to walk/jog and resistance training programs in the elderly. Med Sci Sports Exerc 1991; 2:1194–1200.

26. Matheson GO, McIntyre JG, Taunton JE, Clement DB, Lloyd-Smith R. Musculoskeletal injuries associated with physical activity in older adults. Med Sci Sports Exerc 1989;21:379–385.

27. Thompson PD. Cardiovascular hazards of physical activity. Exerc Sport Sci Rev 1982;10:208–235.

28. Panush RS, Stemmed C, Caldwell JR, et al. Is running associated with degenerative joint disease? JAMA 1986;255:1152–1154.

29. Lane NE, Bloch DA, Hubert HB, et al. Running, osteoarthritis and bone density: initial 2-year longitudinal study. Am J Med 1990;88:452–459.

30. Nichols JF, Omize DK, Peterson KK, Nelson KP. Efficacy of heavy-resistance training for active women over sixty: muscular strength, body composition, and program adherence. J Am Geriatr Soc 1993;41:205–210.

31. Fiatarone MA, Marks EC, Ryan ND, Meredith CN, Lipsitz L, Evans WJ. High-intensity strength training in nonagenarians:effects on skeletal muscle. JAMA 1990;263:3029–3034.

32. Buskirk ER. Exercise, fitness, and aging. In: Bouchard C, Shepard RJ, Stephens T, Sutton J, McPherson B, eds. Exercise, fitness, and health. A consensus of current knowledge. Champaign, IL: Human Kinetics 1990:687–695.

9/ Thromboembolism in the Elderly

Harold J. Welch, Thomas F. O'Donnell, Jr.

The elderly are particularly susceptible to thromboembolic disease commonly seen in hospitalized patients. Often compromised by chronic medical and surgical illnesses, they frequently have little reserve to compensate for the acute cardiorespiratory insult inflicted by a pulmonary embolus (PE). Older patients with long-standing chronic venous insufficiency as a result of deep vein thrombosis (DVT) have significant problems in caring for their swollen, ulcerated lower limbs. This may be due to severe peripheral arterial disease or generalized debilitation preventing the wearing of elastic compression stockings, cardiorespiratory disease preventing the elevation of the legs, or the social problems prevalent in the older population.

It is estimated that there are 600,000 cases of PE per year in the United States and approximately 200,000 deaths directly attributable to PE. Clinically significant PE are usually from the iliac, femoral, or pelvic veins. Unfortunately, the diagnosis of DVT is made in less than half of patients before their PE. Primarily because DVT is often silent and PE often fatal, emphasis must be placed on prevention, especially in the high-risk elderly patient.

ETIOLOGY

The basic etiologic factors in venous thrombosis originally described by Virchow in 1856 are still pertinent today. Those factors are (a) stasis of blood flow, (b) injury to the vessel wall and (c) hypercoagulable state of blood (1). Thrombus formation usually originates in a valve cusp sinus where eddy currents produce relative stasis. This thrombus is primarily composed of fibrin and red blood cells, and thus this "red clot" differs from the "white clot" composed of platelets and fibrin typically seen in arterial thrombosis.

Clot formation is a result of many complex reactions between the blood and vessel wall. The intrinsic clotting pathway is initiated when the blood contacts a nonendothelial surface, resulting

in activation of factor XII. The extrinsic pathway is stimulated when tissue thromboplastins are released by injured cells. Platelets are activated to adhere and aggregate by several complex reactions. The vascular endothelium, a heterogeneous, actively functioning surface, normally prevents thrombus formation, through the action of heparinoids and prostaglandin, but actively participates in thrombogenesis when stimulated to do so.

STASIS

Stasis of blood alone does not cause clotting when blood is in contact with normal endothelium. However, a localized hypercoagulable state occurs in static blood secondary to the accumulation of activated coagulation factors and the incapacity of the blood to mix inhibitors of the activated coagulation factors. Stasis results from immobility and/or obstruction to blood flow, situations frequently seen in the elderly. Inactivity due to infirmity or poor muscle function promotes stasis in the older patient (2), but more commonly, immobilization results from chronic illness, postoperative state, orthopedic traction, stroke, or obesity. The effect of immobilization is illustrated by the fact that limbs paralyzed by stroke have a four to nine times higher rate of DVT than nonaffected limbs, while lower extremities in paraplegic patients have an equal risk of DVT (3, 4).

Obstruction to blood flow can be extrinsic or intrinsic. Extraluminal compression by tumors, lymph nodes, hematomas, and large aortic aneurysms can result in stasis. Intrinsic obstruction may be the result of a previous thrombus, an intraluminal web, or a tumor invading the vein, such as a clear cell renal cancer. Indwelling venous catheters can cause partial obstruction but are more likely to serve as a nidus for thrombosis. Patients with congestive heart failure and elevated venous back pressures will have decreased peripheral venous flow, a common problem in the elderly. Chronic venous insufficiency with its attendant venous reflux, poor muscle pump function, and venous pooling also contribute to venous stasis. Increased blood viscosity, seen in patients with polycythemia vera, dysproteinemias, and erythrocytosis may result in decreased venous flow. Anesthesia and surgery results in significantly decreased flow in the iliofemoral venous system.

VESSEL WALL INJURY

Endothelial injury occurs with extraluminal forces and intraluminal irritants. The former include twisting and stretching often seen in hip and knee surgery and thermal injury resulting from electrocoagulation or the acrylic glue used in total joint replacement, frequent procedures in the aged. Agents that can damage the endothelium include contrast agents, chemotherapeutic drugs, and circulating immune complexes. Injured endothelium exposes the subendothelial collagen to circulating blood, which initiates clotting via platelet adhesion and recruitment, in addition to activating the extrinsic and intrinsic coagulation systems.

HYPERCOAGULABLE STATES

While the primary hypercoagulable states are usually inherited, deficiencies of certain factors can be acquired. Patients with inherited deficiencies of protein C, protein S, antithrombin III, heparin cofactor II, plasminogen, and other factors are commonly afflicted with thrombotic episodes prior to age 50. Acquired deficiencies are seen in hepatic failure, nephrotic syndrome and chronic renal failure, shock, and disseminated intravascular coagulation (DIC).

Secondary hypercoagulable states are seen with surgery and trauma, pregnancy and oral contraceptive use, sepsis, heart failure, obesity, and malignancy. Tumor cells from the breast, colon and vagina can produce factor X activation, while multiple myeloma, mucin-secreting adenocarcinoma, and promyleocytic leukemia cells secrete tissue thromboplastin. Many cancer patients will have decreased fibrinolytic activity with low levels of antithrombin III and increased concentrations of fibrinogen, and factors V, VIII, IX, and X. These patients will frequently develop superficial vein thrombosis, venous thrombosis in unusual locations, and thrombosis resistant to anticoagulant therapy.

As the preceding sections have illustrated, the geriatric patient is at higher risk for thromboembolism because of several possible mechanisms, although definite etiologies have yet to be identified. The decreased fibrinolytic activity and

venous dilation seen in the elderly, in conjunction with decreased mobility and associated disease states, all contribute to the higher incidence of venous thrombosis.

DIAGNOSIS

Any patient with a swollen extremity should be suspected of having a deep venous thrombosis and evaluated accordingly. Physical examination is notoriously unreliable in diagnosing DVT. Pain, swelling, and erythema are just as likely to occur in patients without DVT as in those who actually do have a DVT. Additionally, physical findings of swelling, tenderness, and Homan's sign are also likely to be present in those who do not have DVT but have another cause of their symptoms (5). Thus, Homan's sign, or calf pain with dorsiflexion of the foot, the classic historical sign for DVT, is a useless test. The clinician should recognize extensive iliofemoral venous thrombosis that produces phlegmasia cerulea dolens, manifested by prominent swelling, mottling, and cyanosis, which can lead to gangrenous changes and limb loss.

If deep venous thrombosis is suspected, the patient should undergo one of several diagnostic tests, depending on availability (Fig. 9.1). The current test of choice for the diagnosis of DVT is duplex ultrasound scanning. It is readily available, noninvasive, low (if any) risk, provides good evaluation from the tibial/calf veins to the iliac veins as well as the subclavian vein, and is highly accurate when performed by a competent examiner. Disadvantages are that duplex scanning is highly operator dependent, can be time consuming, and is relatively expensive. Another advantage of duplex scanning lies in its ability to define other causes of the patient's symptoms, such as Baker's cyst, aneurysm, abscess, and hematoma.

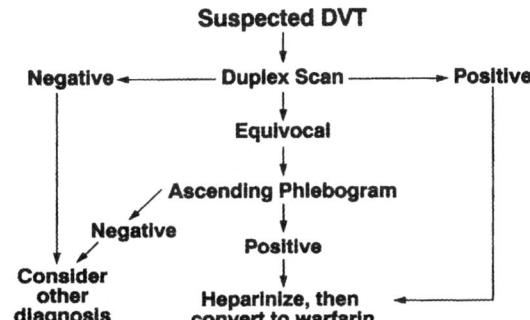

Figure 9.1.   Decision tree in suspected deep vein thrombosis.

By contrast, other noninvasive tests have more limitations. Air plethysmography, impedance plethysmography, and strain-gauge plethysmography are all limited by their ability to accurately diagnose calf and popliteal vein DVT, although they are quite accurate for iliofemoral DVT. A positive plethysmographic study combined with the clinical impression of DVT should provide the basis for treatment. Previously, many studies were done with ^{125}I-labeled fibrinogen, but this test is poor in diagnosing proximal DVT and takes 36 to 48 hours to perform, thus it is rarely used today in clinical situations.

Ascending phlebography is the "gold standard" for the diagnosis of DVT, but it is invasive and not without risk. The injected contrast material may cause an allergic reaction, renal failure, or thrombophlebitis. If the duplex scan is equivocal or unavailable, then phlebography should obtained, but it is no longer the test of choice.

PE is suspected in any patient at risk for DVT and who exhibits dyspnea, tachypnea, tachycardia, or hypoxia on arterial blood gas examination. A chest x-ray and electrocardiogram are often normal after an acute PE, although some changes may be present. If PE is considered, then the patient should undergo either a ventilation/perfusion (V/Q) scan or a pulmonary arteriogram. Clinical impression and a high-probability V/Q scan are fairly accurate in diagnosing a PE, just as a normal scan is in excluding a PE (6). With an indeterminant V/Q scan and an equivocal clinical picture, the clinician must decide to treat or proceed with the gold standard diagnostic test, i.e., pulmonary arteriography. This decision must be determined by the patient's ability to undergo pulmonary arteriography versus the risks of anticoagulation. If the patient is stable enough to have a pulmonary arteriogram and the decision between anticoagulation or a caval filter must be made, then the patient should proceed directly to arteriography. If the arteriogram is positive for PE, the patient can have a filter placed at the same time, if necessary.

MANAGEMENT

Patients presenting with a swollen, tender extremity who are at high risk for DVT should immediately be started on heparin if there are no contraindications (Table 9.1). A delay in diagnostic testing would mean a delay in treatment for those patients who truly have DVT, while there is little risk for a few hours of heparin, which can be stopped if the diagnosis is not a DVT. Anticoagulant treatment for isolated calf vein DVT in

Table 9.1
Contraindications for Heparinization

Relative	Absolute
Thrombocytopenia	Recent CNS, eye surgery (6 weeks)
Bleeding diatheses	Heparin sensitivity
Gastrointestinal ulceration	Major surgery within 48 hours
Severe hypertension	
History of cerebral bleeding	
Recent major surgery	
Recent major trauma	

the outpatient is controversial. Some advocate full treatment with heparin and warfarin (7), whereas others advise frequent duplex scanning with treatment only for evidence of proximal clot propagation (8). We feel treatment is reasonable in a patient with low risk for bleeding, to prevent postthrombotic damage to the critical popliteal and calf vein valves.

After drawing a baseline prothrombin time (PT), partial thromboplastin time (PTT), and platelet count, initial treatment for DVT is an intravenous bolus of 75 to 100 units per kilogram of heparin, followed by a continuous intravenous drip through an infusion pump at 1000 units per hour. Four hours after the initial bolus, a repeat PTT is checked and the heparin infusion adjusted to obtain a PTT level approximately two times normal. Patients are kept at bed rest with leg elevation for 3 to 5 days. Warfarin sodium is usually given to those who can take oral medication on the second or third day of treatment at an initial dose of 10 mg, although some start warfarin simultaneously with heparin therapy.

Thromboplastin reagents used to measure the PT have different sensitivities; those sensitivities are compared to a standard reference thromboplastin by the International Sensitivity Index (ISI). Although not adopted by many North American institutions, the International Normalized Ratio (INR) system correlates the measured PT with the ISI of the particular thromboplastin reagent. Thus, after initiation of warfarin therapy, PTs are measured daily until the proper level of anticoagulation is reached. For DVT or PE, that level is an INR of 2.0 to 3.0, or 1.3 to 1.5 times control using North American thromboplastin.

Heparin therapy is maintained until the PT is therapeutic, which usually takes 3 to 10 days. The patient can be discharged when the symptoms subside, and the PT is monitored twice weekly until a stable warfarin dose is determined, after which the PT is checked less frequently. Warfarin therapy is maintained for 3 months; longer treatment has shown increased risk of bleeding without decreasing the recurrence of DVT or prevention of PE. Long-term anticoagulant therapy is indicated for patients with hypercoagulable conditions or at high risk for recurrent thrombosis.

Thrombolytic therapy is indicated for extensive thrombosis of the iliofemoral system. These patients are monitored in an intensive care unit or on a ward experienced with lytic therapy in conjunction with a vascular specialist or hematologist. While thrombolytic therapy has been shown to decrease the incidence of postthrombotic changes in several prospective studies, very few patients with DVT are eligible for lytic therapy. Most patients with DVT have a contraindication for thrombolytic therapy, primarily recent surgery. Those patients undergoing thrombolytic therapy are at risk for bleeding, particularly the elderly. Surgical thrombectomy is considered in patients with iliofemoral and/or inferior vena cava thrombosis who develop phlegmasia cerulea dolens or venous gangrene.

The risk of anticoagulant therapy can be considerable, especially in the elderly. The primary risk of bleeding occurs in 7 to 14% of patients (9) and depends on the magnitude and duration of anticoagulation therapy. Age over 65 has been identified as an independent risk factor for major bleeding complications. Anticoagulation therapy should be considered with extreme caution in patients with contraindications or who have a history of falls, alcohol abuse, and poor compliance. Patients deemed unsuitable for anticoagulation therapy should have prophylactic interruption of their inferior vena cava with a percutaneously placed filter, to prevent massive PE. Additional treatment for those unsuitable for heparin and warfarin may include intravenous dextran or oral aspirin and dipyridamole.

If bleeding occurs while on heparin, the infusion should immediately be stopped, and if necessary, the heparin should be reversed with protamine sulfate given intravenously in a dose of 1 mg per 100 units of circulating heparin. Bleeding on warfarin therapy with an elevated PT is treated with infusion of fresh frozen plasma and vitamin K injection. Allergic reactions to heparin occur in less than 5% of cases; cessation of the infusion and symptomatic medical treatment is indicated. Heparin-induced thrombocytopenia (HIT) can result in significant morbidity and mortality, paradoxically with thrombotic events more often than bleeding, and usually manifests with decreased platelet counts approximately 8 days

after the start of heparin. Thus, platelet counts should be checked at least every 2 to 3 days. A decrease to less than 100,000 platelets should preclude testing for HIT, and if positive, cessation of all heparin, including flushes and heparin-coated catheters.

Continued anticoagulation for those patients who require it has been effected with several agents, though experience is limited. Low-molecular-weight heparins and heparinoids have been shown to have lower or no cross-reactivity with the heparin-dependent antiplatelet antibodies. Ilioprost (prostaglandin I_2, prostacyclin) will prevent heparin-induced platelet aggregation and has been successful in preventing HIT upon reexposure to heparin. Dextran, aspirin, and dipyridamole can also be used to prevent platelet aggregation. Hirudin and hirudin fragments, which are thrombin inhibitors, are other promising agents.

Warfarin-induced skin necrosis most often affects middle-aged or elderly women and is manifested initially by local erythema and intense pain, followed within 72 hours by dark, hemorrhagic blisters and skin necrosis. It can occur at any time during warfarin therapy and most often affects areas with ample subcutaneous fat, such as the breasts. The pathophysiologic mechanism is thought to be due to a coagulopathy secondary to depletion of vitamin K–dependent factors. Treatment is not standardized, but cessation of warfarin and initiation of heparin should be performed. Steroids have not proven helpful, but intravenous dextran may be beneficial.

Patients who are not able to receive anticoagulation therapy and those that have a PE while therapeutically anticoagulated should undergo placement of an inferior vena cava filter. Additionally, patients with poor cardiorespiratory reserve, who would not tolerate a PE, should have a filter placed prophylactically. Further indication for cava filter placement includes complications of anticoagulation therapy and those patients who have free floating thrombi. Recent advances in the filters' design have led to easier placement, usually percutaneously via a femoral or jugular approach. The primary complications associated with caval filters are malpositioning of the filter in the wrong location during insertion, and late migration of the filters. Thrombosis of the inferior vena cava occurs from 0 to 18% in late follow-up.

UPPER EXTREMITY DEEP VEIN THROMBOSIS

Thrombosis of the axillary or subclavian vein in the elderly is often secondary to an inciting cause, as opposed to the "effort thrombosis" often seen in younger patients. The most likely cause today is an indwelling central venous catheter serving as a nidus for thrombus formation. Other causes include surgical trauma (mastectomy, axillary dissection), radiation therapy, and infusion of agents injurious to the venous endothelium, such as chemotherapeutic drugs or contrast agents. While PE from upper extremity DVT is rare, it is not impossible, thus these veins must be considered a source for PE if no lower extremity source is identified. Patients usually respond well to treatment of upper extremity DVT, with infrequent sequelae. Treatment consists of anticoagulation with heparin and warfarin, if not contraindicated, and elevation of the arm. Removal of an indwelling catheter on the side of the DVT is also indicated. If symptoms of swelling persist, they can often be alleviated with the use of an elastic compression sleeve.

PREVENTION

Prophylaxis for venous thromboembolism is currently underutilized (10), but with several options available to use in the prevention of DVT, failure to do so is inexcusable, especially in today's medicolegal environment. The simplest method is early mobilization and ambulation when possible. In those patients confined to bed by illness or traction, other methods may be used alone or in combination. Mild elevation of the foot of the bed 10 or 15° helps with venous emptying and preventing stasis. While mild graduated compression stockings have been shown to decrease the incidence of DVT and PE, they must be properly applied and fitted, lest they roll down and act as a superficial tourniquet. The best prophylaxis is afforded with the use of graded pneumatic compression boots that gently squeeze the flow of blood from the ankle to the thigh. In addition to inducing venous flow and preventing stasis, they also increase fibrinolytic activity. Their primary drawback is that many patients regard them as a nuisance, and they end up on the floor at the bedside.

Pharmacologic prophylaxis is very common and proven beneficial especially in the perioperative period. Subcutaneous injections of heparin, 5000 units every 8 or 12 hours, reduces the risk of DVT threefold. The risk of significant bleeding is low with this regimen, but hematomas at the injection sites are not uncommon. Many orthopedic surgeons use low-dose warfarin perioperatively, but there are several disadvantages with this. First, it is harder to reverse if there is bleeding, and secondly, the initiation of warfarin therapy creates a temporary hypercoagulable state because of a relative decrease in circulating protein C. Low-molecular-weight dextran 70 and dextran 40 have also been used to prevent DVT. Dextran is less effective in the prevention of DVT than is heparin, but equally effective in the prevention of PE. It must be used with caution, as there is a small but definite risk of anaphylaxis, and because dextran is a volume expander, it may cause congestive heart failure, especially in the frail, elderly patient. Aspirin has been shown to be ineffective in preventing DVT and PE and should not be used as prophylaxis. While all prophylactic methods with the exception of aspirin decrease the incidence of DVT and PE when used correctly, low-dose heparin therapy is the most effective pharmacologic approach.

REFERENCES

1. Virchow R. Neuer Fall von todlicher Emboli der Lungenarterie. Arch Pathol Anat 1856;10:225.
2. Schina MJ, Neumeyer MM, Healy DA, Atnip RG, Thiele BL. Influence of age on venous physiologic parameters. J Vasc Surg 1993;18:749–752.
3. Warlow C, Ogston D, Douglas AS. Deep vein thrombosis of the legs after strokes. Br Med J 1976; 1:1178–1181.
4. Bors E, Conrad CA, Massell TB. Venous occlusion of the lower extremities in paraplegic patients. Surg Gynecol Obstet 1954;99:451–454.
5. O'Donnell TF, Abbott WM, Athanasoulis CA, Millan VG, Callow AD. Diagnosis of deep venous thrombosis in the outpatient by venography. Surg Gynecol Obstet 1980;150:69–74.
6. The PIOPED Investigators. Value of the ventilation/perfusion scan in acute pulmonary embolus. Results of the prospective investigation of pulmonary embolus diagnosis (PIOPED). JAMA 1990; 263(20):2753–2759.
7. Lohr JM, Kerr TM, Lutter KS, Cranley RD, Spirtoff K, Cranley JJ. Lower extremity calf thrombosis: to treat or not to treat? J Vasc Surg 1991;14:618–623.
8. Solis MM, Ranval TJ, Nix ML, et al. Is anticoagulation indicated for asymptomatic postoperative calf vein thrombosis? J Vasc Surg 1992:16:414–419.
9. Hirsh J. Heparin. N Engl J Med 1991;324:1565–1574.
10. Anderson, FA, Wheeler HB, Goldberg RJ, Hosmer DW, Forcier A, Patwardhan NA. Physician practices in the prevention of venous thromboembolism. Ann Intern Med 1991;115:591–595.

10/ Pulmonary Problems in the Elderly

C.B. Sherman, T. Skovrinski

AGING OF THE LUNG

To begin discussing the major pulmonary diseases of the elderly, an understanding of the expected age-related changes in the respiratory system is necessary. Anatomically, there is diffuse enlargement of the distal airspaces and a reduction in chest wall compliance (1). These alterations are largely responsible for the "normal" decreased expiratory flow rates found in most older individuals. Aging is also associated with loss of cough effectiveness and reduction in mucociliary clearance, both of which may predispose the elderly to recurrent lung infections. Furthermore, decreased lung volumes, increased work of breathing, and mild hypoxemia develop with age.

CHRONIC OBSTRUCTIVE PULMONARY DISEASE (COPD)

ASTHMA

Asthma can be defined as reversible airflow obstruction. The disease is a common problem in the elderly. The prevalence of active asthma or persistent wheezing in individuals 65 to 74 years of age is nearly twice that in teenagers (10.4% vs. 5.7%, respectively) (2). Morbidity and mortality rates also appear to be much greater in those over the age of 65 years than in younger asthmatics (3).

The above rates for asthma may underestimate the problem because the disease often goes unrecognized and/or undertreated once diagnosed in the elderly. The tendency of older patients to attribute respiratory symptoms, especially cough, wheeze, and shortness of breath, to aging alone may partially explain the underreporting. Moreover, physicians often confuse asthma with other common diseases of the aged such as chronic bronchitis, emphysema, heart failure, aspiration pneumonia, and tracheobronchial tumors. Furthermore, clinicians are still reluctant to use standard asthma therapy in the old because of presumed but unproven greater side effects.

Elderly asthmatics differ from their younger counterparts in several ways. Although the severity of disease appears to be the same, the aged, in general, report fewer respiratory symptoms and less family or personal history of atopy (4). Typically, an older asthmatic will complain of recurrent episodes of shortness of breath rather than cough or episodic wheezing, the more common symptoms of younger asthmatics. Elderly asthmatics also tend to require more continuous treatment of their disease and are less likely to experience complete disease remission (5).

The physical examination and laboratory findings are similar among all asthmatics, regardless of age. Wheezing is usually heard on lung auscultation. Pulmonary function testing frequently demonstrates air trapping with mild airflow obstruction, partially reversing with bronchodilator administration. Expiratory flow measures (FEV_1 and FEF_{25-75}) may be markedly reduced if chronic bronchitis or emphysema are concurrently present. The elderly are capable of performing methacholine challenge testing and should undergo such testing if baseline lung function is normal and clinical suspicion of asthma exists. Chest roentgenography typically shows hyperinflation but is otherwise normal.

Treatment of asthma in the elderly is similar to the therapy recommended for younger asthmatic groups. Inhaled or oral steroids remain the mainstay of therapy; however oral steroids are reserved for those individuals with more severe disease. Second-line drugs include inhaled anticholinergic agents (e.g., ipratroprium bromide) and inhaled or oral long-acting β-2 selective agonists (e.g., albuterol). Since β-receptor function declines with age (6), anticholinergic therapy may be preferred. Theophylline, once the only medication available for airflow obstruction, has a limited role in asthma management in the elderly. In this age group, theophylline is an exceeding difficult drug to manage because of its reduced metabolic clearance and numerous potential drug interactions.

Specific modifications of this treatment plan are often required for the elderly. Written lists of medications and dosing schedules and the use of less expensive medications are necessary to ensure compliance. The use of a spacer device with all metered dose inhalers (MDIs) is important to maximize the effectiveness of the inhaled medications. At times, because of concurrent diseases, especially arthritis, the aged may not be able to use an MDI at all and must rely on nebulizer therapy. Proper attention to anxiety and depression is paramount, since emotional instability may lead to disease denial and undermedication or overuse of medication.

CHRONIC BRONCHITIS/EMPHYSEMA

Chronic bronchitis is clinically defined as cough and phlegm production for 3 months of the year for 2 consecutive years. The pathophysiological changes include mucous gland hypertrophy and excess mucus secretions, which often lead to mechanical obstruction of the distal airways. Emphysema is a pathological diagnosis, confirmed by findings of destruction of the alveolar-capillary network as well as dilation of distal airways. Cigarette smoking remains the most important risk factor for developing these obstructive lung diseases.

The prevalence of chronic bronchitis and emphysema increases with age and can be explained by several factors. Cumulative pack-years for those elderly who smoke cigarettes may reach considerable magnitude by the sixth or seventh decade of life. Furthermore, the aged often have lifelong exposures to other COPD risk factors, including air pollution and environmental tobacco smoke. Epidemiologic studies have shown that lung function declines with age, starting around the age of 30, and therefore individuals over the age of 65 are more susceptible to the effects of these risk factors, because of less lung reserve.

As seen in asthma, chronic bronchitis and emphysema are often underdiagnosed in the elderly. At times, both physicians and their elderly patients incorrectly assume that respiratory symptoms are caused by aging alone. Also, secondary symptoms of weight loss and fatigue, more common in patients with COPD than other chronic diseases, may be attributed solely to depression. The diagnosis of these diseases is readily made, however, by finding spirometric reductions in the FEV1/FVC ratio ($<70\%$) or in midexpiratory flow ($<65\%$ of predicted) in association with cough, phlegm production, or dyspnea and hyperinflation on chest roentgenography. Of course, mild con-

gestive heart failure, acute or subacute respiratory infections (especially occult aspiration), and anxiety disorders can mimic the symptoms of chronic bronchitis or emphysema.

Management of COPD in the elderly takes a multistep approach. Smoking cessation is essential. Older smokers who stop have been shown to have reduced risk of mortality not only from COPD but also from myocardial infarction and smoking-related cancers (7). The nicotine patch technique is promising as a cessation tool; however, the elderly may be prone to myocardial ischemia with higher doses of the nicotine patch and therefore require more monitoring than their younger smoking counterparts. Unlike in asthma, long-acting β-2 selective agonists and anticholinergic agents are the mainstay of bronchodilator therapy and should be administered using an MDI and spacer device. Again, nebulizer therapy may be required in certain elderly individuals who are unable to use the MDIs. Inhaled steroids are useful if a bronchospastic component has been identified. Theophylline may be helpful in those elderly patients with severe airflow obstruction and resultant respiratory muscle dysfunction, since studies have shown a beneficial effect on diaphragmatic function. However, side effects of tremor, nausea, palpitations, and agitation limit the use of theophylline in the aged. Supplemental oxygen is mandatory to prevent cor pulmonale in patients with $PaO_2 < 55$ mm Hg or oxygen saturation $< 88\%$ at rest.

In addition to these medications, clinicians need to focus on other aspects of care. Good nutrition is essential in maintaining respiratory mechanics and preventing respiratory infection. Exercise is important to safeguard against deconditioning, which may further limit functional capacity in the elderly with obstructive lung disease. Finally, older patients with COPD should receive the pneumococcal vaccine and yearly influenza vaccinations, unless contraindicated by previous reactions or other comorbid conditions.

PNEUMONIA

Pneumonia is still one of the leading causes of death in the elderly (8). Persons over 65 years of age are particularly vulnerable to this infectious process since they often have ineffective immunologic responses, loss of cough effectiveness, and reduction in mucociliary clearance. In addition, the severity of disease is usually increased in the aged because of coexisting illnesses such as COPD, cerebrovascular disease, and malignancy (9).

The diagnosis of pneumonia may be quite elusive in older patients. The cardinal manifestations of pneumonia (i.e., fever, cough, and chest pain) may be absent, and mental confusion, malaise, or general deterioration may be the only clues to the diagnosis. Also, the elderly may not fully cooperate during auscultation of the lungs; therefore, an elevated respiratory rate, tachycardia, or hypotension may be the only pertinent findings on physical examination. The aged may fail to show distinct infiltrates on a chest radiograph because of preexisting lung disease and may not be able to mobilize any sputum, further complicating the clinical evaluation. Furthermore, clinical features of malignancy, congestive heart failure, and pulmonary embolism can often mimic those of pneumonia in this age group. Therefore, those caring for the elderly must maintain a high index of suspicion to make the diagnosis of pneumonia.

Chest roentgenography and examination of sputum remain the two most important diagnostic studies for pneumonia in the elderly. No radiographic pattern is sufficiently specific to establish a diagnosis; however, some roentgenographic findings are more frequently associated with certain pathogens. For example, segmental or lobar consolidation, cavitation, and/or ipsilateral effusions suggest infections with *Streptococcus pneumoniae*, Staphylococcus aureus or *Haemophilus influenzae*, whereas a diffuse reticulonodular interstitial appearance is more often seen with "atypical" pneumonias due to respiratory viruses, *Mycoplasma pneumoniae*, or *Legionella pneumophila*.

When appropriately collected, stained, and examined, sputum samples have a high degree of diagnostic accuracy. Finding fewer than 5 squamous epithelial cells/high power field, more than 25 leukocytes/high power field, and characteristic alveolar macrophages confirms that the specimen is adequate for analysis (10). *S. pneumoniae* is identified on sputum examination as lancet-shaped Gram-positive diplococci, *S. aureus* as clusters of Gram-positive cocci, *H. influenzae* as pleomorphic pale-staining Gram-negative rods, and *Klebsiella pneumoniae, Escherichia coli,* or *Pseudomonas aeruginosa* as large Gram-negative rods. The Ziehl-Nielsen stain can identify up to 40% of cases of active pulmonary tuberculosis, whereas direct fluorescent antibody (DFA) tests can locate Legionella species in sputum specimens. Blood and sputum cultures may be used to verify the initial microscopic sputum impression and help determine antibiotic susceptibilities.

When expectorated sputum is not readily available for analysis, nasotracheal suctioning or sputum induction using aerosolized hypertonic saline may be used. Other, more invasive studies that can be undertaken for specimen retrieval include fiberoptic bronchoscopy combined with lavage, brushing, and endo- or transbronchial biopsies, CT-guided percutaneous needle aspiration of the pulmonary parenchyma, or open lung biopsy, either by thoracoscopy or limited thoracotomy. When dealing with the more common pneumonias, these invasive procedures are rarely indicated in the geriatric population.

In general, therapy for pneumonia in the aged consists of administering appropriate antibiotics, providing adequate hydration, using supplemental oxygenation, and instituting chest physiotherapy and postural drainage when sputum mobilization is ineffective. Important treatment errors to avoid in the elderly include providing inadequate nutritional support, suppressing respiratory efforts with sedatives and hypnotics, and overly aggressive fluid administration resulting in pulmonary edema, especially in those with concurrent cardiovascular disease.

The clinician can be guided in antibiotic choice by the origins of the pneumonia (e.g., community acquired, hospital or institutionally acquired, or aspiration induced) because the types of pathogens found in each group vary greatly. Far and away the most frequent cause of community-acquired pneumonia in the elderly is *S. pneumoniae*, which readily responds to penicillin therapy. The second most common cause is *H. influenzae*, which is effectively treated with ampicillin or cefuroxime if β-lactamase-producing strains are suspected. Less common community-acquired pathogens include *Moraxella catarrhalis* and *S. aureus*, which also respond to cefuroxime, and *L. pneumophila* and *M. pneumoniae*, which are effectively treated with erythromycin. Gastrointestinal distress and the fluid load required to give erythromycin make the newer azithromycin and clarithromycin appealing alternative therapies.

Hospitalized elderly, especially those requiring intensive care settings, are prone to develop pneumonias caused by Gram-negative organisms such as *Klebsiella* spp., *E. coli*, *Proteus mirabilis*, and *Pseudomonas aeruginosa*. Mixed infections with aerobic and anaerobic organisms are also seen, especially in patients known to aspirate. Residents of extended-care facilities are also prone to Gram-negative infections. The preferred treatment for hospital or institutionally acquired pneumonias is a broad-spectrum penicillin such as mezlocillin or piperacillin. Imipenem or a third-generation cephalosporin is a reasonable alternative. An aminoglycoside should be added if there is a strong suspicion of pseudomonas pneumonia, despite the increased risk of nephrotoxicity in the elderly. Peak and trough serum levels of the aminoglycoside must be obtained to avoid renal injury.

The elderly are also at risk for aspiration pneumonia because they often have medical conditions that impair consciousness or interfere with swallowing mechanisms. Typically, the course of this type of pneumonia is indolent and a mixture of anaerobic and aerobic pathogens is involved, including bacteroides, fusiform species, streptococci, and S. aureus (11). Expectorated sputum may not be reliable to establish the microbiologic etiology of the infection, because of oral contamination. Nonetheless, most patients do well with cefoxitin or clindamycin treatment directed against the usual anaerobic organisms and staphylococci.

A special case of aspiration pneumonia worthy of mention is lipoid pneumonia, which is the result of chronic aspiration of lipid-based substances. The elderly are particularly prone to this type of pneumonia because of their excessive use of mineral oil for chronic constipation and their proclivity for esophageal dysfunction. A history of exposure to oil-based substances and findings on sputum analysis of lipid-laden macrophages or sudan stain–positive material confirm the diagnosis. Prevention remains the mainstay of management.

INFLUENZA

Influenza and tuberculosis are particularly devastating illnesses in the elderly and deserve special mention. Influenza pneumonia often occurs in community epidemics, developing 1 to 2 days after the onset of flulike symptoms. Secondary pneumonias caused by S. pneumonieae or S. aureus commonly follow an influenza infection. Major clinical features of influenza pneumonia include dry cough, dyspnea, malaise, and lack of signs of consolidation on physical examination. The chest radiograph often shows perihilar interstitial infiltrates, but these findings are nonspecific. A presumptive diagnosis may be made on the basis of the clinical presentation and the epidemiologic setting. Viral isolation or serological confirmation is required for precise diagnosis, but the results of these tests are rarely available in time to be of clinical value.

Treatment for influenza pneumonia consists mainly of supportive measures and therapy for any concurrent bacterial infection. There are newer antiviral agents available (e.g., amantadine and aerosolized ribavirin) that can modify the course of the illness in select patients. The influenza vaccine remains the most effective method for reducing the incidence of pneumonia and is recommended for all persons over the age of 65 years.

TUBERCULOSIS

Newly acquired pulmonary tuberculosis or reactivation of previous disease is rapidly becoming a significant public health problem in those over 65 years of age, especially for individuals living in nursing homes (12). *Mycobacterium tuberculosis* is transmitted by the respiratory route from an actively infected person with pulmonary tuberculosis to a susceptible host not previously infected with the organism. Primary infection usually is manifested only by the development of a positive tuberculin skin test. Occasionally the patient develops clinical evidence of disease (e.g., fever, nonproductive cough, and infiltrates on chest radiograph). Pleurisy with effusion is a less common manifestation of primary tuberculosis. Primary infection is usually self-limited, but hematogenous dissemination seeds multiple organs, and latent foci are established which may become sites for delayed reactivation.

Overall, 5 to 15% of infected, but not ill, individuals will develop overt disease at some time in their lives. The elderly are particularly susceptible because they often have underlying diseases that depress the cellular immune response. Reactivation begins insidiously with night sweats or chills and fatigue. Physical examination may be unremarkable or may show dullness and rales in the upper lung fields, occasionally with amphoric breath sounds. Chest radiographs may show infiltrates in the posterior segment of the upper lobes or apical segments of the lower lobes, with or without cavitation.

Active tuberculosis should be treated with at least two drugs (13). The preferred regimen is daily isoniazid, rifampin, and pyrazidamide for 2 months, followed by 4 months of isoniazid and rifampin. A 9-month regimen of isoniazid and rifampin can also be effective. These drugs can be supplemented with ethambutol or other agents, depending on the severity of illness and likelihood of isoniazid- and rifampin-resistant strains. Close monitoring for drug toxicity in the elderly is especially important.

INTERSTITIAL FIBROSIS

Interstitial fibrosis is a condition characterized by inflammation of the alveolar walls, associated with progressive fibrosis of the interstitium. It may occur as an isolated entity, namely idiopathic pulmonary fibrosis (IPF), or in connection with a number of other diseases, particularly rheumatoid arthritis (RA), systemic lupus erythematosus (SLE), progressive systemic sclerosis (PSS), and Goodpasture's disease (14). In addition, occupational or environmental exposures to inorganic dust (e.g., asbestos, silica, coal dust, and beryllium), organic dust (e.g., wood and grain dusts), or microbial antigens (e.g., thermophilic actinomycetes) can cause parenchymal scarring and restrictive lung disease. Furthermore, many of the medications used by the elderly are also potential causes of interstitial disease (e.g., amiodarone, diphenylhydantoin, nitrofurantoin, sulfonamides, penicillamine, methotrexate, and many of the chemotherapeutic agents). Less common causes of lung fibrosis in this age group include sarcoidosis and chronic eosinophilic pneumonia. Hydrostatic and nonhydrostatic pulmonary edema, viral or "atypical" pneumonias, and lymphangitic spread of malignancy may mimic interstitial fibrosis in their presentation and must be considered.

Nonproductive cough, dyspnea (especially on exertion), and constitutional symptoms of fatigue and weight loss are the most frequent early manifestations of interstitial fibrosis. Fever, if present, is almost always low grade; high-grade fevers should trigger a workup for an infectious cause such as tuberculosis, *Legionella*, or influenza. The presence of dysphagia and Raynaud's syndrome suggest that PSS may be the cause of the interstitial fibrosis. Likewise, arthralgias and photosensitivity should trigger an evaluation for SLE.

On physical examination, clubbing and basilar crackles are the most common findings. Other useful observations include joint swelling (e.g., rheumatoid arthritis), uveitis (e.g., sarcoidosis), and distended neck veins and a summation gallop (e.g., congestive heart failure).

Several studies can be used by the clinician to confirm the diagnosis of interstitial fibrosis. As a first step, a chest roentgenogram should be obtained and compared with previous films, if available. Early in the disease, a ground-glass appearance at the bases is seen; with more advanced disease, honeycombing with thickened alveolar septum and surrounding cystic air spaces is present. In those cases in which the clinical suspicion is great but the chest roentgenogram shows minimal increased interstitial markings, high-resolution chest CT scanning may be useful in confirming the diagnosis.

Pulmonary function testing is most helpful in following the disease course and measuring response to treatment. Reductions in lung volumes, especially total lung capacity and functional residual capacity, with intact flow rates and a normal FEV_1/FVC ratio are characteristic findings. A reduction in the diffusing capacity, a measure of the alveolar-capillary surface area, and oxygen desaturation with exercise are more sensitive markers of early interstitial damage.

Certain other laboratory tests are more helpful in determining the specific disease process responsible for the fibrosis. Serum antibodies to offending antigens, such as pigeon serum or thermophilic actinomycetes, can confirm a diagnosis of hypersensitivity pneumonitis. A positive rheumatoid factor or antinuclear antibody (ANA) is useful in establishing a diagnosis of RA or SLE, respectively. However, caution is needed when interpreting the ANA titer because it rises with age and may also be elevated in association with IPF. An abnormal urinalysis may be found in SLE or Goodpasture's disease.

Bronchoscopy with bronchoalveolar lavage (BAL) and transbronchial biopsy or open lung biopsy may, at times, be necessary to establish the diagnosis. These more invasive tests are particularly important in individuals with clinical progression and a nondiagnostic initial evaluation. Bronchoalveolar lavage and transbronchial biopsy are likely to make the diagnosis of granulomatous diseases, infections, or metastatic tumors to the lung, but they have limited sensitivity for all other potential causes of interstitial fibrosis. Therefore, thoracoscopy, a newer technique in which a fiberoptic instrument is inserted into the pleural cavity, or limited thoracotomy may be required to obtain diagnostic lung tissue.

Treatment encompasses removing the individual from identified causative exposures, using immunosuppressive medications to prevent further interstitial damage, and correcting hypoxemia with supplemental oxygen. Early therapeutic intervention, especially for those elderly with IPF, is currently recommended. Steroids are the mainstay of treatment but have been disappointing in their ability to alter the natural history of many of the interstitial diseases. If steroids are ineffective, cyclophosphamide or azathioprine can be tried, either as single therapy or as part of a regimen including steroids. Individual schedules are necessary in the elderly because of drug side effects. For example, prednisone therapy may aggravate existing osteoporosis, hypertension, diabetes mellitus, and peptic ulcer disease.

LUNG CANCER

Most cases of lung cancer occur in patients over 65 years of age, many of whom are former or current cigarette smokers (15). Major risk factors for bronchogenic carcinoma include cigarette smoking, occupational exposures (e.g., asbestosis, nickel, arsenic), air pollution, idiopathic pulmonary fibrosis, and to a lesser extent, genetic predisposition. Unfortunately, despite intensive research efforts, the overall 5-year survival rate for all patients with lung cancer is currently estimated to be only 13%, compared with 7% in 1963 (16). Thus, prevention through smoking cessation remains the most effective strategy.

Elderly patients with lung cancer usually have symptoms that are caused by the primary tumor or its metastases. Cough is the most common symptom but unfortunately is often attributed to cigarette smoking or aging, thereby delaying the diagnosis. Thus, a change in the character of the cough, especially if hemoptysis is reported, should trigger an evaluation for lung cancer. Other symptoms include a fixed wheeze caused by endobronchial obstruction, dyspnea, chest pain, and/or hoarseness. A much smaller group of patients may present with such diverse symptoms as flushing, diarrhea, or confusion caused by bioactive substances secreted by certain tumors.

The diagnostic workup for individuals suspected of having lung cancer is fairly straightforward. Chest radiographs and chest CT scans are important first tests that can both define the extent of disease and guide the often necessary, more invasive diagnostic procedures. For proximal tumors, bronchoscopy with brushings and biopsy is indicated for tissue confirmation; peripheral lesions are better approached through CT-guided transthoracic needle biopsy. Mediastinoscopy or thoracotomy may be necessary if the aforementioned procedures are nondiagnostic.

Therapy for lung cancer depends on the type and stage of the carcinoma. Surgical resection is the treatment of choice for all stage I or II non–small cell carcinomas, provided that pulmonary function is adequate. Contraindications to surgery include extrathoracic metastatic disease, positive contralateral, mediastinal or suprahilar nodes, malignant pleural effusion, or involvement of the laryngeal nerve. Age alone is *not* a contraindication to surgery. Radiation therapy is used primarily for locally advanced non–small cell carcinomas and for palliation of symptomatic metastasis (e.g., those causing bone pain, hemoptysis, or endobronchial obstruction) (17). Small cell carcinomas are usually treated with chemotherapy, using cisplatin and etoposide. Cyclophosphamide, doxorubicin, and vincristine may also be tried. Cisplatin/etoposide or cisplatin/mitomycin/vinblastine combinations have occasionally been used for advanced non–small cell lung cancers. Side effects to the various chemotherapeutic agents are common in the elderly but can be minimized by close monitoring. Most importantly in the elderly, the aggressiveness of lung cancer treatment must be guided by the patient's concerns for quality of life.

REFERENCES

1. Verbeken EK, Canberghs M, Mertens I, Clement J, Laumeryns JM, Van de Woestijne KP. The senile lung: comparison with normal and emphysematous lungs. Chest 1992;101:800–809.
2. Evans R, Mullally DI, Wilson RW, et al. National trends in the morbidity and mortality of asthma in the US. Chest 1987;91:655–745.
3. Braman SS. Asthma in the elderly patient. Clin Chest Med 1993;14:1–10.
4. Lee HY, Stretton TB. Asthma in the elderly. Br Med J 1972;4:93–95.
5. Braman SS, Corrao WM, Kaemmerlen JT. The clinical outcome of asthma in the elderly: a 7 year follow-up study. Ann NY Acad Sci 1991;629:449–450.
6. Ullah MI, Newman GB, Saunders KB. Influence of age on response to ipratropium and salbutamol in asthma. Thorax 1981;36:523–529.
7. US Department of Health and Human Services. The health benefits of smoking cessation. US Department of Health and Human Services, Public Health Service, Centers for Disease Control, Center for Health Chronic Disease Prevention and Health Promotion, Office on Smoking and Health, 1990, DHHS Publication no. (CDC) 90–8416.
8. Gleckman RA. Pneumonia: update on diagnosis and treatment. Geriatrics 1991;46:49–56.
9. Harrison BDW. Community-acquired pneumonia in adults in British hospitals in 1982–1983: a survey of aetiology, mortality, prognostic factors and outcome. Q J Med 1987; 239:195–220.
10. Baigelman W, Chodosh S. Sputum 'wet preps': window on the airways. J Respir Dis 1984;5:59.
11. DePaso WJ. Aspiration pneumonia. Clin Chest Med 1991;12:269–280.
12. Yoshikawa TT. Tuberculosis in aging adults. J Am Geriatr Soc 1992;42:178–187.
13. Van Scoy RE, Wikowske CJ. Antituberculosis agents. Mayo Clin Proc 1987;62:1129–1136.
14. Young KR, Merrill WW. Interstitial lung diseases in the elderly patient. Clin Geriatr Med 1986;2:385–410.
15. O'Rourke MA, Crawford J. Lung cancer in the elderly. Clin Geriatr Med 1987;3:595–623.
16. List ND. Perspectives in cancer screening in the elderly. Clin Geriatr Med 1987;3:433–445.
17. Shaw EG, Boumer JA, Foote RL, et al. Role of radiation therapy in the management of lung cancer. Mayo Clin Proc 1993;68:593–602.

11/ Peripheral Artery Disease in the Elderly

Adrian S. Dobs

Atherosclerosis in the lower extremity has a peak incidence about 10 years after the development of coronary artery disease (CAD). Thus, peripheral artery disease (PAD) is primarily a disease of the elderly, and as numbers of older individuals increase in both size and proportion, this condition will become an increasingly important medical problem. By the year 2040, the elderly are expected to compose 22% of the United States population, i.e., 67 million will be over the age of 65 years (1).

The development of PAD is commonly associated with loss of mobility and increased dependency, which potentially worsens comorbidities and drains the health care community of resources. While previously the domain of surgeons, advances in the diagnosis and treatment of peripheral artery disease have now placed geriatricians into key roles in the management of PAD patients.

This chapter discusses the clinical diagnosis, epidemiology, pathogenesis, and treatment of PAD. There is particular emphasis on risk factors associated with the development of the disease, to underscore its possible prevention.

CLINICAL DIAGNOSIS

HISTORY

The diagnosis of PAD can often be made on clinical grounds with a routine history and physical examination. Intermittent claudication is characterized by a cramping pain that occurs during walking and is relieved by rest. Calf pain is common with arterial narrowing in the femoropopliteal distribution; buttock, hip, and thigh pain suggests aortoiliac disease. As the stenosis extends more proximally and involves longer segments of vessels, rest pain may begin. A standardized questionnaire developed by Rose for the World Health Organization has been a useful tool in determining the presence of intermittent claudication (2). Many epidemiologic studies of PAD

use the Rose questionnaire as well as the noninvasive procedures discussed below.

The diagnosis can be difficult in an older population, in which many may not exhibit early symptoms of lower extremity atherosclerosis, such as claudicating pain, since they have voluntarily restricted their activity because of other physically related limitations. The incidence of intermittent claudication is greater in those 70 years or younger. Unfortunately, the elderly may present with lower leg numbness, coldness, cyanosis, or pallor, which may progress quickly to ulceration or gangrene. In addition, lower extremity pain can be misdiagnosed as other diseases commonly encountered in elderly patients, i.e., musculosketetal syndromes such as myositis, tendinitis, sciatica, lumbosacral radiculopathy related to canal spinal stenosis, or obliterative arthritis of the lumbosacral vertebrae.

PHYSICAL EXAMINATION

A thorough examination should include palpation of arterial pulses, auscultation for bruits, and observation for trophic signs of ischemia. Mild cases of PAD may be associated with dry, scaly, and shiny atrophic skin; diminished hair growth; thickened, brittle toenails; or subcutaneous atrophy in an extremity, associated with absent or weak arterial pulses. Tendon xanthomas are a sign of hypercholesterolemia.

NONINVASIVE PROCEDURES

New technologies make it possible to diagnose peripheral arterial disease with greater accuracy using noninvasive procedures, thus allowing physicians to assess a patient's condition at an early stage. Noninvasive methods of diagnosis are based upon a physiologic measure of function, rather than an anatomic change. Objective methods involve segmental blood pressure determination in the legs, using Doppler probes. The ankle/brachial index (ABI) has been recommended by the American Heart Association as a simple measure of PAD (3). The ratio can be obtained at the bedside by measuring systolic blood pressures at the arm (brachial artery at the elbow) and ankle (anterior and posterior tibial arteries immediately above the ankle). One problem in the assessment of PAD incidence in the general population, however, is the variance in the procedure for measuring ABI and the interpretation of the results. With a value of 1.0 or greater being normal, many accept <0.8 as mild, <0.6 as moderate, and <0.4 as severe PAD. Hiatt defined abnormal as <0.94 and found ABI a sufficient measure of PAD in a general population (4). An ABI below 0.9 has been shown to be up to 95% sensitive in detecting angiogram-positive disease (5).

This method is even more helpful when used before and after exercise (6, 7). It can be misleading however in the presence of increased collateral circulation, a finding common in patients with diabetes mellitus (DM). Time to relief from claudicating pain or time to reactive hyperemia provides further information (8). Unfortunately, there can be artifactually elevated distal segmental blood pressures in the elderly who have rigid and/or calcified vessels. These high values can cause falsely elevated ABI values, thus obscuring underlying disease. Duplex scanning provides a dynamic functional assessment of flow. This technique is available in most vascular labs. A more direct noninvasive assessment of atherosclerosis, it can verify dynamic blood flow and localize potential areas of stenoses along the major arteries of the legs (9). Another method uses plethysmography, a pressure tracing to estimate volume flow through the distal segments.

As mentioned above, subjects with increased collaterals, such as diabetics, may in fact have a normal ABI. The addition of exercise to the Doppler study adds some sensitivity to the physician's diagnosis. Five minutes on a treadmill at 2.0 mph or the occlusion of arterial blood flow with a blood pressure cuff may provide enough mild metabolic stress to provide objective evidence of ischemic claudication. In addition, one can document the time for the ABI to return to prestress levels in subjects with PAD. A postexercise ABI below 0.73 and a postreactive hyperemia ABI below 0.78 is highly suggestive of disease (4).

In research settings, high-resolution real-time B-mode ultrasound is used to directly measure the thickness of the arterial wall. In a study of 170 individuals, this method accurately detected PAD in symptomatic patients (10). In the Atherosclerosis Risk in Communities (ARIC) Study, popliteal intimal wall thickness was associated with an increased prevalence of CAD (11).

Noninvasive ultrasound measures also have the potential of providing an easily accessible measure of atherosclerosis. Once the technique is standardized, ultrasonography may become an efficient and inexpensive tool to document atherosclerosis.

INVASIVE PROCEDURES

Arteriography of the lower extremities is generally considered the gold standard in the diagnosis of PAD because it produces the most accurate assessment of lumen diameter. It is necessary to document the anatomy in this way if percutaneous angioplasty or bypass surgery is considered (see treatment section). Although generally safe, angiography is an invasive procedure that carries with it, though unlikely, the complications of dye allergy and subsequent renal impairment.

Angiography is limited, however, by the fact that it documents lumen diameter, i.e., blood flow. This procedure fails to provide information on the thickness of the arterial wall or the actual tissue perfusion. In the near future, intimal-medial wall thickness may be measurable using external-beam B-mode ultrasound or intravascular ultrasound during angiography.

PREVALENCE OF DISEASE

The incidence and prevalence of the disease varies profoundly with the criterion used for diagnosis and the population studied. The Rose Questionnaire to identify intermittent claudication is known to underestimate the prevalence of PAD (12, 13). Noninvasive testing detects two to five times more disease than the Rose Questionnaire (13).

The prevalence of intermittent claudication has been reported to be as low as 0.3% in the U.S. population (14) or as high as 14.4% of men in a geriatric health fair program (15). In men and women aged 55 to 74 years, intermittent claudication was observed in 4.5% of those examined (95% confidence interval (CI): 3.5–5.5%). In a middle-aged, Finnish population, 2.1% of men and 1.8% of women reported typical symptoms of intermittent claudication (16). Because general population screening was not feasible until recently, because of the invasive nature of the testing, conclusive epidemiologic studies are still under way. Even with the advent of noninvasive examination correlations to PAD, however, incidence studies are still skewed because most participants in the studies are patients complaining of intermittent pain or discomfort.

Asymptomatic atherosclerosis affecting the lower limbs may be more common in the population than claudication. As mentioned above, this may be particularly true for an older population. In a study conducted in Edinburgh, in subjects 55 to 74 years of age, the prevalence of intermittent claudication was 4.5% (95% CI: 3.5–5.5%). Significant impairment of blood flow in asymptomatic people occurred in 8.0% (95% CI: 6.6–9.4%). In addition, a further 16.6% (95% CI: 14.6–18.5%) in the 55 to 74 group presented with clinically abnormal blood flow (17). Of these, 9% had an ABI <0.9 and 7.6% had reactive hyperemia pressure reduction 20% (17). Thus, actual intermittent claudication is rare compared with asymptomatic disease states.

Using even broader clinical criteria for the diagnosis of PAD, such as decreased pulses, Aronow et al. evaluated the prevalence of PAD in unselected elderly patients, mean age 82 years, in a long-term health care facility. PAD was found in 34% of 244 men and 23% of 625 women ($P < .005$) (18). This corroborated data from a study conducted in Framingham in which the biennial incidence rate was 7.1/1000 men and 3.5/1000 women, i.e., women lagged about 10 years behind men, with a decreasing gap with increasing age (19).

Prevalence of peripheral arterial disease varies significantly with age. In the Basel study, prevalence at age 20 to 24 years was 0.4%, compared with 7.5% in those 60 to 64 years of age (20). The 5-year cumulative incidence was 4% in men 35 to 44 and 18% in those over 65 years (20). In a Danish study, PAD was noted in 14% of 60-year-olds (13). Criqui et al. found similar trends; prevalence rates increased from 3% in those under 60 to over 20% in those 75 and older (12). Using an ankle/brachial systolic blood pressure ratio less than 0.96, half of an elderly population 68 to 92 years of age had lower limb arterial disease (21). Institutionalized elderly are particularly prone to have PAD; 88% of New York nursing home residents had abnormal ABI values, which continued to worsen into the 10th decade (22).

Though intermittent claudication has been observed equally in men and women, there may be a slight preponderance of asymptomatic disease in males (17). Although not all studies concur (16), gender may be another factor determining the epidemiology of PAD. In fact, the disease rarely occurs in young women (20). The male-to-female prevalence ratio in an elderly population was 1.27

(12), with male predominance decreasing with increasing age above 70 years (23).

Thus, while there are correlations between various studies, the actual incidence and prevalence of PAD is difficult to assess at this time because various tests are used with various resulting interpretations. However, the various studies do illustrate the general trends of PAD affliction, such as a variance with age and possibly gender.

PATHOGENESIS

PATHOPHYSIOLOGY

Atherosclerosis is a systemic disease beginning as a raised focal plaque lesion within the intimal layer of the arterial wall (24). Plaques are distributed in a segmental pattern throughout the body, commonly in the aortic bifurcation, the common iliac bifurcation, the common femoral, the popliteal, and the proximal portions of the tibial vessels. Characterization of the injury initiating damage to the arterial wall is unclear. The development of atherosclerosis may begin with endothelial damage, followed by increased uptake of lipids by macrophages, and calcium and fibrin deposition. This can progress to a complicated lesion that can impinge on the lumen and impair blood flow or ulcerate and act as a source for clot formation.

Clinical symptoms arise from alterations in blood flow, caused by the development of stenoses within the arterial lumen or acute blockages from clot formation. Although collateral circulation may help compensate in the larger more proximal arteries, there are relatively few collateral vessels in the more distal vessels, especially the distal popliteal and proximal tibial arteries. Studies show that these vessels are particularly susceptible to damage in diabetics (25).

DISEASE PROGRESSION

Although noninvasive diagnostic methods can detect early changes in blood flow in the lower extremity, clinical disease usually begins with intermittent claudication or cramping pain with walking. This can progress to ischemic rest pain, the development of ulcers, and ultimately, gangrene. Symptoms of intermittent claudication generally occur in one-third of patients with proven arterial stenosis, and only about 25% of claudicants will deteriorate. Therefore, in most situations, PAD can behave as a stable disease (26).

Not surprisingly, the rate of disease progression depends on the presence of other afflictions. Smoking has a major influence on the course of the disease. Joananson and Ringqvist found a stabilization of ABI over a 5-year period in nonsmokers, compared with smokers, who displayed a constant deterioration (27). Furthermore, quitting smoking also reduced the rate of amputation as a treatment of PAD (28).

Although the presence of DM predicts the development of PAD, it may not alter disease progression. In a study evaluating subjects already diagnosed with PAD, disease progression was identical in the diabetic and nondiabetic groups (29).

Diseases in Other Vascular Beds

In most population-based studies of atherosclerosis, the prevalence of disease in different vascular beds is comparable. Subjects with intermittent claudication are several times more likely to have CAD and cerebrovascular disease (CVD) than is the general population (19). Based on history and/or a resting electrocardiogram, subjects with intermittent claudication have a CAD prevalence rate of 35 to 60% (30, 31). By coronary angiography, 90% of patients with PAD had evidence of CAD, with 57% having stenoses 70% (32). In the Edinburgh Artery Study, asymptomatic subjects with evidence of decreased blood flow during noninvasive testing had a relative risk of 1.6 (95% CI: 1.3–1.9) of having evidence of ischemic heart disease, compared with the normal population (17). Interestingly, this study found that in many patients, the ABI was lower in the left leg than the right, suggesting a unilateral predisposition to disease (17).

The correlation between PAD and CVD is less clear. Prevalence rates vary from 0.5 to 56% (33, 34). These differences may be due to methods of diagnosing CVD and/or differences in the study population. Finally, the prevalence of abdominal aortic aneurysms in PAD patients is twice that in the general population (35).

Mortality

PAD is a strong predictor of subsequent mortality. In most studies, symptomatic PAD doubles the mortality risk (16, 36). Not surprisingly, subjects with more severe manifestations of the disease had increased mortality risk. The lower the ABI, the higher the association with increased mortality (37, 36). In subjects with ABI less than 0.85, the relative risk for total mortality associated with PAD was 2.36 (95% CI: 1.6–3.48). Death from any cause was four to five times higher for both men and women compared with controls when PAD was documented with noninvasive methods (26, 12).

As is the case with disease progression, mortality rates in patients with PAD also vary, depending on other comorbidities. Subjects with cardiovascular disease will clearly have increased total mortality. Smoking increases mortality 3-fold in subjects with symptomatic PAD, compared with nonsmokers (16, 17). Diabetes will double the mortality risk (37); hypertension may increase (16) or be unrelated to mortality rates (38). Criqui et al. found no independent relationship between hypertension and subsequent mortality (12).

The specific cause of death for patients afflicted with PAD is usually cardiovascular. The cause of death was a myocardial infarction in 35 to 70% of patients with PAD (37, 12). The risk of death from cardiovascular causes was nearly 3-fold higher in men with claudication than in those without the complaint (16). However after adjusting for coronary heart disease, claudication had no independent effect on mortality in men (16). Other common causes of death include cerebrovascular disease, occurring in 7 to 17%, and ruptured aneurysms or visceral infarction in 10% of subjects (30).

RISK FACTORS

A great deal more research has focused on potential risk factors associated with the development of CAD than that of PAD. Many assume that these same factors would play a role in the pathogenesis of disease in other vascular beds. In fact, data from the Framingham study suggest that the traditional cardiovascular risk factors are stronger predictors of PAD than they are of CAD. One explanation for this observation is that stenosis may be more important in the pathogenesis of PAD than carotid or coronary disease, in which embolization is a major factor (10).

Most early studies dealt with symptomatic forms of the disease (16, 19). More recently, noninvasive methods have been used to evaluate risk factors and their associations with early or asymptomatic disease (13). These studies are crucial because early disease may be more highly correlated with cardiovascular risk factors than with later stages of the PAD, e.g., when there is increased calcification within the atherosclerotic plaque.

Remember, when reviewing risk factors associated with PAD, few studies have specifically looked at the relationship of risk factors in an elderly population. In a study of about 300 subjects ages 68 to 92 years, traditional cardiovascular risk factors predicted PAD, although the associations were weak (21). The risk factors discussed below include gender, smoking, DM, hypertension, hyperlipidemia, clotting factors, and obesity.

Gender Differences

Prevalence data cited above indicate that men are more likely to develop PAD. However, this gap decreases with age; thus elderly women are at increased risk of PAD (19).

Smoking

Cigarette smoking and DM have been strongly associated with PAD. In a 30-year follow-up study of 5080 subjects of the original Framingham study, cigarette smoking, elevated blood sugars, and hypercholesterolemia were associated with intermittent claudication ($P < .001$) (39). Other studies have reported a prevalence rate 2.4 times control for men and 2.9 times for women who had a history of smoking (18). In an elderly population, smoking was strongly associated with those who developed PAD (21). In a population-based study of 10,000 middle-aged individuals, even former smokers had increased arterial intimal-medial wall thickness, compared with those who never smoked (40).

Diabetes Mellitus

Numerous studies have found DM to be a risk factor for PAD. Claudication is 2.4 times more prevalent in men and 3.0 times more prevalent in elderly women who were diabetic than in nondiabetics (18). In addition, foot gangrene was also found 17 times more commonly in diabetics (41). Similarly, a diabetic has a 5- to 6-fold increased likelihood of undergoing an amputation as a treatment for PAD (41).

The reasons for the correlation between DM and PAD are multifactorial. The premature atherosclerosis observed in diabetic subjects has been attributed to hyperlipidemias, hyperinsulinism, and/or glucose toxicity. Hyperlipidemias are very common in diabetes, particularly hypertriglyceridemia and a combined hyperlipidemia with elevations in both serum triglycerides and LDL-C.

Hyperinsulinism is commonly observed in both insulin-treated and non-insulin-treated dependent diabetes. Elevated serum insulin levels have been associated with smooth muscle cell proliferation, hypertension, and atherosclerosis. Recently, hyperinsulinism has been observed as part of a constellation of symptoms, such as abdominal obesity, hypertension, hypertriglyceridemia, and glucose intolerance. This constellation of symptoms has been termed syndrome X (42). To date, there is no documentation that insulin per se is a risk factor for PAD. However, its increased association with cardiovascular risk factors implicates it as a potential pathological factor.

Whether impaired glucose tolerance, as opposed to true DM, is a risk factor for PAD is controversial. The Framingham data suggest it increases the risk for intermittent claudication by as much as 8.6 times (19).

Hypertension

Systolic blood pressures have been correlated with the presence of PAD in several studies. Hypertension was significantly associated with PAD in both elderly men and women (18) and in the Framingham population, with relative risks of 2.5 in men and 3.9 in women (19). In an elderly population, systolic blood pressure was one of the strongest predictors of PAD (21). In the ARIC population, systolic blood pressure does directly predict popliteal artery wall thickness (40). However, hypertension was shown to be an inconsistent predictor of intermittent claudication in a middle-aged Finnish population (43).

Hyperlipidemia

Most studies suggest that changes in serum lipids predict the development of PAD. This has been true in both case-control and longitudinal studies. Elevated serum cholesterol levels predicted claudication in the Framingham and Danish population (13, 19). Similarly, hypercholesterolemia is a risk factor in both elderly men and women (18).

There is debate however on which of the lipoproteins exert the greatest influence. Early thickening in the popliteal wall using ultrasound was associated with elevated serum LDL, total cholesterol, and triglyceride levels in a population-based study of about 10,000 people in the ARIC Study (40). Although not statistically significant, a trend suggested that lower serum HDL levels were associated with increased popliteal wall thickness (40). Others found that HDL levels were inversely correlated with PAD (18, 21, 44, 45).

In contrast, hypertriglyceridemia has been found fairly consistently in risk factor analysis (13, 44), although not in all studies (16, 18). Hyperlipidemias associated with intermediate-density lipoproteins (such as Fredrickson and Levy's type III) have been consistently correlated with an increased frequency of both CAD and PAD (46).

Clotting Factors

Serum fibrinogen (40, 47), hematocrit (47), and blood viscosity (47) have been consistently associated with the presence of PAD in case-control studies. However, this may be confounded by smoking.

Obesity

Weight may be a relatively weak risk factor in the development of PAD, confounded by the presence of DM and/or hyperinsulinism. Obesity was a risk factor for PAD in elderly women, but not men (18). In the Framingham study, Metropolitan Life Insurance relative weight was inversely associated with intermittent claudication in men and was not predictive in women (39). In a population above 68 years of age, body mass index was inversely associated with PAD (21).

TREATMENT

MEDICAL

The mainstay of primary treatment of subjects with PAD has been exercise. Although it is generally accepted that short-term physical training improves walking tolerance, here have been few controlled studies. Of 91 male patients followed over 2.5 years, those who complied with the regimens prescribed showed improvement (48). In a study of nondiabetic patients with occlusive arterial disease, exercise did not have a significant effect on disease progression.

Pharmacological treatment of intermittent claudication has been rather disappointing. Randomized clinical trials have shown some efficacy, such as an increase in pain-free walking time, with compounds that reduce blood viscosity (pentoxifylline) and those that promote vasodilation (nafrdrofuryl, buflomedil, ketanserin) (49). It is not clear how useful these drugs are in long-term studies.

The most promising work involves aggressive use of lipid-lowering drugs. Several studies have reported atherosclerotic regression in the lower extremity after aggressive lipid-lowering therapy. The Cholesterol Lowering Atherosclerosis Study (CLAS) treated hyperlipidemic patients with niacin and a bile acid sequestrant. Using computerized quantitative analysis of coronary and lower extremity angiograms, the authors documented disease regression in both coronary arteries (50) as well as in the femoral artery (51). Although the data are not as conclusive as those for CAD, the National Cholesterol Education Program has advocated aggressive lipid-lowering for subjects with PAD to a serum LDL level $\leq$ 100 mg/dL (52). Lipid-lowering medications are generally well tolerated by both younger and older patients. Very few data are available on the use of lipid-lowering drugs in subjects over 75 years of age. In general, the geriatrician should feel comfortable using any of the commonly used drugs in subjects less than that age. The treatment of older individuals for hyperlipidemias should be based on their risk profile, overall health, and willingness to comply with follow-up.

SURGICAL

It is estimated that reconstructive surgery to improve blood flow is performed in 1 to 10% of subjects with intermittent claudication (30). Amputation may be required in 1 to 5% (30). The perioperative stroke rate in patients undergoing surgery for PAD is high. By noninvasive testing, a high-grade carotid stenosis or occlusion was noted in 62 (39%) of 160 patients waiting for surgery (34). Postoperative neurological complications occurred in seven (4%) subjects after PAD surgery. Unfortunately no direct relationship was noted between the physical examination for bruits, severity of disease, and the incidence of perioperative stroke (34).

Percutaneous transluminal angioplasty and bypass grafting are useful procedures for revascularizing the lower limb. Data on long-term patency are not yet available. Most studies have shown that these procedures reduce the rates of amputations (30). However, a recent report has questioned their long-term benefits (53).

PREVENTION

As the U.S. population ages, PAD will become a leading cause of increased morbidity and mortality. Age has the strongest association with the extent and severity of atherosclerosis. Risk factor modification to prevent the development and/or progression of PAD may delay the onset of symptomatic disease. As presented above, smoking cessation, physical exercise, and lipid lowering are assumed to slow the progression of PAD. However, much of this is unproven in an elderly population.

We need to improve methods of diagnosis and treatment. Since PAD is associated with increased CAD mortality, identifying elderly subjects with PAD can identify those at high risk for cardiovascular mortality and morbidity. By identifying these patients early we can help them get the treatment they need to live a better life. With the discovery of PAD progression by noninvasive tests, especially the ABI index, geriatricians now stand at the forefront in the battle against peripheral arterial disease.

Acknowledgment. Appreciation is given to Mukesh Prasad for help and review of the manuscript.

REFERENCES

1. Vogt M, Wolfson S, Kuller L. Lower extremity arterial disease and the aging process: a review. J Clin Epidemiol 1992;45:529–542.
2. Rose G, Blackburn H, Gillium RF, et al. Cardiovascular survey methods. WHO Monogr Ser 1982;56:ed 2.
3. Prineas RJ, Harland WR, Janzon L, et al. Recommendations for use of non-invasive methods to detect atherosclerotic peripheral arterial disease in population studies. Circulation 1982;65:1561A–1566A.
4. Hiatt WR, Marshall JA, Baxter J, et al. Diagnostic methods for peripheral arterial disease in the San Luis Valley Diabetes Study. J Clin Epidemiol 1990;43:597–606.
5. Bernstein EF, Fronek A. Current status of non-invasive tests in the diagnosis of peripheral arterial disease. Surg Clin North Am 1952;62:473–487.
6. Carter SA. Response of ankle systolic pressure to leg exercise in mild or questionable arterial disease. N Engl J Med 1972;287:578–82.
7. Laing SP, Greenhalgh RM. Standard exercise test to assess peripheral arterial disease. Br Med J 1980;280:13–16.
8. Baker JD. Post stress Doppler ankle pressure. Arch Surg l978;113:1171–1173.
9. Jager KA, Phillips DJ, Martin RL, et al. Non-invasive mapping of lower limb arterial lesions. Ultrasound Med Biol 1985;11:515–521.
10. Smullens SN, Raines JK, O'Leary DH, et al. Multicenter validation study of real time (B mode) ultrasound, arteriography, and pathology: IV. Comparison of B mode ultrasonic imaging with arteriography in lower extremity arteries. In: Glagov S, Newman WP, Schaffer SA, eds. Pathobiology of the human atherosclerotic plaque. New York: Springer-Verlag, 1990:785–797.
11. Burke GL, Evans GW, Riley WA, Sharrett AR, Barnes RW, et al. Increased carotid wall thickness associated with prevalent disease: the ARIC study. Circulation 1991;84(2):335.
12. Criqui M, Fronek A, Barrett-Connor E, Klaub MR, Gariel S, Goodman D. The prevalence of peripheral arterial disease in defined population. Circulation 1985;71:510–515.
13. Schroll M, Munck O. Estimation of peripheral arteriosclerotic disease by ankle blood pressure measurements in a population study of 60-year-old men and women. J Chronic Dis 1981;34:261–269.
14. Holland WW, Raftery EB, McPherson P, et al. A cardiovascular survey of American east coast telephone workers. Am J Epidemiol l967;85:61–71.
15. Hale WE, Marks RG, May FE, et al. Epidemiology of intermittent claudication: evaluation of risk factors. Age Aging 1988;17:57–60.
16. Reunanen A, Takkunen H, Aromaa A. Prevalence of intermittent claudication and its effect on mortality. Acta Med Scand 1982;211:249–256.
17. Fowkes FGR, Housley E, Riemersma R, Cawood E, Macintyre C, et al. Edinburgh Artery Study: prevalence of asymptomatic and symptomatic peripheral arterial disease in the general population. Int J Epidemiol 1991;20(2):384–392.
18. Aronow WS, Sales FF, Etienne F, Lee NH. Prevalence of peripheral arterial disease and its correlation with risk factors for peripheral arterial disease in elderly patients in a long term health care facility. Am J Cardiology. 1988;62:644.
19. Kannel WB, McGee DL. Update on some epidemiologic features of intermittent claudication. The Framingham Study. J Am Geriatr Soc 1985;33:13–18.
20. Widmer LK, Biland L, DaSilva A. Risk profile and occlusive peripheral arterial disease (OPAD). Proc 13th Int Congress of Angiology, Athens, 1985.
21. Mangione DM, Hawley MS, Norcliffe D. Lower limb arterial disease: assessment of risk factors in an *elderly* population. Atherosclerosis 1991;91:137–143.
22. Paris SE, Libow LS, Halperin JL, et al. The prevalence and one-year outcome of limb arterial obstructive disease in a nursing home population. J Am Geriatr Soc 1988;36:607–612.
23. Rose GA, Ahmeteli M, Checcacci I, et al. Ischemic heart disease in middle aged men. Prevalence comparisons in Europe. Bull WHO 1968;38:885–895.
24. Velican C, Velican D. The precursors of coronary atherosclerotic plaques in subjects up to 40 years old. Atherosclerosis 1980;37:33–46.
25. Menzoian JO, LaMorte WW, Paniszyn CC, et al. Symptomatology and anatomic patterns of peripheral vascular disease: differing impact of smoking and diabetes. Ann Vasc Surg 1989;3:224–228.
26. Kallero KS. Mortality and morbidity in patients with intermittent claudication as defined by venous occlusion plethysmography. A ten year follow-up study. J Chronic Dis 1981;34:455–462.
27. Joananson T, Rigqvist I. Morality and morbidity in patients with intermittent claudication in relation to the location of the occlusive atherosclerosis in the leg. Angiology 1985;36:310–314.
28. Juergens JL, Barker NW, Hines EA. Arteriosclerosis obliterans: review of 520 cases with special reference to pathogenic and prognostic factors. Circulation 1960;21:188–195.
29. Osmundson PJ, O'Fallon WM, Zimmerman BR, et al. Course of peripheral occlusive arterial disease in diabetes. Vascular laboratory assessment. Diabetes Care 1990;13:143–152.
30. Dormandy J, Mahir M, Ascady G, et al. Fate of the patient with chronic leg ischaemia. J Cardiovasc Surg 1989;30:50–57.
31. Malone JM, Moore WS, Goldstone J. Life expectancy following aortofemoral arterial grafting. Surgery 1977;81:551–555.
32. Hertzer NR, Beven EG, Young JR, et al. Coronary artery disease in peripheral vascular patients. A classification of 1000 coronary angiograms and results of surgical management. Ann Surg 1984;199:223–233.
33. Hughson WG, Mann JI, Tibbs DJ, et al. Intermittent claudication: factors determining outcome. Br Med J 1978;1:1377–1379.
34. Turnipseed WD, Berkoff HA, Belzer FO. Postoperative stroke in cardiac and peripheral vascular disease. Ann Surg 1980;192:365–368.
35. Shapira OM, Pasik S, Wasserman JP, et al. Ultrasound screening for abdominal aortic aneurysms in

patient with atherosclerotic peripheral vascular disease. J Cardiovasc Surg 1990;3l:170–172.

36. Howell MA, Colgan MP, Seeger RW, et al. Relationship of severity of lower limb peripheral vascular disease to mortality and morbidity: a six year follow-up study. J Vasc Surg 1989;9:691–697.

37. McKenna M, Wolfson S, Kuller L. The ratio of ankle and arm arterial pressure as an independent predictor of mortality. Atherosclerosis 1991;87:119–128.

38. Joananson T. Ringqvist I. Changes in peripheral blood pressures after five years of follow-up in non-operated patients with intermittent claudication. Acta Med Scand 1986;220:127–132.

39. Stokes J III, Kannel WB, Wolf PA, Cupples LA, D'Agostino RB. The relative importance of selected risk factors for various manifestations of cardiovascular disease among men and women from 35 to 64 years old: 3 years of follow-up in the Framingham Study. Circulation 1987;75(suppl V)(V-65,V-73).

40. Dobs AS, Nieto FJ, Barnes R, Sharrett AR, Ko WJ, Szklo M. Risk factors for popliteal artery thickness in the Atherosclerosis Risk in Communities (ARIC) Study. Circulation 1993;88:261.

41. Kozak GP, Rowbotham JL. Diabetic foot disease: a major problem. In: Kozak GP, Hoak CS, Rowbotham JL, et al., eds. Management of diabetic foot problems. Philadelphia: WB Saunders, 1984.

42. Reaven GM. Role of insulin resistance in human disease. Diabetes 1988;37:1595–1607.

43. DaSilva A, Widmer LK, Zeigler HW, et al. The Basel Longitudinal Study: report on the relation of initial glucose level to baseline ECG abnormalities, peripheral artery disease and subsequent mortality. J Chronic Dis 1979;32:797–803.

44. Pomrehn P, Duncan B, Weissfeld L, Wallace RB, Barnes R, et al. The association of dyslipoproteinemia with symptoms and signs of peripheral arterial disease. The Lipid Research Clinics Program Prevalence Study. Circulation 1986;73(suppl I):I-100,I-107.

45. Beach KW, Brunzell JD, Conquest LL, Strandness DE. The correlation of arteriosclerosis obliterans with lipoproteins in insulin-dependent and non-insulin-dependent diabetes. Diabetes 1979;28:836–840.

46. Mahley RW, Rall SC Jr. Type III hyperlipoproteinemia (dysbetalipoproteinemia): the role of apolipoprotein E in normal and abnormal lipoprotein metabolism. In: Scriver CR, Beaudet AL, Sly WS, Valle D, eds. The metabolic basis of inherited disease. 6th ed. New York: McGraw-Hill, 1989;18:614–618.

47. Hell KMD, Balzereit A, Diebold U, et al. Importance of blood viscoelasticity in arteriosclerosis. Angiology 1989;40:539–546.

48. Cronenwett JL, Warner KG, Zelenock GB, et al. Intermittent claudication. Current results of non-operative management. Arch Surg 1984;199:430–436.

49. DeFelice M, Gallo P, Masotti G. Current therapy of peripheral obstructive arterial disease. The non-surgical approach. Angiology 1990;41:1–11.

50. Blankenhorn DH, Nessim SA, Johnson RL, Sanmarco ME, Azen SP, Cashin-Hemphill L. Beneficial effects of combined colestipol-niacin therapy on coronary atherosclerosis and coronary venous bypass graft. JAMA 1987;257:3233–3240.

51. Blankenhorn DH, Azen SP, Crawford DW, et al. Effects of colestipol-niacin therapy on human femoral atherosclerosis. Circulation 1991;83:438–447.

52. National Cholesterol Education Program (NCEP) Expert Panel on Detection, Education, and Treatment of High Blood Cholesterol in Adults. JAMA 1993;269(23):3015–3023.

53. Tunis SR, Bass EB, Steinberg EP. The use of angioplasty, bypass surgery and amputation in the management of peripheral vascular disease. N Engl J Med 1991;325:556–562.

12/ Clinical Geropsychiatry

Susan W. Lehmann, Peter V. Rabins

While most older people are mentally healthy, persons over age 65 are vulnerable to the same spectrum of psychiatric disorders as are younger people (1). Community epidemiologic studies have indicated that prevalence rates for major depressive disorder, panic disorder, and substance use disorders are lower in the elderly. However, the prevalence of phobic disorders does not change with age, and the prevalence of cognitive disorders and their associated psychiatric morbidity sharply increase with age.

Psychiatric problems in the elderly are more common in certain settings. For instance, anxiety and depressive disorders are common among patients in medical clinics, while confusional states (delirium) are seen in approximately 25% of hospitalized patients on medical and surgical services. In nursing homes and long-term care facilities, over 50% of residents have been found to suffer from some sort of psychiatric problem (usually dementia), and behavioral problems as well as depression are common. In all, there is a need for careful attention to psychiatric symptoms in the elderly, since compassionate and appropriate treatment will improve overall functioning as well as quality of life.

EVALUATION

History

The evaluation of the older adult with a possible mental disorder begins, as does any medical evaluation, with a careful history. If the patient is accompanied by family members, it is helpful to meet with the family as well as the patient to facilitate obtaining a complete history and data base. The history should focus on a thorough assessment of the reason for the appointment including a careful determination of when symptoms first appeared, how they have progressed over time, and accompanying features. In addition the complete history should include the following:

1. *Family psychiatric history.* The clinician should inquire whether any blood relatives, especially first-degree relatives, have ever suffered from a mental disorder or alcoholism or have been hospitalized in a psychiatric facility.
2. *Prior psychiatric history of the patient.* This should include any prior contact with psychiatrists or therapists, prior psychiatric hospitalizations, or previous treatment by any medical professional for mood problems or "bad nerves."
3. *Medical history.* It is important to detail all prior hospitalizations and surgeries, and current medical conditions that continue to be a focus of treatment.
4. *Medications.* This should be a complete list of all medications, both prescription drugs and over-the-counter medications being taken by the patient, including dosages. Because many medications prescribed for a variety of medical conditions have psychiatric side effects, it is helpful to inquire about the length of time the patient has taken the medication and to pay particular attention to changes in medications prescribed shortly before the onset of the current psychiatric symptoms.
5. *Personal history.* This will include information about the patient's family of origin, siblings, childhood history, schooling (especially highest level of education obtained), work history, adjustment to retirement, sexual history, marital history, and children. It is also important to inquire about the patients' current living situation, including with whom they live as well as the type of home (i.e., house vs. apartment, rented or owned). This is also a good time to ask about any structured aspects of the home that may pose problems for the patients, such as stairs, second-floor bathrooms, and tub/showers.
6. *Patterns of alcohol use.* Problems of alcohol use and abuse occur in the elderly as in younger persons and may be underlying symptoms of anxiety, depression, irritability, memory loss, sleep complaints, sexual complaints, or paranoia. It is necessary to obtain information on what type of alcohol is consumed, how frequently, and how much and to inquire about early-morning "shakes," blackouts, alcohol-induced seizures, and prior episodes of detoxification or treatment.

Mental Status Examination

The heart of the psychiatric evaluation is the mental status examination. For the psychiatrist

125

the mental status examination is the here-and-now data-gathering equivalent of the physical examination. It allows a systematic examination of the major aspects of the patient's current mental state. Depending on the nature of the presenting complaint and the cooperativeness of the patient, certain areas of the mental status examination may be emphasized, while others may be only touched upon briefly. The complete mental status examination, however, always includes attention to the following areas.

1. *General appearance.* This includes observation of neatness and personal hygiene, eye contact during the interview, and any abnormal movements, tremors, tics, or unusual behaviors.
2. *Speech.* This refers to the form and structure of the patient's verbal language. It includes attention to the rate, rhythm, and volume level of the patient's speech and whether the patient's use of language is coherent, goal-directed, logical, and easy to follow. Does the patient seem to jump from one idea to another with little connection between ideas? This is described as "loosening of associations" and in an extreme form may be called "flight of ideas." Some patients may have trouble sticking to the topic at hand and exhibit a tendency to wander off track ("tangentiality") but can be redirected back to the issue being discussed. Obsessional patients may be inclined to the overinclusive in detail ("circumstantiality"), sometimes losing sight of the forest for the trees.
3. *Mood.* The assessment of mood involves both an ascertainment of the patient's subjective description of his or her current mood state and the clinician's objective observations of how the patient's mood appears. Some depressed elderly patients report that they don't feel depressed yet will appear tense, anxious, sad, or withdrawn.
4. *Suicidal ideation.* It is important to ask any patient with a sad mood about suicidal thoughts. Contrary to popular myths, asking about suicidal thoughts does not increase the likelihood that a patient will follow through on such ideas. We distinguish between "passive suicidal ideation" (i.e., wishing one were dead or would die) and "active suicidal ideation" (i.e., planning self-harm). Many depressed patients express passive wishes for death yet for personal, religious, or family reasons are adamant that they would never attempt suicide.
5. *Abnormal thought content.*
   a. *Hallucinations* are sensory experiences that are perceived in the absence of a sensory stimulus. Auditory and visual hallucinations are most common, but tactile and olfactory hallucinations also occur in some disorders.
   b. *Delusions* are idiosyncratic, fixed, false beliefs that an individual holds that are not culturally determined or shared. Paranoid delusions and delusions of persecution are most common. Manic patients may have grandiose delusions about themselves and their abilities.
   c. *Obsessive thoughts* are intrusive, repetitive, unwanted *ideas* that an individual cannot stop from coming to mind.
   d. *Compulsions* are intrusive, repetitive, unwanted *behaviors* that an individual cannot stop from doing, though they seem unnecessary, excessive, or foolish. Some examples are compulsive hand washing or checking behaviors.
   e. *Phobias* are excessive specific fears that cause an individual to avoid the dreaded situation.
6. *Cognitive Assessment.* Every psychiatric evaluation of the older patient should include an assessment of cognitive functioning. Depending upon the nature of the initial presenting complaint and the cooperativeness of the patient, this assessment may be fairly brief or very detailed and focused. A basic cognitive screening should include the following areas of assessment: level of alertness, attentiveness, orientation, short- and long-term memory, attention and concentration, naming ability and language comprehension, and abstract reasoning. If significant cognitive impairment is detected in one or more of these areas, further neuropsychological testing and/or laboratory testing may be warranted.

SPECIFIC CONDITIONS

Anxiety Disorders

The word *anxiety* refers to feelings of tension and distress that are distinct from sadness and usually lack a stressful stimulus of sufficient severity to explain the feeling state. It often has both somatic (physical) and psychological components. *Generalized anxiety disorder* is a condition marked by excessive worry and anxiety persisting for 6 months or more. It is accompanied by signs and symptoms of motor tension including muscle aches or soreness, a feeling of restlessness, a feeling of shakiness, and reports of easy fatiguability. In addition there are feelings of being "on edge," having difficulty concentrating, having difficulty falling asleep, and being more irritable. At least three of these additional symptoms of muscle tension must be present along with the subjective distress of constant worry to make the diagnosis of generalized anxiety disorder. *Panic disorder* is diagnosed when the patient reports discrete recurrent episodes (attacks) of intense fear and somatic anxiety symptoms which are both unprovoked and unexpected. The associated somatic symptoms include palpitations, sweating, trembling, shortness of breath, chest discomfort, lightheadedness, or abdominal distress. It is common for panic attacks to occur repeatedly in certain circumstances, e.g., when in a grocery store. *Specific phobias* are clearly delineated fears of objects or situations that an individual realizes are unrealistic but nevertheless can not resist. They sometimes occur in concert with panic attacks.

The anxiety disorders are among the most common psychological problems identified in mental health surveys. Nonpharmacologic and pharmacologic therapies are equally effective. Desensitization (gradually exposing the patient to the source of distress) coupled with relaxation is often effective. The most effective pharmacologic therapy involves the use of the tricyclic antidepressants. There is no evidence that one antidepressant is better than another. While drugs with high anticholinergic properties such as imipramine are often used in the young, medications with less anticholinergic activity, such as nortriptyline, are suggested in the elderly.

Benzodiazepine compounds are also effective in treating anxiety disorders. However, because of their addictive potential they are generally not prescribed as a first-line therapy. Short-acting benzodiazepines have more abuse and addiction liability than longer-acting compounds (e.g., clonazepam), but the longer-acting compounds are more likely to accumulate and lead to sedation, functional impairment, and drowsiness. Buspirone is nonaddicting but appears to be less effective in the treatment of anxiety than benzodiazepines or antidepressants. If symptoms are severe and immediate relief desirable, the clinician may choose to initiate treatment with both an antidepressant and benzodiazepine and taper the benzodiazepine several weeks after the tricyclic drug begins to work.

Mixed Anxiety and Depression

Symptoms of anxiety and depression frequently cooccur in the same patient. The clinician should make an effort to determine which is primary and to focus treatment on that set of symptoms. In the authors' experience, depression is more frequently the primary disorder, but this is a controversial issue. Features in the history that suggest that depression is primary include a previous history of a depressive episode, a family history of depressive episodes, diurnal mood variation, and the presence of self-blame, guilt, and hopelessness. While anxiety disorders can begin de novo in late life, it is much more common for a depressive episode to appear for the first time in an older person. Because tricyclic antidepressants are effective in both, they should be the first-line treatment when the clinician is unsure which is primary.

Mood Disorders

Mood disorders are the most frequently clinically diagnosed and the most treatable psychiatric disorders in older people (2). They encompass a spectrum of disorders ranging from adjustment disorder (in which an identified psychosocial stressor provokes a mild depressive reaction that impairs functioning) to psychotic major depression with hallucinations and/or delusions.

Major depression is characterized by a persistent diminution in three spheres of functioning: (a) mood, (b) vital sense (a measure of one's sense of well-being and energy), and (c) self-attitude (self-confidence). Depressed patients tend to have a more negative self-assessment than is usual for them, may be self-blaming, or can have excessive feelings of guilt, regret, or worthlessness. Patients with major depression experience loss of energy, disturbed sleep (usually insomnia and early morning awakening), diminished appetite and weight loss, difficulty thinking and concentrating, and a loss of interest or pleasure in activities that were once enjoyed. Ruminant thoughts of death and suicidal thoughts may occur during the course of a major depression. Elderly patients who are depressed often complain of physical rather than psychological distress. Up to one-third of older people who suffer from major depression do not describe their mood as depressed. Rather they focus on feelings of weakness, lack of energy, and lack of motivation. Somatic complaints (including headaches, GI disturbances, and body aches) are common. Occasionally, hallucinations and delusions occur. Such hallucinations and delusions tend to have a depressive theme and are consistent with a low mood, for example, the persecutory delusion that one deserves punishment, the delusion that one has no money, clothes, or insurance, and the delusion that one has a terrible illness that doctors cannot find.

Major depression can first occur at any point in the life span. It may occur as a single episode, but recurrence is common. The etiology of major depression is complex and involves genetic, neurochemical, and psychological factors. While genetic transmission is poorly understood, it is clear that affective (mood) disorders tend to run in families and that there is a higher prevalence of affective disorders among first-degree relatives of depressed individuals. The neurochemistry of depression continues to be an active area of research, focusing on abnormalities in adrenergic and serotonergic neurotransmissions in the brain. Many commonly prescribed medications, including steroids, reserpine, methyldopa, anti-

Parkinsonian drugs and β-adrenergic blockers, can cause depression. Depression is especially common in diseases of the brain. For example, 30 to 60% of poststroke patients experience a clinically significant episode of depression within 6 months to 2 years of the stroke. The incidence of poststroke depression has been found to be greatest among patients with strokes affecting the left anterior cerebral hemisphere (3). While a major depression can occur in the absence of any precipitating event, psychological issues such as recent loss (i.e., job, independence, social supports) and chronic medical illness play a contributing role in many cases. Regardless of whether psychological factors provoke a depressive episode, they clearly can affect its course and outcomes. Supportive psychotherapy is an important part of the treatment of depression in conjunction with appropriate pharmacotherapy.

The psychopharmacologic treatment of major depression has advanced considerably in recent years, and there are many effective antidepressant medications available. Older persons do best when given antidepressants with the least anticholinergic activity; therefore, nortriptyline, desipramine, and trazodone are favored for older people. Many of the newer selective serotonin reuptake–inhibitor (SSRI) medications, fluoxetine, sertraline, and paroxetine, have minimal anticholinergic properties and are well tolerated by older patients. However, SSRIs can impair sleep, even when taken in the morning. If this occurs, the addition of trazodone at bedtime can improve sleep. Monoamine oxidase inhibitors can be given to older patients if prescribed cautiously and may be indicated for difficult cases when other medications have failed. All antidepressants must be taken for a minimum of 6 to 8 weeks at an appropriate doses before efficacy can be determined.

Another effective treatment for serious depression is electroconvulsive therapy (ECT) (1). For severe cases of depression, ECT may be the first-line treatment of choice, especially if the patient is refusing to eat and is at risk for dehydration. In other cases, it may be used after one or two antidepressant trials have failed to adequately improve symptoms. There is no age limit to ECT, although several medical conditions may present relative contraindications that need to be evaluated on a case-by-case basis. These include recent myocardial infarction, coronary artery disease, hypertensive cardiovascular disease, bronchopulmonary disease, and venous thrombosis. The only absolute contraindication for ECT is increased intracranial pressure because ECT causes a rise in cerebrospinal fluid pressure that could lead to herniation.

Dysthymic disorder is a chronic depressive condition lasting 2 years or longer, marked by a persistently low mood more days than not, and at least two of the following: appetite change, insomnia, low energy, low self-esteem, poor concentration or difficulty making decisions, or hopelessness. It may be a milder depressive disorder than major depression in severity of individual symptoms, but the chronicity of the depressive symptoms can be disabling and demoralizing to the patient and may contribute to lowering functional capacities. In addition, some patients with dysthymic disorder go on to develop a major depressive episode at a later time. In older people, dysthymic disorder often develops in the setting of physical disability, multiple medical problems, isolation, and loneliness. Sometimes the symptoms may progress to a frank major depression. Many patients with a dysthymic disorders may respond to treatment with an antidepressant. Supportive psychotherapy is a vital component of treatment, with the goals of increasing social contacts, activity level, and improving self-esteem and outlook through an empathic therapeutic relationship.

Grief is not a mental disorder, and depressive symptoms are considered to be part of the normal bereavement process. Although individuals vary in their response to losing a loved one, we recognize that there are common predictable phases to the grief process. The initial response lasts several days and is characterized by shock, disbelief, and emotional numbing. This is often followed by feelings of anger and frustration. Usually these initial reactions give way to a prolonged period of fluctuating despair, mourning, and wishing to be with the deceased. During the first 3 to 6 months following the death of a loved one, insomnia is common, as are frequent episodes of tearfulness, anxiety symptoms, and a loss of interest or pleasure in activities once enjoyed. Usually, the intensity of symptoms begins to remit after the first 6 to 12 months; strong feelings of loss and mourning continue for 1 to 2 years, longer for some people. In addition, intense emotional feelings tend to return on the anniversary of the loved one's death and birthday and at holiday times.

It is unclear at what point a bereaved person should be referred for professional help or counseling. For most bereaved persons, the support of family, friends, and clergy are sufficient to help them through the grieving process. For some people, local widow/widower support groups are helpful in adjusting to life without a spouse and increasing social contacts. When the bereaved person is overwhelmed by grief symptoms and unable to begin to return to usual activities or if grief is complicated by panic attacks, delusions, or suicidal thoughts, referral for psychiatric evaluation is indicated. Grief may trigger a full major depressive episode. While feelings of sadness, disruption of sleep, and loss of motivation and interest may be part of an uncomplicated grief syndrome, feelings of guilt, worthlessness, hopelessness, and suicidal ideation are not part of grief and should signal concern that a major depression has developed that needs treatment as outlined above.

Personality Disorder

Personality is defined as the set of enduring traits that makes each individual unique. Traits are universally shared characteristics on which individuals differ. They include patterns of perceiving and relating to oneself and one's social environment. For example, all people can be rated on their tendency for tidiness. People vary widely in this tendency, but for each individual, a certain degree of tidiness (or lack thereof) is characteristic. Personality disorders are diagnosed when an individual falls at the extreme end of the normal distribution on a set of traits that commonly occur together. Personality disorders are enduring, inflexible, and maladaptive patterns of inner experience and behavior. For example, *histrionic personality disorder* is diagnosed when an individual exhibits provocativeness, self-dramatization, emotional lability, and self-centeredness and frequently engages in attention-seeking behaviors. *Antisocial personality disorder* is associated with repeated illegal actions, impulsivity, frequent lies, consistent irresponsibility, lack of remorse, and a lack of care concern toward others. *Obsessive-compulsive personality disorder* is characterized by extreme perfectionism, rigidity, emotional inexpressiveness, excessive preoccupation with rules and details, and inflexibility. *Dependent personality disorder* is characterized by an excessive need to be taken care of by others, which leads to difficulty making independent everyday decisions. These individuals lack self-confidence in their judgment or abilities to do things on their own, and they often go to excessive lengths to obtain reassurance or support. To receive a diagnosis of personality disorder, problems in these realms must be lifelong. Thus in the elderly, a diagnosis of a personality disorder must reflect a pattern of behavior that has been present throughout adulthood and which has caused problems for the individual throughout his or her life.

Personality disorders can complicate the care of the medically ill. Patients with histrionic personality disorder or prominent histrionic traits are likely to present physical symptoms in a dramatic fashion, to demonstrate marked emotional lability, and to be provocative and demanding. Conversely, patients with obsessive-compulsive personality disorder may underreport symptoms, have very high expectations of their physicians, be inflexible, be unable to make decisions, and to have difficulty accepting the lack of clear guidelines that sometimes occurs in medical conditions.

The physician who is aware that a personality disorder is underlying a problematic patient's behavior can avoid or alleviate problems by considering the patient's predispositions. Patients with prominent obsessional traits often need detailed discussions of proposed procedures and an extensive and specific discussion regarding the steps that are to be taken, the order in which they are to be taken, and the implications of the most likely outcomes. For the histrionic patient, on the other hand, an extensive detailed discussion is often overwhelming. While all patients need to be given options and clear descriptions, patients with histrionic features often do best when information is presented with a reassuring, calm tone, a concise description of alternatives, a direct acknowledgment of emotional distress ("I know this is upsetting but let me present the alternatives before we discuss them"), and more frequent, short visits. Patients with dependent personality disorder will have difficulty following through with recommendations on their own initiative and will do better if important persons in their social support network are made part of the treatment process.

Psychotic Symptoms

Hallucinations (perceptions without a stimulus occurring in any of the five senses) and delusions (false ideas that are unshakable and persistent) can occur in many medical and psychiatric disorders. The first step in their assessment is to determine whether a cognitive impairment (delirium or dementia) is present. The importance of this step is twofold. First, cognitive disorder is a common cause of hallucinations and delusions, and second, this recognition leads to the appropriate medical evaluation.

Hallucinations and delusions can also be caused by depression, schizophrenia, and delusional disorder. After a primary cognitive disorder has been ruled out, the next step is to assess for the presence of a mood disorder. Self-deprecation, self-blame, hopelessness, loss of interest in usually enjoyed activities, somatic preoccupations, and complaints of sad mood all suggest the possibility that major depression is the cause of the psychotic symptoms. *Schizophrenia* and *delusional disorder* are uncommon conditions, occurring in less than 1% of the population. They can present to medical practitioners with isolated somatic delusions (for example, the belief that someone is sending an electrical shock into the body or the belief that a physical illness is present for which there is no evidence). By definition, a *delusional disorder* is characterized by a single delusion occurring in the absence of cognitive impairment, mood impairment, and other psychiatric symptoms. *Schizophrenia* is an illness in which symptoms are present for at least 6 months, hallucinations and social dilapidation are predominant, and mood disorder criteria are not met.

The treatment of psychotic symptoms depends, in part, on the diagnosis of the underlying condition. If the patient is delirious, all attempts should be made to correct the underlying abnormality and to avoid pharmacotherapy unless there are clear indications. So-called neuroleptic, psychotropic, or antipsychotic drugs are the treatment of choice when pharmacotherapy is necessary. In dementia, reorientation and activity therapy should be tried initially. Pharmacotherapy is appropriate when these symptoms increase the likelihood of danger of harm to self or others or cause emotional distress to the patient. In delirium, neuroleptics should be used when extreme agitation, aggression, or fear are present. For mood disorder, several studies demonstrate that delusional major depression responds better to the combination of an antidepressant and neuroleptic than to an antidepressant alone.

Psychiatric Treatment of Irreversible Cognitive Disorders

Dementia and delirium are discussed in detail elsewhere in this book. About 60% of patients with dementia have psychotic symptoms sometime in the course of a dementing illness. These noncognitive symptoms can interfere with the quality of life of the patient and caregiver and are often amenable to treatment. When appropriate, nonpharmacologic environmental therapy is most desirable because of the potential side effects of drugs. Nondrug treatments include providing a structured environment, stimulating the patient at an appropriate level, and providing the level of care that that person needs. When hallucinations and delusions interfere with function, become dis-

tressing to the patient, or are dangerous to others, cautious low-dosage neuroleptic therapy is appropriate.

Between 15 and 30% of patients with dementia also suffer from depression that interferes with function. Antidepressant drugs with low anticholinergic properties (e.g., nortriptyline, desipramine, SSRIs) are recommended. Emotional support for both patient and caregiver is indicated in all cases. The physician should play an important role in educating the family, in managing specific behavioral and noncognitive symptoms, and in helping the families address the social, legal, and financial concerns that they have.

OVERVIEW OF TREATMENT ISSUES

Pharmacotherapy

While older patients can benefit from the same psychopharmacologic agents as younger patients, the clinician must be aware of changes in physiology and pharmacokinetics with age, as well as potential interactions with other medications. As a result, prescribing psychotropic medication for older patients requires special considerations that are discussed in detail in other sources (3). However, some important basic principles are outlined here.

Perhaps the most familiar axiom in prescribing for older adults is "start low and go slow." This means that for just about every medication, be it an anxiolytic, antipsychotic, or antidepressant, one should start at a low dose and titrate the dose upward to a therapeutic dose in a slow and gradual way. A good rule of thumb is to allow at least 3 days between each dosage increase. This allows the patient to adjust to a new medication and to report any troublesome side effects before they become problematic.

Older patients are more sensitive to the anticholinergic effects of medication and therefore more likely than younger patients to develop delirium, constipation, urinary retention, dry mouth, and orthostatic hypotension. For these reasons, medications with the least anticholinergic effects are preferred when a choice of several agents is available.

Another important principle is to choose medications with shorter half-lives. Because of the changes in hepatic metabolism that occur with aging, the half-lives of most pharmacologic agents are prolonged in older people. This increases the likelihood that psychologically active metabolites will accumulate over time and cause toxicity. Obviously, this problem is worsened if the original drug and/or its active metabolite have long half-lives to begin with. Among benzodiazepines, for instance, lorazepam ($t_{1/2} = 16$ hours) or oxazepam ($t_{1/2} = 8$ hours) are better tolerated in older people than is diazepam ($t_{1/2} = 3$ to 4 days). If a longer-acting benzodiazepine is required to manage severe anxiety or withdrawal from benzodiazepines, clonazepam ($t_{1/2} = 1$ to 2 days) is useful.

Lithium carbonate deserves special mention, since it is nearly totally excreted by the kidneys. Because GFR and creatinine clearance decrease steadily with age, older patients are more likely to develop lithium-induced tremor and delirium at lower doses. Furthermore, recent studies seem to indicate that the therapeutic effects of lithium occur at lower blood levels in older patients than in younger ones. For all these reasons, older patients will require lower doses of lithium than younger patients, usually ranging from 150 mg q.d. to 300 mg b.i.d.

In general, the lowest dose of antipsychotic medication needed to control symptoms should be prescribed. In addition to their extrapyramidal and anticholinergic side effects, neuroleptics are more likely to cause tardive dyskinesia in the elderly.

For most antidepressants, on the other hand, patients do best if the medication is within the "therapeutic range," regardless of age. Low-dose antidepressant treatment is likely to be inadequate to treat a major depressive episode. Because of wide variability among older individuals in hepatic metabolism, it is impossible to predict the dose of antidepressant needed to achieve a therapeutic level, but often it is the same as for much younger persons. As for younger people, it is important to give an antidepressant an adequate trial length (6 to 8 weeks minimum) at a therapeutic dose before deciding that the medication trial was a failure and changing to another antidepressant. Indeed, there is some evidence that for at least some antidepressants, such as fluoxetine, a longer trial period of 6 to 8 weeks may be necessary to achieve maximum therapeutic benefits.

Finally, as with all medications, it is important to consider potential drug interactions. Fluoxetine, for example, increases serum levels of digoxin and coumadin and other protein-bound drugs. Tricyclic antidepressant medications and neuroleptics have hypotensive effects that can compound the effects of antihypertensive medications. Nonsteroidal antiinflammatory drugs increase the plasma level of lithium and put an older patient at risk for lithium toxicity. Thus, the older patient must be carefully monitored while being treated with psychotropic medications to avoid both undertreatment and toxicity.

Psychotherapy

Individual Psychotherapy. Contrary to many prevailing myths, older patients do benefit from psychotherapy in the treatment of a variety of disorders (4). For patients with depression, anxiety, and bereavement, psychotherapy is an important part of treatment, even when pharmacotherapy is indicated. Older people can experience significant improvement in self-esteem, self-awareness, adaptation, and personal satisfaction through psychotherapy. No one psychotherapeutic methods works best with older people. We recommend a pluralistic approach that emphasizes life review and a focus on specific issues of concern. Many individuals benefit from a focus on the development of problem-solving skills. Some patients benefit from a return to an active, creative life. Also, patients with anxiety disorders and phobias may benefit from a more cognitive-behavioral approach that stresses the importance of positive problem solving and teaches relaxation techniques.

Marital Therapy. Marital or couples therapy is helpful for older people in several circumstances. Retirement and late-life illnesses can dramatically alter the dynamics of a marital relationship. Spouses who were used to busy, but relatively independent, work lives may find it an adjustment to being home together most of the time. Roles may change as one spouse does more or less of the cooking, shopping, and housekeeping chores. If one spouse is unable to drive because of health problems, this can put limitations on the lifestyles of both partners. Retirement also means living on a fixed income for most people, and these new financial constraints may pose an additional burden. In short, the reality of living "the golden years" often does not meet the expectations for this time of life. This may result in disappointment or resentment, especially if one spouse blames the other for preventing the fulfillment of the retirement dream. In addition, problems can develop between widowed or divorced elders involved in new relationships. Issues such as whether to live together or marry, how to combine finances, and how to deal with each other's adult children can put a strain on the relationship. While couples issues may be the presenting focus for treatment, usually they are not. Rather, these issues may emerge as the patient is beginning treatment for depression or anxiety. Short-term marital therapy can be very useful in defusing stressful situations, improving communications between partners, and fostering a more healthy adaptation to the couple's changing way of life.

Family Assessment. Often other family issues come to light during the course of assessment and treatment of the older patient. For some, decreased functional abilities or illness result in increased dependence on adult children. This may necessitate moving in with adult children or moving closer geographically. When an elderly person develops a dementia and/or other disabling medical illnesses, the spouse or adult child may become a primary caregiver and need to assume new responsibilities for the impaired person's personal and financial care. Older patients may find that their grown children need them in new or different ways, for example, because of illness or divorce on the part of the adult children.

These and other situations can produce family conflicts and stress. It is very helpful to meet with all involved family members at least once to assess how various family members relate to one another, solve problems, deal with their changing family dynamics, and address the needs of the impaired elder person. These meetings can also be useful for educating the family about the impaired older person's medications and illness, for mobilizing family and community resources, and for identifying others in the immediate family who may be in need of additional support or counseling.

Barriers to Treatment

There are many reasons why older people often do not get the psychological treatment they need (5). One common reason is that older people themselves are reluctant or resistant to seeing a psychiatrist because of feelings of embarrassment and negative attitudes. While education is slowly changing society's outlook on mental illness and mental health care, older people who grew up in during the Depression or earlier may still believe one should solve one's own problems and "pick oneself up by the boot straps." To such individuals, seeking help for psychological problems is viewed as a sign of personal weakness. Other contributors to elders not receiving care for emotional problems include the negative attitude of their physician; the focus by patient, family, or physician on medical issues; and lack of transportation. These issues are best overcome by discussing them openly and reviewing the reasons a person is reluctant to seek help.

REFERENCES

1. Jenike MA. Geriatric psychiatry and psychopharmacology: a clinical approach. Chicago: Year Book Medical Publishers, 1989.
2. Blazer DG. Depression in late life. 2nd ed. St. Louis: Mosby, 1993.
3. Lipsey JR, Robinson RG, Pearlson GD, et al. The dexamethasone suppression test and mood following stroke. Am J Psychiatry 1985;142:318–323.
4. Myers WA. New techniques in the psychotherapy of older patients. Washington: American Psychiatry Press, 1991.
5. Waxman HM, Carner EA, Klein M. Underutilization of mental health professionals by community elderly. Gerontologist 1984;24:23–30.

13/ Alcohol and Other Drug Abuse in Older Patients

Alan A. Wartenberg, Ted D. Nirenberg

The abuse of alcohol and other drugs in Western society is extremely common, with prevalence rates of approximately 15% for alcohol abuse and 5% for other drugs (1, 2). It is clear that such use is only occasionally detected by physicians, although abusers are more likely to be seen in the medical setting, whether inpatient (3) or outpatient (4). In older individuals, the diagnosis is even more rarely suspected, diagnosed, treated or referred (5, 6). While there is a tendency for drinking to decrease with age (7, 8), and although estimates of the prevalence of alcoholism or problem drinking among older persons range between 2 and 10%, studies of elderly hospital patients find much higher rates, ranging from 8 to 70%, depending on diagnostic criteria used and the subpopulation under study (9–11). A recent report indicated that among elderly who have used alcohol in the past year, over 25% have responses suggesting or positive for alcoholism on a reliable screening instrument (12). A study showed that the national prevalence of alcohol-related hospitalizations of elderly persons was 54.7 per 10,000 men and 14.8 per 10,000 women, with an estimated total cost of more than $233 million (13).

Physicians, nurses and other health care professionals have received little training in the recognition and management of patients with alcohol and other drug abuse (14). We are particularly unlikely to entertain these diagnoses when the patients do not fit our stereotypic view of what an alcohol or other drug abuser looks like. We are also rarely trained in issues of prescription drug abuse and in judicious prescribing when alcohol and other drug abuse can or should be suspected.

The older patient presents special issues in the recognition and management of alcohol and other drug abuse. There have been few studies of treatment efficacy in this population (15, 16), and frequently treatment recommendations are based on studies of younger individuals, which may not be generalizable to the older patient. Presentation may be atypical, and management decisions may be affected by the other medical and/or psychiatric issues common in the elderly.

NATURAL HISTORY

Alcohol

Clinical observations have led to the classification of elderly problem drinkers and alcoholics on the basis of whether alcohol problems began earlier or later in their life: early vs. late onset (17, 18). Efforts at classification attempt to capture more variation in drinking patterns by including categories for drinkers whose problems are transient or intermittent throughout their lifetime or those that may vary over time with respect to the quantity and consequences of drinking (19).

Dunham has argued that there are at least four distinct drinking patterns that may pose problems for elderly drinkers—heavy, moderate, light, and infrequent—and that there is considerable movement in and out of drinking patterns throughout a drinker's lifetime (20). The age cutoff used to delineate late-onset alcohol problem drinking typically ranges from 40 to 60 years (21). Late-onset problem drinking has been reported to account for between 28 and 40% of elderly problem drinkers found in clinical samples (22). Early-onset drinkers frequently have had previous medical problems related to their drinking, and many have had hospitalizations earlier in life for treatment of medical sequelae, detoxification, or rehabilitation. There is often a strong family history of alcohol abuse, and both the first use of alcohol and the onset of problematic use may have been early in life. Such individuals may present with episodes of intoxication, a withdrawal syndrome, or serious medical sequelae, including. trauma. The family is often devastated by extreme dysfunction, with resentment on the part of spouse or caretaker, siblings, children and friends for years of abuse.

Alcohol and other drug abuse may be problematic on the part of other family members as well. The patient is likely to minimize or deny problems and be resistant to accepting help. The addition of an organic brain syndrome, generally secondary to alcohol abuse but potentially due to other causes (e.g., multiple infarctions, hypothyroidism, vitamin B_{12} deficiency, syphilis, or Alzheimer's disease), may further complicate management. Patients may be cognitively incapable of understanding their situation and of accepting the necessary help, but be competent enough to make decisions regarding their care.

The epidemiologic literature on risk factors predicting vulnerability to late-onset alcohol problems is limited (11). Several studies report that late-onset alcoholics are less likely to have a family history of alcohol abuse and are less likely to experience alcohol-related legal or social problems than early-onset alcoholics (23, 24) and that early alcohol problems are not good predictors of later alcohol abuse (25).

Some evidence suggests that late-onset alcohol problems are a maladaptive response to common personal, social, and environmental stressors that are correlates of the aging process. For example, the loss of self-image associated with cessation of employment, either inside or outside the home, and/or loss of youth, health, and mobility may leave the older individual with significant feelings of anxiety and depression, with an inadequate support system to deal with the losses. Crises such as grief and bereavement due to loss, social isolation, unwanted residential change, death of a spouse or child, financial distress, fear of crime, loneliness, and even pressure from peers in some retirement communities to increase alcohol intake all have been posited as plausible causal factors for late-onset alcohol problems (26). Fear of physical abuse and abandonment by caregivers may particularly affect women and be a factor in their alcohol and other drug abuse. The onset of depression and anxiety may lead to use of alcohol to "self-medicate" (27), which may ultimately lead to increasing tolerance, withdrawal, and continued use of alcohol to avoid withdrawal. Alcohol may be used by the patient who finds that it decreases the severity of an essential or head-bobbing tremor or that it allows them to sleep. Continued use in this setting may again lead to problematic use.

In the individual with late-onset alcohol problems, the family may be more functional and able and willing to assist in the treatment process. It is less likely that other members of the family will have been adversely affected by the individual's alcohol use, and they are more likely to enter into a therapeutic alliance with the physician or therapist. The patient may be more willing to admit that the alcohol use has become problematic and to accept help.

Although metabolism of alcohol is not particularly affected by age, the volume of distribution may change because of reduction in body fat, allowing more of a dose of alcohol to reach the brain (28, 29). In addition, the aging brain may be more susceptible to the effects of alcohol (30).

Older individuals may find that the amount of alcohol that they could easily tolerate when they were younger results in adverse effects. The older patient may present because of such adverse consequences as falls with increased incidence of fracture and subdural hematoma, anemia, gastritis with and without hemorrhage, alcoholic liver disease, pancreatitis, alcohol amnestic syndrome, or early dementia. Alcohol use may increase blood pressure, and the patient may present with late-onset or labile hypertension or hypertension that is difficult to control. The reader is referred to reviews of the medical consequences of alcohol and other drugs (31, 32).

Sedative-Hypnotics

Anxiety disorders and insomnia are common in older persons, and a substantial number of prescriptions for anxiolytic and soporific drugs are used in this population. Normal changes in sleeping patterns may be troublesome, and the physician who fails to take a complete sleep history or inquire into sleep hygiene may be more likely to prescribe hypnotics. While benzodiazepines have become the primary class of prescribed agents, use of barbiturates, meprobamate, chloral hydrate, and other barbituratelike drugs is not uncommon (33).

While most patients for whom sedative-hypnotics are prescribed may take them safely and effectively over a long period of time, abuse and dependence may occur in some patients, particularly those with underlying alcohol abuse or personality disorders. The individual abusing such drugs may develop tolerance over time, gradually increasing the number of doses per day or increasing the amount of each dose. This often results in calls to physicians' offices for refills of prescriptions prior to visits and ultimately may result in claims of lost prescriptions, stolen pills, loss of pills in the toilet, etc. Patients seeking additional drugs may visit multiple physicians, emergency departments, or walk-in clinics. Increasing use of sedatives may result in retrograde or anterograde amnesia, deterioration of personal hygiene, confusion, lethargy, or obtundation. "Automatic" behavior, in which the patient may not remember taking the medication because of its amnestic effects, may result in taking multiple doses with serious adverse consequences.

Patients who are using other CNS depressants, such as alcohol or opioids, may experience additive or synergistic effects with sedatives, and greater caution should be exercised in prescribing. In the alcohol-abusing patient, the concomitant use of benzodiazepines or other sedatives may result in more rapid deterioration and can have serious effects, including risks of respiratory depression, aspiration, pneumonia, falls, and motor vehicle and other accidents. As with alcohol, some patients who develop sedative-hypnotic abuse may be those with long-standing histories of chemical dependency, while others may develop problems later in life, secondary to other problems associated with aging or losses in their lives. The natural history and presentation may vary considerably depending on the nature of onset as well as medical and psychiatric comorbidities.

Opioids

Abuse of illicit opioids, particularly heroin, is extremely rare in patients over 60, although patients with long-standing opioid abuse may occasionally survive into old age. Opium smoking may be seen in older individuals in Oriental cultures, and with increased immigration to the United States from Southeast Asia, these patients may be seen.

Licit opioid abuse is more commonly seen in the elderly. The increase in painful conditions, particularly arthritis and low back pain, may result in prescriptions for oral opioids with abuse potential. As with sedative-hypnotics, abuse occurs in a minority of patients, but the results of such abuse may be serious for patient and family. Fear of abuse has often led to underprescribing of opioids for painful conditions, particularly cancer and other intractable pain. The patient with a prior history of alcohol or other drug abuse and patients with certain psychiatric syndromes may be more likely to abuse opioids and other drugs.

Clinicians working with chronic pain patients usually find that patients can be maintained on a stable dose of opioids for long periods of time, with little or no escalation of dose or problematic use (34). There appears to be relatively little tolerance

to the analgesic effects of opioids; dose increases of 10 to 20% per year are common. On the other hand, tolerance to the mood-altering or euphoriant effects of opioids occurs rapidly, and with it the need to escalate dose. Patients may believe that they are increasing the dose to combat pain, but it is more likely that they are receiving relief of intrapsychic rather than somatic pain.

Increases in dose lead to the same issues as with sedative-hypnotics, including frequent refills, excuses of lost pills or prescriptions, or "doctor shopping." In addition, since the dominant form of opioid prescription is for combinations containing aspirin or acetaminophen, toxicity from these agents may occur. High-dose opioids may result in personality changes, irritability, sedation, and accidental trauma. With propoxyphene, pentazocine, and meperidine, CNS stimulation with seizures and delirium may occur.

Other Drugs

Abuse of cocaine and other stimulants is extremely rare in the elderly, as is abuse of psychotomimetic drugs or inhalants. Prescription of amphetamines or methylphenidate for depression may rarely result in abuse and toxicity. Use of cannabis may occur, particularly with individuals with prior histories of such use, and occasionally cannabis may be self-prescribed to combat nausea from chemotherapy or to treat glaucoma. The elderly may take high-dose aspirin or nonsteroidal antiinflammatory drugs without medical supervision to treat pain, sometimes with serious medical consequences, including gastrointestinal hemorrhage, acid-base disturbances, confusion, or delirium (35). Use of multiple medications with anticholinergic effects is common in the elderly, and while not generally related to abuse, it may result in behavioral changes and presentations with memory impairment, agitation, confusion, or delirium.

Drug-drug interactions, as well as interactions with alcohol, tobacco, and even food products are very common, particularly in the elderly, where polypharmacy is common, and reduction in renal and/or hepatic clearance, decrease in body weight and/or fat, displacement of one drug from protein binding sites by another, and other factors may make such interactions more common and more problematic (36, 37). A careful history of drugs prescribed by all of the patient's physicians, as well as prescribed drugs obtained from other sources (a family member's or friend's medication), over-the-counter drug use, tobacco use, and dietary history, including recent gain or loss of weight, may be required in detecting problems related to drug-drug interaction.

DIAGNOSIS

The diagnosis of chemical dependency, like most others in clinical medicine, should be largely based on history. The criteria in the *Diagnostic and Statistical Manual* of the American Psychiatric Association, 3rd edition-revised (DSM-IIIR) are widely accepted (38). The fourth edition (DSM-IV) is in the process of release. Three of the nine criteria are required for a diagnosis of a substance use disorder (Table 13.1).

The CAGE questionnaire (39) may be helpful (*C*ut down on use; *A*nger if use brought up; *G*uilt over use; need for *E*yeopener.) Although it has not been specifically validated in older populations, there is evidence that suggests that it may be at least a useful screening tool in older populations (40). A positive response to two of the CAGE questions is associated with sensitivity and specificity in the 90% range in younger patients, but it must be stressed that this is a screening instrument, and definitive diagnosis should be based on more comprehensive evaluation. The addition of posi-

Table 13.1
Diagnostic Criteria for Psychoactive Substance Dependence[a,b]

At least three of the following
1. Substance taken in larger amounts or over longer period than intended.
2. Persistent desire or one or more unsuccessful efforts to cut down or control substance use
3. A great deal of time spent in activities necessary to obtain the substance or recovering from its effects
4. Frequent intoxication or withdrawal symptoms when expected to fulfill major role obligations, or fulfilling them when use of substance is hazardous (i.e., driving under the influence)
5. Important social, occupational or recreational activities given up or reduced because of substance use
6. Continued substance use despite knowledge of having a persistent or recurrent social, psychological or physical problem that is caused or worsened by use
7. Marked tolerance: need for increased (50%) amounts of substance in order to achieve desired effect, or reduced effect from using the same amount[b]
8. Characteristic withdrawal symptoms when substance use is stopped or reduced[b]
9. Substance is taken to relieve or avoid withdrawal symptoms

[a]American Psychiatric Association. Diagnostic and Statistical Manual of Mental Disorders. 3rd ed. Rev. Washington, DC: American Psychiatric Association, 1987.
[b]May not apply to cannabis, phencyclidine, hallucinogens.

tive responses to the following questions—Was your last drink within 24 hours of the interview? and Do you think you have ever had a drinking problem?—may add to the positive predictive value of the CAGE questions (41). The Michigan Alcoholism Screening Test (MAST), which is widely used, may have less utility than the CAGE in the elderly (42). One group has found that the short MAST (sMAST) may be more sensitive as a screening tool than the CAGE or standard MAST in older persons (43).

A complete substance use history should be obtained, asking questions in a calm, nonjudgmental, and open-ended way. Emphasis should be on specific questions on quantity and frequency of use, including problematic binge drinking. Specific questions such as "what day did you last drink alcohol?" and "how much did you drink that day?" may be useful. Asking whether the number of drinking occasions per week or month and the amount of drinks per occasion are typical or have changed over time may also be informative. Specific questions regarding doses of prescribed drugs and whether such doses are ever exceeded, as well as asking about frequency of refills, should be part of the history.

Many, if not most, patients will be quite open about their substance use when asked directly about their history. For patients who seem evasive, it may be very useful and even essential to obtain information from signficant others, whether family, friends, or neighbors. The patient may minimize or categorically deny problems, while others in the patient's system may be in a better position to give accurate information. Resistance on the part of the patient to answer questions or allow interviews of significant others should raise the clinician's level of suspicion and should be met with persistent efforts to obtain the needed information. Confidentiality issues may limit the ability to obtain needed information, and the clinicians should be sure of their legal footing in problematic cases.

The presence or history of certain medical/social problems should prompt the physician to further explore the possibility of substance abuse, even though the patient may deny such a problem. For example, a past history of gastrointestinal hemorrhage, unexplained abdominal pain, pancreatitis, liver dysfunction, or frequent unexplained somatic complaints, presence of anxiety, or affective disorders may be suggestive and should also lead the clinician to obtain a comprehensive substance use history.

Mental status changes, history of family dysfunction, divorce, frequent job changes, or geographic moves should alert the clinician to further assess the possibility of substance abuse. One of the most immediate and clinically convenient ways of assessing a person's present blood alcohol concentration (BAC) is to use a breath alcohol test. A reliable and valid measure of alcohol and/or drug use is essential, since clinicians' judgment of patients' states of intoxication is poor, probably because of the phenomenon of tolerance. A BAC of more than 100 mg/100 mL in an individual who shows no signs of inebriation (sustained nystagmus, dysarthria, ataxia, lability of mood, sedation) or a BAC of 250 mg/100 mL in a conscious patient indicates significant tolerance and suggests a diagnosis of alcohol dependence, as well as predicting the likelihood of a significant abstinence syndrome.

Sedative-hypnotics produce a picture similar to that of alcohol, but blood levels are more difficult to obtain. Benzodiazepine and barbiturate levels can be measured in serum but may not be immediately available. Patients who state that they are taking medication as prescribed but have serum levels far above what should be expected are probably taking medication beyond the prescribed dose. Similarly, high serum levels in a patient showing no signs of toxicity suggest dependency. Abuse of butabarbital-containing drugs for headache has become quite common; measurement of butabarbital serum levels and/or acetaminophen or salicylate levels may be definitive.

The patient who abuses opioids may show considerable tolerance and have few if any signs of toxicity. However, pupillary miosis should be seen if the drug was recently used. While levels of most opioids cannot be easily measured in serum, urine toxicology studies can provide a qualitative result. Serum salicylate or acetaminophen levels can be useful in the patient taking combination analgesic products and serve to alert the clinician to the need for separate treatment. Patients presenting with sedation or obtundation, with pupillary miosis and slowed respiration, must be assumed to have opioid intoxication. Abuse of mixed agonist-antagonists, such as pentazocine, propoxyphene, and meperidine, may present with CNS stimulation, including seizures and delirium.

Because polysubstance use has become so common, it is advisable to obtain a qualitative urine toxicology screen in any patient suspected of chemical dependency. This should be done before treatment with any psychoactive drug. Clinicians should familiarize themselves with the use and limitations of toxicology studies (44), particularly if there are any legal ramifications to the urine drug testing. Drug testing should be used as one

component of the comprehensive assessment because false-positive and false-negative results are possible. Patients' use may be in amounts below the limits of detection, patients may be using a prescribed medication with metabolites that cross-react as other drugs on assays, or the patient may adulterate or substitute the urine sample. While positive urine toxicology studies may alert the clinician to unsuspected use of sedative-hypnotics, opioids, or other drugs, a negative study does not exclude such use.

TREATMENT
ROLE OF THE PRIMARY CARE PROVIDER

If a chemical dependency diagnosis is made or suspected, it is incumbent upon the clinician to determine the risk of an abstinence or withdrawal syndrome (45, 46). Well-intentioned advice to a patient to "cut down" or quit alcohol or abrupt discontinuation of a benzodiazepine prescription after evidence of misuse or abuse may result in a patient suffering withdrawal symptoms such as seizures, delirium, and/or a hyperautonomic syndrome, which in many patients, particularly the elderly, may have disastrous consequences. The level of tolerance and the patient's prior experiences in discontinuing drug use are good predictors of the likelihood of an abstinence syndrome.

The older patient may have fewer hyperautonomic signs and symptoms, leading to diagnostic confusion when a seizure or delirium supervenes. When a hyperautonomic state occurs, it may result in angina or myocardial infarction in patients with preexisting coronary heart disease, exacerbation of hypertension with possibility of stroke, diabetes going out of control, or hypoxia and collapse in the patient with underlying chronic obstructive pulmonary disease. Withdrawal of short-acting benzodiazepines or other sedative hypnotics may be similar to alcohol withdrawal syndrome. With barbiturates and barbituratelike drugs, status epilepticus may occur, and delirium may be particularly severe. Opioid withdrawal also may cause a hyperautonomic state, although generally less severe than that with alcohol or sedative hypnotics.

In general, the older patient should be treated in a medically managed or monitored setting, since morbidity and mortality may be higher. A complete medical evaluation must be done, with laboratory studies appropriate to the clinical setting: CBC, electrolytes, blood sugar, BUN/creatinine, chemistry panel with liver function tests, total protein and albumin, uric acid, calcium, and phosphorus. Serum magnesium levels should be obtained in most cases, since hypomagnesemia is common and predisposes to seizures and cardiac arrhythmias. All patients should be given adequate doses of thiamine; generally, 100 mg intramuscularly should be given initially, and then similar doses intramuscularly should be given daily until the patient is taking oral medication. Failure to give adequate thiamine supplementation may result in irreversible Wernicke-Korsakoff syndrome, with permanent neurologic/cognitive disability. Supplementation of other vitamins and minerals may be needed, and other nutritional supplementation should be considered in the debilitated elderly patient.

An ECG and chest x-ray may be obtained if not done recently, particularly if underlying coronary disease is of concern or if tuberculosis or aspiration may be present. Tuberculosis skin tests and controls should be done in patients at risk who have not been recently tested. Further studies, including B_{12} and folic acid levels, CT or MRI, and EEG, may be needed if a seizure has occurred or to exclude intercurrent problems. HIV disease may occur in the elderly, and risk behaviors should be discussed, including blood transfusion and organ transplantation (including corneal) done before widespread HIV antibody testing.

Abstinence syndromes should be treated in consultation with those with experience, particularly with older patients. Benzodiazepines are generally equally effective in the treatment of withdrawal, but because of concern of drug accumulation, long-acting drugs should be used cautiously, since they may result in protracted toxicity, including respiratory depression, aspiration, pneumonia, or intoxication with mood lability, combative behavior, confusion, and injury to self or others.

Short-acting drugs, particularly lorazepam, are preferred. Oxazepam, with a longer latency, produces a "choppier" course. If short-acting drugs are not given with adequate frequency, breakthrough withdrawal, with serious consequences, may occur (47, 48). If shorter-acting drugs are used, the drug should be initially given as often as every 3 to 4 hours, and generally not less than every 6 hours. The dose should be tapered over a longer period of 5 to 7 days. Care should be taken to reduce the dose of the drug rather than the interval, to decrease the likelihood of long periods of reduced drug levels.

Patients using sedative hypnotics should have the dose tapered over 10 to 21 days, depending on the dose and duration of use. Since this withdrawal may have more severe consequences and since many clinicians have less experience with its management, referral to a chemical dependency program where there is more experience is recommended. A variety of regimens may be used (45, 46, 49, 50). Conversion to the equivalent dose of a long-acting benzodiazepine such as chlordiazepoxide, diazepam, or clonazepam is generally recommended, with careful observation and withholding of doses if there is evidence of oversedation. If the patient is using a barbiturate or barbituratelike drug, conversion to phenobarbital in divided doses with a gradual taper is recommended (50).

Patients using minor opioids can generally be treated by tapering the dose of the medication they are taking, in a supervised setting. Shorter-acting drugs such as codeine, hydrocodone, or oxycodone, can generally be tapered over 5 to 10 days. Combination products may need to be avoided because of the salicylate or acetaminophen present. The patient with higher dose use or use of major opioids (e.g., hydromorphone, oxymorphone) may be switched to a longer-acting drug, such as methadone or MS-Contin, and tapered over a longer period of time. This should be done in consultation with someone with pain management and/or substance abuse expertise and again is preferably done in a specialized setting.

For patients who use opiates for pain reduction, effective treatment of the underlying pain problem with alternative therapies must be undertaken, or it is unlikely that the detoxification will be successful. Use of nonsteroidal antiinflammatory drugs; antidepressants; anticonvulsants; physical measures such as heat, ultrasound, or diathermy; and special procedures such as nerve blocks, TENS units, and acupuncture may be needed. In some cases, provision of adequate opioid analgesia in less abusable forms, such as transdermal fentanyl patches, may be appropriate.

PSYCHOSOCIAL TREATMENT

Most studies of treatment have been carried out with younger patients; there have been few systematic studies of treatment in the elderly. Overall, the elderly receive a disproportionately large number of prescriptions for psychoactive drugs. When they present at the physician's office with psychosocial issues, the elderly receive less counseling than other age groups, and they are more likely to receive psychoactive medications. Psychosocial issues must be addressed with patients whose alcohol or other drug abuse began later in life, often as a response to life stresses or losses, and treatment should concentrate on improvement in their social support network. Increased family visits, reentry into the job market, use of "elder cabs" to provide transportation to organized activities, volunteer activities (e.g., teaching their skills to younger unemployed or those starting businesses, involvement in child day-care), and visiting nurse and homemaker services may all serve to decrease the chance of returning to chemical dependency or help to detect relapse early, so that it may be promptly addressed.

The traditional forms of treatment in younger patients, including techniques to decrease denial, minimalization, and rationalization, have generally involved group techniques that are quite confrontational. Such techniques may not be appropriate in older individuals. Putting older individuals with late-onset dependency together with younger patients may both frighten and alienate them; hearing information on illicit drugs, criminal activities, domestic violence, AIDS, and other issues may increase their conviction that they are in the wrong place and do not share a common problem with many others in the group.

One-to-one therapy, groups consisting of older individuals, resocialization efforts, and consideration of psychopharmacologic measures (e.g., antidepressants) may all be of value in the older patient (51). Family therapy is particularly important, since family members may be dismayed by the appearance of chemical dependency in an older relative and may feel guilt or project blame. In the patient with long-standing chemical dependency who has survived to old age, there may be very significant family issues; treatment approaches for such patients may need to be more like those used in a younger population.

While in many cases, patients do well with social referral and/or one-to-one therapy, in some cases self-help or mutual-help programs may be useful for both patients and family. Alanon, Families Anonymous, and NarAnon are groups for the significant others of patients with chemical dependency. It should be stressed to family and friends that their involvement in such groups is for their own benefit, not necessarily the recovery of their affected relative. Alcoholics Anonymous may be a source for individual and group support, and the twelve steps of the recovery program, as well as its "spiritual" nature, may appeal to many older persons. The physician may be of help in locating appropriate meetings, sponsors, or involvement in other self-help groups, such as Rational Recovery.

PREVENTION AND EARLY INTERVENTION

Health care professionals have an important role to play in the prevention of chemical dependency, both in the patient population at large and in the elderly (52, 53). The clinician should have a complete history, regularly updated, which includes information on the use of alcohol and other drugs, as well as the medical, psychiatric, and social problems that may be related to substance abuse. Early intervention may allow resolution of the problem before severe comorbidities and individual and social dysfunction occurs. The clinician can also be a resource to the patient in suggesting more functional coping strategies, such as stress reduction techniques, proper diet, exercise, and recreational activities. Availability of substance abuse educational material in the physician's waiting area may give patients permission to discuss their own personal issues with the clinician. Physicians should be particularly careful in their prescribing practices, so as to not facilitate or even create iatrogenic chemical dependencies.

REFERENCES

1. Knupfer G. The prevalence in various social groups of eight different drinking patterns, from abstaining to frequent drunkenness: analysis of ten U.S. surveys combined. Br J Addict 1989; 84:1305–1318.
2. Myers JK, Weissman MM, Tischler GL, et al. Six-month prevalence of psychiatric disorders in three communities: 1980–1982. Arch Gen Psychiatry 1984;41:959–957.
3. Bristow MF, Clare AN. Prevalence and characteristics of at-risk drinkers among elderly acute medical inpatients. Br J Addict 1992;87:291–294.
4. Cleary PD, Miller M, Bush BT, Warburg MM, Delbanco TL, Aronson MD. Prevalence and recognition of alcohol abuse in a primary care population. Am J Med 1988;85:466–471.
5. Finlayson RD, Hurt RD, Davis LJ, Morse RM. Alcoholism in elderly persons: a study of the psychiatric and psychosocial features of 216 inpatients. Mayo Clin Proc 1988;63:761–768.
6. Miller F, Whitcup S, Sacks M, Lynch PE. Unrecognized drug dependence and withdrawal in the elderly. Drug Alcohol Depend 1985;15:177–179.
7. Barnes GM. Alcohol use among older persons: findings from a western New York State general population survey. J Am Geriatr Soc 1979;27:244–250.
8. Adams WL, Garry PJ, Rhyne R, Hunt WS, Goodwin JS. Alcohol intake in the healthy elderly. J Am Geriatr Soc 1990;38:211–216.

9. Atkinson RM. Aging and alcohol use disorders: diagnostic issues in the elderly. Int Psychogeriatr 1990;2:55–72.

10. Gomberg ESL. Drugs, alcohol and aging. In: Kozowski LT, Annis HM, Cappel HD, et al., eds. Research advances in alcohol and drug problems, vol. 10. New York: Plenum, 1990:171–213.

11. Douglas R. Aging and alcohol problems: opportunities for socioepidemiological research. In: Galanter M, ed. Recent developments in alcoholism, vol. 2. New York: Plenum, 1984.

12. Laforge RG, Nirenberg TD, Lewis DC, Murphy JB. Problem drinking, gender and stressful life events among hospitalized elderly drinkers. Behav Health Aging, in press.

13. Adams WL, Yuan Z, Barboriak JJ, Rimm AA. Alcohol-related hospitalizations of elderly people: prevalence and geographic variation in the United States. JAMA 1993;270:1222–1225.

14. Lewis DC, Niven RG, Czechowicz D, Trumble JG. A review of medical education in alcohol and other drug abuse. JAMA 1987;257:2945–2948.

15. Schuckit MA, Atkinson JH, Miller PL, Berman J. A three-year follow-up of elderly alcoholics. J Clin Psychiatry 1980;41:412–416.

16. Miller NS, Belkin BM, Gold MS. Alcohol and drug dependence among the elderly: epidemiology, diagnosis, and treatment. Compr Psychiatry 1991; 32:153–165.

17. Zimberg S. Two types of problem drinkers: both can be managed. Geriatrics 1974;29:135–138.

18. Hartford JT, Samorajski T. Alcoholism in the geriatric population. J Am Geriatr Soc 1982;30:18–24.

19. Dunham RG. Aging and changing patterns of alcohol use. J Psychoactive Drugs 1981;13:143–151.

20. Atkinson RM, ed. Alcohol and alcohol abuse in old age. Washington, DC: American Psychiatric Press, 1984.

21. Rosin AJ, Glatt MM. Alcohol excess in the elderly. Q J Stud Alcohol 1971;32:53–59.

22. Atkinson RM, Turner JA, Kofoed LL, Tolson RL. Early versus late onset alcoholism in older persons: preliminary findings. Alcoholism (NY) 1985;9:513–515.

23. Bienenfeld D. Alcoholism in the elderly. Am Fam Physician 1987;36:163–169.

24. Vaillant GE. The natural history of alcoholism: causes, patterns and paths to recovery. Cambridge, MA: Harvard University Press, 1983.

25. Institute of Medicine. Prevention and treatment of alcohol problems: research opportunities. Report of a study by a committee of the IOM. Division of Mental Health and Behavioral Medicine. Washington, DC: National Academy Press, 1989.

26. Alexander F, Duff RW. Social interaction and alcohol use in retirement communities. Gerontologist 1988;28:632–638.

27. Liepman MR, Nirenberg TD, Porges R, Wartenberg A. Depression associated with substance abuse. In: Cameron OG, ed. Presentations of depression. New York: John Wiley & Sons, 1987:131–167.

28. Gambert S. Substance abuse in the elderly. In: Lowinson JH, Ruiz P, Millman RR, Langrod JG, eds. Substance abuse: a comprehensive textbook. 2nd ed. Baltimore: Williams & Wilkins, 1992:843–851.

29. Vogel-Sprott M, Barrett P. Age, drinking habits and the effects of alcohol. J Stud Alcohol 1984;45:517–521.

30. Lister RG, Eckardt MJ, Weingartner H. Ethanol intoxication and memory: recent developments and new directions. In: Galanter M, ed. Recent developments in alcoholism. Vol 4. New York: Plenum, 1987:111–126.

31. Wartenberg AA, Liepman MR. Medical complications of substance abuse. In: Lerner WD, Barr W, eds. Hospital-based treatment of substance abuse. New York: Pergamon Press, 1990:49–68.

32. Novick DM. The medically ill substance abuser. In: Lowinson JH, Ruiz P, Millman RR, Langrod JG, eds. Substance abuse: a comprehensive textbook. 2nd ed. Baltimore: Williams & Wilkins, 1992:657–674.

33. Closser MH. Benzodiazepines and the elderly: a review of potential problems. J Subst Abuse Treat 1991;8:35–41.

34. McGivney WT, Crooks GM. The care of patients with severe chronic pain in terminal illness. JAMA 1984;251:752–757.

35. Hoppman RA, Peden JG, Ober SK. Central nervous system side effects of non-steroidal anti-inflammatory drugs: aseptic meningitis, psychosis and cognitive dysfunction. Arch Intern Med 1991;151:1309–1313.

36. Miller NS. The pharmacology of interactions between medical and psychiatric drugs. In: Miller NS. The pharmacology of alcohol and drugs of abuse and addiction. New York, Springer-Verlag, 1991:279–289.

37. Wartenberg AA. Drug-drug interactions in the pharmacotherapy of addiction. In: Miller NS, Gold M, eds. The phamacotherapy of addiction. New York: Marcel Dekker, 1994, in press.

38. American Psychiatric Association. Diagnostic and Statistical Manual of Mental Disorders, Third Edition, Revised. Washington, DC: American Psychiatric Association, 1987.

39. Ewing JA. Detecting alcoholism: the CAGE questionnaire. JAMA 1984;252:1905–1907.

40. Jones TJ, Lindsey BA, Yount P, Soltys R, Farani-Enayat B. Alcoholism screening questionnaires: are they valid in elderly outpatients? J Gen Intern Med 1993;8:674–678.

41. Cyr MG, Wartman SA. The effectiveness of routine screening questions in the detection of alcoholism. JAMA 1988;259:51–54.

42. Sobell LC, Cellucci T, Nirenberg TD, Sobell MB. Do quantity-frequency data underestimate drinking-related health risks: Am J Public Health 1982;72:823–828.

43. McGann KP, Marion GS. Screening for alcoholism in the elderly: the validity of the brief screening measures. Subst Abuse 1992;13:188–195.

44. Schwartz RA. Urine testing in the detection of drugs of abuse. Arch Intern Med 1988;148:2407–2412.

45. Wartenberg AA. Detoxification of the chemically dependent patient. RI Med J 1989;72:451–456.

46. Sellers EM, Naranjo CA. New strategies for the treatment of alcohol withdrawal. Psychopharmacol Bull 1988;22:88–92.

47. Hill A, Williams D. Hazards associated with the use of benzodiazepines. J Subst Abuse Treat 1993;10:449–452.

48. Mayo-Smith MF, Bernard D. Late onset seizures in alcohol withdrawal. J Addict Dis 1993;12:188 [abstract 34a].

49. Smith DE, Wesson DR. A phenobarbital technique for withdrawal of barbiturate abuse. Arch Gen Psychiatry 1971;24:56–61.

50. Sullivan JT, Sellers EM. Treating alcohol, barbiturate and benzodiazepine withdrawal. Rational Drug Ther 1986;20:1–9.

51. Curtis JR, Geller G, Stokes EJ, et al. Characteristics, diagnosis and treatment of alcoholism in elderly patients. J Am Geriatr Soc 1989;37:310–316.

52. Wallack L. Practical issues, ethical concerns and future directions in the prevention of alcohol-related problems. J Prim Prevent 1984;4:199–224.

53. Noel NE, McCrady BS. Target populations for alcohol abuse prevention. In: Miller PM, Nirenberg TD, eds. Prevention of alcohol abuse. New York: Plenum, 1984:55–94.

14/ Evaluation and Management of the Confused, Disoriented, or Demented Elderly Patient

William Reichel, Peter V. Rabins

One of the most common problems facing the physician today is evaluating and managing the elderly patient with cognitive and behavioral disturbances. This chapter focuses mainly on three neuropsychiatric disorders: the patient with acute confusion, disorientation or delirium; the patient with dementia or generalized cognitive loss; and the patient with an emotional or psychiatric disorder. Of course, there are often mixed forms or combinations of each of these clinical entities. Proper diagnosis of these specific neuropsychiatric disorders is essential to making specific treatment plans.

Additional recent information and perspectives on the etiology and new potential pharmacological therapies of the most common form of dementia—Alzheimer's disease—are contained in Chapter 15, Alzheimer's Disease: Biological Aspects.

The physician evaluating a person who complains of memory difficulty must identify correctly individuals with minor age-related memory impairments. These do not require an extensive evaluation but should reflect minor nondisease-related changes.

AGE-RELATED COGNITIVE DECLINE

What was previously called "benign senescent forgetfulness" and "age-associated memory impairment" (1) is now called "age-related cognitive decline" (2, 3). This condition is characterized by complaints of difficulty thinking while carrying out activities of daily life, supported by evidence of mild impairment on psychological performance tests. Symptoms must be present for 6 months and develop gradually. It is characterized by difficulty in remembering names of individuals on meeting them, misplacing spectacles or keys, difficulty remembering tasks to be performed, and

difficulty in remembering telephone numbers. No etiology can be identified, and the symptoms do not meet criteria for dementia, organic amnestic syndrome (severe isolated memory disturbance), or depression.

DELIRIUM OR ACUTE CONFUSIONAL STATE

The elderly patient often presents with acute confusion, delirium, disorientation, or other behavioral alterations (Table 14.1). When this is accompanied by an altered level of consciousness, that is, by a diminution in the clarity of awareness of the environment, a diagnosis of delirium is made (4). Previously known as "acute brain syndrome," delirium is often accompanied by four features: acute onset and fluctuating course, inattention, disorganized thinking, and altered level of consciousness (4). The diagnosis of delirium by the Confusion Assessment Method (CAM) of Inouye and associates, shown in Table 14.1, requires the presence of the first two features and either of the last two. The CAM criteria are highly sensitive and specific. Abrupt or rapid change in patients from their customary state of sensorium, intellectual function, or consciousness should be investigated thoroughly for a possible organic disorder.

The problem may result from almost any physical ailment or drug problem. For example, heart attack, dehydration, urinary tract infection, pneumonia, fecal impaction, pulmonary embolism, gastrointestinal hemorrhage, and many types of drug intoxication and drug withdrawal all cause delirium or acute confusional states. Such confusional states are often transient and reversible. The elderly patient with relatively recent changes in mental status is not suffering from dementia or chronic brain syndrome (Table 14.2), which is characterized by the gradual deterioration of

Table 14.1
The Confusion Assessment Method (CAM) Diagnostic Algorithm[a,b]

Feature 1.	Acute onset and fluctuating course
	This feature is usually obtained from a family member or nurse and is shown by positive responses to the following questions: Is there evidence of an acute change in mental status from the patient's baseline: Did the (abnormal) behavior fluctuate during the day, that is, tend to come and go, or increase and decrease in severity?
Feature 2.	Inattention
	This feature is shown by a positive response to the following question. Did the patient have difficulty focusing attention, for example, being easily distractible; or having difficulty keeping track of what was being said?
Feature 3.	Disorganized thinking
	This feature is shown by a positive response to the following question: Was the patient's thinking disorganized or incoherent, such as rambling or irrelevant conversation, unclear or illogical flow of ideas, or unpredictable switching from subject to subject?
Feature 4.	Altered level of consciousness
	This feature is shown by any answer other than "alert" to the following question: Overall, how would you rate this patient's level of consciousness? (alert, [normal], vigilant [hyperalert], lethargic [drowsy, easily aroused], stupor [difficult to arouse], or coma [unarousable])

[a]The diagnosis of delirium by CAM requires the presence of features 1 and 2 and either 3 or 4.
[b]From Inouye SK, van Dyck CM, Aleissi CA, et al. Clarifying confusion: the Confusion Assessment Method. A new method for detection of delirium. Ann Intern Med 1990:113:941–948.

intellectual function, memory, or cognitive ability in a normally alert individual. In making the diagnosis of dementia, it is necessary to document intellectual decline and loss of memory over a period of months to years.

An illustration of an acute confusional state might be a 75-year-old woman who took care of her household, performing all her usual duties until 3 days prior to her presentation to a hospital emergency room. She appeared confused, agitated, and restless. There were no other medical complaints, but an electrocardiogram revealed an anteroseptal myocardial infarction. Following an initially difficult course in a coronary care unit, she improved and at the time of discharge showed no signs of mental dysfunction.

DEMENTIA

In contrast, a case of dementia is exemplified by an 80-year-old man who presents with a 2-year history of gradually developing memory loss and inability to care for himself. The family has been concerned about his recent failure to recognize his own relatives and an increased tendency to wander astray. Examination demonstrates that he is markedly forgetful, not remembering conversa-

tions from one minute to the next. He has no recall of recent events, although recall of events in the remote past is fair. Neurologic examination is normal. His affect is not blunted, and he appears very pleasant.

In the symptoms/sign complex of dementia (called chronic brain syndrome in DSM-I), the patient initially may experience diminishing ability to concentrate and recall recent events. As the illness progresses, judgment becomes impaired and conversation difficult. Family members may be the first to notice the disorder, but the gradual course of the disease often permits patients some insight into their condition. Irritability, anxiety, or depression may develop. They may become unable to perform usual occupational or household duties. Eventually, remote memory may be affected, and patients can no longer recognize family members or friends. In the final stages, patients are rendered totally incapable of caring for themselves.

TESTING COGNITIVE FUNCTION

It is imperative in testing for dementia that the physician or other health professional evaluate the intellectual functions of the patient. Remote

Table 14.2
Differential Diagnosis and Treatment of Delirium (or Acute Confusional State) and Dementia

	Delirium or Acute Confusional State	Dementia
Differential diagnosis:		
	May be secondary to	Causes include
	Myocardial infarction	Alzheimer's disease (dementia of the Alzheimer's type)
	Dehydration	Vascular dementia
	Pneumonia	Myxedema
	Ischemia mainly in basilar-posterior cerebral artery territory	Hyper/hypoparathyroidism
	Fecal impaction	Acquired immune deficiency disease
	Gastrointestinal hemorrhage	Pernicious anemia
	Electrolyte imbalance	Folic acid deficiency
	Urinary tract infection	Chronic hepatic encephalopathy
	Pulmonary embolism	Chronic drug intoxication
	Heart failure	Chronic subdural hematoma
	Occult malignancy	Brain tumor
	Drug intoxication	General paresis
	Drug withdrawal	Parkinson's disease
	Alcohol intoxication	Wilson's disease
	Alcohol withdrawal or abstinence states	Cushing's/Addison's disease
		Normal pressure hydrocephalus
	Other hidden medical problems	Pick's disease
		Huntington's chorea
		Creutzfeldt-Jakob disease
		Punchdrunk syndrome or dementia pugilistica
		Depression
Treatment		
	Proper recognition and management of the underlying medical disorder or drug problem	Proper recognition and management of the underlying neurologic disorder
		Recognition and treatment of associated medical and behavioral disorders
	Reassurance, frequent reorientation, good lighting, moderately stimulating environment	Family support

memory is preserved to a greater degree than recent memory. Impairment of remote memory carries a graver prognosis than the loss of recent memory alone. The mental acuity of the elderly individual is also affected by socioeconomic factors and the accessibility of interpersonal communication and audiovisual stimuli, such as newspaper, radio, or television. In the absence of sufficient exposure to the external environment, it may be quite difficult for the elderly patient to answer common test questions, such as the date or the names of current political figures.

The Mini-Mental State Examination, developed by Folstein et al. (5), is an easily administered screening examination that measures orientation, memory, concentration, and language (Table 2.4, Chapter 2). Another instrument, the Short Portable Mental Status Questionnaire, developed by Pfeiffer (6), provides a screening examination that tests short- and long-term memory, capacity to perform serial mathematical tasks, and orientation. It is easy to perform and score, is portable, and requires little time to administer (Table 2.5, Chapter 2).

In addition, it is imperative that the health professional be able to verify the answers provided by the patient to questions in the mental status examination. This goal is usually accomplished with the aid of the children, spouse, or other relatives or friends of the patient. If such substantiation is not possible, a different type of test becomes necessary. Asking the patient to repeat a short series of words or numbers in a limited time framework may be particularly efficacious, although this test evaluates a different form of memory. The health professional should also ask questions about home and work that can be verified by family. Questions about recent news or sporting events or even the weather can be very revealing. It is rare that a cognitively normal individual would not know the name of the current president.

DIFFERENTIATING EMOTIONAL DISORDER FROM DEMENTIA

In the interview, the health professional must differentiate dementia from functional or emotional disturbances that resemble dementia. An individual experiencing depression after the loss of a spouse may present the appearance of dementia. On further examination, it becomes evident that the patient is extremely depressed. Hidden depression should be considered in the evaluation of all patients with apparent dementia.

It can be difficult to differentiate between dementia accompanied by some reactive depression and depression with some cognitive loss secondary to the depression. There are occasional situations in which it is simply too difficult to separate these two entities. When faced with this dilemma, a therapeutic trial with an antidepressant medication is useful to separate dementia and depression. However, in most cases, with skillful interviewing technique, the physician should be able to determine what diagnostic category or cluster is predominant. The cluster of symptoms and signs is usually clear. The physician's interviewing skills should, in most cases, determine whether he or she is dealing principally with a loss of intellectual capacity, with a functional disorder, or with some mixture of both.

A great deal of attention has been given to the condition called "pseudodementia" (7). Wells made the point that in the past, the diagnosis of pseudodementia had been made largely after the unanticipated recovery of a patient who had previously been diagnosed as suffering from dementia. According to Wells, early recognition of pseudodementia allows the prediction of improvement or recovery in contrast to the negative prognosis of most patients with dementia. Wells (7) noted that in pseudodementia, the history of previous psychiatric dysfunction is common. In pseudodementia, the onset of the illness can usually be dated with precision, and the symptoms are of short duration before medical help is sought. The patient usually complains to a greater degree of cognitive loss in pseudodementia than in dementia and will communicate a strong sense of distress. Rabins et al. (8) also demonstrated that dementia due to depression can be recognized by its subacute onset, occurrence in persons with a past history of depression, coexistence with hypochondriacal depressive preoccupations, and weight loss.

IMPORTANCE OF DIFFERENTIATING VARIOUS NEUROPSYCHIATRIC DISORDERS

It is by means of a thorough history, interview, and physical examination that the various types of neuropsychiatric disorders may be differentiated. Is this syndrome representative of a delirious or acute confusional reaction with diminished alertness and recent onset caused by medical illness or drug toxicity? Does the history reveal a gradual and progressive decline in the intellectual function and memory? Is the presenting disorder chiefly functional or emotional, a disorder of affect, such as in the case of an elderly patient with recent onset of depression? It is essential for the physician to understand the underlying illness in order to be of benefit to the patient who presents with a neuropsychiatric disturbance. Treatment of the acute confusional state, dementia, or functional illness is based upon the proper recognition and management of the underlying problem. Of course, there are also mixed combinations of these three types of disorders. In mixed cases, the treatment is based upon the proper recognition and management of the several underlying problems.

COMMON DISEASE STATES THAT CAUSE DEMENTIA

A careful consideration of the causes of dementia is appropriate (Table 14.2) In the past, many thought that most cases of dementia were arteriosclerotic in origin. In fact, it is now known that less than one-fourth of all dementia is vascular. The elderly demented individual merits complete evaluation to determine the cause of this problem. The most common form of dementia (approximately 60% of cases of organic dementia in the elderly) is Alzheimer's disease, also called dementia of the Alzheimer's type in DSM-IV. The second most common cause is vascular dementia (9), which comprises approximately 20% of the cases of dementia in the elderly. Some patients show clinical and pathologic features of both Alzheimer's disease and vascular dementia.

SENILE DEMENTIA OF THE ALZHEIMER TYPE

Alzheimer's disease is characterized by memory loss and a deficit of at least one other cognitive skill (10). At an ultrastructural level, the neuropathologist finds senile plaques and Alzheimer's neurofibrillary tangles. Alois Alzheimer first presented his clinical and neuropathologic findings regarding a 51-year-old woman at a meeting of the South West German Society of Alienists in Tübingen in November 1906. His report was noted by title only in the *Neurologisch Zentralblatt* in 1906 and more fully in the *Allgemeine Zeitschrift für Psychiatrie* in 1907. The woman's symptoms consisted of suspiciousness, loss of memory, and disorientation. Within 5 years, she suffered severe dementia and death. Her brain was found to be atrophied, and using a method of silver impregnation, a specific clumping and distortion of the cortical neurofibrils was noted, which is now associated with Alzheimer's name.

The senile, or neuritic, plaque consists of a group of degenerating nerve processes including axons and dendrites surrounding an amyloid core. The neurofibrillary tangle is an intracellular lesion consisting of a tangled mass of abnormal cytoplasmic fibrils. Both neurofibrillary tangles and neuritic (senile) plaques are found in small numbers in the hippocampus of most elderly individuals, but they are found with increased frequency in both the neocortex and hippocampus in patients suffering Alzheimer's disease. A more detailed account of the neurobiology of Alzheimer's disease is contained in Chapter 15, Alzheimer's Disease: Biological Aspects.

In diagnosing different types of dementia, the diagnostic imaging techniques of the brain, such as computerized tomography (CT) and magnetic resonance imaging (MRI) are important in the diagnosis of vascular dementia, normal pressure hydrocephalus, brain tumor, and subdural hematoma. The choice between MRI and CT may depend on availability of technologies, cost, and other circumstances. MRI is more sensitive than CT for detection of small infarcts, brainstem atrophy, and mass lesions, but there is greater hazard of overdiagnosis of equivocal findings that are detected by MRI's increased sensitivity. Furthermore, the MRI is significantly more expensive. The MRI and CT scan provide information regarding the degree of atrophy of the brain, but this information is not diagnostic of Alzheimer's disease.

Although the CT scan and MRI were originally believed to provide an accurate assessment of the degree of atrophy of the brain, it is clear that dementia remains a clinical syndrome; the diagnosis must be based on history, evaluation of mental and behavioral status, and the evaluation of the total clinical picture. There are patients with radiographic signs of atrophy and no dementia. In these individuals, the radiographic findings may represent gross pathologic alterations but are not accompanied by the ultrastructural changes of Alzheimer's disease. Conversely, there are patients with dementia with absence of cerebral atrophy as noted by diagnostic imaging. Huckman et al. (11) pointed out that absence of brain atrophy in the demented patient should alert the physician to a potentially treatable cause of dementia. Ford and Winter (12) suggested that CT evidence of cortical atrophy in the elderly should not be accepted as evidence of dementia; specifically, the presence or absence of brain atrophy should not preclude a vigorous search for potentially reversible causes of dementia, nor should radiologic findings of atrophy or ventricular enlargement be considered pathognomonic of dementia. We do not yet have good longitudinal data on the MRI and CT scan of the brain in an aging population. More information will be required in the future to determine the usefulness of these techniques in the diagnosis of clear-cut Alzheimer's disease in the elderly population.

Very hopeful in obtaining longitudinal data are the efforts of the Consortium to Establish a Registry for Alzheimer's Disease (CERAD), which includes the work of investigators at 28 university medical centers as well as a network of international CERAD sites. Patients followed at the CERAD programs received standardized history and physical examination, MRI, neuropsychological testing, and ultimately autopsy examination. The testing instruments have been modified when insights during the course of the investigation have shed some new light; for example, regarding behavioral disorders seen in Alzheimer's disease. We can look forward with great expectations to the achievements of this important longitudinal process (13–15).

The diagnosis of Alzheimer's disease is based on clinical judgment. Perhaps the best criteria for Alzheimer's disease are found in the report of the NINCDS-ADRDA Work Group (10) that sets criteria for probable, possible, and definite Alzheimer's disease, as well as a classification of Alzheimer's disease for research purpose that includes features such as familial occurrence and onset before the age of 65 (see Table 14.3).

VASCULAR DEMENTIA

Vascular dementia may occur after repeated cerebrovascular accidents or as the result of

Table 14.3
Criteria for Clinical Diagnosis of Alzheimer's Disease[a]

I. The criteria for the clinical diagnosis of PROBABLE Alzheimer's disease include

Dementia established by clinical examination and documented by the Mini-Mental Test. Blessed Dementia Scale or some similar examination, and confirmed by neuropsychological tests

Deficits in two or more areas of cognition

Progressive worsening of memory and other cognitive functions

No disturbance of consciousness

Onset between ages 40 and 90, most often after age 65

Absence of systemic disorders or other brain diseases that in and of themselves could account for the progressive deficits in memory and cognition

II. The diagnosis of PROBABLE Alzheimer's disease is supported by

Progressive deterioration of specific cognitive functions such as language (aphasia), motor skills (apraxia), and perception (agnosia)

Impaired activities of daily living and altered patterns of behavior

Family history of similar disorders, particularly if confirmed neuropathologically

Laboratory results of

Normal lumbar puncture as evaluated by standard techniques

Normal pattern or nonspecific changes in EEG, such as increased slow-wave activity

Evidence of cerebral atrophy on CT with progression documented by serial observation

III. Other clinical features consistent with the diagnosis of PROBABLE Alzheimer's disease after exclusion of causes of dementia other than Alzheimer's disease, include

Plateaus in the course of progression of the illness

Associated symptoms of depression, insomnia, incontinence, delusions, illusions, hallucinations, catastrophic verbal, emotional, or physical outbursts, sexual disorders, and weight loss

Other neurologic abnormalities in some patients, especially with more advanced disease and including motor signs such as increased muscle tone, myoclonus, or gait disorder

Seizures in advanced disease

CT normal for age

IV. Features that make the diagnosis of PROBABLE Alzheimer's disease uncertain or unlikely include

Sudden, apoplectic onset

Focal neurologic findings such as hemiparesis, sensory loss, visual field deficits and incoordination early in the course of the illness

V. Clinical diagnosis of POSSIBLE Alzheimer's disease

May be made on the basis of the dementia syndrome, in the absence of other neurologic, psychiatric, or systemic disorders sufficient to cause dementia, and in the presence of variations in the onset, in the presentation, or in the clinical course

May be made in the presence of a second systemic or brain disorder sufficient to produce dementia, which is not considered to be *the* cause of the dementia

Should be used in research studies when a single, gradually progressive, severe cognitive deficit is identified in the absence of other identifiable cause

VI. Criteria for diagnosis of DEFINITE Alzheimer's disease are

The clinical criteria for probable Alzheimer's disease

Histopathologic evidence obtained from a biopsy or autopsy

VII. Classification of Alzheimer's disease for research purposes should specify features that may differentiate subtypes of the disorder, such as

Familial occurrence

Onset before age 65

Presence of trisomy-21

Coexistence of other relevant conditions such as Parkinson's disease

---

[a]From McKhann G, Drachman D, Folstein M, Katzman R, Price D, Stedlan EM. Clinical diagnosis of Alzheimer's disease: report of the NINCDS-ADRDA Work Group under the auspices of Department of Health and Human Services Task Force on Alzheimer's disease. Neurology 1984; 34:939–944.

chronically diminished blood flow (9). The symptoms of vascular disease are episodic, based on the history of recurrent stroke. The neurologic findings of vascular disease are unilateral signs of motor weakness, sensory loss, or reflex change. Hypertension and/or diabetes are often present, and MRI and CT may demonstrate multiple small subcortical infarcts. Repeated episodes of cerebral infarction are thought to be requisite for arteriosclerotic dementia. Gross examination of the brain shows evidence of cerebral softening secondary to the vascular insults.

PSEUDOBULBAR PALSY

The syndrome of pseudobulbar palsy may be found in the hypertensive patient who has suffered a series of small strokes. It is characterized by an unchanging facies with sporadic outbursts of laughter and weeping, and moderate dysarthria and dysphagia. Signs of a bilateral upper motor neuron paralysis can be found on neurologic examination.

OTHER CAUSES OF DEMENTIA

As mentioned previously, Alzheimer's disease and vascular dementia are the two most common causes of intellectual loss. According to autopsy findings, approximately 60% of cases of organic dementia in the elderly are associated with the neuropathologic findings of Alzheimer's disease, and approximately 20% are due to cerebrovascular disease. Other causes of dementia include myxedema, chronic drug intoxication, folic acid deficiency, pernicious anemia, Huntington's disease, Parkinson's disease, acquired immune deficiency syndrome. Pick's disease, Lewy body disease, Wilson's disease, and Creutzfeldt-Jakob disease (Table 14.2). Obviously, depression, folic acid deficiency, myxedema, chronic drug intoxication, and pernicious anemia are potentially reversible causes of dementia.

NORMAL PRESSURE HYDROCEPHALUS

In 1965, Adams, Fisher and Hakim (16) described a new entity, normal pressure hydrocephalus, and suggested that it was surgically correctable. More often, the cases presenting with gait disturbance have responded better to shunting procedures, and shunting of patients with the presence of dementia has not been as beneficial. The reader is referred to the discussion of this entity in Chapter 18, Neurological Disorders in the Elderly.

ACQUIRED IMMUNE DEFICIENCY SYNDROME

Depending on the total clinical picture, particularly with the presence of risk factors for Human Immunodeficiency Virus infection, the clinician should consider requesting tests for human immunodeficiency viral antibodies. As this disorder grows in epidemic proportions, we can expect to see more elderly who develop not only the immunodeficiency syndrome, but an encephalopathy with dementia as a consequence of infection.

SEARCHING FOR REVERSIBLE DISEASE

It is clear that there are certain correctable forms of dementia in the elderly, but only 2 to 3% of persons presenting for assessment of memory difficulty are found to have a potentially reversible cause. The physician must decide which cases of dementia are worth investigating for any of these possible causes, such as myxedema or normal pressure hydrocephalus. Failure to recognize a correctable cause may result in the establishment of an irreversible or end-state dementia. The physician may not wish to undertake a major evaluation if the situation offers little hope of correction. In an 85-year-old individual with a 4-year history of severe dementia and other serious illnesses and a history of absolutely poor general function preceding the onset of dementia, one may not feel compelled to aggressively pursue a major diagnostic workup. But certainly the physician should at all times be alerted to the possibility of a correctable disorder. Good judgment becomes the final arbiter in determining the appropriate extent of diagnostic evaluation. The tell-tale signs of myxedema, a history of recent head trauma, or the presence of low serum concentrations of vitamin B_{12} or folate would be signals for the practicing physician that the patient's dementia might be reversible (Tables 14.2 and 14.4).

It is difficult to prescribe a cookbook formula for the evaluation of reversible dementia. If the physician is alerted to the possibility of a correctable disorder, then good judgment, common sense, and clinical acumen will determine the extent of diagnostic assessment. It is most helpful if the physician has known the patient over a period of time.

A physician, integrating all available history, mental status examination, physical examination, laboratory, and other clinical information, will recognize certain clusters suggesting reversible or irreversible dementia. Gait disturbance, dementia, and urinary incontinence suggest normal pressure hydrocephalus. Recent head trauma, even without change in consciousness,

Table 14.4
Evaluation of Possible Reversible Dementia

Historical questions of diagnostic importance
    Duration and progress of illness
        Long-term
        Recent
        Recent on top of long-term
    Slow insidious progression versus step-wise progression
        Medication and alcohol use
    Gait disturbance and urinary incontinence
    Previous cerebrovascular accidents, head injury, subarachnoid hemorrhage, subdural hematoma
    Emotional or behavioral history
        Depression
        Paranoia
        Sensory deprivation
        Agitation
        Lethargy/listlessness
    Family history of dementia
    Other major associated illnesses
        Cardiovascular
        Pulmonary
        Hepatic
        Malignancy
        Neurologic
Complete physical examination
Basic diagnostic studies
    Psychologic or mental status evaluation
    Complete blood count
    Chemistry profile
    Chest x-ray
    Urinalysis
    Electrocardiogram
    Magnetic resonance imaging or CT brain scan
    Electroencephalogram
    Thyroid function studies
    Serologic test for syphilis
    Serum folate level
    Serum vitamin B_{12} level
Special examinations in selected cases
    Cisternal scan
    Lumbar puncture
    Heavy metals and or toxicology screening
    Blood ammonia level

suggests subdural hematoma. A fluctuating state of consciousness, inconsistent neurologic findings, a markedly slow electroencephalogram, and a negative MRI or CT scan suggest a metabolic encephalopathy. Dementia, ataxia, and peripheral neuropathy suggest the possibility of chronic alcoholism. Some seemingly benign conditions in the elderly, such as hearing loss or sleep deprivation, may mimic the presence of dementia.

Table 14.4 describes various tests that are useful in assessing the patient for reversible dementia. The history is of major diagnostic importance.

It is helpful if family members or other significant individuals can assist in providing a good history. Is the problem long-term or recent? Is it recent on top of a more long-term problem? How rapidly is the problem progressing? Is there history of head trauma? Gait disturbance? Urinary incontinence? Recent or past emotional disturbance, such as depression? Family history of dementia? Other major associated illness, such as cardiovascular or hepatic disease? Significant medications and/or alcohol use? Drug use remains one of the most common problems causing both acute confusional states and dementia.

In checking the psychologic or mental status evaluation, a screening test such as the Mini-Mental State Examination or the Short Portable Mental Status Questionnaire (as described previously) is useful. It can also be useful in following cognitive status over time.

Complete blood count with indices; chemistry profile, including serum calcium, electrolytes, liver function, glucose, blood urea nitrogen and creatinine; chest x-ray; urinalysis; and electrocardiogram are basic diagnostic studies of dementia. At this time, MRI or CT brain scan, electroencephalogram (EEG), thyroid function test, serologic test for syphilis, and serum folate and vitamin B_{12} levels are also indicated. (The EEG is most valuable in the diagnosis of a metabolic encephalopathy; if normal, the EEG certainly tends to exclude a metabolic or drug-induced encephalopathy and suggests the possibility of depression.) In selected cases, heavy metal screens, toxicology screens, cisternal scan, lumbar puncture, blood ammonia, and medication levels (e.g., digoxin or theophylline) might be indicated. Again, it is very difficult to reduce this type of judgment to a fixed algorithm or protocol in a cookbook fashion.

Single photon emission CT (SPECT), a CT nuclear medicine scan, initially provided hope for an accurate test for the diagnosis of dementia that would be easily clinically available (17). While the role of SPECT scanning has not been fully evaluated, it does not appear to have adequate sensitivity to accurately identify early dementia.

IRREVERSIBLE DEMENTIA: HELPING THE PATIENT AND FAMILY

What can be offered to the patient with dementia in which reversible causes are not apparent? Here the physician and other health professionals face a complex and difficult situation. Although cure is not possible, the health professional can do much to improve the patient's and family's condition. Previously, many patients with dementia were committed to state mental institutions. At present, with prudent evaluation provided by either the physician or specialized geriatric evaluation services, one could hope to maintain patients in their own homes with certain supports, in the community at a nursing home, or in a daycare program. The physician caring for the dementia patient must consider the patient, the caregiver, and the community (18, 19). The behavior of the patient with dementing illness may be burdensome for the family or caregiver, as well as for the physician. There has been increased attention to the handling of behavioral symptoms in Alzheimer's disease, including wandering, catastrophic reactions (uncontrolled agitation precipitated by task failure), communication disorders, waking at night, depression, delusions, paranoia, and agitation (19, 20). The caregiver may easily focus on the most burdensome symptoms, but a more detailed profile of the patient's behavior may be gained by the caregiver's completing the Functional Dementia Scale (Table 14.5) (21).

It is estimated that depressed mood occurs more often than a full-fledged depressive disorder in Alzheimer's disease (22). The depressed mood is often unrelated to the patient's awareness of intellectual impairment.

Important considerations in the evaluation include the presence of firearms and gas ovens in the home. Does the patient wander and get lost? Are there children in the family or in the neighborhood who might be harmed by the patient? How are medications handled in the home? Can they be locked up and dispensed under the control of another adult? The health of the relative or relatives of the elderly demented patient is extremely important. Is the health of the spouse holding up under the stress of caring for the patient? Is there a physician and/or nurse providing care to the patient? Finally, financial affairs must be considered, and it may fall upon the family and personal physician to raise and resolve issues of guardianship and incompetency.

Medications, including over-the-counter products, should be brought in at the time of the first examination and need to be reviewed periodically. It is always helpful if one knows the basis for the patient's being started on such medications as digoxin, thyroid medication, or phenytoin. One is always reluctant to discontinue medication that has been in use for 15 or 20 years. In any case, the physician should attempt to reduce medications that seem unnecessary. Certain drugs, such as phenytoin, may have to be discontinued on a gradual, or tapered, basis.

One should be cautious in the use of psychotropic medications in dementia. Adverse effects may occur, including worsening of the patient's mental status, resulting in chronic oversedation with additional complications of dehydration, pneumonia, and bed sores. A vicious cycle of worsening of the patient's mental status, triggering further use of medications and restraining devices, should be avoided.

Social interaction should be made to help patients maintain their orientation. Newspapers, calendars, clocks, and radio and television can help. The patient's name and the names of significant others should be used in conversation, in addition to reinforcing other aspects of time and location.

Most of all, the patient with dementia needs a physician who will take charge of complicated medical, social, and emotional problems. Patients with Alzheimer's disease may have other serious medical problems. Many of these can be handled by the personal physician; certain problems may require referral to other physicians or health professionals. The diagnosis of medical illness in persons who are already demented can be a major challenge.

Although the physician is alert to the various behavioral symptoms that present in Alzheimer's disease, alternative medical problems such as fecal impaction, urinary tract infection, or electrolyte imbalance should always be excluded. The physician and other health professionals caring for the patient should be aware of falls, visual and hearing deficits, alcohol and tobacco use, nutrition, and motor vehicle use and accidents.

If possible, the physician should include patients in discussions about their care. Their perspective should be sought in the early phase of a dementing illness. Overreliance on antipsychotic medications and physical restraints should be avoided (23). Physicians and health professionals should be sensitive to the effect of the dementia on the individual's self and identity (24). Many chronic illnesses result in disruption of self-image with negative attitudes about one's self, restricted social behavior with increased isolation, and the feeling of being a burden to loved ones (25). Certainly in the early stages of a dementing illness, some patients will be able to understand explanations of their illness (26). The patient may be brought into discussions of arrangements that will be necessary as the illness progresses. The patient may be competent to execute a living will and durable power of attorney.

Most patients can be evaluated for dementia on an outpatient basis. Some will benefit from

Table 14.5
Functional Dementia Scale[a]

| Patient _____ |
| Observer _____ |
| Position or relation to patient _____ |
| Facility _____ Date _____ |

Circle one rating for each item:

    1. None or little of the time   3. Good part of the time
    2. Some of the time   4. Most or all of the time

1. Has difficulty in completing simple tasks on own (e.g., dressing, bathing, arithmetic)	1	2	3	4
2. Spends time either sitting or in apparently purposeless activity	1	2	3	4
3. Wanders at night or needs to be restrained to prevent wandering	1	2	3	4
4. Hears things that are not there	1	2	3	4
5. Requires supervision or assistance in eating	1	2	3	4
6. Loses things	1	2	3	4
7. Appearance is disorderly if left to own devices	1	2	3	4
8. Moans	1	2	3	4
9. Cannot control bowel function	1	2	3	4
10. Threatens to harm others	1	2	3	4
11. Cannot control bladder function	1	2	3	4
12. Needs to be watched so does not injure self (e.g., by careless smoking, leaving the stove on, falling)	1	2	3	4
13. Destructive (e.g., breaks furniture, throws food trays, tears up magazines)	1	2	3	4
14. Shouts or yells	1	2	3	4
15. Accuses others of doing him/her bodily harm or stealing his/her possessions when the accusations are not true	1	2	3	4
16. Is unaware of limitations imposed by illness	1	2	3	4
17. Becomes confused and does not know where he/she is	1	2	3	4
18. Has trouble remembering	1	2	3	4
19. Has sudden changes of mood (e.g., gets upset, is angered or cries easily)	1	2	3	4
20. If left alone, wanders aimlessly during day or needs to be restrained to prevent wandering	1	2	3	4

[a]From Moore JT, Bobula JA, Short TB, Mischell M. A functional dementia scale. J Fam Pract 1983; 16:499–503. Adapted by permission of Appleton & Lange.

evaluation or assessment as an inpatient in the hospital. A great deal of help can be provided to the family by explicitly discussing the question of placement in a long-term care facility. The physician can help assess the patient's various problems, including wandering, agitation, and incontinence, and the family's ability to cope with these problems. By addressing such specific problems as incontinence, depression, or sleeplessness, the physician may relieve some of the burden of the illness, even though the degree of dementia is unchanged.

The physician may help provide counseling or referral for psychotherapy when family problems are evident. Referral of the family for often-needed legal and financial guidance may be necessary. It is very helpful if the physician can make home visits to provide support for the family, in addition to arranging nursing visits or the services of homemak-

ers or home health aides if needed. As part of the home visit, the physician will better understand the patients' actual environments and help advise on eliminating barriers and maximizing the patients' independence in their environments. The physician plays a key role in working with the family or caregiver by providing support and helping the family cope effectively with the long-term stress in caring for the patient.

A study carried out in Maryland (27, 28) demonstrated the plight of the caregiver of patients with dementing illnesses and noted significant service gaps. Using survey instruments designed for 16 target populations in Maryland (caregivers, physicians, nursing homes, educational institutions, public and private service agencies, insurance companies, etc.), the study showed significant need in the areas of respite care out of the home and information and referral services. A highlight of the survey findings was the overwhelming judgment from all categories of respondents that in-home respite care was not adequately provided. Overall, those who reported inadequacy of the service outnumbered those who deemed it adequate by 10:1. Among caregivers, the ratio catapulted to over twice that magnitude. By more than a 3:1 ratio, respondents judged adult day-care provisions to be inadequate.

In the Maryland report (27, 28) caregivers often were frustrated by the lack of information from physicians. The Maryland study also noted that legal and financial matters are often overlooked. In another study, many caregivers also reported the lack of information from physicians (29). Of 219 families, only three reported that physicians had arranged a visit or conference to discuss the diagnosis. In 84% of the families studied, no specific recommendations had been made regarding difficult behavioral symptoms or community services that might be utilized.

Caregivers of demented patients may be elderly themselves. One-fourth of all caregivers are 65 to 74 years of age, and 10% of caregivers are over 75 years of age (30). Women comprise the majority of caregivers (30, 31). Many women are burdened with the "36-hour day," torn between impaired parent and adolescent child and career or job and family (19, 31). The Maryland study graphically describes the burden of the caregiver.

Understanding the impact of dementia on the family is of the greatest importance (32). The family faced with caring for a member with dementia will experience feelings of anger, depression, fatigue, guilt, and shame. The family may be struggling to cope with the behavioral problems of their loved one. Families may be troubled by a poor understanding of the disease; isolation and a trapped feeling; anger and fear about the patient's behavior; feelings of loss of self-identity; role reversal (where the adult child now is taking care of the parent in place of the parent looking after the child); fears about heredity; and simply handling a condition that has become unmanageable. Of course, the family having difficulty coping with such problems is similar to other families in crisis (33). There are similarities of families caring for the dementia patient with those families facing the care of a family member with chronic schizophrenia, substance addiction, cancer or mental retardation. In all these situations, increasing the family's support system will be beneficial (34). Caplan (34) makes the point that families and individuals can be helped in mastering most types of stressful situations by receiving social support.

The physician and other health professionals are in a key position to help family members caring for patients with dementia. These families often turn to physicians for evaluation, advice, and emotional support. There are a number of appropriate interventions that can be readily provided to families experiencing the significant stress of becoming caregivers to a family member with dementia. All these interventions should maximize the patient's level of functioning and quality of life for both the patient and the family or caregiver.

A number of important functions in the physicians' management of dementia can be suggested (19, 35–37). Physicians should provide specific information to the family about the nature of dementing illness. Physicians can help the family understand that even the best efforts of health professionals may not lead to the patient's improvement. They can instruct the family to let the patient do all that he or she is able to do and encourage the family to increase the patient's activities. They can point out to the family ways to balance the patient's needs with the family's needs, e.g., encouraging the family to use community services, including adult day-care centers, or home health aides or sitters in the home. They can teach the family to use more effective ways of communicating with the patient (e.g., offering the patient a simplified message rather than overloading the patient with instructions or complex series of tasks) and to avoid logical arguments when these are no longer effective, but instead to respond to the emotional tone of the patient's message, rather than to the content (37).

A national support group for patients with dementia and their families is the Alzheimer's Association, which has a network of over 200 chapters across the country. The national headquarters are located at 919 North Michigan Avenue, Suite 1000, Chicago, IL, 60611-1676. Families may get information by calling 1-800-272-3900.

Barnes et al. (35) described a support group for caregivers consisting of 12 spouses and 3 adult children of Alzheimer's patients. This group met biweekly for sixteen 90-minute sessions. Group participation was especially helpful for spouses who function as primary caregivers. Participation resulted in their feeling greater support and less isolation and helped members deal with many of the feelings brought about by the illness. The sessions also helped spouses to become more aware of their own needs and regain some feeling of self-identity. Barnes and associates offer much useful advice in developing a support group for families caring for Alzheimer patients.

A handbook that should be of great help to all families dealing with the problem of dementia is *The 36-Hour Day: A Family Guide to Caring for Persons With Alzheimer's Disease, Related Dementing Illness, and Memory Loss in Later Life*, by Nancy Mace and Peter Rabins (19). Not only families dealing with this problem but health professionals, too, will find an abundance of useful information in this book. Other useful literature for families includes *Guidelines for Dignity*, a provider's guide to caring for a person with Alzheimer's, and the companion *Family Guide*, which addresses issues families should consider when selecting care in any residential setting. Both can be ordered through the Alzheimer's Disease and Related Disorders Association or its local chapters (for further information, call 1-800-272-3900).

Many families would like to avoid the use of long-term-care facilities. Physicians, of course, should use the prescription for a nursing home as cautiously as a prescription for cardiac medication or an antibiotic. However, many patients with Alzheimer's disease eventually reach a point in which they are simply not manageable in terms of their need for 24-hour/day, 7 day/week nursing care, medical interventions, and other safety considerations as far as their custodial care. When a family tells the physician early on that they never want their relative to be placed in a nursing home, it is important for the physician to tell the family that their loved one might conceivably some day require care in a nursing home facility.

A recent innovation in nursing home care has been the establishment of special units for the care of Alzheimer's patients (38, 39). These units benefit persons with dementia by allowing appropriate resources to be concentrated in one area and by allowing an interested skilled staff to focus its efforts on a group of individuals most needy of their services. There is much intense research interest at this time on specialized units for Alzheimer's patients, examining the pros and cons of such units.

Other innovative care approaches for those with dementia and their families include in-home visiting nurse or aide services. These allow the family to have some relief from care and provide for stimulation of the ill person. Day-care centers are an important addition to the health delivery system. Many now serve both cognitively impaired and well elderly. These units provide stimulation and activity for the ill person and respite for the family. Cefalu and Heuser (40) address the increased need for such adult day-care for the demented elderly, the relief that adult day-care provides to caregiving families, criteria for patients who would benefit from adult day-care, and the financial barriers in obtaining this service.

Throughout the United States, geriatric assessment programs are being developed in many cities. These are associated with hospitals or long-term-care facilities, county health departments, and even as independent organizations. In many hospitals, geriatric assessment programs are part of a full spectrum of geriatric services, including home care, day-care, information and referral services. There should be little difficulty in most metropolitan areas for a physician to find consultative support from a specialized geriatric evaluation service as a means of helping both dementia victims and their family members or caregivers.

In summary, in the case of irreversible dementia, patients should be maintained, if at all possible, in their own homes or in the community. Establishing a constant and familiar environment is most helpful, in addition to trying to maximize the patient's level of functioning. The impact of the patient's illness on the family or caregiver should be kept in mind. The family or caregiver could be helped through increased social support. Interventions should result in family members feeling less isolated and should improve the quality of life for both the patient and family or caregiver.

REFERENCES

1. Crook R, Bartus RT, Ferris S, Whitehouse P, Cohen GD, Hershon S. Age-associated memory impairment: proposed diagnostic criteria and measures of clinical change. Devel Neuropsychol 1986;2:261–276.
2. Tucker GJ, Caine ED, Folstein MF, Grant I, Liptzin B, Popkin MK. Introduction to background papers for the suggested changes to DSM-IV: cognitive disorders. J Neuropsychiatry Clin Neurosci 1992;4:360–368.
3. Caine ED. Should aging-associate cognitive decline be included in DSM-IV? J Neuropsychiatry Clin Neurosci 1993;5:1–5.
4. Inouye SK, van Dyck CH, Alessi CA, Balkin S, Siegal AP, Horwitz RI. Clarifying confusion: the Confusion Assessment Method. A new method for detection of delirium. Ann Intern Med 1990;113:941–948.
5. Folstein MF, Folstein SE, McHugh PR. Mini-mental state. A practical method for grading the cognitive state of patients for the clinician. J Psychiatr Res 1975;12:189–198.
6. Pfeiffer E. A short portable mental status questionnaire for the assessment of organic brain deficit in elderly patients. J Am Geriatr Soc 1975;23:433–441.
7. Wells CE. Pseudodementia. Am J Psychiatry 1979;136:895–900.
8. Rabins PV, Merchant A, Nestadt G. Criteria for diagnosing reversible dementia caused by depression. Br J Psychiatry 1984;144:488–492.

9. Roman GC, Tatemichi TK, Erkinjuntti T. et al. Vascular dementia: diagnostic criteria for research studies. Report of the NINDS-AIREN International Workshop. Neurology 1993;43:250–260.

10. McKhann G, Drachman D, Folstein M, Katzman R, Price D, Stedlan EM. Clinical diagnosis of Alzheimer's disease: report of the NINCDS-ADRDA Work Group under the auspices of Department of Health and Human Services Task Force on Alzheimer's disease. Neurology 1984;34:939–944.

11. Huckman MS, Fox J, Topel J. The validity of criteria for the evaluation of cerebral atrophy by computed tomography. Radiology 1975;116:85–92.

12. Ford CV, Winter J. Computerized axial tomograms and dementia in elderly patients. J Gerontol 1981;36:164–169.

13. Morris JC, Heyman A, Mohs RC, et al. The Consortium to Establish a Registry for Alzheimer's Disease (CERAD). Part I. Clinical and neuropsychological assessment of Alzheimer's disease. Neurology 1989;39:1159–1165.

14. Mirra SS, Heyman A, McKeel D, et al. The Consortium to Establish a Registry for Alzheimer's Disease (CERAD). Part II. Standardization of the neuropathologic assessment of Alzheimer's disease. Neurology 1991;41:479–486.

15. Davis PC, Gray L, Albert M, et al. The Consortium to Establish a Registry for Alzheimer's Disease (CERAD). Part III. Reliability of a standardized MRI evaluation of Alzheimer's disease. Neurology 1992;42:1676–1680.

16. Adams RD, Fisher CM, Hakim S. Symptomatic occult hydrocephalus with normal cerebrospinal fluid pressure. A treatable syndrome. N Engl J Med 1965;273:117–126.

17. Bonte FJ, Ross ED, Chehabi HH, Devous MD. SPECT study of regional cerebral blood flow in Alzheimer disease. J Comput Assist Tomogr 1986;10:579–583.

18. Gallo JJ, Franch MS, Reichel W. Dementing illness: the patient, caregiver, and community. Am Fam Physician 1991;43:1669–1675.

19. Mace NL, Rabins PV. The 36-hour day: a family guide to caring for persons with Alzheimer's disease, related dementing illnesses, and memory loss in later life. Revised Ed. Baltimore: Johns Hopkins University Press, 1991.

20. Teri L, Rabins P, Whitehouse P, et al. Management of behavior disturbance in Alzheimer's disease. Current knowledge and future directions. Alzheimer's Dis Relat Disorders 1992;6:77–88.

21. Moore JT, Bobula JA, Short TB, Mischell M. A functional dementia scale. J Fam Pract 1983;16:499–503.

22. Wragg R, Jeste D. Overview of depression and psychosis in Alzheimer's disease. Am J Psychiatry 1989;146:577–587.

23. Sloane PD, Mathew LJ, Scarborough M, et al. Physical and pharmacologic restraint of nursing home patients with dementia. Impact of specialized units. JAMA 1991;265:1278–1282.

24. Cohen D. The subjective experience of Alzheimer's disease: the anatomy of an illness as perceived by patients and families. Am J Alzheimer's Care Relat Disorders Res 1991;6:6–11.

25. Charmaz K. Loss of self: a fundamental form of suffering of the chronically ill. Sociol Health Illness 1983;5:168–195.

26. Drickamer MA, Lachs MS. Should patients with Alzheimer's disease be told their diagnosis? N Engl J Med 1992;326:947–951.

27. Reichel W, Franch MS, Solon J. Survey research guiding public policy in Maryland: a case of Alzheimer's disease and related disorders. Exp Gerontol 1986;21:439–448.

28. Reichel W, Franch MS, Beacham E. Alzheimer's disease and related disorders: a growing challenge. Maryland Med J 1986;35:927–932.

29. Chenoweth B, Spencer B. Dementia: the experience of family caregivers. Gerontologist 1986;26:267–272.

30. Stone R, Cafferata GL, Sangl J. Caregivers of the frail elderly: a national profile. Gerontologist 1987;27:616–626.

31. Brody EM. Women in the middle: their patient care years. New York: Springer, 1990.

32. Rabins PV, Mace NL, Lucas MJ. The impact of dementia on the family. JAMA 1982;248:333–335.

33. Kushner HS. When bad things happen to good people. New York: Schocken Books, 1981.

34. Caplan G. Mastery of stress: psychosocial aspects. Am J Psychiatry 1981;138:413–420.

35. Barnes RF, Raskind MA, Scott M, Murphy C. Problems of families caring for Alzheimer patients: use of a support group. J Am Geriatr Soc 1981;29:80–85.

36. Eisdorfer C, Cohen D. Management of the patient and family coping with dementing illness. J Fam Pract 1981;12:831–837.

37. Reifler BV, Wu S. Managing families of the demented elderly. J Fam Pract 1982;14:1051–1056.

38. Coons DH. Specialized dementia care units. Baltimore: Johns Hopkins University Press, 1991.

39. Mace N. Do we need special care units for dementia patients? J Gerontol Nurs 1985;11:37–38.

40. Cefalu CA, Heuser M. Adult day care for the demented elderly. Am Fam Physician 1993;47:723–724.

15/ Alzheimer's Disease: Biological Aspects

Lisa N. Geller, John Delfs, Peter V. Rabins, William Reichel

EPIDEMIOLOGY

Any possible understanding of the etiology of senile dementia of the Alzheimer type must be based on solid epidemiologic information. Genetic theories and an understanding of environmental risk factors, including the possible roles of head injury, viral infection, trace elements such as aluminum, and other causal hypotheses demand a reliable epidemiologic data base.

A wide range of prevalence rates has been reported for senile dementia of the Alzheimer type. Worldwide, approximately 4% of persons over 65 years of age have a severe form of senile dementia, and about 10 to 20% have mild forms. Prevalence rises sharply with age such that for individuals over 85 years of age, 20% have a severe form of Alzheimer's disease (1–3), meaning that there likely will be large increases in the number of persons with Alzheimer's disease in the future. One present estimate is that 1% of the population has senile dementia at age 65 years, 10% at age 75 years, and 25 to 30% at age 85 years. A community-based study in East Boston, Massachusetts, reported a prevalence of over 47% in persons over 85 years (4). As life expectancy is increasing (principally because of the decrease in the death rate from heart disease and stroke), a spiraling increase can be expected in the number of elderly with Alzheimer's disease in each decade past 60 years (5).

Some studies, using data from hospitals and long-term care institutions, have shown a predominance among women and among persons of low socioeconomic status. Others have shown an equal prevalence among men and women and have criticized the use of information largely gathered from institutional experience. Very little is presently known about Alzheimer's disease according to race, rural versus urban, nationality in nations other than western Europe and the United States, and other cross-cultural comparisons.

A number of studies show that the clinical diagnosis of Alzheimer's disease is confirmed pathologically approximately 90% of the time when strict criteria such as those proposed by the NINCDS-ADRDA committee or the DSM-IV are used. However, the clinical diagnosis of vascular dementia is much less accurate, and it may be more common than previously thought (6). Furthermore, approximately 10% of patients with dementia do not meet pathological criteria for either Alzheimer's disease or vascular dementia, the two most common causes of dementia. Studies done during the 1970s and 1980s suggested that vascular dementia was more common in Japan than in the U.S. (7) or Western Europe. More recent epidemiologic studies in Japan report lower rates of the diagnosis of vascular dementia and higher rates of Alzheimer's disease (8). It is unclear whether this is a change in diagnostic practice or a change in the epidemiologic pattern of the disorder.

BIOLOGICAL ASPECTS OF ALZHEIMER'S DISEASE

Alzheimer's description in 1906 of senile plaques and neurofibrillary tangles associated with dementia laid the groundwork for contemporary research. Recently, attention has been directed to several possible etiologic factors, including neurotransmitters, the acute phase response, estrogens, and genetics. These aspects will be considered individually, even though the extent to which they play a role in the disease as well as the extent to which they may interact are not yet clear.

NEUROTRANSMITTER-RELATED STUDIES

In 1976, Davies and Maloney (9) reported a significant reduction in the activity of choline acetyltransferase in the cerebral cortex of patients with "senile dementia of the Alzheimer type" in comparison with age-matched normal individuals. This finding has been confirmed by others. There is a correlation between the change in neurochemical activity and cognitive loss and brain pathology, particularly the number of neuritic plaques seen at autopsy. In contrast, reduction in the activity of choline acetyltransferase is not noted in multi-infarct dementia or depression (10). The decrease in choline acetyltransferase suggests a potential role for replacement therapy.

Whitehouse, Price, and colleagues (11, 12) found that the nucleus basalis of Meynert (located in the basal forebrain) from patients with Alzheimer's disease demonstrated substantially fewer neurons than that of age- and sex-matched controls. Since the nucleus basalis provides diffuse cholinergic input to the neocortex, loss of this neuronal population may represent an important anatomic correlate of the markedly reduced activity of choline acetyltransferase in Alzheimer's disease. This demonstration of selective degeneration of nucleus basalis of Meynert neurons may provide the first documentation of loss of a transmitter-specific neuronal population in a major disorder of higher cortical function. Whether nucleus basalis cell death leads to neocortical deficits remains unanswered; however, more recent evidence now favors other initial sites for the disease, including the cortex (13) and the hippocampus (14). Since cholinergic activity in Alzheimer's disease is diminished, it is logical to try to increase acetylcholine synthesis, prevent its breakdown, or both. In this regard, Alzheimer's disease might be compared to Parkinson's disease as far as the hope of chemical manipulation.

Other neurotransmitter deficits identified in Alzheimer's disease include norepinephrine, serotonin, somatostatin, and corticotrophin-releasing factor (13). This suggests that replacement strategies might have to combine several drugs or that individual patients will require different treatment regimens based on their pattern of deficits. (The reader is referred to Chapter 4: Drugs and the Elderly for a more thorough discussion of cognitive-enhancing medications.) Physicians will be faced with many episodes in which family members and caregivers will make demands for the use of drugs that are receiving attention in the public press as possible cures for this illness. The dilemmas created by multiple pharmacologic interventions are only some of the quandaries in which practicing physicians and other health professionals will find themselves in understanding the many discoveries and claims about the biology of Alzheimer's disease.

SENILE PLAQUES AND NEUROFIBRILLARY TANGLES

The two definitive neuropathological findings of Alzheimer's disease, amyloid plaques and neurofibrillary tangles, have been the focus of an enormous research effort. The amyloid plaque is an extracellular structure composed primarily of β-amyloid protein and α_1-antichymotrypsin. The amyloid protein appears to be an abnormal product derived from the amyloid precursor protein (APP). The normal function of APP is not known, although its structure is consistent with that of a membrane receptor. Some studies have shown that the β-protein is toxic to cells, leading to the suggestion that this protein is the causative agent in Alzheimer's disease (15).

Amyloid plaques in Alzheimer's disease are found in several areas of the brain but are most prominent in those areas associated with memory, such as the hippocampus and neocortex. Knowledge of the β-amyloid protein and APP have raised the hope of diagnostic tests for Alzheimer's disease. Van Nostrand, Benson and associates have reported a reduction in the levels of an APP derivative in the cerebrospinal fluid of persons with familial Alzheimer's disease (FAD), compared with their unaffected siblings. β-Amyloid appears to be produced and secreted in a variety of other tissues including blood (16). The protease inhibitor α_1-antichymotrypsin, a component of amyloid plaques, is specifically induced in β-amyloid peptide amyloidoses (17).

The other major neuropathologic feature of Alzheimer's disease, neurofibrillary tangles (NFTs), is shared with other neurodegenerative disorders. Studies now have shown NFTs to be composed principally of tau, a normal component of neurons that binds to microtubules (18). In the NFT of Alzheimer's disease, phosphates are abnormally attached to tau, resulting in the pathologic tangle structure. Research continues to focus on the mechanisms that cause hyperphosphorylation of tau and result in NFTs.

IMMUNE SYSTEM INVOLVEMENT

The involvement of the immune system in Alzheimer's disease has been postulated for some years. Immunoglobulins and complement components have been reported to be associated with amyloid plaques (19). Reactive microglia, which are the macrophages of the brain, have been localized around amyloid plaques as have reactive astrocytes (20). The presence of these cells is consistent with the theory of an acute phase response as discussed below. Various humoral antibodies directed against Alzheimer's disease tissue and specifically against cholinergic neurons have been reported in Alzheimer's disease patients. Whether an immune response would be involved as a primary inducing factor in Alzheimer's disease or is a response to preexisting damage is not clear.

THE ACUTE PHASE RESPONSE

The acute phase response is an inflammatory response to physiologic stress that has been described primarily in the liver (21) and may involve the immune system. The hypothesis has been advanced that the amyloidogenesis of Alzheimer's disease results from the acute phase response elicited when certain areas of the brain are subjected to stress, whether biologic or environmental in origin (22, 23). A major component of the amyloid plaques, α_1-antichymotrypsin is an acute phase protein that appears to be specifically upregulated in β-amyloidoses (17). Based on the model for the acute phase response in liver, this theory would prescribe roles for interleukin-1 (IL-1), IL-6, tumor necrosis factor, and perhaps nerve growth factor in Alzheimer's disease. Indeed, IL-1 has been reported to increase the amount of APP mRNA in culture cells (24).

OXIDATIVE DAMAGE

Oxidative stress has been suggested to play a role in the etiology of Alzheimer's disease (25). Reactive oxygen metabolites can be generated by microglia in culture and may play an important role in the acute phase response (26). Clues indicating a role for oxidative damage in Alzheimer's disease include reports that cells from Alzheimer's disease patients may be more sensitive to damage by reactive oxygen metabolites (27) and increased levels of enzymes indicative of oxidative stress. These results have led some to suggest a therapeutic role for antioxidants such as vitamin E.

ESTROGEN

Considerable interest has been focused on a possible role for estrogen in Alzheimer's disease. Animal studies have shown that cholinergic neurons of the basal forebrain contain estrogen receptors (28). This information coupled with primarily anecdotal accounts of reduced incidence of Alzheimer's disease in postmenopausal women undergoing estrogen therapy has led to the suggestion that estrogen deficiency may constitute a risk factor for Alzheimer's disease. However, some studies (29) report no consistent evidence of a positive effect of estrogen on cognitive function. Nevertheless, these studies raise the possibility of therapeutic or preventive implications that remain to be tested.

GENETICS OF ALZHEIMER'S DISEASE

There is no question that there is a genetic component to some cases of Alzheimer's disease. The most striking genetic evidence is apparent in early-onset cases of the disease. Nearly all early-onset Alzheimer's disease has been linked to genetic causes and has an autosomal dominant mode of transmission. A small number of the early-onset cases are caused by several mutations on chromosome 21 (30). These mutations lie in the APP gene that is responsible for the production of the β-amyloid protein, a major component of the senile plaques. This finding on chromosome 21 is of particular interest because all persons with Down syndrome (trisomy 21) who survive to the third or fourth decade develop the pathology of Alzheimer's disease, and many develop clinical dementia prior to death.

Even more striking, over 70% of early-onset familial Alzheimer's disease cases that have been studied have been linked to chromosome 14 (31–34). Although several candidate genes have been identified on chromosome 14, none have yet been definitively identified as the cause of Alzheimer's disease in these families.

Some late-onset familial Alzheimer's disease has been linked to a locus on chromosome 19. Current linkage evidence suggests that the chromosome 19 gene is close to the gene encoding apolipoprotein E (35), a plasma protein involved in the transport of cholesterol and other lipids. The apolipoprotein E4 allele has been implicated as a risk factor in late-onset familial Alzheimer's disease, those homozygous for the apo E4 allele being at highest risk (36). Some investigators have reported the presence of apolipoprotein E-like immunoreactivity in amyloid plaques, and Wisniewski and colleagues (37) have reported that apolipoprotein E can interact with the amyloid protein, which may suggest a mechanism of action in Alzheimer's disease (38). Although the question of what proportion of late-onset Alzheimer's disease has a genetic etiology remains controversial, the most common genetic form appears to be linked to apo E.

In addition to the chromosome 14, 19, and 21 loci, a fourth locus for familial Alzheimer's disease is suggested by studies of families of Volga-German descent with no linkage to chromosomes 14, 19, and 21 in their pedigrees.

Except for age of onset and rate of progression, the pathology and clinical presentation among these different genetic entities are indistinguishable. It is evident that there are multiple causes of Alzheimer's disease resulting in a similar end-stage appearance.

ENVIRONMENTAL FACTORS IN ALZHEIMER'S DISEASE

VIRAL THEORIES

Several slow virus diseases, kuru and Creutzfeldt-Jakob disease in man and scrapie in sheep, are of some interest as far as insights they may offer into the dementing process, and in the past they have been proposed as models for Alzheimer's disease. The reader is referred to the report by Gajdusek and colleagues (39) reviewing Creutzfeldt-Jakob disease, kuru, scrapie, and transmissible mink encephalopathy. However, although these encephalopathies are interesting, there is no convincing evidence that there is any relationship between slow viruses and Alzheimer's disease.

ALUMINUM AND OTHER TRACE ELEMENTS

Although studies since 1973 have reported increases in aluminum levels in the brains of Alzheimer's disease patients (40), the role of aluminum in Alzheimer's disease is still not established. Further work will be necessary to determine whether aluminum plays any role in this degenerative process. Zinc may have a significant physiologic interaction with amyloid, as may copper. Whether these metals play a role in the development of Alzheimer's disease remains a question.

HEAD INJURY

Head injury resulting in "punch drunk" syndrome or dementia pugilistica appears to result in a syndrome that is indistinguishable pathologically from Alzheimer's disease (41, 42). Similarly, a history of severe head trauma such as concussion has been reported to be a risk factor for Alzheimer's disease (43). Elucidation of the mechanisms by which these processes are involved in the etiology of Alzheimer's disease remains an important area of future research.

POTENTIAL THERAPEUTIC AGENTS

Many therapeutic possibilities have been considered. The most recent pharmacologic focus has been on tacrine hydrochloride (Cognex), an acri-

dinamine derivative that has received full approval from the Food and Drug Administration. Clinical reports suggest that tacrine has, at best, a low efficacy (44–48). Tacrine appears to improve cognition in a minority of Alzheimer's victims with mild to moderate dementia. Unfortunately, there is no conclusive evidence from controlled trials that tacrine use will result in significant long-term improvement or in long-term prevention of decline. In addition, tacrine can cause hepatic changes, particularly elevations in serum alanine aminotransferase activity, focal necrosis, and granulomatous hepatitis. In the presence of liver toxicity, the dosage should be reduced or the drug stopped. Hepatic toxicity has been reversible with discontinuation of tacrine in virtually all cases thus far. In addition to the hepatic changes, other side effects include nausea and drug interactions. Tacrine is only the first of an array of drugs based on the neurotransmitter aspects of Alzheimer's disease that are expected to appear in trial stage. The practicing physician will be faced regularly with pressures from loving and distraught families to use tacrine and any other new products that emerge from this line of research. In each case, the risk-benefit ratio must be carefully considered for the individual patient.

Given the involvement of the cholinergic system in Alzheimer's disease, it is also important for the physician to consider the question of possible harmful effects of anticholinergic drugs, including tricyclic antidepressants and neuroleptics. A host of medications with anticholinergic properties are used in daily practice. Their use must be individually evaluated and appropriately limited in this patient population.

As mentioned above, the tantalizing but unsubstantiated role of estrogen deficiency in the degenerative process of Alzheimer's disease may someday lead to new treatment. The production of destructive oxygen radicals (possibly related to an immune response component to the disorder) may also be another mechanism in the disease process amenable to therapy. Therefore, the possible therapeutic use of estrogen replacement therapy in postmenopausal women as well as the use of antioxidants such as vitamin E and the use of nonsteroidal antiinflammatory agents may provide hope for preventing or slowing the progress of Alzheimer's disease. Several of these agents are currently under clinical study.

ETHICAL CONSIDERATIONS

Our present understanding of Alzheimer's disease is somewhat disjointed. As discoveries are made in understanding the full biologic picture of Alzheimer's disease, there will be increasing pressure to use new preventive or therapeutic agents, even for marginal benefit. At the same time, physicians must bear in mind their role as a source of helping the patient while avoiding doing harm. The physician must be concerned if agents that are approved for use possess low efficacy and demonstrate significant side effects. The physician must also question the fast-emerging research findings that are sometimes too rapidly translated into new therapies. Therefore, the physician must work hard at monitoring developments in the field.

Another major area of ethical concern is the role of diagnostic tests that may become available, almost certainly before sound therapeutic modalities are available. It is easy to imagine the psychological and social turmoil that will be engendered by the ability to determine that a fetus, a young adult, or a middle-aged adult may eventually develop Alzheimer's disease. It is therefore important to distinguish between testing asymptomatic individuals who, regardless of age, may have positive tests for certain genetic or other biological factors, and testing individuals who are in the early stages of dementia and who may therefore benefit from a differential diagnosis of, for example, vascular dementia. This is emphasized by current NIH guidelines, which recommend professional counseling for patients before and after genetic testing.

CONCLUSION

Although still in the infancy of understanding the causal factors in Alzheimer's disease, various beachheads have been established. By virtue of the genetic information available, it is clear that Alzheimer's disease is the end-stage of more than one basic etiology. Many different physiologic mechanisms and molecules have been implicated. The next decade should see enormous progress in understanding this devastating process. With an improved understanding of etiologic factors, specific preventive or therapeutic measures should become available.

Physicians will be obligated to sort out different physiologic hypotheses and therapeutic interventions regarding Alzheimer's disease. In medical and scientific journals, and in the lay press, physicians will read that Alzheimer's disease has its origin in a wide array of genetic and environmental factors. Wurtman (49) has compared the different pathophysiologic hypotheses to the tale of six blind men and the elephant. The original story (50) of the six blind men reads:

Once upon a time a king gathered some blind men about an elephant and asked them to tell him what an elephant was like. The first man felt a tusk and said an elephant was like a giant carrot: another happened to touch an ear and said it was like a big fan: another touched its trunk and said it was like a pestle; still another, who happened to feel its leg, said it was like a mortar; and another, who grasped its tail, said it was like a rope. Not one of them was able to tell the king the elephant's real form.

It is likely that with the convergence of major scientific discoveries, the true "elephantness" of Alzheimer's disease will soon be understood.

REFERENCES

1. Brody JA. An epidemiologist views senile dementia—facts and fragments. Am J Epidemiol 1982;115:155–162.
2. Brody JA. An epidemiologist's view of the senile dementias—pieces of the puzzle. In: Wertheimer J, Marois M, eds. Senile dementia: outlook for the future. New York: Alan R Liss, 1984:383.
3. Jorm AF, Korten AE, Henderson AS. The prevalence of dementia: a quantitative integration of the literature. Acta Psychiatr Scand 1987;76:465–479.
4. Evans DA, Funkenstein HH, Albert MS, et al. Prevalence of Alzheimer's disease in a community of older persons: higher than previously reported. JAMA 1989;262:2551–2556.
5. Jorm AF. The epidemiology of Alzheimer's desease and related disorders. London: Chapman and Hall, 1990.
6. Skoog I, Nilsson L, Palmertz B, Andreasson L-A, Svanborg A. A population-based study of dementia in 85-year-olds. N Engl J Med 1993;328:153–158.
7. Endo H, Yamamoto T, Kuzuya F. Predispositions to arteriosclerotic dementia and senile dementia in Japan. Book of abstracts of the XIIIth International Congress of Gerontology, New York, July 12–17, 1985:163.
8. Hasegawa K, Homma A, Imai Y. An epidemiological study of age-related dementia in the community. Int J Geriatr Psychiatry 1986;15:122–120.
9. Davies P, Maloney AJF. Selective loss of central cholinergic neurons in Alzheimer's disease. Lancet 1976;2:1403.
10. Perry EK, Tomlinson BE, Blessed G, Bergmann K, Gibson PH, Perry RH. Correlation of cholinergic abnormalities with senile plaques and mental test scores in senile dementia. Br Med J 1978;2:1457–1459.
11. Whitehouse PJ, Price DL, Clark AW, Coyle JT, DeLong NR. Alzheimer disease: evidence for selective loss of cholinergic neurons in the nucleus basalis. Ann Neurol 1981;10:122–126.
12. Whitehouse PJ, Price DL, Struble RG, Clark AW, Coyle JT, DeLong MR. Alzheimer's disease and senile dementia. Loss of neurons in the basal forebrain. Science 1982;215:1237–1239.
13. Perry RH. Recent advances in neuropathology. Br Med Bull 1986;42:34–41.
14. de Leon MJ, Golomb J, George AE, et al. The radiologic prediction of Alzheimer disease: the atrophic hippocampal formation. Am J Neuroradiol 1993;14:897–906.

15. Hardy JA, Higgins GA. Alzheimer's disease: The amyloid cascade hypothesis. Science 1992;256:184–185.
16. Selkoe DJ. The molecular pathology of Alzheimer's disease. Neuron 1991;6:487–498.
17. Abraham CR, Shirahama T, and Potter H. α_1-Antichymotrypsin is associated solely with amyloid deposists containing the β-protein. Amyloid and cell localization of α_1-antichymotrypsin. Neurobiolol Aging 1990;11:123–129.
18. Kosik K. Alzheimer's disease: a cell biological perspective. Science 1992;256:780–783.
19. McGeer PL, Akiyama H, Itagaki S, McGeer EG. Immune system response in Alzheimer's disease. Can J Neurosci 1989;16:516–527.
20. Rozemuller JM, Eikelenboom P, Stam FC, Beyreuther K, Masters C. A4 protein in Alzheimer's disease: primary and secondary events in extracellular amyloid deposition. J Neuropathol Exp Neurol 1989;48:674–691.
21. Heinrich PC, Castell JV, Andrus T. Interleukin-6 and the acute phase response. Biochem J 1990;265:621–636.
22. Vandenabeele P, Fiers W. Is amyloidogenesis during Alzheimer's disease due to an IL-1-/IL-6-mediated 'acute phase response' in the brain? Immunol Today 1991;12:217–219.
23. Potter H, Nelson RB, Das S, Siman R, Kayyali US, Dressler D. The involvement of proteases, protease inhibitors, and an acute phase response in Alzheimer's disease. Ann NY Acad Sci 1992;674:161–173.
24. Forloni G, Demicheli F, Giorgi S, Bendotti C, Angeretti N. Expression of amyloid precursor protein mRNAs in endothelial, neuronal and glial cells: modulation by interleukin-1. Mol Brain Res 1992;16:128–134.
25. Harman D. Free radical theory of aging: a hypothesis on the pathogenesis of senile dementia of the Alzheimer's type. Age 1993;16:23–30.
26. Evans PH. Free radicals in brain metabolism and pathology. Br Med Bull 1993;49:577–587.
27. Piersanti P, Tesco G, Latorraca S, Piacentini S, Sorbi S, Amaducci L. Alzheimer skin fibroblasts susceptibility to oxygen radical damage. Neurobiol Aging 1992;13:81–111.
28. Toran-Allerand CD, Miranda RC, Bentham WD, et al. Estrogen receptors colocalize with low affinity nerve growth factor receptors in cholinergic neurons of the basal forebrain. Proc Nat Acad Sci USA 1992;89:4668–4672.
29. Barrett-Connor E, Kritz-Silverstein D. Estrogen replacement therapy and cognitive function in older women. JAMA 1992;269:2637–2641.
30. Mullan M, Crawford F. Genetic and molecular advances in Alzheimer's disease. Trends Neurosci 1993;16:398–402.
31. Schellenberg G, Bird T, Wijsman E, et al. Genetic linkage evidence for a familial Alzheimer's disease locus on chromosome 14. Science 1992;258:668–671.
32. Mullan M, Houlden H, Windelspecht M, Fidani L, Lombardi C, Diaz P, et al. A major locus for familial early onset Alzheimer's disease is on the long arm of chromosome 14, proximal to α-antichymotrypsin. Nature Genet 1992;2:340–343.
33. Van Broeckhoven C, Backhovens H, Cruts M, et al. Mapping of a gene predisposing to early-onset Alzheimer's disease to chromosome 14q24.3. Nature Genet 1992;2:335–339.
34. St George-Hyslop P, Haines J, Rogaev E, et al. Genetic evidence for a novel familial Alzheimer's disease locus on chromosome 14. Nature Genet 1992;2:330–334.
35. Corder EH, Saunders AM, Strittmatter WJ, et al. Gene dose of apolipoprotein E type 4 allele and the risk of late onset families. Science 1993;261:921–923.
36. Poirier J, Davignon, J, Bouthillier D, Kogan S, Bertrand P, Gauthier S. Apolipoprotein E polymorphism and Alzheimer's disease. Lancet 1993;342:697–699.
37. Wisniewski T, Golabek, A, Matsubara E, Ghiso J, Frangione B. Apolipoprotein E: binding to soluble Alzheimer's β-amyloid. Biochem Biophys Res Comm 1993;359–365.
38. Strittmatter C, Wisgraber KH, Huang DY, et al. Binding of human apolipoprotein E to synthetic amyloid β peptide: isoform-specific effects and implications for late-onset Alzheimer disease. Proc Nat Acad Sci USA 1993;90:8098–8102.
39. Gajdusek DC, Gibbs CJ, Asher DM, et al. Precautions in medical care of and in handling materials from patients with transmissible virus dementia (Creutzfeldt-Jakob disease). N Engl J Med 1977;297:1253–1258.
40. Edwardson JA, Candy JM, Ince PG, et al. Aluminium accumulation. β-Amyloid deposition and neurofibrillary changes in the central nervous system. In: Chadwick DJ, Whelan J, eds. Aluminium in biology and medicine. Ciba Found Symp 169. Chichester: Wiley, 1992:165–185.
41. Roberts GW. Immunocytochemistry of neurofibrillary tangles in dementia pugilistica and Alzheimer's disease: evidence for common genesis. Lancet 1988:1456–1458.
42. Roberts GW, Allsop D, Bruton C. The occult aftermath of boxing. J Neurol Neurosurg Psychiatry 1990;53:373–378.
43. Mortimer JA, Van Duijn CM, Chandra V, et al. Head trauma as a risk factor for Alzheimer's disease: a collaborative re-analysis of case-control studies. Int J Epidemiol 1990;20(suppl 2):S28–S35.
44. Eagger SA, Levy R, Sahakian BJ. Tacrine in Alzheimer's disease. Lancet 1991;337:989–992.
45. Davis KL, Thal LJ, Gamzu ER, Davis CS, Woolson RF, Gracon SI, Drachman DA, et al. A double-blind, placebo-controlled multicenter study of tacrine for Alzheimer's disease. N Engl J Med 1992;327:1253–1259.
46. Farlow M, Gracon SI, Hershey LA, Lewis KW, Sadowsky C, Dolan-Ureno J. A controlled trial of tacrine in Alzheimer's disease. JAMA 1992;268:2523–2529.
47. Knapp MJ, Knopman DS, Solomon PR, et al. A 30-week randomized controlled trial of high-dose tacrine in patients with Alzheimer's disease. JAMA 1994;271:985–991.
48. Winker MA. Tacrine for Alzheimer's disease. JAMA 1994;271:1023–1024.
49. Wurtman RJ. Alzheimer's disease. Sci Am 1985;252:62–71.
50. Bukkyo Dendo Kyokai. The teaching of Buddha. 72nd rev. ed. Tokyo: Kosaido Printing, 1984:75.

16/ Older Adults with Developmental Disabilities and Chronic Mental Illness

Marilyn Adlin

This chapter describes two relatively new populations of elderly persons, aging persons with developmental disabilities (DD) and older adults with chronic mental illness (CMI). Improvements in health care and federally mandated community integration over the past 25 years have resulted in a growing and more visible population of elderly persons with these special needs residing within society. Previously, many adults with mental retardation and CMI had reduced life expectancy and spent much of their lives within public institutions or as unseen inhabitants of families dedicated to lifetime caregiving. As a result, aging among these individuals has not been a primary concern for those caring for the elderly. With residential relocation from state institutions to community-based facilities many health care providers find themselves faced with the challenge of providing medical care for, and advising the service sector on, appropriate health care planning for older individuals in these two groups. For these older patients, age-associated medical and social problems may be superimposed on lifelong disabilities further encumbering evaluation and treatment.

Beginning in 1963 with the passage of the Mental Retardation Facilities and Community Mental Health Centers Construction Act (Public Law 88–164), federal legislation has sought to replace use of state hospitals with less restrictive community-based services. Few of the first community programs were developed to meet the needs of the older mentally ill or developmentally disabled adult, and as a result, the initial outcome of this policy for many elderly persons with mental retardation and mental illness was nursing home placement (1). Between 1969 and 1973 the percentage of inpatients over the age of 65 in state and county mental hospitals declined 36% while the number treated in nursing homes increased 101% (2). In 1987, the Nursing Home Reform Act (OBRA, 1987) was passed to ensure that the chronic mentally ill and developmentally disabled were not merely transitioned from one institutional setting to another. This law required preadmission screening and active treatment for individuals of any age found to have mental illness or a developmental disability. Individuals without physical disorders were to be excluded from the nursing homes (3). However, insufficient funding and limited availability of community services for older adults with these conditions has limited implementation of this legislation, creating conflicts for many practitioners.

Aging persons with CMI and those with DD, while separate groups, share some characteristics. In the past, both groups were susceptible to long-term institutionalization and treatment with psychotropic medication. In addition, both groups may be poorly equipped as they approach old age, with weak social supports, diminished capacity to report changes in their own health status, and dependency on public assistance. Physical and biologic changes associated with aging may be seen prematurely in both groups because of long-term effects of medications and institutional care. Medical problems in both of these populations are frequently overlooked as well.

Knowledge of these populations is limited, and published literature is scarce. Most of the literature on mental illness in the elderly addresses the more common diagnoses of dementia and depression, while studies on the developmentally disabled concentrate on children and adolescents. Research in these areas has increased over the past decade, but comprehensive longitudinal studies in both populations are badly needed. In this chapter, aging issues for developmentally disabled and chronically mentally ill older persons are discussed and suggestions for optimizing health care delivery are made.

DEFINITIONS

Despite similarities between the two groups, individuals with DD and persons with CMI represent two distinct populations. Only a small percentage of individuals have both conditions or what is referred to as a "dual diagnosis" (4). Identifying the correct group to which an individual belongs is crucial to providing appropriate health care and services. The following definitions will be used to distinguish between these two populations.

DEVELOPMENTAL DISABILITY

The federal definition of a developmental disability is a severe, chronic disability of a person which (a) is attributable to a mental or physical impairment or a combination of mental and physical impairments; (b) is manifested before the person attains the age of 22; (c) is likely to continue indefinitely; (d) results in substantial functional limitations of major life activities; and (e) reflects the person's need for a combination of special services that are usually lifelong. By this definition only disabilities that have an onset before adulthood are considered developmental. Examples include mental retardation, cerebral palsy, Down syndrome, autism, and epilepsy. The etiology for the disability can vary and may be genetic or due to pre- or postnatal influences such as infection, toxicity, trauma, or hypoxia. The lifelong nature and/or genetic origins of the disability may place the individual at greater risk for additional age-associated disability than the general population because of a variety of environmental, social, psychological, physical, and biologic factors discussed below.

CHRONIC MENTAL ILLNESS

No uniform definition for chronic mental illness exists. Definitions vary widely depending upon the source. The term CMI is often used synonymously with chronic schizophrenia. However, it is also used in a broader, nondiagnostic sense to denote individuals who have had a long stay in a mental hospital or who might have been chronically hospitalized in a psychiatric facility if not for deinstitutionalization policies of the past two decades (2). In general, it describes individuals with a psychiatric disorder who also have functional limitations in social, vocational, or self-care areas (3). Examples include organic mental disorder, chronic affective disorder, personality disorder, paranoid and other psychoses, as well as schizophrenia. For this discussion, we will focus primarily on individuals with severe mental illness with onset before old age, who have spent a major portion of their life in a psychiatric facility.

In most individuals with CMI, the onset of mental illness occurs in adulthood, with near normal family and educational experiences up to that time. Most patients with schizophrenia manifest symptoms by the age of 35, although emergence has been noted in all age groups, including initial onset in the elderly. The course of mental illness may include intervals of relative wellness interrupted by periodic exacerbations. Successful outcomes for the mentally ill may be related to the character of the premorbid personality (1) and adequacy of social supports (2). Mental illness is now widely considered to be primarily of organic etiology with genetic origins, influenced by environmental stressors.

DEVELOPMENTAL DISABILITIES

POPULATION CHARACTERISTICS

A notable increase in life expectancy over the past 50 years for persons with DD has increased this population faster than the general elderly population. In 1935, the average age at death for institutionalized persons with mental retardation was 14.9 and 22.0 years for males and females, respectively; by 1980, these figures had increased to 58.3 and 59.8 (5). When life expectancies and mortality rates for individuals with Down syndrome are discounted, current life expectancies and mortality rates approach those found in the general population. These improvements in life expectancy can be largely attributed to improvements in health care and the national move toward deinstitutionalization.

It is difficult to estimate the actual size of the elderly population with DD. The definition for "aged" varies in studies of developmentally disabled adults, partly because of evidence of premature aging in some subpopulations (e.g., Down syndrome, cerebral palsy, severe mental retardation). At this time, 55 is generally accepted as the onset of "old age" among persons with DD, although individual variations occur. Additionally, older persons with DD are difficult to identify unless they are receiving formal services. It is estimated that up to 60% of persons with DD have never received services and are therefore unknown to the service sector. Considering these limitations, it is currently believed that the population of persons in the United States over the age of 55 with DD will be approximately 500,000 by the year 2000 (6).

SOCIAL ISSUES

Deinstitutionalization. The transition from a public institution to a community residential setting may initially be difficult for elderly individuals who have spent most of their adult lives in a state facility. State institutions were widely used to provide training for mentally retarded individuals and relief to families from the burden of care. Prevailing social attitudes at the time resulted in prolonged segregation, and many of these older individuals have lost contact with family members and depend on formal support mechanisms to live within the community. Studies have shown that older adults are able to transition from institutional life to community residence as well as (and in some cases better than) their younger peers. In addition, it has been demonstrated that the quality of life dramatically improves for older individuals placed in the community and that new social and living skills can be acquired even at advanced age (4).

Aging Caretakers. Most persons with DD remain with their families until their parents are no longer able to provide care for them. It is estimated that almost 80% of individuals with DD live with their families. Parents, particularly mothers, may benefit from the role of lifelong caregiver, compared with age-matched peers (4, 5). Adult children with disabilities may provide assistance to some elderly parents including help with household chores and companionship.

As aging parents become ill or disabled or die, out-of-home placements increase. In many cases, aging parents never expected their disabled child to outlive them and thus are poorly prepared to cope with this transition. Past encounters of the family with the service system may have been unsatisfactory, with inadequate community placement options, long waiting lists, and frequently changing policies. For these reasons, planning is often delayed until the health of the parent deteriorates substantially or until death suddenly creates a placement crisis. Placements in these urgent situations are more likely to be to nursing homes and other institutional settings than to more homelike residential care. Advanced planning is invaluable in these situations. Older adults with a developmental disability may have lived with their parents for 50 to 60 years and may be poorly equipped with the social and community skills necessary to easily transition to a residential setting within the community. Despite advanced age, most older adults with DD can eventually adjust to community living as well as younger persons with disabilities.

Adults with DD usually do not marry, and when they do, they rarely have children to provide supportive assistance as they age. Sibling relationships become increasingly important for this group (4). Parents may assume that siblings of their disabled child will provide caretaking or guardianship upon their death. Estate planning, trusts, and wills may reduce burdens for caregiving siblings.

Other sources of social support such as friends, other relatives (including nieces and nephews), co-workers, staff members, church members, and volunteers are also important to persons with DD. Older adults with DD may need assistance in forming and maintaining these relationships. Correspondence or telephone contact can be very beneficial when time or distance precludes regular visiting.

Long-Term Planning. Retirement, guardianship, and residential needs are important areas to be considered in long-range planning for aging persons with DD (7). Formal daytime programming for persons with DD has used a sheltered workshop format with vocational training as a goal. Retirement requires initiating alternative leisure activities, including integrating clients into existing senior programs to ensure that the individual has something to "retire to." In some cases, individuals may be reluctant to give up employment, which was not available to them earlier in their life, or the social relationships within the work environment.

Residential planning should take into account the age-associated onset of additional disability or deteriorating health to prevent unnecessary moves to more restrictive nursing home environments. Greater in-home medical services increase the ability of older adults to age in a familiar environment. Long-term planning and health care decisions need to include the developmentally disabled adult who, with appropriate provision of information, can often express important preferences.

PSYCHOLOGICAL ISSUES

Behavioral Problems. One of the most frequent concerns of health and service providers caring for persons with DD is the development of challenging behaviors. Factors that may precipitate observed changes in usual behavior include a change in health status, an environmental change, or emotional stress. Belligerent behavior, inappropriate acting out, withdrawal, or declining functional skills may indicate an underlying medical problem or be secondary to isolation or sensory losses. Limitations in communication and expressive language skills may hinder more appropriate self-reporting of physical or emotional distress. Inappropriate sexual expression may result from insufficient education about sexuality (8).

Emotional Expression. Older adults with DD, isolated in institutional or home environments during much of their lives, may be emotionally constricted because of limited training in identifying and expressing emotions. Despite advancing age, many individuals with DD can improve their ability to express emotion with modeling and encouragement, leading to an improved ability to cope with the stresses of aging.

Depression. Elderly persons with DD have experienced many of the same losses as their peers in the general population and appear to be as susceptible to late-onset depression (5). Loss of parents is usually accompanied by sudden and traumatic residential changes that may be perplexing to an individual with diminished comprehension. Grieving may be suppressed by well-intentioned family and staff who attempt to "protect" the mentally retarded adult, frequently excluding them from funerals and other opportunities for mourning. As a result, grieving may be delayed for years and can contribute to depression. Depression in persons with DD can present as profound and sudden loss in functional skills. Adults with DD seem to respond well to antidepressants, and improvements in functional capabilities can be dramatic with treatment. Encouraging emotional expression and reminiscence may assist in the grieving process (9).

Developmental Stage. Cognitive testing can be used to determine cognitive strengths and weaknesses of the older adult with DD and may assist in the diagnosis of dementia. Older adults with DD may never have had formal testing or test results may be outdated. Current formal cognitive testing assists care providers in adjusting programming to the developmental age and level of understanding of the client. Strategies for managing or responding to specific behavior problems can be enhanced when it is known whether the adult developmentally perceives interactions from a 2-year-old, 4-year-old, or adolescent perspective. Developmentally appropriate approaches to challenging behaviors can be far more effective than the negative reinforcements for inappropriate behaviors traditionally used, particularly in the institutional setting. Testing may also identify previously undetected areas of cognitive strength that can be useful in augmenting functional skills as age-associated sensory or mobility deficits result in limitations.

Dementia. Dementia may be overdiagnosed in individuals with DD. Other conditions such as sensory losses, depression, sleep apnea, pain, or physical discomfort may present with behavioral changes and functional declines and mistakenly be attributed to Alzheimer's disease (AD).

CHRONIC MENTAL ILLNESS

POPULATION CHARACTERISTICS

Mortality rates for individuals with mental illness are greater than those for their peers in the general population. Outpatients with a psychiatric diagnosis are twice as likely as other outpatients to die in a 1-year period (2). Of all persons born in 1920 or earlier, half died before reaching old age (10). Mortality in young and middle-aged schizophrenics may be two to three times that of the general population, while mortality for schizophrenics over age 65 may more closely resemble that of the general population (1). Death from suicide is a major factor in this excess mortality, as are inadequate health care and poor health behaviors. We can expect growth in this population with improved health care.

The course of mental illness as it extends into old age can be quite variable, leading to a heterogeneous population of individuals with CMI. Favorable evolution of schizophrenia has been noted in approximately two-thirds of cases, with complete and lasting remission in a quarter of these (1). Improvements in symptoms with age may represent an alteration in symptomatology from overt manifestations of schizophrenia (hallucinations, bizarre behavior, etc.) to more covert ones (withdrawal, passivity, poverty of speech, etc.), which may lead to better social adjustment in some cases (10). Social and environmental factors may be more important than biologic ones in determining long-term outcomes. In some cases, however, schizophrenics continue to have florid symptoms with accompanying assaultive and destructive behavior into old age.

Prior to the deinstitutionalization policy, the population of elderly with CMI was easier to identify, as most resided in state hospitals. Current estimates put the number of elderly CMI at roughly 2 million. Approximately 500,000 chronically mentally ill elderly reside in nursing homes.

SOCIAL ISSUES

Deinstitutionalization. As state mental hospital admissions decreased between 1970 and 1984, admissions to private psychiatric hospitals and psychiatric units in general hospitals increased, indicating that outpatient services have not replaced inpatient services for this population as was the original intention of deinstitutionalization policies (3). Many poorly functioning mentally ill elderly were relocated to nursing homes from psychiatric hospitals. In 1977, 50% of nursing home residents were noted to have psychiatric histories. Those in the community may reside in congregate care, in single-room occupancy hotels, in board-and-care homes, or with family members.

Homelessness. Among the homeless, three groups have been identified: the deinstitutionalized, the chronically homeless, and the temporarily homeless. The American Psychiatric Association estimates that between 25 and 50% of homeless individuals are severely mentally ill (11). The proportion who are elderly is not known but will undoubtedly be increasing as this population ages.

Social Support. Social support reduces the risk for hospitalization and institutionalization in individuals with CMI (2). Unfortunately, many elderly CMI have small social networks. Years of caregiving burden and periods of long hospitalization may diminish family contact and limit friendships. Those able to live in the community rely heavily on family support from spouses, children, and siblings.

PSYCHOLOGICAL ISSUES

Depression. It is not unusual for individuals with CMI to experience depression (or become clinically depressed), requiring the addition of antidepressants to current antipsychotic medication. Lack of social support may place individuals at greater risk for nontreated depression. Symptoms may be falsely attributed to the onset of dementia, delaying treatment.

HEALTH CARE

Older adults with mental retardation and CMI experience the same common, age-associated, physical changes as other elderly persons, including sensory losses, immobility, incontinence, mental status changes, cardiovascular disease, and malignancy. Medical conditions and symptoms, however, are frequently undetected or incorrectly treated as behavioral problems or exacerbations of psychiatric illness. Studies of psychiatric patients have identified serious undiagnosed conditions including infection, neoplasm, drug reactions, diabetes, and cardiovascular disease in up to 20% of individuals studied (10). Sensory losses

have been identified in over half of older mentally retarded individuals presenting to a referral clinic, and in 50% of these cases care providers were unaware of any existing deficits (4). Loss of functional skills or nonspecific behavioral changes may be the only apparent symptoms of physical illness. Mentally ill and mentally retarded individuals infrequently verbalize pain or discomfort and may instead withdraw, appear confused, or become agitated, resulting in misinterpretation of symptom manifestations. For example, exertional angina may appear as a refusal to participate, and incontinence may be attributed to a volitional objection to toileting. A careful evaluation for physical problems is needed when changes in behavior or level of functioning are noted, to prevent delay of treatment of potentially reversible conditions and inappropriate use of psychotropic drugs.

Perhaps the greatest limitation in evaluating the health of aging persons with DD and CMI is difficulty in obtaining accurate health histories. Communication difficulties hinder self-reporting, and information about health status may be scarce and poorly documented. Individuals may reside in environments where direct care staff may be unavailable (single-occupancy hotels) or inconsistent (group homes) or with elderly relatives with diminished observational skills. Frequent residential moves may result in few potential reporters with knowledge of past medical history. Family members and direct care staff may be unaware of symptoms or of normal aging changes. Treatment for potentially reversible conditions may be delayed, increasing the risk of premature nursing home placement. Health professionals can improve symptom reporting by teaching observational skills to care providers and encouraging good recording of health behaviors. Improved symptom reporting improves health care and reduces the need for costly and inconvenient laboratory testing. Regularly administered, objective, functional assessment measures are useful for early detection of functional declines, an important and sometimes only indicator of disease in this population.

PSYCHOTROPIC DRUGS

One of the major differences between individuals with DD and persons with CMI is the appropriateness of psychotropic drug use (4). While phenothiazine medication, beginning in the 1950s, has proven to be extremely effective in treating debilitating hallucinations and delusions in the mentally ill, it was also widely used for behavioral manipulation of mentally retarded individuals, even when environmental alterations and behavioral programming have been found to be far superior. Challenging behaviors in both groups can look very similar, consisting of aggressive outbursts, noncompliance, withdrawal, and self-abusive or self-mutilating activities. In individuals with mental illness these behaviors may originate from delusional thinking and hallucinatory rumination, while for persons with mental retardation these behaviors are more likely a product of diminished comprehension and a means of interacting with the environment in which they are placed. Limitations in funding for mental health services for both mentally retarded and mentally ill may result in overreliance on drugs when behavioral modes and therapy may be effective.

Regardless of the appropriateness of past neuroleptic use, both groups may have been prescribed these medications for more than three decades without the current understanding of their side effects. Consequently, many now experience tardive dyskinesia, severe chronic constipation and megacolon, intellectual impairment, blunted affect, poverty of speech, and parkinsonism (4, 10). Tardive dyskinesia impairs gait and posture, increases risk for aspiration, and can lead to malnutrition. As a partial result, elderly with CMI have twice the death rate from respiratory and digestive disorders than the general population. The elderly are more prone to tardive dyskinesia, not only because of physiologic changes but also because they have been exposed to implicated medications for longer periods. Lower doses of phenothiazines have been shown to reduce adverse effects and improve social functioning (4). In the elderly, altered pharmacokinetics reduce dose requirements. Neuroleptic medication should be avoided if possible, especially in the developmentally disabled, where behavioral programming can be substituted with better efficacy.

SPECIAL POPULATIONS

Certain subgroups among those with DD have been noted to experience differential aging (4).

Mild-to-Moderate Mental Retardation (MR).   Individuals in this group seem to have reduced risk of certain malignancies and heart and lung disease because of limited exposure to smoking, alcohol, and overeating within protective institutional environments. Overall this group may appear to be healthier because of a greater survivorship of the healthier individuals in this group.

Severe and Profound MR.   Persons with MR in the severe-to-profound range experience a shortened life expectancy because of the high prevalence of additional chronic medical problems such as scoliosis, dislocated hips, respiratory disease, chronic otitis media, and vision and hearing deficits (12). Their medical needs can be successfully met within community settings (13).

Epilepsy.   Persons with lifelong histories of use of antiseizure medication are at increased risk for osteoporosis and may experience more fractures as they grow older. Exercise, calcium, and vitamin D may assist in reducing this risk.

Down Syndrome.   Life expectancy for persons with Down syndrome has increased dramatically over the past 50 years, from 9 years of age in 1929 to approximately 55 years today (4). Previously, deaths among those with Down syndrome were attributed to respiratory and other types of infectious disease, malignancy (childhood acute leukemia), and congenital heart disease. Today the primary causes of death in persons with Down syndrome are stroke, dementia, and infection. Individuals with Down syndrome experience several conditions associated with premature aging including hypothyroidism, presbycusis, cataracts, obstructive sleep apnea, immune senescence, osteoarthritis, bunions, and AD. At autopsy, 100% of persons with Down syndrome age 40 or above have the neuropathological changes (neurofibrillary plaques and tangles) associated with AD. However, only 40% of persons with Down syndrome develop clinical symptoms of AD, with onset generally after age 50 (14). Because of the wide-spread belief that all or most persons with Down syndrome will develop AD, changes in behavior or function may mistakenly be attributed to AD rather than to the underlying causes (e.g. depression or other illnesses).

Cerebral Palsy.   Older persons with cerebral palsy (CP) have earlier age-specific mortality, which is related to the coexistence and level of MR. When evaluating persons with CP, it is difficult to determine what is related to general aging, what is pathological aging, and what may be related to preventable secondary conditions. Some persons with CP experience increasing problems with mobility as they age, because of pain syndromes from degenerative joint disease caused by overuse of an irregular joint. In addition, persons with CP may experience increased difficulty with speech, ventilation, swallowing, eating, and urinary incontinence as they age. Sensory losses may be more prevalent than in the general population and, when present, may magnify existing disability.

SUMMARY

The current cohort of elderly persons with CMI and those with DD have experienced dramatic changes in the health care system as a result of social policies. Many spent much of their earlier life within institutional settings and have faced the challenge of integrating into the community at an already advanced age. In delivering health care, it is important to approach these groups in a systematic manner. As health care providers, it is our responsibility to encompass these special populations in our aspiration to provide high-quality care for all aging individuals.

REFERENCES

1. Miller NE and Cohen GD. Schizophrenia and aging. New York: Guilford Press, 1987.
2. Light E, Lebowitz BD, eds. The elderly with chronic mental illness. Baltimore: Springer, 1991.
3. Gatz M, Smyer MA. The mental health system and older adults in the 1990s. Am Psychol 1992; 47(6):741–751.
4. Sutton E, Heller T, Factor A, Hawkins BA, Seltzer GB, eds. Older adults with developmental disabilities: toward community integration. Baltimore: Paul H Brookes, 1993.
5. Janicki MJ, Seltzer MM, eds. Aging and developmental disabilities; Challenges for the 1990's. Washington, DC: Special Interest Group on Aging, American Association on Mental Retardation, 1991.
6. Janicki MP, Wisniewski HM. Aging and developmental disabilities: issues and approaches. Baltimore: Paul H Brookes, 1985.
7. Berkobien R. A family handbook on future planning. Arlington, TX: Association for Retarded Citizens of the United States, 1991.
8. Heighway S, Kidd Webster S, Shaw M. Stars: skills training for assertiveness, relationship-building and sexual awareness. 2nd ed. Madison, WI: Wisconsin Council on Developmental Disabilities, 1990.
9. Wadsworth JS, Harper DC. Grief and bereavement in mental retardation: a need for a new understanding. Death Studies 1991;15:281–292.
10. Strome TM. Schizophrenia in the elderly: what nurses need to know. Arch Psychiatr Nurs 1989;3:47–52.
11. Koegel P, Burnam MA, Farr RK. The prevalence of specific psychiatric disorders among homeless individuals in inner city Los Angeles. Arch Gen Psychiatry, 1988;45(12):1085–1092.
12. McDonald EP. Medical needs of severely developmentally disabled persons residing in the community. Am J Mental Deficiency 1985;90:171–176.
13. Minihan PM, Dean DH. Meeting the needs of health services of persons with mental retardation living in the community. Am J Publ Health 1990;80:1043–1048.
14. Dalton AJ, Wisniewski HM. Down's syndrome and the dementia of Alzheimer's disease. Int Rev Psychiatry 1990;2:43–52.

17/ The Therapeutic Milieu

Social-Psychological Aspects of Treatment

Dorothy H. Coons

This chapter examines the social-psychological aspects of treatment and their influence on the quality of life and care in treatment facilities for the elderly. It emphasizes the need for innovation and creativity in designing environments for the "old, old" who will make up in increasing numbers the population of the future. With the increase in the very old will come a dramatic swelling in the number of people at risk of developing dementia (1).

The chapter examines the four major components of the milieu: the program and opportunities that are available to residents, the staff, the physical environment, and the residents themselves. A comparison of the design of a therapeutic milieu is made with that of custodial treatment. To define and develop the implications and impact of each mode clearly, the author presents the two systems as though they were discrete and opposing models; although, in reality, treatment facilities often incorporate elements of both custodial care and a therapeutic milieu in varying degrees.

CUSTODIAL CARE

Custodial care has been the predominate model for long-term care facilities for a number of years. An outgrowth of the medical style of operation practiced in acute care hospitals, it is now viewed by many health care professionals as inappropriate and nontherapeutic for elderly persons in need of residential treatment. Custodial care focuses on meeting the physical needs of residents and on providing for their physical health and safety. Daily routines concentrate on caretaking, and in some facilities staff members are discouraged from developing social relationships with residents. The focus is upon getting the daily tasks, such as bathing, feeding, and toileting, completed on schedule. In facilities that are un-

derstaffed, the daily tasks become routinized to an assembly-line style of operation.

Social and psychological needs in the traditional setting are largely ignored, and the program actively fosters dependency. The system ignores the differences among residents and provides no mechanisms to accommodate personal preferences. The strict routines and rigid schedules discourage flexibility needed to accommodate individual lifestyles and wishes. Staff learn quickly that it is not acceptable to adjust bathing schedules, for example, to follow earlier patterns of residents. Coercion and control are frequently used in efforts to get essential jobs done. The only role available to residents in custodial care is that of "sick, old patient."

The roles that are essential in giving meaning to life, such as family member, homemaker, friend, and religious being, are not fostered, and the program offers no opportunities for those roles to be maintained. The expectations and assumptions of staff are that the impaired person is no longer capable of establishing relationships or continuing tasks related to everyday life beyond the activities of daily living, and even some of those tasks are done by staff to save time.

The behavioral expectations for residents in the role of patient are that they will respond in sick ways. When this role is emphasized, it is assumed that residents will be dependent, confused, withdrawn, sometimes incontinent, forgetful, or even bizarre, and they may respond to these expectations because this is one way to get attention. It is sometimes easier for staff to cope with ill and inappropriate behavior than with normal, well behavior in a setting where people are expected to be sick. Only the exceptional person will resist the numbing influence of the total environment, and that exceptional person is likely to be labeled "a behavioral problem" and treated very critically.

The custodial environment makes no effort to respond to individual needs and abilities. Activities are often repetitious, even childlike, and staff are not trained to focus on the special interests and skills of residents. Staff use the same approaches constantly, even though they may be upsetting and ineffective.

One of the most blatant flaws in our system of long-term care has been the consistency with which facilities have been built making no provisions for privacy. Even newly built units are offering few if any private rooms. Two-, three-, and four-bed rooms with only divider curtains to give visual privacy are constant reminders to individuals that they are sick and that their world has shrunk to a single hospital bed.

The environment offers little that is sensory or socially stimulating. The drab, sterile environments of many custodial settings are constant reminders of sickness. They are institutional rather than homelike. They often make no provision for personal possessions and memorabilia that help residents maintain a sense of identity and help staff to understand the history and dimensions of the individual. Architectural designs in the past have incorporated features that resemble the acute care hospital—the long double-loaded corridors, multiple sleeping rooms, and the large nursing stations with high divider walls separating residents from staff—all features reminding older persons that they are sick and require care.

Many traditional settings make no effort to group residents according to needs and capacities. The wide mix of persons from the very alert to those who have severe cognitive impairment leads to many problems among residents and makes it impossible for staff to design a strong, supportive milieu that accommodates both those who are able to function independently and those who are in need of much help and care.

The custodial environment offers little staff support or assistance with problem solving. The traditional setting follows the hierarchical system in which orders are handed down from above, and there are seldom opportunities to exchange ideas among staff, to get help with difficult situations, or to get information from those who are working directly with residents. Staff burnout and high turnover rates are common problems (2). The custodial environment discourages innovation, change, and experimentation. Routines become firmly entrenched, and suggestions for change are often considered by staff to be a criticism of the way they are currently functioning. Innovative ideas are often viewed as unsafe or as possible infringements on regulatory measures.

Staff shortages, rigid job descriptions, an inflexible hierarchy of authority, red tape, and paperwork are common products of the custodial system. They provide the staff of many long-term care settings with high-pressure, low-reward jobs. The qualities for which the traditional system rewards staff, such as efficient performance of custodial responsibility or cleanliness and quietness, may actually contribute to the tedium characteristic of these jobs.

THE THERAPEUTIC ENVIRONMENT

The therapeutic milieu encompasses the total environment, and therefore all parts need assessment and often alteration to ensure that all foster well-being. While each part has its own influence on the life of the individual, the milieu fulfills its greatest potential for therapeutic impact only when all of its components mirror the therapeutic milieu. In fact, it may be rendered impotent if staff assume a highly custodial stance or the program lacks challenge and stimulation (3). The following criteria form the basic concepts in designing a therapeutic environment.

The therapeutic milieu offers opportunities and experiences for the individual to maintain continuity with the past and assume, to the fullest extent possible, the social roles normally available in the outside community.

Roles prescribe the patterns of behavior that are socially acceptable for each position or function in a group or society. If, for example, the only available role is "frail sick patient," the individual will conform to the expectation embodied in that role. If, however, a number of normal social roles that had meaning to the individual in earlier life, such as citizen, friend, family member, religious being, consumer, worker, or volunteer, are available, and the individual is encouraged to choose freely among them, behavior will be varied and far more positive and healthful than that prescribed by the sick patient role. These roles enable even the very frail to respond and to function in an environment that is nurturing and enabling.

Each role needs to be considered and plans developed to provide residents with access and opportunities for involvement in those that are crucial to each resident's sense of individuality. For example, residents are often deprived of the opportunity to continue in the role of religious or spiritual being in facilities that are not church affiliated. For many of the elderly, worship and membership in religious life have provided strength and meaning to their lives for years. Without this opportunity they feel they are living in an alien world. Concerned facilities offer a chapel or chaplaincy services or a nondenominational worship service as a bridge to the residents' religious or spiritual life, so essential to their sense of well-being and completeness.

The therapeutic milieu offers maximal autonomy and freedom of choice to the individual and provides environmental flexibility to accommodate individual needs and wishes.

The assumption in the therapeutic milieu is that elderly residents are capable of making choices and of determining what is appropriate and desirable for their well-being. It offers, to the greatest extent possible, individual choices in times to get up or go to bed or bathe, selection of food, choices of dress, and whether or not to participate in activities. Flexible daily routines allow for adjustment to the special needs of residents and their individual lifestyles.

Two of the most drastic infringements on autonomy are the use of physical restraints and the overuse of drugs. Both forms of control are infantilizing and dehumanizing practices that strip the elderly person of freedom, personality, and dignity. Research has provided evidence that physical restraints are not only degrading but are ineffective in reducing falls and accidents (4).

In the therapeutic milieu, there is individualization in staff approaches, in the opportunities for involvement, and in elements of the physical environment.

When staff adopt an individualized approach, they are able to adjust expectations and methods to each individual's abilities, needs, moods, and preferences. They recognize that one set of norms, one style of approaches, and unvaried activities will not be effective with everyone. The effective program of opportunities enables residents to use their existing capabilities, to continue interests and skills that were rewarding to them in earlier life, and to select from a variety of options the activities that are most appealing at the moment.

The physical environment also needs to be individualized with each person's room furnished with personal furniture and memorabilia to help the individual maintain continuity with the past, a sense of ownership, and to the extent possible, a feeling of home.

The therapeutic milieu recognizes the individual's right to privacy and fosters human dignity.

Few people would argue against the individual's right to privacy, but our systems of acute care and long-term care have for years fostered physical environments by the building of multiple sleeping rooms that make privacy essentially impossible. Multiple-person sleeping rooms also offer few or no opportunities for having private possessions. Many bathing and toileting practices in treatment settings are shattering to human dignity.

Staff in traditional settings are faced with a challenge of how to provide privacy and help each person to live with dignity. The selection of roommates is crucial, and if residents are involved in the decision making, the situation may be more acceptable to them. Families can be encouraged to individualize the small space available to each person by hanging family pictures or other personal memorabilia, but these are only token gestures.

Persons who are responsible for accrediting or designing facilities need to establish priorities that place privacy and human dignity as primary goals in long-term care. Until this happens, nursing homes in this country will continue to be looked upon as situations to be dreaded and places of last resort.

The therapeutic milieu provides good health care and a health-fostering and sensory-stimulating environment.

Good medical care is absolutely essential in the therapeutic milieu, requiring ready access to physicians who are knowledgeable in geriatric medicine and sensitive to the physical and cognitive changes that may be occurring in elderly residents and which they may no longer be able to describe. There is also a need for close monitoring of medications for side effects or excessive dosages that may gradually cause behaviors and symptoms resembling dementia or other illnesses. Staff must be trained to be alert to special physical problems residents may be having such as pain, impactions, or problems with eating.

The health-fostering environment provides the essential supports and cues that help the older person to remain as independent as possible. It also makes every effort to deemphasize the features that are constant reminders of sickness.

Many new designs are now offering smaller and more intimate units that are manageable, homelike, and attractive. Single sleeping rooms surround small dining areas, activity space, and lounges that are appealing, easily visible, and accessible. Nursing stations are discarded or disguised, and there are no clearly defined barriers separating residents from staff. This new approach to design provides a milieu that discards the reminders of illness and creates an appealing and comfortable living situation.

The therapeutic milieu creates opportunities for fun, humor, and enjoyment.

Perhaps the truly exceptional milieu is distinguished from others by the frequency with which laughter and humor are shared by staff and residents. The ambience that exists and the pleasure that occurs when they enjoy incidents or situations together create an environment that is health fostering and wholesome. Staff need to be taught that residents are never the objects of the humor. It is the sharing of funny situations and light-hearted activities that creates a climate of warmth, friendship, and togetherness. It may be one of the tragedies of our long-term care system that light-heartedness and fun are often considered inappropriate behaviors for staff and a waste of staff time.

OTHER CONSIDERATIONS IN CREATING A THERAPEUTIC MILIEU

HOMOGENEITY OF THE RESIDENT POPULATION

The assumption here is that the environment has the potential for being the most therapeutic and health fostering when it is designed for a population that is homogeneous with respect to needs and degrees of impairment. An environment, for example, designed to care for cognitively impaired persons often provides services, care, and protection that are inappropriate for the alert elderly person, even though that person may have a number of chronic diseases. No single environment can meet the needs of both the mentally frail and the alert older person. It is the sickest person for whom the limits are often established. Doors are locked, materials and equipment are not available for maximum independence, and activities are often inappropriate and degrading for the alert person. If, on the other hand, the focus is on the alert person, the cognitively impaired are often neglected or ignored.

It is particularly challenging and rewarding to apply the therapeutic concepts described in this chapter to special dementia units. As in other settings, the goals are to create a milieu that will enable each resident to function maximally and get satisfaction from life. Well-trained staff in such settings recognize that impaired persons have little or no control over their behavior. Staff

are undemanding and accepting, and their focus is upon establishing an environment that will give residents opportunities for fun and enjoyment. Emphasis is not on behavioral management but upon providing a positive and supportive milieu that helps residents relax and enjoy the activities and companionship that are offered. The result is a decided reduction in the frequency and intensity of difficult behaviors (5–7).

There needs to be a degree of homogeneity, however, in setting up special dementia units. Too frequently the diagnosis of Alzheimer's disease is considered sufficient in selecting the population for special units. It must be recognized that those in the early and middle stages of dementia have far different capacities and needs than those in the latter stages, and environmental factors need to be planned accordingly.

REVISION OF STAFF ROLES

Staff responsibilities in the therapeutic milieu extend beyond mere custodial care and medical treatment to the establishment of an environment that enables the elderly to live with dignity and with a sense that others care about and value them. Staff members act as friends, therapists, and teachers rather than caretakers. All staff members share knowledge and participate in decision making as it relates to the treatment program.

The quality of human relationships in any milieu becomes the major factor in defining the character and climate of the setting. Staff, therefore, hold the key to determining whether the elderly will live in an enabling environment in which they have opportunities to assume responsibilities for decisions about their own lives or in an environment in which the residents lose all power and gradually the capacity to take responsibility. In a therapeutic milieu, staff give clear messages of warmth and understanding in their communication with residents and illustrate in their relationships that they recognize the value and the capacities of each individual.

Enhancing the independence and self-actualization of residents through environmental intervention becomes the primary responsibility of all staff members in a therapeutic milieu. All are actively involved in planning, providing treatment, and developing opportunities. These new responsibilities are less easy to describe than custodial ones (bathe patient, make bed, maintain a toileting schedule). In general, an aide's job will shift from doing tasks for the residents to assisting residents or teaching them the essential skills they need to perform the tasks themselves. Through modeling and training, supervisors provide aides with the knowledge and communication skills they need to become teachers and enablers rather than caretakers.

STAFF TRAINING

Staff training plays a major role in changing a treatment setting from custodial care to a therapeutic milieu. Staff need to be taught the essentials in health care and how to assist residents in activities of daily living, topics that are a part of many training programs. Staff also need to be taught, however, the technique of task breakdown so that they can help residents function as long as possible. They need to learn how to examine their approaches and communication styles, how to share tasks and activities with residents, and how to help residents maintain identity and a sense of autonomy. Training also needs to include methods for developing a cohesive and effective team that is able to provide support and give help in problem solving (8).

This expanding of staff roles, knowledge, and skills helps to increase job satisfaction and encourages growth. The total milieu becomes increasingly supportive and wholesome for both staff and residents as staff become more innovative and creative.

Training has been found to be most effective and conducive to change when the participants represent a broad cross-section of institutional staff—physicians, administrators, nurses, social workers, physical and occupational therapists, activity directors, aides, and housekeeping personnel. This enables staff and employees at all levels to gain a better understanding and appreciation of others' responsibilities. It can create a climate in which staff learn to work as a team rather than at cross-purposes and in which each person can have influence over the action taken.

Consideration of effective teaching methodology is especially important when the trainees represent a wide range of institutional personnel. The use of a variety of teaching methods—lectures, audiovisual materials, simulations, skill exercises, fantasies, and role playing—enables each person to gain from the methods that provide the best learning experiences for him or her.

PHYSICAL SETTING

The therapeutic setting is attractive and homelike and is designed to accommodate sensory changes and physical and social needs. It provides the materials and equipment essential for self-suf-

ficiency and for the enhancement of the life of the elderly residents (9, 10).

A therapeutic physical environment, in its use of color and such "unhygienic" but warming elements as carpeting, curtains, pictures, and artifacts, shifts the emphasis from a sterile sickroom to one focusing on wellness. It provides residents easy access to equipment and materials essential for self-care and for involvement in activities of personal interest. This leads to greater independence and a sense of self-reliance and communicates staff confidence in residents.

The therapeutic milieu must include opportunity for each individual to have privacy—both auditory and visual—but not isolation. This includes territory over which single individuals hold the rights and can carry out those activities that they do not wish to share with others. The behavior of all people is influenced by the physical environment in which they find themselves. Whenever people are able to exert some control over the way their environment is designed, they organize space and possessions in ways that best meet their own special needs.

As a normal part of the aging process, gradual changes may occur in the sensory systems of vision, hearing, touch, taste, and smell. These changes take place at different rates both among individuals and for different senses in the same individual. The ultimate result of decreased sensory activity can be diminished ability to function in the physical environment, since the cues that give us the information we need about our environment are perceived through our senses. If the cues are not clear enough or are not organized in an understandable way, the person adapting to sensory changes can be left without the information needed to function at maximal capacity. A colorful, stimulating, well-lighted environment and landmarks or prominent features marking a particular locality can help a person remain oriented.

PROGRAM OF ACTIVITIES AND OPPORTUNITIES

The program of the therapeutic milieu incorporates all of the activities that make up the fabric of each person's day, including self-care to the extent possible, choices in daily life that accommodate individual differences and contrasting lifestyles, and those activities that enable the elderly to continue to get pleasure from life and maintain contact with family and friends and the greater community.

The specifics of the program in a therapeutic milieu will vary to meet the needs of the elderly residents and, at the same time, take into account the potential of staff and the resources existing at the particular institution. One constant, however, is the climate produced by the implementation of a therapeutic program. It fosters, enables, and supports individual worth, and is aimed toward helping each resident and staff member achieve a maximal degree of success.

The opportunity-filled therapeutic program fosters a sense of individual worth and of normalcy, affirmation, and achievement. It generates a spirit of community through mutually recognizing and accommodating needs, and it demands recognition of the residents' human rights to satisfaction and dignity in their lives. Because the therapeutic milieu is a total, integrated view, this climate invades all aspects of the institution, not just some specially designated therapeutic segment. Clearly, it is a 24-hour need that is always with the resident and not something that happens only in craft classes or at a weekly group meeting.

The therapeutic milieu defines the long-term care facility as fundamentally a "home" that accommodates the diversity of individual needs and desires. Good medical care and treatment are essential and should aid, not impede, a favorable life. In the hospital version of long-term care, medical treatment becomes an end in itself. In the therapeutic milieu, as in the outside community, medical treatment becomes the means by which the individual is able to maintain the energy and capacity for continued life satisfaction.

Within the context of the therapeutic milieu, the variety of programs that meet resident needs, fit within available resources, and utilize staff and residents' abilities is unlimited. A program designed with sensitivity and in response to resident ideas and individual differences can build a life, even for the very frail, that has meaning and worth.

RESIDENTS IN A THERAPEUTIC MILIEU

The residents in a therapeutic milieu are provided with opportunities to be involved in a variety of social roles and through their participation become effective agents in their own treatment and that of other residents.

In the therapeutic environment, the life space of residents is extended beyond their own bed, room, or dining area to include the whole facility and all of the residents and staff. Residents no longer limit their concern to the routine of their own bodily functions, taking medicines, and reporting ailments. In the enlarged environment with its multiple non–sick role opportunities, res-

idents manage their own affairs and their own expectations of what satisfaction will be derived from the day's activities and social transactions. The resident is in contact with other residents and often shares interests and activities with them.

In the roles of friend, leader, teacher, consumer, volunteer, worker, religious being, and so on, the resident links the current life patterns with those of the past. Value and reward systems, long established, can still be retained, and continuity of personality is uninterrupted.

In a therapeutic milieu, residents are encouraged to select their own programs according to their wishes, for self-determination is a precious privilege of all persons. As in any society, this free selection operates with a set of built-in expectations: being up and dressed, taking care of one's possessions and living space, and being on hand for meals. But beyond these normal everyday expectations, the individual residents spend their time as they choose.

Motivating residents who have experienced years of traditional institutional life can be a major hurdle in implementing programs. Yet research data from various projects of the Institute of Gerontology at the University of Michigan demonstrate that residents, even those long deprived of activity, will become intensively and consistently involved if motivated. Several necessary conditions for this have been discussed. For example, activities need to have relevancy and value for the older person. The depressed or withdrawn person may need time to consider what is involved and may require help and encouragement from staff to return step by step to the life of an active participant. Many residents have lost confidence in their own abilities, but a well-trained and optimistic staff and a careful selection of activities to ensure success can help older persons begin to test their abilities to cope with new and different expectations and opportunities.

The extent to which the elderly in treatment settings can continue in social roles varies, of course, with the functioning level and energy of individuals. The objectives are to enable persons to get pleasure from each day and continue relationships and involvement to the greatest extent possible.

THE CHANGE PROCESS

Converting a custodial facility to one that is therapeutic and strongly supportive to both residents and staff is a challenging and often difficult process, but the results are highly rewarding. In implementing changes, well-established and tested principles of management apply to treatment settings as well as to industry. For example, staff at all levels need to participate in the planning after they have grasped the fundamentals of the changes to be instituted. This involvement increases the participants' understanding of the new program, and it ensures that maximal expertise, awareness, and insight have gone into the decisions. If staff are involved in finding solutions to the inevitable problems that arise in making changes, even some of the most resistant staff will support plans that they have helped to formulate (11).

The sequencing and pacing of program implementation are crucial. Introducing too many changes and too many programmed activities simultaneously can bring chaos. Reasonable goals need to be set and sufficient time allowed to test out each phase of programming.

Even best laid plans will go awry, however, without strong leadership. The leader's role throughout is one of support, encouragement, clarification, and training. It is the leader who can model behavior, demonstrating that it is rewarding and exciting to work with the elderly, that follow-through is essential in effective programming, and that staff at all levels are valued and essential members of the team. It is the leader, too, who can establish a climate in which it is safe to test out new techniques and programs and fail and in which the failure itself becomes a learning experience to insure the effectiveness of future efforts.

The style of administration is crucial in introducing new approaches and programs. In the traditional style of management that discourages innovation, the objective of administrative persons is control. They rely on giving orders to bring about any change, impose discipline, and function within a clearly defined hierarchy. In contrast, the strong leaders' objective is change. They rely on facilitating and teaching to alter practices, act as role models, encourage creativity and involvement of others, and are open to the ideas and opinions of others (12–14).

The support of the administration is fundamental to change. With such administrative support, new policies can be planned and clarified, existing practices can be reviewed and altered, new programs and methods can be tested as needed, and the total system can be modified to advance therapeutic objectives. Transformation to a new system is likely to appear risky to staff members who may not feel that it represents a change for the better or who see the change as a threat to their authority. The administration must assure staff and provide them with essential supports to help them feel comfortable with the transition.

CONCLUSION

The predictions for the future are overwhelming. With the steady increase in the numbers of elderly persons over the next several decades and the corresponding growth in the proportions of dementia victims, this country is faced with a challenge in long-term care unlike any in the past. The system can meet the increasing demands by refining assembly-line methods that are dehumanizing, frightening, and dreaded by elderly persons and their families, or the system can explore new and better ways of caring for the elderly that will, over the next decades, develop nurturing environments that will demonstrate to the elderly that they are a truly valued and cherished segment of our society.

REFERENCES

1. U.S. Congress, Office of Technology Assessment. Losing a million minds: confronting the tragedy of Alzheimer's disease and other dementias, OTA-BA-323. Washington, DC: U.S. Government Printing Office, 1987.
2. Diamond T. Making gray gold. Chicago: University of Chicago Press, 1992.
3. Birren JE, Lubben JE, Rowe JC, Deutchman DE, eds. The concept and measurement of quality of life in the frail elderly. New York: Academic Press, 1991.
4. Frengley JD, Mion LC. Incidence of physical restraints on acute general medical wards. J Am Geriatr Soc 1986; 34(8):565–568.
5. Coons DH, ed. Specialized dementia care units. Baltimore: Johns Hopkins University Press, 1991.
6. Friedman A, Robinson A. Wesley Hall: a special life. A 29-minute film or videotape. Innerimages Productions. Distributed by Terra Nova Films, Chicago, 1986.
7. Mace NL. Dementia care: patient, family, and community. Baltimore: Johns Hopkins University Press, 1990.
8. Coons DH, Metzelaar L. A manual for trainers of direct service staff in special dementia units. Ann Arbor: University of Michigan, 1990.
9. Cohen U, Weisman GD. Holding on to home. Baltimore: Johns Hopkins University Press, 1991.
10. National Center on Housing and Living Arrangement for Older Americans. Homelike attributes of dementia special care units. Ann Arbor: College of Architecture and Urban Planning, University of Michigan, 1993.
11. Boling TE, Vrooman DM, Sommers KM. Nursing home management: a humanistic approach. Springfield, IL: Charles C Thomas, 1983.
12. Aburdene P, Naisbitt J. Megatrends for women. New York: Villard Books, 1992.
13. Dobyns L, Crawford-Mason C. Quality or else. Boston: Houghton Mifflin, 1991.
14. Walton M. The Deming management method. New York: Perigee Books, 1986.

18/ Neurologic Diseases in the Elderly

Joseph H. Friedman

Although neurologic disorders in the elderly are a major cause of disability and nursing home placement, it is often unclear where normal aging ends and pathology begins (1, 2). Mild memory deficits are common but do not necessarily indicate incipient Alzheimer's disease. Slowing down, stooping posture, and minor deficiencies in balance may be the result of normal aging, not Parkinson's disease. Loss of strength and atrophy of muscles do not mean motor neuron disease. But such declines could presage disease. Noting the demarcation between normal aging and disease may or may not be in the patient's best interest, but knowing how to recognize the distinction is always important.

In this chapter, the major causes of neurologic decline in the elderly are each considered briefly. The emphasis is on diagnosis, particularly where early recognition may alter outcome.

STROKE

Stroke is the third leading cause of death in the U.S. (3) and is second only to Alzheimer's disease as a neurologic cause for nursing home placement. Although stroke rates have been declining steadily over the past few decades, the incidence of stroke doubles each decade after the age of 55 (3) (Fig. 18.1).

Risk factors for stroke include age, male gender, hypertension, coronary artery disease, left ventricular hypertrophy, cigarette smoking, congestive heart failure, diabetes, and atrial fibrillation. A transient ischemic attack (TIA), defined as an episode of neurologic dysfunction presumed to be due to ischemia, lasting under 24 hours and leaving no residual deficit, is a special risk factor that immediately increases the risk of a stroke to 5% the first week, 10% the first month, 20% within 1 year, and 35% within 5 years.

Strokes can be classified into two major categories, ischemic and hemorrhagic. In the former, loss of adequate blood flow leads to ischemic necrosis in a vascular territory. In the latter, a blood vessel, usually on the arterial side, ruptures, leaking blood into the brain or subarachnoid space. Ischemic strokes are more common, but the ratio of the different types varies in different ethnic groups, with Afro-Americans having a much higher rate of cerebral hemorrhages than Caucasian Americans. Death rates from stroke vary with ethnicity as well. The mortality rate from stroke in Afro-Americans is almost twice that in whites.

Ischemic strokes may be caused by embolus, thrombus, or diminished perfusion. Emboli may be of arterial origin, generally from the carotid arteries or heart. In rare cases, right-to-left shunts in the heart allow venous emboli to bypass the filtration system of the pulmonary circulation and cause strokes. In general, large artery strokes (i.e., strokes in the distribution of the middle, anterior, or posterior cerebral arteries) are usually embolic. Thrombotic strokes, caused by atherosclerosis-induced stenosis and obstruction, can occur in the intracranial vessels but usually involve the internal carotid or the vertebrobasilar system. As a result of occlusion in the neck, the distal blood supply becomes insufficient and infarction occurs.

Since management of focal ischemia in different locations is different, recognizing distributions, at least crudely, is crucial. Large vessel strokes are most often seen in the territory of the middle cerebral arteries. On the dominant side, these strokes cause aphasia, homonymous field cuts, more weakness of face and arm than of leg, and a mild hemisensory loss. On the nondominant side, the aphasia is replaced by denial or neglect. When the frontal lobe eye movement region is involved, the eyes will be deviated to the side of the lesion, away from the side of the weakness. Anterior cerebral infarctions affect the leg primarily, with various mental status abnormalities. The posterior cerebral artery territory encompasses the thalami, the medial temporal lobes, the occipital pole, and the visual association regions. Pos-

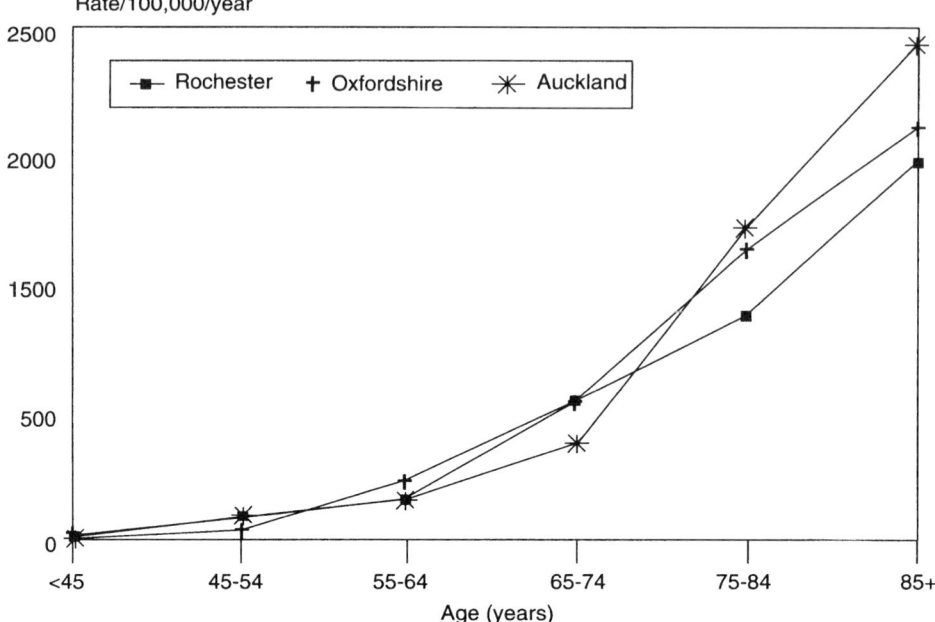

Figure 18.1. Age-specific incidence rates for stroke in three populations. (Used with permission of Lea & Feb-iger and JP Broderick, MD. From: Barclay M. Clinical geriatric neurology. Philadelphia: Lea & Febiger, 1993.)

terior cerebral infarction usually causes a hemi-anopsia but may cause profound sensory deficits from thalamic involvement or memory deficits from medial temporal lobe infarction. Remember that the two posterior cerebral arteries arise from a single basilar artery, so that blockage of the basilar near its bifurcation can cause bilateral signs. The middle and anterior cerebral arteries arise from the carotids, so events in these territories point to carotid or more proximal disease, whereas posterior cerebral abnormalities imply a vertebrobasilar source. Remembering this anatomy makes test ordering more relevant. A diagnosis of a posterior circulation event makes a carotid evaluation of limited value.

Brainstem infarctions, caused by vertebrobasilar ischemia, are diagnosed by finding lower motor neuron cranial nerve abnormalities such as disconjugate eye movements, pupillary abnormalities, facial weakness involving the upper as well as the lower face, an asymmetric gag reflex, weakness of masticatory muscles on one side, or crossed signs. Most brainstem strokes cause a cranial abnormality on one side and a bodily deficit on the other; supratentorial deficits always cause deficits on the same side. Crossed findings always imply a brainstem localization.

Lacunar infarcts are small, fairly round strokes that occur deep in the brain and brainstem, due primarily to chronic changes in the ar-

teriolar blood vessel secondary to hypertension but probably also due to emboli.

Lacunar syndromes are legion. From a very small set of syndromes initially described only a short time ago, the number of lacunar syndromes increased dramatically with improved imaging. Fisher, who first described the syndrome, noted over 20 different ones a decade ago, even before MRI became commonly available and refined our knowledge further. The most common lacunar syndromes are pure motor and pure sensory deficits, typically affecting the whole half of the body, face, arm, and leg, but with numerous variants. Although lacunes are associated with hypertension and are often due to progressive stenosis of small arteriolar lumens, a revisionist view of these strokes has considered them (depending on their location) as being sometimes related to carotid disease, just as large vessel strokes are. This change has led to changes in our management, discussed below.

Hemorrhages into brain parenchyma are primarily due to chronic hypertension or cerebral amyloid angiopathy. Hypertensive hemorrhages occur in the putamen, thalamus, cerebellum, and pons. The importance of recognizing the typical locations is that a hemorrhage in one of these locations in a hypertensive requires no further evaluation. Hemorrhages do not typically occur in these locations as a result of an acute episode of hypertension but only as the result of chronic hypertension. Thus emergency treatment of hypertension is rarely necessary for stroke prevention. Cerebral amyloid angiopathy (CAA) is a newly recognized entity that is age related and bears an unclear but definite association with Alzheimer's disease. This pathological change, without associated hypertension, causes lobar hemorrhages, which are located closer to the brain periphery than hypertensive hemorrhages. Unfortunately these patients are subject to repeated lobar hemorrhages in different locations and to infarcts as well. This amyloid is unrelated to systemic amyloidosis.

Mortality following stroke is now about 17%, down from 33% in 1950, because of better care in the immediate poststroke period. The risk factors for ischemic stroke can often be modified, even in the elderly, and thus alter outcome. For example, treatment of hypertension, including isolated systolic hypertension reduces stroke risk in patients over 60 (4). Identifying carotid-distribution transient ischemic attacks or minor strokes, including lacunes, should lead to a carotid evaluation and endarterectomy if stenosis is greater than 70% on the appropriate side and the patient is a surgical candidate. The management of symptomatic stenosis under 70% is currently under investigation. Also under investigation is a comparison between endarterectomy and medical management for asymptomatic carotid stenosis. This is important because asymptomatic carotid stenosis occurs in about 5% of the elderly and is often found when patients undergo angiography for coronary artery disease. The very infirm and those with severe deficits, dementia, or limited life expectancy are not endarterectomy candidates, and hence carotid studies are not indicated.

For patients who have had ischemic events but are not candidates for endarterectomy, aspirin, in doses of 325 to 1300 mg daily, or ticlopidine, reduce risk a modest amount. Although many physicians use "baby" aspirin to reduce the risk of gastric problems, there are few data to support this low dose (5). Dipyrimidole has been shown to be ineffective, both alone and in combination with aspirin, in reducing stroke risk, so its use is discouraged.

Cerebral hemorrhages from hypertension or CAA are evacuated only when the hemorrhage is causing herniation and is located in the nondominant hemisphere. Cerebellar hemorrhages are often evacuated early to prevent edema in the posterior fossa from compressing the brainstem. For the evacuation to be helpful, intervention must occur before the patient has been comatose for more than a few hours. Subsequent care is supportive, as risk factors are reduced. There is no role for steroids.

Management of acute ischemic stroke is debated. The role of heparinization is unclear and has not been properly studied. Often its use is justified by its relative safety and the hope that it may prevent stroke extension. More important is attention to blood pressure, which should not be lowered acutely because of the brain's loss of normal autoregulation, which puts the patient at risk for stroke extension. Steroids are of no use in cytotoxic edema, the type that follows ischemic infarcts. Most elderly patients have suffered sufficient atrophy to accommodate considerable edema without risk of herniation anyway. Attention to airway management, pulmonary toilet, and prevention of deep vein thrombosis, decubital sores, and contractures is crucial.

Management after the acute period has ended should include rehabilitation when feasible. Patients awaiting endarterectomy, which usually is performed several weeks after a stroke, should be either on antiplatelet agents or Coumadin until the procedure. Those candidates with carotid territory events who are not endarterectomy candidates should be treated with antiplatelet therapy forever, barring complications. Patients with posterior circulation ischemic events are generally maintained on Coumadin for 1 to 3 months then switched to an antiplatelet agent. The rationale is that posterior vessel thrombi, unlike anterior ones, tend to propagate.

EPILEPSY

Epilepsy, defined as recurrent unprovoked seizures, is almost as common a problem for the elderly as stroke, and as with stroke, incidence increases with age (6). Epilepsy can be broadly categorized into partial and generalized seizures. Partial seizures begin in a localized region of the brain; generalized seizures begin synchronously over the whole cortex. Most common in adults, including the elderly, are partial seizures with secondary generalization, that is, seizures that begin electrically in one location but spread rapidly to involve the whole brain.

Partial seizures are themselves divided into simple partial seizures, in which consciousness is not impaired, and complex partial seizures, in which patients have motor, somatosensory, special sensory (smell, taste), autonomic, or psychic symptoms. The most common examples of simple partial seizures are clonic jerking of an arm or face, transient burning, or paresthesias in a focal body part. Complex partial seizures, commonly called absence seizures, psychomotor seizures, or temporal lobe seizures because most (70 to 80%) originate there, involve alteration but not loss of consciousness. Patients may appear as if in a trance or intoxicated and often perform "automatisms," purposeless movements such as lip smacking, blinking, arm raising, or hand rubbing lasting a few seconds to a couple of minutes, following which they may return to normal or may be confused for a few minutes.

Generalized seizures involve the whole body without focality. It is usually not possible to distinguish secondarily generalized from primary generalized seizures on clinical grounds alone. In adults, these are typically tonic-clonic or clonic and occasionally tonic alone. In the most common form the patient suddenly, without warning, stiffens as the tonic phase begins, often emitting a cry, which is due to a sudden inspiration, and remains stiff for a few seconds, then begins to jerk as the clonic phase sets in. This may end the seizure or be followed by an additional tonic phase. Seizures rarely last more than 2 minutes but are followed by a period of stupor and confusion lasting minutes to several hours, especially in the elderly. An aura before the apparent ictus actually marks the onset of the seizure and always indicates a focal onset.

Oftentimes patients are evaluated for episodes of neurologic dysfunction that were unwitnessed and for which scant information is available. The differential diagnosis for unwitnessed spells are syncope, seizures, TIA, intoxication, and psychogenic spells. TIA and partial seizures can be difficult to tell apart. In general, partial seizures last under 2 minutes, whereas TIAs usually last more than 15. Ischemic symptoms are usually negative: an absence of feeling, a "deadness" or "wooden feeling" or weakness; seizures usually produce positive phenomena such as movement, stiffening, burning, or tingling. Unwitnessed loss of consciousness is a more difficult problem (7), complicated by the common occurrence of myoclonus or even true seizures induced by hypotension. Psychogenic spells are rare as new phenomena in the elderly and should be considered only when spells are lengthy or bizarre or a known psychosocial precipitant exists.

The elderly with new-onset seizures need an evaluation to rule out a metabolic derangement and a structural brain abnormality. An EEG may be necessary, especially if the diagnosis is in doubt, but in clear-cut cases when a decision has been made to treat the patient and the drug choice would not be altered by the EEG, the test takes on academic interest only. If a single unprovoked seizure occurs, the risk of a second spell is only about 30%, so a decision to not treat is justifiable (8).

Certainly two or more unprovoked seizures require treatment, the drugs of choice being phenytoin, carbamazepine, and valproic acid. All three drugs are effective for the major convulsive types but to a lesser degree in complex partial seizures than in generalized seizures. Anticonvulsant drug (ACD) levels should be routinely monitored shortly after starting and then at regular intervals, such as every 4 to 6 months if all metabolic conditions remain stable.

The question of stopping ACD after seizures have been controlled has been studied over the past few years. Most patients in remission can have their medications discontinued after being seizure-free 2 to 5 years, but older patients are more likely to suffer relapses than the younger or patients with a known cause. Abnormal EEGs increase the risk of recurrence, as do abnormal neurologic evaluations.

GAIT DISORDERS

Gait changes with aging include a shorter stride and broader base, with decreased pelvic rotation, and mild slowing. Balance also declines with age but may be disease related (1, 2). Gait dysfunction may be due to mechanical problems such as deformed joints, arthritis, focal or diffuse weakness, deafferentation from a neuropathy, vestibular or visual impairment, or abnormalities in the central nervous system integration (9). Patients will often be able to identify the problem, especially when it is pain. A sore foot, ankle, knee, or hip is easily identified as a major problem. A patient will walk in a way that induces minimum pain. This frequently involves a slow walk, stiff limbs, quick shift of position, use of supportive devices to distribute weight, asymmetric jerky movements, or limping. Asymmetric leg lengths cause a subtle limp and result in scoliosis.

Symmetric leg weakness causes gait changes that depend on the location of the weakness. Proximal weakness, when mild, causes difficulty getting out of a chair, and when severe, may lead to a waddling gait. Quadriceps weakness causes stiffening of the knees as if the knees were ankylosed in extension. This is because very little strength is required to maintain posture with the knee extended, whereas a great deal of strength is required to walk with even a slight degree of knee flexion. Anterior calf weakness causes a foot drop. The leg is lifted high off the ground, depending on severity, to avoid tripping. Gastrocnemius weakness causes a reduced stride length and loss of "bounce," as the weak foot cannot push off the ball of the foot.

Sensory problems are more difficult to recognize and require formal evaluation of position and tactile sensation. With increasing loss of peripheral sensation, vision assumes increasing importance for compensation. A sensory-impaired gait is ataxic, with a wide base and inability to walk in a straight line, and the steps are high and slapping.

The most common central nervous system gait problems are due to strokes, cervical myelopathy, and parkinsonism (9). The typical stroke causes a diminished arm swing and a stiff leg on the affected side. The leg tends to circumduct mildly. A cervical myelopathy causes a "spastic" gait. There may be a decreased arm swing, and the legs tend to be extended at knee and ankle so that the legs circumduct. There is a tendency to walk on the toes with the feet tending toward, or even past, the midline. A parkinsonian gait is characterized by stooped posture, diminished arm swing, decreased stride length, decreased elevation of the feet (causing shuffling), turning "en bloc" without a pivot, and postural instability. Cerebellar ataxic gait is a "drunken gait." The base may be wide, and the patient lurches forward. There is a tendency to lose balance, and the arms may be abducted for stability. Sometimes the base is normal but the patient veers to one or both sides.

Cervical myelopathy, generally caused by spondylosis, a narrowing of the spinal canal from arthritic bony development, may present as a gait disorder. As a result of cord compression in the neck, patients develop a slowly progressive spastic gait along with bladder spasticity, manifest as urinary urgency and frequency. If the cervical spondylosis compresses nerve roots, then one sees focal wasting and diminished reflexes in the upper limbs while the legs are pathologically hyperreflexic.

Very often the problems are multiple, and emphasis must be placed, of course, on treatable aspects. For example, knee or hip replacements can dramatically improve gait in Parkinson patients with severe arthritis. Plastic braces for foot drops prevent falls. Recognition of weakness may lead to treatment of polymyositis, peroneal palsy, or lumbar spondylosis. Starting medications for Parkinson's disease or stopping sedative drugs, which impair balance, can improve function and reduce the risk of falling.

PARKINSON'S DISEASE

Parkinsonism refers to the syndrome of akinetic-rigidity. Parkinson's disease (PD) and drug-induced parkinsonism, the two most common parkinsonian syndromes, cannot be distinguished by clinical criteria. Many other parkinsonian syndromes exist and are briefly described below.

PD affects about 1% of the American Caucasian population above the age of 65, with a male predilection of about 1.5:1. It is considerably less common among the Afro-American population for unknown reasons. Its cause is unknown. Median age of onset is about 60, but since life expectancy has become relatively normal since the develop-

Table 18.1
Neurologic Gait Disorder Pattern

	Posture	Base	Armswing	Balance	Description
Parkinsonian	Stooped/tilted	N			Small shuffling steps, hips and knees flexed
Cerebellar	N	Or N arms abducted			Staggering, "drunken"
Hemiparetic side	N	Mild	On weak side	N or	Stiff leg on paretic side with circumduction "Scissoring," toe walk, legs stiff
Spastic	N	N			
Footdrop	N	N or	N	N	High steps, weak foot drags
Sensory	N		Arms abducted		Staggering, "drunk"; much better with eyes open
Myopathic	N or hyperlordotic	N	N	N	Waddling, knees stiff

ment of levodopa, most patients with the disease are elderly.

PD is a syndrome consisting of four cardinal features: slowness of movement, tremor at rest, rigidity, and postural abnormalities. Patients are statuesque. They blink and swallow less than normals (hence the drooling) and have a "masked" facial expression, all elements of akinesia. Coupled with this is a variable degree of slowness caused both by a delay in initiating movements and by slowness in completing the movement. The tremor occurs at rest, often continues during sustension of posture, but resolves with movement. About 80% of patients have tremor, which usually affects the fingers (pill rolling) or hands but may involve the jaw, lips, tongue, or feet. It only rarely involves the head, so the presence of a head tremor should raise the question of essential tremor or torticollis. Tone is assessed with the patient relaxed and may be increased at some or all joints. Cog wheeling is not a sine qua non of the disorder but is common. The postural abnormality of PD is basically one of flexion. With increasing disease, patients become more flexed at all joints, causing the appearance of exaggerated old age. Balance is affected, so the risk of falling increases substantially. Parkinsonian gait is distinctive (see above). Other changes that occur are micrographia, urinary urgency, hypophonia, frequent stuttering, and difficulty initiating sounds. Depression occurs in about 50% of cases, and while there is debate about the depression being "reactive" or intrinsic to the disease, each patient should be assessed for this problem, as it is amenable to therapy. Dementia ultimately occurs in about 30% of patients, often due to concomitant Alzheimer's or vascular disease, although in a significant percentage the PD is the only identifiable cause. PD has a variable course, with many patients incapacitated within a few years and others requiring only minor lifestyle alterations after 10 years.

Treatment of PD currently rests on medications regulating the balance of dopamine and acetylcholine. Levodopa is the single best drug, and virtually every patient requires it at some point. It is used because dopamine does not cross the blood-brain barrier. It is normally present in the brain during the synthesis of dopamine and occurs after the rate-limiting enzyme. Levodopa helps almost all PD patients, but the degree of response varies from the mild to the miraculous. Unfortunately, more than half the patients on levodopa develop complications of therapy after 5 years. These are generally mild dyskinesias, but marked clinical fluctuations, dystonia, and erratic responses to the drug also occur.

Drugs that directly stimulate the dopamine receptors, the dopamine agonists, pergolide and bromocriptine, are useful adjuncts to levodopa but do not replace it. Clinical experience has shown that patients who fail to respond to levodopa also fail to respond to dopamine agonists. Anticholinergic drugs are useful for tremor and rigidity but are not helpful for slowness, gait dysfunction, and balance, which are often the disabling features of the disease. The anticholinergics also are poorly tolerated by the elderly, and the adverse effects of confusion, memory dysfunction, urinary retention, and worsened constipation are likely to occur. Amantadine, a dopamine-enhancing drug, is sometimes helpful. By itself, it is usually well tolerated but loses effect within a month or two. As a supplement to levodopa, it may be useful longer. Finally, the only medication for PD that has a proposed "protective" effect of slowing down disease progression, selegiline (deprenyl) probably does not do this. It is approved for use in the United States for "wearing off," a problem with levodopa not producing clinical benefits lasting through the next dose.

As the illness progresses, fewer intact neurons in the substantia nigra survive, so the response to levodopa and the other drugs declines. Thus, patients who survive a long time or who have rapidly progressive disease may reach a stage of being essentially unresponsive to medications.

DRUG-INDUCED PARKINSONISM

Drug-induced parkinsonism is caused by medications that interfere with dopamine. In most cases these are dopamine receptor blockers. The antipsychotic drugs are the major offenders but antiemetics such as prochlorperazine (Compazine) and droperidol (Inapsine) as well as the gastrointestinal motility enhancer metoclopramide (Reglan) may cause parkinsonism or worsen PD. The clinical effects are identical, even to the point of being asymmetric, just as in PD. Unfortunately older patients may be exquisitely sensitive to the adverse effects and even on low doses of these drugs may develop disabling parkinsonism. These parkinsonian effects can be disabling and may take months to resolve after stopping the drug.

Drug-induced parkinsonism may respond to amantadine or anticholinergics. In the elderly, amantadine is the drug of choice because of its better side-effect profile. Unfortunately, a sizable percentage of patients don't respond to either.

Other causes of parkinsonism are distinctly less common. Progressive supranuclear palsy

(PSP) is an akinetic syndrome named after the eye movement abnormality in which patients lose the ability to look down and up voluntarily while maintaining normal eye movement brainstem reflexes (doll's eyes maneuver). There is usually no tremor in this disorder, and the facial expression is more quizzical than masked, although it is quite akinetic. Patients frequently exhibit axial dystonia with an opisthotonic posture, but many remain fairly erect or even stooped. Slowness and poor balance, coupled with an inability to look down, lead to increasing numbers of falls. Medications are rarely helpful, although the usual PD medications are always worth trying. Striatonigral degeneration is a progressive akinetic rigid syndrome that might mimic PD except for a poor response to levodopa. Normal pressure hydrocephalus (NPH) and multiple infarct (atherosclerotic parkinsonism) state cause a form of "parkinsonism from the waist down."

NORMAL PRESSURE HYDROCEPHALUS (NPH)

NPH is a syndrome usually defined by the clinical triad of dementia, gait dysfunction, and urinary incontinence associated with communicating hydrocephalus. From the first description in 1965 until recently, its place of importance in the etiologies of dementia and gait difficulty in the elderly has undergone radical revision (10). For a time it was considered an extremely important cause of reversible dementia, but it has now assumed its rightful place as a rare disorder.

The syndrome comes in two variants: symptomatic and idiopathic. The symptomatic type has, by definition, a known cause, such as meningitis or subarachnoid hemorrhage. These patients improve with shunting, most of the time. The cases that lack a known precipitant are idiopathic. The frequency of occurrence of the idiopathic form is about 1 case per million per year. Since there is no known pathology associated with NPH, diagnosis rests on improvement with shunting.

The gait of NPH has been described with many confusing terms such as "ataxic" and "apractic." Studies have shown however that the gait generally looks like "Parkinson's from the waist down." The term "magnetic gate" is accurately descriptive, as the feet may appear to be stuck to the ground. The urinary dysfunction is of the hyperactive type, with urgency and frequency. The dementia is less well characterized, leading to major diagnostic problems. The only test that has been helpful in diagnosing NPH is spinal fluid drainage. A variety of other tests have fallen out of favor, and the most commonly ordered test, cister-

nography, has never been shown to be of value. Complicating the diagnosis is the observation that the longer the syndrome has been present, the more severe the dementia and the less likely the patient is to improve. Onset of dementia before gait dysfunction also predicts a poor outcome. These patients may have other causes for their dementia.

As with all illnesses, the earlier the treatment, the better the outcome. Improvement may be immediate or evolve over days to weeks. Complications unfortunately are common and include subdural hematomas, seizures, strokes, and shunt malfunctions. For reasons not understood, many patients have only transient improvement.

In most series, under 50% of patients improve with shunting, and complications of surgery occur in about 30%. Shunting works best in patients who primarily have a gait disturbance with little dementia. The presence of urinary incontinence is not a major predictor of shunt response.

OTHER MOVEMENT DISORDERS

Aside from parkinsonism, the most common movement disorder is tremor. Senile tremor is an outdated term for "essential" or "benign familial tremor." This tremor usually affects the arms but also may involve the head or voice. Other body parts such as tongue, lips, legs, and eyebrows may be involved, but considerably less often. The hand tremor is not present at rest but is seen with sustained postures and movements. Although the tremor is usually hereditary, it is so variable in different generations that it can be missed. The tremor responds in most cases to alcohol, primidone, propranolol, or phenobarbital but rarely resolves entirely. Anxiety worsens the tremor; alcohol and other anxiolytics ameliorate tremor partly via this mechanism. Primidone should be initiated at 25 mg at night, as older people are extremely sensitive to the nausea and dizziness it induces. Doses above 300 mg of primidone or 320 mg of propranolol are usually not helpful. When the tremor is severe, surgical intervention using thalamotomy should be considered. However surgery improves only the contralateral tremor, and bilateral surgery markedly increases the risks of adverse effects.

Akathisia, the syndrome of restlessness, is another neuroleptic-induced movement disorder. This may occur early, within minutes to hours of the first dose, or after weeks. The patient develops an uncomfortable, irresistible urge to move. Since geriatric patients usually receive neuroleptics because of behavioral problems associated with dementia, akathisia must be looked for by the clinician. The patient may be unable to explain the problem. It should always be considered when behavior worsens after starting a neuroleptic. In such cases, stopping the offending agent and starting propranolol or an anticholinergic is indicated.

HEADACHES

Headaches can be divided into those with a serious or a benign prognosis. In younger adults, benign headaches are far more common than serious ones, with tension headaches, migraines of various types, and mixtures of the two constituting the vast majority. New-onset headaches in the elderly however should always be considered serious, with brain tumor, subdural hematoma, temporal arteritis, and sinusitis being the major considerations. Migraines and tension headaches may continue into old age but do not usually begin then. Headaches also frequently occur from systemic illness, such as infections outside the nervous system, pulmonary disease, and endocrinopathies. Sinus headaches may not be accompanied by fever and purulent discharge. They tend to be most severe on awakening, when the sinus is full, and improve during the day as it drains. Tumor headaches are usually relatively mild, with an insidious onset but relentless progression. Tumors generally don't cause pain until they have grown fairly large or cause hydrocephalus. Tumors cause deficits as a function of location. Subdural hematomas, on the other hand, usually do produce deficits by the time headaches occur, since they are located over the cortex. A history of significant head trauma may not be present. The headache of temporal arteritis is usually a temporal region pain and tenderness associated with other signs and symptoms (see rheumatology chapter). Subarachnoid hemorrhages produce the same symptoms as in the younger population, the "thunderclap" headache, with the typical history of the sudden onset of the "worst headache of my life." Meningitis produces headache with fever and usually neck stiffness, although indolent infections such as fungal infections and tuberculosis may not initially cause meningismus.

Evaluation of new-onset headaches, even with a normal neurologic examination, should involve a brain CT scan with contrast, to better identify tumors and subdural hematomas, a lumbar puncture if meningitis is a consideration, an erythrocyte sedimentation rate determination, or sinus x-rays. EEG and MRI are not usually indicated, as the former is of extremely limited sensitivity and the increased cost of MRI over CT is not offset by its greater sensitivity.

LOW BACK PAIN

Low back pain is common in all adults and is mainly of musculoskeletal origin. Neurogenic pain is due to cord or nerve root impingement, which is primarily due to disk or degenerative joint disease. Disk disease is less common in the elderly than in the younger population, because of chemical changes in the disk with aging. The disk develops an increasingly thick calcified perimeter as the nucleus pulposus slowly dehydrates and becomes less viscous. This makes the disk less likely to rupture or deform.

Lumbar stenosis, due to progressive bone growth from arthritis or previous surgery, causes a progressive radiculopathy or "claudication syndrome." The radiculopathies tend to involve more than one nerve root, often on both sides, in contrast to disk disease, which only rarely causes bilateral symptoms and uncommonly involves two or more roots. Back pain is the major symptom, with associated radicular pain, numbness, tingling, weakness, sensory and reflex changes in affected nerve distributions. A high-level stenosis involving the cauda equina, which is usually located at about L1, may cause bladder symptoms as well. High lumbar stenosis may cause a syndrome analogous to leg claudication but is actually due to intermittent compression of the cauda equina, not ischemia. After standing or walking, there is progressive numbness or weakness of one or both legs, sometimes associated with objective changes on neurologic examination, such as diminished reflexes.

While lumbar stenosis can often be managed conservatively, surgery may be necessary and can be tolerated even by the elderly.

VERTIGO AND DIZZINESS

Dizziness is a common symptom often used to connote vertigo, hypotension with near or presyncope, poor concentration, impaired thinking or balance, and many other ill-defined symptoms. It is important to attempt to accurately define the symptom, as hypotension implicates the cardiovascular system and vertigo an inner ear disturbance, whereas poor concentration and impaired thinking could be drug effect, psychomotor seizures, or depression.

Vertigo, the sensation of movement, is an extremely unpleasant sensation. It is a common symptom of the elderly but is rarely of neurologic origin (11). The history usually localizes the problem. The absence of associated brainstem complaints such as diplopia, limb ataxia, weakness, numbness, or dysarthria makes a brain problem unlikely. Gait ataxia is not a useful symptom for distinguishing the locus of the problem, since it occurs with inner ear disturbances (spin yourself around several times to set up a current within your semicircular canals and try to walk) and cerebellar or brainstem dysfunction. Patients with true vertigo feel as if they or the room is spinning or as if they are on a boat. They should have nystagmus when symptomatic (12).

Eighth nerve or labyrinthine induced nystagmus is usually rotary, with the eyes turning clockwise or counterclockwise, and the nystagmus direction usually doesn't change whether looking left or right. Cerebellar nystagmus is horizontal and does change direction with direction of gaze. Central nystagmus may be profound without vertigo, whereas vertigo should always be accompanied by nystagmus. Central vertigo does not abate with repeated head movements; peripheral vertigo does. Central vertigo appears immediately with head movements; peripheral vertigo is delayed by a few seconds.

The importance of distinguishing central (i.e., brainstem) vertigo from eighth nerve or end organ dysfunction lies in the significance of the problem and then the management. A central etiology would point to an ischemic or neoplastic cause and would require a brain MRI for diagnosis, whereas most causes of peripheral vertigo are benign and transient and can be managed with symptomatic therapy such as an antivertiginous medication.

NEUROMUSCULAR DISEASES

It is accepted as normal for the elderly to develop increased thresholds for touch, vibration, and deep pain; diminished ankle jerks; mild orthostatic hypotension; decreased thermal regulation; decreased muscle bulk; and loss of strength. Thus, normal involutional changes of aging mimic neuromuscular diseases, making the recognition of a pathological change difficult.

Diabetes mellitus (DM) is the most common cause of neuropathy, ultimately affecting over 50% of diabetics. It causes primarily a distal sensory-motor and autonomic neuropathy. Most commonly patients experience decreased distal sensation, loss of ankle jerks, and a variable loss of autonomic regulation. With time, over half of diabetic men develop impotence from erectile dysfunction. Weakness from the distal neuropathy occurs only rarely.

DM also causes a variety of less common neuropathic processes. Small fiber neuropathy primarily affects unmyelinated small-diameter nerves that transmit pain and temperature sensation, causing a burning dysesthetic sensation (often with a relative paucity of abnormalities on nerve conduction studies). The syndrome of a mononeuritis multiplex, in which a single large nerve is affected, most commonly affects the femoral nerve, causing proximal leg weakness, loss of the knee jerk, and decreased sensation on the anterior thigh. It also may affect other nerves, including cranial nerves. A diabetic third nerve palsy, with weakness or paralysis of all third nerve functions except for the pupil, causes retroorbital pain, ptosis, and diplopia. Recognition of this "pupil sparing third nerve palsy" precludes the need for an angiogram to exclude an aneurysm. The sixth nerve as well as somatic nerves may be affected, but much less often.

Diabetes also makes nerves more subject to other neuropathic processes, so that diabetics are more prone to Bell's palsy, carpal tunnel syndromes, and other compression neuropathies. Diabetes also causes a syndrome of subacute or acute proximal leg weakness, generally in patients over 50, associated with back pain and weight loss. Since it is often the presenting feature of the DM, it is usually initially attributed to epidural cord compression from metastatic cancer.

Other causes of peripheral neuropathy are considerably less common. Alcoholic and nutritional neuropathies must be considered. Chronic uremia typically causes distal sensory neuropathy. Chronic ischemic neuropathy occurs in over 50% of people with intermittent claudication. Collagen vascular diseases generally cause a mononeuritis multiplex when affecting peripheral nerves but may cause symmetric distal neuropathies. Paraneoplastic syndromes, Guillain Barré; syndrome, and benign monoclonal gammopathies are relatively rare. Hypothyroidism generally causes greater problems outside the peripheral nervous system before it affects the peripheral nerves.

How to approach the elderly patient with a peripheral neuropathy depends on the situation. It is important to evaluate for treatable causes. This should involve a history checking for potential toxins such as megavitamins, chemotherapy agents, and chemical exposures; testing for diabetes, vitamin B12, folate, thyroid functions, and monoclonal gammopathies; and an ESR and ANA to screen for collagen vascular disorders. Electrodiagnostic studies may be helpful for prognosis and occasionally for diagnosis but are often disappointing.

Myopathies are uncommon at all ages but especially in the elderly. Occasionally, mild forms of hereditary myopathies may not be discovered until old age, but most myopathies, other than the inflammatory ones, present in a much younger population. Polymyositis and dermatomyositis are conditions of progressive weakness without apparent cause that occur at all ages and are of most concern. Patients develop progressive weakness, usually more proximal. This may be associated with achiness but often without any complaint to indicate the inflammatory nature of the condition. Diagnosis rests upon the muscle biopsy. About 20% of the polymyositis patients have an associated collagen vascular disorder, and a higher percentage of older patients with dermatomyositis have a malignancy. The other syndromes of progressive muscle weakness of most concern in the elderly are endocrinologic. Hypo- and hyperthyroidism, hyper- and hypoadrenalism, and acromegaly should be considered in older patients with progressive weakness and no evidence of a peripheral neuropathy.

Diseases of neuromuscular function such as myasthenia gravis and Eaton-Lambert syndrome are exceedingly rare and may not be encountered even after years of geriatric practice.

TUMORS

Tumors affect the central or peripheral nervous system. The peripheral nerves are usually affected by compression and only rarely by a paraneoplastic syndrome. The only common primary tumors of nerves are acoustic neuromas and neurofibromas. Tumors affecting the brain are metastatic, primary, or of meningeal origin. Clinically these present as a result of their location and growth rate. Tumors in clinically silent areas will grow large before being recognized. The clinical presentation is slowly progressive neurologic focal dysfunction, headache, weight loss, malaise, and loss of interest, but sometimes with an abrupt neurologic deficit simulating a stroke or a TIA.

Meningiomas are far more common in the elderly than in other age groups and are often seen in as an incidental finding in autopsies or brain scans of the elderly. Since these are usually very slow growing, they can usually be followed via imaging without operation. When they cause dysfunction via compression or seizures, they are surgically removed.

Primary and metastatic brain tumors typically develop in the cerebral hemispheres, with only a minority appearing in the cerebellum or brainstem. Primary tumors are not very responsive to radiation or chemotherapy. While these interventions prolong life while improving quality of life, the choice of treatment must be individualized. Steroids arc helpful if edema is present but should not be used in its absence. While many physicians prescribe anticonvulsants when a brain tumor is diagnosed, there are few data to support this approach. Most neurooncologists recommend anticonvulsants only after a seizure has occurred. This approach should be more firmly adhered to in the elderly, in whom anticonvulsant side effects and drug interactions are more likely to occur and the difficulty of monitoring drug levels is greater. Whether a brain lesion is primary or secondary can only be definitively answered with a biopsy. Brain imaging is often "almost diagnostic," but the clinical situation will determine how important tissue diagnosis is.

Epidural cord compression from metastatic cancer is an extremely important clinical problem, since failure to recognize it will lead to a marked loss in quality of life. Most patients with this problem experience progressive back pain in a single location before neurologic symptoms begin (13). Pain is usually radicular, with numbness or a constricting-band-like sensation around the chest or abdomen. Weakness and numbness develop next, along with urinary retention. In the setting of a known primary cancer, the new development of back pain should trigger concern. About 10 to 15% of patients present with this problem, which can be distinguished from benign compression fractures only with imaging. About 80% of plain x-rays of the spine will show abnormalities suggestive of cancer. The occurrence of epidural cord compression is one of the few neurologic emergencies and should be treated with high-dose steroids before definitive diagnosis if the deficit is progressing. MRI or myelography are the tests of choice. Treatment is usually nonsurgical, with radiation and steroids. Surgery is reserved for radiation treatment failures, those with an unknown diagnosis, and possibly those with rapidly progressive loss of neurologic function.

NEUROLOGICAL TESTING

There is no doubt that neurologic tests are overordered and that the changing financial climate of health care will soon limit this. It is crucial to understand what results a test might provide before ordering it. Brain MRI is more sensitive for identifying structural brain lesions than CT but is considerably more expensive. It is most useful for identifying lesions in the posterior fossa (brainstem and cerebellum) where bone artifact reduces the utility of CT. It is also helpful for identifying small lesions, such as pituitary region tumors and multiple small infarcts. Identifying small infarcts may be helpful in assessing patients for shunting for NPH where large ventricles may occur secondary to brain volume loss, in which case shunting won't help. For identifying tumors, MRI with gadolinium enhancement surpasses CT with contrast, but unless a clinical decision rests entirely on the best imaging study possible, CT is usually adequate. MRI is helpful in visualizing demyelination, but this is rare in the elderly aside from AIDS. Brain MRI is important in assessing neurologic sequelae of AIDS, where HIV encephalopathy and progressive multifocal leukoencephalopathy are seen on MRI but not CT.

CT is helpful in assessing presumed strokes for two reasons: (a) to rule out alternative structural etiologies such as neoplasms, which can mimic strokes or TIA and (b) to evaluate for hemorrhage, which will guide a decision for potential anticoagulation. Usually there is no need for a second CT scan, even if the first was obtained before the infarct appeared on the scan, other than to document the location and size of the stroke, establishing a baseline for the future.

EEG is useful for seizure evaluation, especially when the diagnosis is unclear, and should always be obtained if seizure medications are to be discontinued after a remission. An EEG with epileptiform activity should be cause for reassessing the decision to halt therapy. The EEG is not helpful in the assessment of headache or dizzy spells, and its use should be discouraged because unrelated abnormalities are often detected, leading to further unwarranted studies. EEG is helpful in diagnosing brain death and may be useful for prognosis in coma assessment.

Spinal fluid analysis is mandatory for evaluation of meningitis and encephalitis before antibiotics are started. For patients without focal deficits or other evidence to suggest a possible brain abscess, a lumbar puncture (LP) should not be significantly delayed for a brain imaging study. CSF should also be obtained for evaluation of subarachnoid hemorrhage if the brain CT is negative, which occurs in about 10% of cases.

Myelography has been largely supplanted by MRI but may be required when an MRI will cause unacceptable delay in treatment, when the problem cannot be localized to a particular region, or when spinal fluid and an imaging study are both required, as may occur with carcinomatous meningitis. Occasionally it may be desirable to instill oil-based myelogram dye, which never is absorbed, to follow the response of epidural metastases to radiation treatment.

Evoked potentials are measures of brain or brainstem responses to peripheral stimulation. Brainstem auditory evoked responses test the hearing pathway and are helpful in the evaluation of brainstem auditory pathways. Since conduction above the acoustic nucleus requires a response here, deafness precludes testing. Vestibular nerve dysfunction will have no effect on this test. Somatosensory evoked potentials test sensory pathways and may be useful for evaluating spinal cord function. Visual evoked responses primarily test the optic nerve, which is only rarely affected in the elderly.

Nerve conduction studies test nerve function in superficial motor and sensory nerves and are useful for evaluating peripheral neuropathies. Small, brief electrical shocks are applied to the skin over a nerve, and a response is measured in a muscle or over a sensory nerve. The electromyogram (EMG) involves recording electrical activity from a needle electrode inserted into a muscle. It is used to evaluate denervation and myopathy. Although EMG can distinguish acute and chronic conditions, it cannot distinguish causes. This is the job of the electromyographer, who chooses which muscles to test to make a diagnosis. F and H waves are electrical stimulation tests that assess electrical reflexes and thus test the sensory and motor nerve proximal to the stimulus. These are particular useful in the early diagnosis of Guillain-Barré syndrome.

Isotope cisternography is still used by some for the evaluation of NPH but is of no proven benefit. Nuclear brain scan has occasionally been used to help diagnose herpes simplex encephalitis when the brain CT is negative, but MRI is undoubtedly a more sensitive test.

Duplex carotid ultrasonography is helpful in evaluating extracranial carotid disease, producing both a flow velocity curve and an image of the blood vessels. In centers where duplex studies are reliable, they can be used to screen for stenosis in patients with carotid territory ischemic events. Transcranial Doppler studies can be performed to assess flow in the major vessels in the circle of Willis but cannot produce an image. Transcranial Doppler studies are used in assessing the vertebrobasilar system.

Angiography is used to assess the carotid before endarterectomy and to show aneurysms following subarachnoid hemorrhage. MRI angiograms (MRA), which do not require arterial dye, have improved in quality in recent years and may soon replace standard arteriograms. The utility of MRA varies with the center at which the test is performed.

Single positron emission tomography (SPECT) is a nuclear technique that illustrates blood flow to regions of the brain. Labeled isotopes have been developed to illustrate neurotransmitter receptor changes as well. SPECT scans are of some value in evaluating ischemic disease, Alzheimer's disease, and a few other neurodegenerative disorders, but they should not be considered routine at this time (14).

Positron emission tomography (PET) scanning is still primarily a research technique. Using radioactive isotopes one can determine blood flow and metabolic, neurotransmitter, and neurotransmitter receptor status. It is currently useful in localizing epileptic foci before surgery and in the evaluation of ischemia. It may also prove useful in the evaluation of neurodegenerative diseases.

REFERENCES

1. Potvin AR, Syndulko K, Tourtellotte WW, Lemon JA, Potvin JH. Human neurologic function and the aging process. J Am Geriatr Soc 1980;28:1–9.
2. Critchley M. Neurologic changes in the aged. J Chronic Dis 1956;3:459–477.
3. Biller J, ed. Cerebrovascular disorders in the 1990's. Clinics in Geriatric Medicine 1991;7(3). Philadelphia: WB Saunders, 1991.
4. Petrovitch H, Vogt TM, Berg KG. Isolated systolic hypertension: lowering the risk of stroke in older patients. Geriatrics 1992;47:30–38.
5. Dyken ML, Barnett HJM, Easton JD, Fields WS, et al. Low-dose aspirin and stroke. "It ain't necessarily so." Stroke 1992;23:1395–1399.
6. Hauser WA. Seizure disorders: the changes with age. Epilepsia 1992;33(suppl 4):S6–S14.
7. Hoefnagels WAJ, Padberg GW, Overweg J, et al. Syncope or seizure? The diagnostic value of the EEG and hyperventilation test in transient loss of consciousness. J Neurol Neurosurg Psychiatry 1991; 54:953–956.
8. Van Doselaar CA, Geerts AT, Schimsheimer RJ. Idiopathic first seizure in adult life: who should be treated? Br Med J 1991;302:620–623.
9. Sudarsky L. Geriatrics: gait disorders in the elderly. N Engl J Med 1990;322:1441–1446.
10. Vanneste J, Augustijn P, Dirvin C, Tan WF, Goedhart ZD. Shunting normal pressure hydrocephalus: do the benefits outweigh the risks? A multicenter study and literature review. Neurology 1992;42:54–59.
11. Kroenke K, Lucas CA, Rosenberg ML, et al. Causes of persistent dizziness. A prospective study of 100 patients in ambulatory care. Ann Intern Med 1992;117:898–904.
12. Drachman DA, Hart CW. An approach to the dizzy patient. Neurology 1972;22:323–334.
13. Byrne TN, Waxman SG. Spinal cord compression. Philadelphia: FA Davis, 1990.
14. Devous MD. Comparison of SPECT applications in neurology and psychiatry. J Clin Psychiatry 1992;53(ll suppl):13–19.

19/ Rehabilitation and the Aged

Gregg A. Warshaw, John B. Murphy

The philosophy, clinical approach, and therapeutic interventions of rehabilitation medicine can be of benefit to many older adults. Those recovering from an acute illness and/or having chronic illness are at risk of developing disabilities and functional loss. Eighty-six percent of adults over age 65 have at least one chronic condition, and 53% of those over age 75 are limited in at least one activity of daily living (ADL) (1).

Rehabilitation is an approach to care provided by a team of professionals. Although physicians specializing in physical medicine and rehabilitation, physical therapists, and occupational therapists are most closely identified with rehabilitation practice, the rehabilitation approach is applicable to older patients being cared for by geriatricians, primary care physicians, orthopaedists, neurologists, nurses, psychologists, social workers, and most other health care professionals. Principles of successful rehabilitation include

- A comprehensive approach that incorporates physical, emotional, and social parameters in the care process.
- A team effort that is multidisciplinary in membership and interdisciplinary in process.
- A continuous and ongoing intervention that is not time limited.
- A focus on function, whether it be lost function that may be restored (restorative therapy) or remaining function that needs to be modified and strengthened to accommodate other disability (maintenance therapy) (2).

A useful model of disease progression and functional loss has been promulgated by the World Health Organization. When a disease becomes symptomatic at the organ level, the individual is aware of an *impairment*. Examples of impairments include sensory loss, muscle weakness, and joint pain. *Disabilities* are the functional consequences of impairments. Examples of disabilities include difficulty walking and the inability to perform personal care. A disadvantage resulting from a disability is a *handicap*. A handicap limits or prevents the fulfillment of a role that is normal for the affected individual. The nature and severity of a handicap are determined by the interaction of the adaptation of the person to the social and environmental surroundings and the adjustments made by society to accommodate the impaired individual. Buildings or public transportation inaccessible to a person in a wheelchair may result in a handicap (1, 3). Whereas in the traditional medical model physicians are trained to interact at the level of disease, rehabilitation occurs at all levels (disease, impairment, disability, and handicap).

Although rehabilitation medicine offers hope of reducing disability and handicap among older adults, research in this area is limited (1). A few studies have documented the benefits of inpatient assessment and rehabilitation (4, 5) and the application of geriatric and rehabilitation principles to specific clinical problems (6–8). These studies need replication in other settings and with a broader range of patients.

In this chapter we review the rehabilitation process and the use of teams, the settings in which rehabilitation can occur, and the prescription of assistive devices. We also discuss specific approaches to stroke, hip fracture, Parkinson's disease, arthritis, and amputation, as well as the role of the primary care physician in the rehabilitation process.

ASSESSMENT

Rehabilitation focuses on restoring and maintaining functional ability; thus, assessment of the patient must be functionally oriented. The optimal process is interdisciplinary, involves all disciplines relevant to a particular case; identifies not just disease, but impairments, disabilities, and handicaps; involves physical, mental, and social spheres; and results in the establishment of objective goals. The assessment and goal-setting processes need to be individualized, capitalize on the patient's strengths and abilities, and be designed to restore or make adaptive changes to foster independence. The family and social network should be involved, and assessment should be ongoing, not static, with goals regularly reassessed.

In a given case, all rehabilitation disciplines involved will have a discipline-specific focus to their portion of the comprehensive assessment. The physician's physical assessment should include the traditional medical history and physical as well as a functional assessment of ADLs, Instrumental ADLs (IADLs), and mobility. Observing the patient perform functional tasks such as eating, dressing, putting on glasses, and combing hair will help identify diseases, impairments, disabilities, and handicaps not previously recognized. A patient's apraxia, hemineglect, or visual field cut, which may have been missed by a standard examination, will become apparent in the functional assessment. The patient's problem list should include functional (e.g., incontinence, impaired mobility) as well as traditional medical problems, and the rehabilitation team should address each problem. Also, sexual function should not be overlooked as part of the rehabilitation assessment and program for the older patient.

Sensory impairments, very common among older persons, have an impact on all aspects of the rehabilitation process. Unfortunately, even moderate and severe impairments can go unrecognized or untreated. Early identification of such impairments is particularly important because obtaining a hearing aid, low-vision aid, or glasses may take time, and the absence of such assistive devices may slow or preclude progress in a rehabilitation program.

The assessment of mental function should cover both psychological and cognitive function. In assessing mood, the clinician should have a high index of suspicion for depression, common and very treatable among rehabilitation populations. Cognitive function is particularly important with the older patient, as the prevalence of dementia rises dramatically with age (9, 10). Standard mental status tests such as the Mini-Mental State Examination (MMSE) (11) or more lengthy and sensitive measures are essential components of the comprehensive rehabilitative assessment. A patient's cognitive ability influences all aspects of rehabilitation including eligibility, choice of setting, assessment, goal setting, therapeutic interventions, and outcome. Although some persons with severe dementia may not be candidates for rehabilitation, many cognitively impaired individuals and their families benefit greatly from the rehabilitation process. Thus, cognitive impairments

per se are not necessarily a reason to exclude a patient from rehabilitation.

An older person's family and social network are essential in the design and implementation of a rehabilitation program. Care should be taken to realistically assess the strengths and weaknesses of the patient's social network. Financial resources must also be assessed, because the availability of family and friends as well as paid home health care workers will greatly influence the rehabilitation goals and outcomes.

REHABILITATION SETTINGS

Rehabilitation can occur in a variety of settings and can range from care provided by a single discipline to that offered by many disciplines. When more than one discipline is involved, care can be provided in both multidisciplinary and interdisciplinary models. The site and number of disciplines involved depend upon the needs and resources of the patient. An interdisciplinary model is preferred in all but the most straightforward cases. Table 19.1 outlines the range of settings where rehabilitation is provided as well as general criteria for patients cared for in the respective settings. Table 19.2 lists and briefly describes the roles of various rehabilitation professionals.

Acute inpatient hospital rehabilitation generally requires that a patient tolerate and need 3 or more hours of therapy per day and that the patient would benefit from involvement of two or more rehabilitation disciplines (e.g., physical therapy and occupational therapy). This "3-hour rule" is just a guideline that has been used by many intermediaries as a proxy for the complexity of the case, and it is not an absolute necessity. The acute hospital rehabilitation setting is the ideal and most intensive setting for the most medically complex patients. However, the older deconditioned patient may not tolerate such intensive therapy, and a skilled nursing facility (SNF) or home-care program may be more appropriate in some cases.

The classic example of a patient ideally suited for an SNF is the individual recovering from a hip fracture who needs skilled physical therapy on a daily basis but does not need additional rehabilitation disciplines. Patients with more complex needs requiring multiple rehabilitation disciplines and interdisciplinary care who cannot tolerate the intensity of an inpatient program can also be served in an SNF. Care provided in an SNF does not preclude return to an acute hospital setting when the patient can tolerate 3 hours of therapy a day.

Table 19.1
Rehabilitation Settings and Characteristics

Settings	Characteristics
Acute inpatient hospital (Hospital unit or freestanding hospital)	• Requires 2 or more disciplines • Generally 3 hours of therapy/day • Medicare coverage same as for other types of acute hospitalization
Skilled nursing facility (SNF)	• Skilled therapy 5 times/week • Less than 3 hours per day • One or more disciplines • Medicare covers 20 days in full, and days 21–100 partially
Home care program	• Patient must be homebound • Single or multiple therapies • Limited Medicare coverage • Adequate social supports required
Outpatient Comprehensive outpatient rehabilitation facility (CORF)	• Complexity requires an interdisciplinary process • Multiple disciplines involved • Adequate social resources required • Limited Medicare coverage
Individual therapies	• Limited number of disciplines • Less complex cases • Adequate social resources required • Limited Medicare coverage

Table 19.2
Rehabilitation Professionals

Professional	Role
Physiatry (Physical Medicine–trained MD)	Evaluates patient, integrates assessment data, determines potential, coordinates rehabilitation plan
Primary care physician	Manages acute and chronic medical care
Rehabilitation nurse	Integrates medical, nursing, rehabilitation plan
Physical therapist	Addresses mobility, strength, range of motion
Occupational therapist	Addresses activities of daily living and self care
Speech pathologist	Addresses communication, swallowing
Psychologist and neuropsychologist	Diagnosis/treatment of mood, behavioral and cognitive conditions
Social worker	Works with family, patient, financial counseling, discharge planning
Nutritionist	Assess nutrition status, diet plan
Pharmacist	Reviews medication use
Audiologist	Provides hearing assessment and treatment
Vocational counselor	Evaluates work potential, provides training
Recreational therapist	Assists with hobbies, leisure activities, motivation
Orthotist/prosthetist	Makes and fits orthopaedic aids

Home care programs are best suited to individuals who have adequate social resources and are medically stable. The unavailability of cumbersome equipment (e.g., whirlpool, tilt table) in the home can be a limiting factor, however. Reimbursement for home treatment may also require that the patient be "homebound."

In the outpatient setting, a Comprehensive Outpatient Rehabilitation Facility (CORF) is ideal for providing care to the patient who requires multiple disciplines and an interdisciplinary team process. Obviously social support and transportation resources need to be sufficient to allow daily travel to the CORF and to provide a safe home environment. Individual therapies provided on an outpatient basis are the appropriate alternative when a single discipline is all that is required.

Medicare covers acute hospital inpatient rehabilitation (as it does for any other medical problem). However, many primary private health insurance programs have significant limitations and require preauthorization for rehabilitation services. Medicare covers SNF care fully for 20 days and partially for days 21 to 100. Most supplemental insurance policies pick up a portion of the deductible but do not extend coverage beyond 100 days. Home care programs requiring skilled therapies are covered by Medicare for a limited duration. CORF programs and individual therapies on an outpatient basis are also covered by Medicare, with a limit on the total dollar amount of therapy that can be provided per incident or illness.

ASSISTIVE DEVICES

Assistive devices are used to relieve pain and maintain or restore function. Patients with functional losses who perceive a need for an assistive device need help choosing appropriate equipment. Assistive devices that address problems with hearing, vision, mobility, and most ADLs and IADLs are available. Most require patient education and training for proper use. Physical and occupational therapists can assist the physician, patient, and family in the selection and proper use of available products. Table 19.3 is a brief summary of selected assistive devices.

Deciding which is the most appropriate device and teaching the patient its appropriate use are probably beyond the scope of the average primary care physician. However, many older persons use canes for which they were never appropriately evaluated, and as many as 75% may be using the wrong type of cane, using a cane in ill repair, using the device improperly, or using an improperly sized device. Thus, the primary care physician who sees a patient with a cane should ascertain that it is in good repair (rubber tip, no cracks, etc.), that it is the right size (height of greater trochanter), and that the patient uses it properly (e.g., for osteoarthritis, that the patient advances cane at the same time as the affected hip but holds the cane on the contralateral side).

STROKE

The rehabilitation of stroke patients is an enormous challenge because the condition is common and the functional consequences are often serious. About 25% of stroke sufferers die by 1 month poststroke, and 40% are dead by 1 year (16). Survivors with cerebral infarction show some improvement at 2 to 3 weeks when the cerebral edema has resolved. In general, 50% of expected functional recovery occurs by 1 month, 75% at 3 months, 90% at 6 months, and nearly 100% at 1 year (17). Overall, 80% of survivors will attain independent ambulation, and two-thirds become independent in ADLs (18).

The rehabilitation approach to the older stroke patient may be supportive, preventing complications while spontaneous recovery occurs, or more active, involving intensive rehabilitation therapy. The effectiveness of aggressive stroke rehabilitation therapy and its relative contribution to recovery of function, compared with spontaneous recovery, is controversial. It is also unclear whether intensive rehabilitation is most beneficial immediately poststroke or at 2 to 4 weeks after the initial event when spontaneous recovery may allow for more intensive therapy.

The clinical approach to stroke is usually divided into three phases: acute (admission to 48 hours), subacute (48 hours to 3 months), and chronic (3 months and after). During the acute phase, the patient is stabilized, and a functional assessment is initiated. Management of the acute phase of stroke is discussed in Chapter 18.

After stroke patients are stabilized, it is helpful to identify those with the best chance of benefiting from intensive rehabilitation. Although a number of negative prognostic indicators have been identified (Table 19.4), early prognostication is unreliable for the individual patient. Older age has not been shown to be an independent predictor of poor outcome, although many older stroke patients also have comorbidities that can affect recovery.

Rehabilitation treatment for the stroke patient derives from an ongoing team assessment. The physical therapist's focus is on strength, endurance, and mobility. Motor recovery frequently follows a predictable sequence: initial flaccid paralysis, then flexor pattern synergy (flexion with movement), then extensor pattern synergy, then flexor selection, and lastly, extensor selection. Although this sequence can vary from case to case, it is helpful to recognize that certain patterns can be capitalized on to assist with particular activities (e.g., extensor synergy and walking) (12). Treatment begins with bed mobility and progresses to balance training and sitting. Ambulation requires adequate strength and trunk stability. Patients with severe impairments may begin walking in parallel bars and then be advanced to walkers or canes. If weakness in the lower leg is present, an ankle-foot orthosis (short leg brace) can promote more efficient ambulation by insuring fixed dorsiflexion at the ankle and minimizing toe dragging in the swing phase of gait.

The occupational therapist addresses upper extremity function and the ability to perform ADLs, IADLs, and visual spatial perception deficits. Maintenance of range of motion in the affected upper extremity is essential to avoid the

Table 19.3
Selected Assistive Devices

Functional Problem	Device	Comments
Bathing	"Soap on a rope" Long-handled back sponge Tub seat or bench Grab bars Hand-held shower hose	• Will help when reaching is impaired; these aids require adequate grip strength and range of motion • Allows for safe sitting in the bathtub; reducing the risk of falls during transfers is crucial; tub transfer bench bridges the tub side with two legs in the tub and two legs beside the tub
Toileting	Raised toilet seat Versa frames Bedside commode	• Toilet seat should be 20 inches from the floor; handrails can be attached to the wall or a free-standing frame can be used
Oral Care	Tooth brush grip	
Dressing	Reaching devices (Fig. 19.1) Long shoe horns Button hooks (Fig. 19.1) Sock donners Velcro closures Elastic shoe laces Clothes hook (Fig. 19.3)	• Aids in picking things off the floor • Helps with hand weakness or loss of agility; sock aid helps if hip flexion is limited; Velcro substitutes for buttons or shoelaces • Aids in dressing
Grooming	Electric razor Tilt mirror Built-up grips on handles	
Eating	Built up grips High-edged plates and nonskid pads Rocker knives Cups with lid	• Grips help with arthritis or decreased strength • Keeps food on plate and plate on table • Allows one-handed food cutting • Useful for spilling that occurs with intention tremor
Mobility Orthoses	Foot Ankle-foot (AFO) Knee-ankle-foot (KAFO)	• Modified shoes and lifts • Plastic shell or metal brace used for mild limb weakness (foot drop) after stroke; aids weight bearing or alignment • Aids knee support; with or without hinge
Canes	Hemicane or hemiwalker Tri or quad cane Standard cane	• A four-point frame that provides considerable support to the hemiplegic patient; all canes held on the side opposite involved leg • More support than single-point cane; come with wide or narrow base • Pistol grip is best; with tip positioned on ground; elbow is flexed 25°
Walkers	Standard Roller	• Rubber tips; need to lift when moving; helps with weakness or imbalance if grip strength is poor, but can be fitted with platform grip attached to forearm, proximal strength is adequate • Front, three- or four-wheel models; can have brakes and cargo baskets; provides help with balance, but less support than standard walker; can help patients with Parkinson's disease, unstable gait, or person with limited cardiorespiratory reserve for whom lifting would intolerably increase work (e.g., COPD, CHF)
Wheelchairs	Standard Powered	• Provided if limited endurance or inability to walk; need to be carefully fitted: seat width, arm height, seat cushion, foot rests; folding models available • Expensive, require physiatry input
Scooter		• A three-wheeled electric scooter can help with mobility over long distances

[a]Adapted from Erickson RV. Principles of rehabilitation. In: Beck JC, ed. Geriatric review syllabus. New York: American Geriatrics Society, 1991:73–88.

Table 19.4
Predictors of Poor Functional Outcome after Stroke[a]

Preexisting or new impairment in cognitive function
History of a previous stroke
Coexistent symptomatic cardiovascular disease
Large lesion on computed tomography
Initial coma
Perceptual-spatial deficit
Aphasia
Neglect or denial syndrome
Impaired proprioception
Multiple neurologic deficits
Incontinence 2 weeks after stroke
No motor return 1 month after stroke

[a]Modified from Kemp B, Brummel-Smith K, Ramsdel S. Geriatric rehabilitation. Boston: College-Hill Press, 1990.

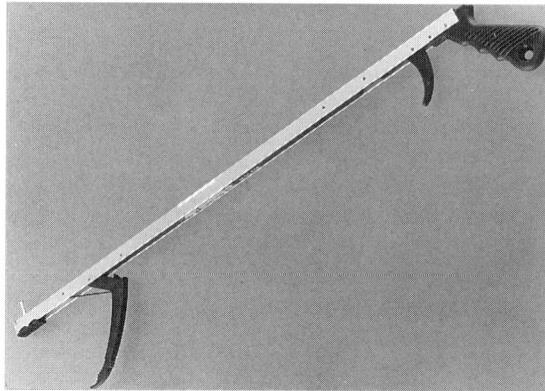

Figure 19.1. Reacher. Used to pick up objects from the floor when hip flexion is limited.

development of a painful shoulder or contractures. When distal upper extremity spasm is present, wrist splints are prescribed. To avoid shoulder subluxation, transfers are managed without additional stress on the shoulder joint, and pillows and arm boards are used to support the affected arm. These positioning techniques maintain the humeral head in its proper position when the muscles usually responsible for this alignment are flaccid. Dressing aids, such as clothes reachers, button hooks, sock donners, and Velcro closures may be prescribed (Figs. 19.1–19.3). Feeding aids, such as rocker knives and plate guards, can be helpful.

Impairment of language function can be the most frustrating consequence of stroke. Dysarthria and aphasia require assessment by a speech pathologist. Communication boards can be provided to help patients with expressive aphasia make their wishes known. The speech pathologist can also help rehabilitation team members communicate with the patient.

A number of complications may interfere with functional recovery from stroke (Table 19.5). Identification and aggressive treatment of these potential problems is important during both active rehabilitation and maintenance therapy. For example, a shoulder-hand syndrome (reflex sympathetic dystrophy) can result in severe pain-poststroke. Early therapy can reduce the risk for, and impact of, this syndrome. Adequate range of motion of the shoulder joint, isometric muscle exercises, and elevation to reduce edema can help. If the syndrome progresses, oral steroids and stellate anesthetic blocks may help relieve the pain.

Clinical depression occurs in as many as 60% of stroke patients, and if unrecognized and un-

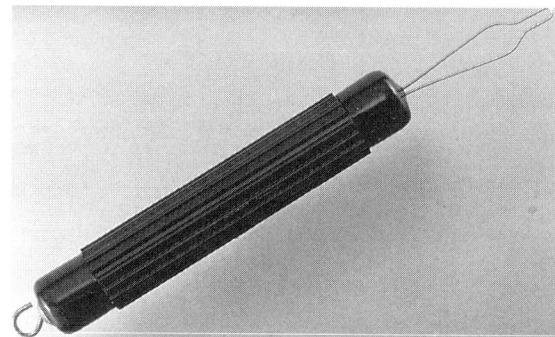

Figure 19.2. Button hook. Allows a person with decreased manual dexterity or strength to button clothing.

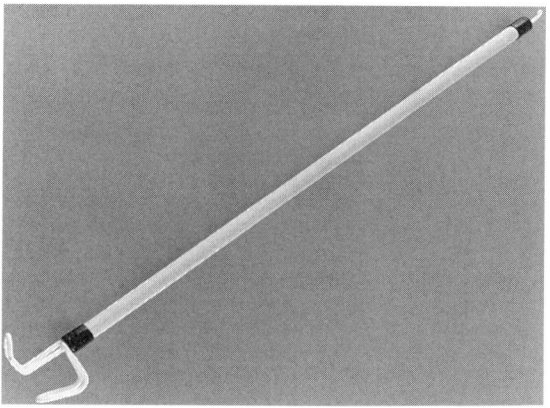

Figure 19.3. Clothes hook. Used to unhook Velcro straps, pull off socks, or a variety of other actions.

Table 19.5
Poststroke Complications That May Impair
Functional Recovery[a]

Medication toxicity
Sensory deprivation syndrome
Cognitive impairment
Depression
Aphasia
Dysphagia
Spasticity
Contractures
Shoulder problems
Pressure sores
Urinary incontinence
Constipation and fecal incontinence
Peripheral nerve palsies
Poor adjustment to disability
Caregiver withdrawal or burnout

[a]Modified from Kemp B, Brummel-Smith K, Ramsdel S. Geriatric rehabilitation. Boston: College-Hill Press, 1990.

treated, it can interfere with rehabilitation. Dysphagia is common and can result in aspiration, malnutrition, and dehydration. The speech pathologist working with nursing and nutrition staff can often prevent complications by designing an appropriate plan for feeding.

HIP FRACTURE

Two-hundred and fifty-thousand hip fractures occur each year in the United States, and the incidence of femoral neck fractures is rising by about 40% per decade (19). During the year following the fracture, 20% of patients spend time in a nursing home, and 10 to 20% die. Postoperative care and rehabilitation can affect outcome (8). Mental status and the patient's prefracture functional status are also important predictors of functional recovery. Rapid return to ambulation (by 2 weeks) is another good predictor of successful outcome. During the past decade, reimbursement from Medicare and other payers has shifted the location of hip fracture rehabilitation from the hospital to the outpatient, nursing home, and home settings (20).

Hip fractures are classified into three major categories according to anatomic location: femoral neck (subcapital or intracapsular), intertrochanteric, and subtrochanteric. Femoral neck fractures place the blood supply to the femoral head at risk, resulting in a higher incidence of avascular necrosis. Intertrochanteric fractures usually unite, but they are associated with significant blood loss and more early complications than femoral neck fractures. Subtrochanteric fractures are less common in the older patient, result from very significant force, and are more difficult to repair.

The fracture site and the surgical technique chosen for repair greatly affect the course of rehabilitation. In the older patient, a stable repair that allows for early weightbearing is crucial to avoid postoperative complications and deconditioning. Occult or impacted femoral neck fractures can be treated with internal fixation with multiple pins, leading to early ambulation. In most older patients with displaced femoral neck fractures, prosthetic replacement is the best option, reducing the risk of necrosis of the femoral head and nonunion and allowing for immediate weightbearing. Although intertrochanteric fractures can be treated with traction for 4 to 8 weeks, operative repair with a compression screw and plate allows for early weightbearing with a walker.

Avoidance of medical complications in the immediate postoperative period is imperative. Warfarin therapy reduces the occurrence of deep venous thrombosis (10 mg before surgery, 5 mg evening after surgery). Attention to removing bladder catheters quickly postoperatively will help avoid urinary tract infections. Adequate skin care requires exemplary nursing care. A 4-inch or better egg-crate mattress is required, and heel protectors may be helpful. Sedative drugs should be avoided, and analgesics should be monitored closely.

Most orthopaedic surgeons recommend specific weightbearing (WB) orders for hip fracture patients. These can include non-WB, touch down WB (10 to 15% body weight on limb), partial WB (30%), 50% WB, and full WB (75 to 100%). There is considerable controversy in orthopedic medicine concerning the rate of progression of the degree of weightbearing versus fracture healing (19). Many surgeons are quite cautious with older patients, which can result in unnecessary delay in postoperative mobilization. Partial weightbearing is also very difficult for some older patients to implement, leaving the physical therapist withholding treatment while awaiting more liberal orders from the attending surgeon. The older patient with a preexisting cognitive deficit may be unable to participate in any therapy that involves degrees of weightbearing. They may not be able to learn or remember to apply less than full weight. Thus, it is important to choose an operative repair that allows the earliest possible full weightbearing in this population.

PARKINSON'S DISEASE

Parkinson's disease (PD) is a chronic progressive disorder that is uncommon before age 50 and has an increasing incidence through the eighth decade. Rehabilitation has not been shown to retard the progression of the illness. However, rehabilitation efforts can lessen the impact of the illness by helping an individual maximize functional abilities and maintain independent function for as long as possible (23, 24). Therapy can usually be provided in the outpatient setting and should begin early in the course of the illness. Unfortunately, pharmacologic interventions are usually emphasized, and physical interventions are often overlooked. Physical and occupational therapists as well as speech pathologists should be consulted early in the course of the illness.

The physical therapist should focus on body alignment, gait, strength, and range of motion (ROM) exercises, as well as transferring. Patients should be taught to look up and consciously lift their toes during the swing phase of gait. Their feet should be wide apart (12 to 15 inches), and they should concentrate on lengthening their step. A program of regular exercises can improve or maintain strength and range of motion as well as prevent contractures. Group exercise programs can also help prevent the social isolation common in patients with Parkinson's disease. The patient should avoid rubber-soled shoes, which tend to stick when the patient walks, and canes, which are difficult for the person with a typical parkinsonian posture. When a PD patient needs a walker, it should have front wheels. A pickup walker is inappropriate for a person who has difficulty initiating motions (such as repeatedly picking up the walker) and the person with retropulsion, where the motion of picking up a walker may cause backward falling.

The occupational therapist can enhance the patient's independence in performing ADLs. To simplify dressing routines it can be helpful to use Velcro closures or zippers and over-the-head shirt rather than buttons. Slip-on shoes with elastic shoelaces can also be helpful. Adaptive equipment can be used to assist with eating. If the patient is poorly coordinated, large-rimmed dishes or plate guards as well as weighted plates and cups can help minimize handicap. Environmental aids such as grab rails in the bathtub and near the toilet, a raised toilet seat, and raising the back legs of chairs by 1 to 3 inches to facilitate rising from a chair are also helpful.

The speech pathologist can help with communication and swallowing. Hypokinetic dysarthria is common in PD, and therapeutic efforts designed to improve respiration by teaching the patient diaphragmatic breathing exercises can improve the volume of sound and the number of words spoken per breath. The prevalence and type of swallowing disorders associated with PD varies. Nonetheless, individualized swallowing and stimulation techniques taught by a speech pathologist may be beneficial.

Hospitalization for intercurrent illnesses poses a particular risk for PD patients. Emphasis should be placed on avoiding bed rest while continuing exercise programs during hospitalization. Should hospitalization or an intercurrent illness result in a significant decline in functional status, treatment in an acute hospital or SNF-level rehabilitation unit may be necessary.

ARTHRITIS

The goals of therapy for any arthritic condition are to improve or maintain functional ability and relieve or minimize pain. Physical therapies address both goals and should begin early in the course of a symptomatic disease. Nonpharmacologic interventions need to be individualized to the specific patient, the specific arthritic condition, and the stage of the disease. Rheumatologic conditions are dynamic, and thus periodic monitoring and reevaluation are necessary to adjust treatment as the condition progresses. Therapeutic interventions include rest, exercise, orthotics, assistive devices, and heat and cold modalities as well as patient and family education.

Local rest of inflamed joints reduces pain and inflammation and may prevent contracture (25). Short rest periods to interrupt daily activities lasting more than 30 minutes (energy conservation program) have been shown to increase physical activity level in patients with rheumatoid arthritis (RA) (26). Systemic rest should be reserved for times when the patient with RA has multiple inflamed joints and fails to respond to conventional pharmacologic and nonpharmacologic interventions. It may also be of benefit to patients with polymyalgia rheumatica (PMR) during the acute phase of their illness. However, systemic rest can lead to deconditioning and should be used cautiously.

Exercise programs for patients with arthritis can increase or maintain ROM, strengthen muscles, increase endurance, and improve the biomechanical function of joints (25). Exercise programs should take into account the degree of joint inflammation or effusion, the condition of surrounding muscle, the patient's overall endurance, mechanical derangement of the joint, and other comorbid illnesses.

Therapeutic heat and cold modalities have been used to provide relief of pain and promote increased range of joint motion. However, no controlled trials in the use of these modalities have been conducted (27). The use of cold seems most appropriate for the acutely inflamed joint. Cold can decrease pain and cause relaxation of surrounding spastic muscles. Later, in the subacute period when inflammatory pain is subsiding and stiffness is present, either cold or superficial heat may be appropriate.

Splints and orthotics are used to unweight joints, stabilize joints, decrease joint motion, or support joints in a position of maximal function and to increase joint motion (i.e., dynamic splint). Orthotics for the upper extremity are mainly confined to the wrist and hand and include resting splints, functional wrist splints, thumb post splints, ring splints, and dynamic splints. They are most commonly used in RA and carpal tunnel syndrome. Orthotics of the lower extremity are most useful for the foot and ankle and much less so for the knee. Shoes with a wide toe box can be used for the wide forefoot, cock toes, and hallux valgus deformity seen in RA and osteoarthritis (OA).

OA, the most common type of arthritis found in older individuals, can result in significant pain and disability. The hip, knee, foot, and carpal carpometacarpal joint are frequently involved joints that can result in disability. Given the joints commonly affected and OA's primarily noninflammatory nature, rehabilitation of OA patients is somewhat different than that of RA patients.

Hip OA rehabilitation management involves relieving weightbearing stress by use of an appropriate assistive device (e.g., cane), stretching exercises to maintain ROM, and strengthening hip musculature. Jogging can cause undue joint stress and should generally be avoided, whereas swimming is an optimal exercise. Bicycling is also acceptable. Unilateral hip disease has a high association with increased leg length on the affected side, and a lift for the opposite shoe is indicated if there is more than a 1/4-inch length discrepancy.

OA of the knee can result in restricted ROM, contractures of the joint capsule and hamstring, an unstable joint, and valgus or varus deformity. Patients should avoid using a pillow under the knee at night because this encourages knee and hip flexion contractures. A functionally important goal is to maintain knee extension, because more than a 10° flexion contracture results in less than optimal knee biomechanics and increases stress with weightbearing. For strengthening, non-weightbearing quadriceps isometric exercises should be done twice daily by patients with OA of the knee. This is particularly important for the

patient with OA who is hospitalized with an intercurrent illness. Rising from a toilet or chair that is too low can increase joint stress and should be avoided by using appropriate height chairs and raised toilet seats.

OA commonly results in hallux valgus with or without bunions, hallux rigidus with cocked toes, metatarsal head calluses, and abrasions on the dorsum of the toes. Thus, a properly fitting wide toe box shoe is essential.

The carpometacarpal joint is frequently affected by OA. Using a thumb post splint to immobilize the thumb in a functionally abducted position relieves pain and allows performance of functional activities.

Strengthening exercises are also important in the rehabilitation management of RA, but care must be taken to avoid aggravating the inflamed joint. Brief isometric exercises performed with joints in the least painful posture (usually mid-joint range) can allow for strengthening with the least harm. A 6-second maximal contraction twice daily for each muscle group is adequate to maintain strength (26). Progressive ROM exercises can be used to maintain or regain ROM in the patient with RA. However, care must be taken to avoid aggravating inflamed joints, and it must be recognized that once subluxation or dislocation has occurred no exercises will restore alignment.

When pharmacologic and nonpharmacologic interventions fail to relieve pain or restore function, surgery should be considered for OA of the hip and knee, and to a lesser extent, for RA. Rehabilitation can enhance the outcome of surgery in many situations, and the involvement of the appropriate rehabilitation professionals should occur early, preferably preoperatively.

AMPUTATION

A review of the rehabilitation of the older amputee is beyond the scope of this chapter. However, an ageist bias about whether or not to prescribe a prosthesis for the older patient is not justified. Rehabilitation programs for older amputees are successful, even in the face of other disabilities and comorbidities (28–30). Wheelchair locomotion may be appropriate for all but the shortest distances for the patient with severe medical problems or the bilateral amputee, but a prosthesis may still be beneficial from the standpoint of transfers, standing, and cosmetics. In some cases, where ambulation is not a goal, a prosthesis may allow the otherwise bed-bound patient to get out of bed to a chair, commode, or wheelchair. This is because the stand pivot transfer made possible by the prosthesis may be safer and require much less assistance than a sliding board transfer or a total lift, which would otherwise be necessary.

PRIMARY CARE PHYSICIAN

The primary care physician plays a key role in the rehabilitative care of the older patient. The nature of the role may vary depending upon the specific condition, the phase of the illness, the setting, and regional variations in available resources and standard practices. Regardless, the primary care physician needs to function to some extent as a team leader. This role may be explicit in some situations in which, for example, the primary care physician is the designated team leader on an inpatient rehabilitation unit. However, more often the role is implicit, such as in the SNF, home care, or outpatient setting. As the team leader, no matter how explicit the role is, the primary care physician needs to coordinate services, facilitate an interdisciplinary process, and use function as the bench mark for establishing goals, monitoring progress, and assessing outcomes. When teams are well established, the role is relatively straightforward. However, when this is not the case, the task can be cumbersome, time consuming, and unreimbursed. Nonetheless, it is essential for good patient outcomes. Furthermore, when done well it is extremely gratifying for the patient, the family, the rehabilitation professionals, and the primary care physician.

REFERENCES

1. Cole TM, Edgerton VR, eds. Medical rehabilitation research: report of the Task Force. Bethesda, MD: National Institutes of Health, 1990:29.
2. Erickson RV. Principles of rehabilitation. In: Beck JC, ed. Geriatrics review syllabus. New York: American Geriatrics Society, 1991:73–88.
3. World Health Organization (WHO). International classification of impairments, disabilities and handicaps. Geneva: World Health Organization, 1980:184.
4. Applegate WB, Miller ST, Graney MJ, Elam JT, Burns R, Akins DE. A randomized, controlled trial of a geriatric assessment unit in a community rehabilitation hospital. N Engl J Med 1990;322:1572–1578.
5. Rubenstein LZ, Josephson KR, Wieland GD, English PA, Sayre JA, Kane RL. Effectiveness of a geriatric evaluation unit: a randomized clinical trial. N Engl J Med 1984;311:1664–1670.
6. Granger CV, Hamilton B, Gresham G. The stroke rehabilitation outcome study: part I. Arch Phys Med Rehabil 1988;59:506–509.
7. Granger CV, Hamilton B, Gresham G. The stroke rehabilitation outcome study: part II. Arch Phys Med Rehabil 1989;70:100–104.
8. Kennie DC, Reid J, Richardson IR, Kiamari AA, Kelt, C. Effectiveness of geriatric rehabilitative care after fractures of the proximal femur in elderly women: a randomized clinical trial. Br Med J 1988;297:1083–1086.
9. Evans DA, Harris F, Albert MS, et al. Prevalence of Alzheimer's disease in the community population of older persons. JAMA 1989;262:2551–2556.
10. Skoog I, Nilsson L, Palmertz B, et al. A population based study of dementia in 85-year-olds. N Engl J Med 1993;328:153–158.
11. Folstein MF, Folstein SE, McHugh PR. Mini-Mental State: a practical method for grading the cognitive state of patients for the clinician. J Psychiatr Res. 1975;12:189–198.
12. Brummel-Smith K. Rehabilitation. In: Ham R, Sloane P, eds. Primary care geriatrics. 2nd ed. St. Louis: Mosby Yearbook, 1992:137–161.
13. Friedmann LW, Capulong ES. Specific assistive aids. In: Williams TF, ed. Rehabilitation in the aging. New York: Raven Press, 1984:315–344.
14. Wasson JH, Gall V, MacDonald R, Liang MH. The prescription of assistive devices for the elderly: practical considerations. J Gen Intern Med. 1990;5:46–54.
15. Wilson GB. Progressive mobilization. In: Sine RD, Liss SE, Roush RE, Holcomb JD, Wilson G, eds. Basic rehabilitation techniques. 3rd ed. Rockville, MD: Aspen Publishers, 1988:132–136.
16. Bonita R. Epidemiology of stroke. Lancet. 1992; 339:342–344.
17. Caronna JJ. Cerebrovascular diseases. In: Kelley WN, ed. Textbook of internal medicine, 2nd ed. Philadelphia: JB Lippincott, 1992:2166.
18. Kelly J. Stroke rehabilitation for elderly patients. In: Kemp B, Brummel-Smith K, Ramsdel S. Geriatric rehabilitation. Boston: College-Hill Press, 1990.
19. Bonar S, Tinetti M, Speechly M, Cooney L. Factors associated with short- versus long-term skilled nursing facility placement among community-living hip fracture patients. J Am Geriatr Soc 1990; 38:1139–1144.
20. Pryor GA, Williams DR. Rehabilitation after hip fractures: home and hospital management compared. J Bone Joint Surg. 1989;71:471–474.
21. Kane RL, Ouslander JG, Abrass IB. Essentials of clinical geriatrics. 2nd ed. New York: McGraw Hill, 1989:230.
22. Goldstein TS. Geriatric orthopaedics: rehabilitative management of common problems. Gaithersburg, MD: Aspen Publishers, 1991:39–55.
23. Gauthier L, Dalziel S, Gauthier S. The benefits of group occupational therapy for patients with Parkinson's disease. Am J Occup Ther. 1987;41:360–364.
24. Palmer SS, Mortimer JA, Webster DD, et al. Exercise therapy for Parkinson's disease. Arch Phys Med Rehabil 1986;67:741–747.
25. Hicks J, Gerber L. Rehabilitation of the patient with arthritic and connective tissue disease. In: Delisa JA, et al. Rehabilitation medicine: principles and practice. 2nd ed. Philadelphia: JB Lippincott, 1993:1047–1081.
26. Gerber L, Furst G, Shulman B, et al. Patient education program to teach energy conservation behaviors to patients with rheumatoid arthritis. Arch Phys Med Rehabil 1987;68:442–45.

27. Swezey RL. Rehabilitation in arthritis and allied conditions. In: Kottke FJ, Lehmann JF, eds. Krusen's handbook of physical medicine and rehabilitation. 4th ed. Philadelphia: WB Saunders, 1990: 679–716.
28. Clark GS, Blue B, Bearer JB. Rehabilitation of the older amputee. J Am Geriatr Soc 1983;31:439–448.
29. Wolf E, Lilling M, Ferber I, Marcus J. Prosthetic rehabilitation of elderly bilateral amputees. Int J Rehabil Res. 1989;12:271–278.
30. O'Connell PG, Gnatz S. Hemiplegia and amputation: rehabilitation in the dual disability. Arch Phys Med Rehabil. 1989;70:451–454.

20/ Gastrointestinal Disease in the Aged

Richard A. Norton

Of the symptoms that bring patients of all ages to their physicians, digestive complaints are very common. Elderly patients share this pattern. In 300 ambulatory patients over 65 years of age, Sklar (1) found that large subgroups had the digestive symptoms listed in Table 20.1. Each of these groups is discussed in this chapter.

The basic processes of digestion and absorption and the functions of the liver do not ordinarily show deterioration with advancing age. In older patients, however, the diagnosis of organic disease may be more difficult, and this raises concerns for the practicing physician. For example, there may be decreased acuity of pain sensation during the early progression of organic disease. This change in appreciation of tissue injury may delay the warning system as a peptic ulcer develops. Wroblewski and Ostberg found ulcers in 2504 patients aged 60 to 98, but only 18% had abdominal pain (2). Acute appendicitis may be overlooked by the older patient and remain inapparent to the clinician until after perforation has occurred. Studies confirm that appendicitis is still the most common cause of the surgical acute abdomen for all age groups (3).

THE ESOPHAGUS

Among the complaints that bring the older patient to the doctor's office, one of the commonest is heartburn. Careful study usually reveals a weak gastroesophageal sphincter, with or without a hiatus hernia, and esophagitis may be demonstrable. Many variants of this problem may occur, with some complications. The pain of acid reflux may be intense and may mimic angina pectoris or even the pain of an acute myocardial infarction. Esophagitis may be severe enough to result in esophageal stricture, or it may produce islands of gastric-type mucosa in the lower esophagus, called Barrett's anomaly. This latter condition is thought to be premalignant, so regular surveillance by endoscopy and biopsy is indicated.

The mere presence of a hiatus hernia, together with a competent gastroesophageal sphincter, does not justify surgical repair. Because of the generally good results of medical therapy, even a hiatus hernia that produces reflux of gastric secretions into the esophagus very rarely needs an operation.

Other causes of esophagitis include irradiation, overuse of alcohol, caustic substances, and infectious agents (fungal, viral, and bacterial).

Evaluation of the patient with severe heartburn calls for upper gastrointestinal endoscopy, with biopsy of any areas of mucosa that appear to be abnormal. An alternative is traditional upper gastrointestinal x-ray study, using double-contrast technique. If doubt still exists after these studies, manometric study of the lower esophageal sphincter should be done, looking for other disease entities, such as scleroderma.

Treatment for heartburn consists of mechanical measures with weight control, smaller meals, elevation of the head of the bed at least 6 inches on blocks, no food within 2 hours of retiring, and also control of gastric acidity (antacids, H2-blockers, or omeprazole).

Management of the patient with a symptomatic esophageal stricture includes tests to exclude malignancy, usually by upper endoscopy, followed by bougienage. Treatment with dilators (bougies) may need to be repeated at monthly or longer intervals, but the patient whose symptoms are stable usually does not require repeat endoscopic study except each year or two.

When an elderly patient presents with difficulty swallowing, and there is marked dilatation of the body of the esophagus, two main diagnoses need to be considered: (a) achalasia and (b) dilatation due to an infiltrating carcinoma from the cardia of the stomach. While x-ray study is very helpful, the diagnosis must be made by endoscopy with multiple biopsies.

Achalasia presents as a new disease only infrequently in persons over 50, but it may be treated

Table 20.1

Symptom	Patients (N)	(%)
Functional bowel distress	93	31.0
Peptic ulcer disease	37	12.3
Inflammatory bowel disease	36	12
Diverticular disease	34	11.3
Neoplasms of the digestive tract	33	11
Hiatal hernia	25	8.3
Cholelithiasis, symptomatic	9	3
Miscellaneous, including liver	33	11
Total	300	100

as in younger patents. Vigorous stretching of the cardia with a pneumatic instrument is usually successful when carried out by an experienced gastroenterologist. When this does not produce good results after two or three procedures a few weeks apart, a surgical procedure should be considered, such as the Heller esophagomyotomy. This involves incising the circular muscle layer of the lower esophagus, and it usually has a high rate of success.

Adenocarcinoma of the esophagus usually starts in an area of chronic involvement by Barrett's esophagus. Other conditions associated with the development of this carcinoma include caustic burns, achalasia, cigarette smoking, and alcoholism. It may be detected by biopsy at an early stage if endoscopic surveillance is carried out on a regular basis. If the cancer is advanced at the time of diagnosis, there is a disappointingly low 5-year survival rate of less than 20% (4). The choices for treatment include radiation therapy or surgical excision, but usually not both. For palliation of a patient with inoperable carcinoma, a stent may be placed through the tumor, allowing improved swallowing of secretions and feedings. Other measures for palliation include endoscopic use of laser energy to enlarge the lumen by removing pieces of tumor, intraluminal radiation therapy, and cauterization with diathermy equipment during endoscopy. Esophagogastrectomy may be an effective form of palliation.

Squamous cell carcinoma of the esophagus is more frequently found than adenocarcinoma in the U.S. Risk factors are high in those who smoke or drink alcohol to excess and for patients with caustic strictures or achalasia. Rates are higher for men than for women and higher for blacks than for whites. Diagnosis begins with diagnostic imaging and is confirmed by endoscopic biopsy. Surgical treatment of this condition by esophagogastrectomy has led to a 5-year survival of about 6% (5), and the survival after treatment with radiation is about the same (6). Early reports of improved survival using chemotherapy with radiation and surgery involve small series, so the future use of this form of treatment is in doubt.

A troublesome symptom is the "lump in the back of the throat," which often follows emotional stress. When organic disease has been ruled out, a diagnosis of globus sensation may be made, formerly called "globus hystericus." The physiologic basis for this can be demonstrated to the patient as a provocative test. The patient should be coached to swallow several times over a few minutes, and as the supply of saliva is depleted, the action of the back of the tongue during swallowing is lubricated less and less adequately. Friction then produces the feeling of an obstructing lump. The treatment is to demonstrate this, then advise keeping a cup of water or juice handy, and in general, swallowing less frequently. For most patients, this is fully effective in relieving the symptoms. A different group of patients may develop globus sensation as a result of reflux of stomach acid into the lower esophagus, so this possibility should be investigated.

A Zenker's diverticulum, also known as a pharyngoesophageal diverticulum, is a pouch that is directed posteriorly just above the upper esophageal sphincter. Some are tiny and asymptomatic, but others are large and tend to empty their contents when the patient is horizontal, with reflux into the airway, possible pneumonia, and even lung abscess. Since the condition results from a hypertensive or poorly coordinated relaxation of the upper sphincter, surgical weakening of the sphincter is usually effective. It may be combined with removing the diverticulum or inverting it so that it tends to empty easily (7). A diagnostic clue is that some patients become aware that they are regurgitating food that they had swallowed many hours previously.

Several conditions in the elderly population call for an alternative to the ordinary route of swallowing food and fluid. These include esophageal carcinoma, brainstem stroke, and advanced muscular dystrophy, resulting in severe dysphagia with aspiration and inability to maintain adequate hydration and nutrition. After the diagnosis is made, management of the immediate problems of feeding and hydration can be made easier by insertion of a percutaneous endoscopic gastrostomy (PEG). This procedure has replaced the surgical placement of a gastrostomy feeding tube. It avoids the problems of maintaining a nasogastric tube in place for a prolonged period. It is placed endoscopically through the patient's left upper abdominal wall under light intravenous sedation. The patient may be admitted for a night of observation afterward or sent home, as conditions require (8). When the underlying condition improves, as may occur with a brainstem stroke, the PEG may be removed after a few weeks.

STOMACH

Many drugs may induce gastritis, including ethanol, aspirin and other nonsteroidal antiinflammatory drugs (NSAIDs), iron salts, potassium chloride, antineoplastic medications, and caustic chemicals. Because of the widespread use of NSAIDs for joint symptoms, the incidence of ulcer disease in the aging population has been increasing (9). It is possible to decrease the tendency toward gastritis by adding the synthetic prostaglandin misoprostol to the antiinflammatory drug regimen.

The incidence of type B gastritis (gastritis not associated with reflux) increases with age, and exceeds 75% in individuals over 50 years old. This phenomenon may reflect chronic infection with *Helicobacter pylori*, an organism now thought to be causally related not only to gastritis but also to gastric and duodenal ulcers (10). The complications of bleeding, obstruction, and pain may become disabling or even life-threatening. When a duodenal ulcer is present, the pain may awaken the patient between 1:00 and 3:00 AM, a helpful clinical sign. Food or antacids usually relieve the pain quickly, and so do H2-blocking agents or omeprazole. Gastric mucosal biopsy should be carried out to look for the presence of *Helicobacter pylori*. If it is present, the patient should receive antibiotics, since the ulcer tends to recur, even with antacid therapy, unless the organism has been eliminated (11). The preferred regimen in 1994 consists of 3 weeks of Pepto-Bismol 2 tablets four times a day, metronidazole 250 mg three times a day, and tetracycline 1 to 2 g daily in divided doses. Until symptoms subside, an H2-blocker or omeprazole should be continued. If there is a gastric ulcer, repeat x-ray study or endoscopy should be done at intervals of 4 to 6 weeks until the ulcer is completely healed.

The incidence of gastric cancer has been falling dramatically in all industrialized countries since about 1950. The reason is not clear (12). Those who do develop the disease usually present with pain, digestive tract bleeding, loss of appetite, or with more subtle symptoms. Screening by either x-ray or endoscopy will generally show the lesion, and biopsy for a definitive diagnosis by endoscopy is essential. Clinical types of adenocarcinoma are (*a*) polypoid, (*b*) ulcerating, and (*c*) infiltrating (linitis plastica). The most important factor in the outcome of surgical treatment is the stage of the tumor. Five-year survival rates for patients operated upon range from 7.4 to 16.5% (13). Chemotherapy for metastatic disease usually leads to partial responses and seems not to affect survival.

Gastric outlet obstruction usually arises from either a channel ulcer that has scarred the pylorus or from infiltration by a gastric carcinoma. Diagnosis of carcinoma, even with endoscopic biopsy, may be difficult, since biopsies may miss the malignant cells that are located deep in the tissue.

Therapy for benign pyloric stricture requires surgical bypass for most patients (gastrojejunostomy), and the outcome is very favorable.

Failure of the stomach to empty may also result from a failure of normal motility, known as gastroparesis. In approximate order of frequency, the causes include (*a*) bowel surgery in the immediate postoperative period, (*b*) diabetic neuropathy, (*c*) infiltrating carcinoma, or (*d*) idiopathic.

Fortunately, there is reasonably good medical treatment for gastroparesis: The patient may take oral metoclopramide before meals, with a good chance for improvement. Side effects in elderly patients include tardive dyskinesia and akathisia, also gynecomastia. These have been found in 10 to 20% of patients in some studies. Cisapride is another stimulant of gastric motor activity and can be given on the same schedule. This drug is attractive because of its relative lack of side effects. Erythromycin is another prokinetic drug being studied for use in gastroparesis (14).

SMALL BOWEL AND PANCREAS

One of the most common causes of diarrhea in elderly patients is lactose intolerance, involving as many as one-third of white persons and two-thirds of persons of Asian, African or Latin American ancestry. Whenever there is even a small possibility of this condition being present, it is useful to test for it with a lactose breath test, since treatment with a lactose-free diet is effective, and the patient welcomes the improvement in symptoms. A less quantitative, but inexpensive, test can be carried out by the patient at home: On an empty stomach the patient drinks a glass of milk that has been allowed to warm up to room temperature. If significant flatulence, pain, or diarrhea in any combination occurs within 2 hours, the test is considered positive for lactose intolerance. Nutritional counseling can then focus on making the diet as low in lactose as possible. Prepared foods may have lactose cooked in sauces, and many patients obtain good protection by simply swallowing a tablet or two of lactase before each meal. Others treat their milk with lactase powder that is available over the counter.

Inflammatory bowel disease, including Crohn's ileitis, Crohn's colitis and idiopathic ulcerative colitis may occur in older patients, although new onset after age 60 is not common. Evaluation involves exclusion of other disease entities by blood and stool studies, x-ray examination, and endoscopy with biopsy.

Treatment of inflammatory bowel disease has as a goal controlling the inflammatory process, since a "cure" is not at present a possibility. In general, the disease may be suppressed by prednisone in the short run and by other agents in the long run, such as 5-aminosalicylates or 6-mercaptopurine. Still other agents are under study, such as cyclosporine, chloroquine, and FK-506 (16). Surgery is best reserved as a last resort. Recurrence of active disease after surgery for Crohn's disease may be seen in 65% or more in some series.

Elderly patients with diarrhea offer a diagnostic challenge. A useful outline for evaluating diarrhea follows.

1. *Is there microbial infection of the small or large bowel?* Stool study for parasitic and bacterial pathogens usually settles this matter. If there is an infection , it can be treated specifically.
2. *Is there localized disease of the rectum and colon?* Useful procedures are rectal examination, flexible sigmoidoscopy and barium enema, or total colonoscopy. If disease is found, it can be treated at this point.
3. *Is there significant steatorrhea?* A 72-hour stool collection with laboratory estimation of fat content gives the most dependable answer to the question. The patient must have been on a 100-g fat diet for at least 3 days before and during the collection. Steatorrhea is defined as more than 7 g fat per 24 hours of stool output. Qualitative study of a single stool specimen may be used as a screening test, but this tends to be inaccurate unless the patient has been taking at least 60 g of fat per day.
4. *If steatorrhea is present, is the small bowel capable of absorbing nutrients (especially fats)?* This can be evaluated by a d-xylose test, since the carbohydrate xylose is absorbed in approximately the same portion of the small bowel as fat. If the small intestine is diseased, further study should lead to appropriate treatment. Examples are celiac sprue, extensive involvement by scleroderma, or advanced Crohn's ileocolitis.
5. *If steatorrhea is present, and small bowel absorption is normal, the pancreas may be responsible.* It may fail to produce adequate enzymes for lipolysis within the lumen of the small bowel. This diagnosis may be confirmed by giving a therapeutic trial of oral pancreatic enzymes and monitoring the stool fat output. Treatment is discussed below under pancreatic disease.
6. *Is there bacterial overgrowth in the upper small intestine?* This may be determined by barium study of the small bowel, looking for diverticula in this area. A lactulose-hydrogen breath test may confirm the bacterial origin of steatorrhea (16). Treatment with courses of an antibiotic like tetracycline (e.g., daily for 1 week out of each month) should give good results.

COLON AND RECTUM

In caring for older patients, diverticular disease is a challenge. Diverticulosis is defined as the presence of "pockets" or diverticula in the wall of the colon but without any demonstrable inflammation. The condition apparently results from high intraluminal pressures that have forced sacs of mucosa into the wall. The pockets occur most often in the sigmoid region but may be found in any part of the colon. *Diverticulitis* refers to the presence of diverticula accompanied by inflammation manifested by abdominal pain (usually in the left lower quadrant), tenderness, a palpable swelling of the tissues, and sometimes fever. Evaluation during an acute attack takes the form of ultrasound or computed tomography to look for other disease entities or complications such as abscess formation. When treatment with antibiotics has led to a decrease in inflammation, barium enema or colonoscopy may be carried out. Some patients have repeated attacks and eventually become candidates for resection of the involved segment of colon.

The major health problem involving the colon and rectum in the older population is adenocarcinoma, so screening for this condition is a matter of great concern for physicians. At present, there is no consensus as to the best and most cost-effective method of screening, except for annual rectal examination of every patient and guaiac testing of the stool, which are recommended by the American Cancer Society. The use of cards for stool-testing by patients at home is widespread, and the method may supplement other techniques. Some physicians carry out flexible sigmoidoscopy on a regular basis for patients over a specific age, such as 50 or 60, as recommended by the American Cancer Society, but this has not been universally adopted as a standard. When a member of the family has been found to have colonic carcinoma, a complete evaluation of the patient's colon should be carried out, either by colonoscopy or by barium enema and flexible sigmoidoscopy.

When a patient reports rectal bleeding or when the stool is shown to contain blood by chemical test, the usual course is to arrange for complete study of the colon and rectum, either by total colonoscopy or by combined sigmoidoscopy and barium enema x-ray study. Hemorrhoids are the most frequent source of rectal blood loss. When other potential sites of bleeding have been excluded, the hemorrhoids should be treated by a medical program (keeping the stool soft, using sitz baths, etc.). If the problem persists, the hemorrhoids may be coagulated by infrared technique, an outpatient technique that has a high rating for effectiveness and safety (17). If polyps are present, they should be removed endoscopically and examined histopathologically. Follow-up at regular intervals by colonoscopy is indicated. Colonoscopic study may reveal fragile, superficial blood vessels known as arteriovenous malformations, or angiodysplasia (18). For patients in whom these lesions are prominent and a likely cause of blood loss, electrocautery treatment through the endoscope will often reduce the rate of hemorrhage, even to the point of eliminating it for a period of time. Diverticulosis of the colon may be a site of significant bleeding, but this is not usually the cause of occult blood in the stools.

Constipation is a common problem for the aged (see Chapter 5). If there is an abrupt change in bowel habits, the colon should be studied to exclude anatomic lesions such as carcinoma. Medical treatment of idiopathic constipation consists of increased physical activity, a trial on a moderately high fiber diet, and agents such as psyllium, magnesium citrate, or magnesium hydroxide. Less desirable agents include mineral oil and irritant laxatives.

Rectal prolapse may occur in the older population, usually related to multiple episodes of severe constipation with straining at stool. Medical management consists of keeping the stool soft and gently reducing the prolapse when it occurs. If this is not successful, a surgical repair should be considered.

Fecal incontinence plagues many older patients. Evaluation is needed to see if there is an anatomic problem, including a neurologic deficit, or fecal impaction. If the latter is revealed by digital rectal examination, disimpaction should be followed by an active program to prevent recurrence. Treatment of a weak sphincter by exercises several times a day to strengthen the anal sphincter muscle may be successful. The patient is coached to "squeeze your bottom, as if you were trying to hold back a bowel movement." The diet may also be regulated to produce a firmer stool.

Antidiarrheal medication such as loperamide may add to the effectiveness of this program.

The diagnosis and management of the irritable bowel syndrome requires some finesse. By definition, this is a group of symptoms involving dysfunction of the intestinal tract but no organic abnormality. At some point it is necessary to carry out tests to make sure that tumors, specific infections, and other disease processes are absent. Patients bring functional digestive problems to their doctors' office every day, and the challenge is to sort out the functional symptoms from the equally troublesome organic ones and to treat them effectively. What are the clues for the clinician that the problem is more likely to be functional? (a) It arises soon after the most stressful events of the patient's life and disappears soon after. (b) It does not awaken the patient during the night. (c) The patient has psychological stress of at least a medium level. (d) The symptoms do not fit any of the usual organic disease patterns. (e) Absence of anemia, occult blood in stools, or weight loss. These clues are not hard-and-fast rules, of course.

Which tests are of most value? With most digestive symptoms, such as chronic diarrhea or abdominal pain, sigmoidoscopy and stool examination for pathogens are of great help. Other presenting symptoms and signs call for further examinations.

For treating the patient with the irritable bowel syndrome, a positive approach is very helpful: "You have gone through careful testing, and here is what we have found: Your intestinal tract is anatomically normal, but you have a disorder that makes it contract in an uncoordinated manner. As a result, you have pain (or diarrhea, or constipation, etc.)." After some discussion, it is important to add, "You appear to be free of serious diseases . . . such as cancer." The patient often gives an audible sigh of relief.

A list of practical suggestions for the patient with irritable bowel syndrome follows:

1. *Foods allowed:* baked or broiled meat, fish, poultry; any cooked fruits and vegetables
   Avoid: fried, fatty, or ice-cold foods and fluids
   Note: When you have been free of symptoms for at least 2 weeks, you may reintroduce foods that have been excluded, but only one per day.
2. Drink a cup of comfortably hot water upon arising and continue this every 2 hours until supper. The water need not be boiling hot. You may add flavoring to it.
3. For severe discomfort, apply local heat to the abdomen, with a hot water bottle or a heating pad, one to three times a day.

4. Get regular physical exercise. This is best if you select a form of exercise that you enjoy. A minimum schedule is 20 minutes of vigorous exercise twice a week. Better is 30 to 60 minutes every day or two.
5. Eat slowly. Chew carefully. Take enough time for a leisurely meal.

LIVER DISEASE

The differential diagnosis of jaundice is of great concern in elderly patients, as it is in younger ones. Fortunately, diagnostic imaging and laboratory technology have advanced to a large degree, making this more swift and precise.

A blood sample will determine the bilirubin, alkaline phosphatase, and aminotransferase levels. Obstruction of the biliary tree leads to elevation in the alkaline phosphatase, about three- to fivefold, while hepatocellular disease such as hepatitis leads to elevation in the aminotransferases, usually fivefold. It is not possible to determine the site of obstruction of biliary obstruction from the blood tests alone.

When jaundice is present, the clinician makes use of noninvasive tests first and then as necessary turns to the invasive ones. The history, including a careful listing of medications, and physical examination, aided by blood studies, will usually establish or exclude hepatocellular disease. Percutaneous needle liver biopsy may be necessary to complete this phase of diagnosis.

If cholestasis, the elevation of serum bilirubin and alkaline phosphatase, is apparently the problem, the next step is determining the site of obstruction. An ultrasound study of the liver and pancreas usually shows whether the biliary tree is dilated and whether there is a tumor mass. Other relatively noninvasive procedures are computerized tomography (CT scanning) and hepatobiliary scintigraphy (HIDA and similar scanning).

Invasive studies such as endoscopic retrograde cholangiopancreatography (ERCP) and percutaneous transhepatic cholangiography (PTC) may be needed to confirm the diagnosis. With either of these, it may be possible to carry out some treatment such as removing stones or placing a stent to allow preoperative drainage of bile.

Hepatitis is no more frequent in the elderly than in the young, and the clinical course may be milder (19). As with other disorders, when the course of hepatitis becomes complicated, the morbidity and mortality tend to rise steeply in the older patient.

BILIARY DISEASE

Older patients are especially at risk for tumors of the biliary tract and also for cancers of the pancreas that invade and obstruct the bile ducts. ERCP may allow removal of stones or bypassing obstructing neoplasms. Biliary stones are moderately common in North America and Western Europe; at least 20% of women over 40 years of age have gallstones, and 10% of men. Only a fraction of persons who have gallstones, however, ever have abdominal pain that is clearly related to the stones. Friedman and associates found that approximately two-thirds of persons with gallstones never have symptoms (20).

When characteristic pain or jaundice (or both) occur and the patient and the physician agree that removal is indicated, a plan must be drawn up that includes the possible courses of action, with the benefits, costs, and risks of each.

1. **Conventional surgical cholecystectomy,** with common duct exploration if indicated (with jaundice or elevated alkaline phosphatase). Before laparoscopic removal became available, open cholecystectomy was the best procedure for resolving the patient's problem. Low morbidity and mortality became routine throughout Western surgical circles. It remains the procedure of choice in difficult or complicated situations, such as uncertain diagnosis, impacted stones, etc. The disadvantages are the larger amount of tissue trauma, the longer incision, more pain, and longer recovery period.
2. **Laparoscopic cholecystectomy.** The big advantages are the short hospital stay and the early return to full activity. It may require longer operating room time than the conventional operation. The surgeon may have to convert to a conventional incision during the procedure.
3. **Extracorporeal shock wave lithotripsy.** This treatment focuses pulses of ultrasonic energy on the gallstones from a source outside the body. A program for long-term lowering of the cholesterol level in the bile must follow the treatments, such as daily oral ursodiol. This procedure is still experimental and is performed in only a few teaching centers under a defined protocol. Because it is somewhat painful, sedation is necessary. The recurrence rate has been high. Altogether, it has waned in popularity over the past few years.
4. Long-term oral ursodiol treatment alone. This program has limited appeal except for patients with few or no symptoms and with major contraindications for any invasive procedures. When treatment ends, the recurrence rate is 10 to 15% per year (21).
5. "**Do nothing.**" This means continuing to observe with no specific therapy. Some people will tolerate enormous amounts of pain rather than go through a surgical operation, and there will always be patients whose symptoms disappear and do not return.

What should the clinician tell patients who have asymptomatic gallstones, with no symptoms referable to biliary disease at all? Since there is at least a 67% chance that they will never have pain or other symptoms, a reasonable argument is to leave the stones where they are (20). The patient whose anxiety level is high (and now is higher because of the abnormality) may need more counseling, but the risk-benefit ratio strongly favors waiting and watching. Even in elderly patients, the mortality and morbidity of cholecystectomy is reasonably low when the procedure is indicated.

PANCREATIC DISEASE

Acute pancreatitis in a nonalcoholic, otherwise healthy elderly person is usually traceable to one or more gallstones in the common bile duct, possibly impacted. There is recent good evidence that endoscopic treatment within the first 24 hours of admission leads to fewer complications and lower mortality (22). This procedure is ERCP, with the option of opening the ampulla of Vater to extract stones so the pancreatic duct can drain normally. The endoscopic sphincterotomy is carried out with a "knife" that consists of a wire on one side of the tip of a slender plastic catheter. When the tube is properly placed under endoscopic vision in the orifice of the ampulla, an electrical current is passed through the wire so that the local tissue is both cut and cauterized. Bleeding is usually minor, although aberrant arteries in the duodenal wall occasionally bleed when cut. The stones can be extracted with a variety of instruments, including tiny rubber balloons, wire baskets, and heavy wire snares that can crush the stones.

Other causes of acute pancreatitis include trauma, bowel infarction, alcoholic overuse, and many groups of drugs, including sulfonamides and thiazides. Levels of lipase tend to remain elevated longer than those of amylase, so that lipase levels should be determined when a suspicion of pancreatitis persists. Acute pancreatitis in a nonalcoholic elderly patient without gallstones suggests the presence of pancreatic cancer.

Chronic pancreatitis resulting from overuse of alcohol or from unknown causes may produce little or no pain, and the resulting scarring may leave the gland incapable of secreting adequate amounts of proteolytic and lipolytic enzymes into the pancreatic juice. Weight loss is moderate to severe, as is weakness and fatigue, due to the nutritional deficiency. Diagnosis may follow the algorithm above in the discussion of diarrhea, and treatment would then consist of adding pancreatic extract to the patient's program. It may be difficult for the patient to ingest enough extract

to overcome the steatorrhea, so some regimens call for taking two or three tablets before, during and again after each meal. Once the treatment plan is in place and working, however, there is usually gratifying weight gain and return of the patient's baseline energy and sense of well-being.

Pancreatic cancer usually produces epigastric pain, often radiating to the midback, and precedes jaundice by up to 3 months. The pain is often vague, poorly localized, and made worse by eating. Lying curled up on one's side may give relief. Weight loss follows and, later, jaundice from biliary obstruction. Diagnosis was formerly difficult, but with the advent of ERCP as well as abdominal ultrasound and computed tomography, the patient's problem can usually be localized precisely. Needle biopsy of the pancreatic mass may be guided by ultrasound or by CT scanning. The ERCP is likely to demonstrate a "double duct sign," meaning that the same malignant tumor has invaded at least two ducts (biliary or pancreatic or both). Treatment has not advanced at the same pace, and the standard measures of surgery, chemotherapy, and radiation therapy have resulted in only very modest improvement in survival. The prognosis remains poor.

Acknowledgment. The author is grateful to Drs. George Dickstein, David Johnston, Tamsin Knox, and Robert Russell for helpful suggestions on this chapter.

REFERENCES

1. Sklar M. Gastrointestinal diseases in the aged. In: Reichel W, ed. Clinical aspects of aging. 2nd ed. Baltimore: Williams & Wilkins, 1983:206–217.
2. Wroblewski M, Ostberg H. Ulcer disease among geriatric inpatients with positive faecal occult blood test and/or iron deficiency anemia: a prospective study. Scand J Gastroenterol 1990;25:489–495.
3. Peltokallio P, Tykka H. Evolution of the age distribution and mortality of acute appendicitis. Arch Surg 1981;116:153–156.
4. Silverberg E, Boring CC, Squires TS. Cancer statistics. CA 1990;40:9–26.
5. Earlam R, Cunha-Melo JR. Oesophageal squamous cell carcinoma: II. A critical view of radiotherapy. Br J Surg 1980;67:457–461.
6. Ellis FH Jr. Surgical palliation: esophageal resection—a surgeon's opinion. In: Delarue NC, Wilkins EW Jr, Wong J, eds. International trends in general thoracic surgery. Vol 4: Esophageal cancer. St. Louis: CV Mosby, 1988:375–381.
7. Bowdler DA, Stell PM. Surgical management of posterior pharyngeal pulsion diverticula: inversion versus one-stage excision. Br J Surg 1987;74:988–990.
8. Ponsky JL. Percutaneous endoscopic gastrostomy. In: Yamada T, ed. Textbook of gastroenterology. Philadelphia: JB Lippincott, 1991:2596–2601.
9. Papp JP. Management of upper gastrointestinal bleeding. Clin Geriatr Med 1991;7:255–264.

10. Graham DY, Malaty HM, Evans DG, et al. Epidemiology of Helicobacter pylori in an asymptomatic population in the United States: effect of age, race, and socioeconomic status. Gastroenterology 1991; 100:1495–1501.

11. Hentschel E, Brandstatter G, Dragosics F, et al. Effect of ranitidine and amoxicillin plus metronidazole on the eradication of Helicobacter pylori and the recurrence of duodenal ulcer. N Engl J Med 1993;328:308–312.

12. Howson CP, Hiyama T, Wynder EL. The decline in gastric cancer; epidemiology of an unplanned triumph. Epidemiol Rev 1986;8:1–27.

13. Faivre J, Justrabo E, Hillon P, et al. Gastric carcinoma in Cote d'Or (France), a population based study. Gastroenterology 1985;88:1874–1879.

14. Janssens J, Peeters TL, Vantrappen G, et al. Improvement of gastric emptying in diabetic gastroparesis by erythromycin. N Engl J Med 1990; 322:1028–1031.

15. Korelitz BI. Where do we stand on drug treatment for ulcerative colitis? (editorial) Ann Intern Med 1992;116:692–694.

16. Kerlin P, Wong L. Breath hydrogen testing in bacterial overgrowth of the small intestine. Gastroenterology 1988;95:982–988.

17. Ambrose NS, Morris D, Alexander-Williams J, et al. A randomized trial of photocoagulation or injection sclerotherapy for the treatment of first- and second-degree hemorrhoids. Dis Colon Rectum 1985; 28:238–240.

18. Boley SJ, DiBiasi A, Brandt LJ, et al. Lower intestinal bleeding in the elderly. Am J Surg 1979; 137:57–64.

19. Zauli D, Crespi C, Fusconi M, et al. Different course of acute hepatitis B in elderly adults. J Gerontol 1985;40:415–418.

20. Friedman GD, Kannell WB, Dawber TR. The epidemiology of gallbladder disease: observations in the Framingham Study. J Chronic Dis 1966;19:273–292.

21. Hofmann A. Medical dissolution of gallstones by oral bile acid therapy. Am J Surg 1989;158:198–204.

22. Tan S-T, Lai ECS, Mok FPT, et al. Early treatment of acute biliary pancreatitis by endoscopic papillotomy. N Engl J Med 1993;328:228–232.

21/ Infectious Disease Problems in the Elderly

Glenys O. Williams, Gerald J. Jogerst

The combined burdens of diseases that accompany aging, changes caused by the aging process, and reduced immunocompetence imperil elderly patients with infections and challenge their physicians. The mortality rate for the elderly with serious infections is higher than that for younger people (1–3). For those who recover, morbidity is prolonged (1, 4). Hospital admissions are more frequent in old age, and the invasive procedures that are increasingly used often lead to infection. An acute infection in an older person living at home may trigger the crisis that leads to hospital, then nursing home admission. Thus the most frail patients come to live in a closed environment, exposed to more sources of infection than they were in the community. Disease processes, such as pneumonia, are caused by a variety of different organisms, depending on the setting in which they occur. Choice of antibiotics is complicated because many cause serious adverse reactions in the elderly. Finally, treatment decisions may be clouded by ethical questions about prolonging the life of patients who are incapacitated by physical or mental illness.

RESPONSE OF OLDER PATIENTS TO INFECTION

Aging is a state of immune dysregulation (5). There is involution of the thymus and altered T cell–mediated immunity, but also increased antibody production to self-antigens. Diminished cell-mediated immunity results in the reactivation of dormant infections such as herpes zoster and tuberculosis. Influenza deaths after age 65 are increased, and the antibody response to influenza vaccine is decreased (5). Spouse caregivers of demented persons are significantly more likely to have upper respiratory tract infections than are controls (6), showing that medical problems cannot be separated from psychosocial needs in infected older patients.

Early recognition of infection in the elderly is difficult because patients underreport symptoms, the presentation is often vague or atypical, and symptoms are difficult to assess (7). Pain may be poorly localized or absent, as in appendicitis, or it may be confused with preexisting conditions, as in septic arthritis (4). Change in mental state is common in acute infections; for example, altered mental status and unexplained leukocytosis are manifestations of bacteremia (8). If symptoms are unnoticed by patients or caregivers, delay in diagnosis contributes to the high mortality rate. Cognitively impaired patients are at particularly high risk.

Fever in older patients may not be high enough to cause concern because the basal body temperature is low. Fever can also be masked by drugs such as aspirin and corticosteroids (9), delayed, or missed if temperatures are not taken in the evening. Castle et al. (10) recommend lowering the threshold for recognition of fevers to 99 or 100°F (oral temperature) in nursing home residents with a change in function, to assist in early recognition of infections. If the febrile response is absent in an elderly patient with a serious infection, it is a predictor of higher mortality. A review of elderly with fever of unknown origin found that 36% had infections such as endocarditis, intraabdominal abscess, and tuberculosis (11).

URINARY TRACT INFECTIONS

Infections in the vulnerable aging urinary tract are the commonest cause of fever in patients over 65 and the most frequent cause of bacteremia (7). There are multiple predisposing factors. The female introitus is colonized with fecal flora, estrogen deficiency causes atrophic urethritis, bladder contractility is reduced, and bladder emptying is affected by commonly prescribed drugs such as β-blockers and anticholinergics. Urinary incontinence is common in elderly women, who may restrict fluids to reduce urine flow, thus also reducing bacterial washout from the bladder. Resumption of sexual activity may be a factor in some women. Bacteria adhere more readily to the uroepithelial cells of elderly men. Obstruction of the urinary tract, most often by benign prostatic hypertrophy, sets the stage for stasis and infection. Indwelling and condom catheters, whatever the reason for their use, put the patient at high risk.

Obtaining urine for testing can be difficult. Non–clean catch samples may be easier to obtain and as reliable on culture as catheterized samples in women aged 30 to 90 years (12). Condom catheters with leg bag are useful in incontinent men; patients must be checked often, so that the specimen can be refrigerated as soon as possible (13). Urine specimens can be obtained from indwelling catheters that have been in place for a short time by inserting a sterile needle and syringe into the catheter; after 30 days, urine should be obtained from a newly inserted catheter because more bacteria will be found in the old catheter than in the bladder (14).

Providing high-quality care in nursing homes is a challenge, given the difficulty of obtaining diagnostic workups in some facilities, the special problems of the patient population, and the choice of some patients and families to refuse hospitalization. Zimmer et al. introduced criteria for starting antibiotics in cases of proven or suspected urinary tract infection (15). When laboratory results are not immediately available, he requires fever of 100°F on the day of drug order plus (a) gross hematuria or pyuria, (b) costovertebral or suprapubic tenderness, (c) urinary frequency of recent onset, or (d) burning or pain on urination. If there is no fever, any two of the four symptoms listed (a-d) must be present (15). While waiting for culture results in cases of presumed lower tract infection in ambulatory and institutionalized patients, treatment with trimethoprim-sulfamethoxazole tablets or liquid is appropriate for patients who are not seriously ill. Single-dose treatment should not be used for the elderly because their infections are usually complicated. It is important to maintain adequate fluid intake during acute infections, even in patients with reduced renal concentrating ability. Long-term antibiotic prophylaxis may be indicated when more than four symptomatic episodes occur in 1 year and in the presence of chronic bacterial prostatitis.

ASYMPTOMATIC BACTERIURIA

The prevalence of asymptomatic bacteriuria is high, 25% in patients older than 80 years (16), yet there is a high rate of spontaneous resolution. Treatment can eliminate bacteriuria in 64% of nonhospitalized elderly women for periods up to 6 months (17) and may reduce the rate of symptomatic infections, but there is a high rate of early recurrence in hospitalized and institutionalized patients (18). Treating nursing home patients produces no short-term benefits, the potential for adverse reactions to antibiotics, and the danger of growth of resistant organisms (19). It is generally agreed that asymptomatic bacteriuria should not be treated (16, 18, 21).

PYELONEPHRITIS

Acute symptomatic pyelonephritis is a serious infection in which 61% of hospitalized elderly patients have bacteremia and 26% develop septic shock (fever, altered mental status, and systolic blood pressure <90 mm Hg) (22). Diagnosis may be difficult and delayed. Patients must be hospitalized if they cannot drink fluids adequately, take medications, have an uncertain social situation, are severely ill, have underlying illness, or have decreased renal reserve (23, 24). Most adult women with pyelonephritis do well as outpatients, with oral therapy such as trimethoprim-sulfamethoxazole, but there is no evidence that elderly patients with underlying illness or decreased renal function can be safely treated at home (24). Male patients and those with poor response to treatment need urgent workup to identify any obstruction and prevent renal damage.

CATHETERS AND INFECTION

The incidence of catheter-associated urinary tract infections increases at a rate of up to 10% per day after insertion. Bacteriuria appears early, and by 30 days, 85% of indwelling catheters with closed drainage systems are infected, and organisms and sensitivities change every few weeks. Antibiotic treatment is reserved for infections causing systemic symptoms and fever. Meatal care, scheduled catheter changes, intermittent irrigation, and systemic antibiotics are expensive, are time-consuming for nurses, and do not reduce the rates of infection.

SKIN AND SOFT TISSUE INFECTIONS

Skin and soft tissue infections are particularly troublesome in nursing home patients. They caused 14% of the cases and more than half of the deaths from bacteremia in one long-term care facility study (7).

HERPES ZOSTER

Herpes zoster or shingles is caused by reactivation of latent varicella zoster virus (VZV) in older patients who had chickenpox when young. Common complications are scarring, secondary infection, and postherpetic neuralgia. If the ophthalmic nerves are affected, blindness may result. Disseminated herpes zoster and central nervous system involvement may occur in immunosuppressed patients, in those with leukemia or lymphoma, and in cellular immunodeficiency. Diagnosis may be difficult in the preeruptive stage when fever, malaise, and burning pain are the only symptoms, but the appearance of typical vesicles on a red base in a dermatomal distribution, usually in the thoracic region, is readily recognized. Direct immunofluorescence for VZV antigens applied to smears obtained from vesicles is the best available test, but laboratory confirmation of diagnosis is rarely necessary.

Acyclovir, 800 mg, five times daily for 7 days, reduces the extent and duration of the rash and pain severity (25, 26), but it is expensive and does not prevent neuralgia. Intravenous acyclovir for 7 days is recommended for immunosuppressed patients and for ophthalmic zoster. There is no proof that oral steroids reduce pain or the incidence of postherpetic neuralgia. Symptomatic treatment begins with scheduled analgesics. Topical treatments such as gentle washing and calamine lotion or aluminum acetate (Burow's solution) may relieve discomfort. Postherpetic neuralgia is difficult to manage. Nortriptyline is useful for chronic pain, but the anticholinergic side effects are undesirable in elderly patients. Carbamazepine and levodopa may be helpful. Topical capsaicin cream applied three to four times daily to healed lesions is a counterirritant, promising for pain relief but very costly. Transmission of herpes zoster infection in nursing homes is prevented by scrupulous attention to hand washing while the lesions are open. Immunosuppressed patients, staff, and family members who have not had chickenpox should be separated from the infected resident (26). Varicella-zoster immune globulin can be used early for high-risk contacts.

PRESSURE SORES

Pressure sores are an important and expensive source of infection. Prevention is essential. It includes careful attention to the mattress, preferably one of the newer varieties of air mattress; turning the patient every 2 hours; optimal nutrition (protein, vitamin C, and zinc supplements); and cleanliness (27). Occlusive dressings should be changed daily on stage II ulcers to prevent infection. Bactericidal solutions, especially those containing iodine, are best avoided because they interfere with wound healing. Cellulitis, underlying osteomyelitis, and sepsis resulting from stage III and IV ulcers need urgent treatment with intravenous antibiotics that cover aerobic and anaerobic bacteria, even before culture results are available (27). When determining whether a pressure sore is infected, it is important to distinguish reddened skin, recently healed, from inflamed, hot, tender skin accompanied by systemic signs of infection. There is no consensus on the need to culture these wounds.

PARASITIC INFECTIONS

Parasitic infections may become more prevalent in the future because parasites are more common due to the spread of AIDS, the population over 65 is increasing, and the elderly are relatively immunodeficient, making them more susceptible. Crowded cities in the warm southern United States are likely to be the locations of these infections (28).

Scabies epidemics in nursing homes are a common problem in geriatric practice. Patients present with itching and scratching, especially at night. The typical rash occurs in skin folds such as the wrist, between fingers, elbow, axilla, groin, waist, and genitalia. Norwegian scabies is an aberrant host response by elderly patients with reduced immune system activity; there is little pruritus, and the rash is widespread with hyperkeratotic lesions, crusting, and scaling. This form is highly contagious because thousands of mites infest each patient. Transmission is by contact, linens, and gait belts (29). Diagnosis is by skin scraping over a suspected burrow.

Permethrin 5% cream (Elimite), the safest treatment for older patients, is applied to the whole body, and washed off after 8 to 14 hours (30). Side effects include temporary itching and burning. Bed linens and clothes must be laundered, and hand washing emphasized. The nails of patients and staff must be cut short. All persons in close contact with the patient should be treated to avoid a widespread epidemic. These infestations cause intense anxiety among institution staff.

METHICILLIN-RESISTANT STAPHYLOCOCCUS AUREUS

Methicillin-resistant *Staphylococcus aureus* (MRSA) is responsible for considerable inappropriate fear and for denied admission to long-term care facilities. It is not a superbug, but it is resistant to most antibiotics (31). Debilitated patients, especially males with pressure sores, urinary incontinence, current antibiotic use, presence of an intravenous line, recent hospitalization, or nasogastric intubation are at high risk (32). Treatment with intravenous vancomycin is recommended for symptomatic infected patients. Colonization alone does not usually warrant treatment, but transfer of information between hospital and nursing home is important when a patient is admitted or discharged with a positive culture, to prevent the infection from spreading (31). Meticulous hand washing and gloving are adequate for infection control. Colonized patients must not share rooms with high-risk patients; the greatest risk of nosocomial transmission is from MRSA-positive patients with copious secretions, such as sputum and drainage from large infected decubiti (32). High-risk patients should have screening cultures done on admission to nursing homes. Recommended sites for these cultures are pressure sores, the nose, ostomy sites, and sputum (32).

OTHER SKIN AND SOFT TISSUE INFECTIONS

Bacterial conjunctivitis is common and recurs, especially affecting elderly patients who have dry eyes and chronic blepharitis. Artificial tears are necessary, but if the solution contains preservative, it should not be used more than every 4 hours, to avoid preservative toxicity. This treatment is combined with lid hygiene: warm soaks, baby shampoo scrubs, and antibiotics such as trimethoprim sulfate/polymyxin B sulfate (Polytrim) ophthalmic solution or sulfacetamide 10% (Sulamyd) solution or cream. Meibomian gland dysfunction responds to tetracycline 250 mg twice daily (33). Ectropion and entropion, frequently found in old age, are also predisposing factors for infection and may need surgical revision if severe.

Malignant otitis externa occurs in the elderly, particularly in diabetics. It is a necrotizing infection, caused by *Pseudomonas aeruginosa*, which may spread to the temporal bone, meninges, and brain. The discharge is greenish and foul-smelling, and there is ear pain. Parenteral gentamicin with a β-lactam agent is recommended, and surgery may be necessary (34). Oral agents such as ciprofloxacin and rifampin may be effective for moderate infections in the future.

Skin tears are common on the thin-skinned arms of the institutionalized elderly. Cleaning with saline solution and application of a nonstick polyurethane membrane synthetic dressing (Te-

gaderm, Bioclusive) is usually sufficient. It is customary but not necessary to apply topical antibiotics as a preventive measure. If localized bacterial cellulitis supervenes, oral therapy with erythromycin, dicloxacillin, or a cephalosporin is usually appropriate. More severe and widespread cellulitis is life-threatening in the elderly and should be treated accordingly. Culture results from superficial infections are rarely accurate but are useful if there is an epidemic.

GASTROINTESTINAL INFECTIONS

Host resistance of the gastrointestinal tract is maintained by acid secretion from gastric mucosa and by lymphoid tissue. In old age, gastric acidity declines, and the amount of lymphoid tissue decreases, but it is not clear why the elderly have increased susceptibility to, and increased mortality from, conditions such as infectious diarrhea. Most deaths from appendicitis and cholecystitis occur in the elderly, partly because abdominal pain and tenderness are minimal or absent. Diagnostic delays, reluctance to perform surgery, the presence of underlying disease, and postoperative complications may contribute to the high mortality rate for elderly patients with these and other intraabdominal infections such as diverticulitis and intraabdominal abscess (35).

ACUTE SUPPURATIVE PAROTITIS

Acute suppurative parotitis occurs in critically ill, dehydrated elderly patients, probably because of reduced flow of saliva and stasis leading to infection from oral flora. Gram-negative bacilli and *S. aureus* have been identified as causative organisms. Cultures are taken from discharge at the opening of Stensen's (parotid) duct, and treatment is started when the results of a Gram's stain are available. Attention to oral hygiene and stimulation of salivary flow may prevent this infection.

FOOD-BORNE INFECTIONS

A Centers for Disease Control (CDC) study found that in food-borne disease outbreaks in nursing homes, nontyphoidal *Salmonella* infection caused 81% of the deaths, with a case-fatality ratio 10 times higher than that for outbreaks in different settings (3). Other infectious agents commonly found include *S. aureus* (26%), Norwalk agent virus, *Clostridium difficile* (associated with antibiotic therapy), and *Clostridium perfringens*. *Escherichia coli* 0157:H7 infections can cause the hemolytic uremic syndrome and hemorrhagic colitis (36). The danger, as in infants, is dehydration, with the added risk in the elderly that volume depletion can lead to myocardial infarction or stroke. Bacteremia, endarteritis, and endocarditis may be caused by *Salmonella* spp. Abdominal examination is necessary to check for signs of other intraabdominal conditions, particularly in patients unable to describe their symptoms. It is also important to rule out fecal impaction with overflow diarrhea. A good indicator of hypovolemia in the elderly is hypotension, a more reliable sign than decreased skin turgor when the skin is inelastic. Stool cultures and smears for white blood cells should be sent if diarrhea does not resolve rapidly, if the patient is in a nursing home, or if the stool contains blood.

For basically healthy ambulatory patients who are able to take fluids and also for nursing home patients who are very ill but do not wish to be hospitalized, dehydration can often be satisfactorily treated orally or by enteral tube (37). One or two 8-ounce glasses of electrolyte solution after each bowel movement are recommended. Some starchy food should be allowed because it helps the absorption of water and nutrients. Bismuth subsalicylate (Pepto-Bismol) may reduce the duration of diarrhea. Antibiotics are not indicated in self-limited infections such as Norwalk virus and rotavirus, but they should be considered for diarrhea due to *Shigella, Salmonella, Campylobacter jejuni,* invasive *E. coli, Vibrio parahaemolyticus,* and *Yersinia enterocolitica* (37). It may be necessary to discontinue diuretics temporarily to conserve fluid.

Epidemics and death from food-borne disease are preventable if food handlers are properly trained, but in nursing homes the presence of patients with dementia and fecal incontinence adds to the danger. Shell eggs, poultry, and salads are the most frequent vehicles of infection (3). An active infection-control program in each institution helps to educate all staff and identify and deal with outbreaks rapidly.

MENINGITIS

The problem in older patients is not the frequency of infection (1 in 450,000 per year over age 60); the problems are delayed diagnosis, the urgent need for aggressive treatment, and the high risk of complications and mortality. Predisposing conditions are sinusitis, diabetes mellitus, alcohol abuse, neoplastic disease, steroid therapy, and recent neurosurgery (38). An elderly patient with fever, confusion, coma, and/or headache is very likely to have bacterial meningitis. Nausea, vomiting, and neck pain are also common (2), and fre-

quently there are respiratory symptoms due to pneumonia or sinusitis. On examination, nuchal rigidity must be differentiated from cervical osteoarthritis, in which flexion is usually retained while lateral flexion and rotation are restricted. Look for focal neurologic deficits, seizures, and change in mental status (38). Organisms found most frequently in cerebrospinal fluid are *Streptococcus pneumoniae, Listeria monocytogenes, S. aureus, Enterobacter,* and *Pseudomonas.*

Until a specific diagnosis is made, intravenous ampicillin with a third-generation cephalosporin is appropriate therapy. Treatment should be continued for 10 to 14 days for all cases except those caused by Gram-negative bacilli, for which 3 to 4 weeks is recommended (2).

ENDOCARDITIS

Once a disease of the young, endocarditis is increasingly affecting older people. High-risk patients are those who have prosthetic heart valves and invasive devices or procedures, particularly if they involve the male urinary tract. The mortality is high in the elderly, and those who recover may have permanent cardiovascular or neurologic disabilities (1). Symptoms are vague and frequently include weakness, malaise, change in mental state, and musculoskeletal pains, with or without fever. A new regurgitant murmur may be heard. Cardiac failure and vascular phenomena such as petechiae, splinter hemorrhages, hematuria, and other peripheral emboli must be looked for. Neurologic signs, aphasia, and hemiplegia are more common than in the young. Any elderly patient with unexplained fever for 1 week should have blood cultures drawn, which may be positive intermittently. Streptococci, followed by staphylococci, are the most frequent causative organisms. Endocarditis caused by enterococci is likely to be secondary to urinary tract infection; *Streptococcus bovis* is an indicator of gastrointestinal disease, often colorectal carcinoma.

Empiric antibiotic treatment with intravenous penicillin G, ampicillin, nafcillin, or oxacillin and gentamicin are indicated immediately for critically ill patients, until organism identification is available. Stable elderly patients may remain untreated until there is a specific microbiologic diagnosis (1).

The 1990 American Heart Association recommendations for the prevention of bacterial endocarditis advise antimicrobial treatment during perioperative periods only, with oral amoxicillin (erythromycin or clindamycin in penicillin-allergic patients) for upper body procedures. Parenteral antibiotics are recommended for high-risk patients undergoing lower body procedures (39).

SEPSIS

Patients of advanced age are devastated by sepsis. They are more likely to acquire it, and they are more likely to die. Nosocomial and nursing home–acquired infections are the most lethal. More often than the young, the elderly develop Gram-negative and Gram-positive bacteremia as complications of pyelonephritis, pneumococcal pneumonia, and salmonella enteritis/colitis. Fifty percent of bacteremic patients in long-term care die within 24 hours despite treatment (7). The difference in the mortality rate between these patients and those with community-acquired sepsis may reflect the number of underlying diseases and age-related changes. Colonization of the oropharynx by Gram-negative organisms is found in 19% of healthy elderly and 23% of nursing home residents (40), and it predisposes to Gram-negative pneumonia. The sources of infection in long-term care patients are the urinary tract (56%), skin (14%), and respiratory system (10%) (7); in the community, infections originate in the urinary tract (34%), biliary tract (20%), and lungs (13%) (41). The highest mortality is from sepsis due to skin infections (57%), which often originate from pressure ulcers (41). Organisms most frequently responsible in long-term care are *E. coli, Proteus* spp., *Klebsiella* spp., and *S. aureus* (7); in the community, the most frequent organisms are *E. coli, Klebsiella* spp. and *S. pneumoniae* (41, 42). Early presentation is subtle, usually with malaise, altered mental state, and chills or fever. The outcome for afebrile septic patients was invariably fatal in one study (8). Tachypnea, tachycardia, and unexplained leukocytosis are frequent findings (8). Hypotension indicates early septic shock. Sepsis due to biliary tree infection can present with rigors, vomiting, and abdominal discomfort (41). Urinary tract symptoms are often absent (41), but a traumatic catheter-related event may precede the onset of sepsis (43). Cultures must be done immediately, even if the patient is already on antibiotics (8).

Initial empiric treatment must be broad and consider the possible source of the infection. It should include coverage for Gram-negative organisms and *S. aureus,* especially in patients 85 or older (44). Third-generation cephalosporins, imipenem/cilastin, ticarcillin/clavulanate, and combinations of these drugs with an aminoglycoside, aztreonam, or a parenteral quinolone are suitable choices (45). Volume replacement and frequent monitoring are essential, and a vasoactive drug, such as dopamine, is indicated for septic shock. Monoclonal antibodies may reduce the mortality in patients with Gram-negative bacteremia and shock.

SEPTIC ARTHRITIS

Most elderly patients with septic arthritis have underlying osteoarthritis, rheumatoid arthritis, or gout and are accustomed to painful joints. Under these circumstances, it is not surprising that diagnosis is often delayed. Besides arthropathy, other predisposing factors for infection are minor trauma and steroid injections into the joint. Pain in a prosthetic joint must also arouse suspicion of an infection. Restricted movement, erythema, and warmth are frequently found, but fever, leukocytosis, and elevated erythrocyte sedimentation rate are not always present (4). The most commonly infected joint is the knee, followed by the hip and foot. Infection is usually due to *S. aureus,* found in synovial fluid obtained by aspiration or surgical drainage or in blood culture.

Parenteral antibiotics are generally given for 4 to 6 weeks. Most elderly patients with septic arthritis do not recover full function of the joints (4).

RESPIRATORY INFECTIONS

Pneumonia combined with influenza is the leading infectious cause of death, the fifth leading cause of death overall, and the fourth leading cause of hospitalization in persons 65 years and older (46). Mortality rates from pneumonia in the elderly depend on both the patient's underlying diseases and the bacterial etiology. The elderly person's place of residence is associated with the number and severity of disease processes, the functional capabilities of the person, and the type of microbial exposures. Therefore mortality rates vary with the environment in which the elderly live. Rates vary from 24 to 33% for elderly in American and British community-based studies to 5.7 to 8% in younger adults (47). Mortality for hospital-acquired pneumonias is 36 to 40%; for nursing home pneumonia, it approaches 40% (47). Concomitant disease is the principal risk factor for pneumonia in the elderly. Because of coexisting illness, most older persons require hospitalization and have longer lengths of stay than young patients. There are two peaks of mortality, one occurring within 24 hours of admission and a second late in hospitalization, caused by Gram-negative superinfections (48). Mortality is associated with systolic hypotension, increasing hypoxemia, urinary incontinence, alcoholism, and absence of fever. Antibiotic therapy does not seem to change mortality rates in the first 36 hours of illness (41).

The clinical manifestations and responses to pneumonia are influenced by age-related alterations in lung structure and function. Aging produces several changes in the body's ability to acquire oxygen. Reduced compliance of the chest wall leads to increased muscular work and thus a higher energy cost for each respiration. Ventilation-perfusion imbalance increases with aging, leading to decreased arterial oxygen saturation. Slowing of the mucociliary apparatus and a decreased cough mechanism result in reduced clearance of the tracheobronchial tree. The collapse of small airways and loss of elasticity further increase the risks of infection. However, the many chronic diseases and malnutrition associated with aging may have a more profound effect on the risk for and the outcome of pneumonia than do pulmonary or immunologic aging.

GENERAL CONSIDERATIONS

The elderly pneumonia patient may be acutely ill or only show a recent subtle decline in function. The severity of the illness, the site of the encounter, and the wishes of the patient influence the management approach. Certain general principles, however, apply no matter what the situation is at presentation.

The clinical features of pneumonia may consist of an insidious deterioration of functional abilities without evident fever, cough, or purulent sputum. Berman et al. reported that during a 6-month period, 50 of 65 instances of functional decline in elderly patients were associated with subsequent infection (49). Sudden deterioration of, or slow recovery from, a preexisting disease such as stroke or congestive heart failure can indicate pneumonia. The physical examination is frequently nonspecific, but accurate measurement of the respiratory rate is a valuable diagnostic aid. McFadden reported that 19 of 21 patients diagnosed with lower respiratory tract infections had respiratory rates above 25 breaths a minute on the day of diagnosis (50). The rise in respiratory rate preceded the clinical diagnosis by 3 to 4 days (50).

The initial diagnostic evaluation should include complete blood count, glucose, electrolytes, BUN, and creatinine. Leukocytosis remains a reliable finding. Harper and Newton reported that 73% of their elderly pneumonia patients developed leukocytosis with a left shift (51). Although the chest x-ray is the "gold standard" for the diagnosis of pneumonia, it may be negative initially and become positive following rehydration. Radiographic findings may be overshadowed by underlying disease. Congestive heart failure, malignancy, atelectasis, and adult respiratory distress syndrome (ARDS) may obscure or be mistaken for pneumonia. Chronic obstructive pulmonary disease (COPD) may lead to incomplete consolidation. Sputum cultures should be obtained, if possible, but limited to specimens with Gram's stain showing more than 25 white blood cells (WBCs) and fewer than 10 epithelial cells per high power field. Two sets of blood cultures are recommended; approximately 7% of these cultures are positive (52). Arterial blood gas determinations are needed to assess for hypoxemia and hypercapnia. Diagnostic thoracentesis may be indicated for Gram's stain, culture, and cytology of pleural effusions.

Treatment begins with the stabilization of any life-threatening conditions such as hypoxia, dehydration, hypotension, severe anemia, or cardiac dysrhythmias. After laboratory specimens are obtained, parenteral antimicrobials should generally be administered for 7 days, followed by a week of oral antibiotics after the patient is clinically stable. Supportive care with adequate nutrition, hydration, mobilization, and skin care is essential. The proper management of other acute or chronic illness must be coordinated with the treatment of pneumonia. The use of aminoglycosides in patients with renal insufficiency or the use of penicillins with high sodium content (ticarcillin disodium) in patients with congestive heart failure may be inappropriate.

The community, nursing home, and hospital settings are a convenient way to consider the presentation and treatment of pneumonia. Remember that we treat individuals, not settings. The 80-year-old person living in her own home, who is bedridden with severe COPD and requires around the clock caregivers, would need attention similar to that of the nursing home patient rather than an independent community dweller. Home therapy with parenteral antibiotics is an option for this patient.

COMMUNITY-ACQUIRED PNEUMONIA

The cause of community-acquired pneumonia (CAP) is confirmed in approximately 50% of elderly patients (52, 53). *S. pneumoniae* accounts for 40 to 60% of the established cases of acute bacterial pneumonia. Clinical and radiographic presentations are diverse, but pneumococcal infections present as bronchopneumonia more often than as a lobar consolidation. Other bacteria to be considered in CAP are *Haemophilus influenzae* (especially in COPD patients), enteric Gram-negatives (in debilitated hosts), *Legionella pneumophila* (widely varied incidence) and mycoplasma (uncommon and generally mild illness). *S. aureus, Moraxella (Branhamella) catarrhalis,* and anaerobes are also contributing causes of CAP. Mixed bacterial or bacterial/viral infections must also be considered.

A major consideration in CAP is the site for treatment. Can the patient safely stay at home or is hospitalization required? Hospitalization is usually easiest for the physician, but this may be neither the patient's wish nor in his or her best interest. If the person has been functioning well at home and has no evidence of worsening chronic diseases, home treatment should be considered if the patient has (*a*) desire for home care, (*b*) pneumonia limited to one lobe, (*c*) good oxygen saturation without labored breathing, (*d*) good nutritional status and adequate hydration, (*e*) an adequate caregiver, (*f*) appropriate transportation to the hospital in case of clinical decline, (*g*) ability to be closely followed in the office or with home visits, and finally, (*h*) capability of taking the appropriate antimicrobial agent at home.

Because of the severity of acute lower respiratory tract infections and the dramatic age-related rise in mortality rates (especially in bacteremic patients), empiric antimicrobial therapy is initiated before the causative pathogen is isolated. The clinical setting and the patient characteristics at the time of diagnosis provide insight into which organism is the most probable cause of the pneumonia and affect choice of antibiotics. For clinically stable patients with CAP and a sputum Gram's stain demonstrating a predominant organism, treat accordingly. If good sputum is unavailable or a predominant organism is not identified, a second-generation cephalosporin (cefuroxime or cefotetan) is a reasonable first choice. Alternative agents include trimethoprim-sulfamethoxazole, amoxicillin-clavulanate (both available orally), ampicillin-sulbactam, and ticarcillin-clavulanate. The clinically unstable patient who may be immunosuppressed or has recently been on antibiotics requires combination antibiotic therapy regardless of Gram's stain results. A first- or second-generation cephalosporin (cefazolin or cefuroxime) plus an aminoglycoside is a rational first choice. Alternatives include a third-generation cephalosporin (ceftriaxone or ceftizoxime) with or without an aminoglycoside. Erythromycin and, in severe cases, rifampin should be added if there is any suspicion of *Legionella.*

NURSING HOME PNEUMONIA

Elderly residents of chronic care facilities have a reported incidence of pneumonia two to four times that of the noninstitutionalized. Infection accounts for 27% of transfers to acute care hospitals from nursing homes, and nearly one-half of these infections involve the respiratory tract (47). In the nursing home as in the hospital, patients are exposed to increasingly virulent organisms during a time of high vulnerability. Debilitated persons may not be able to give an interpretable history, and caretakers may not notice functional decline, especially if the patient is sedated or has serious neurologic disease. Up to 40% of nursing home patients with pneumonia are afebrile (54). These factors delay presentation to the physician. Frequent monitoring of residents, by measuring function and accurate respiratory rates, could lead to earlier recognition and treatment of pneumonia.

Pneumonia in the nursing home is likely to be a Gram-negative infection because of increased Gram-negative colonization in debilitated patients with multiple medical illnesses. Garb et al. (55) reported that antibiotic therapy was more common in the nursing home than in the community. A higher incidence of *Klebsiella* and *S. aureus* pneumonia was seen in nursing home patients (40% and 26%) than in CAP patients (less than 10% and 14%) (55). *S. pneumoniae* and *H. influenzae* together account for up to 40% of bacterial pneumonias in the institutionalized elderly (56). Mixed flora infections secondary to aspiration are frequent in nursing home pneumonia. Using transtracheal aspiration in radiographically confirmed pneumonia, Bentley reported 50% of infections to be associated with mixed flora (57).

Nursing home–acquired pneumonia may be treated in the nursing home if the patients are not severely ill or if they refuse hospitalization through advance directives or direct communication of their autonomous decision to the physician. Antibiotic therapy with oral agents used for community-acquired pneumonia would be appropriate for patients who are mildly to moderately ill (49). The severely ill patient should be treated as a person with a nosocomial pneumonia. If MRSA is present in the nursing home, vancomycin may have to be added to the treatment protocol (58). Ciprofloxacin has activity against MRSA, but many strains are resistant to this antibiotic (59).

NOSOCOMIAL PNEUMONIA

Nosocomial infection results from underlying illnesses as well as from therapeutic interventions. Patients in the hospital typically have impaired host defenses and therefore are most likely to be colonized with Gram-negative organisms.

Colonization, aspiration, recent surgery (especially thoracoabdominal surgery), and the use of mechanical ventilation devices are all associated with hospital-acquired pneumonia.

The primary cause of nosocomial pneumonia is Gram-negative bacilli. *P. aeruginosa* is present in approximately 30% of mechanically ventilated patients (60). Other etiologic agents include *S. aureus,* mouth anaerobes, and *S. pneumoniae. L. pneumophila* is also a consideration, and clinicians should know if it is present in the hospital water supply. Mixed flora infections secondary to aspiration may be the most common cause of nosocomial pneumonia but are difficult to document without invasive procedures (61). Bronchoscopy with a culture specimen obtained using a protected brush is often necessary to guide therapy in patients not responding to empiric treatment.

While awaiting culture results, empiric therapy for the clinically stable patient is a third-generation cephalosporin or second-generation (cefuroxime) plus piperacillin. Intravenous erythromycin, ceftazidime, and an aminoglycoside should be instituted in the patient with rapidly progressive pneumonia. Ceftazidime is recommended because it provides better coverage of Gram-negative bacilli, including *P. aeruginosa.* The use of vancomycin is also a consideration in hospitals with a high incidence of MRSA. If aspiration is suspected, a good choice is a third-generation cephalosporin and clindamycin.

When a hospitalized elderly patient with pneumonia deteriorates, a decision must be made whether to transfer the patient to the intensive care unit (ICU). Certain characteristics of the patient may help in this decision. A patient's desire for aggressive measures combined with a good premorbid functional status and a single-system failure (lung) help predict a positive outcome from ICU treatment. Keep in mind that patients with severe pneumonia may be destined to die and that intensive care and antibiotics may not change this outcome.

Pneumococcal immunization given at the time of a routine checkup or at discharge from the hospital is an underutilized ounce of prevention that could eliminate the need for pounds of cure (62).

VIRAL INFECTIONS

Viruses are often not considered in the differential diagnosis of respiratory infection in the elderly, but data suggest that viral agents cause a significant number of the cases of pneumonia. Morales (63) reported on respiratory tract infections in geriatric medical wards and found that 17% were caused by bacterial pathogens, and 27% were definite viral illnesses. The death rates for the two groups were similar. In adult patients hospitalized with community-acquired pneumonia, 4 to 19.5% of the cases have been associated with viral agents, most commonly with influenza type A (64). Although viral pneumonia in the elderly is most commonly due to influenza, respiratory syncytial virus, parainfluenza virus, adenovirus, cytomegalovirus, varicella-zoster and herpes simplex virus are also causative agents.

Influenza is the most common serious viral infection afflicting the elderly. The symptoms of influenza may not be typical. Cough, headache, and pneumonia are common in the older adult; but sudden onset of chills, fever, myalgias, and coryza are less frequent (65). Secondary bacterial pneumonia is extremely common, especially that caused by *S. pneumoniae, S. aureus* and *H. influenzae.* Influenza case-fatality rates in nursing home patients can be as high as 30%. Trivalent influenza vaccine is 30 to 70% effective in reducing clinical manifestations of disease and 60 to 90% effective in decreasing mortality in nursing home residents (66).

Amantadine, 100 mg daily, may reduce the clinical manifestations and duration of influenza A illness if started soon after the onset of symptoms. Confusion and disorientation are troublesome side effects of amantadine, and the dose needs to be reduced in the presence of renal disease. Amantadine chemoprophylaxis is 70 to 90% effective in preventing infections with influenza A but is of no benefit in preventing influenza B (67).

TUBERCULOSIS

Rates of tuberculosis increase with advancing age, and deaths due to *Mycobacterium tuberculosis* are also the highest in persons 65 years and older. The incidence of tuberculosis in nursing home residents is up to 10 times higher than that in elderly community dwellers, although up to 90% of tuberculosis in the elderly occurs outside chronic care institutions. (68).

The clinical diagnosis of tuberculosis in older patients is difficult. A significant number of patients manifest atypical complaints or exhibit only minor pulmonary symptoms. Weight loss or functional decline may be the only diagnostic clue. Any person suspected of tuberculosis should have a chest radiograph. In geriatric patients, pulmonary tuberculosis is not limited to the upper lobes. Reinfection in particular may involve middle and lower lobes as well as pleura. Infection may present as lobar pneumonia, bronchopneumonia, cavities, or interstitial infiltrates and may be bilateral. Culturing remains the standard procedure for definitive diagnosis of tuberculosis. Three fresh morning sputum specimens are recommended, but bronchoscopy may be required if sputum cannot be obtained.

The five tuberculin unit skin test is the primary screening test for tuberculosis. The predictive value of tuberculin skin testing for identifying infection with *M. tuberculosis* declines with advancing age. Remember the booster phenomenon when interpreting skin test results. Waning skin test reactivity is boosted by applying a second antigen challenge. It is important to apply the second skin test within 2 weeks after the initial negative skin test to ensure accurate interpretation of the response and to avoid identifying future positive skin test results as conversions when they are the result of the booster effect. All patients in chronic care facilities should therefore receive a two-step tuberculin skin test with controls on admission to eliminate interpretive confusion of future test results (69). Immunizations with BCG may affect skin test specificity, but this effect wanes after 10 years (70).

Treatment of active tuberculosis in older patients is the same as that for the general adult population. Isoniazid 300 mg daily and rifampin 600 mg daily for 9 months is commonly used. Since most older adults would have acquired their *M. tuberculosis* infection prior to the availability of modern chemotherapy, primary drug resistance of tubercle bacilli should be rare. Older patients receiving isoniazid are at increased risk for hepatitis. They should be monitored for symptoms of hepatitis and have serum glutamic oxaloacetic transaminase (SGOT) levels determined at 1, 3, and 6 months of therapy. If SGOT rises five times above the upper limit of normal or symptoms of hepatitis occur, isoniazid and rifampin should be discontinued. Isoniazid may be restarted at 50 to 100 mg per day after SGOT returns to normal levels. Doses may be gradually increased over several weeks, with careful monitoring for liver abnormalities. Isoniazid must be stopped and an alternative regimen used if SGOT elevation recurs. Pyridoxine (vitamin B_6) 50 mg daily is recommended to minimize the peripheral neuropathy associated with isoniazid.

Persons who have a positive tuberculin skin test and are at high risk for tuberculosis should receive preventive therapy with isoniazid (71). Residents of nursing homes are a high-risk group in whom the benefit of chemoprophylaxis outweighs the risk of isoniazid toxicity (72). A 12-month course of isoniazid 300 mg daily is 90% effective and must be monitored closely.

UNDERUSED PREVENTIVE MEASURES

Finally, it is important to reemphasize the prevention of unnecessary illness and death due to infectious disease. For example, the consequences of missed opportunities for vaccination were stressed in a CDC report of a fatal case of tetanus in an elderly woman gardener who had numerous prior contacts with the health care system but was not vaccinated against tetanus (73). Primary health care providers are urged to use every opportunity to review the vaccination status of their patients (73). Ensuring that every elderly patient has a primary tetanus-diphtheria immunization series, annual influenza immunization, and a pneumococcal pneumonia vaccination would do much to reduce the consequences of these infections.

REFERENCES

1. Terpenning MS. Infective endocarditis. Clin Geriatr Med 1992;8(4):903–912.
2. Gorse GJ, Thrupp LD, Nudleman KL, Wyle FA, Hawkins B, Cesario TC. Bacterial meningitis in the elderly. Arch Intern Med 1984;144:1603–1607.
3. Levine WC, Smart JF, Douglas LA, Bean NH, Tauxe RV. Foodborne disease outbreaks in nursing homes, 1975 through 1987. JAMA 1991;266:2105–2109.
4. Cooper C, Cawley MID. Bacterial arthritis in the elderly. Gerontology 1986;32:222–227.
5. Ben-Yehuda A, Weksler M. Host resistance and the immune system. Clin Geriatr Med 1992;8(4):701–711.
6. Kiecolt-Glaser JK, Dura JR, Speicher CE, et al. Spousal caregivers of dementia victims; longitudinal changes in immunity and health. Psychosom Med 1991;53:345–362.
7. Setia U, Serventi I, Lorenz P. Bacteremia in a long-term care facility. Spectrum and mortality. Arch Intern Med 1984;144:1633–1635.
8. Gleckman R, Hibert D. Afebrile bacteremia. A phenomenon in geriatric patients. JAMA 1982;248:1478–1481.
9. Norman DC, Toledo SD. Infections in elderly persons. An altered clinical presentation. Clin Geriatr Med 1992;8(4):713–719.
10. Castle SC, Norman DC, Yeh M, Miller MD, Yoshikawa TT. Fever response in the elderly. Are the older truly colder? J Am Geriatr Soc 1991;39:853–857.
11. Esposito AL, Gleckman RA. Fever of unknown origin in the elderly. J Am Geriatr Soc 1978;26:498–505.
12. Immergut MA, Gilbert EC, Frensilli FJ, Globe M. The myth of the clean catch urine specimen. Urology 1982;17:339–340.
13. Nicolle LE, Harding GKM, Kennedy J, McIntyre M, Aoki F, Murray D. Urine specimen collection with external devices for diagnosis of bacteriuria in eld-

erly incontinent men. J Clin Microbiol 1988; 26:1115–1119.

14. Grahn D, Norman DC, White ML, Cantrell M, Yoshikawa TT. Validating urinary catheter specimen for diagnosis of urinary tract infection in the elderly. Arch Intern Med 1985;145:1858–1860.

15. Zimmer JG, Bentley DW, Valenti WM, Watson NM. Systemic antibiotic use in nursing homes. A quality assessment. J Am Geriatr Soc 1986;34:703–710.

16. Boscia JA, Kobasa WD, Knight RA, Abrutyn E, Levison ME, Kaye D. Epidemiology of bacteriuria in an elderly ambulatory population. Am J Med 1986; 80:208–214.

17. Boscia JA, Kobasa WD, Knight RA, Abrutyn E, Levison ME, Kaye D. Therapy vs no therapy for bacteriuria in elderly ambulatory nonhospitalized women. JAMA 1987;257:1067–1071.

18. Nicolle LE, Mayhew JW, Bryan L. Outcome following antimicrobial therapy for asymptomatic bacteriuria in elderly women residents in an institution. Age Ageing 1988;17:187–192.

19. Nicolle LE, Mayhew WJ, Bryan L. Prospective randomized comparison of therapy and no therapy for asymptomatic bacteriuria in institutionalized elderly women. Am J Med 1987;83:27–33.

20. Boscia JA, Kaye D. Asymptomatic bacteriuria in the elderly. Clin Geriatr Med 1988;4(1):57–70.

21. Abrutyn E, Boscia JA, Kaye D. The treatment of asymptomatic bacteriuria in the elderly. J Am Geriatr Soc 1988;36:473–475.

22. Gleckman R, Blagg N, Hibert D, Hall A, Crowley M, et al. Acute pyelonephritis in the elderly. South Med J 1982;75:551–554.

23. Hooton TM, Stamm WE. Management of uncomplicated urinary tract infection in adults. Med Clin North Am 1991;75(2):339–357.

24. Safrin S, Siegel D, Black D. Pyelonephritis in adult women: inpatient versus outpatient therapy. Am J Med 1988;85:793–798.

25. Morton P, Thompson AN. Oral acyclovir in the treatment of herpes zoster in general practice. NZ Med J 1989;102:93–95.

26. Straus SE, moderator. NIH conference. Varicella-zoster virus infections: biology, natural history, treatment and prevention. Ann Intern Med 1988; 108:221–237.

27. Braun JL, Silvetti AN, Xakellis GC. What really works for pressure sores. Patient Care 1992;26:63–83.

28. Albright JW, Albright JF. Aging of immunity to animal parasites. Geriatr Focus 1993;3:4.

29. Degelau J. Scabies in the nursing home. Clin Rep Aging 1989;3:1–4.

30. Yankosky D, Ladia L, Gackenheimer L, Schultz MW. Scabies in nursing homes: an eradication program with permethrin 5% cream. J Am Acad Dermatol 1990;23:1133–1136.

31. Oklahoma State MRSA Working Group in conjunction with Oklahoma State Department of Health. Recommendations for the transfer of patients colonized with antibiotic resistant bacteria between facilities and the control of methicillin-resistant Staphylococcus aureus in acute and extended-care facilities. Oklahoma City: Oklahoma State Department of Health, May 1990.

32. Murphy S, Denman S, Bennett RG, Greenough WB, Lindsay J, Zelesnick LB. Methicillin-resistant Staphylococcus aureus colonization in a long-term care facility. J Am Geriatr Soc 1992;40:213–217.

33. Nelson JD. Managing the dry eye. Postgrad Med 1989;85:38.

34. Pollack M. Pseudomonas aeruginosa. In: Mandell GL, Douglas RG, Bennett JE, eds. Principles and practice of infectious diseases. 3rd ed. New York: Churchill Livingstone, 1990:1680.

35. Norman DC, Yoshikawa TT. Intraabdominal infections in the elderly. J Am Geriatr Soc 1983;31:677–684.

36. Carter AO, Borczyk AA, Carlson JAK, et al. A severe outbreak of Escherichia coli 0157-H7-associated hemorrhagic colitis in a nursing home. N Engl J Med 1987;317:1496–1500.

37. Bennett RG, Greenough WB III. Diarrhea: a ubiquitous disease in older persons. Clin Rep Aging 1987;1(6):1–9.

38. Roos KL. Meningitis as it presents in the elderly: diagnosis and care. Geriatrics 1990;45:63–75.

39. Dajani AS, Bisno AL, Chung KJ, et al. Prevention of bacterial endocarditis. Recommendations by the American Heart Association. JAMA 1990;264: 2919–2922.

40. Valenti WM, Trudell RG, Bentley DW. Factors predisposing to oropharyngeal colonization with gram-negative bacilli in the aged. N Engl J Med 1978; 198:1108.

41. Esposito AL, Gleckman RA, Cram S, Crowley M, McCabe F, Drapkin MS. Community-acquired bacteremia in the elderly: analysis of one hundred consecutive episodes. J Am Geriatr Soc 1980;28:315–319.

42. Whitelaw DA, Rayner BL, Wilcox PA. Community-acquired bacteremia in the elderly: A prospective study of 121 cases. J Am Geriatr Soc 1992;40:996–1000.

43. Gleckman R, Blagg N, Hibert D, et al. Catheter-related urosepsis in the elderly: a prospective study of community-derived infections. JAGS 1982;30:255–257.

44. Meyers BR, Sherman E, Mendelson MH, et al. Bloodstream infections in the elderly. Am J Med 1989;86:379–384.

45. Bender BS. Sepsis. Clin Geriatr Med 1992;8(4):913–924.

46. Centers for Disease Control. Hospitalizations for the leading causes of death among the elderly—United States, 1987. MMWR 1990;39(43):777–779.

47. Ely EW, Haponik EF. Pneumonia in the elderly. J Thorac Imaging 1991;6(3):45–61.

48. Andrews J, Chandrasekaran P, McSwiggan D. Lower respiratory tract infections in an acute geriatric male ward: a one-year prospective surveillance. Gerontology 1984;30:290–296.

49. Berman P, Hogan DB, Fox RA. The atypical presentation of infection in old age. Age Aging 1987; 16:201–207.

50. McFadden JP, Price RC, Eastwood HD, Briggs RS. Raised respiratory rate in elderly patients: a valuable physical sign. Br Med J 1982;284:626–627.

51. Harper C, Newton P. Clinical aspects of pneumonia in the elderly veteran. J Am Geriatr Soc 1989; 37:867–872.

52. Marrie TJ, Durant H, Yates L. Community-acquired pneumonia requiring hospitalization: five-year prospective study. Rev Infect Dis 1989; 11(4):586–599.

53. Marrie TJ, Haldane EV, Foulkner RS, et al. Community-acquired pneumonia requiring hospitalization: is it different in the elderly? J Am Geriatr Soc 1985;33(10):671–680.
54. Marrie TJ. Pneumonia. Clin Geriatr Med 1992; 8(4):721–734.
55. Garb JL, Brown RB, Garb JR, et al. Differences in etiology of pneumonias in nursing home and community patients. JAMA 1978;240:2169–2175.
56. Bentley DW. Bacterial pneumonia in the elderly. Hosp Pract 1988;23:99–116.
57. Bentley DW. Bacterial pneumonia in the elderly: clinical features, diagnosis, etiology, and treatment. Gerontology 1984;30:297–307.
58. Hsu CC, Macaluso CP, Special L, et al. High rate of methicillin resistance of *Staphylococcus aureus* isolated from hospitalized nursing home patients. Arch Intern Med 1988;148(3):569–570.
59. Wolfson JS, Hooper DC. Fluoroquinolone antimicrobial agents. Clin Microbiol Rev 1989;2(4):378–424.
60. Fagon JY, Chastre J, Domart Y, et al. Nosocomial pneumonia in patients receiving continuous mechanical ventilation. Am Rev Respir Dis 1989; 139:877–884.
61. Fein AM, Feinsilver SH, Niederman MS. Atypical manifestations of pneumonia in the elderly. Clin Chest Med 1991;12(2):319–336.
62. Fedson DS, Harward MP, Reid RA, et al. Hospital-based pneumococcal immunization: epidemiologic rationale from the Shenandoah Study. JAMA 1990; 264(9):1117–1122.
63. Morales F, Calder MA, Inglis JM, et al. A study of respiratory infections in the elderly to assess the role of respiratory syncytial virus. J Infect 1983; 7:236–247.
64. Crossley KB, Thurn JR. Nursing home-acquired pneumonia. Semin Respir Infect 1989;4(1):64–72.
65. Cate TR. Clinical manifestations and consequences of influenza. Am J Med 1987;82(suppl 6A):15–23.
66. Saah AJ, Neufeld R, Rodstein M, et al. Influenza vaccine and pneumonia mortality in a nursing home population. Arch Intern Med 1986;146:2353–2357.
67. Centers for Disease Control. Prevention and control of influenza. Recommendations of the Immunization Practices Advisory Committee. MMWR 1992; 41(No RR-9):1–17.
68. Stead WW, Dutt AK. Tuberculosis in elderly persons. Annu Rev Med 1991;42:267–276.
69. Finucane TE, for the Clinical Practice Committee of AGS. The American Geriatrics Society statement on two-step PPD testing for nursing home patients on admission. J Am Geriatr Soc 1988;36:77–78.
70. Snider DE Jr. Bacille Calmette-Guerin vaccinations and tuberculin skin tests. JAMA 1985;253(23): 3438–3439.
71. Centers for Disease Control. Screening for tuberculosis and tuberculous infection in high-risk populations and the use of preventive therapy for tuberculosis infection in the United States. Recommendations of the Advisory Committee for Elimination of Tuberculosis. MMWR 1990;39(No RR-8):1–12.
72. Yoshikawa TT. Tuberculosis in aging adults. J Am Geriatr Soc 1992;40:178–187.
73. Centers for Disease Control. Tetanus fatality—Ohio, 1991. MMWR 1993;42(8):148–149.

22/ HIV Infection in Older Persons

Tom J. Wachtel, Michael D. Stein

EPIDEMIOLOGY

The AIDS epidemic in the United States has affected primarily young adults because the prevalence of behaviors that result in infection with HIV is higher in that age group. Indeed, industrialized nations are still experiencing the epidemiologic pattern in which 80 to 90% of HIV transmission is attributable to male homosexual contact or intravenous drug usage (IDU) (1). However, with a 10.4% proportion of cases in persons 50 years of age or above, geriatricians cannot ignore the epidemic (2).

Blood transfusion is the mode of transmission in only 1% of aged 13 to 49, but grows to 6% of patients aged 50 to 59, 28% of patients aged 60 to 69, and 64% of patients aged 70 or above (2). Other changes that can be attributed to blood transfusion as the dominant mode of transmission include the proportion of women, increasing with age from 6% of those aged 50 to 59 to 13% of those aged 60–69 and 29% of patients 70 and above, and the proportion of white persons, increasing with age from 56% (age 13 to 49), 63% (age 50 to 54), 70% (age 60 to 69) to 82% (age 70 and above).

Blood transfusion is a very efficient mode of inoculation, with each contaminated unit associated with a 90% probability of infection (1). Most of the transfusion-acquired HIV infections in one study occurred during coronary bypass surgery (3). Both nonwhites (4) and women (5) are less likely to be subjected to this type of surgery in the United States. Since the introduction in 1985 of routine screening of blood products for antibodies to HIV, it is estimated that the risk for contracting HIV by transfusion is now lower than 1:150,000 per unit transfused (6).

PRIMARY CARE OF HIV-INFECTED OLDER PERSONS

HISTORY

Up to the age of 70, homosexual contact is the most common mode of transmission (2); therefore,

questions about sexual activity are important. In our experience, older people are willing to discuss these sensitive areas. Questions specifying high-risk sexual activities should be asked directly and nonjudgmentally. A positive history of sexually transmitted disease should be considered a marker for HIV infection.

Equally important is a history of transfusions between 1978 and 1984. An estimated 20,300 persons over age 50 received transfusions contaminated with HIV (7). Since the incubation period between inoculation and a diagnosis of AIDS is estimated to average 8 to 10 years (8, 9), we can expect additional cases over the next few years as elderly persons transfused during the early 1980s become symptomatic. Indeed, elderly people with HIV infection have lower CD4 counts at the time of diagnosis (183 ± 140 cells/mm^3 in persons over age 55 compared with 402 ± 248 cells/mm^3 in persons under age 40) and more frequently present with AIDS at the time of diagnosis (36 vs. 5%), both observations suggesting that the diagnosis of HIV infection is delayed in older persons (3).

The injection of illicit drugs should be discussed openly but the yield of this area of inquiry generally will be lower than in younger persons.

The review of systems should focus on constitutional symptoms (weight loss, fever, night sweats, fatigue), decreased physical or mental function, pain and specific symptoms such as lymphadenopathy, rashes, oral lesions, headaches, decreased vision, cough, dyspnea, recurrent pneumonias, abdominal pain, diarrhea, recurrent vaginal discharge, and abnormal bleeding (10).

PHYSICAL EXAMINATION

The patient's weight should be recorded at each visit. The oral cavity is often the site of early manifestations of HIV infection. These include herpetic lesions, thrush, bacterial periodontitis, hairy leukoplakia (plaques on the side of the tongue), and nodules, which may represent Kaposi's sarcoma or lymphoma. The skin can also be involved early in the course of HIV infection; common skin disorders in HIV infection include viral infections (herpes simplex, herpes zoster, molluscum contagiosum, human papilloma virus) fungal infections (candidiasis, cryptococcosis), bacterial infections (staphylococcus, syphilis) and noninfective disorders (seborrheic dermatitis, psoriasis, pruritic papules, Kaposi's sarcoma, and drug reactions).

The lymph node groups should be examined; generalized lymphadenopathy may be the only manifestation of HIV disease. Lymph node biopsy should not be routine but should be considered if a single lymph node is rapidly enlarging, if the patient has "B type symptoms" of lymphoma, or if confirmation of a diagnosis of fungal or mycobacterial disease is needed.

The pulmonary and cardiovascular examination should be documented for baseline purposes, together with liver and spleen size. The genitalia and rectum should be examined for the presence of any sexually transmitted disease. In women, recurrent *Candida* vaginitis is considered a marker of HIV disease, and the increased risk of cervical cancer in HIV-infected women calls for Pap smears every 6 months.

The nervous system is involved in as many as 80% of patients with HIV disease, because the AIDS virus itself and many of the complicating opportunistic infections (e.g. *Cryptococcus*) or malignancies (e.g. lymphoma) have an affinity for it. Therefore, a careful baseline neurologic examination is important and should include cranial nerve, motor, sensory, cerebellar, and reflex testing. HIV infection has been recognized as an important cause of dementia in older individuals (11). In one study, HIV encephalopathy was diagnosed in 24% of patients above 55 years of age, compared with only 9% of patients under the age of 40 (3). Therefore, a formal mental status examination should be performed every 3 to 6 months in all elderly persons with HIV infection.

DIAGNOSTIC STUDIES (Table 22.1)

Testing for HIV is clearly the first step in the diagnosis of HIV infection. The actual ordering of an HIV test should always be preceded by pretest counseling. Test recipients should be advised that testing can be performed anonymously at various testing sites or that it can be performed confidentially in the doctor's office. People have many misconceptions about the test. They should be told that a positive test does not imply AIDS, but rather infection with the virus that causes AIDS, and while they may remain asymptomatic for many years, they are contagious and must be taught how the virus is transmitted. Test recipients also should be told that while very accurate, predictive value of a positive test can be low if the pretest probability is low (i.e., in low-risk persons).

The physician must be aware of specific laws that exist in each state regarding the reporting of test results, the notification of partners, and the limits of confidentiality. False-negative tests may occur early in the course of infection, during the window of seroconversion. Therefore, persons participating in HIV risk activities may need to be retested. Causes for false-positive test results include chronic liver disease, autoimmune diseases, multiple myeloma, and infection with other retroviruses. Test results should always be given in person, which allows patients to ask questions and express feelings, as well as the development of a management plan.

Most laboratories perform the ELISA and Western blot tests sequentially on a specimen submitted for HIV testing. The ELISA test is extraordinarily sensitive (99.5%) but less specific (98%). The Western blot test, used for confirmation of a positive ELISA, is less sensitive (98%) than the ELISA test, but very specific (99.7%). Other tests for HIV infection include radiofluorescent antibody (RFA) and polymerase chain reaction (PCR).

The CD4 helper lymphocyte is a direct target of HIV, and its count is the most widely used indicator of a patient's level of immunodeficiency. The CD4 count is currently used to guide decisions regarding antiretroviral therapy and prophylaxis against opportunistic infections. Because there is variability in CD4 results depending on laboratory expertise, intercurrent infection, or time of day the specimen is drawn, treatment decisions should be based on several values.

Many staging systems have been suggested, the most widely used being the CDC classification system for HIV infection (12). In the clinical setting, we find it more useful to stratify patients into four groups according to the CD4 count. This stratification allows predictions of prognosis and vulnerability to specific HIV-related disorders. Having more than 500 CD4 cells/mm^3 indicates a robust immune system, and patients with such counts are almost always asymptomatic. Below 500 and above 200 cells/mm^3, patients are usually asymptomatic but susceptible to bacterial and minor fungal infections; they should be treated with antiretroviral therapy aimed at postponing the onset of symptomatic disease. Below 200 cells/mm^3, antiretroviral therapy is continued, and pro-

Table 22.1
Management of Older Persons with HIV Disease

	CD4 = 750 cells/mm^3	CD4 = 350 cells/mm^3	CD4 = 70 cells/mm^3
Routine physical examination	Every 3 to 6 months	Every 3 months	Monthly
HIV test	Once	Once	Once
Pelvic examination/Pap	Every 6 months	Every 6 months	Every 6 months
Cognitive testing	Every 6 months	Every 3 months	Monthly
CBC	Every 3 to 6 months	Monthly	Monthly
BUN and/or creatinine	Yearly	Every 3–6 months	Every 3–6 months
Transaminase, alkaline phosphatase	Yearly	Every 3–6 months	Every 3–6 months
Syphilis serology	Once	Once	Once
CD4 count	Every 6 months till <600, then every 3 months	Every 3 months	Every 3 months
PPD	Yearly	Yearly	Yearly
CXR	Baseline	For pulmonary symptoms or as otherwise needed	For pulmonary symptoms or as otherwise needed
Pneumococcal vaccine	Once	Once	Once
Influenza vaccine	Yearly	Yearly	Yearly
Antiretroviral therapy	No	Yes	Yes
PCP prophylaxis	No	No	Yes
MAI prophylaxis	No	No	Yes

phylaxis against opportunistic infections is suggested. Patients with fewer than 200 cells/mm^3 should be protected against *Pneumocystis carinii* pneumonia (PCP). Below 100 cells/mm^3, patients usually have advanced disease and are most susceptible to opportunistic infections; at this point, consideration is given to substitution or addition of other antiretroviral treatment (didanosine (ddI) and zalcitabine (ddC)), prophylaxis against additional opportunistic infections, and closer patient monitoring.

Other diagnostic studies should include complete blood counts, renal function tests, liver function tests, baseline hepatitis serology, baseline syphilis serology, skin testing for anergy and tuberculosis, and a baseline chest roentgenogram. Substantial consensus exists for planning the following care and laboratory testing of individuals, depending on CD4 count (13). Cancer screening should be offered as recommended for other patients of similar age, except for Pap smears, which should be obtained every 6 months.

TREATMENT

The reader is referred to specific textbooks on AIDS for the management of opportunistic infections and malignancies (14). This section deals principally with the management of HIV disease in the primary care setting.

Antiretroviral Therapy

Three drugs are currently FDA approved as antiretroviral agents, and all three inhibit viral reverse transcriptase: zidovudine (AZT), ddI, and ddC. AZT is the most widely used and the accepted first-line agent. It may be initiated in patients with CD4 counts of 500 cells/mm^3 or less. The standard dose is 200 mg orally three times daily. The most common side effects, nausea, headache, restlessness, and insomnia, usually decrease over time and are managed symptomatically. Intractable headaches, gastrointestinal distress, or myositis may require drug discontinuation. Many patients receiving AZT develop macrocytosis, and its absence may suggest noncompliance. Severe anemia can occur and require a lower dosage of AZT or the addition of erythropoietin. Viral replication continues, and the disease advances in spite of AZT therapy, perhaps as a result of viral resistance to AZT.

After 12 to 24 months using AZT, patients may continue AZT or have an additional medicine added or substituted. DdI is usually administered to adults at a dose of two 100-mg tablets twice daily, and substituted for rather than added to AZT. Indeed, HIV resistance to AZT may wane, thus allowing reintroduction of AZT at a later date. The major adverse reactions to ddI are pancreatitis and peripheral neuropathy. DdC on the other hand is recommended for use with AZT. The recommended dose on adults is 0.75 mg t.i.d., and like ddI, it is associated with peripheral neuropathy.

Pneumocystis carinii Pneumonia Prophylaxis

When the CD4 count falls below 200 cells/mm^3, oral sulfa-trimethoprim (Bactrim, Septra) is recommended at a dose of one double-strength tablet daily or every other day. This regimen has been shown to be more effective than aerosolized pentamidine (15), which should be reserved for patients who develop toxic reactions (usually a rash) to sulfa-trimethoprim. Aerosolized pentamidine is administered monthly at a dose of 300 mg. Oral dapsone 50 mg/day may be as effective as aerosolized pentamidine in the primary prevention of PCP (and, like bactrim, may have the additional benefit of preventing toxoplasmosis), although it has been less well studied in clinical trials.

Prophylaxis for MAI and Fungal Infections

At CD4 cell counts below 100 cell/mm^3, patients are most susceptible to opportunistic infections. At this time, many clinicians offer additional forms of prophylaxis. Rifabutin (300 mg/day) and clarithromycin (500 mg/day) may prevent *Mycobacterium avium-intracellulare* infection (MAI), a progressive systemic infection characterized by fevers, diarrhea, and weight loss (16). Similarly, fluconazole (100 to 200 mg/day) has been used to prevent two infections: *Cryptococcus* and candidiasis.

VACCINATION

All patients with HIV infection should be given pneumococcal vaccination once, as early in the course of illness as possible, to increase the likelihood that the patient will develop protective antibodies. Indeed, bacterial infections, while not AIDS-defining illnesses, play an important role in the morbidity and mortality of patients with HIV disease. Influenza vaccination should be given yearly for the same reason. Hepatitis B vaccination should be reserved for patients whose personal behavior places them at risk for infection, and who show no laboratory signs of previous immunity. Of course, tetanus vaccination should be up to date (every 10 years) as in all adults.

Table 22.1 displays the routine diagnostic and therapeutic measures that the authors use as guidelines for the management of all elderly persons with HIV infection.

COURSE OF ILLNESS

The prognosis of HIV disease is considerably worse in persons over 50 years of age than in younger persons (17, 18). Many studies on prognosis are flawed by inaccurate information on the date of seroconversion and the finding that older people with HIV infection are diagnosed later in the course of infection (2, 3). Nevertheless, the information available from cohorts of HIV-infected hemophiliac patients and blood transfusion recipients indicates rather convincingly that survival time after an AIDS diagnosis is inversely related to age (19), that the period between inoculation and an AIDS diagnosis is inversely related to age (19), and that infection in older adults progresses to subclinical immunodeficiency more rapidly than in younger adults (20). A recent study from Canada indicated a mean time from AIDS diagnosis to death of 6.3 ± 5 months in patients above age 55 and 16.5 ± 9 months in patient under age 40 (3). Causes of death in older patients with AIDS are similar to those described in younger patients (3, 21), with opportunistic infections and bacterial infection leading the list in all age groups.

Finally, quality of life is important to consider in patients with HIV disease as it is in any terminal illness. We have shown that it can be reliably measured with the Medical Outcomes Study Instrument (22), which explores six dimensions of well being: physical function, role functions, social function, mental health, health perception, and pain. All other known parameters being equal, older age is associated with lower quality of life scores in all the dimensions measured by the instrument. In addition, equally important, was the finding that symptoms are the strongest correlates of well-being, suggesting that aggressive management of patient complaints in HIV disease can achieve a positive impact on quality of life.

REFERENCES

1. Holmes KK. The changing epidemiology of HIV transmission. Hosp Pract 1991;26:153–178.
2. Ship JA, Wolff A, Selik RM. Epidemiology of acquired immune deficiency syndrome in persons aged 50 or older. J Acquired Immune Deficiency Syndrome 1991;4:84–88.
3. Ferro S, Salit IE. HIV infection in patients over 55 years of age. J Acquired Immune Defic Syndr 1992; 5:348–355.
4. Johnson PA, Lee TH, Cook EF, Rouan GW, Goldman L. Effect of race on the presentation and management of patients with acute chest pain. Ann Intern Med 1993;118:593–601.
5. Ayanian JZ, Epstein AM. Differences in the use of procedures between women and men hospitalized

for coronary heart disease. N Engl J Med 1991; 325:221–225.

6. Cumming PD, Wallace EL, Schorr JB, Dodd RY. Exposure of patients to human immunodeficiency virus through the transfusion of blood components that test antibody negative. N Engl J Med 1989; 321:941–946.

7. Peterman TA, Lui KJ, Lawrence DN, Allen JR. Estimating the risks of transfusion-associated acquired immmunodeficiency syndrome and human immunodeficiency virus infection. Transfusion 1987;27:371–374.

8. Medley GF, Anderson RM, Cos DR, Billard L. Incubation period of AIDS in patients infected via blood transfusion. Nature 1987;328:719–721.

9. Bacchetti P, Moss AR. Incubation period of AIDS in San Francisco. Nature 1989;338:251–253.

10. Lynn LA. Primary care for HIV infection. Hosp Pract 1992;27:48–64.

11. Philip GW, Mungas D, Pomeranz S. AIDS as a cause of dementia in the elderly. J Am Geriatr Soc 1988; 36:139–141.

12. Centers for Disease Control. MMWR 1992; 41(RR18):1–29.

13. Stein MD, O'Sullivan P, Rubenstein L, Weller P, Wachtel T. The ambulatory care of HIV-infected persons: a survey of physician practice patterns. J Gen Intern Med 1992;7:180–186.

14. Sande MA, Volberding PA. The medical management of AIDS. 3rd ed. Philadelphia: WB Saunders, 1992.

15. Schneider MME, Hoepelman AIM, Karel J, Schattenkerk KME, Nielsen TL, Van Der Graaf Y, et al. A controlled trial of aerosolized pentamidine or trimethoprim-sulfamethoxazole as primary prophylaxis against Pneumocystis carinii pneumonia in patients with human immunodeficiency virus infection. N Engl J Med 1992;327:1836–1841.

16. Horsburgh CR. Mycobacterium avium complex in acquired immunodeficiency syndrome. N Engl J Med 1991;324:1332–1338.

17. Piette JD, Mor V, Fleishman JA. Patterns of survival with AIDS in the United States. Health Serv Res 1991;26:75–95.

18. Sutin DG, Rose, DN, Mulvihill M, Taylor B. Survival of elderly patients with transfusion-related acquired immunodeficiency syndrome. J Am Geriatr Soc 1993;41:214–216.

19. Stehr-Green JK, Holman RC, Mahoney MA. Survival analysis of hemophilia-associated AIDS cases in the United States. Am J Public Health 1989; 79:832–835.

20. Goedert JJ, Kessler M, Aledort LM, et al. A prospective study of human immunodeficiency virus type 1 infection and the development of AIDS in subjects with hemophilia. N Engl J Med 1989; 321:1141–1148.

21. Stein M, O'Sullivan, Wachtel T, Fisher A, Mikolich D, et al. Causes of death in persons with human immunodeficiency virus infection. Am J Med 1992; 93:387–390.

22. Wachtel T, Piette J, Mor V, Stein M, Fleishman J, Carpenter C. Quality of life in persons with human immunodeficiency virus infection: measurement by the medical outcomes study instrument. Ann Intern Med 1992;116:129–137.

23/ Nutrition and Health in the Elderly

B. Lynn Beattie, Victoria Y. Louie, Johanna Dwyer

Mark Twain said, "The only way to keep your health is to eat what you don't want, drink what you don't like, and do what you'd druther not." Nutrition, health, and aging are related, and in recent decades, choices of food and drink have made healthy eating easier. The objective of this chapter is to provide some understanding of the role of nutrition in aging, health, and disease, along with some practical guidelines for assessment and thoughtful intervention. We hope that these comments are more useful than Mark Twain indicated, since "nutrition is the environmental factor most subject to human control in contributing to the health of the aging and aged" (1).

Fries (2) speculated that the goal of a long and vigorous life may be attainable as a result of the compression of morbidity from chronic disease into the very latter part of human life. However, it appears that increasing longevity is usually accompanied by fair or poor health and limited activity, especially in the ninth and tenth decades of life (3). There is evidence in North America today that mortality from "lifestyle diseases," such as heart disease and stroke, is declining (4–6). Is personal responsibility for health producing the impact? How much of this responsibility is related to nutrition?

Exton-Smith (7) observed that individual dietary patterns in most old people remain similar to those that have been acquired by habit established at a younger age. Nutritional health education is, therefore, an early responsibility in life. There is a great need for longitudinal studies and standardized surveys that measure dietary intake and incorporate clinical examination and laboratory investigation to develop meaningful descriptions of the specific nutritional needs of the elderly population. The American Dietetic Association position statement emphasizes the relationship between nutrition, aging, and health (8). The "association supports comprehensive nutrition services for the elderly as an integral component of the continuum of health care." Good health with increased physical activity stimulates appetite and thereby promotes better intake of nutrients.

Aging brings progressive loss of tissue function along with possible accumulation of diseases, including osteoporosis, atherosclerosis, cancer, obesity, diabetes mellitus, and hypertension. Application of current knowledge of nutritional risk factors may influence the impact these diseases have on our society. Hazzard (9) commented in legal prose:

Whereas all age-related diseases are (by definition) time-dependent; and
Whereas all such processes are multifactorial in origin; therefore:
Single modality intervention late in life is unlikely to yield appreciable benefit;
Intervention should be multifactorial and begin at an early age.

NUTRITION AND LONGEVITY

Knowledge of the relationships between nutrient intake and duration of life span is expanding. Dietary restriction in laboratory animals can be brought about by reducing daily intake of a nutritionally adequate diet (one that supports maximal growth), intermittently feeding a nutritionally adequate diet (e.g., feeding every second, third, or fourth day), and feeding ad libitum a diet containing insufficient amounts of protein to support maximal growth (10).

McCay et al. (11, 12) showed that although growth was retarded, the life span of rats was increased with dietary restriction. Masaro (13) notes from animal studies that food restriction retards the aging process, extending the life span and altering the rate of increase in age-specific mortality. This is apparently due to energy restriction, not restriction of a specific nutrient(s). The mechanism may involve a reduced rate of production of reactive oxygen molecules, an increased ability to scavenge them, increased ability to repair molecular damage, or a combination thereof. Whether these findings have applicability to human aging is debated. A cohort of individuals (following vegetarian diets and health-conscious lifestyles) from Germany have been followed longitudinally (11 years), and mortality from all causes was reduced by half, compared with the general population (14). Factors other than diet, such as abstinence from smoking and selection bias, no doubt played a role.

There is an urgent need for research into levels of specific nutrients and eating patterns that will optimize physical and mental development in youth, physiologic performance during adulthood, and retention of health and vigor in senescence. This research needs to be extended from laboratory animals to man.

NUTRITION AND AGING

With aging, physiologic changes may affect ingestion and enjoyment of food. The sense of taste changes with aging. The number of taste buds on the lateral surfaces of the tongue that detect sweet and salty tastes decrease, leaving the central taste buds, which identify sour and bitter tastes, to predominate. The sense of smell tends to decline also, and the combined loss of gustatory and olfactory senses may lead to less interest in food. Decreased salivary flow, poor dentition, and decreased power of mastication that accompany the aging process may limit the amount and variety of foods eaten. The superimposition of various pathological conditions may emphasize these physiologic changes.

Ingestion may be hampered by the edentulous state, gingival lesions, mucous membrane erosions, or difficulty swallowing. The most common age change in the digestive tract with nutritional implications is achlorhydria (15), as it occurs in 25% of subjects over age 60. Lactase deficiency may also increase with aging, but to date no systematic study has been undertaken.

Digestion tends to be slower with aging. There is a reduced capacity to regulate metabolism, hormonal induction of enzymes requires more time, and reduced numbers of hormone receptors are evident on cell surfaces. These factors may be increasingly significant in the face of pathological changes such as hiatus hernia, reflux, and/or atrophic gastritis. Absorption appears to be little affected by aging, but many factors including quality of nutrients, the presence of medications, and the presence of various disease states may affect this function.

The cumulative effects of the changes of aging are more prominent as the years go on. Pathology may be superimposed. Awareness of both kinds of change is necessary when assessing nutritional vulnerability.

DIETARY SCREENING

The need for screening for those at risk of malnutrition is now well accepted, although there is less unanimity on how best to do it. The principles of the Canadian Task Force on the Periodic Health Examination have included screening for risk of malnutrition in the elderly, based on prudence. Historical information related to tobacco use, alcohol use, physical activity, and loneliness are some of the items physicians are to include (16). The American Academy of Family Physicians, the American Dietetic Association, and the National Council on Aging, Inc. are promoting the Nutrition Screening Initiative (NSI) in the United States (17). The focus is on the elderly, seen to be the single largest demographic group at disproportionate risk of malnutrition and potentially amenable to preventive strategies. The NSI is aimed at enhancing public awareness. A checklist, "DETERMINE your nutritional health," has been devised for the older person or the caregiver of those thought at risk of poor nutrition. Nutritional screen I by a social service or health care professional is recommended. If necessary, it is followed with screen II, which includes laboratory work and is completed by a health care professional in a medical setting. The innovations of NSI are that it grew from consensus of a multidisciplinary group and there is an emphasis on preserving the function of the individual. From screens I or II, targeted interventions are made.

Horwath (18), in a comprehensive review, noted that the two factors most consistently associated with poor dietary intake in the elderly were low social status and, among men only, living alone. Niewind et al. (19) determined that use of dentures reduced overall food variety and that living situations, particularly living alone, exerted negative influences on food variety.

Dwyer (20) commented on the important convergence of prevention and treatment measures as various groups review the importance of dietary intervention, and further outlined 12 steps involving medical, nutrition, and behavioral science skills for achieving lasting dietary change and relevant impact on chronic disease (21). Crucial to dietary change is the application to primary care and continuing patient education (22). McNutt (23) suggested that educational methods such as focus groups and student (e.g., patient) as teacher are two techniques that could be relevant to the needs of the older person. Stanek et al. (24) surveyed nurses practicing in long-term care facilities and found that just over 60% indicated that the quality and quantity of their nutritional education was sufficient, underlining again the importance of health professional education. Similarly, physician education in nutrition has been limited.

ASSESSMENT OF NUTRITIONAL STATUS

Nutrition assessment and intervention are essential components of nutrition services and integral to the continuum of health care for the elderly (8, 23, 25). Nutritional status is the health condition of an individual as influenced by his or her intake and utilization of nutrients. Its assessment requires the corroboration of data from clinical, dietary, anthropometric, and biochemical evaluations. Simultaneous use of these techniques serves to substantiate and increase the sensitivity by which individuals at risk for protein-calorie malnutrition, nutrient deficiencies, or overnutrition may be identified. In the elderly, the assessment of nutritional status is complicated by age-related changes in routinely measured parameters and by lack of appropriate standards for interpretation of most measurements.

CLINICAL HISTORY

When addressing nutritional assessment, it is important to assess attitude and interest in life and the activities of daily living. The role physical disabilities may play in either procurement or preparation of foods is significant. Problems in ingestion and digestion must be addressed. Noteworthy are food avoidances and preferences. A history of bone fracture(s) or abdominal surgery may be relevant. A complete drug history, including prescribed medications, over-the-counter medications, and laxatives, is necessary. Bowel and urinary habits may influence personal eating habits. The health of nails, hair, and skin and the predisposition to infection and ability to heal are important indicators of nutritional and general health.

The physician may assess nutritional risk through review of clinical status by history, physical examination, and assessment of the general intake of the major food groups. Baker et al. (26) studied the effectiveness of clinical evaluation of nutritional status, and examiners agreed in 81% of cases. This clinical evaluation correlated well with objective measures, although the oldest patient was only 76 years of age. Subsequent referral to a dietitian for a more extensive dietetic history is indicated when risk is evident and when intervention is recommended.

DIETARY ASSESSMENT

Dietary assessment is important as an indicator of nutritional status. It offers the most practical means of predicting an individual's nutritional risk. The estimated food and nutrient intake of an individual is evaluated against appropriate dietary standards.

There are a number of methods developed for the collection of data on food intake. The 24-hour recall provides a retrospective account of foods actually consumed in the previous 24 hours. It is a simple and rapid means of obtaining information at an interview. Because the accuracy of the information obtained depends on memory capabilities, the 24-hour recall may yield unreliable data from older individuals, particularly older men. Nevertheless, the method is a tool for securing information on food and mean nutrient intakes of large groups of 50 or more individuals, although it tends to underestimate caloric intake (27).

A more extensive diet history, which attempts to describe the general pattern of food usually consumed over a period of time, also can be recalled at an interview. The method incorporates the 24-hour recall, but it uses a checklist of predetermined foods to ensure the completeness of recalled information and subsequently verifies the data against a 3-day record of actual food intake.

Generally, more-accurate data presume a well-defined dietary pattern, and while the extensive dietary history takes into account seasonal variation in food intake, it is time consuming, it requires skilled interviewers, and it depends on the recall abilities of subjects.

The method that affords the greatest accuracy is the weighed food record, which records present intake of foods through accurate weighing and correction for plate wastes.

Direct observation of the elderly at mealtimes may be the method of choice for the collection of food consumption data (28). This method may be limited to institutions and nursing homes and to the study of individuals or small groups. Brown et al. (29) have suggested a videotape method for evaluation studies.

Following data collection, the actual nutrient intake is interpreted by comparison with the dietary standard. The standards of adequacy applied have varied from 100% of the Recommended Dietary Allowances (RDAs)/Recommended Nutrient Intake (RNIs), to 67%, to as low as 40% (30). This makes comparison of survey data difficult and recommendations for individuals arbitrary.

Dietary assessment often depends on recall and good interview techniques. Presence of a relative or significant other and use of a checklist may be helpful. Data collected are compared against the RDAs/RNIs as the nutritional standard.

CLINICAL ASSESSMENT

Clinical evaluation involves assessment of the mouth, skin, hair, eyes, nails, lower extremities, and various organs and systems.

Angular stomatitis or cheilosis may be associated with niacin, riboflavin, or pyridoxine deficiency, but both are seen with ill-fitting dentures. Poor oral hygiene and periodontal disease produce changes that are indistinguishable from deficiency glossitis and gingivitis. The raw appearance of the tongue with filiform papillary atrophy is associated with niacin deficiency, and a magenta color reflects riboflavin deficiency, although irritants, systemic antibiotics, and uremia are possible causes for the discoloration. Soft and spongy bleeding gums indicate ascorbic acid deficiency or poor oral hygiene. The condition of the skin may reflect an individual's nutritional status. Dry, inelastic skin may be associated with aging alone, dehydration, or follicular hyperkeratosis of vitamin A deficiency; nasolabial seborrhea with lack of pyridoxine; and skin lesions of the exposed parts of the body with niacin deficiency. Dryness, thickening, and opaqueness of the conjunctivae are observed with progressively advanced vitamin A deficiency. Pale mucous membranes and cupping of the nails suggest inadequate iron. Lack of luster, depigmentation, and easy "pluckability" of the hair may accompany protein deficiency. Edema of the extremities may be associated with thiamine lack or protein deficiency from many causes. Enlargement of the liver or the thyroid, petechiae, ecchymoses, and other nonspecific findings should be considered in the overall assessment.

Clinical assessment is highly subjective, and physical signs may indicate multiple nutrient deficiencies, nonnutritional influences, or combinations.

ANTHROPOMETRY

Anthropometry is a useful, noninvasive means of evaluating nutritional status from measurements of body composition. It allows the assessment of an individual's muscle mass (protein) and energy reserve (fat). The most common measurements are height, weight, triceps skinfold thickness, and upper arm circumference.

Accurate estimates of height are important for use in computing several indices of nutritional status. Standing height may be obtained by direct measurement or by measurement from crown to heel in the supine position (31). The presence of kyphosis or flexion contractures of the legs may invalidate these estimates. Age-related bone loss also contributes to progressive loss in stature. Alternate means of predicting full adult height, such as knee-to-ankle ratios, have been proposed, but these must be validated for all heights and races (32).

Body weight should be measured under standard conditions to minimize errors introduced by diurnal variation, clothing, different weighing scales, and other considerations such as dressings, casts, or artificial limbs. Appropriate standards of weight for height in the elderly are limited. The 1983 Metropolitan Height and Weight Tables show the average weights of younger men and women associated with the lowest mortality. Average weights of the elderly up to age 74 years have been compiled by Frisancho (33) as percentile distributions based on data from the first and second National Health and Nutrition Examination Surveys. There are questions about whether the standard applies to all races and if the criteria for assigning frame size are justified (32). Another index of nutritional status based on height and weight for the estimation of body composition is the Quetelet or Body Mass Index (BMI). The BMI (weight (kg)/height (m²)) is an index of obesity. Weight may be measured against the Age-Specific Gerontology Research Center Recommendations (34), although these have been criticized by some investigators as being too heavy. The Canadian Guidelines for Healthy Weights have been developed for adults 20 to 65 years of age. A target BMI is recommended, and a continuum related to potential of health problems below and above acceptable levels; a BMI between 20 and 25 is a good weight for most people. How this standard applies to those over 65 has not yet been ascertained. Arbitrarily, weight 20% above the desirable weight is considered as evidence of overnutrition, while weight that is 20% or more below the desirable weight is considered presumptive of undernutrition (35). Information on the rate and extent of weight loss/gain as well as the current weight relative to the usual body weight and the average weight for the population provides some estimate of the presence or risk of developing malnutrition. At present, the soundest weight recommendation for health is an attempt to maintain healthful weights in young adulthood with no more than a 10- to 15-pound weight gain with aging. Sustained losses of as little as 10 to 15 pounds can improve morbidity and mortality of those who gain more. Knowledge of weight loss of 5% or more in 6 months or less is significant. A keen eye to fit of clothing and belt tightening is helpful in raising awareness. Roy et al. (36) emphasized the significance of weight loss of greater than 6% in preoperative assessment predicting postoperative complications.

The Creatinine Height Index (CHI) estimates muscle protein by comparing the 24-hour creatinine excretion of an individual with that of the standard healthy individual of the same height. This tool is most practical in a research setting and may lack validity in older adults.

Bioelectrical impedance is a relatively new, economical, inexpensive and simple but as yet insufficiently standardized technique for assessing lean body mass and fatness. Recently, attention has been drawn to skeletal muscle function. Jeejeebhoy (37) has demonstrated that the force-frequency curve of the adductor pollicis muscle, obtained by stimulating the ulnar nerve at the wrist, is a sensitive and specific measure of nutrient intake or withdrawal. This technique is not affected by age and disease and has the advantage of being useful for ill or sedentary individuals.

Recording serial weight measurements remains the most practical way to assess significant fluctuations in nutritional status or change in chronic disease states. Age- and gender-specific standards must be applied when using standards. Measures of muscle strength, including ability to rise from seating and to use kitchen implements, are keys to evaluation.

LABORATORY ANALYSIS

Laboratory evaluation provides an objective means of assessing nutritional status. The selective use of biochemical analysis provides data to substantiate clinical judgment and dietary evaluation. The measurements may not accurately identify a subclinical deficiency state, but they may have prognostic value.

The initial laboratory evaluation should include hemoglobin, hematocrit, red cell morphology, WBC with differential, total protein, and albumin determinations. Further evaluation, when indicated, should include serum iron, transferrin, red blood cell folate, serum cobalamin, calcium, phosphorus, alkaline phosphatase, urea, creatinine, and serum lipid determinations. Finally, specific tests may be indicated. These would include urinary vitamin levels, studies of absorptive capacity, measurement of trace elements, and assessment of the immune system. Michel et al. (38) recommend plasma thyroxine-binding prealbumin and retinol-binding protein levels as truer indicators of subclinical malnutrition and of response to enteral and parenteral nutrition. Detsky et al. (39) suggested that clinical judgment with serum albumin concentrations could best predict nutritionally associated complications in surgery. Klonoff-Cohen et al. (40) demonstrated that serum albumin decreased and globulin increased in a longitudinal study of community-living elders. Reduced serum albumin was associated with increased 3-year mortality. Practically, clinical status and weight changes are most useful.

Care must be taken in interpreting results of some of the vitamin and trace mineral assessments. Serum (plasma) ascorbate levels, for example, are likely to reflect recent dietary intakes of vitamin C and not the state of the body's reserve of the vitamin. With vitamin C deprivation, serum ascorbate levels fall rapidly to near zero while reserves in other tissues are depleted only 50% (41). Because the white blood cell ascorbate levels relate to tissue stores of the vitamin, the levels fall more slowly, and only when the reserve is down to 20% of normal do symptoms of scurvy occur. Ascorbic acid saturation tests, which determine the extent of tissue saturation, may be used for corroboration when presumptive evidence of deficiency is present.

Zinc is involved in enzymatic reactions that are predominantly intracellular. Plasma zinc levels are a poor measure of body zinc content, and a small shift from intracellular fluids may markedly increase the plasma concentration. Although low plasma zinc is found in zinc deficiency states, it may be associated with low serum albumin states, infection, trauma, myocardial infarction, neoplasm, or low-dose estrogen treatment. Zinc levels can be measured in hair samples, but valid results are difficult to ascertain. More recently, leukocyte zinc content has been suggested as a better index of zinc status. Goode et al. (42) developed techniques for the isolation of polymorphonuclear and mononuclear cells for zinc analysis to overcome the problems of the influence of differential leukocyte count on total leukocyte zinc. A single observation may not be relevant to zinc status. Complex cellular phenomena appear to control zinc levels. Serial measurements, after zinc supplementation, may indicate a therapeutic response. Further studies are required to evaluate the effects of zinc supplementation on cellular immunity, one of the integral roles for zinc function.

Radiological studies and bone densitometry may reveal significant bone changes including osteoporosis and osteomalacia. Other studies, such as those of the gastrointestinal tract and kidney, may point to specific problems.

Laboratory or radiological evaluation may confirm suspicions based on clinical and dietary history and physical examination or may be used to monitor clinical management.

DIETARY STANDARDS

The RDAs (43) in the United States have been defined by the Food and Nutrition Board of the National Academy of Sciences of the United States as the levels of intake of essential nutrients considered, on the basis of available scientific knowledge, to be adequate to meet the known nutritional needs of practically all healthy persons. In Canada, similar values are the RNIs (44).

The RDAs and RNIs reflect the current knowledge derived from epidemiologic findings, food consumption patterns, animal research, and metabolic studies on nutrient requirements, and they are subject to periodic revision. Set above the average physiologic requirement, the levels cover variations in the needs of nearly all individuals in each category of the population (45). The probability is high that an individual's needs will be met and dietary deficiency be unlikely when nutrients are consumed at the recommended level (46). The RDAs/RNIs are not guaranteed to represent complete nutrient needs for any one individual, particularly when additional demands are engendered by illness, injury, or surgery.

The standards in the United States and Canada differentiate energy requirements only for age groups under 50 years. Fewer calories are required to maintain the basal metabolic rate in the older individual, but there are few quantitative data, and age-associated adjustments in calorie intake are not absolute (10). Current assumptions are that even though caloric requirements decrease after age 50, most nutrient levels should remain relatively constant, with the exception of a decrease in iron for postmenopausal women. With accumulated information, there is every reason to believe that more-specific recommendations can be made for those aged 51 and over, and relevant modification to the RDAs/RNIs is in order.

Leverton (47), in her commentary "The RDAs Are Not for Amateurs" pointed out that effective application of the RDAs requires understanding, skill, restraint, and even tolerance. She noted that their existence has been a potent factor in coordinating and directing dietary planning and nutritional teaching. She cautioned against the use of the RDAs as the basis for fabricated, contrived, or synthetic foods.

The RDAs/RNIs are given in terms of nutrients, and these can be hard to interpret because we eat foodstuffs composed of various combinations. Thus, food groups that will supply the nutrients must be identified. The revised "Dietary Guidelines for Americans" and similar "Canada's Guidelines for Healthy Weights" and Nutrition Recommendations (48) for Canadians outline the basic principles of a sound diet: eat a variety of foods; maintain desirable weight; avoid too much fat, saturated fat, and cholesterol; eat foods with adequate starch and fiber; avoid too much sugar; avoid too much sodium; and if you drink alcoholic beverages, do so in moderation. The challenge for the aging population is to maintain nutrient content with a decrease in the amount of energy or calories related to physical activity.

ENERGY

Energy sources are protein, carbohydrate, and fat. For the elderly, there is controversy about the most appropriate balance between them and the amounts needed. Young (49) emphasizes the energy balance equation:

$$\text{Stored energy} = \text{energy intake} - \text{energy expenditure.}$$

Energy is required for basal metabolic rate, physical activity, and thermogenesis. The FAO/WHO/UNU 1985 (50) procedure for estimating energy needs is based on kilograms of body weight. To date, energy requirements for the elderly are essentially the same as those for younger individuals. Clearly "research is required on actual levels of energy expenditure, on the metabolic responses to altered energy intakes and on the significance of different energy sources in relation to maintenance of body composition and function" (49).

PROTEIN

With decrease in lean body mass (muscle), there is a decline in the muscle contribution to protein metabolism. Further, a redistribution in total protein synthesis occurs, with the metabolically active visceral organs making a more important contribution to nitrogen metabolism.

Munro and Young (51) showed that with similar and adequate protein intake, the total rate of albumin synthesis in the elderly is less than that in younger adults. Gersovitz et al. (52) noted in a 30-day metabolic nitrogen balance study that where energy intake approximates requirement, the current RDA is inadequate for male and female subjects 70 years of age and above. Young and Pellett (53) reviewed available information and concluded that a somewhat higher recommendation for protein should be made for the elderly. The daily intake should be not less than 12 to 14% of caloric intake. Recently, speculation regarding the role of protein intake in kidney dysfunction in those with already compromised status has been raised. With current knowledge, however, protein intake restriction should probably be limited to patients in mid to late chronic renal failure.

RDAs for protein in the elderly are uncertain. The decrement in lean body mass and altered rate of protein synthesis with increasing age enhance the uncertainty. Requiring further investigation are the data showing that older people, particularly those with chronic disease, may need more protein to achieve nitrogen balance (51) than do young adults.

CARBOHYDRATES

There is evidence that glucose tolerance changes with increasing age. It is estimated that approximately 20% of the elderly over age 80 years have diabetes mellitus, predominantly type II, non-insulin-dependent (54). However, advancing age alone may account for only 1 to 6% of the variances in insulin response among the elderly. Other age-related environmental factors such as obesity, physical inactivity, and use of potentially diabetogenic drugs may play significant roles.

Treatment of diabetes in the elderly is similar to that for younger diabetics (57). Diet remains the cornerstone of therapy to achieve euglycemia in both insulin- and non-insulin-dependent diabetes (IDDM and NIDDM, respectively). The recommended diet provides, as proportions of total calories, 55 to 60% carbohydrate, <30% total fat, and 12 to 20% protein. The dietary prescription is consistent with the fundamentals of good nutrition as outlined in the RDAs, the Dietary Guidelines for Americans, and the recommendations of the American Heart Association and the National Cancer Institute (55). Attempts should be made to alter lifestyle within an acceptable degree to encourage compliance with diet (56). Diet should be complemented by exercise within the limits of individual capacity.

With respect to diet, maintenance of healthful weights is the priority, despite the difficulties related to limited availability of standards for the elderly. It is not known whether elderly diabetics tend to be more overweight than healthy nondiabetic elderly subjects. Rosenthal et al. (57) have emphasized that institutionalized elderly diabetics are more commonly underweight. Total calories may first be aimed at weight reduction but must be adjusted once this has been achieved. As with all prescriptions, adequate follow-up and education are important. (Refer to Chapter 35 for a more complete discussion of diabetes mellitus in the elderly patient.)

Although different carbohydrate-containing foods elicit variable glycemic responses in individuals with IDDM and NIDDM, studies have shown that the glycemic effect of a single food is mitigated when it is consumed as part of a complete meal. In most individuals, modest amounts of sucrose or other refined carbohydrates may be acceptable, contingent on metabolic control and body weight. The revised Exchange Lists for Meal Planning (58) will facilitate menu planning for a high-carbohydrate, high-fiber, fat-modified diet.

FATS

The risk of CHD (coronary heart disease) increases with elevated total cholesterol (TC) and other factors including smoking, hypertension, diabetes (59), and possibly coffee consumption (60), inactivity, and obesity. Decreasing the risk of CHD must address all risk factors, not just TC alone. Chapter 24 reviews lipid abnormalities in the elderly.

It is reasonable to recommend modification of lifestyle and treatment for known risk factors including obesity, hypertension, and diabetes. The availability of highly effective drugs such as reductase inhibitors, which decrease cholesterol production, and the interest of the pharmaceutical companies in these products, which may be presented to 15 to 20% of the population estimated to have hypercholesterolemia, provide a major challenge to the medical community. The availability of these drugs must not preclude appropriate dietary and lifestyle management.

For prevention of CHD in later life (after 65 years), maintaining TC as low as is realistic is a goal. Dietary prudence and lifestyle modifications in middle age may well reduce the burden of atherosclerosis in older age.

The ideal diet aims at reducing the intake of saturated fatty acids and cholesterol and maintaining desirable body weight. There is controversy about substituting carbohydrates, monounsaturated fatty acids, or polyunsaturated fatty acids for saturated fatty acids, but moderate introduction of all three may be viable. The National Institutes of Health (NIH) Consensus Development Panel (61) recommended a diet that provides 30% of energy as fat, divided equally between saturated (S), polyunsaturated (P), and monounsaturated fats, and limits cholesterol intake to 250 to 300 mg/day. Further dietary restrictions may be necessary to achieve the desired blood cholesterol levels in individuals. The suggested guidelines are consistent with those of the American Heart Association (62) and the National Cholesterol Education Program. Modest restrictions of total fat intake at a P:S ratio of >1 appears most effective in lowering LDL without a concomitant rise in VLDL or a similar fall in HDL. The cholesterol-lowering effects of n-6 polyunsaturates (63) and monounsaturated fats (64) as substitutes for saturated fats are established.

Minor modifications in eating patterns probably provide the best chance of obtaining optimal mean concentrations of cholesterol and low-density lipoproteins. This focus must be supported by other factors including restricted smoking and increased physical activity. Specific dietary restriction may be recommended for individuals with hyperlipidemic states. No studies to date demonstrate the effectiveness of attempting to lower serum lipids in the elderly. However, the potential benefit of this approach should not be precluded.

WATER

The aged, through custom or distaste, may consume less than optimal quantities of water (65). It is often more acceptable in soups, juices, tea, coffee, soft drinks, or milk products. The water content of diets has received increased attention with respect to its effect on utilization of other nutrients, but such effects have not been investigated in controlled studies in aged men.

Thirst responses tend to be impaired with increasing age (66, 67), and temperature regulation is less efficient in the elderly. These two homeostatic malfunctions, together with high ambient temperature, impaired mental function, or drugs such as chlorpromazine, may quickly lead to dehydration that may be fatal.

A daily intake of at least 1500 mL of fluid is recommended. Monitoring of diuretic therapy, prevention of unintentional diuresis from drugs, such as Dilantin, the tetracyclines, and some oral hypoglycemics, and ambient temperature control

is necessary. In institutions, provision of fluid in bedside containers does not ensure adequate hydration. These liquids must be actively offered at frequent intervals by concerned staff. Consistent adequate fluid intake is a preventive measure for constipation, a very common problem in the elderly.

Water is an important nutrient for every age group, especially the elderly. Awareness of changes in homeostatic regulation for the elderly and monitoring and controlling factors such as environment and drugs can prevent significant morbidity.

CALCIUM AND PHOSPHORUS

The current RDA and RNI for calcium in adults over 50 years is 800 mg/day. The level of dietary intake that meets the calcium requirement remains a controversial issue (68, 69). Whether calcium deficiency is a major cause of osteoporosis is central to the controversy (68, 70). Previous estimates were erroneously based on metabolic studies performed in young adults at zero calcium balance. In elderly men and women, there is an age-related reduction in calcium absorption, caused by impaired production of 1,25-dihydroxy vitamin D or secondary to relative hyperparathyroidism (71, 72).

Recent studies estimated the daily calcium allowances to be 1000 mg for estrogen-replete women and 1500 mg for estrogen-deprived women as a result of hormonal changes across menopause (73). The NIH Consensus Development Conference on Osteoporosis recommended that the calcium allowance for premenopausal and untreated postmenopausal women be increased accordingly (74). Similarly, the 1985 RDA Committee proposed higher recommendations: 800 mg for men and 1000 mg for women of ages 55 and older.

Heaney (69) is provocative in his review of information available to date, stating that there is benefit in providing adequate calcium, 1000 to 1500 mg, and vitamin D, 400 to 800 IU (10 to 20 μg), or both, to prevent osteoporotic fractures. It must be noted that the margin of safety for vitamin D (oral) is narrow, and concurrent consumption of fortified foods and supplement has been observed to cause hypercalcemia (44).

Osteoporosis is a heterogeneous, multifactorial disorder and is discussed in Chapter 31. Calcium deficiency, possibly exacerbated by vitamin D deficiency, may contribute to the pathophysiology of bone loss by reducing the maximal adult bone mass accumulated at skeletal maturity. Lower initial bone mass coupled with age-related bone loss results in reduced bone mass and increased fracture risk (75).

Inclusion of milk, dairy products, and calcium-rich foods is an important consideration throughout life (see Table 23.1). Recker and Heaney (76) concluded that milk and milk products recommended as sources of calcium may have an advantage as they do not suppress bone remodeling as severely as does calcium carbonate. Recker (77) suggested that calcium absorption from carbonate is impaired in achlorhydria and may not be the ideal supplement. Other available supplements include the gluconates and calcium-citrate-malate, an increasingly used food additive.

Preventive measures against osteoporosis must be begun early in life to ensure that the maximal bone mass is attained at skeletal maturity. Both weight-bearing physical activities and calcium nutrition play some role in the complex bone physiology. It is controversial whether calcium supplements or exercise can prevent age-related bone loss and osteoporosis, but it is reasonable to presume need for maintenance of calcium intake at least at current RDA/RNI recommendations throughout life.

VITAMINS

Vitamins are hormones as well as enzymes. Vitamin D acts as a hormone, while B vitamins act as coenzymes, combining with protein apoenzymes, to form holoenzymes. The cellular capacity for vitamins is saturated at levels of the vitamin in the range of the RDAs/RNIs. Undesirable effects of megadoses of vitamins have been recorded (78). Vitamins A, D, niacin, and B6 have been implicated, and possibly ascorbic acid as well.

Baker et al. (79) examined vitamin profiles in elderly institutionalized individuals and in healthy volunteers and detected subclinical vitamin deficits, particularly for B vitamins. They have recommended (80) parenteral multivitamin supplementation to bring levels to normal in some cases.

Drinka and Goodwin (81) reviewed the prevalence and consequences of vitamin deficiency in the nursing home. There appeared to be an increased requirement, particularly for some water-soluble vitamins, in a number of studies, and meeting the RDA in that substance in the diet was not adequate. They concluded that administration of an inexpensive multiple vitamin containing the RDA would be prudent in addition to placing the more debilitated residents on generic supplements containing several times the RDA of water-soluble vitamins. Donald et al. (82) studied community-living individuals between 65 and 74 years of age, and 41% of men and 67% of the women used supplements. The use of supplements of vitamins A and B_{12}, folacin, and zinc eliminated nutritional risk (defined by probability analysis), and calcium supplements reduced nutritional risk in both males and females.

Vitamin supplements at RDA/RNI levels are recommended for the frail elderly and for vulnerable individuals who have inadequate intake, disturbed absorption, or increased tissue requirements. Special consideration should be given to supplementation in nursing homes. Megavitamin consumption is questionable, and potential toxicity may ensue (83).

SALT

Carruthers (84) expressed concern that physicians and their patients have accepted too readily the option of long-term medication for hypertension rather than the review and revision of nutritional habits. He maintained that there is unequivocal evidence of a clear correlation between obesity and hypertension and focused on the association between high sodium intake and excessive caloric intake.

The control of dietary salt intake may be offset by the presence of sodium in many foodstuffs and medications. Fast foods and processed foods such

Table 23.1
Calcium Content of Some Foods[a]

Food Sources	Quantity	Calcium (mg)
Dairy products		
Low-fat (2%) milk	250 ml	314
Skim milk	250 ml	318
Buttermilk	250 ml	300
Cheddar cheese	45 g	324
Swiss cheese	45 g	432
Processed cheese	45 g	277
Cottage cheese, low-fat	250 ml	142
Yogurts, plain low-fat	175 ml	348
Ice cream	125 ml	92
Nondairy products		
Red kidney beans	250 ml	102
Soya beans	250 ml	115
Broccoli	1 stalk	158
Nuts	125 ml	175
Brazil nuts	125 ml	128
Salmon, with bones	100 g	258
Sardines, with bones	7 medium	393
Scallops	6	115
Tofu (processed with calcium sulfate)	125 ml	145

[a]Modified from Pennington JAT, Church HN. Bowes and Church's food values of portions commonly used. 14th ed. New York: Harper & Row, 1984.

as canned soups are notorious for salt content. Medications also may add substantial salt intake.

Awareness of the potential preventive aspects of limiting salt in the diet should be maintained. Restaurants and fast-food outlets should use less salt; customers should be allowed to determine their own salt preference. Not salting food discourages the expectation of saltiness, and because the taste preference for sodium diminishes after a few months of restriction, good adherence is achievable (85). Hypertensive patients should use less salt. The effectiveness of thiazide therapy in hypertension is enhanced by reduced salt intake.

FIBER

The human digestive tract does not contain enzymes necessary for the breakdown of dietary fiber. Aging, growth, food preparation, and hydrochloric acid in the stomach affect the cellular structure of plant material, leaving the fiber constituents: cellulose, hemicellulose, pectin, gums, mucilages, and lignin. These constituents pass through the small intestine to the colon, where they are acted on by intestinal bacteria.

The Expert Advisory Committee on Dietary Fibre (86) indicated that there are four specific physiologic effects for different types of dietary fiber: (a) regularizing colonic function, (b) normalizing serum lipid levels, (c) attenuating the postprandial glucose response, and (d) (perhaps) suppressing appetite.

As little as 2 to 4 g of dietary fiber can alter bowel behavior. Ten to 15 g of fiber affect stool volume, possibly by increasing bulk from water absorption. This amount of fiber promotes peristalsis and decreases transit time. It produces fatty acid and sequesters bile salts in the small intestine, with a subsequent additional cathartic effect. Dietary fiber supplementation, particularly for institutionalized individuals, is a popular mode for alleviating constipation (87).

The type and amount of fiber ingested may influence colonic bacterial flora and possibly decrease colonic cancer risks (88). Lack of fiber has been implicated in diverticular disease. Hypocholesterolemic function has been attributed to gelling fibers (86), but overall it is thought that changes in steroid excretion may be attributable to other mechanisms as well. Existing studies show that serum cholesterol-lowering effects are modest at best.

The potential of fiber for influencing carbohydrate absorption and insulin response curves in management of diabetes mellitus is being considered. Anderson and Sieling (89) reported favorable results of high-carbohydrate, high-fiber diets on glucose metabolism on older diabetic patients. They noted that patients who have well-controlled diabetes mellitus on oral agents or who are taking less than 40 units of insulin respond especially well. The major diabetes associations now agree that there may be definite benefits from increasing the consumption of carbohydrate foods high in fiber (86).

Dietary fiber in very large amounts may have untoward effects by decreasing the apparent digestibility of other nutrients or by causing abdominal distress through increasing intestinal transit time. It may bind trace elements, making them unavailable for absorption.

The role of dietary fiber is not yet defined clearly enough to transpose with assurance the clinical and experimental studies to physiologic needs (90). Fiber content of a variety of foods is included in Table 23.2. The equivalent of up to 10 g of bran per day to the diet has been recommended for maintenance of normal bowel function. This supplement must be accompanied by adequate fluid intake.

MALNUTRITION

Malnutrition is a sequitur of disease whether physical, metabolic, emotional, or attitudinal (91). Malnutrition in the broad sense may describe populations either undernourished or overnourished. Acute illness and accidents require immediate attention to nutrition as well as other factors if needless morbidity and mortality are to be avoided.

O'Hanlon and Kohrs (30) reviewed 28 surveys assessing the intake of older Americans. They found that food energy and calcium were most frequently below standards, and protein and niacin were most frequently adequate. They noted difficulties in comparing results of studies because of differences in methodology and standards used. Horwath (18) reviewed 90 surveys of community-dwelling elderly and noted that calcium, zinc, magnesium, vitamin B_6, folate, and potassium were least adequately supplied. Ryan et al. (92) surveyed individuals at home between 65 and 98 years of age. They noted that over 20% skipped lunch and over 40% of men had intakes of vitamins A and D, calcium, and zinc significantly below the RDA, and over 40% of women had intakes of vitamin E, calcium, and zinc below the RDA.

OVERNUTRITION

Obesity is the common form of overnutrition. For most adults, a gain in weight is associated

Table 23.2
Dietary Fiber Content of Selected Foods (% of fresh weight)

Food	Fiber Method[a]			
	HPB	AOAC	Englyst	Moisture
White bread	1.84	2.11	1.78	40.4
Whole wheat bread	5.43	5.18	3.89	40.8
Oatmeal	9.82	9.25	7.29	11.1
Rice	0.85	1.96	0.5	29.5
Corn kernels	2.08	2.06	1.57	73.4
Baked potatoes	2.07	2.56	1.54	72.3
Celery	1.46	1.67	1.52	94.3
Broccoli	2.21	2.57	2.25	91.8
Carrots	2.71	2.95	2.72	88.4
Onions	1.45	1.42	1.40	91.6
Green beans	1.97	2.12	1.93	93.7
Peanuts	7.50	7.28	5.71	1.3
Orange	1.82	1.71	1.75	86.7
Apple	1.77	1.83	1.67	87.5

[a]Adapted from Scientific Review Committee. Nutrition recommendations: the report of the Scientific Review Committee. Ottawa: Canadian Government Publishing Centre, 1990:35.

with a gain in excess fat. There is progressive loss of lean body mass and increase in fat with increased age. The rate of fat accumulation is slower in physically active individuals. Moderating calorie intake and maintaining physical activity levels are the keys to successful weight control.

Andres (93) has concluded that the major population studies of obesity and mortality fail to show that overall obesity leads to greater risk of early mortality. He recommends, therefore, a need for reappraisal of advice on the subject of obesity and research into the possible associated benefits of moderate obesity. On the other hand, the Framingham Study (94) showed a clear relationship between weight (obesity) and coronary artery and cerebrovascular disease.

Kushner (95), after reviewing publications related to body weight and mortality, concluded that excess body weight is associated with increased mortality but that the relationship is modified by fat pattern, gender, and age. Lifestyle issues (cigarette smoking, alcohol consumption, and physical activity) are modifiable risk factors. Changes in body weight (fluctuations related to dieting) may affect mortality, although the data are difficult to interpret.

Paganini-Hill et al. (96) concluded that individuals at least risk for significant osteoporosis and hip fracture are those who tend to be overweight. The role of adipocyte production of estrogen is entertained. De Waard (97) has suggested that perhaps calorie restriction and weight loss would be an adjunct to hormonal or chemotherapy for breast cancer in obese postmenopausal women.

He based this on the assumption that diet and/or nutritional status contain promoting factors for breast cancer.

One should be cautious when advising overweight healthy elderly people to lose weight, and be conservative about weight goals. Individuals with high blood pressure or diabetes mellitus, however, will likely benefit by weight loss. Very restrictive diets of 600 to 1000 calories should seldom be considered for elderly people, particularly those who participate in physical activities. A 1200 to 1500 calorie diet may be preferable, allowing a flexible meal pattern that is adequate in the RDAs/RNIs. Vitamin and mineral supplements should be considered for sedentary individuals who require more caloric restriction.

UNDERNUTRITION

Many interrelated factors contribute to the nutritional vulnerability of the elderly, including physical, psychological, socioeconomic, and cultural considerations. For many, aging is coping with losses. Loved ones and contemporaries die or live significant distances away. Retirement may impose loss of social and economic status. Inflation may add to this burden. Declines in physical and mental health may restrict activity, particularly that associated with procurement and preparation of food. Any combination of isolation, relocation, loneliness, depression, economic constraint, and disability may lead to loss of appetite, impaired quality and variety of available foods, and subsequent marginal status. The advent of an acute episode such as bereavement or physical illness may tip the balance in favor of overt malnutrition.

Health care workers and other professionals as well as families should be aware of risk factors that may lead to malnutrition and should be alerted to the need for preventive intervention. The NSI material noted earlier in this chapter is a tool for awareness and education. Housebound individuals are often already known to health and social service agencies. Help with shopping, assistance in preparing meals, Meals on Wheels programs, luncheon clubs, and day centers are some measures that can be taken. "Health foods" and dietary supplement use should be monitored because such products tend to needlessly erode purchasing power and do not guarantee a balanced diet.

PROTEIN CALORIE MALNUTRITION

The definition of protein energy undernutrition is the loss of lean body mass (protoplasm, extracellular fluid, and bone) and adipose tissue because of inadequate intake of amino acids and calories. Existing amino acids are oxidized as fuel or catabolized for other purposes instead of being used for protein synthesis. With decreased intake, there is depletion of triglyceride in adipose tissue and decreased protoplasmic protein in muscle, liver, kidneys, gastrointestinal tract, pancreas, and skin. Weight loss occurs but may be masked by edema. For individuals in acute care situations, the problems may be immediate. It has been estimated that 25 to 50% (98) of patients in hospital for 2 weeks or longer suffer protein calorie malnutrition. The elderly are particularly vulnerable, in hospital and at home. Linn (99) observed that malnourished hospitalized patients are at high risk for long-term health problems, probably through continued or recurring episodes of malnutrition. Implied with malnutrition is a greater susceptibility to infection together with impaired mechanical, cellular, and humoral immunologic defenses.

A prominent nutrition problem in patients who are chronically or seriously ill is not that they cannot eat but that they do not willfully eat enough. Frequent encouragement with deference to personal preferences may not be adequate intervention, and special enteral or parenteral measures may be needed. The physiologic advantage of enteral nutrition is maintenance of structural and functional integrity of the small intestine. The use of enteral feeding solutions that are more nearly nutritionally complete than most intravenous solutions may be considered, and there are many choices (100).

Bastow et al. (101) described the benefits of supplementary nasogastric tube feeding after fractured neck of the femur in a group of elderly patients on an orthopaedic service. Although one in five of the subjects did not tolerate the tube feeding, treatment was associated with improvement in anthropometrics and, importantly, in clinical outcome, with shorter rehabilitation time and hospital stays. Mowe and Bohmer (102) underlined that despite the potential of relevant interventions, undernutrition continues to be unrecognized, especially in elderly patients in acute care. Nutritional variables were correlated with risk of developing infection or other major morbid complication or death in a geriatric rehabilitation unit (103).

Bernard and Rombeau (104) reviewed aspects of nutritional support for elderly patients including oral liquid supplementation, enteral feeding by tube, and parenteral feeding. There are many commercially available enteral feeding solutions. Because of the vast array and the expense of providing these substances, it may be useful for institutions to have a formulary with one standard meal replacement formula, one high-protein meal replacement formula, two hypercaloric formulas, and one elemental diet plus a protein, fat, and carbohydrate module. This approach will lessen the confusion from the many choices. Potential complications of enteral feeding and their management should be understood. Reading mixing and diluting instructions for enteral feeding is mandatory (105). Total parenteral nutrition may be a consideration in specific patients, but it is beyond the scope of this chapter.

Identification of individuals at risk for malnutrition is important whether they are at home or in acute or long-term institutions. The frail elderly are especially vulnerable. Prevention requires attention to nutritional status. Treatment of acute medical or surgical illness requires early intervention, possibly with enteral nutritional supplements, to modify or prevent the downhill course of nitrogen depletion.

NUTRITION AND DEMENTIA

Dementia and nutrition has several aspects: (a) the role of nutrient deficiencies in the development of dementia, particularly Alzheimer's disease and other syndromes of impaired cognition; (b) the role of nutrients in the treatment of dementia, particularly Alzheimer's disease and potentially reversible cognitive impairment (B_{12}, thiamine); (c) the potential for malnutrition due to self-neglect in some cases of dementia; (d) the potential for malnutrition due to high energy use in some individuals with dementia.

Many amino acids are precursors for neurotransmitters including tyrosine, tryptophan, threonine, histidine, and choline. Vitamin precursors include A, B_6, B_{12}, thiamine, niacin, riboflavin, C, D, E, and folic acid. The role of amino acid and vitamin deficiencies in dementing disorders has been evaluated (106), but their effects in the pathogenesis of Alzheimer's disease are uncertain. The role of minerals including aluminum in the development of Alzheimer's disease remains controversial. The use of supplements such as choline and lecithin has not been shown to be effective in treating the dementia or slowing down the disease. In vascular dementia, diet may play a role through effects on blood pressure and related risk factors, and nutritional control may alter progress of this type of dementia. Studies to date have suggested that individuals with vascular dementia tend to have less weight loss than those with Alzheimer's disease (106).

Another common dementia is due to alcohol excess. Abstinence and good nutrition including thiamine replacement may have a positive effect on this form of dementia. In clinical situations however, there is a group of patients who may well have complex pathogenesis with an early history of alcohol excess and then, despite withdrawal from alcohol, go on to have a progressive dementing disorder of the Alzheimer's type.

Loney et al. (107) suggested that in dementia, the disease itself does not affect nutrition, but secondary effects such as neglect and forgetting mealtimes, decreased motor skills, depression, paranoid reactions, and eating nonfoodstuffs or spoiled food may be more relevant. Malnutrition is more likely to be found in newly institutionalized (demented) individuals and is reversible, although unfortunately the dementia remains.

Monitoring weights is crucial (106, 108) among demented individuals. Rheaume et al. (109) used a pedometer to measure daily miles (despite some difficulties encouraging demented individuals to keep these in place) and presumed walking at a speed of 3 miles per hour. They found that the pacing group walked 3.9 ± 0.4 miles/day, and the sedentary group of demented individuals walked 2.4 ± 0.9 miles/day. From their calculations, they determined that pacers required an additional 1600 cal/day. Appetites may increase, but energy intake is seldom adequate, and ongoing weight loss is frequent.

Gray (106) has suggested a number of strategies for dealing with provision of adequate nutrition in demented individuals, including the need to understand behavioral and functional changes associated with the disorder (attention to energy requirements, olfactory and gustatory changes, difficulties with chewing and swallowing, and the often time-consuming and emotionally draining task of assisting with feeding). Dietary supplements may be in order to bolster energy requirements.

NUTRITION AND THE INSTITUTIONAL MILIEU

The need for institutionalization is often precipitated by a deterioration in the capacity for self-care or the loss of caretakers. Very few elderly view placement in an institution as an ideal alternative living arrangement. The loss of independence and privacy and the inability to assume previous lifestyles make the adjustment more difficult. Adaptive capacities may be diminished by illness.

The food service in an institution has the monumental task of providing attractive and nutritious meals that are pleasing to the palate. The quality of food service in any institution is constrained by budgetary restrictions necessitated by spiraling food and labor costs. Nevertheless, a dietitian's skills can be used to translate the resident's nutritional needs into an individualized plan.

Retraining residents to feed themselves should be encouraged whenever possible. Follow-up is critical to any plan to do this. In this case, observation of meal service allows the dietitian, nurse, or other staff to evaluate actual intake and alter the diet if necessary. Table 23.3 identifies some nutrient intake problems and possible solutions to be considered.

Food acceptance itself is a complex reaction determined by the physiologic, psychological, biochemical, social, educational, and sensory reactions of individuals moving in a framework of race, religion, tradition, economic status, and environmental conditions. Some degree of dissatisfaction is inevitable. Food preferences fall into distinct patterns, and knowledge of these patterns for an institutionalized group may minimize dissatisfaction and increase consumption.

Barr et al. (110) studied nutrient intakes of a group of women over 80 in a care facility. They found that only 75% of the food provided was consumed, with mean intake of vitamin C, iron, niacin, and riboflavin adequate compared with RDAs/RNIs, but average intakes of protein,

Table 23.3
Problems of Nutrient Intake and Potential Solutions[a]

Problems	Potential Solutions
Poor appetite and poor intake	Reassess eating capabilities and diet consistency
	Provide small portions, more frequent meals
	Tailor diet to personal preferences and food intolerances
	Offer selective menu
	Capitalize on breakfast, usually the best-eaten meal
	Consider use of high-caloric-density supplements or complete meal-replacement formulas
	Schedule aperitifs
	Allow sufficient time for meals
	Maintain oral hygiene and personal grooming
	Plan seating arrangements for compatibility
	Appeal to the senses by describing the aroma, taste, and visual appeal of a meal
	Remove from other residents with highly objectionable eating habits
	Establish patient rapport
	Maximize comfort and tolerance by proper positioning and management of pain and energy level
	Encourage use of dining room to increase socialization
	Encourage families to bring in favorite home-cooked or ethnic foods
	Use outings and catering activities to encourage participation
Low energy level	Keep food warm by using heat-retaining dishes
	Use high-caloric-density supplements
	Offer smaller portions, more frequent feeding
	Place liquids and beverages in paper cups and styrofoam
	Set up tray by making foods easily accessible, e.g., removing lids and opening packaged items; spreading butter and jam
	Allow sufficient time for meals by providing early trays
	Assist with feeding as necessary
Impaired vision	Ensure lighting is adequate
	Orient to tray or table setting
	Help set up tray
	Place food in reach
	Place tray in field of vision
Mastication	Assess need for dentures
	Ensure properly fitting dentures
	Modify food consistency, avoiding pureed whenever possible
	Offer pureed as a last resort
Hemiparesis	Offer bite-size portions, finger foods
Poor hand-to-mouth coordination	Help set up tray; place beverage to resident's functional side
	Use mechanical aids or adapted eating utensils
Dysphagia	Suction excess saliva before meals
	Allow sight and smell of food to stimulate salivation and prepare swallowing reflex
	Seat in an upright position with the head flexed slightly forward
	Encourage thorough chewing of food
	Offer solid foods—soft, moist, full-bodied, and held together well, e.g., fish, souffle, canned pears, ripe bananas
	Exclude pureed, sticky, stringy, grainy, acidic, or dry foods
	Provide thickened fluids, e.g., tomato juice, fruit nectar, eggnog
	Serve jello, sherbet, frozen juice, etc. if imbibing fluids is a problem
	Serve cold foods cold and hot foods hot to stimulate the senses
	Suggest exercise to improve swallowing, e.g., sucking on ice chips, frozen fruit juices

Table 23.3—*continued*
Problems of Nutrient Intake and Potential Solutions[a]

Problems	Potential Solutions
Objectionable behavior	Permit staff to role model desirable behaviors
	Seat according to compatibility and level of function
	Allow ample time to eat and provide flexible times of meal service
	Maintain calm, relaxed atmosphere; reduce background noise; minimize distraction by serving one food at a time
	Provide special plates and adapted utensils to maintain independence
	Encourage peer interaction and support
	Offer praise and encouragement for improvements

[a]The authors acknowledge contribution of members of the Gerontological Practice Group of the British Columbia Dieticians' & Nutritionists' Association, B. C., Canada.

calcium, vitamin A, thiamine, and zinc were lower than the standards. Advanced age was negatively correlated with overall dietary adequacy.

Mealtime tends to be a reference for the time of day for some individuals and may be the highlight activity of the day for others. Intake of food produces a psychologic need for social interchange. Many times the feeding situations in early life have a strong influence. The first sustained human contact and socially important transaction is feeding. It makes the world dependable, comforting, satisfying, and nonthreatening (111).

For the institutionalized aged, food may again become a symbol of security. The patient may reject food to manipulate the staff or concerned family. Staff attitudes may inadvertently promote dependency. Staff must be encouraged to patiently accommodate individual needs. If food on trays is attractively presented and judiciously chosen, monitoring of returns on trays may indicate a spectrum of problems from quality of food preparation to failure to address mental and physical handicaps of consumers. Table 23.4 describes considerations for planning institutional food services.

Asplund et al. (112) assessed psychogeriatric institutionalized patients. They found energy and protein undernutrition in 30% and obesity in 4% of the patients. Undernutrition did not correlate with duration of stay and was less frequent in subjects with their own teeth than in edentulous individuals. Because food intake was similar in patients with and without undernutrition, possible interactions between malnutrition and chronic psychiatric disorders in the elderly were considered, such as "generalized dysmetabolism" in handling of substrates. Morgan et al. (113) observed that women in a psychiatric hospital suffering from severe dementia weighed 15

kg less as a group than a comparison group of active elderly women living in the community consuming a similar calorie intake. The role of occult disease in the institutionalized group is uncertain.

Anderson (114) compared a group of institutionalized veterans with a group of clinic patients. The greatest dietary difference between the clinic and domiciliary patients was not related to the use of dentures. Findings suggested that regardless of earlier diet, older persons in institutions will eat nutritionally important foods if given the opportunity. Staff attitudes are important for institutional food services. If staff expect old people to be dependent and conforming (111), they may inadvertently extinguish independence. There is a nutritional bill of rights (American Dietetic Association 1976) in which the resident has a right to be as independent as possible in eating.

Institutional food is simply not everyone's home-cooked meal. The residents can be involved in menu revision. They may be solicited for menu suggestions and feedback once these are implemented. A representative of the dietary department should be identified to whom the resident may direct criticism and communicate changing food preferences. The dietitian or delegate must maintain a high profile to establish, observe, direct, encourage, and educate residents, families, and staff. Training dietetic and food service staff to monitor and note tray returns as part of their cleanup procedure is an asset.

NUTRIENT DRUG INTERACTIONS

Lamy (115) suggested that food-drug interactions are probably more common than indicated in the literature. Some associations between nutritional status and drugs include reduced albu-

Table 23.4
Components of Institutional Food Service and Considerations for Planning[a]

Component	Consideration for Planning
Menu design	Provide attractive meals based on the four food groups to meet the nutritional needs of residents
	Consider day-to-day variations in color and visual appeal, texture, consistency, size, shape, and flavor combination in each meal
	Survey ethnic, religious, and regional preferences
	Note personal preferences on residents' menus when a selective daily menu is not available and update
	Plan for longer menu cycle; 4 or more weeks is more desirable
	Consider the type of meal pattern, the number of food items offered, and the times meals are served, e.g., a choice of three-meal-a-day plan; four-meal plan consisting of a continental breakfast, late morning brunch, main meal in the late afternoon, and a substantial snack in the evening; or five-meal plan
	Choose a meal pattern that will be compatible with the sleeping habits of residents (i.e., early risers, early retirers)
	Ensure that no more than 15 hours elapse between the last meal of one day and the first meal of the following day
	Adjust menu to reflect holiday items, special occasions, and social activities
	Offer alternatives compatible with therapeutic dietary modifications
	Semiannually review menu on the basis of quality review standards, production efficiency, and cost factor
	Revise menu to incorporate seasonal fruits and more economical food items
	Establish daily feedback for updating of preferences, assessing acceptability of menu selection, and monitoring of residents' nutritional intake
	Select china for stability and ease of eating; consider use of plate guards and rimmed plates
Type of meal service and staffing	Family-style dining, i.e., delivery of bulk food to be distributed
	Buffet—smorgasbord service, self-served selection
	Encourage socialization of dietary staff with residents during mealtimes to provide individual attention and maintain rapport
	Adopt a policy for dietary and nondietary staff to help with serving, tray returns, etc.
Atmosphere of dining room	Create a comfortable homelike environment and subdued painted walls and good lighting
	Partition room with mobile dividers for intimacy
	Provide soft, nonobtrusive background music
	Arrange for attractive table setting that highlights the season and special events or themes
	Group no more than six residents around small tables
	Make tables available for singles or couples
	Position tables for ease of movement
	Offer choice of seating companion to stimulate socialization
	Base seating arrangements on the need for supervision, assistance, and level of orientation
	Encourage use of dining room for group-related cooking activities
	Minimize background noise emanating from television, trolley, clatter of cutlery and plates, and staff talk and consider use of thick wall hangings, baffles, and padded placemats
	Separate noisy and difficult residents and those with objectionable table manners

Table 23.4—*continued*
Components of Institutional Food Service and Considerations for Planning[a]

Component	Consideration for Planning
Food-related activities	Meal preparation, baking session
	Men's group; Ladies' friendship tea
	Reminiscence group (to discuss favorite, traditional, "by-gone" foods)
	Pub nites, family nites
	Outings to restaurants
	Outdoor picnics, barbecue
	Champagne breakfast
Cooking facility for residents' use	Small kitchenette with storage facilities
	Sink, stove, oven, refrigerator
	Electric kettle, toaster, pots, and pans
	Plates, bowls, teacups, and saucers
	Supply of tea, coffee, sugar, cream, bread, butter, cheese, cookies, milk, juice

[a]Modified from Beck C. Dining experiences of the institutionalized aged. J Gerontol Nurs 1981;7:104–107; Davies L, Holdsworth MD. An at-risk concept used in homes for the elderly in the United Kingdom. J Am Diet Assoc 1980;76:264–267; Mahaffey MJ, Mennes ME, Miller BB. Food service manual for health care institutions. Chicago: American Hospital Association, 1981.

min with consequences for highly protein-bound drugs (antimicrobials, cardiac drugs), changes in microsomal liver enzymes with alterations in effects of drugs metabolized in the liver (digitoxin, tricyclics), effects on urinary pH with change in the excretion patterns of drugs (urinary antimicrobials), and altered absorption (chelation of iron, calcium) (116, 117).

Many commonly used drugs affect vitamin and mineral status (118, 119). The elderly, particularly those with chronic illness, may be vulnerable to subclinical deficiencies. Drugs may stimulate (tricyclic antidepressants) or depress (digoxin) appetite and thereby induce over- or undernutrition.

Ethanol has many effects. It can stimulate appetite as an aperitif. Excessive ethanol ingestion may impair pyridoxine or folate metabolism or promote zinc and magnesium losses.

Pharmacotherapy in the elderly is a common situation. Awareness of potential drug-food interactions may allow interventions that will preclude undesirable side effects.

DIET AND CANCER

Farber (120) reviewed some aspects of nutrients and cancer. Diet may influence the incidence of cancer in some sites, such as the colon, breast, and endometrium. Carcinogens may occur in food as natural substances, as contaminants, or as products of food preparation methods. Balducci et al. (121) suggested that dietary prevention of cancer may be effective in advanced age and that the dietary guidelines of the National Academy of Sciences should be implemented in this population.

Micronutrients have a role in the endogenous formation of carcinogens. Dietary amines or drugs such as oxytetracycline or chlorpromazine, for example, can react with nitrous acid generated in the stomach to form nitroso compounds. These compounds are carcinogenic to laboratory animals. They may be effectively inhibited by dietary ascorbic acid and vitamin E. Fiber content plus vitamins C and E are being considered as modulators of carcinogens generated in the feces.

Plumlee et al. (122) reviewed the harmful effects of cooking methods that produce carcinogens (e.g., benzo[a]pyrene). They described their process for setting priorities for food items to be tested for possible mutagen information when cooked.

Weisburger (123) addressed the role of the food type, quality, and mode of cooking in the etiology of carcinoma in the gastrointestinal tract and endocrine-sensitive organs. If current concepts are correct, risk for gastric cancer can be reduced by ensuring that appropriate amounts of food containing vitamin C are eaten with each meal and by reducing salt, which acts as an adjuvant. Reduced intake of fried foods and fat will lower risk for colon, breast, and prostate cancer. These and other observations have led to dietary recommendations by the American Cancer Society.

Nutritional strategies are now incorporated into management plans for cancer patients. The effects of the disease on appetite, digestion, and other factors as well as nausea, vomiting, and anorexia, which frequently accompany radiotherapy and chemotherapy, require ongoing monitoring, prevention, and intervention (100).

The promotion and prevention of carcinogenesis by micronutrients is an intriguing field ripe for study. Cancer patients require attention to specific strategies to promote adequate nutrition in treatment programs.

SUMMARY

Consumption of a nutritionally adequate, balanced, and tasty diet is recommended for optimal health. This must be individualized to suit each person's needs and preferences. Intakes of energy (calories) rich foods low in nutrients is discouraged. Dietary standards must be continuously monitored, and the relation between nutrition, environment, and lifestyle must be researched more thoroughly.

Education and personal responsibility for health are lifetime pursuits. Knowledge and application of the principles of good nutrition may go a long way toward enhancing prospects for successful aging. We should not be misled by extremists, lay or professional, who would consign us to a life of spartan diets and galley-slave exertion as a recipe for long life. Moderation has been touted for generations as a prescription for good health. There is no current evidence that this advice is out of date.

REFERENCES

1. Justice CL, Howe JM, Clark HE. Dietary intakes and nutritional status of elderly patients. Study in a private nursing home. J Am Diet Assoc 1974; 65:639–646.
2. Fries JF. Aging, natural death, and the compression of morbidity. N Engl J Med 1980;303:130–135.
3. Disability and health: characteristics of persons by limitation of activity and assessed health status, United States, 1984–1988. In Advance Data from vital health statistics of the National Center for Health Statistics. Number 197, May 21, 1991.
4. Garraway WM, Whisnant JP, Furlan AJ, Phillips LH, Kurland LT, O'Fallon WM. The declining incidence of stroke. N Engl J Med 1979;300:449–452.
5. Morgan PP, Wigle DT. Medical care and the declining rates of death due to heart disease and stroke. Can Med Assoc J 1981;125:953–954.
6. Walker WJ. Changing United States life-style and declining vascular mortality: cause or coincidence? N Engl J Med 1980;297:163–165.
7. Exton-Smith AN. Malnutrition in the elderly. Proc R Soc Med 1977;70:615–619.
8. American Dietetic Association. Position of the American Dietetic Association: nutrition, aging and the continuum of health care. J Am Diet Assoc 1993;93:80–81.
9. Hazzard WR. Aging and atherosclerosis: interactions with diet, heredity and associated risk factors. In: Rockstein M, Sussman C, eds. Nutrition, longevity and aging, Proceedings of Symposium on Nutrition, Longevity and Aging, Miami. New York: Academic Press, 1976:143.
10. Barrows CH, Kokkonen GC. Relationship between nutrition and aging. In: Draper HH, ed. Advances in nutritional research, vol 1. New York: Plenum, 1977:253.
11. McKay CM, Crowell MF, Maynard LA. The effect of retarded growth upon the length of life span and upon the ultimate body size. Nutrition 1989;5:155–171. (Reproduction of classic 1936 paper.)
12. McKay CM, Sperling G, Barnes LL. Growth, ageing, chronic diseases and life span in rats. Arch Biochem 1943;2:469–479.
13. Masoro EJ. Retardation of aging processes by food restriction. an experimental tool. Am J Clin Nutr 1992;55:1250S–1252S.
14. Chang-Claude J, Frentzel-Beyme R, Eilber U. Mortality pattern of German vegetarians after ll years of follow-up. Epidemiology 1992;3:395–401.
15. Lemming JT, Webster SPG, Dymock IW. Gastrointestinal system. In: Brocklehurst JC, ed. Textbook of geriatric medicine and gerontology. Edinburgh: Churchill Livingstone, 1973:321.
16. Canadian Task Force on Periodic Health Examination. Periodic (vs. annual) health examination. Can Med Assoc J 1979;121:3–45, 1984;130:4–16, 1986;134:724–727, 1988;138:618–626.
17. White JV, Dwyer JT, Posner BM, Ham RJ, Lipschitz DA, Wellman NS. Nutrition screening initiative: development and implementation of the public awareness checklist and screening tools. J Am Diet Assoc 1992;92:163–166.
18. Horwath CC. Nutrition goals for older adults: a review. Gerontologist 1992;31:811–821.
19. Niewind AC, Krondl M, Lau D. Relative impact of selected factors on food choices of elderly individuals. Can J Aging 1988;7:32–47.
20. Dwyer JT. Dietary change; convergence of prevention and treatment measures. Top Clin Nutr 1991; 6:42–49.
21. Dwyer JT. Steps to take in primary care for achieving lasting dietary change. Top Clin Nutr 1991; 6:1–10.
22. Frankle RT, Owen AL. Nutrition in the community. The art of delivering services. 3rd ed. St Louis: Mosby, 1993:226–251.
23. McNutt KW. New perspectives to meet nutrition information needs of the older consumer. Geriatr Clin North Am: Nutrition in Older Persons 1987; 3:289–295.
24. Stanek K, Powell C, Betts N. Nutritional knowledge of nurses in long-term health care facilities. J Nutr Elderly 1991;10:35–48.
25. Dzajka-Narins DM, Kohrs MB, Tsui J, Nordstrom J. Nutritional and biochemical effects of nutrition programs in the elderly. Clin Geriatr Med 1987; 3:275–287.
26. Baker JP, Detsky AS, Wesson DE, et al. Nutritional assessment: a comparison of clinical judgment and objective measurements. N Engl J Med 1982;306:969–972.
27. Shoeller DA. How accurate is self reported dietary intake? Nutr Rev 1990;48:373–379.
28. Brogdon HG, Alford BB. Food preferences in relation to dietary intake and adequacy in a nursing home population. Gerontologist 1973;13(3):355–357.
29. Brown JE, Tharp TM, Dahlberg-Luby EM, et al. Videotape dietary assessment: validity, reliability and comparison or results with 24-hour dietary re-

calls from elderly women in a retirement home. J Am Diet Assoc 1990;90:1675–1679.

30. O'Hanlon P, Kohrs MB. Dietary studies of older Americans. Am J Clin Nutr 1978;31:1257–1269.

31. Gray DS, Crider JB, Kelley C, Dickinson CC. Accuracy of recumbent height measurement. JPEN 1985;9:712–715.

32. Kohrs MD, Czajka-Narins DM. Assessing the nutritional status of the elderly. In: Young EA, ed. Nutrition, aging, and health. New York: Alan R Liss, 1986:25.

33. Frisancho AR. New standards of weight and body composition by frame size and height for assessment of nutritional status of adults and the elderly. Am J Clin Nutr 1984;40:808–819.

34. Morley JE, Silver AJ, Fiatarone M, Mooradian AD. Geriatric grand rounds: nutrition and the elderly. J Am Geriatr Soc 1986;34:823–832.

35. Butterworth CE, Weinsier RL. Malnutrition in hospital patients: assessment and treatment. In: Goodhard RS, Shils ME, eds. Modern nutrition in health and disease, Philadelphia: Lea & Febiger, 1980:667.

36. Roy LB, Edwards PA, Barr LH. The value of nutritional assessment in the surgical patient. JPEN 1985;9:170–172.

37. Jeejeebhoy KN. Common modes of assessment of nutritional status. Front Clin Nutr 1992;1:1–6.

38. Michel L, Serrano A, Mait RA. Nutritional support of hospitalized patients. N Engl J Med 1981; 304:1147–1152.

39. Detsky AS, Baker JP, O'Rourke K, et al. Predicting nutrition-associated complications for patients undergoing gastrointestinal surgery. JPEN 1987; 11:440–446.

40. Klonoff-Cohen H, Barrett-Connor EL, Edelstein SL. Albumin levels as a predicator of mortality in the healthy elderly. J Clin Epidemiol 1992;45:207–212.

41. Hodges RE, Hood J, Canham JE, Sauberlich HE, Baker EM. Clinical manifestations of ascorbic acid deficiency in man. Am J Clin Nutr 1971;24:432–443.

42. Goode HF, Penn ND, Kelleher J, Walker BE. Evidence of cellular zinc depletion in hospitalized but not in healthy elderly subjects. Age Ageing 1991; 20:345–348.

43. Food and Nutrition Board, National Research Council. Recommended dietary allowances. 10th ed. Washington, DC: National Academy of Sciences, 1989.

44. Scientific Review Committee. Nutrition recommendations: the report of the Scientific Review Committee. Ottawa: Canadian Government Publishing Centre, 1990.

45. Harper AE. Recommended dietary allowances: are they what we think they are? J Am Diet Assoc 1974;64:151–156.

46. Beaton GH. Uses and limits of the use of the recommended dietary allowances for evaluating dietary intake data. Am J Clin Nutr 1985;41:155–164.

47. Leverton RM. The RDAs are not for amateurs. J Am Diet Assoc 1975;66:9–11.

48. Canada. National health and welfare. Report of an expert group convened by Health Promotion Directorate Health Services and Promotion Branch. Canadian guidelines for healthy weights. Ottawa: Canadian Government Publishing Centre, 1988.

49. Young VR. Energy requirements in the elderly. Nutr Rev 1992;50:95–101.

50. FAO/WHO/UNU. Energy and protein requirements. Report of a Joint FAO/WHO/UNU Expert Consultation. WHO Tech Rep Ser 74. Geneva: WHO, 1985.

51. Munro HN, Young VR. Protein metabolism and requirements. In: Exton-Smith AN, Caird FE, eds. Metabolic and nutritional disorders in the elderly. Chicago: A. John Wright & Sons, 1980:13.

52. Gersovitz M, Motil K, Munro HN, Scrimshaw NS, Young VR. Human protein requirements: assessment of the adequacy of the current recommended dietary allowance for the dietary protein in elderly men and women. Am J Clin Nutr 1982;35:6–14.

53. Young VR, Pellett PL. Protein intake and requirements with reference to diet and health. Am J Clin Nutr 1987;45(suppl 5):1323–1343.

54. Bennett, PH. Diabetes in the elderly: diagnosis and epidemiology. Geriatrics 1984;39:37–41.

55. American Diabetes Association. Nutritional recommendations and principles for individuals with diabetes mellitus. Diabetes Care 1987;10:126–132.

56. Wheeler ML, Delahanty L, Wylei-Rosett J. Diet and exercise in noninsulin dependent diabetes mellitus: implications for dieticians from the NIH Consensus Development Conference. J Am Diet Assoc 1987;87:480–485.

57. Rosenthal MJ, Hartnell JM, Morley JE, et al. UCLA geriatric grand rounds: diabetes in the elderly. J Am Geriatr Soc 1987;35:435–447.

58. Franz MJ, Holler H, Powers MA, Wheeler ML, Wylie-Rosett J. Exchange lists: revised 1986. J Am Diet Assoc 1987;87:28–34.

59. Grundy SM. Cholesterol and coronary heart disease: a new era. JAMA 1986;256:2849–2858.

60. LaCroix AZ, Mead LA, Liang KY, Thomas CB, Pearson TA. Coffee consumption and the incidence of coronary heart disease. N Engl J Med 1986; 315:977–982.

61. NIH Consensus Development Conference. Lowering blood cholesterol to prevent heart disease. Arteriosclerosis 1985;5:404–412.

62. Goto AM, Bierman EL, Connor WE, et al. Recommendations for the treatment of hyperlipidemia in adults. Circulation 1984;69:1067A–1090A.

63. Nestel PJ. Polyunsaturated fatty acids (n-3, n-6). Am J Clin Nutr 1987;45(suppl):1161.

64. Grundy SM. Monounsaturated fatty acids, plasma cholesterol, and coronary heart disease. Am J Clin Nutr 1987;45(suppl):1168–1175.

65. Watkin DM. Nutrition for the aging and the aged. In: Goodhart RS, Shils ME, eds. Modern nutrition in health and disease. Philadelphia: Lea & Febiger, 1980:781.

66. Leaf A. Dehydration in the elderly. N Engl J Med 1984;311:791–792.

67. Phillips PA, Rolls BJ, Ledingham JGG, et al. Reduced thirst after water deprivation in healthy elderly men. N Engl J Med 1984;311:753–759.

68. Nordin BEC, Polley KJ, Need AG, Morris HA, Marshall D. The problem of calcium requirement. Am J Clin Nutr 1987;45:1295–1304.

69. Heaney, RP. Thinking straight about calcium. N Engl J Med 1993;328:503–505.

70. Gordan GS, Vaughan C. Calcium and osteoporosis. J Nutr 1986;116:319–322.

71. Heaney RP. Calcium intake, bone health, and aging. In: Young EA, ed. Nutrition, aging, and health. New York: Alan R Liss, 1986:165.

72. Riggs BL, Melton III LJ. Involutional osteoporosis. N Engl J Med 1986;314:1676–1686.

73. Heaney RP, Recker RR, Saville PD. Menopausal changes in calcium balance performance. J Lab Clin Med 1978;92:953–963.

74. NIH Consensus Conference. Osteoporosis. JAMA 1984;252:799–802.

75. Melton JL III, Wahner HW, Richelson LS, O'Fallon WM, Riggs BL. Osteoporosis and the risk of hip fracture. Am J Epidemiol 1986;124:254–261.

76. Recker RR, Heaney RP. The effect of milk supplements on calcium metabolism, bone metabolism and calcium balance. Am J Clin Nutr 1985;41:254–263.

77. Recker RR. Calcium absorption and achlorhydria. N Engl J Med 1985;313:70–83.

78. Herbert V. The vitamin craze. Arch Intern Med 1980;140:173–176.

79. Baker H, Frank O, Thind I, Jaslow SP, Louria DB. Vitamin profiles in elderly persons living at home or in nursing homes, versus profile in healthy young subjects. J Am Geriatr Soc 1979;27:444–450.

80. Baker H, Frank O, Jaslow SP. Oral versus intramuscular vitamin supplementation for hypovitaminosis in the elderly. J Am Geriatr Soc 1980;28:42–45.

81. Drinka PJ, Goodwin JS. Prevalence and consequences of vitamin deficiency in the nursing home. a critical review. J Am Geriatr Soc 1991;39:1008–1017.

82. Donald EA, Basu TK, Hargreaves JA, Thompson GW, et al. Dietary intake and biochemical status of a selected group of older Albertans taking or not taking micronutrient supplement. J Can Diet Assoc 1992;53:36–39.

83. Chandra RK, Imbach A, Moore C, Skelton D, Woolcott D. Nutrition of the elderly. Can Med Assoc J 1991;145:1475–1487.

84. Carruthers SG. Nutrition and hypertension. J Can Diet Assoc 1980;41:274–281.

85. Kaplan NM. Non-drug treatment of hypertension. Ann Intern Med 1985;102:359–373.

86. Report of the Expert Advisory Committee on Dietary Fibre to the Health Protection Branch. Health and Welfare Canada. Minister of National Health and Welfare. Canada, 1985.

87. Sandman PO, Adolfsson R, Hallmans G, Nygren BS, Nystrom L, Winblad B. Treatment of constipation with high-bran bread in long-term care of severely demented elderly patients. J Am Geriatr Soc 1983;31:289–293.

88. Freeman HJ. Dietary fiber and colonic neoplasia. Can Med Assoc J 1979;121:291–296.

89. Anderson JW, Sieling B. High-fiber diets for diabetics: unconventional but effective. Geriatrics 1981;36:(5)64–72.

90. Anderson JW. Health implications of wheat fiber. Am J Clin Nutr 1985;41:1103–1112.

91. Watkin DM. Logical bases for action in nutrition aging. J Am Geriatr Soc 1978;26:193–202.

92. Ryan, AS, Craig LD, Finn SC. Nutrient intakes and dietary patterns of older Americans: a national study. J Gerontol 1992;47:M145–M150.

93. Andres R. Effect of obesity on total mortality. Int J Obes 1980;4:381–386.

94. Dawber TR. The Framingham Study: the epidemiology of atherosclerotic disease. Cambridge: Harvard University Press, 1980.

95. Kushner RF. Body weight and mortality. Nutr Rev 1993;51:127–136.

96. Paganini-Hill A, Ross RK, Gerkins VR, Henderson BE, Arthur M, Mack TM. Menopausal estrogen therapy and hip fractures. Ann Intern Med 1981; 95:28–31.

97. De Waard F. Premenopausal and postmenopausal breast cancer: one disease or two? JNCI 1977; 63:549–552.

98. Heymsfield SB, Bethel RA, Ansley JD, Nixon DW, Rudman D. Enteral hyperalimentation: an alternative to central venous hyperalimentation. Ann Intern Med 1979;90:63–71.

99. Linn BS. Outcomes of older and younger malnourished and well-nourished patients one year after hospitalization. Am J Clin Nutr 1984;39:66–73.

100. Dwyer J. The spectrum of dietary and nutritional approaches to cancer. Nutrition 1989;5:197–199.

101. Bastow MD, Rawlings J, Allison SP. Benefits of supplementary tube feeding after fractured neck of femur: a randomized controlled trial. Br Med J 1983;287:1589–1592.

102. Mowe M, Bohmer T. The prevalence of undiagnosed protein-calorie undernutrition in a population of hospitalized elderly patients. J Am Geriatr Soc 1991;39:1089–1092.

103. Sullivan DH, Patch GA, Walls RC, Lipschitz DA. Impact of nutrition status on morbidity and mortality in a select population of geriatric rehabilitation patients. Am J Clin Nutr 1990;51:749–758.

104. Bernard MA, Rombeau JL. Nutritional support for the elderly patient. In: Young EA, ed. Nutrition, aging, and health. New York: Alan R Liss, 1986:229.

105. Posner GF, Hickisch SM. Dilution factors for commercial enteral formulas. J Am Diet Assoc 1984; 84:1219–1220.

106. Gray GE. Nutrition and dementia. J Am Diet Assoc 1989;89:1795–1802.

107. Loney LA, Hutton JT, Stewart JR, Spallholz JE. Nutritional concerns for patients with Alzheimer's disease. Texas Med 1987;83:40–43.

108. Litchford MD, Wakefield LM. Nutrient intakes and energy expenditures of residents with senile dementia of the Alzheimer's type. J Am Diet Assoc 1987;87:211–213.

109. Rheaume Y, Riley ME, Ladislav V. Meeting nutritional needs of Alzheimer patients who pace constantly. J Nutr Elderly 1987;7:43–52.

110. Barr SI, Chrysomilides SA, Willis EJ, Beattie BL. Nutrient intakes of the old elderly: a study of female residents of a long-term care facility. Nutr Res 1983;3:417–431.

111. Beck C. Dining experiences of the institutionalized aged. J Gerontol Nurs 1981;7:104–107.

112. Asplund K, Normark M, Pettersson V. Nutritional assessment of psychogeriatric patients. Age Ageing 1981;10:87–94.

113. Morgan DB, Newton HMV, Schorah CJ, Jewitt MA, Hancock MR, Hullin RP. Abnormal indices of

nutrition in the elderly: a study of different clinical groups. Age Ageing 1986;15:65–76.

114. Anderson EL. Eating patterns before and after dentures. J Am Diet Assoc 1971;58:421–426.

115. Lamy PP. The elderly and drug interactions. J Am Geriatr Soc 1986;34:586–592.

116. Lamy PP. Drug interactions and the elderly—a new perspective. Drug Intell Clin Pharmacy 1980; 14:513–515.

117. Lamy PP. Nutrition and the elderly. Drug Intell Clin Pharm 1981;15:887–891.

118. Roe DA. Therapeutic significance of drug-nutrient interactions in the elderly. Pharmacol Rev 1984; 36(suppl 2):109S–122S.

119. Roe DA. Therapeutic effects of drug-nutrient interactions in the elderly. J Am Diet Assoc 1985; 85:174–181.

120. Farber E. Chemical carcinogenesis. N Engl J Med 1981;305:1379–1389.

121. Balducci L, Wallace C, Khansur T, Vance RB, Thigpen JT, Hardy C. Nutrition, cancer, and aging: an annotated review. I. Diet, carcinogenesis, and aging. J Am Geriatr Soc 1986;34:127–136.

122. Plumlee C, Bjeldanes LF, Hatch FT. Priorities assessment for studies of mutagen production in cooked foods. J Am Diet Assoc 1981;79:446–449.

123. Weisburger JH. Mechanism of action of diet as a carcinogen. Cancer (Phila) 1979;43:1987–1995.

24/ Lipid Abnormalities in the Elderly

Roy Verdery, Jan Busby-Whitehead

This chapter provides an introduction to lipid and lipoprotein metabolism and its abnormalities in general, since the mechanisms that regulate lipid and lipoprotein levels in older people are the same as those found in younger people. Effects of genetics, environment, diseases, and drugs on lipid and lipoprotein levels are described with particular emphasis on those aspects that are different in older individuals. The relationship of lipid and lipoprotein levels to risk of atherosclerosis in older people is discussed. Finally, the steps to be used in evaluating clinically significant elevations in lipid and lipoprotein levels and designing their treatment to reduce risks of atherosclerosis and subsequent coronary and cerebrovascular disease are considered in detail.

LIPIDS AND LIPOPROTEINS

The clinically important plasma lipids are triglycerides and cholesterol. Triglycerides are nonpolar fats made up of a glycerol molecule to which three fatty acids have been esterified. Triglycerides primarily carry energy derived from food to storage sites in fatty tissues of the body. Cholesterol is a polar lipid that is a necessary part of all cell membranes. Because it is able to help form emulsions, cholesterol is combined with proteins and phospholipids to help carry triglycerides from their sites of origin in the intestine and liver to storage sites in the fatty tissues of the body. Much cholesterol in the blood, however, is in the form of cholesterol esters. These nonpolar lipids, formed by esterification of cholesterol with a fatty acid, are found in highest concentration in those lipoproteins that are associated with increased risk for atherosclerosis.

Lipoproteins are particles containing nonpolar lipids that are kept in solution by association with specific proteins (apolipoproteins) and polar lipids, including phospholipids and unesterified cholesterol. The biggest lipoproteins, chylomicrons and very low density lipoproteins (VLDL), are the carriers of triglycerides synthesized from dietary fat and carbohydrates. Chylomicrons are synthesized in the intestine and VLDL are synthesized in the liver. Both are degraded in peripheral tissues by the action of lipoprotein lipase (LPL). Clinically, chylomicrons and VLDL are most important as carriers of dietary energy. By themselves they are not risk factors for atherosclerosis. However, high levels of chylomicrons appear to cause acute pancreatitis, and high levels of VLDL are associated with poor glucose control in diabetics.

The products of chylomicron and VLDL metabolism include chylomicron remnants, intermediate-density lipoproteins (IDL), low-density lipoproteins (LDL), and LP(a). These products of chylomicron and VLDL metabolism are associated with increased risk for atherosclerosis. Thus, clinically, chylomicron remnants, IDL, LDL, and LP(a) are the "bad" lipoproteins.

LDL are the lipoproteins that carry most of the cholesterol in the blood. In most people, elevated LDL levels are the most significant lipoprotein risk factors for development of atherosclerosis. These elevated levels lead to accumulation of cholesterol in atherosclerotic plaques. LDL also appear to be part of the cause of progression of early plaques (fatty streaks) to complex calcified plaques. The mechanisms by which LDL cause atherosclerosis are only partially understood. Several factors play roles in this process: (a) direct infiltration of LDL into the arterial wall where they are taken up by cells, stimulating pathologic changes in the arterial wall, (b) increased transport and atherogenicity of certain LDL subfractions, and (c) oxidation of LDL forming LDL that are especially atherogenic. The goal of the National Cholesterol Educational Program (NCEP) is to reduce LDL levels in all people who have elevated cholesterol levels (1). Strategies to change levels of especially atherogenic dense LDL may be developed in the next few years.

High-density lipoproteins (HDL) are intermediaries in triglyceride metabolism. In population studies, high levels of HDL are associated with reduced risk for atherosclerosis. The mechanism for the inverse relationship of HDL to risk of atherosclerosis is unclear. High levels of HDL are associated with low levels of chylomicrons, VLDL, chylomicron remnants, IDL, LDL, and LP(a) because of their role in the intermediary metabolism of these other lipoproteins. Conversely, in "syndrome X" as identified by Reaven, low levels of HDL are associated with high levels of triglyceride-rich lipoproteins (along with high blood pressure and insulin resistance) (2). In people with a genetic deficiency of lecithin cholesterol acyltransferase (LCAT), low levels of HDL and abnormal HDL are associated with reduced removal of unesterified cholesterol from peripheral tissues. The association of high HDL with low atherosclerosis rates, the importance of hypercholesterolemia in experimental atherogenesis, the role of HDL and LCAT in removal of cholesterol in LCAT deficiency, and experimental evidence for a role of HDL in cholesterol transport from cells to lipoproteins in vitro has led to the hypothesis that HDL is somehow responsible for removal of cholesterol from peripheral tissue and prevention of the accumulation of cholesterol in arteries, which eventually leads to atherosclerosis. This so-called reverse cholesterol transport is the prevailing hypothesis regarding the mechanism of HDL in protecting against atherosclerosis (3).

EFFECTS OF GENETICS ON LIPID AND LIPOPROTEIN LEVELS

Genetic abnormalities in the apolipoproteins, cell receptors that bind apolipoproteins, and enzymes that regulate lipoprotein metabolism affect the levels of all lipoproteins (4, 5). Genetically high levels of chylomicrons caused by LPL deficiency are associated with increased risk for pancreatitis. Genetically high levels of VLDL, IDL, and LP(a) caused by low levels of LPL, isoforms of apolipoprotein E, and genetic differences in apolipoprotein LP(a) are associated with increased risk of atherosclerosis (6). Genetically low levels of chylomicrons, VLDL, chylomicron remnants, IDL, LDL, and LP(a) found in people with abetalipoproteinemia are associated with deficiencies in fat-soluble vitamins, particularly vitamin E. Genetically high levels of HDL caused by either increased rates of synthesis of HDL apolipoproteins or decreased levels of cholesterol ester transfer protein (CETP) are associated with low rates of atherosclerosis. Genetically low levels of HDL have been found in six different conditions. About half of these are associated with high

rates of atherosclerosis, while the rest are associated with low or normal rates of atherosclerosis. However, low levels of HDL are also associated with corneal opacities and, in the case of LCAT deficiency, are associated with increased incidence rates of kidney disease.

In general, the effects of genetic abnormalities in lipid and lipoprotein metabolism have not been studied in aging people. Homozygous familial hypercholesterolemia, one of the best studied genetic diseases affecting LDL levels, is associated with premature atherosclerosis and early mortality. Relatively few elderly people are heterozygous for familial hypercholesterolemia, suggesting that presence of this gene is also associated with shorter life spans (7). Similar studies have shown a relative low prevalence of the apolipoprotein E3 phenotype in older people. Apolipoprotein E3 is another genetic abnormality that, in the homozygote state, is associated with marked increased risk for atherosclerosis. Hence, this phenotype also appears to shorten life when present in the heterozygote state. Small family studies of people who are extremely long lived have suggested that genetically increased HDL levels may be associated with particularly long life. However, because these studies were not longitudinal, it is not possible to exclude the possibility that very old people have especially high HDL levels possibly caused by changes in metabolism such as declining androgen levels in men.

In addition to abnormalities that affect the quantity of lipoproteins, genetic abnormalities commonly affect the structure and metabolism of lipoproteins. As mentioned above, LCAT deficiency leads to low HDL levels and the presence of HDL of unusual sizes. Relatively unusual disk-shaped HDL are also found in LCAT deficiency. The specific apolipoprotein E isoform, apolipoprotein E3, is associated with increased levels of IDL, in part because the clearance of lipoproteins containing this isoform of apolipoprotein E is decreased. LP(a) is a genetically complex lipoprotein that is structurally similar to plasminogen. It has been suggested, on the basis of studies in vitro, that LP(a) may be atherogenic because of its ability to inhibit thrombolysis, a property that would be under complex genetic control.

EXERCISE, BODY COMPOSITION, AND DIET

Three environmental factors that are under direct control of individuals affect lipid and lipoprotein levels: exercise, diet, and body fat. However, because of the effects of exercise and diet on body fat, these three factors are not independent modulators of lipid and lipoprotein levels.

In general, exercise increases HDL levels and decreases levels of triglyceride-rich lipoproteins, chylomicrons, and VLDL. To a lesser extent, exercise decreases LDL levels. People with higher percentage body fat, particularly those with concomitant glucose intolerance, have relatively high levels of VLDL and LDL. Reducing the percentage body fat by exercise and diet and increasing the relative amount of muscle, decreases triglycerides, particularly VLDL triglycerides, and increases HDL levels. The major metabolic regulator that is affected by changing percentage body fat is LPL activity. LPL increases with exercise, decreasing percentage body fat and increasing percentage muscle mass.

The effects of diet on lipid and lipoprotein levels have been the subject of extensive studies performed over the last 20 years. From a clinical point of view, the major dietary effects on lipid and lipoprotein levels are due to total calories in the diet, total cholesterol in the diet, relative amounts of saturated and transunsaturated fatty acids in the diet, and relative amounts of omega-3 fatty acids in the diet. Decreasing the total calories and total fat in the diet decreases chylomicron, VLDL, chylomicron remnant, IDL, and LDL levels. Similarly, decreasing the amounts of cholesterol, saturated fatty acids, and transunsaturated fatty acids also decreases the levels of atherogenic lipoproteins. Under certain circumstances, however, decreasing total cholesterol intake also decreases total HDL levels, especially when saturated fatty acids are replaced by complex carbohydrates and polyunsaturated fats in the diet. The role of omega-3 fatty acids, principally found in fish oils, on atherogenesis is actively under investigation. Increasing intake of omega-3 fatty acids appears to decrease serum clotting rates and may decrease acute cardiac and cerebrovascular disease. However, ingesting large amounts of fish oil can increase triglyceride levels and decrease HDL levels in some people.

DISEASES AFFECTING LIPOPROTEIN LEVELS

Diseases that affect lipoprotein levels primarily include endocrine and inflammatory diseases. Hypothyroidism and diabetes lead to elevated lipid and lipoprotein levels. Inflammatory diseases generally lead to lower lipid and lipoprotein levels. Hypothyroidism is well known to cause increased cholesterol levels. Principally, LDL are elevated. Thyroid replacement normalizes cholesterol levels. A lipid-lowering drug that is presently out of favor because of its side-effect profile is reverse T3, an analogue of the active thyroid hormone triiodothyronine. Diabetes is well known to lead to increased triglyceride levels and secondarily increased cholesterol levels. In diabetics who are poorly controlled, the principal lipoprotein that is elevated is VLDL. Good diabetic control normalizes triglyceride levels and reduces cholesterol levels proportionately. In fact, the relationship of triglyceride levels to diabetic control is so close that diabetics with elevated triglycerides must be evaluated for poor control. The importance of diabetes in lipoprotein metabolism is also apparent in "syndrome X," in which hypertriglyceridemia, low HDL levels, hypertension, and insulin resistance occur together.

In general, inflammatory diseases decrease both triglyceride and cholesterol levels. Typically, VLDL, LDL, and HDL are all decreased. Occasionally VLDL is increased because of deficiencies in LPL while LDL and HDL are decreased because of direct effects of inflammation, probably inhibiting hepatic lipoprotein production. In severe inflammatory conditions, acquired LCAT deficiency occurs, leading to relative elevations in unesterified cholesterol. Recovery from the cause of inflammation, e.g., acute arthritis, pneumonia, or myocardial infarction, leads to normalization of lipoprotein levels. The effect of inflammation on lipoprotein levels is so marked that lipoprotein levels measured immediately after a myocardial infarction (MI) are not reliable. Evaluation of post-MI patients for secondary prevention strategies must be delayed until 2 to 3 months after the myocardial infarction.

EFFECTS OF DRUGS ON LIPID AND LIPOPROTEIN LEVELS

Several different categories of drugs, particularly hormones and antihypertensive agents, affect lipid and lipoprotein levels. Thyroid medications decrease cholesterol, primarily LDL levels. Estrogens, in general, lower LDL levels and raise HDL levels. In fact, the beneficial effect of estrogens on LDL and HDL makes estrogen treatment one of the first considerations in treating dyslipoproteinemias in older women, because of its combined beneficial effects on both bone and lipid metabolism. In contrast to estrogen, testosterone and other androgens increase LDL and decrease HDL levels. A clinically important aspect of this is the effect of anabolic steroids on lipid levels. People taking anabolic steroids often have profoundly low HDL levels.

Thiazides, particularly thiazide diuretics, increase LDL levels. Population studies have shown that people taking β-blockers also have increased LDL levels. Specific lipid-lowering drugs work via a variety of mechanisms. These drugs are discussed in the section on modifying lipoprotein risk factors for atherosclerosis.

AGE-ASSOCIATED CHANGES IN LIPID AND LIPOPROTEINS

Age-associated changes in lipid and lipoprotein levels have been studied both longitudinally and cross-sectionally (8, 9). In general, total and LDL cholesterol levels increase with age until approximately age 55 to 65 in men, after which they show a slight decrease. In women, however, the increase in cholesterol and LDL primarily occurs after the menopause, and the peak occurs about 10 years later than in men, between ages 65 and 75. In men, HDL levels decrease significantly at puberty. After this decrease, HDL levels in men remain relatively low, compared with those in women, until late in life. In men, HDL levels increase slightly after the age of 65 or 75 in association with decreasing levels of testosterone. HDL levels in women are fairly constant throughout life, although there is a slight decrease after menopause. Age-associated changes in triglyceride levels and the prevalence of "syndrome X" have not been described.

LIPID AND LIPOPROTEIN LEVELS AND THEIR RELATIONSHIP WITH HEART DISEASE

The major clinical reason to measure cholesterol, triglyceride, and lipoprotein levels is to evaluate and modify risk for heart disease and stroke (10). Elevated levels of atherogenic lipoproteins are associated with increased risk for atherosclerosis and, consequently, increased risk of cardiovascular and cerebrovascular disease. The primary goal in changing these risk factors is to decrease the risk of myocardial infarction and stroke.

There are three major prevention strategies: primary prevention, secondary prevention, and atherosclerosis regression. Primary prevention is accomplished by modifying risk factors before disease develops and is addressed mostly to young and middle-aged people under the age of 65 (1, 11). Secondary prevention is accomplished by reducing risk factors after an event caused by atherosclerosis such as myocardial infarction or stroke. Regression of atherosclerosis has been demonstrated recently using noninvasive techniques to image arteries and determine degrees of atherosclerosis before myocardial infarction or stroke. Regression appears to be achievable by ag-

gressively lowering levels of atherogenic lipoproteins and eliminating other risk factors. Vigorous treatment in this fashion may reduce atherosclerosis long before effects on incidence of myocardial infarction and stroke can be demonstrated (12).

In discussing lipid and lipoprotein risk factors for cardiovascular and cerebrovascular disease, it is critical to realize that other risk factors may be more important than lipid and lipoproteins (13, 14). The most significant reversible risk factor is smoking. Smoking cessation has beneficial effects on subsequent cardiovascular and cerebrovascular disease much sooner than lowering levels of atherogenic lipoproteins. Similarly, uncontrolled hypertension causes greater short-term risk for cardiovascular and cerebrovascular disease than elevated lipid and lipoprotein levels. Finally, certain diseases, such as uncontrolled diabetes, need to be addressed at the same time as elevated lipid levels are addressed.

The basic premise for modifying lipid and lipoprotein risk factors for coronary and cerebrovascular disease is that data from primary prevention, secondary prevention, and regression trials carried out primarily in younger people apply in general to older people (15). There are no data suggesting that the mechanisms regulating lipid and lipoprotein levels that operate in younger people are at all different in older people. The few clinical trials that have been carried out in older people have shown no difference in the effect of modifying lipid and lipoprotein levels on reducing risk for development of atherosclerosis and subsequent coronary and cerebroarterial disease (16–19). The primary results of these intervention trials suggest that reducing cholesterol levels, particularly LDL cholesterol levels, will reduce the incidence of new coronary artery disease, symptoms (e.g., angina), and events (e.g., MI) (20). The same statement holds true for reducing triglyceride levels, although this effect is not as pronounced for reasons still unknown. The primary lipoprotein that has been decreased in these trials is LDL. However, reduced levels of LDL also are accompanied by reduced levels of chylomicron remnants, IDL, and LP(a). Reducing LDL cholesterol levels does not actually reduce the death rate; rather, it decreases the incidence of new cardiac and cerebrovascular events. Thus, while life is not necessarily prolonged, active life expectancy is prolonged because of the reduced rate of disabling heart attacks and strokes.

Secondary prevention and reversal of atherosclerosis have not been as well studied as primary prevention but can be accomplished by decreasing the same atherogenic lipoprotein levels that are lowered in primary prevention (13). In secondary prevention, people who have already had a myocardial infarction are vigorously treated for all of their risk factors including elevated levels of lipids and atherogenic lipoproteins. In such secondary prevention trials, a beneficial effect is seen in approximately 5 years. People who have had heart attacks and whose lipid and lipoprotein levels are vigorously treated have a lower incidence of second heart attacks, and this reduced incidence can be seen within 5 years of beginning the secondary prevention.

Recently it has been shown, using noninvasive techniques to image arteries and measure the degree of atherosclerosis, that very vigorous treatment of hyperlipidemias along with modifying other risk factors can reduce the amount of atherosclerosis in large vessels. Reversal of atherosclerosis is accomplished in part by lowering the cholesterol level to less than 160 mg/dL using a combination of strict diet, often a vegetarian diet, and lipid-lowering drugs. Reversal can be seen in less than 5 years, which suggests that a rapid beneficial effect on clinical endpoints such as new symptoms or coronary or cerebrovascular events will eventually be described.

Based on the observation in population studies that high HDL levels are associated with lower risk for coronary and cerebrovascular disease, it is expected that raising HDL levels would also reduce the risk of heart attack or stroke. However, there are no interventions that specifically raise HDL levels, and this idea has not been tested. Modalities that raise HDL levels include those that lower triglyceride, cholesterol, and atherogenic lipoprotein levels. Moreover, elevated HDL levels are associated with relative leanness and increased exercise tolerance. (Reducing body fat and increasing exercise tolerance has benefits to most people's feeling of well-being and, therefore, those things that raise HDL levels are generally beneficial). An exception to this is alcohol. Although it has been reported that modest intake of alcohol raises HDL levels, excessive alcohol intake is deleterious and can be life threatening.

It is important to consider treatment of dyslipoproteinemias in the context of other diseases that individual patients might have. This is especially important in older people because of the greater prevalence of chronic diseases that shorten life or drastically limit life, such as untreatable metastatic cancer and advanced, end-stage Alzheimer's disease. Primary prevention of coronary and cerebroarterial disease does not show beneficial effects in fewer than 5 to 10 years. Therefore a rule of thumb is that patients with

less than 10 years life expectancy will not benefit from primary prevention of atherosclerosis by reducing cholesterol levels. People in this category include those with cancer or end-stage heart, lung, or other organ disease, and the very old. The average life expectancy of someone 65 years old is about 17 years; therefore, a person of this age should be considered a candidate for primary prevention. However, the life expectancy of men in the United States decreases to 10 years by the age of about 73; in women, the life expectancy decreases to 10 years by the age of about 78. Therefore, men over the age of 75 and women over the age of 85 are probably not candidates for primary prevention of atherosclerosis by reduction of cholesterol levels unless they are in exceptionally robust good health.

Actuarial estimates of the effect of preventing heart disease by reducing lipid levels suggest that no more than 2 to 3 years can be added on to life expectancy by vigorous treatment of hypercholesterolemia. Thus, it is probably not correct in general to treat lipid and lipoprotein risk factors in people over these ages even though such treatment may delay a heart attack or stroke by a few years (21). These arguments, however, are based on actuarial estimates and on the assumption that the average patient will have an average life expectancy. These arguments do not hold up when it can be established that a particular patient will have more than an average life expectancy. Thus, an 85-year-old man or woman in perfect health with no familial predisposition to other life-threatening diseases who might live until the age of 100 or more might benefit from primary prevention of atherosclerosis even if it is initiated at the age of 85. It is expected, however, that in considering the general population, such individuals are rare and difficult to identify.

Given the effect of vigorous treatment of hypercholesterolemia on quality of life and the possibility that unregulated dietary modifications to lower cholesterol levels can cause dietary deficiencies of, for example, calcium, which would shorten both active life and total life span, vigorous treatment of people over the age of 85 must be considered the exception rather than the rule. A clinical rule of thumb is that people with a short life expectancy, regardless of age, should not be treated for hyperlipidemias.

CLINICAL EVALUATION AND TREATMENT OF LIPID AND LIPOPROTEIN LEVELS

When considering modification of lipid and lipoprotein levels to reduce risk for cardiovascular and cerebrovascular disease, cholesterol level is the most important (22). In general, cholesterol levels over 220 mg/dL should be further studied. The higher the cholesterol level is over 200 mg/dL, the more important it is to perform further evaluation and consider intervention because the risk of cardiovascular and cerebrovascular disease increases directly with the cholesterol level above 200 mg/dL. People with levels substantially over 350 mg/dL are at very high risk for early death.

In actuality, however, the relationship of risk of death to cholesterol level is a U-shaped curve (23). The U-shape appears to be more pronounced in older people than in younger people. While elevated cholesterol levels are associated with increased risk for coronary and cerebrovascular disease, very low cholesterol levels (less than 150 mg/dL) are commonly associated with other life-threatening problems including cancer, acute infection, other inflammatory disease, starvation, and other causes of malnutrition. Hence, a clinician observing an older person with a very low cholesterol level must consider that it may indicate the presence of another disease requiring further evaluation. There is no evidence to suggest that lowering previously elevated cholesterol levels to levels less than 160 mg/dL causes these diseases. It has been speculated, however, that very low cholesterol levels may be associated with depression (24). Whether this is a cause of depression, or an effect of poor food intake occurring during depression, or whether both low cholesterol levels and depression are caused by the same condition (e.g., cancer) remains to be established.

Triglyceride is often measured at the same time as cholesterol in an initial screening. Utility of this without measuring HDL cholesterol levels is limited. Nonetheless, very high triglyceride levels (over 1000 mg/dL) must be immediately evaluated and treated because they are associated with the development of acute pancreatitis. In addition, as mentioned above, very high triglyceride levels should also alert the clinician to the possibility of uncontrolled diabetes. Very high triglyceride levels also occur in nephrotic syndrome, although, by the time triglyceride elevation is seen, the edema of nephrotic syndrome is usually pronounced.

After observing that the cholesterol level is elevated, systemic disease must be ruled out. The two most important diseases affecting older people that are associated with elevated cholesterol levels are hypothyroidism and diabetes. Hypothyroidism is associated with markedly elevated cholesterol levels, sometimes as high as 350 mg/dL.

Most of the elevated cholesterol is in the form of LDL. Both the total cholesterol and LDL levels are rapidly normalized with appropriate thyroid replacement. Uncontrolled diabetes is primarily associated with elevated triglyceride levels. However, since triglyceride-rich lipoproteins also contain cholesterol and since most screening programs measure cholesterol but not triglyceride, it is necessary to consider that a person with newly recognized cholesterol elevation may have previously undiagnosed diabetes or diabetes that is not properly controlled. As in the case of hypothyroidism, proper diabetic control promptly normalizes triglyceride levels and reduces cholesterol levels proportionately.

After ruling out systemic diseases that may be responsible for elevated cholesterol levels, it is necessary to repeat the cholesterol measurement, measure triglycerides, and measure HDL cholesterol levels. From these measurements, LDL can be calculated. The calculation usually used is

$$\begin{aligned} \text{LDL cholesterol} = \ &\text{total cholesterol} \\ &- \text{HDL cholesterol} \\ &- (\text{triglyceride level}/5). \end{aligned}$$

This formula is based on the assumption that in most people, the amount of cholesterol in the triglyceride-rich lipoproteins is equal to 1/5 the triglyceride level when measured in mg/dL. Two different methods are used to assess the LDL level calculated in this way. The method proposed by the National Cholesterol Education Program is to recognize that people with LDL cholesterol levels over 160 mg/dL are at increased risk for developing cardiovascular and cerebrovascular disease. An alternative approach is to calculate the LDL/HDL ratio. Such a calculation takes into account the fact that higher HDL levels are associated with lower risk for cardiac and cerebrovascular disease. Thus, an LDL/HDL ratio above 5 suggests increased risk of these cholesterol-associated diseases.

TREATMENT OF HIGH CHOLESTEROL AND TRIGLYCERIDE LEVELS

Treatment of elevated lipid and lipoprotein levels must begin by establishing purposes and goals of treatment. Age- and disease-dependent life expectancy modifies the goals, since all of the treatments, including dietary modification, have potential adverse side effects and may adversely affect quality of life. The goals and likelihood of accomplishing them must be carefully discussed. Secondly, the goals must address which specific lipids and lipoproteins are going to be modified. Triglyceride lowering uses somewhat different diets and drugs than does cholesterol lowering. In many cases both cholesterol and triglyceride levels are elevated, and certain LDL-lowering diets and drugs can be chosen to lower triglyceride levels as well as LDL cholesterol levels. Finally, in many people it would be advisable to raise HDL cholesterol levels. Drugs and diets that increase HDL levels are not well developed, and lowering cholesterol levels often lowers HDL cholesterol levels as well. While low cholesterol levels found in populations at screening are associated with bad outcome, especially if cholesterol levels below 160 mg/dL are found, there is no evidence that lowering cholesterol levels causes increased morbidity and mortality.

The first goal in modifying cholesterol and triglyceride levels is to modify behavior (25). Initially, all risk factors for cardiovascular and cerebrovascular diseases must be addressed, since many of these are affected directly by behavior. Moreover, risk factors for other problems causing morbidity and mortality must also be addressed. It is important to counsel patients about use of seat belts while driving, prevention of accidents and falls, smoking cessation, control of hypertension, and regulation of diabetes if present (26).

Diet is the first behavior to modify. Generally, trained dietitians help set goals and procedures and should be used whenever possible. The first step is to reduce total caloric intake. The American Heart Association (AHA) Step 1 Diet calls for a 30% reduction in calories. In addition to reducing calories, it is important to reduce intake of cholesterol and saturated fats. It is especially important in older people to pay attention to preventing deficiencies, particularly in fat-soluble vitamins (vitamins A and D) and minerals (e.g., iron and calcium). Iron and calcium deficiency must be prevented, especially when meat intake is specifically reduced. Remember that weight reduction due to improved diet causes other benefits: it improves glucose control, it improves self-image, and it increases physical energy. This can be an important motivational factor in getting people to adhere to diets.

The second behavior to modify is exercise. Increased exercise reduces percentage body fat and increases the percentage lean mass. Concomitant with this, exercise decreases triglyceride levels. Exercise can increase HDL levels somewhat. This effect is most marked in competitive male athletes. As with weight reduction due to diet, increased exercise carries similar benefits: im-

proved glucose control, improved self-image, and increased energy to do important activities.

It is reasonable to consider addition of pharmaceuticals after a 3- to 6-month trial of diet and exercise. It is critical, if pharmaceutical treatment is contemplated, to compare the goals in terms of reducing specific lipids and lipoproteins with the drugs that will be used. Costs and side effects must also be considered. First-line treatment of hypercholesterolemia can be niacin (27), a fibric acid derivative, a bile salt–binding resin, or an HMG-CoA reductase inhibitor (29). First-line pharmaceutical treatment of hypertriglyceridemia includes niacin or a fibric acid derivative. In women who are trying to reduce cholesterol levels, strong consideration should be given to beginning cyclic estrogen therapy, since estrogens in women both lower cholesterol and raise HDL levels.

All of the cholesterol-lowering drugs are associated with side effects. Niacin (nicotinic acid) causes flushing even at low doses, although this can be ameliorated if an aspirin is taken before the nicotinic acid. Fibric acid derivatives cause nausea and other GI symptoms. Bile salt–binding resins cause constipation. HMG-CoA reductase inhibitors cause many GI side effects. In vigorous attempts to reduce cholesterol levels, which are necessary to cause regression of atherosclerosis, the major side effect is elevated liver function tests, especially if several drugs are used. The use of the drug combination lovastatin and gemfibrozil has been discouraged because of reports of associated severe myopathy, rhabdomyolysis, and renal failure.

FOLLOW-UP

Once treatment has been initiated for a patient, annual (or more frequent) follow-up is critical to determine its effectiveness and to monitor side effects. Therapeutic goals must be periodically reviewed. As with all medications used in older patients, both initial and maintenance treatment should be the lowest possible dose necessary to achieve satisfactory results. Particular attention should be paid to possible drug interactions, as polypharmacy is a major cause of morbidity in the older population.

CONCLUSION

Although there are changes in lipid and lipoprotein levels that are associated with aging, metabolism in older people is similar to that in younger people. Thus, high LDL cholesterol levels are "bad" and high HDL cholesterol levels are "good" in older people as they are in younger people. When treating older people for lipid abnormalities, however, the presence of other diseases may modify decisions to treat or not to treat; in addition, there is less time remaining in the lives of older people for treatment to be effective. Since improvement in morbidity or mortality may not be as great in older people, careful attention must be paid to adverse side effects and other things affecting quality of life, even extensive changes in diet. In conclusion, abnormalities in lipoproteins in older people should be carefully evaluated. Treatment decisions, however, must be carefully considered in the light of other medical problems, chronic conditions, and life expectancy.

REFERENCES

1. Goodman DS. The national cholesterol education program: guidelines, status, and issues. Am J Med 1991;90(suppl 2A):32S–55S.
2. Reaven GM. Role of insulin resistance in human disease. Diabetes 1988;37:1595–1607.
3. Gordon DJ, Rifkind BM. High-density lipoprotein—the clinical implications of recent studies. N Engl J Med 1989;321:1311–1316.
4. Thieszen SL, Hixson JE, Nagengast DJ, Wilson JE, McManus BM. Lipid phenotypes, apolipoprotein genotypes and cardiovascular risk in nonagenarians. Atherosclerosis 1990;83:137–146.
5. Rader DJ, Brewer HB. Lipoprotein(a). Clinical approach to a unique atherogenic lipoprotein (clinical conference) (published erratum appears in JAMA 1992:267:1922) JAMA 1992:267:1109–1112.
6. Scanu AM, Lawn RM, Berg K. Lipoprotein(a) and atherosclerosis. Ann Intern Med 1991;115:209–218.
7. Murano S, Shinomiya M, Shirai K, Saito Y, Yoshida S. Characteristic features of long-living patients with familial hypercholesterolemia in Japan. J Am Geriatr Soc 1993;41:253–257.
8. Gofman JW, Young W, Tandy R. Ischemic heart disease, atherosclerosis, and longevity. Circulation 1966;34:679–697.
9. Kronmal RA, Cain KC, Ye Z, Omenn GS. Total cholesterol levels and mortality risk as function of age. Arch Intern Med 1993;153:1065–1073.
10. Grundy SM. Cholesterol and coronary heart disease. Scand J Clin Lab Invest Suppl 1990;199:17–24.
11. Muldoon MF, Manuck SB, Matthews KA. Lowering cholesterol concentrations and mortality: a quantitative review of primary prevention trials. Br Med J 1990;301:309–314.
12. Barth JD, Arntzenius AC. Progression and regression of atherosclerosis, what roles for LDL-cholesterol and HDL-cholesterol: a perspective. Eur Heart J 1991;12:952–957.
13. Grundy SM. HMG-CoA reductase inhibitors for treatment of hypercholesterolemia. N Engl J Med 1988;319:24–31.
14. Harris T, Cook EF, Kannel WB, Goldman L. Proportional hazards analysis of risk factors for coronary heart disease in individuals aged 65 or older. J Am Geriatr Soc 1988;36:1023–1028.
15. Rubenstein C, Romhilt D, Segal P, et al. Dyslipoproteinemias and manifestations of coronary heart disease. The Lipid Research Clinics Program Prevalence Study. Circulation 1986;73(suppl):91–99.
16. Hazzard WR. Dyslipoproteinemia in the elderly. Clin Geriatr Med 1992;8:89–102.
17. Karvonen MJ. Determinants of cardiovascular diseases in the elderly. Ann Med 1989;21:3–12.
18. Aronow WS, Starling L, Etienne F, et al. Risk factors for coronary artery disease in persons older than 62 years in long-term health care facility. Am J Cardiol 1986;57:518–520.
19. Denke MA, Grundy SM. Hypercholesterolemia in elderly persons: resolving the treatment dilemma. Ann Intern Med 1990;112:780–792.
20. Lipid Research Clinics Program. The lipid research clinics coronary primary prevention trial results. JAMA 1984;251:351–374.
21. Oster G, Epstein AM. Cost-effectiveness of antihyperlipemic therapy in the prevention of coronary heart disease. The case of cholestyramine. JAMA 1987;258:2381–2387.
22. Kannel WB, Doyle JJ, Shephard JF, Stamler J, Vokonas PS. Prevention of cardiovascular disease in the elderly. J Am Coll Cardiol 1987;10:25A–28A.
23. Verdery RB, Goldberg AP. Hypocholesterolemia as a predictor of death. A prospective study of 224 nursing home residents. J Gerontol 1991;46:M84–90.
24. Oliver MF. Serum cholesterol—the knave of hearts and the joker. Lancet 1991;2:1090–1095.
25. Stamler J. Risk factor modification trials: implications for the elderly. Eur Heart J 1988;9(suppl D):9–53.
26. Hermanson B, Omenn GS, Kronmal RA, Gersh BJ, and participants in the Coronary Artery Surgery Study. Beneficial six-year outcome of smoking cessation in older men and women with coronary artery disease. N Engl J Med 1988;319:1365–1369.
27. Canner PL, Berge KG, Wenger NK, et al., for the Coronary Drug Project Research Group. Fifteen year mortality in coronary drug project patients: long-term benefit with niacin. Am Coll Cardiol 1986; 8:1245–1255.
28. Grundy SM. Multifactorial etiology of hypercholesterolemia. Implications for prevention of coronary heart disease. Arteriosclerosis Thrombosis 1990; 11:1619–1635.

25/ Principles of Fluid/Electrolyte Balance and Renal Disorders in the Elderly

Kenneth L. Minaker

Normal aging, in the absence of disease, is associated with substantial loss of renal function (1). When added to common disease processes influencing renal performance, the high prevalence of disorders of fluid and electrolyte balance in the elderly is understandable. This chapter outlines the impact of age on the anatomic and functional changes that occur in the aging kidney and emphasizes the adaptive mechanisms responsible for maintaining the constancy of the volume and composition of the extracellular fluid. Management of common fluid and electrolyte disturbances in elderly people and the common disease processes that influence the well-being of elderly individuals are discussed.

ANATOMIC AND PATHOLOGIC CHANGES

Morphologic alterations have been documented in aging glomeruli, tubules, basement membranes, and blood vessels. Aside from the vascular component of these changes, the pathogenesis of these structural abnormalities remains unclear. Many of the anatomic changes have significant functional sequelae of importance to the understanding of illness syndromes (2).

The combined weight of the two kidneys declines from 250–270 g at age 30 to 180–200 g by age 90. There is usually bilateral reduction in kidney size, with the renal capsule often adhering to the renal surface. The aging kidneys show a fine granular appearance of the subcapsular surface. It is notable that decline in renal mass is primarily due to loss of cortical tissues, whose interstitium appears fibrotic.

On microscopic examination the aging kidney demonstrates substantial glomerular sclerosis (3). Detailed study has revealed that less than 10% of the glomerular would be expected to be sclerotic in individuals up to the age of 45 years. In individuals over age 50 years without clinical evidence of primary renal disease or hyperten-

sion, over 95% of individuals had more than 10% sclerotic glomeruli. There do not appear to be differences related to gender. Detailed structural examination reveals thickening of the glomerular tuft and a widening of the extracellular matrix area in the sclerotic glomeruli. A terminal event appears to be global sclerosis. Electron microscopic examination demonstrates loss of epithelial cell foot processes around the shrinking glomerular capillaries and sometimes a redundant Bowman's capsule (5).

The cause of the glomerular sclerosis is currently unclear. The presumption has been that these changes have been related to vascular sclerosis and consequent renal ischemia. Hemodynamic and dietary factors may also be relevant to the changes associated with human aging. In animal studies, hemodynamic, dietary, and genetic factors appear to play a role in the progressive glomerular sclerosis that occurs with aging (6). When superimposed on aging processes, specific illnesses affecting the kidney may accelerate renal deterioration. These illnesses include glomerulonephritis, diabetes mellitus, nephrolithiasis, hypertension, vesicoureteral reflux, trauma, infection, infarction (7–9), or drug reactions, which through immunologic mechanisms cause interstitial nephritis.

A broad spectrum of vascular alterations is seen in the aging kidney. Lesions typical of atherosclerosis in large vessels and hyaline arteriolar sclerosis in smaller arterioles are observed. Medium-size vessels may also show characteristic changes of atherosclerosis. Usually, however, smaller vessels demonstrate irregular thickening of vessel walls because of fibrosis of the intima and the media, occasionally leading to vascular stenosis. In smaller interlobular arteries, fibroelastic intimal thickening is the most characteristic alteration. The most characteristic lesion involving the arterioles is hyaline arteriolosclerosis, characterized by homogeneous hyaline depositions in the intima and media.

These changes, which are predominant in the proximal afferent arterioles, have been mechanistically related to endothelial damage. It is hypothesized that leakage of plasma contents, followed by subendothelial deposition of these molecules in the form of eosinophilic hyaline material, is causal. Further thickening of vessel walls results from extracellular matrix production by neighboring smooth muscle cells. It is believed that the primary reason for the glomerular ischemia and sclerosis is this arteriolar stenosis. Vascular changes described above occur in approximately 15% of humans over age 50 years—a process dramatically accelerated by the presence of hypertension, which increases the chance of these findings to over 97%. It remains unclear whether these small vessel changes contribute to the genesis of hypertension, but they are clearly associated with the decline in renal function observed during aging.

FUNCTIONAL RENAL CHANGES DURING AGING

RENAL BLOOD FLOW AND GLOMERULAR FILTRATION RATE

Substantial information is available about the physiology of renal function with aging because of the relative ease of blood and urine assessment and the availability of good data from which to understand changing renal function with advancing age. The Baltimore Longitudinal Study on Aging has conducted the most rigorous observations in a cross-sequential analysis of a large number of aging individuals. In 1976, a major study of 884 community-dwelling volunteers indicated that there was an accelerating decline in creatinine clearances with advancing age, findings that confirmed earlier cross-sectional studies. This indicated that selective mortality and differences between groups of individuals had no significant impact on the major observation that there was a decline in creatinine clearance with advancing age (10).

Historically, the earliest mechanism thought to explain the decline in glomerular filtration was a documented change in renal blood flow with age. A progressive reduction in renal plasma flow of approximately 10%/decade, from 600 mL/min in young adulthood to 300 mL/min by 80 years of age is well established. Detailed studies indicate a selective loss of cortical flow with relative preservation of medullary flow. Cortical vascular changes outlined earlier probably account for the

patchy cortical defects commonly seen on renal scans in healthy elderly adults. Function parallels the histologic findings. Filtration fraction (the fraction of renal plasma flow that is filtered at the glomerulus) actually increases with advancing age. This is because outer cortical nephrons have a lower filtration fraction than juxtamedullary nephrons, and the aging kidney is composed of relatively more higher-filtering medullary nephrons.

The major clinically relevant renal functional defect arising from these histologic and blood flow changes is a progressive decline after maturity in the glomerular filtration rate (GFR), as estimated by clearance of inulin or creatinine. Age-adjusted normative standards for creatinine clearance have been established. Creatinine clearance is stable until the middle of the fourth decade, at which time a linear decrease of about 8 mL/min/ 1.73 m^2/decade begins. The absence of a reciprocal elevation in serum creatinine associated with the decrease in GFR with age is of major clinical relevance. Muscle mass, from which creatinine is derived, falls with age at roughly the same rate as GFR; thus the rather drastic age-related loss of renal function is not reflected in an elevation in serum creatinine. Thus, serum creatinine overestimates GFR in the elderly. Depressions of GFR severe enough to result in elevation of serum creatinine above 1.5 mg/dL are rarely caused solely by normal aging and thus should be viewed as indicating the presence of renal disease.

While the normative trend is for decline in renal function with advancing age, predicting an individual's performance over time has been more difficult. This is because there is a large variance in renal function at baseline and a large scatter of normative values of GFR progressively over the life span. Lindeman has made more recent observations based on a detailed study of 446 volunteers studied between 1958 and 1981, each with five or more creatinine clearance determinations (11). Lindeman selected three groups of individuals: (a) subjects with any history or laboratory evidence of renal or urinary tract disease; (b) subjects started on diuretics or antihypertensive agents; and (c) approximately 254 normal subjects. The mean decrease in creatinine clearance in the healthiest group was very similar to that observed in the large study published by Rowe.

Examining the detailed patterns of longitudinal changes in renal function in these healthy individuals revealed that one-third of all subjects had a clear decline in creatinine clearance. The middle group showed small but largely insignificant decreases in serial creatinine clearances over time. The remaining one-third showed a subtle but significant increase in creatinine clearance in late life. The factors associated with these differential patterns of renal function over time may, in part, be related to differences in blood pressure; those with the higher pressures experiencing the greatest declines (12, 13). The clinical point related to estimation of glomerular filtration rates with age is to recognize the likelihood of decline in renal function with advancing age and adjust initial management for this probable change. However, in any important circumstance, clinical measures of renal function should be taken and blood values of any important metabolite or medication be routinely evaluated.

The kidney, like other organs, has the capacity to respond to decreasing function. Removing a kidney results in compensatory hypertrophy in the remaining normal kidney. The rates of enlargement of the remaining kidney and the increased function that results are much reduced in the elderly kidney, compared with the young kidney. The number of glomeruli does not increase after birth, and the compensatory enlargement of the kidney is not due to an increase in nephrons, but due to enlargement of individual glomeruli and renal tubules. The dominance of hypertrophy as the major cellular response to unilateral nephrectomy has been well studied. This rate of hypertrophy is more sluggish in elderly animals. In renal transplant donors in their third decade, renal function was increased almost 50% 3 years after they donated a single kidney. In those individuals in their seventh decade, single kidney GFR had increased only 30% (14). Thus, the aging kidney is limited in its ability to compensate for injury or aging (15).

The "adaptive" hyperperfusion and hyperfiltration characterizing renal functional changes with age have been mechanistically studied to clarify the consequences of this state. Unchecked, glomerular capillary membrane disruption occurs, resulting in proteinuria, accumulation of mesangial deposits, and glomerular sclerosis. Hostetter studied the influence of varied amounts of protein on proteinuria and glomerular sclerosis, observing that dietary protein restriction delays significantly the development of these findings (16). Protein is associated acutely with increases in GFR and renal plasma flow, independent of altering cardiac output (17, 18).

Two common illnesses in late life, hypertension and diabetes mellitus, also result in hyperperfusion and hyperfiltration. In the case of diabetes mellitus, good control of the glucose levels reduces the declines in renal function (19). In diabetes-related hypertension, control of the carbohydrate load and protein restriction helps to preserve renal function. The underlying mechanisms for hyperfiltration are complex and may additionally involve intrarenal vascular regulation and growth factors. It is not certain at this time whether protein restriction will have any long-term benefits in individuals aging normally. Further study is necessary in this important area.

SODIUM BALANCE

SODIUM EXCRETING ABILITY

Excessive sodium retention and volume overload are commonly encountered problems in elderly patients. Both the excretory capacity for sodium and the diurnal variation in excretion are influenced by age. Short-term intravenous loading reveals distinct age-related differences in sodium excretion. Following a 2 L normal saline load, individuals older than 40 years excrete less sodium per 24 hours than do race-, sex-, and size-matched subjects below 40 years of age (20). The peak excretory capacity of sodium in the elderly is approximately half of that of young individuals (Fig. 25.1) (21).

Additionally, in the 24-hour period following intravenous sodium loading, elderly individuals excrete at relatively stable rates over a substantial portion of the 24-hour follow-up. Young individuals, however, excrete most of their sodium load promptly, well before the 24 hours of follow-up. However, the elderly can excrete significant

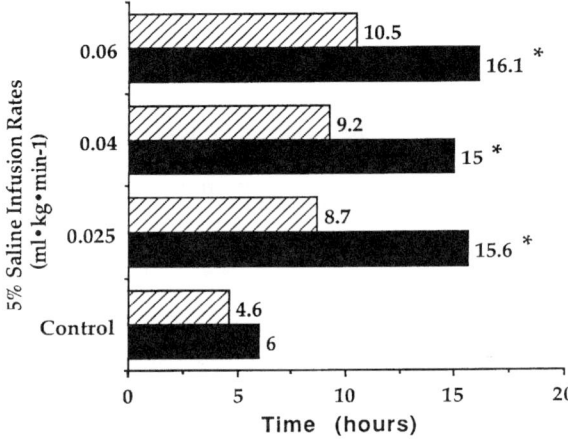

Figure 25.1. Time to excrete 50% of sodium load, young vs. old subjects. Young in *hatched bars*; old in *solid bars*. The time to excrete 50% of the sodium load was significantly longer in the old subjects across all hypertonic sodium loads (*$P < .05$). Control infusion, 0.45% saline at 100 mL/hr for 2 hr.

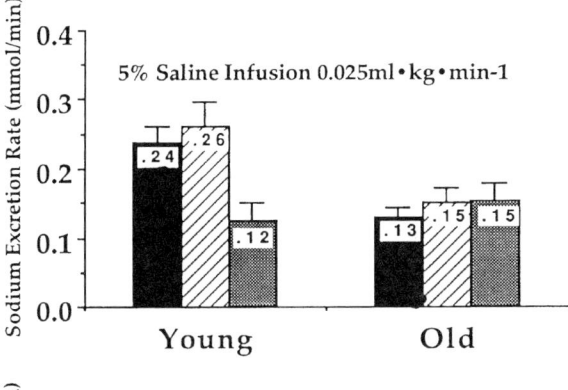

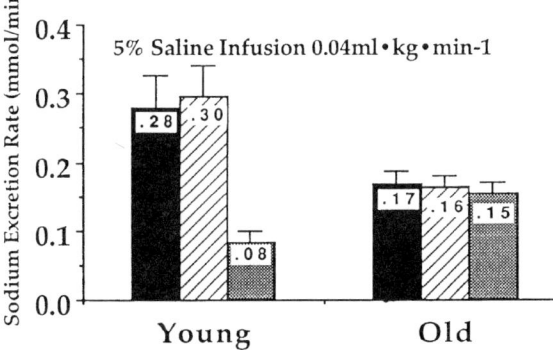

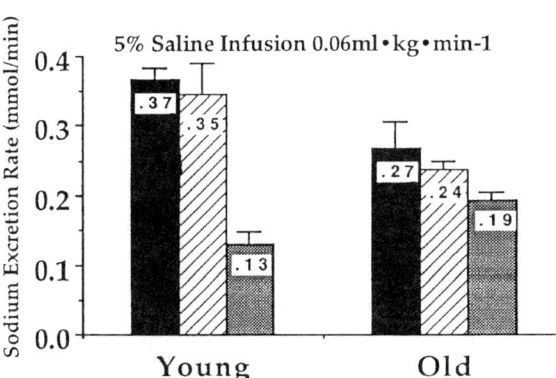

Figure 25.2. Sodium excretion rates, young vs. old at three time periods: *black column*, 8 AM to 4 PM; *hatched bars column*, 4 PM to 12 AM; *gray column*, 12 AM to 8 AM for each of three infusion rates: 5% saline at a rate of 0.025 mL/kg – 1/min – 1; 0.04 mL/kg – 1/min – 1; and 0.06 mL/kg – 1/min – 1. The number in the bar is the sodium excretion rate.

loads of sodium, albeit subjecting themselves to volume expansion for a greatly prolonged time (Fig. 25.2). In addition to demonstrating the restricted maximum capacity of the aged kidney to excrete sodium, these changes are not related to any alteration in creatinine clearance that occurs

as part of the aging process. These data strongly suggest that the loss of sodium excretory capacity with advancing age is primarily a tubular functional change. A final observation of this important study is that the delay in renal sodium excretion is observed across a broad range of sodium loads. This means that during most sodium-intake situations encountered during life, a fairly fixed delay in excretion is observed.

The potential role of additional factors, including intrarenal hemodynamics, renal nerve activity, and activities of the intrarenal β-adrenergic system, renin-angiotensin-aldosterone, dopamine, and prostaglandins has not been elucidated.

SODIUM-CONSERVING CAPACITY

The ability of the aging kidney to conserve sodium in response to reduced salt intake is impaired. Clinical studies have shown that when placed on a very low sodium diet (10 mmol/Na/day), healthy elderly individuals reduce urinary sodium excretion much less promptly than their younger counterparts, but are able over time to come into balance and reduce urinary sodium losses (22). This sluggish response to abruptly impaired sodium intake, such as accompanies surgery or acute illness, can have major clinical consequences and result in substantial overall reduction in extracellular fluid volume.

Clearance studies in young and elderly subjects have shown a decreased distal tubular capacity for sodium reabsorption in elderly individuals (23). Contributors to this distal tubular dysfunction might include anatomic changes in the aging kidney involving the interstitial tissues as well as functional and hormonal changes. There are important age-related alterations in the renin-angiotensin-aldosterone system. Basal plasma renin concentration and activities are decreased by 30 to 50% in elderly subjects in spite of normal levels of renin substrate (24). In response to maneuvers designed to stimulate renin secretion, the age difference in plasma renin activity is further amplified. There is a similar 30 to 50% decrease in plasma aldosterone levels in elderly subjects during recumbency and normal sodium intake, becoming more pronounced during stimulation, which may involve upright posture, sodium restriction, and furosemide administration (25, 26).

The age-related aldosterone deficiency appears to be related to the renin-angiotensin deficiency and not to intrinsic adrenal gland defects. Studies show marked improvement in distal tubular sodium reabsorption with aldosterone administration. Additionally, plasma aldosterone and cortisol responses to corticotrophin infusion are normal in the elderly. Thus, during sodium restriction, impaired angiotensin levels and/or decreased aldosterone response may reduce renal tubular reabsorption in the elderly.

ATRIAL NATRIURETIC PEPTIDE (ANP)

There are striking changes in ANP with aging that have implications for several aspects of fluid and electrolyte balance. Peptides isolated from the cardiac atria cause diuresis, natriuresis, and reduction in blood pressure. The most striking effects of ANP are increases in GFR, free water clearance, and natriuresis, without a corresponding increase in renal blood flow. These effects are believed to be secondary to alterations in intrarenal blood flow and are independent of changes in total renal blood flow or tubular sodium transport (27, 28).

ANP decreases blood pressure by vasodilation and perhaps through direct modulation of baroreceptor reflexes. Cardiac output is decreased by several mechanisms, primarily the basal vasodilatory effect of ANP resulting in lowered cardiac filling pressures. Plasma volume is decreased by ANP-mediated renal effects on sodium and free water loss as well as by a translocation of fluid from plasma to the interstitial space secondary to an increase in capillary permeability. This "edemagenic effect" may be particularly important in elderly persons. Atrial natriuretic peptide also directly antagonizes the components of counterbalancing vasoconstrictive, sodium-retaining hormonal systems, through inhibition of the secretion of aldosterone and vasopressin.

In healthy elderly individuals, atrial natriuretic peptide levels are three to five times higher than those of healthy younger individuals. Baseline ANP levels in clinically stable patients with evidence of cardiovascular disease are twice those seen in healthy elderly individuals. Several possible mechanisms for the increased levels of ANP in the elderly deserve consideration (31): (a) aging is a state of increased effective extracellular fluid volume (this view is supported by the coexisting elevations of ANP and the suppression of renin levels; (b) elevated ANP is secondary to enhanced sensitivity of the atrial afferent system for ANP release; and (c) end-organ resistance to ANP actions induce feedback stimulation of ANP. This would help explain several age-related effects including the decrease in GFR and impaired ability to excrete a sodium load (secondary to resistance

to the renal vascular effects of ANP), the increase in systolic blood pressure (because of resistance to the antagonization of angiotensin-norepinephrine-mediated vasoconstriction of large arteries), and the age-related enhancement of vasopressin secretion with osmotic stimulation (to counterbalance the suppressive effect of ANP on vasopressin secretion). In this regard, preliminary evidence suggests that renal sodium excretion in healthy elderly is relatively resistant to physiologic-range elevations of ANP (32).

While the clinical implications of age-related increases in ANP have not yet been elucidated, several intriguing possibilities deserve careful study. Specifically, the role of ANP in enhancing edema development in elderly people during the daytime, facilitating nocturnal diuresis, has obvious implications for the management of very common clinical problems in this age group.

Another major issue currently under investigation is related to the possible value of ANP levels as predictors of future cardiovascular morbidity or mortality in the elderly. A recently reported prospective study related ANP levels and clinical history to future clinical events in 310 elderly residents of a long-term care facility (Fig. 25.3) (33).

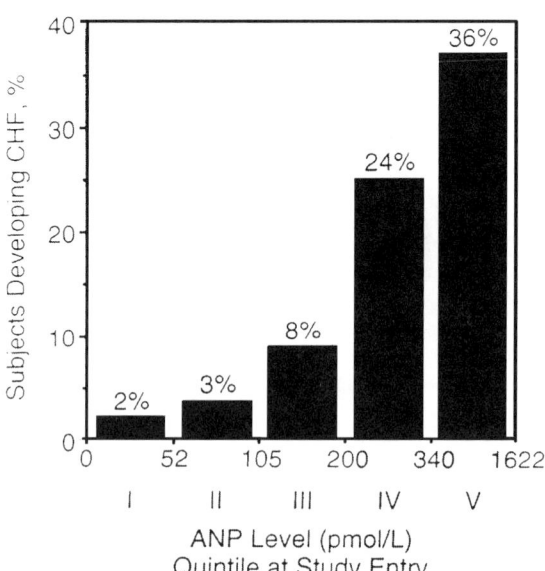

Figure 25.3. Percentage of subjects developing congestive heart failure (CHF) during prospective follow-up by atrial natriuretic peptide (ANP) levels at study entry. The 310 subjects are divided into quintiles by ANP level, with 60 to 64 subjects in each quintile ($P < .001$ for differences in percentage developing CHF among the quintiles by χ^2 contingency analysis).

In this very old, frail, but clinically stable population, 15% of individuals developed at least one episode of congestive heart failure over the course of 1 year. Baseline ANP levels in those developing congestive heart failure were twice as high as the levels in those who did not. While a prior history of heart failure was a strong risk factor for future heart failure within this previously affected high-risk group, elevated ANP levels independently predicted heart failure. For the patients with prior heart failure, the risk of another episode was nearly 75% if ANP was high, whereas the risk fell to 25% if ANP was low. These findings suggest that clinically stable elderly individuals are a physiologically heterogeneous group and that ANP determinations may help in identifying those at greatest risk for clinical decompensation.

POTASSIUM BALANCE

Studies of the effects of aging on renal and extrarenal adaptation to high potassium loads or dietary potassium deprivation in man are lacking. Two different studies, however, have found that total body potassium and total exchangeable potassium decreases with age in both sexes and that the decrease is more marked in women than in men. This decrease may relate to the decrease in muscle mass with advancing age. Over the past several years there has been substantial attention paid to extrarenal potassium disposal.

It has been demonstrated in humans that β-adrenergic mechanisms are responsible for potassium disposal during potassium infusion (34). The study was conducted on healthy individuals across the adult age range, and the authors found no effect of age on the extrarenal potassium disposal or the effect of β-adrenergic blockade.

A second study evaluated the effects of insulin level, β-adrenergic blockade, and age on potassium homeostasis during hyperinsulinemia (35). These investigators showed that increasing steady-state levels of insulin are associated with dose-dependent declines in plasma potassium during the first hour of the insulin infusion but that during second hour of insulin infusion, plasma potassium continued to decline at the lowest insulin doses but began to rise at the highest insulin dose levels. This finding suggests the presence of a regulatory mechanism influencing insulin-mediated alterations in plasma potassium. The effect was not influenced by β-adrenergic blockade or aging. Taken together, these studies suggest that hormonal regulation of extrarenal potassium homeostasis is generally intact in aged persons.

ACID-BASE BALANCE

Baseline indicators of acid-base balance are unchanged with age. Serum pH, PCO_2, and bicarbonate levels remain constant (36). There is, however, a delayed recovery of pH and bicarbonate concentrations following ingestion of an ammonium chloride load by older individuals. Total acid excretion in aging individuals under such stimulation decreases at a rate that parallels the decrease in GFR. Several investigators have also shown reduced excretion of ammonia in elderly subjects, compared with young subjects.

WATER BALANCE

RENAL CONCENTRATING ABILITY

Renal concentrating ability declines with age in humans. In several studies, the maximum urine osmolality, measured following 12 to 24 hours of dehydration, was inversely related to age (37). In one careful study, the maximum urine osmolality was 1109 mOsm/kg in 31 subjects aged 20 to 39 years, compared with 1051 mOsm/kg in 48 subjects aged 40 to 59 years, and 882 mOsm/kg in 18 subjects aged 60 to 79 years (38). The age-related decline in concentrating ability did not correlate with the age-related decline in GFR.

While this age-related deficit in water conservation is easily demonstrated in physiologic studies, it is likely to be of only minor clinical consequence, since substantial reserve concentrating capacity remains. Studies in humans suggest that the concentrating defect is due to an intrarenal defect rather than a failure in osmotic-induced release of AVP (39). Following intravenous infusion of hypertonic saline in young and old individuals, plasma AVP levels rose 4.5 times the baseline in older men and 2.5 times the baseline in younger individuals, despite similar free water clearances. The slope of the plasma AVP concentration vs. serum osmolality curve, an index of the sensitivity of the osmole receptor, was significantly increased in the older subjects. In addition, in the same study, intravenous infusion of ethanol resulted in a progressive decline in plasma AVP levels in the young subjects, but failed to have a similar effect in the older subjects. In contrast to osmotic stimulation, volume-pressure-mediated AVP release has been found to decrease with age and appears to be absent in many healthy elderly people (40). An additional factor that may influence AVP levels and impair water conservation in the elderly is the previously discussed increase in ANP levels. ANP suppresses AVP release in response to hyperosmolality in young and old individuals.

RENAL DILUTING ABILITY

Renal diluting ability is also impaired as a function of age (41). In water-diuresing subjects, minimal urine osmolality is significantly higher (92 mOsm/kg in elderly subjects vs. 52 mOsm/kg in young subjects). Free water clearance is also decreased (5.9 mL/min in elderly subjects vs. 16.2 mL/min in young subjects). The impairment in free water clearance is largely due to the decrease in GFR. However, when the free water clearance is adjusted for GFR, there is, however, still a significant but less substantial decrease in older individuals. Mechanisms for the impaired diluting ability in the elderly have not been well studied but may involve inadequate suppression of AVP release or impaired solute transport in the ascending Loop of Henle.

THIRST IN THE ELDERLY

The age-related impairment in renal concentrating and sodium conserving ability is associated with increased incidence of volume depletion and hypernatremia in the elderly. Under normal physiologic conditions, increased thirst and food intake are natural defense mechanisms against volume depletion and hypernatremia. The deficit in thirst and regulation of fluid intake in the elderly, however, may further contribute to the increased incidence of dehydration and hypernatremia.

Recent studies confirm the long-held clinical observation that thirst and food intake are impaired in the elderly (42). In a series of studies, the osmotic threshold for thirst during hypertonic saline infusion was much higher in healthy elderly subjects than in their younger counterparts, with many apparently normal elders not reporting thirst despite elevations of plasma osmolality to levels over 300 mOsm/kg (43). In studies of water ingestion after intravenously induced hyperosmolality, elderly individuals demonstrate marked reductions (compared with a young group) in their water intake and the rate of return of plasma osmolality to baseline. Finally, the same investigators evaluated the influence of free access to water on prevention of osmolality during hypertonic saline infusion. Despite equivalent increases in plasma volume, the older group displayed significantly less water intake and greater increases in plasma osmolality than did the younger group (44). Clinical studies have also suggested that individuals with a prior history of stroke without the presence of cognitive impairment or evidence of hypothalamic or pituitary dysfunction may also have seriously impaired thirst (45, 46).

CLINICAL DISORDERS

SYNDROMES OF DISORDERED FLUID HOMEOSTASIS

Dehydration

Dehydration is a commonly underdiagnosed condition of the frail elderly. Approximately 1% of all hospital admissions are associated with hypernatremic dehydration in which serum sodium levels exceed 148 mEq/L (47). Isotonic dehydration occurs much more frequently; recent data suggest that perhaps 1 million elderly individuals are admitted per year to acute care hospitals with dehydration as a major component of their clinical picture. In one large study, only 43% of hospitalized patients were hypernatremic on admission; most developed elevated serum sodium level during hospitalization, one-half of them within the first 8 days. The mortality of those who developed hypernatremia during hospitalization approached 50%.

What is difficult in the geriatric population is that almost half of all patients have three or more factors contributing to dehydration. This is consistent with the generally held gerontologic principle that multiple factors usually contribute to illness in the elderly. No matter what the overall clinical precipitant is, evaluation must assess for excessive fluid loss or impaired fluid intake.

Increased Fluid Losses (Table 25.1)

Acute infections, such as pneumonia and urinary tract infections, are common in the elderly, accounting for up to 20% of acute hospitalizations in this population. The associated fever results in increased insensible water loss from sweating, tachypnea, and increased cellular catabolism. Infection of the upper urinary tract may specifically result in reduction of the renal concentrating ability that may persist for weeks following resolution of the infection. Excessive urinary losses of water and sodium are very common in the sick elderly patient.

Continuation of diuretic drug therapy in the elderly patient is an unfortunate yet common and preventable problem. As many as 10% of hospitalized elderly in the United Kingdom are the result of diuretic side effects such as dehydration. In addition to pharmacologic diuresis, obligate diuresis is common to many prevalent illnesses in the elderly. These include the glycosuria of dia-

Table 25.1
Causes of Increased Fluid Loss in the Elderly

Chronic or acute infections
Excessive urinary losses
   Diuretic misuse
   Glycosuria
   Hypercalciuria
   Mannitol
   Radiographic contrast agents
   Elevated blood urea nitrogen
   Diabetes insipidus
      Central (pituitary)
      Nephrogenic
   Hypoaldosteronism
      Addison's disease
      Hyporeninemic hypoaldosteronism
   Suppressed vasopressin
      Phenytoin
      Ethanol
      Postatrial tachyarrhythmia
   Postobstructive diuresis
Gastrointestinal losses
   Upper GI
   Vomiting
   Nasogastric drainage
Lower GI (diarrhea)
   Laxative abuse/bowel preparation
   Infectious/secretory
   Surgical bypass/fistulas
   Ischemic bowel
   Colectomy
Excessive blood loss
Environment-related fluid loss
   Heat wave
   Hypothermia
Compartmental fluid shifts
   Hypoalbuminemia
   Pancreatitis
   Ascites
   Anaphylaxis
   Burns
   Hypertonic peritoneal dialysate

betes mellitus, hypercalciuria of malignancy and hyperparathyroidism. An obligate diuresis may result from renal absorption of excessive blood urea nitrogen (BUN) generated by increased protein catabolism in the gut in the setting of gastrointestinal bleeding or high-protein enteral tube feeding (48).

Central diabetes insipidus is not a common disease in the elderly, but nephrogenic diabetes insipidus is frequently seen in association with the use of drugs such as lithium, demeclocycline, and methoxyflurane anesthesia. Hypoaldosteronism occurs in the setting of Addison's disease with inadequate mineralocorticoid replacement, as well

as in the hyporeninemic state associated with normal aging. This hypoaldosteronism results in impairment in the renal salvage of sodium and water during periods of dehydration. Drugs such as phenytoin and ethanol cause a suppression in the release of vasopressin, resulting in a decrease in tubular reabsorption of water. Alcohol abuse contributing to dehydration is frequently underrecognized in the elderly patient.

Urinary tract obstruction is a common affliction in the elderly male with prostatic hypertrophy (often exacerbated by anticholinergic medication). In the elderly female, postoperative urinary retention is a frequently unrecognized cause of obstructive uropathy. The postobstructive diuresis associated with relief of urinary tract obstruction, is physiologically similar to nephrogenic diabetes insipidus with its inadequate renal responsiveness to vasopressin.

Gastrointestinal losses of fluid occur with vomiting, nasogastric drainage, diarrhea, and bleeding. In addition to the commonly recognized etiology of diarrhea, laxative abuse is often present but unreported in the elderly. As many as 40 to 60% of elderly persons use laxatives regularly, and the elderly patient may experience unrecognized continuation of regularly ordered laxatives and stool softeners in the setting of diarrhea. Older patients are often victimized by aggressive bowel cleansing regimens before radiographic study of the bowel or kidney. A patient with previous intestinal bypass or colectomy is at further risk for dehydration because of reduced gastrointestinal water absorptive capacity.

The elderly are especially prone to heat-related fluid loss from excessive sweating with inadequate volume replacement. The excess mortality seen during prolonged summer heat waves disproportionately affects the elderly. Many older persons have inadequate social and physical protective mechanisms to avoid excessive heat exposure. These same people may suffer from limited access to (or recognition of the need for) salt and water and therefore do not compensate for the increased insensible fluid loss.

Compartmental fluid shifts from conditions such as hypoalbuminemia and pancreatitis often result in a relative intravascular dehydration without clinically obvious sources of fluid loss.

Decreased Fluid Intake (Table 25.2)

Often underappreciated in elderly individuals are conditions resulting in inadequate fluid intake. Patients with physical restraints, restricted mobility, and poor vision may not have free access

Table 25.2
Causes of Decreased Fluid Intake in the Elderly

Limited access to fluids
   Physical restraints
   Mobility restriction
   Poor visual acuity
Fluid restriction
   Preprocedure
   Prevention of incontinence/nocturia/aspiration
   Therapy for edema or hyponatremia
Altered sensorium
   Decreased consciousness level
      Sedatives, neuroleptics, narcotics
      Structural and metabolic CNS insults
      Febrile illness
   Decreased level of awareness
      Dementia, delirium
      Mania, psychosis, depression
Gastrointestinal disorders
   Swallowing disorders
   Bowel obstruction
      Mechanical
      Metabolic
      Ischemic
   Anticholinergic medication
Alteration in thirst mechanism
   Primary adipsia
   Medication-related
      Cardiac glycosides
      Amphetamines
Associated with focal CNS pathology

to fluids. Most frequently underrecognized as being at risk for fluid access problems are patients with deteriorating mobility, vision, or level of consciousness who were independent in their fluid access before becoming ill.

Iatrogenic oral fluid deprivation is commonly ordered before diagnostic or surgical procedures or, inappropriately, for edema, renal insufficiency, or hyponatremia. Self- or caregiver-imposed fluid restriction is common in the older persons prone to urinary incontinence, nocturia, or pulmonary aspiration. Acute and chronic alterations in sensorium are prevalent in the ill elderly patient, with a resulting decrease in perception of the need for, and access to, appropriate fluids.

Gastrointestinal problems, such as swallowing disorders, bowel obstruction, and the underrecognized side effects of medication (nausea, vomiting, early satiety), often preclude adequate oral fluid intake. A common yet infrequently diagnosed cause of bowel obstruction in the elderly is ischemic bowel disease. This condition is exacerbated by dehydration, resulting in a vicious cycle of dehydration and ischemic bowel injury.

A further decrease in thirst perception in the elderly can be precipitated by drugs such as cardiac glycosides and amphetamines (49, 50).

THERAPY FOR DEHYDRATION

Prevention and early intervention are the most effective therapies for dehydration. This strategy can be accomplished by education of patients, families, and health care workers to appreciate the need for early intervention with fluid therapy in the elderly patient prone to dehydration. Specific fluid prescriptions in home, nursing home, or acute care hospital settings can be very helpful toward this end.

For the dehydrated patient, it is essential to establish the causes of fluid loss with history, physical examination, and appropriate laboratory studies and to direct therapy accordingly. Dehydration may be classified as either isotonic or hypertonic. Isotonic dehydration is characterized by loss of equimolar amounts of sodium and water, with resulting dehydration but without change in serum osmolarity. Hypertonic (hypernatremic) dehydration is seen in conditions of primary loss of free water more than sodium and is characterized by hypernatremia and hyperosmolarity.

The severity of fluid loss must be estimated by evaluation of blood pressure, orthostasis, skin turgor (though less useful in elderly persons), and urine output. Very useful is a careful measurement of weight to compare with a baseline weight determined before the most recent illnesses. The serum osmolarity can be measured or estimated within ± 10 mOsm/L by the following formula:

$$\text{Serum osmolarity} = 2\,(\text{Na}) + \text{glucose}/18 + \text{BUN}/2.8$$

where Na is measured in mEq/L and glucose and BUN are measured in mg/dL. If measured osmolarity is significantly greater than the calculated value, the presence of abnormal unmeasured solutes such as ethanol, isopropanol, ethylene glycol, methanol, or mannitol should be considered.

The magnitude of fluid deficits with primarily free water loss (hypernatremic dehydration) can be estimated by the following calculation:

$$\text{Fluid deficit (l)} = \text{desired TBW} - \text{current TBW}$$
$$\text{Current TBW} = 0.5 \times \text{body weight (kg)}$$
$$\text{Desired TBW} = \text{measured serum sodium}/140 \times \text{current TBW}$$

where TBW is the total body water in liters. In the young, water comprises 60% of the body weight, compared with only 50% in the elderly male and 45% in the elderly female. This proportional decrease in water is due to the increase in fat and decrease in lean body mass with aging (51).

Three methods of fluid replacement (oral, subcutaneous, and intravenous) may be used singly or in combination, depending on the setting and the severity of the condition. Oral rehydration is preferred; administration of free water or oral electrolyte solutions developed for use in third world countries is encouraged. Subcutaneous fluids may be very effective, safe, and easily administered, especially in the home or in the nursing home. Three liters of isotonic fluid/day may be delivered through two subcutaneous infusion sites, each dispensing 60 mL/hr. The addition of hyaluronidase (Wydase, Wyeth) may facilitate fluid absorption (52). The abdomen and upper outer aspect of the thighs are the preferred infusion sites. Intravenous fluid replacement is best reserved for the acute care setting in which the dehydrated patient can be closely monitored.

The first step in the therapy of hypernatremic dehydration is correction of hemodynamic collapse, manifested by hypotension, orthostasis, and decreased urine output. Rapid infusions of isotonic saline until these parameters of volume status stabilize constitute initial therapy. The hemodynamically stable patient should have replacement of one-half of the fluid deficit over the first 24 hours. A goal during rapid fluid replacement is to reduce serum osmolarity to 300 at a rate of no greater than 1 mOsm/kg/hr, followed by gradual infusion to correct the total osmolar deficit over the next 48 to 72 hours. The replacement fluid for these patients during this phase is 5% dextrose in 0.5 N saline. Patients with isotonic dehydration (normal or low serum sodium levels) should have isotonic saline as replacement fluid.

In addition to correction of the fluid deficit, ongoing fluid losses must be replaced. These losses average 2 to 3 L/day in the healthy person and may be significantly greater in illness. Continued reassessment of fluid status, including measurement of intake and output, weight, blood pressure, pulse, serum chemistries, and osmolarities, must be done to assure appropriate fluid replacement.

Overzealous rehydration, such as replacement of the entire fluid deficit over 24 hours, may result in death from cerebral edema. Dehydration of brain cells is prevented by the generation of osmotically active solute ("idiogenic osmoles"), thereby setting up an osmotic gradient to retain intracellular water in the face of systemic hyperosmolarity. If plasma hyperosmolarity is corrected too rapidly, there may be excessive movement of water into brain cells, resulting in cerebral edema. The fluid deficits of dehydration may be safely corrected over 72 hours, yet the associated mental status changes may persist for as long as 2 weeks.

HYPERNATREMIA

The incidence of severe hypernatremia among the elderly exceeds one case per hospital per month. Clinical experience suggests that patients likely to present in this manner are institutionalized, cognitively impaired persons who may have impaired thirst mechanisms. They may be receiving sedatives and major tranquilizers that contribute to hypodipsia. Many renal diseases impair urine-concentrating ability and accelerate the age-related decline in GFR. When the GFR decreases below 60 mL/min, urinary concentrating ability is significantly limited.

Obstructive uropathy secondary to prostatic hypertrophy, chronic pyelonephritis, renal amyloidosis, and the tubulointerstitial diseases associated with excretion of Bence Jones protein in multiple myeloma are conditions frequently seen in patients of advanced age; all of these conditions further reduce renal concentrating ability. Chronically ill elderly patients are at risk for protein-calorie malnutrition and sodium depletion, both of which further reduce medullary tonicity. The cerebral result of hypertonicity may be brain shrinkage, capillary hemorrhages, and permanent neurologic injury if deficits are severe and prolonged.

Data on the rate at which hypernatremia can be corrected in elderly patients are lacking. Rapid correction of hypertonicity to a serum osmolality of approximately 300 mOsm/kg is suggested; this can be followed by a more gradual repletion of free water deficits over 48 hours (54–56).

HYPONATREMIA

Although age-related alterations of the maximal diluting capacity of the senescent kidney are less than the decreases of concentrating ability, the most commonly encountered electrolyte disturbance among elderly individuals is hyponatremia. Eleven percent of elderly patients in a 638-bed geriatric service were found to have serum sodium concentrations below 130 mEq/L. Sixty-one percent of those individuals were symptomatic, albeit with nonspecific complaints. It has been suggested that symptoms are determined by both the magnitude and rate of development of hyponatremia. Subclinical brain edema occurs after a 7% increase in brain water (at sodium concentrations below 125 mEq/L). The results can be seizures or permanent neurologic injury.

Age has been implicated in the syndrome of idiopathic excess vasopressin secretion, in which volume status is generally euvolemic to slightly volume expanded. In this syndrome, the mechanism causing the hyponatremia is known as "vasopressin leak," in which vasopressin continues to be released at a time when it should be completely suppressed. It is seen in the absence of conditions or medications commonly associated with the syndrome of inappropriate vasopressin secretion. Both anesthesia and surgery predispose older persons to hyponatremic states. The usual cause is sustained vasopressin secretion plus the administration of hypotonic fluids. Chlorpropamide-induced hyponatremia secondary to prolonged stimulation of vasopressin release occurs in 4% of the general clinic population, yet advanced age is the dominant feature of the cases of severe hyponatremia associated with this drug. Other conditions with protean manifestations in the elderly, such as tuberculosis and hypothyroidism, are commonly associated with hyponatremia and excess vasopressin release. Diuretics, especially thiazides, impair free water excretion. In one series, diuretics were identified as causative in 64% of elderly patients admitted with hyponatremia.

The diagnostic approach to hyponatremia is first the assessment of the underlying osmolar state. If hyponatremia results when another osmotically active solute occupies the extracellular space, water will move from the intracellular space and lower the serum sodium concentration. Hyperglycemia and mannitol cause this form of hyperosmolar hyponatremia. The underlying treatment is obviously to lower the glucose level and to allow the mannitol to dissipate from the system.

In some settings, hyponatremia occurs as a spurious finding because of hyperlipidemia or hyperproteinemia. The low plasma sodium is artifactual because the plasma volume is occupied by lipids or protein. Rarely, occupation of the plasma volume by glycine or mannitol results in this biochemical artifact. When hyponatremia is associated with low osmolality, the next diagnostic step involves determining whether hypovolemia, euvolemia, or hypervolemia is present. Clinical suggestions that hypovolemia is present are postural changes in blood pressure, dryness and wrinkling of the skin, and low jugular venous pressure. Hypervolemia is suggested if edema is present or jugular venous pressure is elevated, and hyperten-

sion may be present. In all three situations, water intake exceeds the capacity of the kidney to excrete water, either because of elevated levels of plasma antidiuretic hormone or poor effective circulating volume leading to low water filtration by the renal glomerulus. In most circumstances producing hypovolemic and hypervolemic hyponatremia, urinary sodium is usually low, whereas in the euvolemic hyponatremias most oftenly caused by antidiuretic hormone excess, the urinary sodium will vary according to the dietary intake.

The symptoms and signs of hyponatremia are varied and include agitation, anorexia, ataxia, motor slowing, altered level of consciousness including coma, muscular cramps, hallucinations, hypothermia, nausea, respiratory depression, vomiting, and seizures.

While all tissues are influenced by hypoosmolality, perhaps the most important organ to be aware of clinically and therapeutically is the central nervous system. Acute lowering of the serum sodium level can lead to cerebral edema, as the osmotic gradient promotes movement of water across the blood-brain barrier into the brain. Adaptation to lowered serum sodium concentration is made possible by movement of fluid from the brain into the spinal fluid because of mechanical pressures and chronically by loss of intracellular osmotic particles.

During treatment, extracellular plasma sodium increases and the brain may become dehydrated. Therefore, rapid correction of hyponatremia may produce serious mechanical and pathologic effects. Perhaps the best characterized is demyelination in the central pons, basal ganglia, internal capsule, and cortex. The clinical features include pseudobulbar palsy, mental status changes, behavioral disturbances, altered level of consciousness, and motor dysfunction. Permanent disability can result in this situation from too rapid correction of hypoosmolar hyponatremia. There still exists some controversy as to the rate of correction of hyponatremia, and in general, it is best to rapidly correct low serum sodium levels to 120 mEq/L and then correct more slowly after this. In this setting, seizures will be avoided.

Treatment of hypovolemic hyponatremia involves repletion of the extracellular fluid volume with normal saline until the blood pressure is stable and correcting the underlying cause of the hypovolemia. In patients with edema associated with the hyponatremia, salt restriction and fluid restriction are standard measures, with administration of hypertonic saline and loop diuretics if severe hyponatremia is present. In patients with euvolemic hyponatremia, fluid restriction is the most conservative therapy, if the clinical situation permits. If there is no response, an infusion of 3% saline at 50 mL/hr with 10 to 20 mg of furosemide can be used to promote free water excretion. In chronic situations, the use of demeclocycline to produce a mild nephrogenic diabetes insipidus may be very helpful (57).

In an acutely symptomatic patient, aggressive therapy is required; the goal is a rise of 3 mEq/L/ hr until the sodium level reaches 120 mEq/L. Hypertonic saline is infused at a rate of 150 ml/hr. Furosemide is employed as described above. In states of chronic hyponatremia, fluid restriction is the primary treatment, with the goal of increasing serum sodium concentration by 0.5 mEq/L/hr. Chronic hyponatremia associated with seizures or coma should be managed as is acute hyponatremia.

SPECIFIC RENAL DISEASES

GLOMERULAR DISEASES

Membranous glomerulonephritis and glomerulosclerosis occur more commonly in elderly than in younger individuals. The common systemic illnesses associated with glomerular disease include diabetes mellitus (in particular, non-insulin-dependent diabetes mellitus), vasculitis, and amyloidosis. In a large study of 277 renal biopsies of individuals over the age of 60 years, approximately one-half of the biopsies revealed primary glomerular disease, 21% revealed secondary glomerular disease, and a variety of miscellaneous causes accounted for the rest.

In the primary glomerular disease category, the commonest pathologic cause was membranous glomerulonephritis, with minimal change disease, focal glomerulosclerosis, membranoproliferative glomerulonephritis, mesangial proliferative glomerulonephritis, crescentic glomerulonephritis, IgA nephropathy, and acute glomerulonephritis accounting for smaller percentages. Among individuals undergoing renal biopsy who were found to have secondary renal diseases, the largest number demonstrated amyloidosis, with diabetic glomerulosclerosis, lupus nephritis, and vasculitis contributing smaller percentages to these secondary illnesses. Almost certainly underrepresented in this series of individuals selected for diagnostic renal biopsy are hypertensive and diabetic individuals in whom renal biopsy was not undertaken to confirm a specific diagnosis.

Nephrotic Syndrome

One of the commonest renal glomerular syndromes in the elderly is hypoalbuminemia, proteinuria with associated edema, and hyperlipidemia. Diabetes mellitus is probably the major clinical cause, but membranous glomerulonephritis, minimal change disease, proliferative glomerulonephritis, focal glomerulosclerosis, and amyloidosis are major contributors to the appearance of nephrotic syndrome in the elderly. The diagnosis of nephrotic syndrome in an elderly diabetic should be assigned only when the diabetes has been of known long duration (beyond 7 to 10 years), vascular disease is clinically evident (including retinopathy or large vessel disease), and no other signs suggest a solitary renal disease. Hypertension and moderately impaired renal function are commonly associated with nephrotic syndrome associated with diabetes mellitus. While the severity of glucose intolerance is not helpful in differentiating diabetic glomerulosclerosis from nondiabetic disease, evidence of proliferative retinopathy is usually associated with diabetic glomerulosclerosis.

Membranous Glomerulonephritis. Approximately 40% of nephrotic syndrome in the elderly is secondary to membranous glomerulonephritis. Most individuals will never have a specific cause determined, but other causes including neoplasm, chronic viremia, and medication induced illnesses provide the bulk of diagnosable illnesses. The clinical profile in the elderly resembles that in the young, with heavy proteinuria and nephrotic syndrome being the presenting findings. It may be awkward to determine whether membranous glomerulonephritis is primary or secondary, and a good history and physical examination are probably the most directly helpful approaches.

Approximately 70% of malignancies associated with nephrotic syndrome have membranous glomerulonephritis as the presenting syndrome (61). Approximately 10% of patients with nephrotic syndrome due to membranous glomerulonephritis have an underlying malignancy. In most cases, the neoplastic process is evident before the onset of the nephrotic syndrome. If no cancer is obvious, a careful evaluation for underlying cancer is indicated in elderly patients with a diagnosis of nephrotic syndrome secondary to membranous glomerulonephritis.

A fairly common complication of membranous glomerulonephritis (up to 50% of cases) is renal vein thrombosis. Individuals with this diagnosis show no change in renal function but may develop symptoms of pulmonary emboli. Clinically, these individuals have very low serum albumin concentrations. The long-term outlook for this condition includes approximately one-third of individuals developing progressive renal impairment over the ensuing 3 years and approximately one-fifth undergoing spontaneous remission. The remaining patients will have an intermediate clinical profile. Because of this relatively benign outlook, only patients with urinary protein excretion exceeding 10 g/day, elevated serum creatinine levels, severe disease, and definite tubulointerstitial lesions with fibrosis on renal biopsy should be treated. Treatment with steroids is predominantly designed to temporarily improve renal function. Agents such as chlorambucil and cyclophosphamide have produced complete or partial remissions in the younger population. Therapy is likely to benefit the elderly but with an increased likelihood of complications of these treatments.

Minimal Change Disease. Approximately 20% of elderly patients with nephrotic syndrome have minimal change disease (62). Usually renal function is stable, and there is a rapid onset of heavy proteinuria. This illness has a relatively benign prognosis and is steroid responsive. Approximately 90% of older individuals will respond to oral steroid therapy within 4 months. Perhaps one-third will have relapses of their illness, in which case oral cyclophosphamide in conjunction with lower doses of prednisone may be helpful. Other primary glomerular lesions such as focal and segmental glomerulosclerosis, membranoproliferative glomerulonephritis, and mesangial proliferative glomerulonephritis are found in less than 10% of elderly individuals.

Amyloidosis. Rheumatoid arthritis and malignancies (most commonly multiple myeloma) are the leading causes of amyloidosis in the elderly. Perhaps 13% of patients who require renal biopsy for a diagnosis of nephrotic syndrome are found to have amyloidosis. Other clinical findings, including carpal tunnel syndrome, unexplained congestive heart failure, conduction defects, organomegaly, postural hypotension, and capillary fragility should increase the suspicion that primary amyloidosis is present. Progression to renal failure and renal vein thrombosis is common. Treatment with alkylating agents and prednisone has generally proven to be unsatisfactory (63).

Rapidly Progressive Glomerulonephritis (RPG)

When rapidly progressive renal failure leading to end-stage renal disease occurs over several months in association with urine sediment findings suggesting a glomerulonephritis, rapidly progressive glomerulonephritis may be the answer. The syndrome occurs in approximately 15% of patients undergoing renal biopsies for a diagnosis of their kidney disease. This autoimmune disease may be associated with anti-glomerular basement membrane antibodies, deposits of IgG in the glomerular capillaries, and circulating immune complexes accompanied by low serum complement levels. A variant type may have little in the way of immune deposits but occur in the context of a vasculitic picture. This is indeed perhaps the most common type of RPG in the elderly. Whether RPG is primary or secondary is largely determined by the dominance of the renal findings in the overall clinical picture. Hypersensitivity angiitis, cryoglobulinemia, systemic lupus erythematosus, infectious endocarditis, Wegener's granulomatosis, and necrotizing vasculitis secondary to drugs or cancer are the most common causes (64).

Hematuria and Proteinuria

Hematuria and proteinuria in the older patient are relatively common and occasionally can occur without an apparent cause. The correct approach in evaluating such patients involves a thorough urologic evaluation, abdominal ultrasonography to exclude polycystic kidney disease, and consideration of a broad differential diagnosis of renal diseases. While there may be a slight tendency for protein excretion to increase with age, excretion in the elderly does not exceed 150 mg/day. Excretion of more than 30 µg/min of albumin in the urine is usually associated with underlying diabetes mellitus or hypertensive nephrosclerosis. A correct approach is to quantitate the underlying proteinuria and evaluate the patient for a paraprotein through quantitative immunoglobulins. When a diagnosis is not apparent, patients should be followed for evidence of renal dysfunction and progressive proteinuria, at which time renal biopsy is indicated. When proteinuria and hematuria occur together, renal disease is suspected, and renal evaluation should be full.

Tubulointerstitial Nephropathy (TIN)

With advancing age there is an increase in interstitial volume, cellular infiltration, and fibrosis. The number of tubules decreases with age, paralleled by reduced volume and length of the proximal tubules and an increase in the number of diverticula in the distal convoluted segment of the renal tubule. These anatomic changes are associated with a reduced ability to maximally concentrate the urine, generate free water, conserve sodium, resorb glucose, and excrete an acid load (65–69). With senescence contributing to decreased homeostatic reserve related to tubulointerstitial function, it is understandable that given reduced reserve, the elderly are more apt to display TIN when compounded with an illness that also affects the same portion of the kidney.

The causes of tubulointerstitial nephritis are antibiotics, infections, and systemic diseases, primarily metabolic, vasculitic, and malignant diseases. Medications can produce lesions characteristic of this syndrome through direct injury or from hypersensitivity. Most cases are secondary to drug hypersensitivity. The first-noted group included antibiotics including sulfonamide, penicillin, cephalosporin, and rifampin. The second commonest group of agents are the nonsteroidal antiinflammatory drugs and a variety of other related drugs including diuretics such as furosemide, thiazides, and other agents including diphenylhydantoin, cimetidine, captopril, allopurinol, and triamterene (70, 71). With drug-induced TIN the nature of the sensitizing antigen is not clear but may well involve drug/local tissue interaction that is the offending immunologic agent (72).

Infection may provoke TIN as a reaction to invasion of the renal parenchyma or it may be the complication of systemic infection presumably of an immunologic nature. In the elderly, the more common form encountered is secondary to urinary tract infection and invasion of the renal parenchyma with bacteria. In the circumstance of acute pyelonephritis, symptoms include fever, shaking chills, flank pain, and dysuria. Positive blood and urine cultures are common. Pathologically, the renal lesions of pyelonephritis are focal, confined to wedge-shaped areas of the central and medial renal parenchyma. A defect in urinary concentration and acidification may be present, which will subside once treatment is successful. If infection is bilateral and severe, a decrement in renal function may be documented.

The two metabolic states associated with older individuals developing TIN are hypercalcemia and hyperuricemia, often occurring in association with lymphoproliferative disorders. This may occur because of tumor burden itself or as a consequence of rapid cell lysis resulting from chemotherapy. Combined with dehydration, the loads of urate and calcium may result in inflammatory reaction as well as concentration of these chemicals in the renal medulla, which may sludge or precipitate. In the clinical circumstances in which this possibility may arise, adequate hydration, alkalization of the urine, and in particular reduction of uric acid by administration of allopurinol prior to chemotherapy is essential. The pathophysiology of hypercalcemia in the production of TIN appears to be vascularly induced, with vasoconstriction being the predominant lesion. In infiltrative diseases associated with malignancy (among which multiple myeloma is the commonest cause), precipitation of myeloma protein in the urine with resultant injury and interstitial edema are the primary features of tubulointerstitial nephritis.

Chronic Tubulointerstitial Nephropathies

The renal lesions usually associated with chronic pyelonephritis have been recognized over the past several decades as also occurring in the absence of obstruction or renal infection. Chronic tubulointerstitial nephropathies have a broad variety of causes including drugs (analgesics, cyclosporine, lithium, and platinum); urinary tract obstruction; hematologic disorders (sickle cell anemia, lymphoproliferative disorders, and multiple myeloma); metabolic disorders (diabetes mellitus, hypercalcemia, and hyperuricemia); vascular disorders (embolic disease); infection (bacterial, fungal, mycobacterial, and occasionally viral); immunologic disorders (transplant rejection, vasculitides, amyloidosis and Wegener's granulomatosis); hereditary disorders (polycystic disease); heavy metal exposure; and others (sarcoidosis, radiation, and unknown).

The major characteristics include atrophy and degeneration and dilation of tubules, primarily in the cortical and medullary areas, which can be patchy. Ultimately, fibrosis results. The primary approach to treatment is to define the underlying cause and recognize that with successful control of the primary cause, progression of renal involvement stops. Renal function may indeed improve. In rare instances, the disease may progress even after removal of the precipitant.

Atherosclerotic Emboli

Cholesterol embolization has increased with advancing age of the population and the increased use of invasive vascular procedures including diagnostic and surgical techniques. This late sequela of atherosclerosis is most common in individuals who have multiple risk factors for atherosclerosis. Migration of emboli to distal organs occurs as cholesterol crystals released from ulcerated plaques travel and lodge in organs downstream. The usual clinical profile is that of an elderly male smoker with evidence of coronary or intraabdominal aortic disease. There may be bruits, prior coronary artery bypass surgery, recent instrumentation of the arterial tree, or a history of transient ischemic attacks or retinal emboli. The most frequent organs involved with cholesterol emboli are the kidneys, spleen, pancreas, gastrointestinal tract, and adrenal glands.

Diagnosis is infrequently made before death and can only be secure when a biopsy specimen shows cholesterol emboli. The clinical picture is often subacute with hypertension, fever, leg and back pain, and livedo reticularis (74). Laboratory examination reveals renal insufficiency, leukocytosis, and elevated eosinophil count. When the disease is more subacute, it is perhaps even more difficult to diagnose until evidence of clear embolization is present. There is no specific treatment for this condition, whose prognosis is poor. Corrective and life-saving surgical procedures are indicated when intraabdominal catastrophes have occurred. Renal dialysis, if necessary, is often only transiently needed.

Diabetes Mellitus

About one-half of all end-stage renal disease occurs in non-insulin-dependent diabetes mellitus, the most common form of diabetes in late life. Four major types of glomerular disease occur in diabetes: intercapillary sclerosis, the fibrin cap lesion, the capsular drop, and intercapillary sclerosis. With end-stage diabetic renal disease, tubular disease with atrophy and interstitial changes suggesting an inflammatory process and fibrosis develop. The clinical characteristics of diabetes in late life include hypertension, proteinuria, and progressive renal dysfunction. The mechanisms for functional changes include vascular disease in the large vessels, nonenzymatic glycosylation of structural proteins, basement membrane abnormalities, and alternations in renal plasma flow because of autonomic and cardiovascular changes.

It has been suggested recently that renal failure can be retarded or limited by careful control of blood sugar levels. While this observation was made in aggressively treated insulin-dependent diabetes mellitus patients, it is hoped that because the underlying pathology in non-insulin-dependent diabetes mellitus is similar, close and careful control of glycemia will be helpful in this more prevalent condition in the elderly population. A secondary treatment approach is to control high blood pressure and to consider restricting protein once renal function has declined. Diabetic individuals are more prone to urinary tract infection, and this must be recognized as an increased risk in diabetic individuals.

Acknowledgment. This work was supported in part by grants AG-00599, AG-04390, and AG-08812 from the National Institute on Aging and Grant RR-01032 from the General Clinical Research Centers Program of the Division of Research Resources, National Institutes of Health. Many thanks for the expert secretarial support from Susan Consoletti.

REFERENCES

1. Davies DF, Shock NW. Age changes in glomerular filtration rate, effective renal plasma flow, and tubular excretory capacity in adult males. J Clin Invest 1950;29:496–507.
2. Bruin JA, Cotran RS. The aging kidney: pathologic alterations. In: Martinez-Maldonado MM, ed. Hypertension and renal disease in the elderly. Cambridge, MA: Blackwell Scientific Publications, 1992; 1:1–9.
3. Kaplan C, Pasternack B, Shah H, et al. Age-related incidence of sclerotic glomeruli in human kidneys. Am J Pathol 1975;80:227–234.
4. Kappel B, Olsen S. Cortical interstitial tissue and sclerosed glomeruli in the normal human kidney, related to age and sex. A quantitative study. Virchows Arch (Pathol Anat) 1980;387:271–277.
5. Heptinstall RH. Hypertension. II. Essential hypertension. In: Heptinstall RH, ed. Pathology of the kidney. Boston: Little, Brown & Co, 1983;181–246.
6. Anderson S, Brenner BM. Effects of aging on the renal glomerulus. Am J Med 1986;80:435–442.
7. McGregor L. Histological changes in the renal glomerulus in essential (primary) hypertension. A study of fifty-one cases. Am J Pathol 1930;6:347–366.
8. Weening JJ, Beukers JJB, Grond J, et al. Genetic factors in focal segmental glomerulosclerosis. Kidney Int 1986;29:789–798.
9. Grond J, Beukers JJB, Schilthuis MS, et al. Analysis of renal structural and functional features in two rat strains with a different susceptibility to glomerular sclerosis. Lab Invest 1986;54:77–83.
10. Rowe JW, Andres R, Tobin J, et al. The effect of age on creatinine clearance in men: a cross-sectional and longitudinal study. J Gerontol 1976;31:155–163.
11. Lindeman RD, Tobin J, Shock NW. Longitudinal studies on the rate of decline in renal function with age. J Am Geriatr Soc 1985;33:278–285.
12. Lindeman RD, Tobin JD, Shock NW. Association between blood pressure and the rate of decline in renal function with age. Kidney Int 1984;26:861–868.
13. Lindeman RD. Hypertension and the kidney. Nephron 1987;47(suppl 1):62–67.
14. Boner G, Shelp WD, Neton M, et al. Factors influencing the increase in glomerular filtration rate in the remaining kidney of transplant donors. Am J Med 1973;55:169–174.
15. Kennedy CG. Effects of old age and overnutrition on the kidney. Br Med Bull 1957;23:67–70.
16. Hostetter TM, Olson JL, Rennke HG, et al. Hyperfiltration in remnant nephrons: a potentially adverse response to renal ablation. Am J Physiol 1981; 9:F85–F93.
17. Brenner BM, Meyer TW, Hostetter TH. Dietary protein intake and the progressive nature of kidney disease: the role of hemodynamically medicated glomerular injury in the pathogenesis of progressive glomerular sclerosis in aging, renal ablation, and intrinsic renal disease. N Engl J Med 1982;307:652–659.

18. Anderson S, Brenner BM. Effects of aging on the renal glomerulus. Am J Med 1986;80:435–442.
19. Zatz R, Meyer TW, Noddin JL, et al. Predominance of hemodynamic rather than metabolic factors in the pathogenesis of diabetic glomerulopathy. Proc Natl Acad Sci USA 1985;82:5963–5967.
20. Luft FC, Weinberger MH, Fineberg MS, et al. Effects of age on renal sodium homeostasis and its relevance to sodium sensitivity. Am J Med 1987; 82(suppl 1B):9–15.
21. Fish LC, Murphy DJ, Elahi D, Minaker KL. Renal sodium excretion in normal aging: decreased excretion rates lead to delayed handling of sodium loads. J Geriatr Nephrol Urol 1994, in press.
22. Epstein M, Hollenberg NK. Age as a determinant of renal sodium conservation in normal man. J Lab Clin Med 1976;87(3):411–417.
23. Macias-Nunez JF, Garcia-Iglesias C, Bonda-Roman A, et al. Renal handling of sodium in old people: a functional study. Age Ageing 1978;7:178–181.
24. Crane MG, Harris JJ. Effect of aging on renin activity and aldosterone excretion. J Lab Clin Med 1976;87:947.
25. Weidmann P, De Myttenaere-Bursztein S, Maxwell MH, et al. Effect of aging on plasma renin and aldosterone in normal man. Kidney Int 1975;8:325–333.
26. Weidmann P, de Chatel R, Schiffmann A, et al. Interrelations between age and plasma renin, aldosterone and cortisol, urinary catecholamines, and the body sodium/volume state in normal man. Klin Wochenschr 1977;55:725–733.
27. Brenner BM, Ballersmann BJ, Gunning ME, et al. Diverse biological actions of atrial natriuretic peptide. Physiol Rev 1990;70:665–699.
28. Weidmann P, Hasler L, Gnadinger MP, et al. Blood levels and renal effects of atrial natriuretic peptide in normal man. J Clin Invest 1986;77:734–742.
29. McKnight JA, Roberts G, Sheridan B, et al. Aging and atrial natriuretic factor. J Hum Hypertens 1990;4:53–56.
30. Clark BA, Elahi D, Fish L, et al. Atrial natriuretic peptide suppresses osmostimulated vasopressin release in young and elderly man. Am J Physiol 1991; 261: E252–E256.
31. Davis KM, Fish LC, Davis KM, et al. Resistance to atrial natriuretic peptide (ANP) in the institutionalized elderly. Gerontologist 1989;29:A6.
32. Clark BA, Fish LC, Davis KM, et al. Resistance to atrial natriuretic peptide (ANP) induced sodium excretion (NaXR) in the elderly. Gerontologist 1988; 28:A141.
33. Davis KM, Fish LC, Clark BA, et al. Atrial natriuretic peptide (ANP) levels in the prediction of congestive heart failure (CHF) in frail elderly. JAMA 1992;267:2625–2629.
34. Rosa RM, Silva P, Young JB, et al. Adrenergic modulation of extrarenal potassium disposal. N Engl J Med 1980;302:431–433.
35. Minaker KL, Rowe JW. Potassium homeostasis during hyperinsulinemia: effect of insulin level, β-blockade, and age. Am Physiol Soc 1982:73–E377.
36. Lindeman RD. Renal hemodynamics and glomerular filtration and their relationship to aging. In: Martinez-Maldonado MM, ed. Hypertension and renal disease in the elderly. Cambridge, MA: Blackwell Scientific Publications, 1992;2:10–25.
37. Lindeman RD, Lee TD, Jiengst MJ, et al. Influence of age, renal disease, hypertension, diuretics, and calcium on the antidiuretic responses to suboptimal infusions of vasopressin. J Lab Clin Med 1966; 68:206–223.
38. Rowe JW, Shock NW, DeFronzo RA. The influence of age on the renal response to water deprivation in man. Nephron 1976;17:270–278.
39. Helderman JH, Vestal RE, Rowe JW, et al. The response of arginine vasopressin to intravenous ethanol and hypertonic saline in man: the impact of aging. J Gerontol 1978;33:39–47.
40. Rowe JW, Minaker KL, Sparrow D, et al. Age-related failure of volume-pressure-mediated vasopressin release. J Clin Endocrinol Metab 1982;661–664.
41. Crowe MJ, Forsling ML, Rolls BJ, et al. Altered water excretion in healthy elderly man. Age Aging 1987;16:285–293.
42. Minaker KL, Fish LC, Rowe JW. Altered thirst threshold during hypertonic stress in aging man. Gerontologist 1985;25:A118.
43. Murphy DJ, Minaker KL, Fish LC, et al. Impaired osmostimulation of water ingestion delays recovery from hyperosmolarity in normal elderly. Gerontologist 1988;28:A141.
44. McAloon-Dyke M, David KM, Clark BA, et al. Age-related failure to defend against hypertonicity. Gerontologist 1990;30:A183.
45. Miller PD, Krebs RA, Neal BS, et al. Hypodipsia in geriatric patients. Am J Med 1982;73:354–356.
46. Rowe JW, Minaker KL, Levi M. Pathophysiology and management of electrolyte disturbances in the elderly. In: Martinez-Maldonado MM, ed. Hypertension and renal disease in the elderly. Cambridge, MA: Blackwell Scientific Publications, 1992;12:170–184.
47. Snyder NA, Feigal DW, Arieff AI. Hypernatremia in elderly patients. Ann Intern Med 1987;107:309.
48. Berenyl M, Straus B. Hyperosmolar states in the chronically ill. J Am Geriatr Soc 1968;17(7):648.
49. Hays RM, Levine SO. Pathophysiology of water metabolism. In: Brenner B, Rector FC Jr, eds. The kidney. Philadelphia: WB Saunders, 1980:105–130.
50. Miller P, Krebs R, Neal B, McIntyre D. Hypodipsia in geriatric patients. Am J Med 1982;73:354.
51. Weitzman RE, Keeman CR. The clinical physiology of water metabolism. Part I: The physiologic regulation of arginine vasopressin secretion and thirst. West J Med 1979;13(5):373.
52. Berger EY. Nutrition by hypodermoclysis. J Am Geriatr Soc 1984;32(3):199.
53. Arieff AI, Guisado R, Lazarowitz VC. Pathophysiology of hyperosmolar states. In: Andreoli TE, Grantham JJ, Rector FC Jr, eds. Disturbances in body fluid osmolality. Bethesda, MD: American Physiological Society, 1997:227.
54. Davis KM, Minaker KL. Disorders of fluid and electrolyte balance. In: Hazzard WR, Andres R, Bierman EL, Blass JP, eds. Principles of geriatric medicine and gerontology. 2nd ed. New York: McGraw-Hill, 1989:1079–1083.
55. Minaker KL, Rowe JW. Disorders of fluid and osmolality regulation (section on Geriatrics). In: Kelley W, ed. Textbook of internal medicine. New York: JB Lippincott, 1989;526(2):2654–2658.
56. Kleinfeld M, Casimir M, Borra A. Hyponatremia as observed in a chronic disease facility. J Am Geriatr Soc 1979;27:156.

57. Davidman M. The management of hypoosmolar states. Ann R Coll Physicians Surg Can 1994; 27(1):90–92.

58. Ramirez G, Saba SR. Primary glomerulonephritis in the elderly. In: Zawado ET Jr, Sica D, eds. Geriatric nephrology and urology. Littleton, MA: PSG Publishing Co, 1985:49–66.

59. Abrass CK. Glomerulonephritis in the elderly. Am J Nephrol 1985;5:409–418.

60. Zech P, Colon S, Pointet P, et al. The nephrotic syndrome in adults aged over 60: etiology, evolution and treatment of 76 cases. Clin Nephrol 1982; 17:232–236.

61. Brueggemayer CD, Ramirez G. Membranous nephropathy, a concern for malignancy. Am J Kidney Dis 1987;9:23–27.

62. Glassock RJ. Glomerular disease in the elderly. In: Martinez-Maldonado MM, ed. Hypertension and renal disease in the elderly. Cambridge, MA: Blackwell Scientific Publications, 1992;15:211–224.

63. Kyle R, Wagoner RD, Holley D. Primary systemic amyloidosis: resolution of nephrotic syndrome with mephalan and prednisone. Arch Intern Med 1982; 142:1445–1449.

64. Fauci AS, Haynes BF, Kat P, et al. Wegener's granulomatosis; prospective clinical and therapeutic experience with 85 patients for 21 years. Ann Intern Med 1983;76–98.

65. Beck LE. Kidney function and disease in the elderly. Hosp Pract 1988;15:75–90.

66. Lindeman RD, Lee TD, Yiengst MJ, et al. Influence of age, renal disease, hypertension, diuretics, and calcium on the antidiuretic responses to suboptimal infusions of vasopressin. J Lab Clin Med 1966; 68:206–222.

67. Epstein M, Hollenberg NM. Age as a determinant of oral sodium conservation in normal man. J Lab Clin Med 1976;87:411–417.

68. Miller JH, McDonald RK, Shock TW. Age changes in the maximal rate of renal tubular reabsorption of glucose. J Gerontol 1952;7:196–200.

69. Adler S, Lindeman RD, Yiengst MJ, et al. Effect of acute acid loading on urinary acid excretion by the aging human kidney. J Lab Clin Med 1968;72:278–289.

70. Blackshear JL, Napier JS, Davidman M, et al. Renal complications of nonsteroidal anti-inflammatory drugs: identification and monitoring of those at risk. Semin Arthritis Rheum 1985;14:163–175.

71. Fialk MA, Romankiewicz J, Perrone F, et al. Allergic interstitial nephritis with diuretics. Ann Intern Med 1974;81:403–404.

72. Ten RM, Torres VE, Milliner DS, et al. Acute interstitial nephritis: immunologic and clinical aspects. Mayo Clin Proc 1988;63:921–930.

73. Dubach UC, Rosner B, Pfister E. Epidemiologic study of abuse of analgesics containing phenacetin. Renal morbidity and mortality (1968–1979). N Engl J Med 1983;308:357–362.

74. Stone WJ, Fogo A. Cholesteral embolization. In: Martinez-Maldonado MM, ed. Hypertension and renal disease in the elderly. Cambridge, MA: Blackwell Scientific Publications, 1992;18:261–271.

26/ Common Lower Urinary Tract Problems in the Elderly

Louis C. Breschi

Since the publication of the third edition of *Clinical Aspects of Aging*, a significant increase in attention both in the medical community and in the national media has focused on two aspects of the lower urinary tract in males. Consequently, a significant portion of this chapter is devoted to the discussion of these two topics, the medical treatment alternatives of benign prostatic hyperplasia (BPH) and the screening and diagnosis of cancer of the prostate. Other perennial problems of the lower urinary tract are also addressed and updated. Urinary infections continue to be a problem in this age group. In addition, the workup of hematuria, female urethral diseases, cystocele, urinary retention in women, prostatitis, and various diseases of the external male genitalia are discussed. Finally, an ever-increasing area of concern for the healthy elderly is the problem of male impotence. This chapter concludes with a review of this topic, the initial evaluation of which is well within the expertise of the primary care physician. The topic of urinary incontinence is addressed in the next chapter.

BENIGN PROSTATIC HYPERPLASIA

BPH is the enlargement of the prostate gland that develops in the aging male. Although the exact cause of BPH is still unknown, it originates very early in life, about the third decade, and nearly all men will develop BPH if they live long enough. However, the current estimates are that only 25 to 35% of men will progress to prostatectomy (1). There has been a significant growth in knowledge in the pathophysiology of BPH in the past 6 years. The previously held notions that the clinical symptoms of BPH are due to a mass-related increase in urethral resistance are too simplistic.

Current research has revealed two major factors in the pathophysiology of BPH (2): the hormonal regulation of prostatic growth and the role of prostatic smooth muscle in obstructive uropathy. The evolving clarification of these two findings has, in turn, opened the area to medical management of symptomatic BPH, but the most important issue for physicians continues to be how to evaluate patients' symptoms to choose the most appropriate form of management.

INVASIVE MANAGEMENT OF BPH

For over 50 years, transurethral resection of the prostate (TURP) has been the "gold standard" by which all other treatments of obstructive uropathy are measured. Until the last 5 years, virtually no other option other than watchful waiting was available. Now, not only are there medical options for treatment of symptomatic BPH, but also a host of invasive alternatives, in various stages of refinement, which may eventually diminish the use of TURPs. The first question to ask, then, is when is an invasive procedure of the prostate generally agreed to be the best choice of treatment.

It is difficult to be dogmatic about anything relating to the constantly changing field of management of prostatic disease. However, as of 1993, current absolute indications for surgical intervention of BPH are acute urinary retention, recurrent urinary tract infections due to urinary stasis, severe hematuria secondary to an enlarged congested prostate, hydronephrosis and renal failure due to prostatic obstruction, and marked bladder instability associated with urge incontinence (3, 4).

At the present time, fewer than 10% of prostatectomies are performed by means of an open incision. This open procedure is used when the prostate gland is unusually large or there is present a large bladder stone or stones not amenable to transurethral manipulation. A urethral stricture or the need to correct an associated bladder

269

problem such as a bladder diverticulum are other indications for an open prostatectomy.

The vast majority of prostatectomies, however, are performed by TURP. In 1991, TURPs were the second most common surgical procedure in the U.S. (after cataract surgery). During 1991, more than 400,000 such procedures were performed. Though later figures are not available at this time, anecdotal experiences would suggest a dramatic decline in TURPs since the availability and discussion of nonsurgical treatments of BPH surfaced. This would also suggest that TURPs were being performed for more situations than the absolute indications mentioned above; and surgical alternatives and invasive therapies are emerging that may also be contributing to the diminished use of TURPs.

The alternative surgical procedures currently being used by some urologists are transurethral incision of the prostate (TUIP), transurethral ultrasound-guided laser-induced prostatectomy (TULIP), and even more recently, visual laser ablation of the prostate (VLAP). TUIP is a procedure in which an incision or incisions are made through the muscle of the bladder neck and, in most cases, through the prostatic capsule. This procedure is applicable for small prostatic glands, usually under 20 g. A TULIP procedure uses ultrasound-guided laser energy transmitted to prostate tissue compressed by inflating an intraurethral balloon. Using cystoscopy and direct visualization, the VLAP procedure appears to be an even less cumbersome use of laser energy to treat prostatic obstruction. All of these alternative measures to TURP claim decreased morbidity and less cost. Thus far, no consensus is at hand.

Three nonsurgical invasive therapies also have their proponents. These are balloon dilation of the prostate, urethral stents, and hyperthermia. Balloon dilation involves dilating the prostatic urethra to between 75 and 90 French size at high pressure. Urethral stents are biocompatible inert mesh that is inserted in the prostatic urethra under direct vision. When approved by the FDA, this modality may offer a suitable alternative to long-term catheterization. The technique of hyperthermia applies heat to the prostate, either transrectally or transurethrally, causing tissue necrosis and shrinkage of the gland.

MEDICAL TREATMENT OF BPH

The burst of information in the last 5 years in the area of nonsurgical management of BPH has had a dramatic impact on the method of care of these patients by urologists. Two types of drug therapies are proving helpful in symptomatic BPH: α-adrenergic blockers and hormonal replacement.

The bladder neck and prostate and its capsule are well supplied with α-receptors that mediate contraction of the prostate. Therefore, α-blockade causes relaxation of the bladder outlet without impairing bladder contractility. The drugs most commonly used for this purpose are prazosin (Minipres), terazosin (Hytrin), and, more recently, doxazosin (Cardura). The advantage of the latter two is the convenience of once-daily doses.

The other major method of medical treatment of BPH is hormonal manipulation. It has been known for at least 50 years that suppressing male hormone decreases prostatic size. Orchiectomy and the use of diethylstilbestrol in the treatment of prostate cancer were two obvious ways of reducing the prostate. Unfortunately, these modalities, as well as the more recently developed drugs for prostatic cancer treatment, such as luteinizing hormone releasing hormone (LHRH) and antiandrogens such as flutamide, all have undesirable side effects.

A newer hormonal therapy category, the 5α-reductase inhibitors, have shown fewer side effects. This class of drugs acts by selectively inhibiting the production of dihydrotestosterone (DHT) without suppressing testosterone levels. Therefore, testosterone-dependent activity such as erectile function, libido, and muscle mass, should not be affected. Instead, there is reduction only of prostate volume and, one hopes, improvement of urine flow (5). The prototype drug in this class is finasteride (Proscar). Currently, the recommended dose of finasteride is 5 mg daily.

In concluding the discussion of treatment of symptomatic BPH, several points need to be made. First, all of the various treatment modalities mentioned should be considered only for *symptomatic* BPH. Though surgical intervention is unlikely in cases of asymptomatic BPH, there may be an increasing tendency to begin medical treatments, particularly with the 5α-reductase drugs, simply on the basis of prostatic enlargement. Until controlled studies demonstrate the safety and efficacy of such prophylactic treatment, it should not be encouraged.

Second, the efficacy of surgical treatment of BPH is not likely to be matched by the newer medical options. The lack of uniform effectiveness, together with individual hypersensitivity to medication, make it necessary to advise patients of the possibility of partial or complete failure of medical treatment. In addition, it is likely that medical treatment will be required indefinitely to maintain a desired level of voiding stability. Thus, future research must explore the comparative cost-benefit ratios of surgical and medical therapies.

Third, all patients should be screened for associated carcinoma of the prostate before any treatment is undertaken for BPH. A digital rectal examination (DRE) along with a prostatic specific antigen (PSA) are the minimum prerequisites before embarking on the management of BPH.

Finally, primary care physicians should not hesitate to use urologic consultation in any uncertain situation, whether in reference to uncertain physical findings or to unclear subjective complaints.

CARCINOMA OF THE PROSTATE

Prostate cancer is the second leading cancer killer in men and the most commonly diagnosed cancer in men. For African American men, the incidence rate is nearly twice that of the general population, and the death rate is up to three times greater (6). The magnitude of this public health problem has been widely reported in the medical literature, as well as in the lay press. This increased public awareness of prostate cancer has placed increased demands on the health care system for early diagnosis and treatment, and the dilemma has now become who to treat aggressively. In fact, the first article (7) to analyze the outcomes of radical surgery, radiation therapy, and watchful waiting, suggests that only selected younger men may benefit from any aggressive therapy. A even more basic problem is the extent of prostate screening that should be carried out. These dilemmas are currently unanswered. Therefore, what will be described in this section is the best course to follow in evaluating the male population at risk.

Two categories of men are at higher risk for carcinoma of the prostate—African Americans and men with a family history of prostatic cancer. Therefore, it appears logical at this time to screen these two groups of men yearly with a DRE and PSA, beginning at age 40. The remainder of the male population should be screened annually beginning at age 50. What is not clear is what age to stop annual screening. Most urologists would agree that screening should stop at age 65 or perhaps 70, but with many variables affecting men at this time in life, the question cannot be answered definitively. However, it is uniformly agreed among urologists that routine screening PSAs in the 80-plus age group are not appropriate. Thus, 70- to 79-year-old men remain as the group for whom no firm guidelines can be given

because of the wide variability of health in this population.

Symptoms pointing to prostatic carcinoma are nonspecific. Most often, cancer of the prostate is found on rectal examination. Probably the next most common complaints associated with cancer of the prostate are rapidly developing urinary retention and skeletal pain associated with metastatic disease. Other lower urinary symptoms such as initial hematuria, urinary frequency, dysuria, bloody urethral discharge, or nocturia are nonspecific. If a suspicious nodule is palpated and the PSA is elevated, prostatic biopsy, with or without rectal ultrasound, is indicated. Ultrasound is usually employed if the area of suspicion is ill defined or small, so as to make blind biopsies less successful. The difficulties occur when either of the screening parameters is abnormal, but not both. In the case of a prostatic nodule in the absence of an elevated PSA, most urologists would rule out the nodule being malignant by at least ultrasound and, most often, biopsy. An even greater dilemma is an elevated PSA in the presence of a benign-feeling prostate gland.

PSA is only produced by the prostate. The dilemma occurs because PSA is produced by both normal and malignant prostatic epithelium. Therefore, elevations of serum PSA may be seen in several nonmalignant processes, including BPH, prostatitis, and prostatic tissue infarction, to name just the most common conditions. To complicate matters further, while the manufacturer of the system used to measure PSA originally described the norms as being 0 to 4 ng/mL, ongoing experience has shown that only a minority of patients (approximately 25%) will have cancer of the prostate when the PSA falls in the range of 4 to 10 ng/mL. And in a current study (8), the authors suggest that the correlation of age and prostatic volume should be used to redefine the upper limits of normal for PSA. These particular data suggest thresholds of 3.5 ng/mL for those 50 to 59 years; 5.4 ng/mL for those 60 to 69 years; and 6.3 ng/mL for those 70 to 79 years of age.

A third screening modality for cancer of the prostate is rectal ultrasound. Combined with DRG and PSA, rectal ultrasound does increase the incidence of diagnosis of cancer; however, its use as a screening modality alone is not as effective as either of the other two modalities of screening. The most appropriate use of transrectal ultrasound is after a urologist determines it is needed, either to rule out a suspicious lesion or to help guide biopsies. The request of ultrasound alone before urological consultation may result in repetition of this examination by the urologist and, furthermore, could be more misleading in interpretation without urological opinion.

In summary, prostate screening is recommended currently on an annual basis for men aged 50 to 70. This screening should include DRE and PSA. For men with a family history of prostate cancer and for African Americans, current sentiment is that prostate screening should begin at age 40. After age 70, no specific guideline other than an annual rectal examination is recommended. If PSAs are done in this age group, their value as a pure screening tool remains uncertain. Transrectal ultrasound is best used to clarify an uncertain finding on either DRE or PSA.

LOWER URINARY TRACT INFECTIONS

Comprehensive studies of urinary tract infections in the elderly have shown a marked increase with advancing age (9, 10) and a 5:1 ratio of women to men. Contributing factors to this rise in the rate of infections include menopause and subsequent hormonal changes, prostatism, increased hypotonia of the bladder musculature, perineal soilage in elderly women, impaired mental status, and the higher incidence of immobile or bedbound patients (11, 12).

Symptomatic urinary tract infections should be treated in patients of any age. Typical symptoms of lower urinary tract infections include dysuria, burning on urination, urgency, frequency, hematuria, nocturia, and suprapubic discomfort. Urinalysis shows pyuria and, at times, hematuria. Symptomatic relief can be provided by use of urinary analgesics (Pyridium) or combination analgesics and antispasmodics (Urised). While urine culture results are pending, the empiric use of an appropriate antibiotic will often have the patient asymptomatic by the time the results of the culture are available.

For the elderly female patient with a first episode or only infrequent episodes of lower urinary tract infection, the first choice of medication is generally from a cost-effective group of antibiotics that includes synthetic penicillins (amoxicillin or ampicillin), sulfamethoxazole/trimethoprim, nitrofurantoins, and doxycycline/tetracycline. In male patients, however, the synthetic penicillins are often of little value. In patients of both sexes with known previous urinary tract infections, the use of second-line, albeit more expensive, drugs should be considered. These drugs include the cephalosporins and the quinolones.

Periodically, success with a single megadose or a 3-day regimen of antibiotics has been reported for acute lower urinary tract infections in women

(13, 14). Drugs used in these regimens have included amoxicillin, sulfamethoxazole/trimethoprim, and more recently, the quinolones (15). An even more recent study, however, suggests that none of these regimens are effective in geriatric women (16).

Catheter-associated urinary tract infections deserve special mention. For many reasons, catheter drainage is prevalent in the elderly, and the presence of bacteriuria with chronic indwelling Foley catheters is unquestioned. In addition, the likelihood of urosepsis in this elderly patient population is significant. Hence, there are two important questions to be answered in the care of the patient with a chronic Foley catheter: What practical methods should be used in daily care of these patients? What is the role, if any, of antibiotic therapy?

All authorities agree that an essential factor in minimizing the likelihood of symptomatic infection is good fluid intake. A minimum of 1.5 L per day is recommended. Likewise, it is not felt that, in general, bladder irrigation with any substance is of any value. Urinary acidification is difficult because of the chronic pyuria created by the foreign body presence of the catheter. There is disagreement about how often to change an indwelling Foley. Some authors would change catheters only if drainage stops (17). But in other than an institutional setting, this is impractical and dangerous. Rather, most recommend changing the catheter at 4- to 6-week intervals.

The other question is the role of antibiotics in the patient with an indwelling Foley. Ideally, if a patient can be successfully managed by the previous steps, it is not necessary to consider antibiotics. But the frequent occurrence of urosepsis with the subsequent need for hospitalization of these patients, continually raises the question of the value of antibiotic suppressive therapy, especially in those patients who have demonstrated recurrent urosepsis. Unfortunately, the medical literature does not provide clear guidance. The author's personal opinion is that the use of sulfamethoxazole/trimethoprim, nitrofurantoins, or occasionally, a quinolone drug in low daily doses is effective in preventing urosepsis in this patient population. This observation has been borne out in nursing home, acute hospital, and community settings. A debilitated and deteriorating patient, however, may well frustrate any management course.

The management of asymptomatic bacteriuria is another controversial topic. Studies are available that plead the importance of bacteriuria and shortened survival (18); there are also studies that support asymptomatic bacteriuria as being a benign condition (9, 10). Management of asymptomatic bacteriuria should include regular follow-up visits, encouragement of good fluid intake (1.5 L daily), and urinary acidification if Gram-negative organisms are present.

HEMATURIA

Hematuria continues to be a cause for serious concern for primary care physicians and a source of frequent referral to urologists. The level of concern varies with whether the hematuria is gross or microscopic, and if microscopic, whether intermittent or persistent.

In the elderly population, gross painless hematuria, whether associated with concomitant anticoagulant therapy or not, deserves a complete urologic workup. This workup should consist of either intravenous pyelography or renal ultrasound, urine for cytology, and in most cases, cystoscopy.

If the hematuria, either gross or microscopic, is associated with urinary symptoms such as dysuria, burning, or flank pain, the suspected condition, such as cystitis, prostatitis, or renal calculus, should be treated. If the suspected primary condition has cleared but the microscopic hematuria persists, then the patient should be referred for urologic evaluation.

In a discussion of microscopic hematuria, one must first define what is normal, and then, if abnormal, whether it is intermittent or persistent. The most commonly accepted upper limit of normal for urinary RBCs is 3 RBCs per high-powered field (19). The screening for microscopic hematuria by dipstick testing alone is not recommended (20). If the patient has only one episode of microscopic hematuria, a complete urologic workup is not indicated. Several episodes of microscopic hematuria, however, should warrant an ultrasound study of the upper urinary tract as well as urine cytology. Because the incidence of epithelial cancer increases with age, performing cystoscopy on the older patient is also usually indicated.

LOWER FEMALE UROLOGIC DISEASES

FEMALE URETHRAL DISEASES

The female urethra is normally 3 to 5 cm in length. In the postmenopausal female, the urethra is subject to various inflammatory and anatomic changes. One common finding in the elderly female is the hypospadiac urethra. In this condition, the urethral meatus has retracted inside the vaginal vault. The more proximal location of the urethral meatus often makes catheterization more difficult. This position of the meatus also predisposes to trauma and ascending urethritis. The recessed urethra may also irritate the distal vagina by emptying urine partially into the vaginal vault (Figs. 26.1 and 26.2).

Another common postmenopausal finding is urethral prolapse. The prolapse may be localized only at the six o'clock position of the urethra. This localized prolapse is often nodular and is referred to as a urethral caruncle. If the prolapse is circumferential, the appearance is similar to a mulberry surface and is deep red. Although usually benign, associated urethral carcinoma has been encountered in this area.

Two other frequent anatomic abnormalities in the elderly female are urethroceles and urethral diverticuli. A urethrocele is a protrusion of the anterior vaginal wall containing the urethra into the vaginal vault. Though usually associated with the loss or weakening of support of the anterior vaginal mucosa, it occurs occasionally because of distal urethral stenosis. A urethral diverticulum is a localized outpouching of the urethra, most often the result of an infection of a periurethral gland. A urethral diverticulum should be considered in one of several situations: the expression of purulent discharge from the urethral meatus during a bimanual vaginal examination; a history of urethral discharge between urinations; and occasionally as a cause of recurrent cystitis.

Urethral stenosis is still another anatomic abnormality found in elderly women. It may be due to postmenopausal estrogen deprivation with secondary tightening of the periurethral tissue, recurring urethritis, or trauma from urethral instruments, or it may be a lifelong condition. Symptoms that suggest urethral stenosis include hesitancy of the urinary stream, straining to void, and a small stream that takes a long time to complete the act of urination.

Senile urethritis is an inflammatory condition of the urethra that occurs often but is only occasionally symptomatic. When symptoms do occur, they are usually irritative, such as burning on urination, or occasionally, frequency. Usually, the urine culture is sterile. Urinary analgesics alone or in combination with antispasmodics are helpful in clearing the symptoms. Topical or systemic estrogen replacement therapy have been found useful in reducing recurrent lower tract infections in postmenopausal women.

DISEASES OF THE FEMALE BLADDER

Prolapse of the anterior vaginal wall is a common finding in the elderly female patient. Mild

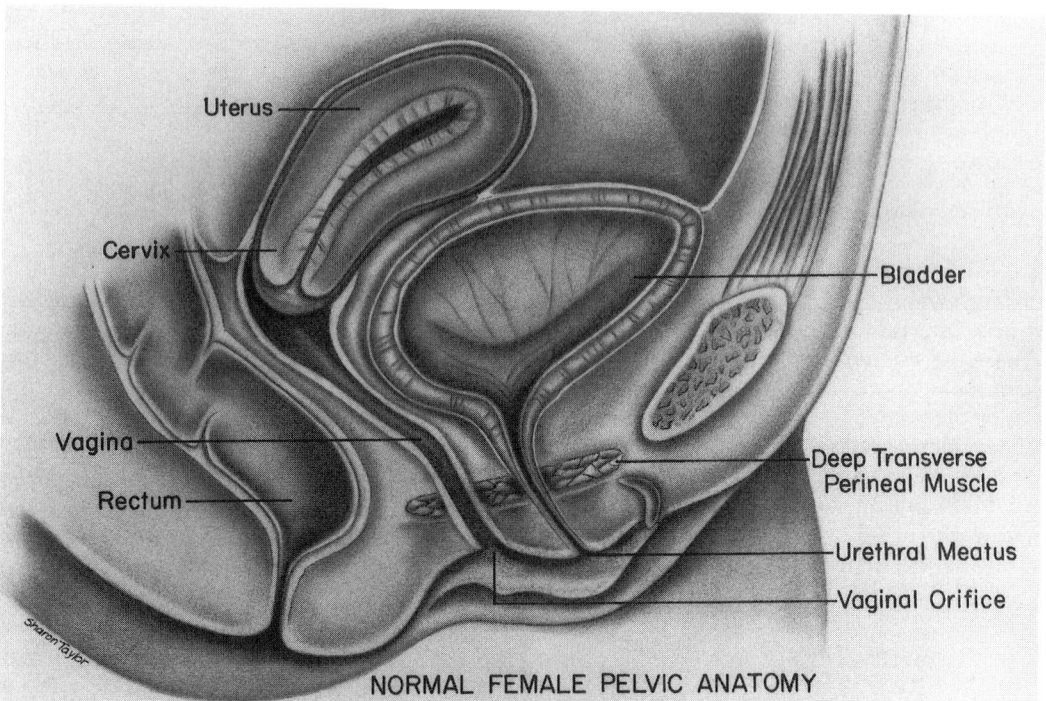

Figure 26.1. The normal anatomic relationship of the urethra and vagina.

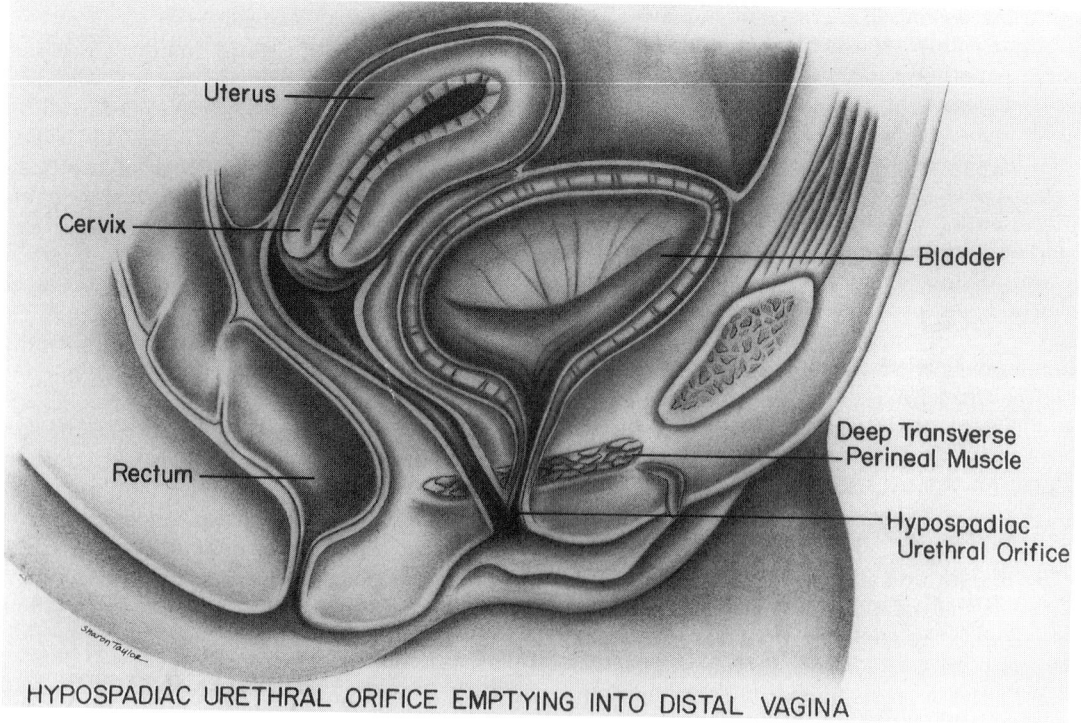

Figure 26.2. The hypospadiac urethra often found in postmenopausal women.

degrees of cystocele are frequently not symptomatic. A woman with a symptomatic cystocele may complain of feeling a mass protruding from the vagina or of feeling heaviness or pulling in the vagina or of difficulty in emptying the bladder. A cystocele may be associated with incontinence, most often stress incontinence. A cystocele without incontinence may be managed by use of a pessary, or, if the patient is an appropriate surgical candidate, by plication of the anterior vaginal wall. When stress urinary incontinence is present along with a cystocele, urethral and bladder neck suspension must be part of any surgical correction.

DISEASES OF THE LOWER MALE URINARY SYSTEM

The topics of BPH and carcinoma of the prostate were addressed extensively at the beginning of this chapter. This section summarizes other common lower urinary problems of elderly men.

PROSTATITIS

It has been estimated that as many as 20% of new patients attending urology clinics have evidence of prostatic inflammation. It is clear that prostatitis is not a single disease. There are three generally accepted categories of prostatitis: bacterial prostatitis, nonbacterial prostatitis, and prostatodynia. Patients with bacterial prostatitis have bacterial infections by culture. Those with nonbacterial prostatitis have evidence of inflammation but no signs of bacterial infection by culture. Prostatodynia describes those patients with symptoms associated with prostatitis, who have no evidence of either bacterial infection or inflammation.

Bacterial infections of the prostate are either acute or chronic and are caused by Gram-negative organisms, most commonly *Escherichia coli, Klebsiella spp.*, and *Pseudomonas spp.* The most common route of infection is by way of the distal urethra. Therefore, if a patient is prone to repeated prostate infections and is not circumcised, circumcision should be strongly considered.

Acute bacterial prostatitis is characterized by sudden onset of fever, chills, perineal pain, urinary frequency, myalgia, and varying degrees of bladder outlet obstruction. Rectal examination reveals an exquisitely tender, swollen prostate gland. If these findings are present, the prostate gland should *not* be massaged, and hospitalization with the use of appropriate i.v. antibiotics should be considered. Once the acute process has been controlled, further outpatient management

of bacterial prostatitis should include 3 to 4 weeks of oral antibiotics and careful follow-up.

Chronic prostatitis is more commonly encountered in the elderly male. Symptoms may include any of the following: burning or dysuria, frequency, suprapubic discomfort, testicular or perineal discomfort, low back pain, increased nocturia, urgency, feeling of incomplete emptying, and arthralgias. The rectal examination may show varying degrees of softness or swelling with or without tenderness. Massaged prostatic secretions are a helpful guide in determining inflammation. It does not however distinguish bacterial from nonbacterial prostatitis. For a culture of prostatic secretions, a urine specimen is obtained following prostatic massage.

The treatment of chronic prostatitis, bacterial or nonbacterial, is associated with varying degrees of success. Patients with chronic prostatitis should be advised of the likelihood of recurrences. The drugs used currently that are most successful in treating chronic prostatitis include trimethoprim/sulfamethoxazole, doxycycline, carbenicillin, and the quinolones. The length of therapy will vary. For an initial episode, treatment for 10 to 14 days will usually be successful. Longer courses of treatment are required when there are recurrent episodes. These courses of treatment are individualized. Treatment could be daily, every other day, one week each month, or on an "as needed" basis for early symptom recurrence. In addition, dietary restrictions are often very helpful. Eliminating colas, beer, and coffee should be recommended. Occasionally, spicy foods and chocolates have also caused ongoing irritation during the treatment of chronic prostatitis.

The role of prostatic massage in the treatment of chronic prostatitis remains controversial. Before the development of more effective antibiotics for treatment of prostatitis, prostatic massage was widely used by both family practitioners and urologists, with varying degrees of success. However, more recently, the value and usage of massage has been questioned and currently has fewer proponents (21).

Prostatodynia describes the syndrome in patients who have some or many of the symptoms mentioned above in bacterial and nonbacterial prostatitis, but who have no objective findings. Occasionally, the prostatic examination is painful to the patient, but there is no softness, and the prostatic secretions are normal. Often, these patients receive antibiotics without any improvement. In these cases, urethral stricture or some other less common bladder condition needs to be ruled out by cystoscopy. Once this has been done, eliminating the dietary items mentioned above should be proposed to the patient. In addition, reviewing with the patient the circumstances surrounding the onset of symptoms may reveal stressful situations that could be contributing to the symptoms.

DISEASES OF THE PENIS

Phimosis, paraphimosis, and balanoposthitis are frequent penile problems encountered in elderly men. *Phimosis* is a tightening of the foreskin around the glans, causing varying degrees of difficulty in retracting the foreskin, including total inability to retract the foreskin at all. *Paraphimosis* describes the condition in which the retracted foreskin becomes trapped and swollen proximal to the corona of the glans (Fig. 26.3). Left untreated, this results in necrosis and infection of the foreskin. Early treatment consists of manual reduction as illustrated in Figure 26.3; advanced cases require surgical reduction and should be considered urologic emergencies. *Balanoposthitis* describes the condition of inflammation of the glans and overlying foreskin. By far, the most common underlying cause for this condition is diabetes. So often is this the case that diabetes should be ruled out in any patient not known to be diabetic who presents with balanoposthitis. The management of balanoposthitis consists of thorough cleansing of the glans and foreskin with mild soap, followed by the application of an antifungal-steroid ointment twice daily. If the balanoposthitis recurs or fails to clear, a circumcision should be performed.

A patient complaining of a "lump" in the penis, curvature of the penis with erection, or painful erections most likely has Peyronie's disease. The condition is not truly a disease but is the development of fibrous plaques that partially surround the cavernous sheath of the penis. Though described for over a century, its cause(s) remain unknown. Very recently, attention has been focused on trauma, usually during vigorous intercourse, as a significant etiologic factor. Treatment of Peyronie's disease remains uncertain and very limited. Some benefit is obtained by the use of vitamin E (400 units twice daily). *p*-Aminobenzoate (Potaba) is probably the most widely used medical treatment. This drug has its greatest benefit in men with plaques that are painful or those who have painful erections. Other treatments that have been tried include ultrasonic treatments, steroid injections, and surgical excision of the plaques.

Carcinoma of the penis constitutes less than 1% of all malignancies that occur annually in the male population of the United States (22). The uncircumcised male is much more likely to develop carcinoma of the penis. In fact, neonatal circumcision essentially eliminates the risk of malignancy. Poor hygiene and genital warts are additional contributing factors in the development of carcinoma of the penis. A large number of these malignancies can be successfully managed by partial amputation or by laser surgery.

DISEASES OF THE SCROTUM AND SCROTAL CONTENTS

Epididymitis

The most frequently encountered acute problem of the scrotum is epididymitis. In the elderly male, epididymitis may follow instrumentation of the urinary tract, including the use of a Foley catheter. A preceding cystitis or prostatitis may also lead to onset of epididymitis. Symptoms include painful hemiscrotum with enlargement and tenderness of the epididymis, often with fever and malaise. Treatment includes bed rest, scrotal support, ice packs until the testis and epididymis are no longer tender, and appropriate oral antibiotics. In diabetics, very close attention is necessary, because progression to abscess formation, though not common, is more likely in this group of men.

Hydrocele

A diffuse, cystic enlargement of the scrotum that transilluminates is diagnostic of a hydrocele. It is usually unilateral. Hydroceles frequently are well tolerated and asymptomatic. Large hydroceles preclude satisfactory palpation of the surrounded testis. If there is concern about the testis, a scrotal ultrasound can be performed to confirm the status of the testis. Good techniques currently exist to perform hydrocelectomy safely and comfortably on those men requiring relief of significant symptoms. They can be done on an outpatient basis using local anesthesia. Careful aspiration of a symptomatic hydrocele may also be tried, but the results are often only temporary.

Spermatocele

Another cystic structure of the scrotum is a spermatocele. This structure also transilluminates. However, a spermatocele is usually located above the upper pole of a clearly palpable testis. Most spermatoceles are asymptomatic, and their main concern is the clarification to the patient of the "lump" present in the scrotum. Occasionally, an enlarging, painful spermatocele will justify surgical removal. This lesion can also be success-

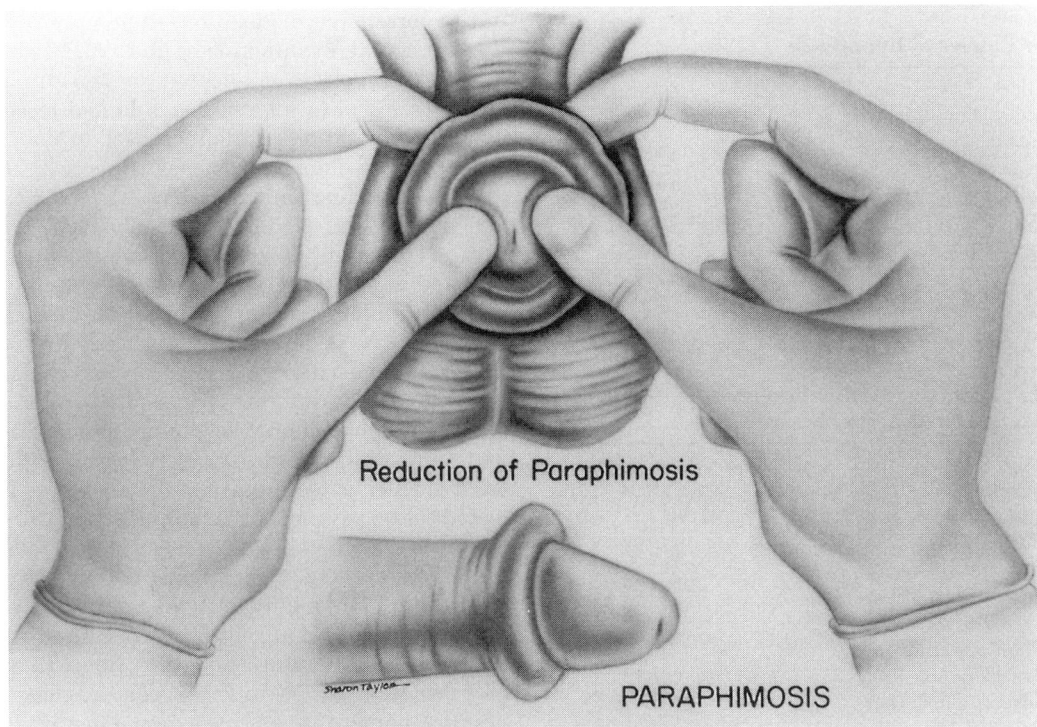

Reduction of Paraphimosis

PARAPHIMOSIS

Figure 26.3. Paraphimosis is the trapping and swelling of the foreskin proximal to the corona of the glans penis. Correction of the paraphimosis is usually done by firm constant pressure on the glans by thumbs, with the forefinger under paraphimosis.

fully removed surgically on an outpatient basis under local anesthesia; however, spermatoceles should not be aspirated.

Cancer of the Testis

Malignancy of the testis is normally a disease of younger men. In elderly males with testicular tumors, the most common types are lymphomas or metastatic carcinomas, including metastatic carcinoma of the prostate.

SEXUAL DYSFUNCTION

The number of men seeking urologic consultation for erectile difficulties has dramatically increased in the last 5 years. In the author's own practice, problems with impotence are the primary or secondary complaint of 40% of new patients over 60 years of age. The upsurge in complaints of this nature is likely due to increased media awareness and to the educational efforts of both professional and nonmedical associations.

The primary causes of impotence are far more often organic than psychogenic. Furthermore, organic impotence in the elderly male often has multiple causes, making the resolution of sexual dysfunction even more difficult. The major causes of impotence are listed in Table 26.1 (23). This list clearly demonstrates the need for a complete medical history. In addition, it is necessary to know if the erections are partial or totally absent, how long the problem has existed, and of course, the current sexual relationship with the patient's partner.

The physical examination should include an assessment of the patient's general health. The abdomen should be examined for aneurysm. The status of femoral and peripheral pulses should be determined. Examining the genitalia to rule out the penile plaques of Peyronie's disease and other structural abnormalities and examining the testes to rule out hypogonadism are obviously important. A good rectal examination, not only to evaluate the prostate, but also to assess the rectal sphincter tone as a quick indicator of altered sacral neurologic status, is also recommended. At times, a more complete neurologic examination may be helpful. Basic laboratory tests that complement the physical examination include routine urinalysis, blood glucose and serum testosterone determinations and perhaps thyroid function tests.

Special attention should be directed at the patient's medications (24). Table 26.2 lists the major

Table 26.1
Major Causes of Impotence

Vascular
Pharmacologic
Hormonal
Diabetes mellitus
Neurologic
Psychogenic
Other limiting medical conditions

Table 26.2
Antihypertensive Medications Associated with Sexual Dysfunction in Males

Diuretics
  Thiazides
  Spironolactones
  Chlorthalidone
Antihypertensives
  α-Adrenergic blockers
    Phenoxybenzamine
    Phentolamine
    Prazosin
  β-Adrenergic blockers
    Propranolol
    Metoprolol
  Central sympatholytics
    Methyldopa
    Clonidine
    Reserpine
  Neurotransmitter depletion
    Guanethidine
  Vasodilators
    Hydralazine
    Minoxidil

Table 26.3
Other Drug Categories Associated with Sexual Dysfunction in Males

Tranquilizers
  Phenothiazines
  Antidepressants
  Antianxiety agents
Anticholinergics
Miscellaneous drugs
  Cimetidine
  Clofibrate
  Digoxin
  Indomethacin
  Lithium carbonate
  Barbiturates
Addictive drugs
  Alcohol
  Nicotine
  Narcotics

antihypertensive medications that may contribute to sexual dysfunction. Table 26.3 lists the other drugs often implicated in this problem. Given this wide range of drugs linked to sexual dysfunction and given the increased use of medication by the elderly, it is easy to see why drugs are often an important part, if not the main cause, of sexual dysfunction in the elderly male.

The treatment of sexual dysfunction should be directed at the underlying cause, if possible. For vascular impotence, operations that reduce venous return, venous arterialization, and techniques to revascularize the corpora have been developed, but with mixed results. Potentially offending drugs should be changed or discontinued. Impotence of androgenic etiology can often be treated with testosterone supplementation. In selected cases, psychological counseling may be very useful. If the diagnosis is unclear, a trial with yohimbine may help.

If the patient's impotence has multiple causes or the underlying cause is otherwise unamenable to treatment, there are several options. Injection of vasoactive drugs into the corpora has been gaining momentum as safer, more effective, more easily administered combinations are developed. The vacuum pump device, an external, nonsurgical method of creating erections, has also rapidly gained wide acceptance. And finally, there is the mainstay of surgical procedures, the penile prosthesis. Because the various types of prostheses and their indications are continually changing, their discussion is beyond the scope of this chapter.

REFERENCES

1. Osterline JE. The origin and development of benign prostatic hyperplasia. An age-dependent process. J Androl 1991;12:348–355.
2. McConnell JD. The pathophysiology of benign prostatic hyperplasia. J Androl 1991;12:356–363.
3. Lepor H, Brower M, McConnell JD, Osterling, JE. What will replace TURP? Contemp Urol 1992;4:30–40.
4. Graverson PH, Gasser TC, Watson JH, Hinman F, Bruskewitz RC. Controversies about indications for transurethral resection of the prostate. J. Urol 1989;141:475–481.
5. The MK-906 Study Group. One year experience in the treatment of benign prostatic hyperplasia with finacteride. Androl 1991;12:372–375.
6. Natarajam N, Murphy GP, Mettlin CJ. Prostate cancer in blacks. J Surg Oncol 1989;40:232–236.
7. Fleming C, Wasson JH, Albertson PC, Barry MJ, Wennberg JE. A decision analysis of alternative treatment strategies for clinically localized prostatic cancer. JAMA 1993;269:2650–2658.
8. Dalkin BL, Almann FR, Kupp JB. Prostate specific antigen levels in men older than 50 years without

clinical evidence of prostatic carcinoma. J Urol 1993;150:1837–1839.

9. Yoshikawa TT. Chronic urinary tract infections in elderly patients. Hosp Pract 1993;28:103–118.

10. Smith IM. Infections in the elderly. Hosp Pract 1982;17:69–85.

11. Nicolle LE, Muir P, Harding GKM. Localization of urinary tract infection in elderly, institutionalized women with asymptomatic bacteriuria. J Infect Dis 1988;157:65–70.

12. Kaye D. Problems concerning bacteriuria in the elderly. Infect Dis 1982;12:4–20.

13. Dontas AS. Management of urinary tract infections in the geriatric patient. Geriatr Med Today 1987; 6:41–53.

14. Rubin RH, Fong LST, Jones SR, et al. Single dose amoxicillin therapy for urinary tract infection. JAMA 1980;244:561–564.

15. Hooton TM, Johnson C, Winter C. Single dose and three day treatment regimens of ofloxin versus trimethoprim-sulfamethoxazole for acute cystitis in women. Antimicrob Agents Chemother 1991; 35:1479–1483.

16. Ford S. New considerations in treatment of urinary tract infections in adults. Urology 1992;39:1–11.

17. Seiler WD, Stalelie HB. Practical management of catheter associated UTIs. Geriatrics 1988;43:43–50.

18. Dontas S. The effect of bacteriuria on survival in old age. Geriatr Urol. 1983;2:74–79.

19. Classock RJ. Hematuria and pigmenturia. In: Massry SG, Classock RJ, eds. Textbook of nephrology. Baltimore: Williams & Wilkins, 1989:491–495.

20. Sutton, JM. Evaluation of hematuria in adults. JAMA 1990;263:2475–2480.

21. Loughlin KR, Whitmore WF. Managing prostate disorders in middle age and beyond. Geriatrics 1987;42:45–56.

22. Schellhammer PF. A concise plan for managing carcinoma of the penis. Contemp Urol 1992;4:13–25.

23. Moxley JE. Impotence in older men. Hosp Pract 1988;23:139–158.

24. Van Arsdalen KN, Wein AJ. Drug induced sexual dysfunction in older men. Geriatrics 1984;39:63–70.

27/ Urinary Incontinence

Jan Busby-Whitehead

Urinary incontinence, defined as involuntary loss of urine, affects over 10 million adults, including 15 to 20% of community-dwelling individuals aged 65 years or older, 35 to 40% of all older patients in acute care hospitals, and 50% of all elderly nursing home residents. Age of 75 years or greater, female gender, immobility, dementia, or a history of gynecologic or urologic surgery are factors that convey the greatest risk for developing incontinence (1–3). Urinary incontinence is an underreported condition. Many patients do not mention their symptoms to a health care provider because they are too embarrassed or because they believe nothing can be done to help them (4). Because urinary incontinence is in fact curable in many and can be rendered more manageable in almost all cases, health care providers should specifically ask about symptoms of urinary incontinence and then provide appropriate evaluation and management of this clinical condition. This chapter discusses the pathophysiology, classification, diagnosis, and treatment of urinary incontinence in the elderly.

PATHOPHYSIOLOGY

Urinary incontinence is not a normal consequence of aging; its presence reflects an underlying disorder that is structural or functional in origin. The lower urinary tract consists of the bladder (detrusor muscle) and the urethra with its internal and external sphincters. The bladder maintains a variable volume up to 400 to 600 mL, yet intravesical pressure remains low prior to voiding. The internal sphincter is formed by the smooth muscle layers of the urethra. In postmenopausal women, its mucosal integrity may be compromised by a decline in estrogen. In older men, the internal sphincter is vulnerable to damage during prostatic resection. The external sphincter is composed of urethral striated muscle that may be voluntarily contracted to interrupt voiding.

Neurologic innervation of the lower urinary tract system is cholinergic (parasympathetic), adrenergic (sympathetic), and somatic. The basic reflex controlling urination occurs through the cholinergic S2–4 sacral nerve roots. β-Adrenergic receptors are located in the bladder dome, while α-adrenergic receptors are found in the bladder neck, bladder base, and proximal urethra. During bladder filling, urine storage is enhanced by (a) stimulation of β-adrenergic receptors, which inhibit cholinergic effects on the bladder and cause relaxation of the bladder dome and (b) stimulation of α-adrenergic receptors, which constrict the bladder neck and internal sphincter. Somatic innervation through the pudendal nerve allows reflex and voluntary contraction of the external sphincter and pelvic floor musculature, which protects against urine loss with sudden increases in abdominal pressure. The reflex inhibition of the striated external urethral sphincter during urination is also mediated by the pudendal nerve.

For normal voiding to occur, intravesical pressure must overcome bladder outlet and urethral sphincter resistance. Continued bladder filling increases cholinergic tone, stimulating the urge to void and, at a higher filling volume, the involuntary contraction of the bladder via the reflex arc. Simultaneously, adrenergic and somatic inhibition occur, allowing relaxation of the internal and external sphincters. Bladder constriction is enhanced while the urethral sphincters and pelvic floor muscles relax. Unless central inhibition occurs, this sequence of events results in normal urination. Central coordination of bladder and sphincter function is primarily inhibitory and occurs through neural linkages of the brainstem to the cerebellum, thalamus, and sensorimotor cortex of the frontal lobes. Normal urination is thus a complicated process requiring the integration of musculoskeletal and neurologic responses to stimuli from the lower urinary tract. If any component of this delicately balanced physiologic mechanism is disrupted, urinary incontinence may occur.

CLASSIFICATION

The initial distinction to be made by the clinician is whether the patient has temporary or established incontinence. Temporary incontinence generally occurs suddenly, is associated with an acute medical or surgical illness or drug therapy (Table 27.1), and is reversible with resolution of the underlying problem. Established incontinence is usually chronic, is not related to acute illness, requires investigation, and may be reversible with proper diagnosis and treatment (8). Some patients with established causes of incontinence may have developed strategies for staying dry, such as staying near toilet facilities. However, the problem may become acute if they become immobile, develop an acute infection, or begin a new medication.

The following section reviews the etiologies and clinical presentations of types of urinary incontinence on the basis of underlying pathophysiology (4): (a) detrusor instability; (b) outlet obstruction; (c) atonic bladder; (d) sphincter insufficiency/pelvic floor weakness; and (e) functional (physical, pharmacologic, psychological, or environmental) barriers. It is important to note that several types of incontinence may be present concurrently.

DETRUSOR INSTABILITY

Detrusor instability results from unsuppressed bladder contractions that are strong enough to overcome bladder outlet resistance and generally result in complete bladder emptying. Detrusor hyperreflexia has been defined by the International Continence Society as detrusor motor instability associated with a neurologic disorder (5). Any insult to the structural integrity of the cholinergic inhibitory centers of the central nervous system or the afferent innervation from the lower spinal cord where the reflex arc is located can cause detrusor hyperreflexia. Alzheimer's disease, cerebrovascular atherosclerosis, multiple sclerosis, Parkinson's disease, spinal cord tumors or transection, and cervical spondylosis (among others) may result in incontinence by this mechanism. It is not known whether the urinary incontinence associated with Alzheimer's disease and stroke is due to direct damage to the central inhibitory pathways or whether these disorders impair the patient's motivation to voluntarily inhibit urination when it is socially inappropriate (6). A subset of patients may have detrusor hyperreflexia with impaired contractility (DHIC) that is associated with a bladder that empties about one-third of its volume (7).

An alternative cause of detrusor instability is increased sensory stimulation that overrides central inhibition. This may result from local, irritating processes such as urinary tract infection, inflammation from radiation or chemotherapy, fecal impaction, or an enlarged prostate. Detrusor instability may also result from frequent low-volume voiding that may be begun by a patient in an effort to avoid an accident, but which leads to increased bladder tone and reduced functional capacity.

The patient with detrusor instability usually presents with symptoms of frequency and nocturia associated with a loss of large urine volumes (>100 mL). An irresistible urge to void is a very common complaint, but up to 20% of persons with detrusor instability will not have this symptom (8). Patients with stress or overflow incontinence may also have urgency, so this symptom is not specific to detrusor instability.

OUTLET OBSTRUCTION

Anatomic obstruction occurs primarily in men because of prostatic hypertrophy, neoplasm, or

Table 27.1
Common Drugs That May Precipitate Urinary Incontinence

Detrusor instability	
Sedatives/hypnotics	Flurazepam
	Diazepam
	Ethanol
Diuretics	Furosemide
	Hydrochlorothiazide
Overflow	
α-Adrenergic agonists	Pseudoephedrine
Antiarrhythmics	Disopyramide
Antispasmodics	Belladonna/
	phenobarbital
	Dicyclomine
Antiparkinson agents	Benztropine mesylate
	Trihexyphenidyl
Calcium channel blockers	Diltiazem
	Nifedipine
Opiates	Diphenoxylate
	Meperidine
	Morphine
Psychotropics	Amitriptyline
	Chlorpromazine
	Imipramine
Sphincter insufficiency	
	Methyldopa
α-Adrenergic antagonists	Prazosin

urethral stricture. Less commonly, in women, urethral stricture or severe bladder prolapse may block urine outflow. A functional obstruction may occur with simultaneous contractions of the bladder and external sphincter. This bladder-sphincter dyssynergia is uncommon in the elderly and occurs primarily in younger patients with spinal cord injury or multiple sclerosis.

The clinical presentation of outlet obstruction is overflow incontinence. Symptoms of frequent postvoid dribbling or urgency may predominate. Patients may have an enlarged, palpable bladder due to urinary retention. They must strain to urinate, and both voluntarily voided and involuntarily lost urine volumes are small.

ATONIC BLADDER

Impaired detrusor tone may result from low spinal cord lesions, diabetic or alcoholic neuropathy, or the use of muscle relaxants, narcotics, or antidepressants that block the cholinergically induced contraction of the bladder. Diabetes mellitus or tabes dorsalis may cause a decrease in sensory input from the bladder; however, central inhibition remains intact, so patients may be able to maintain volitional bladder control by voiding at scheduled times. The patient with an atonic bladder also has symptoms of urinary retention and overflow incontinence as described above.

SPHINCTER INSUFFICIENCY/PELVIC FLOOR WEAKNESS

Almost one-third of all incontinent women have stress incontinence caused by incorrectly positioned (hypermobile) urethra, sphincter insufficiency, and/or reduced support by the pelvic floor musculature of the bladder outlet. Multiple childbirths, gynecologic surgery, and/or decreased estrogen effect on pelvic tissues, vasculature, and urethral mucosa are the most likely causes. Sphincter weakness may also result from local urethral inflammation, neurologic disease, radiation therapy, or sympatholytic drugs. In men, stress incontinence occurs much less frequently, usually in those who have sustained sphincter trauma during prostatectomy. The patient complains of the loss of small amounts of urine with an increase in abdominal pressure from laughing, coughing, straining, lifting, or a change in posture. Nocturia is uncommon, but symptoms of urgency may occur.

FUNCTIONAL

Functional incontinence primarily results from the inability of otherwise continent persons to reach the toilet in time because of physical, pharmacologic, psychogenic, or environmental factors. Joint pain, muscle weakness, immobility, decreased vision, and inability to articulate need are the primary physical causes of functional incontinence. Medications that increase urinary frequency or cause confusion may precipitate functional incontinence as well (Table 27.1). Functional incontinence may also result from lack of motivation (dementia, depression, psychosis) or a history of frequent failure to reach the toilet in time (giving up). Environmental contributors include inconveniently located toilets, obstacles in the path to the toilet, or physical restraints.

The patient with physical limitations may complain of early morning incontinence. Symptoms of incontinence may be fixed in relation to drug dosing intervals. The patient with psychological or cognitive problems may never voice any complaints. Episodes occurring while the patient is en route to a toilet or while restrained in a Geri-chair suggest environmental causes. With functional incontinence, the amount of urine lost per episode may vary.

EVALUATION

The evaluation of the elderly incontinent patient should begin with a careful history directed at understanding the nature, severity, and burden of the problem and identifying the most easily remedied contributing causes of incontinence.

The medical history should focus on urinary symptoms, noting onset and duration of incontinence, frequency, amount of urine lost per episode, and any contributing factors. A bladder or incontinence chart filled out before the patient's visit is an important means of documenting each episode. A more quantitative assessment of urinary incontinence is the standardized pad weighing test, but the sensitivity is low (9).

Incontinence associated with symptoms of coughing, laughing, or posture change suggests stress incontinence, while dysuria and hematuria may indicate infection. A decrease in force of the urine stream and strain with urination denotes obstruction; inability to stop urine flow voluntarily suggests pelvic muscle weakness. A low score on a mental status screening examination suggests dementia, which may cause detrusor instability or indifference to the symptoms, or both.

The past medical history should target history of childbirth, pelvic surgery, cancer, neurologic disease, diabetes mellitus, congestive heart failure, and previous treatment of urinary incontinence. Specific questions should be asked about ambulation, prescription and over-the-counter medication use, alcohol use, or excessive fluid intake. Inquiries should be made about the physical layout of the patient's home, where the patient spends most of the day, and whether impaired mobility limits access to toilet facilities. The patient should bring a bag containing all prescription and nonprescription medications to the clinic.

Physical examination of incontinent patients targets the abdominal, rectal, genital, and neurologic examinations. A palpable bladder strongly suggests overflow incontinence due to outlet obstruction or atonic bladder. The rectal examination may reveal fecal impaction, pelvic mass, or enlarged prostate gland. The size of the prostate, however, does not correlate well with obstruction (10). Assessing perianal sensation and the ability to voluntarily contract and relax the anal sphincter tests lumbosacral innervation. During the pelvic examination, prolapse of urethra, bladder, or uterus or pelvic mass should be sought. Atrophic vaginitis reflects lack of estrogen.

In women, the major diagnostic dilemma is to differentiate detrusor instability from stress incontinence. In men, the primary distinctions to be made are between obstructed and atonic bladder, and/or detrusor instability. Most studies have shown poor correlation between these etiologies and symptoms. The presence of incontinence from several different causes (mixed incontinence) in many older people limits the usefulness of evaluation algorithms based on symptoms and signs alone (11).

DIAGNOSTIC TESTS

Although not well validated in the elderly population, selected laboratory tests and simple tests of urinary tract function have generally been recommended for the evaluation of most incontinent patients (19). Initial diagnostic testing should include urinalysis and urine culture (infection, neoplasm) as well as serum electrolytes, urea nitrogen, calcium, and glucose determinations (renal insufficiency, polyuric syndromes). The urine studies may be obtained in conjunction with measurement of postvoid residual volume (PVR). This is obtained by inserting a 14 French straight catheter into the bladder in sterile fashion 5 to 10 minutes after the patient has voided. Caution is indicated in patients with outflow obstruction, as a single catheterization may cause infection. Pelvic ultrasound, more costly but noninvasive, may be considered for PVR determination. Although the definition of high residual urine volume is controversial, a return of 100 mL or more suggests either obstruction or atonic bladder and is an indication for further urologic evaluation (5).

Clinical tests for stress incontinence in women may be useful. With a full bladder, the patient should cough, laugh, or strain to induce urine leakage. The patient then voids, and the urine volume is measured. To perform the Bonney test, the clinician places a finger just inside the vagina on either side of the urethra while the patient coughs. Pressure against the fingers may be felt, and urine loss may occur. If upward pressure of the fingers stops urine leakage, the test is positive. However, this maneuver may cause urethral occlusion instead and should not be relied upon as a definite indicator of stress incontinence in older women (11).

A bedside bladder filling test has been proposed by several investigators to evaluate bladder capacity and to detect detrusor instability (10, 12). The test is usually performed after catheterization for postvoid residual volume. A 50-mL syringe (without plunger) attached to the catheter is held 15 cm above the pubic symphysis and filled gravitationally in 50-mL increments until the urge to void is noted by the patient. Filling is continued in 25-mL increments until involuntary contractions cause a rise in fluid level in the syringe or the patient complains of severe urgency. In one study of 171 older, mostly female patients, bedside cystometry had a 75% sensitivity and 79% specificity for detrusor instability, compared with multichannel cystometry (13). The accuracy of the test for other conditions or different patient populations is unknown.

FORMAL URODYNAMIC TESTING

Although uncomplicated stress incontinence and detrusor instability as well as acute medical (temporary), metabolic, and functional causes of urinary incontinence can be evaluated and managed by the primary care physician, some patients will need gynecologic or urologic referral for further evaluation and testing. Common urodynamic tests that provide more detailed diagnostic information include urine flowmetry, voiding cystourethrography, multichannel cystometrogram, pressure flow study, urethral pressure profile measurement, and sphincter electromyography (14). Specific findings on history or physical examination that should suggest referral include recent gynecologic or urologic surgery or radiation therapy, recurrent or relapsing urinary tract infection, and evidence of obstruction (pelvic prolapse in women, enlarged or indurated prostate in men). In addition, increased postvoid residual, inability to pass a straight catheter, or failure of therapy for simple stress incontinence or detrusor instability should prompt referral (5).

TREATMENT

Accurate diagnosis of urinary incontinence is essential for selecting the most appropriate form of management. Behavioral, pharmacologic, and surgical therapies are effective in older people. In some cases, a combination of these therapies will be most beneficial. It is generally advisable to begin treatment with the least risk and burden to the patient and caregiver. In all types of incontinence except those characterized by overflow (obstructed or atonic bladder), behavioral techniques should be considered as first-line therapy (14). In the following section, appropriate management for each type of urinary incontinence is discussed.

DETRUSOR INSTABILITY

Treatment of detrusor instability is directed toward decreasing or blocking uninhibited bladder contractions, improving bladder capacity, and prolonging time from symptoms of urgency to voiding. Behavioral techniques useful for this condition include bladder training (or retraining), habit training, and biofeedback. Bladder training uses an educational program, scheduled voiding, and positive reinforcement to train the patient to resist urge sensations, postpone voiding, and urinate on a fixed timetable. A randomized, controlled study in women reported that 75% of the subjects reduced incontinent episodes by half, and 12% became continent (15).

Habit training (timed voiding) also requires that the patient void according to a timetable. With this method, the patient is not taught to resist urge symptoms. In one controlled nursing-home-based trial, 86% of subjects had significantly decreased frequency of incontinent episodes over a 3-month period (16). Prompted voiding, a technique requiring a caregiver to check for wetness at routine intervals and to prompt the patient to void is an effective adjunct to habit training in dependent and cognitively impaired nursing home or home care patients (17).

Bladder-sphincter biofeedback techniques record bladder, vaginal, and rectal pressures or electrical activity and display the information to the patient, who learns to modify these measures by relaxing the bladder and contracting pelvic floor muscles. These procedures require insertion of catheters and a trained technician. However, biofeedback in combination with bladder retraining

has been successfully used in selected patients to teach voluntary inhibition of detrusor contractions, achieving 50% or greater improvement in incontinence. This approach is most successful with patients who are mobile and who have minimal cognitive impairment. Electrical stimulation via the sacral reflex arc has also been used to inhibit detrusor hyperactivity in selected patients (14).

Pharmacologic therapy has proven useful for many patients with detrusor instability. Drugs with anticholinergic and smooth muscle relaxing properties are the most beneficial in this condition, although calcium channel blocking agents, nonsteroidal antiinflammatory drugs, β-adrenergic agonists, spinal synaptic inhibitors, and quaternary ammonium antimuscarinic agents are being tested. Drugs recommended in the Agency for Health Care Policy and Research (AHCPR)'s 1992 Clinical Practice Guideline for Urinary Incontinence in Adults for treatment of detrusor instability are listed in Table 27.2. These drugs have anticholinergic properties, while oxybutynin and dicyclomine also have smooth muscle relaxant properties. Of note, only oxybutynin and flavoxate have been approved officially by the FDA for this use. Flavoxate, a tertiary amine with smooth muscle relaxant properties, is not now recommended because none of the four randomized controlled studies of its efficacy showed significant benefit over placebo (14).

SPHINCTER INSUFFICIENCY/PELVIC MUSCLE WEAKNESS

Behavioral training and biofeedback are also useful for treating this condition. In addition, Kegel's exercises are beneficial for strengthening the pelvic floor muscles, but patients must be taught to avoid the Valsalva maneuver. A series of muscle contractions and relaxations are performed up to 100 times daily for 6 weeks or longer. One study reported improvement in incontinence in 54%, and cure in 16%, of elderly women subjects (18). The use of cone-shaped vaginal weights that are squeezed by the patient may improve the effectiveness of Kegel's exercises in selected patients (19). Electrical stimulation may also be useful for some patients.

Pharmacologic therapy is limited in the treatment of stress incontinence, but may be very effective. The mainstays of therapy are an α-adrenergic agonist (phenylpropanolamine) and estrogen, which enhance muscle contraction through α-adrenergic receptor stimulation. Estro-

Table 27.2
Pharmacologic Therapy for Urinary Incontinence[a]

Type of Incontinence	Drug	Dose	Side Effects
Detrusor instability	Oxybutynin	2.5–5 mg t.i.d.-q.i.d.	Dry skin Blurred vision Constipation Nausea Xerostomia Confusion Increased intraocular pressure
	Dicyclomine hydrochloride	10–20 mg t.i.d.	As above
	Propantheline	7.5–30 mg t.i.d.-q.i.d.	As above
	Imipramine	10–25 mg q.d.-t.i.d.	Fatigue Xerostomia Blurred vision Postural hypotension Dizziness Arrhythmias Nausea
Sphincter insuffi-ciency	Phenylpropanolamine	25–75 mg b.i.d. SR	Anxiety Insomnia Agitation Hypertension Sweating Arrhythmias
	Conjugated estrogens	0.3–1.25 mg q.d. oral 1–2 g topical	Thrombophlebitis Endometrial cancer ? Breast cancer

[a]Effectiveness supported in randomized controlled trials.

gen also has a direct effect on urethral mucosa and periurethral tissues. The doses and side effects of these drugs are shown in Table 27.2. Use of phenylpropanolamine in sustained release form has resulted in improvement of 30 to 60% versus placebo response. If long-term therapy with estrogen is planned, continuous or cyclic methyhydroxyprogesterone should be given simultaneously in doses of 2.5 to 10 mg daily (14).

For women in whom conservative therapy has failed, surgery may be appropriate. For incorrect urethral placement, retropubic suspension of the urethrovesical junction and needle bladder neck suspension are the procedures of choice. Cure rates of 78 to 84% with complication rates of 20% have been reported (14). For intrinsic sphincter deficiency, surgical treatment options include artificial sphincter placement (20), sling placement beneath the urethrovesical junction (21), and periurethral bulking injections with Teflon or collagen (22). Complications related to erosion of artificial sphincters and migration of injected bulking agents limit the usefulness of these procedures in the elderly. In men with urethral insufficiency, the use of a condom catheter should be considered before surgery.

OUTFLOW OBSTRUCTION

For men with moderate to severe obstruction due to prostate enlargement, surgery is the treatment of choice. Transurethral prostatectomy can result in a high cure rate in patients with properly functioning bladders. Women with a significant cystocele may require surgical repair. In these patients, full evaluation including urodynamic testing prior to surgery is essential to rule out coexisting causes of incontinence.

ATONIC BLADDER

Overflow incontinence due to a hyporeflexic bladder is generally poorly responsive to behavioral or pharmacologic therapy. Surgery is not indicated. A cholinergic agonist such as bethanechol (Urecholine) in doses of 10 to 30 mg t.i.d.-q.i.d. should stimulate bladder contraction, but this has not proven effective over the long term (5). In patients with milder dysfunction, scheduled voiding may be useful. In patients with more severe neurologic deficits, intermittent clean catheterization every 2 to 4 hours by the patient or caregiver is the best management. If this is not possible or practical, an indwelling catheter may be necessary. Use of chronic indwelling catheters is generally not encouraged, as complications including urolithiasis, symptomatic bacteriuria, periurethral abscess, and acute pyelonephritis are common. Appropriate management of an indwelling catheter depends upon proper insertion using sterile technique and maintaining a closed, sterile system. Urethral cleansing, routine bladder irrigation, and prophylactic antibiotic therapy should be avoided (23).

FUNCTIONAL

Successful treatment of functional incontinence relies upon recognition that physical, pharmacologic, psychological, or environmental problems exist. Providing the patient with assistive devices such as urinals or bedside commodes; treating depression; addressing hostility; reassessing drug indications, doses, and schedules; eliminating barriers in the path to the toilet; and removing restraints may improve incontinence dramatically. Timed voiding schedules are particularly useful in the cognitively impaired or physically disabled patient.

SUMMARY

Urinary incontinence remains a common, underreported, and costly problem in elderly patients. However, new therapeutic options using behavioral, pharmacologic, and surgical approaches are now available that can lead to symptomatic improvement or cure of this important clinical problem and increased comfort for the patient.

REFERENCES

1. NIH Consensus Development Conference. Urinary incontinence in adults. JAMA 1989;261:2685–2690.
2. Diokno AC, Brock BM, Brown MB, Herzog AR. Prevalence of urinary incontinence and other urological symptoms in the noninstitutionalized elderly. J Urol 1986;136:1022–1025.
3. Sier H, Ouslander JG, Orzeck S. Urinary incontinence among geriatric patients in an acute care hospital. JAMA 1987;257:1767–1773.
4. Wyman JF, Harkins SW, Choi SC, Taylor JR, Fantl JA. Psychosocial impact of urinary incontinence in women. Obstet Gynecol 1987;70:378–381.
5. Ouslander JG. Urinary incontinence. In: Hazzard WR, Andres R, Bierman EL, Blass JP, eds. Principles of geriatric medicine and gerontology. 3rd ed. New York: McGraw-Hill, 1990:1123–1142.
6. Whitehead WE, Burgio KL, Engel BT. Behavioral methods in the assessment and treatment of urinary incontinence. In: Brocklehurst JC. Urology in

the elderly. New York: Churchill Livingstone, 1984:74–91.
7. Resnick NM, Yalla SV. Detrusor hyperactivity with impaired contractile function: an unrecognized but common cause of incontinence in elderly patients. JAMA 1987;257:3076–3081.
8. Resnick NM, Yalla SV, Laurino E. The pathophysiology and clinical correlates of established urinary incontinence in frail elderly. N Engl J Med 1989; 320:1–7.
9. Walsh JB, Mills GL. Measurement of urinary loss in elderly incontinent patients: a simple and accurate method. Lancet 1981;1:1130–1133.
10. Frimodt-Moller PC, Jensen KM-E, Iverson P, et al. Analysis of presenting symptoms in prostatism. J Urol 1984;132:272–274.
11. DuBeau CE, Resnick NM. Evaluation of the causes and severity of geriatric incontinence. Urol Clin North Am 1991;18:243–256.
12. Sutherst JR, Brown MC. Comparison of single and multichannel cystometry in diagnosing bladder instability. Br J Med Clin Res 1984;288:1720–1725.
13. Ouslander J, Leach G, Abelson S, et al. Simple versus multichannel cystometry in the evaluation of bladder function in an incontinent geriatric population. J Urol 1988;140:1482–1486.
14. Urinary Incontinence Guideline Panel. Urinary incontinence in adults: clinical practice guideline. AHCPR Pub. No. 92–0038. Rockville, MD: Agency for Health Care Policy and Research, Public Health Service, U.S. Department of Health and Human Services, March 1992.
14. Fantl JA, Wyman JF, McClish DK, Harkins SW, Elswick RK, Taylor JR, et al. Efficacy of bladder training in older women with urinary incontinence. JAMA 1991;265:609–613.
16. Jarvis GJ. A controlled trial of bladder drill and drug therapy in the management of detrusor instability. Br J Urol 1981;53:565–566.
17. Schnelle JF. Treatment of urinary incontinence in nursing home patients by prompted voiding. J Am Geriatr Soc 1990;38:356–360.
18. Burns PA, Pranikoff K, Nochajski T, Desotelle P, Harwood MK. Treatment of stress incontinence with pelvic floor exercises and biofeedback. J Am Geriatr Soc 1990;38:341–344.
19. Olah KS, Bridges N, Denning J Farrar DJ. The conservative management of patients with symptoms of stress incontinence: a randomized, prospective study comparing weighted vaginal cones and interferential therapy. Am J Obstet Gynecol 1990; 162:87–92.
20. Appell RA. Techniques and results in the implantation of the artificial urinary sphincter in women with type III stress urinary incontinence by a vaginal approach. Neurourol Urodyn 1988;7:613–619.
21. McIndoe GA, Jones RW, Grieve BW. The Aldridge sling procedure in the treatment of urinary stress incontinence. Aust NZ J Obstet Gynecol 1987; 27:238–239.
22. McGuire EJ, Wang SC, Appel R, Webster G, Deridder P, Bennett A. Treatment of urethral incontinence by collagen injection: one year follow-up. J Urol 990;143(4, suppl):224A.
23. Wong ES. Guidelines for prevention of catheter-associated urinary tract infections. Philadelphia: WB Saunders, 1974.

28/ Geriatric Gynecology

Mary C. Ciotti

A woman lives approximately one-third of her life after menopause (1). Although most medical problems that arise will not be gynecologic in origin, it is important to continue to address gynecologic issues and problems as a woman ages. A gynecologic history and pelvic examination should be viewed as a routine part of every woman's general physical examination, particularly since the incidence of all genitourinary cancers increases with age (2).

The average age of menopause in the United States is 51 years. This is largely influenced by a woman's family history. Menopause is the actual cessation of menses. However, approximately 5 years before that time, there is a gradual decrease in follicular function and the ovaries produce less estrogen. This is why some women have hot flashes and symptoms prior to "menopause." This time of decreasing ovarian function is known as the "climacteric" or perimenopause (1).

Hot flashes are one of the most common symptoms of menopause in the United States. The exact cause is unknown but appears to be related to a disturbance of central thermoregulation, signaling a need to lower temperature, which initiates peripheral heat loss and a resultant fall in core temperature. Slightly overweight or obese women are less likely to have hot flashes because of the ovarian and adrenal production of androgens, which are then peripherally converted to estrone by adipose tissue. Conversely, women who are thin or of slight build are more likely to experience hot flashes.

These vasomotor symptoms can occur daily, sometimes at multiple times during the day, but are most common in the evening. Often they interrupt sleep and cause insomnia. Women can experience hot flashes for 2 to 3 years after menopause, and some women experience them as many as 5 years after menopause. Most women report a lessening of the severity of these flushes within 6 to 12 months. Situations that exacerbate hot flashes are emotional upset, stress, hot weather, hot drinks, caffeine, alcohol, warm rooms, and warm beds. Women should be informed of these associations and avoid them when possible.

If a patient is symptomatic and feels that more aggressive measures need to be taken, estrogen replacement therapy will alleviate the vasomotor symptoms. If estrogen therapy is contraindicated or the patient does not want estrogen therapy, Bellergal may be helpful in regards to sleep, but it is a sedative and can be habit forming. The clonidine patch can help reduce vasomotor symptoms. However, the effect of pharmacologic treatments other than estrogen seem to be short-lived. Some patients report diminished symptoms with the use of homeopathic or herbal remedies.

Tissues in the genitourinary tract are quite responsive to estrogen. With the lack of estrogen stimulation, the vagina becomes atrophic with decreased rugae, lubrication, and distensibility. Again, estrogen replacement therapy, either systemic or topical, is helpful for treatment of these complaints, but much of the elasticity of the tissue can be maintained by having regular intercourse. Lubricants such as K-Y Jelly, AstroGlide, and Personal may also help relieve dyspareunia from vaginal dryness.

Hypoestrogenization affects the collagen support of the tissues supporting the bladder, uterus, and rectum and results in pelvic relaxation. Although estrogen replacement does not totally alleviate these problems, it often will increase pelvic structural support, and patients may become less symptomatic. Other ways to prevent further worsening of pelvic relaxation are encouraging the patient to avoid heavy lifting or straining and recommending Kegel's exercise regularly. Increased fiber in the diet should be encouraged, so that a patient does not strain with her bowel movements. Chronic straining to defecate can result in a rectocele or in worsening of an existing rectocele. The bladder and the urethra are estrogen-dependent tissues (3). A woman may develop symptoms of urgency, urinary incontinence, dysuria, and frequency. It is important to rule out urinary tract infections whenever these symptoms persist, as menopausal women are more susceptible to cystitis. However, keep in mind that these symptoms may be secondary to estrogen deprivation of the tissue.

The psychosocial impact of perimenopause and menopause is variable, and much depends upon each woman's personality style, past coping mechanisms, cultural influences, and life situation. Menopause is often perceived as a major life change that causes women to suffer depression and psychiatric complaints. However, research shows that there is not an increase in depressive disorders during this time (4). Women commonly will complain of insomnia, increased temper, decreased libido, and crying spells. This is most likely related to hormonal fluctuations and the decrease in hormonal production. However, it can be exacerbated by the concomitant life changes that often occur and which require major adjustment, such as aging parents, an aging spouse, and children moving back into the home. It is important to differentiate whether the symptoms or changes are due to "menopause," life's situational influences, or an exacerbation of an existing psychiatric syndrome. Treatment can then be geared toward assurance of normalcy, hormonal treatment, psychosocial intervention, and/or psychiatric medication (5). It is also important for health practitioners to view menopause as a normal phase of a woman's life, not as a medical condition characterized by estrogen deprivation that needs medical therapy.

HISTORY AND PHYSICAL EXAMINATION

Gynecologic History

Each woman should be asked about menstrual history, age of menarche, regularity of menstrual cycle, characterization of menses, age of last menses, episodes of postmenopausal bleeding, and a description of menopausal symptoms. It is important to ask at each visit about postmenopausal bleeding and to emphasize the need to inform the practitioner if that should occur. Information about dysplasia, abnormal Pap smears, and date and results of her last Pap smear should be ascertained.

Gynecologic Surgical History.   Ask if the patient has had a hysterectomy and, if so, ascertain if she had removal of her ovaries, uterus, and/or cervix. Women with hysterectomies before the 1960s are more likely to have had a supracervical hysterectomy; therefore the cervix may still remain. Ask whether the hysterectomy was for benign or malignant disease, especially cervical abnormalities, because this will guide you in the need for following a patient with Pap smears and pelvic examinations.

Pelvic Relaxation.   Women with pelvic prolapse may or may not have any symptoms. When symptomatic, some women will complain of a bearing-down sensation, heaviness or pelvic pressure, or a sense of fullness. This may be especially evident when a woman is standing for a long period of time or with heavy lifting, and is generally relieved by sitting or lying down. A woman may actually feel a protrusion of the cervix, uterus, or vaginal wall through the vaginal introitus. She also may complain of internal discomfort during intercourse, which may be secondary to cervical motion during intercourse.

Initial assessment of bladder symptoms should be elicited by asking a woman if she loses urine, especially when she coughs, sneezes, or exerts herself. Determine how often she needs to get up at night to urinate and if she is incontinent. If she answers affirmatively to these inquiries, further evaluation may be warranted (see Urinary Incontinence).

Bowel symptoms such as constipation, diarrhea, changes in stool character, blood in the stools, and soiling of underwear need to be addressed. Each woman should be directly asked if she has difficulty with bowel evacuation. The need to use two fingers in the vagina to push out stool would indicate a symptomatic rectocele (see Types of Pelvic Relaxation).

Sexual History.   Is the patient sexually active? If so, the provider should ask about the frequency of intercourse, patient's satisfaction, use of lubricants, and if there are any specific concerns. A woman experiencing pain during intercourse should be asked to characterize it. If the patient is not sexually active and is involved in a relationship, is her lack of sexual activity related to her partner, the patient, or a combination of factors?

Obstetric History

Information about a woman's obstetric history will give some insight into her risk of pelvic relaxation and problems. Thus, the practitioner should ask about the number of deliveries, mode of delivery (i.e., vaginal vs. cesarean section), and any postpartum complications.

Physical Examination

Positioning.   Positioning the patient for the gynecologic examination can often be the most difficult part of this examination. The lithotomy position is preferred. The patient should empty her bladder before the examination. Have her sit at the end of the table, then place one foot in each stirrup. Have the patient lie back. If she is still not at the end of the table, have her scoot down toward the end of the table. If she is not agile and cannot easily lie back with her feet in the stirrups because of arthritis or physical disabilities, other techniques may be used. One can start by having the patient sit at the edge of the table, pull out the shelf underneath the table, and then ask her to lie back in the supine position. Then pull out the stirrups, place one foot into each stirrup and finally return the shelf back under the table. The patient at this point can be properly placed in the lithotomy position. Pull out the stirrups only as much as needed, minimizing the amount of abduction in the hips. At times it is very difficult for the patient to be flat on her back, and if the patient so desires, one can elevate the table back to have her head slightly higher. Many patients prefer to keep their shoes and socks on during this examination.

Other less optimal ways to perform a speculum and bimanual examination are as follows:

1. *Lateral recumbent position.* The patient lies on her side with both knees bent. An assistant helps hold up the top leg and the examiner inserts the speculum with the handle facing either the patient's back or her abdomen. At that point, the cervix is visualized and the Pap smear obtained. If possible, the patient should be turned over for the pelvic examination (6). If she is unable to this, then the examination can be performed from the lateral recumbent position.
2. *Diamond-shaped position (frog-leg position).* The patient lies on her back with her feet together at the foot of the table, letting her knees fall out to the side, lying close to the table. The speculum is then inserted with the handle up. The bimanual examination can be performed from either the side or the foot of the table (6).
3. *V-shaped position.* The patient lies on her back with both legs straight out to the side, spread out in a V position. One or two assistants are required for this position to support her straightened legs. The speculum is inserted with the handle up. The bimanual examination is done from the side or the foot of the table (6).

Technique. With time and patience, one of the above methods should allow an adequate pelvic examination. An adequate pelvic examination is one in which the vulva is inspected in its entirety, the vagina is inspected, the cervix is visualized and any abnormalities noted, and a Pap smear is obtained if indicated. The bimanual ex-

amination is performed by palpating the vaginal walls as well as the cervix, feeling the uterus and any adnexal masses, and finally, completing a rectovaginal examination.

The vulva should first be inspected by noting hair distribution. Pubic hair decreases, becoming more sparse with menopause. Atrophic changes, leukoplakia, ulcers, or tumors should be considered. Any abnormalities of the vulva should be biopsied. A hand-held magnifying glass sometimes helps to obtain a closer observation of the vulva.

The vagina is examined with the speculum. Often the Pedersen speculum is preferred in older women because with atrophy or lack of intercourse, the introital opening is decreased. Because of decreased lubrication, it is important to lubricate the instruments. If a Pap smear is to be done, the speculum should be lubricated with warm water (K-Y Jelly may affect the accuracy of the Pap smear). If the patient has a large amount of relaxation, a Graves speculum is preferred. The speculum is fully placed into the vagina and opened. The vagina and cervix are inspected. The vaginal rugae are decreased, especially in women not on estrogen and the color becomes a lighter pink. The cervix is often small and pale, and it can become flush with the vaginal wall, making it difficult to distinguish from the vaginal mucosa. Specimens for a Pap smear and cultures are then obtained, if necessary. The vagina should be examined as the speculum is being removed. If an abnormality of the cervix or vagina is noted, biopsy or colposcopy is necessary even if the patient has a normal Pap smear. Any abnormality needs to be referred or evaluated further.

The bimanual examination is performed by placing two gloved fingers into the vagina, palpating the vagina and cervix for abnormalities. The position of the uterus is felt, and any tenderness is noted. The mobility of the uterus and its size also are noted. An attempt should be made to palpate the adnexa. In general, the uterus is smaller, and in postmenopausal women the adnexa should not be palpable, especially if the patient is more than three years postmenopausal (7). If ovaries are palpated, further workup is necessary (see Palpable Postmenopausal Ovary Syndrome).

A rectovaginal examination should be done in all women over 40, to confirm the bimanual examination, to feel for pathology in the posterior cul-de-sac, and to rule out anorectal polyps or tumors. At that time, stool should be tested for heme, but this is not a substitute for obtaining serial stool specimens to check for occult blood.

PELVIC RELAXATION

Pelvic relaxation is a common finding in older women. It is more common in women who have had children; however, it also occurs in nulliparous women. The extent of pelvic floor damage determines the degree of prolapse. Pelvic relaxation usually appears as a combination of uterine prolapse, cystocele, and/or rectocele, although it is possible for each to appear singularly. Some women can have remarkable findings on physical examination and yet be asymptomatic, and others can initially appear to have minimal findings yet are quite symptomatic. Following is a discussion of classification, diagnosis, and possible treatment options.

A grading system is used to describe the amount of relaxation or prolapse. This same system can be used to describe cystocele, rectocele, and uterine prolapse. A *first-degree prolapse* is defined as descent of the structure into the upper two-thirds of the vagina. A *second-degree prolapse* occurs when the structure is at or near the vaginal introitus. A *third-degree prolapse* occurs when the structure is outside of the introitus. *Total procidentia* is complete prolapse of the pelvic organs beyond the vaginal orifice.

A *cystocele* is a protrusion of the bladder into the anterior vaginal wall. The patient may or may not have symptoms of urinary incontinence. A *urethrocele* is a protrusion of the urethra into the vagina, signifying loss of the support of the urethrovesical junction (8). This finding is commonly seen in patients having stress urinary incontinence. Cystocele and urethrocele both can be demonstrated by speculum examination. This can be evaluated by taking the speculum apart and, using only the posterior blade as a retractor, inserting into the vagina, pushing down on the posterior wall of the vagina and observing the anterior wall for a cystocele. Having the patient bear down will be helpful in eliciting the cystocele as well as the urethrocele. A cystocele will bulge forward from the anterior vaginal wall. In the presence of a urethrocele, the urethra will bulge outward, and the urethral meatus often will curl outward around the symphysis. Often a moderate-to-large cystocele is asymptomatic and does not require treatment. However if the patient has distressing pressure symptoms, recurrent cystitis, or incontinence, surgical repair is the most effective treatment. If she does not want surgery or is not a surgical candidate, a pessary may be considered. The rubber doughnut or plastic ring with perforated base may be useful, provided the cystocele is not too large (9).

A *rectocele* is a protrusion of the rectum into the posterior vagina, signifying a relaxation of the fascial support to the rectum (8). This can be diagnosed by taking the posterior blade of the speculum and inverting it, pulling up on the anterior wall of the bladder, and having the patient bear down and observing the rectocele bulge forward. Also, one can demonstrate a rectocele by doing a rectal examination, hooking the finger forward to demonstrate the rectocele pocket. Rectoceles are usually associated with a cystocele and some degree of uterine descent. A small rectocele that is not symptomatic does not need repair. Patients should be told the importance of not straining with bowel movements to prevent further herniation of the rectum through the posterior vaginal wall. Larger rectoceles, particularly those that cause pressure and difficult elimination, should be repaired surgically.

An *enterocele* is a protrusion or herniation of the posterior cul-de-sac (pouch of Douglas) through the uterosacral ligaments (8). This is often difficult to ascertain on physical examination and particularly hard to distinguish from a rectocele.

Uterine descensus or prolapse refers to the descent of the uterus from its normal position high in the vagina. Symptoms include pelvic heaviness, bearing-down, and pelvic pressure or fullness that is usually relieved by sitting or lying down. If a patient is symptomatic and is limiting normal activities, treatment is indicated. The most effective and widely used therapy is surgical intervention, but consideration can be given to fitting a patient with a pessary.

Pessary

Pessaries can be an alternative to surgery for patients who do not want to undergo surgery and would prefer to try less invasive methods or for patients with debilitating disease who are not surgical candidates. They are especially useful in women with uterine prolapse without concomitant marked outlet relaxation. Women with marked pelvic relaxation and prolapse usually have atonic tissues, and a pessary is not helpful because it will not stay in place.

There are many types of pessaries: the ring, Gellhorn, donut, Hodge, and cube types are in common clinical usage, and all come in various sizes (10). The ring pessary and the ring with support are very easy to use and are helpful for treatment of uterine prolapse and cystocele (10). They are very similar to the outer ring of a diaphragm. They are flexible and fit anteriorly behind the symphysis and posteriorly in the posterior fornix. The Hodge is useful in treatment of uterine descensus, especially in women with a retroverted uterus. Like the ring, it also is flexible, although less so. The blunt end fits under the symphysis, and the rounded end encompasses the cervix and fits against the uterosacral ligaments (9). The donut, cube, and Gellhorn are more occlusive and more likely to cause problems with ulceration. They also are more difficult to remove and replace but may be more effective in women with marked relaxation.

When fitting a pessary, it is helpful to have several types and sizes available, for it is similar to diaphragm fitting and is done by trial and error. Once the size is selected and placed, one should ask about discomfort. If it is uncomfortable, it should be removed. If it is not uncomfortable, have the patient bear down to make sure it stays in place. Then have the patient walk around the room. If it comes out, replace with a bigger size or different type. In private, have the patient remove and replace the pessary. Then check for appropriate placement (10).

The patient should return in 3 to 4 days to assess placement and effectiveness. She should not be aware of the pessary when it is in place, and when checked, the pessary should be in the same position it was at the time of placement. Sometimes it is necessary to alter sizes at this visit. Instructions regarding use and hygiene should be given. The pessary should be cleaned with soap and water. If irritation or mild ulceration of the vagina occurs, women can remove the pessary at night and use it only during the day. Women who are not able to manage their own pessary care should be seen every 6 weeks for assessment and evaluation (10). Complications of pessaries do occur, such as ulcerations and vaginitis, and if proper hygiene and management are not maintained, pessaries can become embedded within the vaginal mucosa. Ulcerations can usually be treated with topical estrogen and by discontinuing use of the pessary until healed. In addition, a pessary may become ineffective if the prolapse worsens.

VULVA

As mentioned earlier, all abnormalities of the vulva should be biopsied before beginning therapy. This is to ensure proper therapy and also to prevent missing vulvar cancer, which often presents with pruritus and irritation.

Lichen Sclerosus et Atrophicus (LSA)

Most patients with LSA present with vulvar itching, although some may present with vulvo-dynia. The disease usually spreads toward the perianal area, and the skin appears white and parchmentlike. In the past, testosterone therapy has been the treatment of choice for LSA; however, studies presented at the 11th International Congress of the International Study for the Study of Vulvar Disease concluded that topical steroid therapy was the treatment of choice (11). One study involved 79 patients with biopsy-proven LSA who were treated for 3 months. There was remission of symptoms in 75% of those patients treated with clobetasol, 20% of the testosterone-treated group, 10% in the progesterone-treated group, and 10% in the cream-based preparation group. Of note, the only treatment group that showed a reversal of the histologic changes caused by LSA was the clobetasol group. Therefore, it was concluded that potent topical steroids were the treatment of choice (11).

Squamous Cell Hyperplasia

Squamous cell hyperplasia should also be biopsy proven (12). Often these areas appear red and irritated. Often there are substances that are causing the irritation of the vulva, and initial treatment should be aimed at obtaining a good history to identify substances that might be causing this, such as change in soap, feminine hygiene products, etc. After all possible substances have been removed that would be irritating to the vulva, treatment is geared toward breaking the itch-scratch cycle. This can be done by initial therapy with steroid cream. If itching is severe and the patient is scratching at night in her sleep, the provider may need to consider treatment with an oral antihistamine in addition to steroid cream.

Mixed Dystrophy

It is not uncommon to find a combination of squamous cell hyperplasia and lichen sclerosus et atrophicus (12). Treatment is geared toward breaking the itch-scratch cycle with antipruritics and topical corticosteroids.

Vulvar Intraepithelial Neoplasia (VIN)

VIN is a preinvasive neoplastic process that is often multifocal. A patient with VIN should be referred for colposcopy.

Nevi

Five percent of all melanomas in females arise in the vulva (12). All vulvar nevi should be carefully evaluated, and if suspicious, they should be excised. This can be both diagnostic and curative.

Tinea Cruris Psoriasis

Biopsy is helpful in making the diagnosis of psoriasis. Certainly, one needs to consider this as a differential diagnosis of vulvar itching if the patient has psoriasis on other parts of her body.

Vitiligo

Any area of the body can be involved with vitiligo. No treatment is indicated.

Condyloma Acuminata

Condyloma acuminata, a sexually transmitted viral disease caused by the human papilloma virus (HPV), can affect women of all ages. It can present as very small, flat, confluent, white appearing lesions to large cauliflowerlike lesions (13). One must be very careful in the diagnosis and treatment of condyloma because verrucous carcinoma and VIN can be indistinguishable from condyloma (12). Older women are more likely to have VIN or carcinoma. Diagnosis must be made by biopsy, preferably several, and colposcopy is strongly advised. Immunocompetence should be investigated if an older woman presents with new-onset condyloma or a recurrence, especially if there has not been a change in sexual partner. There are many treatment options including trichloroacetic acid, topical 5-fluorouracil, cryotherapy, or laser. Choosing a particular treatment depends on the extent of the disease. One may need to supplement therapy with estrogen replacement to allow the tissue to heal better.

Vulvovaginitis

Atrophic Vaginitis. The vagina and vulva become atrophic in postmenopausal women not on estrogen therapy. The mucosa thins, becomes devoid of rugae, loses elasticity, and becomes pale pink, in which petechial or ecchymotic spots can be present. There is an increase in pH and a decrease in vaginal secretions. The bacterial flora resembles that of a prepubescent female. Tissue is more likely to be traumatized and break, allowing infection (10).

Often the patient will have itching, burning, discomfort, dyspareunia, and possible vaginal spotting or bleeding due to a very thin vaginal epithelium that has been traumatized. On physical examination, one finds severely atrophic external genitalia and vagina. There is no evidence of an infection, but a thin-appearing vaginal mucosa looks irritated and somewhat traumatized. If a discharge is present, it is most likely to be related to bacterial effects on the atrophic vagina. Bleed-ing associated with atrophic vaginitis is secondary to a break or fissure in the vaginal mucosa. It is sometimes difficult to ascertain whether the bleeding is from the vagina or uterus. If there is any question, an endometrial biopsy should be done.

When advanced mucosal thinning is present and there are no signs of infection, the patient is best treated with estrogen. This can be either topical or systemic. If one chooses to begin treatment with vaginal cream use one-fourth to one-third applicator full nightly for 2 to 4 weeks. The dosage can then be decreased to a maintenance dose of 1 to 2 times per week. Remember that vaginal estrogen therapy can be absorbed systemically and eventually cause endometrial hyperplasia. Its absorption systemically is somewhat erratic, and if one is considering long-term estrogen replacement therapy, it is best given through the oral or transdermal route. If oral estrogen replacement therapy is contraindicated, then vaginal estrogen therapy is as well.

Candidiasis. The patient usually presents with persistent itching, burning, and increased vaginal discharge, which is odorless. It is unusual for a postmenopausal woman to have candidiasis, but certain conditions may predispose a woman to vaginal candidiasis, such as a recent course of antibiotic therapy, immunosuppression, or diabetes mellitus. On wet preparation, one should see hyphae and/or spores. There is not a direct correlation between the number of organisms seen and the signs and symptoms of candidiasis. Treatment is usually initiated with one of the imidazoles, which include clotrimazole (Lotrimin and Mycelex G), miconazole (Monistat), butoconazole (Femstat), and terconazole (Terazol). The effectiveness of these therapies is approximately 90%. Treatment with nystatin (Mycostatin) for a 10- to 14-day course is approximately 80% effective. One may need to consider therapy with an oral preparation such as ketoconazole or fluconazole (13). This can be a very difficult problem to treat, and it is suggested that a patient with recurrent candidiasis have a consultation with a gynecologist.

Trichomoniasis. *Trichomonas vaginalis* is an unusual pathogen in postmenopausal women. The patient may complain of vulvar irritation or pruritus, of feeling wet with a gray, yellowish, or greenish discharge, and of an odor. Trichomoniasis is diagnosed by a wet preparation that shows many WBCs and protozoa. The treatment of choice is metronidazole, 1 g in the morning and 1 g in the evening or 500 mg b.i.d. for 7 days. Also, metronidazole can be given in the intravaginal gel form for 7-day treatment (13).

Bacterial vaginosis. The incidence of *Gardnerella vaginalis* decreases with increased age. Often the patient will complain of a malodorous discharge with varying degrees of vulvar or vaginal discomfort. Adding KOH to the discharge, one smells a fishy odor caused by the release of amines. On wet preparation, clue cells are found. Treatment of bacterial vaginosis is with metronidazole 500 mg b.i.d. for 7 days, single 1-g oral dose, metronidazole gel for 5 days, or clindamycin cream for 7 days (13). Metronidazole is less likely to destroy the normal vaginal flora, and therefore the patient is less likely to experience a yeast infection secondary to antibiotics.

CERVIX

Cervical Cancer

The incidence of cervical cancer increases with age. Approximately 27% of the cases of invasive cervical cancer and 41% of the deaths occur in women over the age of 65. When cervical cancer is diagnosed in older women, it is more likely to be found at a more advanced stage (14). This is in part due to the fact that older women are the least likely to have regular screening using the Pap smear (15). Although it has not been tested prospectively in the United States, several epidemiologic studies show a decrease in the incidence of cervical cancer after the introduction of the Pap smear as a screening test.

Screening Guidelines. Currently, the American Cancer Society, the National Cancer Institute, the American College of Obstetricians and Gynecologists, American Medical Association, American Academy of Family Physicians, and American Medical Women's Association recommend annual Pap smears for all women who are sexually active or have reached the age of 18. Pap smears may then be performed less frequently once three or more annual smears have been normal and if recommended by the physician (16). It is important to note that these groups do not recommend a time to stop screening. Any recommendation to cease screening in women over the age of 60 to 65 is based upon previous regular screening prior to the age of 65 (17).

In the United States, older women are the least likely to have a prior history of consistent Pap smear screening. One study of older, indigent women who received care in a large metropolitan hospital clinic found that 25% had never had a Pap smear, and 75% had irregular screening (18). Any recommendations to decrease screening also should depend upon women having records of their previous smears. Patients are poor historians regarding when they had a previous Pap smear as well as actually knowing whether or not it was normal (19, 20).

Pap Smear

The technique in performing the Pap smear is critical; it is reported that up to 60% of false-negative Pap smears may be due to sampling error (21). The cervix should be completely visualized. It is important to sample the transformation zone. It is usually recommended that two sampling devices be used: a spatula—wooden or plastic—and an endocervical brush. The endocervical brush has been shown to be more effective in sampling the endocervical/transformation zone. As a women ages, the transformation zone regresses higher into the endocervical canal, so at times it is difficult to sample in this area under direct visualization. Here the endocervical brush is very helpful and effective, although it may need to be inserted further into the cervix than one would do with a younger patient.

The cells should then be applied to the slide and fixed immediately. One or two slides can be used, although the most efficient use of resources supports using only one slide when doing a Pap smear. It is important to label the slide appropriately with a patient's name and to note on the cytopathology slip any history of cervical dysplasia, radiation therapy, estrogen use, and concomitant infection. This decreases the chance of having a false-positive Pap smear.

In December 1988, the National Cancer Institute addressed the issue of standardization of cervical/vaginal cytopathology reports and developed the Bethesda system. In 1991, the system was revised and simplified, and criteria were developed for specimen adequacy. The following algorithms for follow-up of abnormal Pap smears are based on the interim guidelines from the Michigan Department of Public Health's Interim Protocol for Cervical Cancer Screening in Women Age 40 and Older using the Bethesda system lexicon. As the title implies, these protocols are undergoing review and revision as our knowledge regarding screening in older women increases. It is important to be aware of possible changes, and as always, any questions should be referred to an expert (22).

Satisfactory Smear, Infectious Agent Identified. If the patient was treated at the time of her Pap smear, then one should follow-up with this patient as usual. If she has not been treated, the patient should be returned to the office, evaluated for infection, and treated if appropriate. The Pap smear does not need to be repeated, because it has been identified as a satisfactory smear.

Satisfactory Smear, Nonobscuring Inflammation. This again is a satisfactory smear. However, there is evidence of inflammation. It may be appropriate to have the patient return for a visit to determine whether the inflammation is due to an infectious agent or atrophic changes. Treat if appropriate.

Obscuring Inflammation. This is not an adequate smear, as inflammation obscures the slide to the point that the cytopathologist does not feel it can be read. The reason for inflammation needs to be investigated and treated, and a repeat Pap smear performed in 3 months. If obscuring inflammation persists after a second treatment and smear, then the patient should be referred for colposcopy.

Uninterpretable Pap Smear Secondary to Atrophic Changes. This will be more prevalent in postmenopausal women who are not on estrogen replacement therapy. If estrogen is not contraindicated, the patient should be treated with topical estrogens for approximately 3 to 4 weeks; approximately 1 to 2 weeks after therapy, the Pap smear should be repeated. If repeat Pap smear is negative, the patient can be screened regularly.

Low-Grade Squamous Intraepithelial Lesion (LSIL). If a patient has LSIL and is considered a high-risk patient, she should be referred for colposcopy. High-risk factors include not having previous routine Pap smears, history of abnormal smears, history of high-risk sexual behavior, HIV positive, or history of DES exposure. If she is at low risk, the Pap smear can be repeated in 3 to 4 months. If the repeat Pap smear is normal, then she should have her Pap smear repeated every 4 to 6 months for 2 years. After three consecutive negative smears, she can change to yearly Pap smears. On the other hand, if the repeat Pap smear shows low-grade SIL, then she should be referred for a colposcopy.

High-Grade Squamous Intraepithelial Lesion (HSIL). All patients with a diagnosis of HSIL should be referred for colposcopy.

Atypical Squamous Cells of Undetermined Significance (ASCUS). High-risk patients should be sent for colposcopy.

ASCUS with Severe Inflammation. Have the patient return for a visit and treat any evidence of infection. Repeat the Pap smear in 3 to 4 months. If the repeat Pap smear is negative, the patient should have repeat Pap smears done every 4 to 6 months for 2 years, and after three

consecutive negative smears, can change to yearly smears. If the repeat smear shows ASCUS, the patient should have colposcopy.

ASCUS Not Qualified or Reactive Process. Repeat Pap smear every 3 to 4 months. After three consecutive smears, the patient can be changed to yearly Pap smears.

ASCUS with Atrophy. If not contraindicated, treat the patient with estrogen therapy. If contraindicated, the patient should probably be sent for colposcopy.

Please note that a patient with any of the above diagnoses of ASCUS who has a repeat smear that shows ASCUS during the 2-year follow-up period should be considered for referral for colposcopy.

Atypical Glandular Cells of Undetermined Significance (AGUS). This may be a precursor of endocervical adenocarcinoma. The patient should be referred to a qualified health care provider for evaluation, which may include colposcopy, endocervical curettage, and possible conization.

Endometrial Cells Present on Smear. If the patient is postmenopausal, this is an abnormal finding, and she should be referred for further evaluation, which should consist of at least endometrial sampling but may include ultrasound, hysteroscopy, or dilation and curettage.

High Estrogen for Age. If the patient is on estrogen replacement therapy, nothing further needs to be done. If she is not on estrogen replacement therapy, the cause of high estrogen for age should be sought.

UTERUS

Endometrial cancer is the most common gynecologic cancer in women. The incidence of endometrial cancer rises sharply after the age of 45 and peaks between the ages of 55 and 69 (2). Fortunately, endometrial cancer is diagnosed at an earlier stage than other cancers and can often be treated by surgical intervention. On the other hand, older women are more likely to be diagnosed in an advanced stage. Vaginal bleeding is usually the first and only symptom of endometrial cancer. Approximately 75% of women will initially present with vaginal bleeding.

If a women has an episode of postmenopausal bleeding, it is imperative to rule out gynecologic cancer. It does not matter whether or not the patient complains of spotting or frank bleeding. Any bleeding needs to be further investigated. There does not seem to be a correlation between the amount of bleeding and the stage of the disease.

Approximately 20% of women with postmenopausal bleeding will have a gynecologic malignancy. The remaining 80% will have a nonmalignant condition such as hyperplasia or atrophic vaginitis (23). Unfortunately, women who are on estrogen replacement therapy may find it difficult to ascertain whether bleeding is a normal side effect of their therapeutic regimen. It is equally important for women who are on estrogen replacement therapy to report any abnormal uterine bleeding and to record their bleeding patterns for at least 1 year after initiation of therapy.

Screening for Endometrial Cancer

There are no tests that are recommended for general screening for endometrial cancer, although the American Cancer Society does recommend that endometrial tissue sampling be performed on women during menopause who are at risk. These are women who are obese, infertile, and anovulatory or those who have a history of abnormal uterine bleeding.

Endometrial Biopsy. The appropriateness of using an endometrial biopsy for detection and diagnosis of endometrial cancer is often argued. Sensitivity ranges between 87 and 100% (24). A recent study by Stovall et al. reported a 97% accuracy rate when using a Pipelle (26). These results are comparable to those obtained when doing a dilation and curettage under general anesthesia (25). The endometrial biopsy is an appropriate first-line evaluation for the woman who has postmenopausal bleeding. If positive results are found on the endometrial biopsy, then this should be acted upon appropriately. If the endometrial biopsy performed in the office is negative, this should be looked upon as an inadequate means of evaluation. This patient should have further evaluation, which could include dilation and curettage, hysteroscopy, and ultrasound evaluation (28).

Ultrasound. As a screening test for endometrial cancer, ultrasound seems to have a low sensitivity. Several studies have indicated that a endometrial thickness greater than 4 to 5 mm in a postmenopausal female is abnormal and should be further evaluated with direct sampling of the endometrium (27).

Pap Smear. The Pap smear is not considered a screening test for endometrial cancer, although endometrial cancers can be detected with the Pap smear. The presence of endometrial cells on the Pap smear of a postmenopausal woman requires further evaluation of the endometrium (22).

In summary, there are no methods that are appropriate for general screening for endometrial cancer at the present time (27, 30). However, practitioners need to ask about postmenopausal bleeding and inform women that this is not a normal occurrence. Women also should be told that this is often an early warning sign of a treatable form of endometrial cancer. Aggressive evaluation should be undertaken in any woman who complains of postmenopausal bleeding. The practitioner also should be mindful of postmenopausal women on estrogen replacement therapy, especially if they are on low doses of progestins. Women who have had breast cancer or are on tamoxifen therapy, women who have other risk factors for endometrial cancer or a past history of colon or breast cancer, and women who have a strong family history of endometrial or colon cancer should be followed closely and offered periodic endometrial biopsies.

OVARY

Although ovarian cancer is the least common of gynecologic cancers, it causes over 50% of all deaths from gynecologic cancer (31). It is a virulent neoplasm and carries a poor prognosis. The 5-year survival rate has not changed much since 1973. The incidence and death from ovarian cancer continue to increase with age. Forty-three percent of all ovarian cancers occur in women over the age of 64. The 5-year survival rate is much poorer for women over the age of 65 (24% vs. 48% for those under the age of 65) (12). Ovarian cancer is found at more advanced stages in older women, and stage for stage, older women have a poorer prognosis (31).

The symptoms of ovarian cancer are often very vague. A history of several months of abdominal discomfort such as bloating and digestive disturbances may suggest ovarian cancer. Unfortunately, all of these can be attributed to more common causes. However, if a woman over the age of 40 complains of persistent gastrointestinal symptoms, one should consider ovarian cancer in the differential diagnosis. Family history of ovarian cancer is one of the more identifiable risk factors for ovarian cancer. However, most women with ovarian cancer have no significant family history or other risk factors. Others identifiably at risk include those with a family history of breast cancer and colon cancer; those who have been diagnosed with endometrial, breast, or colon cancer; and nulliparous women. Women who have had early menarche or late menopause also are at risk (7).

Screening for Ovarian Cancer

Pelvic examination. The pelvic examination is the most available, but yet least reliable, test for screening for ovarian cancer. Unfortunately, by the time a mass has been detected on pelvic examination, an ovarian cancer is more likely to be metastatic.

Palpable Postmenopausal Ovary Syndrome. This syndrome was initially described by Barber in 1971. Women who are 3 years postmenopausal have very atrophic ovaries, and a practitioner should not be able to palpate these on pelvic examination. Thus, further workup would include a second opinion on physical examination findings, ultrasound, and CA 125. If the patient is at least 3 years postmenopause and one finds a palpable ovary, further investigation is needed, although the fact that one can palpate a postmenopausal ovary does not by itself indicate ovarian cancer.

CA 125. CA 125 is a serum tumor-associated antigen. Early reports were very promising. However, it was found that women who had stage I disease were less likely to have an elevated CA 125. In other words, if the CA 125 was elevated, it was more likely that the patient had disseminated disease. CA 125 lacks specificity; however, it is more specific in postmenopausal women (32–34).

Ultrasound. Although ultrasound has a high sensitivity, it is associated with a large number of false positives (35). The false-positive rate is decreased in postmenopausal women. Van Nagel et al. studied 1300 asymptomatic postmenopausal women; 27 had abnormal scans and 2 had cancer. The use of CA 125 when there is an abnormal ultrasound finding improves the specificity of ultrasound (36). To date, there are no long-term studies of the effect on morbidity or mortality.

In summary, the risk of ovarian cancer increases with age. It is found at more advanced stages in older women, and treatment tends to be less aggressive. Currently, there does not seem to be an effective or appropriate screening method that is applicable to the general population. Clinicians need to be vigilant, with a high degree of suspicion regarding older women with abdominal complaints and women who have a history that places them at high risk for ovarian cancer. At present, it may be beneficial to follow such women with CA 125 and ultrasound. However, to date there have been no long-term studies of the effect of these tests.

GENITOURINARY SYSTEM

Urinary Incontinence

Urinary incontinence is a major clinical problem that affects women of all ages, but in particular, older women. The prevalence of incontinence in women is two times that of men. Many of these women have not sought help for this problem. It is a myth that urinary incontinence is a part of normal aging. Although age-related problems may predispose women to incontinence, it is not necessarily a normal consequence of aging. Many causes of urinary incontinence can be cured or at least treated and the symptoms improved. Treatment does not necessarily need to be surgical. It is imperative that health care providers ask about incontinence and provide appropriate evaluation and treatment (37–39).

There are different causes of incontinence. Often the cause can be mixed, which makes evaluation and treatment more difficult. The evaluation is based on history and physical examination. Of the 25% of postreproductive women who have significant incontinence, 20% will have stress incontinence, 20% will have urge incontinence, and 60% will have a combination of the two. Treatment for stress incontinence is primarily surgical. Treatment for urge incontinence is primarily medical. Due to the high incidence of mixed incontinence, it is not surprising that patients who have had previous surgical therapy continue to have problems with incontinence. Therefore, it is important to be thorough in one's workup (40).

Urinary Tract Infections

Asymptomatic bacteriuria is much more common in the older woman. In fact, as many as a third of community-dwelling older women will have asymptomatic bacteriuria (ASB). The urogenital epithelium has decreased resistance to infections, and older women are less likely to respond to a short course of antibiotics. It is more appropriate to treat older women with a 10- to 14-day course of antibiotics and then check for a cure than to treat them with shorter courses (41).

Should one treat asymptomatic bacteriuria? Treatment of ASB does seem to have long-term benefits. There is resolution of the bacteriuria in most cases for at least 6 months and, therefore, a decrease in the incidence of pyelonephritis. Some studies have shown increased survival in women who are treated for asymptomatic bacteriuria. It does seem that the lack of estrogenation of the urothelium does contribute greatly to its lack of resistance to infection. If other etiologies of recurrent urinary tract infections are ruled out, then one might consider a course of estrogen therapy to see whether or not this improves her recurrent urinary tract infections or cystitis. In older women who develop urinary tract infections following coitus, a useful preventive strategy is to have them take 100 mg of Macrodantin after intercourse.

ESTROGEN REPLACEMENT THERAPY

There are many potential benefits of estrogen replacement therapy (ERT). Estrogen relieves vasomotor symptoms of menopause. This may also improve insomnia, which may have a positive effect on irritability and cognitive function. It is effective in the treatment of urogenital atrophy including atrophic vaginitis, dyspareunia, urethritis, and occasional mild forms of incontinence. Estrogen therapy prevents or delays bone loss and reduces the incidence of hip fracture (42), although a recent study indicated that this effect may be limited after age 75 (43). Estrogens have a positive effect on the lipid profile, with an increase in high-density lipoproteins (HDL) and a decrease in low-density lipoproteins (LDL). Studies indicate a significant decrease of 50% in cardiovascular disease (44), although most of these studies are observational studies of women on unopposed estrogen (45).

There also are risks of estrogen therapy. There is a fourfold increase in the incidence of endometrial cancer in women who are on unopposed estrogen (46). Most are found at an early stage and can be treated by surgery; however, this is costly, can cause morbidity, and is an unacceptable risk to many women. This risk can be lowered by the addition of progestins (47). The relationship between breast cancer and postmenopausal estrogen therapy is controversial, as evidenced by the lack of agreement among research studies and meta-analyses (48, 49). At the present time, the risk of breast cancer with 5 years of estrogen therapy with or without progestins seems low; for longer treatment, the data are still too sparse to interpret with confidence (44). There is an increase in the incidence of cholelithiasis, and a patient should be observed for these symptoms. The increased incidence of thromboembolic disease, hypertension, and altered carbohydrate metabolism observed with oral contraceptive use is not seen in postmenopausal therapy because of the lowered dosage (50).

Absolute contraindications to estrogen therapy are a history of breast cancer, endometrial cancer, acute vascular thrombosis with or without pulmonary emboli, neurophthalmologic vascular disease, acute liver disease, chronic impaired liver function, or undiagnosed vaginal bleeding. There are reports of women on estrogen therapy after diagnosis and treatment of breast cancer, stage I endometrial cancer, and a prior history of thrombosis (50). Further discussion of these exceptions are beyond the scope of this chapter and should be thoroughly researched and discussed before instituting such therapy. Relative contraindications include uterine leiomyomata, gall bladder disease, seizure disorders, familial hyperlipidemia, or migraine headaches (50).

Types of Estrogens

Estrogen can be divided into physiologic, natural, and synthetic types. *Physiologic* estrogens are estradiol (E_2), estrone (E_1), and estriol (E_3). These are produced by aromatization of androgenic compounds. The cellular potency of E_2 is greater than that of E_1, which is greater than E_3; however, continuous administration of weak estrogens has the same metabolic effect (51). *Natural* estrogens include conjugated equine estrogens and E_2. Conjugated equine estrogens (CEE) are sulfates or esters of estrone, equilin, and equilenin and are extracted from the urine of pregnant mares. E_2 has been successfully micronized and is active over 24 hours. E_2 taken orally is rapidly converted to E_1 in the gastrointestinal tract. After absorption, it then travels via the portal circulation to the liver, where further conversion to the less active E_3 occurs. Similar levels of E_1 and E_2 are reached when patients receive CEE. However, CEE contains various compounds in addition to E_1 and E_2, such as equilin sulfate, which are metabolized and stored in the adipose tissue and released for several weeks after treatment withdrawal (52). *Synthetic* estrogens are ethynyl estradiol, mestranol, and diethylstilbestrol. They are more potent than natural estrogens and tend to be more hepatotoxic. These estrogens are found in oral contraceptives and are not preferred for estrogen replacement therapy (51).

Route of Administration

Estrogens can be given orally, the most often prescribed method; however, as noted above, these are rapidly converted to the less potent E_1 by conversion in the gastrointestinal mucosa and liver. Efforts to bypass the initial intestinal and liver metabolism have centered around topical applications via vaginal mucosa, oral mucosa, and skin (51). Micronized estradiol is efficiently absorbed through the vaginal mucosa with more physiologic $E_2:E_1$ ratios, however, the levels vary from one day to another.

Transdermal administration of E_2 with a patch provides controlled delivery of estrogen and more physiologic $E_2:E_1$ ratios. All the above-mentioned routes have been shown to increase HDL and decrease LDL. However, to date there have been no epidemiologic studies to compare the cardiovascular risk in menopausal women treated by the nonoral routes (51). One main drawback of the transdermal system is skin irritation. However, regular site rotation decreases the incidence of this reaction.

Progestins

Progestin compounds include micronized progesterone, derivatives of 17-hydroxyprogesterone, and derivatives of 19-nortestosterone. Micronized progesterone is most like physiologic progesterone. It induces a secretory change in the endometrium, stimulates sodium excretion, and is devoid of the androgenic effects on the lipid profile. Derivatives of 17-hydroxyprogesterone, usually given as medroxyprogesterone acetate (MPA), induce a secretory change in the endometrium. MPA does have an androgenic effect at high doses and has been the most widely available and the most extensively studied progestin. Derivatives of 19-nortestosterone also interact with androgenic receptors and have a negative effect on the lipid profile.

The known benefit of adding progesterone to the estrogen therapy is that it decreases the incidence and risk of endometrial hyperplasia and cancer (47). There is controversy as to the possible negative effect progestins might have on the cardiovascular benefits because of its metabolic effect on lipid metabolism. These effects on lipid fractions are dose related. Micronized progesterone does not exert unwanted effects on lipids at the usually recommended doses; medroxyprogesterone has fewer effects on lipoproteins than do the nortestosterone compounds. Norethindrone 1 mg, medroxyprogesterone 10 mg, and oral micronized progesterone 300 mg daily cause minimal or no lipid disturbances (47). The effect of progesterone on osteoporosis continues to be investigated, and results range from no reported effect to promotion of resorption and growth (54). The effect on breast cancer also remains controversial, with some investigators reporting a protective effect (55) and others suggesting that progestins increase the risk (56). At this point, there is not enough evidence to support the use of progestins in women without a uterus.

Initiation of Estrogen Therapy

The decision to place a women on estrogen therapy should be individualized. A thorough history and physical examination should be performed, paying particular attention to menstrual history, risk factors, and contraindications of estrogen therapy. A mammogram should have been performed within the last year and be negative. A decision regarding endometrial sampling should be made before initiation of therapy. If a patient has a history of regular menstrual cycles and then cessation of menses, symptoms of estrogen deprivation, and no risk factors for endometrial hyperplasia, one can start her on estrogen/progestin therapy without endometrial biopsy. If she has a history of irregular menses, intermenstrual bleeding or spotting, heavy periods, obesity, or family history of endometrial cancer, then an endometrial biopsy with negative results should be obtained before initiation of therapy. At that time, what to expect regarding side effects should be thoroughly discussed, with emphasis given to the patient to record bleeding patterns for the first year of therapy and to report any unexpected bleeding. If the patient is on sequential therapy, she should expect to have withdrawal bleeding approximately 2 to 3 days after she stops the progestin. If she is on continuous therapy, she may expect to have some spotting for the first 3 to 6 months, but after she stops spotting, it should not reoccur. She should return in approximately 3 months to reassess this treatment plan. If at that time she has experienced irregular bleeding and an endometrial biopsy was not performed before beginning therapy, one should be done at this time. She should then be seen in 6 to 9 months. If her bleeding pattern is normal, there are no complications, and she wants to continue, one can continue with the present treatment plan.

Treatment Regimen

If the patient has a uterus, the most accepted therapy is a combination of an estrogen and progestin. This can be given either sequentially or continuously. Addition of the progestin in either fashion is effective in decreasing the incidence of endometrial hyperplasia. The most effective method of preventing endometrial hyperplasia is 10 mg of medroxyprogesterone or its equivalent for 12 days of the month (57). A recent study of micronized progesterone suggests that 200 mg for 14 days or 300 mg for 10 days appears adequate to prevent hyperplasia (58). Ten milligrams of medroxyprogesterone for 10 days of the month and 2.5 mg daily are slightly less effective in preventing hyperplasia (57). Estrogens are given for the first 25 days of the month.

Sometimes a patient becomes symptomatic during the time she is not on estrogen, and a decision is made to place her on continuous estrogen. If continuous estrogen is given, one may need to increase the amount or duration of progestins. The author's preference is to begin a patient on sequential therapy for the first year, taking the estrogen daily and the progestin from the first to the twelfth day of the month. The patient should expect withdrawal bleeding on the fourteenth day. If she has had no irregular bleeding after the first year of therapy, she can continue with this regimen. If she would like to try continuous therapy, a switch at this time can be considered. By this time the endometrial lining has become more atrophic, and there should be a decrease in the incidence of irregular bleeding and subsequent need for endometrial biopsy.

Dosages

Daily estrogen:
   0.625 mg conjugated estrogen or
   1.0 mg micronized estradiol or
   0.5 mg 17β-estradiol transdermal patch

Note that most epidemiologic evidence is based on 0.625 mg conjugated estrogen. The effectiveness of lower doses on osteoporosis and cardiovascular disease is not known, although a study using 0.3 mg of conjugated estrogen supplemented with 1500 mg of calcium was effective in the prevention of osteoporosis (59). Persistence of menopausal symptoms indicates that an increase in dose may be helpful. Breast tenderness and headache may indicate overtreatment, and the dose should be decreased.

Daily progestins:
   2.5–5 mg medroxyprogesterone acetate
Sequential progestins:
   10 mg medroxyprogesterone 10–12 days of month or
   200–300 mg micronized progesterone 10–14 days of month

The goal of progestin therapy is to use the minimal dose to prevent endometrial hyperplasia. Many of the bothersome side effects of hormonal therapy, such as irritability, bloating, weight gain, and dysphoria, are secondary to the progestin component. Micronized progesterone seems to have fewer side effects. If a lower dose of progestin is used, an endometrial biopsy should be performed periodically to check for hyperplasia.

Duration of Therapy

There are few guidelines regarding the length of therapy. Information regarding length is needed to achieve beneficial effects; how long the effect lasts after discontinuation is not known. The Consensus Conference on Osteoporosis stated that appropriate duration is unknown but at least 10 years seems reasonable (47). Length of therapy does appear to have an impact on breast cancer risk (44). The reasons and goals of therapy should be reviewed on an annual basis with each patient.

Summary

There are still many unanswered questions regarding hormonal replacement therapy. Currently, much of our knowledge of long-term implications is based on observational studies. There may be bias in some of the studies because of the lack of control for socioeconomic status, compliance, general health, frequency of visits to the physician, and screening tests (60). Ongoing randomized trials should provide this information, but it will be years before these data are available. It does appear that there are benefits that improve the quality of life for many women. For many, the benefits outweigh the risks, especially when one considers the decrease in cardiovascular disease. However, the decision to place a woman on ERT needs to be individualized by assessing her risks, needs, and the possible benefits. The limits of knowledge should be conveyed to each patient, and her treatment reassessed regularly. It is equally important to include counseling regarding lifestyle changes such as exercise, smoking, and diet that also have an impact on quality of life but which carry no risk (45).

REFERENCES

1. Shingleton HM, Hurt WG, eds. Postreproductive gynecology. New York: Churchill Livingstone, 1990.
2. Boring CC, Squires TS, Tong T. Cancer statistics. CA 1993;43:7–26.
3. Bhatia NN, Bergman A, Karram MM. Effects of estrogen on urethral function in women with urinary incontinence. Am J Obstet Gynecol 1989;160:176–181.
4. Avis NE, Burnhill MS, Connell E, et al. Psychosocial implications of the perimenopause. ARHP Clinical Proceedings, July 1993, p 4.
5. Tobias CR, Lewis S. Menopause and depression: cause, assessment, and treatment. Women's Psych Health 1993;2(1):1–2,12–13.
6. Ferreyra S, Hughes K. Table manners: a guide to the pelvic examination for disabled women and health care providers. 2nd ed. San Francisco: Planned Parenthood Association, 1984.
7. DiSaia PJ, Creasman WT. Clinical gynecologic oncology. 3rd ed. St. Louis: CV Mosby, 1989.

8. Beecham CT. Classification of vaginal relaxation. Am J Obstet Gynecol 1980;136:957–958.

9. Jones HW, Jones GS. Novak's textbook of gynecology. 10th ed. Baltimore: Williams & Wilkins, 1981.

10. Brubaker, L. The pessary, an important gynecologic option. Menopausal Med 1994;2(1):1–4.

11. Bracco GL, Carli P, Sonni L, et al. Clinical and histologic effects of topical treatments of vulval lichen sclerosus. J Reprod Med 1993;38:37–40.

12. Friedrich EG. Vulvar disease. 2nd ed. Philadelphia: WB Saunders, 1983.

13. Herbst AL, Michsell DR, Stenchever MA, Droegemueller W. Comprehensive gynecology. 2nd ed. St. Louis: CV Mosby, 1992.

14. Baranovsky A, Myers MH. Cancer incidence and survival in patients 65 years of age and older. CA 1986;36:27–41.

15. Kleinman JC, Kopstein A. Who is being screened for cervical cancer? Am J Public Health 1981;71:73–76.

16. U.S. Preventive Services Task Force. Guide to clinical preventive services: an assessment of the effectiveness of 169 interventions. Baltimore: Williams & Wilkins, 1989.

17. Stenkvist B, Bergstrom R, Eklund G, Fox CH. Papanicolaou smear screening and cervical cancer: what can you expect? JAMA 1984;252:1423–1426.

18. Mandelblatt JS, Faks MC. The cost effectiveness of cervical cancer screening for low-income elderly women. JAMA 1988;259:2409–2413.

19. Mandelblatt J, Gopaul I, Wistreich M. Gynecological care of elderly women: another look at Papanicolaou smear testing. JAMA 1986;256:367–371.

20. Celentano DD. Early detection of cervical cancer in elderly women. In: Yancik R, Yates JW, eds. Cancer in the elderly: approaches to early detection and treatment. New York: Springer, 1989.

21. Koss LG. The Papanicolaou test for cervical cancer detection: a triumph and a tragedy. JAMA 1989; 261:737–743.

22. Interim protocol for cervical screening in women age 40 and older. Recommendations from the Cervical Cancer Advisory Committee. Michigan Department of Public Health, June 1993.

23. Rubin S. Postmenopausal bleeding: etiology, evaluation and management. Med Clin North Am 1987; 71:59–56.

24. Koss LG, Schreiber K, Oberlander SG, et al. Detection of endometrial carcinoma and hyperplasia in asymptomatic women. Obstet Gynecol 1984;64:1–11.

25. Grimes DA. Diagnostic dilation and curettage: a reappraisal. Am J Obstet Gynecol 1982;142:1–6.

26. Stovall TG, Photopulos GJ, Poston WM, et al. Pipelle endometrial sampling in patients with known endometrial carcinoma. Obstet Gynecol 1991; 77:954–956.

27. Archer DF, McIntyre-Seltman K, Wilborn WW Jr, et al. Endometrial morphology in asymptomatic postmenopausal women. Am J Obstet Gynecol 1991; 165:317–322.

28. Gimpelson RJ, Rappold HO. A comparative study between panoramic hysteroscopy with directed biopsies and dilation and curettage. Am J Obstet Gynecol 1988;158:1489–1492.

29. Osmers R, Volksen M, Schauer A. Vaginosonography for early detection of endometrial carcinoma? Lancet 1990;1596–1571.

30. Pritchard KL. Screening for endometrial cancer: is it effective? Ann Intern Med 1989;110:177–179.

31. Yancik R, Ries LG, Yates JW. Ovarian cancer in the elderly: an analysis of surveillance, epidemiology and end results program data. Am J Obstet Gynecol 1986;154:639–647.

32. American College of Obstetricians and Gynecologists. Cancer of the ovary. (ACOG technical bulletin 141) Washington, DC: ACOG, 1990.

33. Bast RC Jr, Klug TL, St. John E, et al. A radioimmunoassay using a monoclonal antibody to monitor the course of epithelial ovarian cancer. N Engl J Med 1983;309:883–887.

34. Mann WJ, Pastner B, Cohen H, Loub M. Preoperative serum CA 125 antigen levels in patients with surgical stage I ovarian adenocarcinoma. J Natl Cancer Inst 1988;80:208–209.

35. Campbell S, Bhan V, Royston P, et al. Transabdominal ultrasound screening for early ovarian cancer. Br Med J 1989;299:1363–1370.

36. VanNagell JR, DePriest PD, Pues LE, et al. Ovarian cancer screening in asymptomatic postmenopausal women by transvaginal sonography. Cancer 1991; 68:458–462.

37. Jolleys JV. Reported prevalence of urinary incontinence in women in a general practice. Br Med J 1988;296:1300–1302.

38. Rowe JW, Besdine RW, Ford AB, et al. Urinary incontinence in adults. Consensus Conference. JAMA 1989;261;2685–2690.

39. Ouslander JG. Urinary incontinence: out of the closet. JAMA 1989;261:2695–2696.

40. Wall LL. The unstable bladder. In: Thompson JD, Rock JA, eds. TeLinde's operative gynecology updates. Philadelphia; JB Lippincott, 1993:1–14.

41. Ostergard D, ed. Gynecologic urology and urodynamics. Baltimore: Williams & Wilkins, 1985.

42. Genant HK, Baylink DJ, Gallagher JC. Estrogens in the prevention of osteoporosis in postmenopausal women. Am J Obstet Gynecol 1989;161:1842–1846.

43. Felson DT, Zhang Y, Hannan MT, Kiel DP, Wilson PWF, Anderson JJ. The effect of postmenopausal estrogen therapy on bone density in elderly women. N Engl J Med 1993;329:1141–1147.

44. Barrett-Conner E. Risks and benefits of replacement estrogen. Annu Rev Med 1992;43:239–251.

45. Rosenberg L. Hormone replacement therapy: the need for reconsideration. Am J Public Health 1993; 83:1670–1673.

46. Judd HL, Cleary RF, Creasman WT. Estrogen replacement therapy. Obstet Gynecol 1981;58:1267–1275.

47. Whitehead M, Lobo RA. Progestogen use in postmenopausal women. Consensus Conference. Lancet 1988;2:1234–1240.

48. Steinberg KK, Thacker SB, Smith J. A meta-analysis of the effect of estrogen replacement therapy on the risk of breast cancer. JAMA 1991;265:1985–1990.

49. Wingo PA, Layde PM, Lee NC, Rubin G, Ory HW. The risk of breast cancer in postmenopausal women who have used estrogen replacement therapy. JAMA 1987;257:209.

50. Speroff L, Glass RH, Kase NG. Clinical gynecologic endocrinology and infertility, 4th ed. Baltimore: Williams & Wilkins, 1989.

51. Sitruk-Ware R, Utian W, eds. The menopause and hormonal replacement therapy. New York: Marcel Dekker, 1991.

52. Hammond CB, Maxon WC. Current status of estrogen therapy for the menopause. Fert Steril 1981; 37:5–25.

53. Ottoson UB, Johansson BG, von Schaultz B. Subfractions of high density lipoprotein cholesterol during estrogen replacement therapy: a comparison between progestins and natural progesterone. Am J Obstet Gynecol 1985;151:746–750.

54. Gallagher JC, Kable WT, Goldgar D. The effect of progestin therapy on cortical and trabecular bone: comparison with estrogen. Am J Med 1991;90:171–178.

55. Gambrel RD. Proposal to decrease the risk and improve the prognosis of breast cancer. Am J Obstet Gynecol 1984;150:119–132.

56. Bergkivist, Adami HO, Persson I, Hoover R, Schairer C. The risk of breast cancer after estrogen and estrogen-progestin replacement therapy. N Engl J Med 1989;321:293–297.

57. Whitehead MI, Hillard TC, Crook D. The role and use of progestogens. Obstet Gynecol 1990;75:59s–80s.

58. Moyer DI, deLingieres B, Driguez P, Pez JP. Prevention of endometrial hyperplasia by progesterone during long term estradiol replacement: influence of bleeding pattern and secretory changes. Fertil Steril 1993;59:992–997.

59. Ettinger B, Genant HK, Cann CE. Postmenopausal bone loss is prevented by treatment with low dosage estrogen with calcium. Ann Intern Med 1987; 106:40–54.

60. Barrett-Conner E. Postmenopausal estrogen and prevention bias. Ann Intern Med 1991;115:455–456.

29/ Breast Cancer

Rebecca A. Silliman, Lodovico Balducci

Breast cancer is a common problem in old age. If diagnosed in its early stages, survival rates comparable to those of women in most younger age groups can be attained (1). As is the case with many other conditions, an incomplete scientific knowledge base and the complicating factors of comorbidity, impaired functional status, and diminished social support together create challenges for the clinician caring for older women with this disease. This chapter focuses primarily on issues related to the management of local disease but briefly discusses screening issues (see also Chapter 2) and the approach to the patient with advanced disease.

EPIDEMIOLOGY

Breast cancer has become increasingly important in older women for three major reasons. First, the incidence of breast cancer increases dramatically with age, growing from about 300 per 100,000 women aged 65 to 69 to over 375 per 100,000 women 85 years of age and older (1). Second, the numbers of women 65 years of age and older and, in particular, the numbers 85 years of age and older are increasing rapidly (2). Third, the age-adjusted incidence of breast cancer is also increasing, in part because of increased use of screening mammography (3, 4). Taken together, these factors have three important consequences: (a) the number of newly diagnosed older breast cancer patients will continue to increase, (b) the average age of women with newly diagnosed breast cancer will continue to rise, and (c) the number of older women who are survivors of breast cancer will become greater.

SCREENING

Although screening mammography has proven efficacy in women 50 to 65 years of age (5), its efficacy in older women remains unproven. Nonetheless, there are several reasons why screening older women makes good clinical sense. First, the

302

positive predictive value of mammography and physical examination is higher in older women than in younger ones (6). Second, as noted earlier, the incidence of breast cancer continues to increase well into old age. Third, life expectancy even at age 85 is over 6 years.

Yet, it is older women, particularly those aged 65 years and above, who are least likely ever to have had a mammogram. Although rates have increased, the proportion of women 65 to 74 years of age surveyed in five communities in California, Massachusetts, New York, North Carolina, and Pennsylvania who reported receiving a mammogram in 1991 was only 35 to 59% (7). While these rates are improved over those in previous years, they are probably optimistic when considering all older women, since the percentage of women who ever have had a mammogram decreases with age (6). This is because physicians tend not to recommend mammographic screening to their older patients and because older women themselves do not believe that such screening is effective (6, 8).

Although information from available clinical studies does not provide guidance about when to stop screening, the recommendations of the Forum on Breast Cancer Screening in Older Women seem most reasonable (9):

1. Clinical breast examination should be performed annually, and mammography should be performed approximately every 2 years for women aged 65 to 74.
2. Clinical breast examination should be performed annually, and mammography should be performed at regular intervals of approximately every 2 years for women age 75 and over whose general health and life expectancy are good.
3. It is prudent for women age 65 and over to perform monthly breast self-examination (BSE) to identify clinical lesions and seek professional care.

Note that these guidelines emphasize the importance of general health and life expectancy in clinical decision making about screening for those women 75 years of age and older. They also emphasize that no one screening modality should be relied upon to the exclusion of others. Neither negative self-examination nor a negative clinical examination should give one a sense of security; mammography is still indicated, and vice versa.

APPROACH TO THE PATIENT WITH NEWLY DIAGNOSED DISEASE

The new diagnosis of cancer at any age is frightening. When coupled with the prospect of having to be seen by up to three or more new physicians (one or more surgeons and medical and radiation oncologists), it may be overwhelming. The primary care physician can play a critical role in cancer care for older patients by answering questions and reviewing the recommendations of specialists, clarifying patient values with respect to the risks and benefits of various treatment options (particularly in light of coexisting comorbidities and functional impairments), and advocating for patients who may be inclined to choose the quickest treatment "just to get it over with." In addition to older patients themselves, family members are likely to be involved in decision making and need to be included in discussions about treatments. Their questions and fears need attention as well.

Meeting both patient and family needs requires a thorough understanding of the best available scientific evidence regarding treatment efficacy, including the gaps in knowledge and the areas of uncertainty.

EARLY-STAGE DISEASE: MANAGEMENT OF THE PRIMARY TUMOR

The 1990 NIH Consensus Development Conference on the treatment of early stage breast cancer concluded that "breast conservation treatment is an appropriate method of primary therapy for the majority of women with stage I and II breast cancer and is preferable because it provides survival rates *equivalent* to those of total mastectomy and axillary dissection while preserving the breast." Here, breast conservation treatment is defined as breast-conserving surgery (e.g., lumpectomy), level I or II axillary node dissection, with postoperative radiation of the breast. In the view of the Consensus Development Conference, total mastectomy should be considered only when the cancer is multicentric or when the cancer and/or breast size would make the cosmetic results unacceptable to patients (10).

Note that these recommendations have been made for all women, regardless of age. While most would agree that, in general, basing treatment recommendations on age alone is inappropriate, generalizing treatment recommendations from studies of younger women may be equally problematic. To date, published large-scale clinical trials of surgical therapy in early-stage disease have not included women over the age of 70 years. For this reason and because patients with major comorbidities are usually excluded from clinical trials, women studied have been, for the most part, free of other diseases. One must presume also that they have been free of functional disabilities, but no clinical trials have gathered either baseline or follow-up functional information (11–15).

Although a lesser surgical procedure is now recommended (breast-conserving surgery) and is likely to result in less postoperative loss of function in older women (16), some women still prefer to have a total mastectomy. For these women, a mastectomy seems to be a more definitive procedure and the loss of a breast of less consequence. Furthermore, it obviates the need for follow-up radiation therapy.

While radiation therapy to the breast is well tolerated by most older women, the need for daily radiation treatments can be daunting. Arranging transportation, coping with long distances to radiation therapy facilities, and/or managing emotional and physical fatigue may not seem worth it. These barriers may sway women into deciding against breast-conserving surgery.

Although recommended and undoubtedly prudent, whether radiation therapy is needed in older women following breast-conserving surgery remains controversial. First, postoperative radiation therapy has not been shown to be effective in preventing the development of systemic disease and prolonging survival (10). Second, it is not clear whether it is effective in preventing disease recurrence in older women, since older women appear to have lower recurrence rates than younger women (13, 17–20).

Partial mastectomy without radiation may be reasonable in those older women for whom a course of radiation would be especially burdensome and in whom a lesser surgical procedure (i.e., breast-conserving surgery) would be especially indicated because of increased perioperative risk. While a few of these patients will develop recurrent disease, their survival will not be compromised, provided that a total mastectomy can be performed at the time of recurrence. Deciding between total mastectomy and breast-conserving surgery, with or without radiation, must take into account body image and upper body function, the logistical difficulties associated with radiation therapy, the emotional impact of disease recurrence, and the ability to tolerate mastectomy surgery at some time in the future (21).

Regardless of the type of surgical procedure chosen, careful attention should be paid to preserving upper body, shoulder, and arm strength and mobility. During the early postoperative period, physical therapy and the judicious use of analgesics will facilitate the preservation of function. This is particularly important when an axillary lymph node dissection is performed, since incisional pain, lymphedema, and paresthesias can all adversely affect upper body function. Axillary dissection is an essential staging procedure when the decision to prescribe adjuvant therapy is based on involvement of the regional lymph nodes. If, however, almost all postmenopausal women with breast cancer receive adjuvant therapy with tamoxifen (see discussion below), then axillary dissection may not be necessary (10, 22).

A final issue related to primary tumor management is the consideration of medical, rather than surgical treatment. In studies comparing the survival of women initially treated with tamoxifen with those surgically treated, survival has been comparable. However, patients treated with tamoxifen alone have had more local progression than those treated surgically (23–25). These findings suggest that tamoxifen alone should be reserved as a treatment option only for women who are too frail to undergo surgery or who simply do not want to have it. One would hope that this would apply to a very small number of patients, since the risks of breast-conserving surgery, in particular, are small.

EARLY-STAGE DISEASE: ADJUVANT TREATMENT

TAMOXIFEN

Unlike the case of primary tumor management, the benefits of tamoxifen in older women (>70 years) are fairly well understood, as older women have been studied in two clinical trials (26, 27) and have been considered separately in a recent meta-analysis of clinical trials worldwide (28). The two randomized trials included women aged 65 to 84 with one or more positive axillary lymph nodes. Although both studies found an increase in disease-free survival in patients treated with tamoxifen, there was no positive effect on overall survival (26, 27).

In contrast, the studies contained in the meta-analysis included 2656 women 70 years of age or greater. Both recurrence and overall mortality rates were lower among these older women treated with tamoxifen. In addition, the magni-

tude of risk reduction, both in terms of recurrence and mortality, was similar across postmenopausal age groups: 50 to 59, 60 to 69, and 70 +. Adjuvant tamoxifen therapy also appears to decrease recurrence and mortality rates in women with estrogen hormone-receptor-poor tumors, although the benefit is less than that in women with hormone-receptor-rich tumors. Finally, tamoxifen is of benefit in both node-negative and node-positive women, although the absolute benefit is greater for those who are node-positive (28).

A minimum of 2 years of treatment with tamoxifen is recommended (10), although longer treatment may delay recurrence (28–31) and promote health in other ways. While tamoxifen is a partial estrogen antagonist, it also has estrogenic effects (32, 33). As a result, it may prevent osteoporosis, lower levels of LDL cholesterol, and prevent contralateral breast cancer (28, 34–36). Although serious complications (e.g., deep venous thrombosis and a form of retinitis) of tamoxifen are rare, hot flashes are common (37).

On balance, treatment with tamoxifen (10 mg b.i.d.) is prudent for most older women with early-stage disease, except those with an excellent prognosis (those with tumors ≤ 1 cm in size). Treatment for longer than 2 years makes sense in women who are not troubled by side effects and who may experience non–breast cancer benefits: those at risk for osteoporosis and coronary heart disease.

CHEMOTHERAPY

The value of adjuvant chemotherapy alone or in conjunction with tamoxifen has not been well studied in women over 70 years of age. Indeed, the meta-analysis of studies worldwide referred to earlier included only 366 women in this age group who received adjuvant chemotherapy. In these women, adjuvant chemotherapy did not appear to be of benefit (38). Chemotherapy may be efficacious in patients with aggressive disease, but this is not known. What is known is that older women are able to tolerate combination chemotherapy when renally excreted drugs are adjusted on the basis of creatinine clearance (39, 40).

METASTATIC DISEASE

Survival rates in older women diagnosed with metastatic disease decrease with age. While the 1-year survival rate for women 65 to 74 years of age is similar to that in the first postmenopausal age decade (55 to 64 years, 61%; 65 to 74 years, 58%), rates decline thereafter to 54% in those 75 to 84 years and 44% in those 85 years of age and older (1). Five-year survival rates across all age groups are uniformly dismal and range from 16 to 20%. These rates provide a compelling argument for a more systematic approach to screening and early diagnosis, especially since the overall average life expectancy at age 75 is 11.7 years and that at age 85 is 6.4 years (41).

While hormonal treatment in these women has only a modest effect on survival, symptom palliation can be achieved in most patients (42, 43). Tamoxifen is recommended as the first line of treatment, regardless of hormone receptor status. Should bony metastases be present, calcium levels should be monitored initially, since transient hypercalcemia can occur. Megestrol acetate or aromatase inhibitors (aminoglutethimide) may be useful when patients relapse.

Although the use of chemotherapy in older women with metastatic disease has not been well studied, recent reports suggest no age-related differences in response rates, time to progression, survival, and toxic side effects (39, 40). These findings have led investigators to advocate enrollment of older women in clinical trials that assess the efficacy of chemotherapy in advanced disease (40). In the interim, older women with life-threatening disease who are receptor-negative and relapse while taking tamoxifen may be candidates for combination chemotherapy (22).

As is the case with all older patients with life-threatening disease, treatment decisions in women with metastatic disease must take into account risk and benefits, especially quality-of-life issues, and patient preferences. End-of-life care, including preferences for site of death and the use of hospice, also needs discussion. Decision making should be iterative; patient and families need to understand that the therapeutic plan can be flexible and change as patient needs change. (See Chapters 59, 63, and 64 for more thorough discussions of these issues.)

VARIATIONS IN BREAST CANCER TREATMENT WITH AGE

There are substantial variations in breast cancer treatment, and these become greater as patients age. Older women have been shown repeatedly to receive less aggressive evaluation and treatment. These patterns are clearest when the experience of women 75 years of age and older and is compared with that of postmenopausal women less than 75. Nonetheless, some studies have also shown increasing differences by decade of age beginning with those from 55 to 64 years of age (44–51).

While some or all of this less aggressive evaluation and treatment may be appropriate for very frail patients, studies that have considered the effects of comorbidity and functional status have not demonstrated that either or both satisfactorily explain the variations observed (47, 49). Physician, patient, and family factors that may explain the variations have not been well studied. Furthermore, at present, there is no evidence that variation in diagnostic and treatment patterns adversely affects patient outcomes. Since patients' overall clinical heterogeneity increases with age, heterogeneity in treatment strategies may be appropriate. Carefully designed studies that examine a range of short- and long-term outcomes in older women are needed to address these issues.

When survival rates of older women with breast cancer are compared with those of younger women with breast cancer, older women fare less well. However, this does not appear to be due to the aggressiveness of the cancer itself or how it is treated. Rather, the main problem is delayed diagnosis and the more common presentation of late-stage disease in old age. After adjusting for other causes of death, older and younger women with early-stage disease have comparable 8-year survival rates.

SUMMARY AND CONCLUSIONS

Although not unique to breast cancer, the care of older women with this disease is complicated by the lack of a complete body of evidence supporting the efficacy of recommended screening or treatments. Physicians can best serve their older women patients by emphasizing the importance of screening and early detection when clinically appropriate. When breast cancer is diagnosed, patient preferences, comorbidity, functional status, life expectancy, risks and benefits of treatment, and family support all need to be taken into account when developing a treatment plan. Given the need for better information on which to base treatment decisions, older patients should be encouraged to participate in studies that will expand our knowledge.

REFERENCES

1. Yancik R, Ries LB, Yates JW. Breast cancer in aging women: a population-based study of contrasts in stage, surgery, and survival. Cancer 1989;63:164–169.
2. Schneider EL, Guralnik JM. The aging of America: impact on health care costs. JAMA 1990;263:2335–2340.
3. Lantz PM, Remington PL, Newcomb PA. Mammography screening and increased incidence of breast

cancer in Wisconsin. J Natl Cancer Inst 1991; 83:1540–1546.

4. Feuer EJ, Wun L-M. How much of the recent rise in breast cancer incidence can be explained by increases in mammography utilization? A dynamic population model approach. Am J Epidemiol 1992; 136:1423–1436.

5. Guide to clinical preventive services: an assessment of the effectiveness of 169 interventions. Report of the U.S. Preventive Services Task Force. Baltimore: Williams & Wilkins, 1989:39–46.

6. Costanza ME, Annas GJ, Brown ML, et al. Breast cancer screening in older women: supporting statements and rationale. J Gerontol 1992;47(special issue):7–16.

7. Coleman EA, Feuer EJ, and the NCI Breast Cancer Screening Consortium. Breast cancer screening among women from 65 to 74 years of age in 1987–88 and 1991. Ann Intern Med 1992;117:961–966.

8. Taplin SH, Montano DE. Attitudes, age, and participation in mammographic screening: a prospective analysis. J Am Board Fam Pract 1993;6:13–23.

9. Breast cancer screening in older women: screening recommendations of the forum panel. J Gerontol 1992;47(special issue):5.

10. NIH consensus conference. Treatment of early stage breast cancer. JAMA 1991;265:391–395.

11. Veronesi U, Saccozzi R, Del Veccio M, Banfi M, Clemente C, De Lena M. Comparing radical mastectomy with quadrantectomy, axillary dissection, and radiotherapy in patients with small cancers of the breast. N Engl J Med 1981;305:6–11.

12. Sarrazin D, Le M, Rouesse J, et al. Conservative treatment versus mastectomy in breast cancer tumors with macroscopic diameter of 20 millimeters or less: the experience of the Institut Gustave-Roussy. Cancer 1984;53:1209–1213.

13. Fisher B, Redmond C, Poisson R, et al. Eight year results of a randomized clinical trial comparing total mastectomy and lumpectomy with or without irradiation in the treatment of breast cancer. N Engl J Med 1989;320:822–828.

14. Veronesi U, Banfi A, Del Vecchio M, et al. Comparison of Halsted mastectomy with quadrantectomy, axillary dissection and radiotherapy in early breast cancer: long-term results. Eur J Cancer Clin Oncol 1986;22:1085–1089.

15. Habibollahi F, Fentiman IS. Breast conservation techniques for early breast cancer. Cancer Treat Rev 1989;16;177–191.

16. Vinokur AD, Threatt BA, Vinokur-Kaplan D, Satariano WA. The process of recovery from breast cancer for younger and older patients: changes during the first year. Cancer 1990;65:1242–1254.

17. Nemoto T, Patel JK, Rosner D, et al. Factors affecting recurrence in lumpectomy without irradiation for breast cancer. Cancer 1991;67:2079–2082.

18. Clark RM, McCulloch PB, Levine MN. Randomized clinical trial to assess the effectiveness of breast irradiation following lumpectomy and axillary dissection for node-negative breast cancer. J Natl Cancer 1992;84:683–689.

19. Kantorowitz DA, Poulter CA, Sischy B, et al. Treatment of breast cancer among elderly women with segmental mastectomy or segmental mastectomy plus postoperative radiotherapy. Int J Radiat Oncol Biol Phys 1988;15:263–270.

20. Veronesi U, Luini A, Del Vecchio M, et al. Radiotherapy after breast-preserving surgery in women with localized cancer of the breast. N Engl J Med 1993;328:1587–1591.

21. Lichter AS. Conservative treatment of primary breast cancer: how much is required? J Natl Cancer Inst 1992;84:659–660.

22. Balducci L, Schapira DV, Cox CE, Greenberg HM, Lyman GH. Breast cancer of the older woman: an annotated review. J Am Geriatr Soc 1991;39:1113–1123.

23. Robertson JF, Ellis IO, Elston CW, Blamey RW. Mastectomy or tamoxifen as initial therapy for operable breast cancer in elderly patients: 5-year follow-up. Eur J Cancer 1992;28A:908–910.

24. Gazet JC, Markopoulos C, Ford HT, et al. Prospective randomized trial of tamoxifen versus surgery in elderly patients with breast cancer. Lancet 1988; 1:679–681.

25. Bates T, Riley DL, Houghton J, et al. Breast cancer in elderly women: a Cancer Research Campaign trial comparing treatment with tamoxifen and optimal surgery with tamoxifen alone. The Elderly Breast Cancer Working Party. Br J Surg 1991; 78:591–594.

26. Castiglione M, Gelber RD, Goldhirsch A. Adjuvant systemic therapy for breast cancer in the elderly: competing causes of mortality. J Clin Oncol 1990; 8:519–526.

27. Cummings FJ, Gray R, David TE, et al. Adjuvant tamoxifen vs. placebo in elderly women with node-positive breast cancer: long term follow-up and causes of death. J Clin Oncol 1993;11:29–35.

28. Early Breast Cancer Trialists' Collaborative Group. Systemic treatment of early breast cancer by hormonal, cytotoxic, or immune therapy: 133 randomised trials involving 31 000 recurrences and 24 000 deaths among 75 000 women. Part 1. Lancet 1992; 339:1–15.

29. Fisher B, Brown A, Wolmark N, Redmond C, Wickerham DL, Wittliff J. Prolonging tamoxifen therapy for primary breast cancer. Ann Intern Med 1987; 106:649–654.

30. Falkson HC, Gray R, Wolberg WH, Gillchrist KW, Harris JE, Tormey DC. Adjuvant trial of 12 cycles of CMFPT followed by observation or continuous tamoxifen versus four cycles of CMFPT in postmenopausal women with breast cancer. An Eastern Cooperative Oncology Group Phase III Study. J Clin Oncol 1990;8:599–607.

31. Jordan VC. Overview from the International Conference on Long-term Tamoxifen Therapy for Breast Cancer. J Natl Cancer Inst 1992;84:231–234.

32. Love RR. Tamoxifen therapy in primary breast cancer: biology, efficacy, and side effects. J Clin Oncol 1989;7:803–15.

33. Jordan VC. Estrogen receptor mediated direct and indirect antitumor effects of tamoxifen. J Natl Cancer Inst 1990;82:1662–1663.

34. Fornander T, Rutqvist LE, Sjoberg HE, Blomqvist L, Mattsson A, Glas U. Long term adjuvant tamoxifen in early breast cancer: effect on bone mineral density in postmenopausal women. J Clin Oncol 1990;8:1019–1024.

35. Love RR, Mazess RB, Barden HS, et al. Effects of tamoxifen on bone mineral density in postmenopausal women with breast cancer. N Engl J Med 1992;326:852–856.

36. Love RR, Wiebe DA, Newcomb PA, Cameron L, Leventhal H, Jordan VC. Effects of tamoxifen on cardiovascular risk factors in postmenopausal women. Ann Intern Med 1991;115:860–864.

37. Love RR, Cameron L, Connell BL, Leventhal H. Symptoms associated with tamoxifen treatment in postmenopausal women. Arch Intern Med 1991; 141:1842–1847.

38. Early Breast Cancer Trialists' Collaborative Group. Systemic treatment of early breast cancer by hormonal, cytotoxic, or immune therapy: 133 randomised trials involving 31 000 recurrences and 24 000 deaths among 75 000 women. Part 2. Lancet 1992; 339:71–85.

39. Gelman RS, Taylor SG. Cyclophosphamide, methotrexate and 5-fluorouracil chemotherapy in women more than 65 years old with advanced breast cancer: the elimination of age trends in toxicity by using doses based on creatinine clearance. J Clin Oncol 1984;2:1404–1413.

40. Christman K, Muss HB, Case LD, et al. Chemotherapy of metastatic breast cancer in the elderly. The Piedmont Oncology Association experience. JAMA 1992;268:57–62.

41. Manton KG, Stallard E. Cross-sectional estimates of active life expectancy for the U.S. elderly and oldest-old populations. J Gerontol 1991;46:S170–182.

42. Pritchard RI, Sutherland DJA. The use of endocrine therapy. Hematol Oncol Clin 1989;3:765–806.

43. Ziegler LD, Buzdar AU. Recent advances in the treatment of breast cancer. Am J Med Sci 1991; 301:337–349.

44. Allen C, Cox EB, Manton KG, Cohen HJ. Breast cancer in the elderly: current patterns of care. J Am Geriatr Soc 1986;34:637–642.

45. Samet J, Hunt WC, Key C, Humble CG, Goodwin JS. Choice of cancer therapy varies with age of patient. JAMA 1986;255:3385–3390.

46. Chu J, Diehr P, Feigl P, et al. The effect of age on the care of women with breast cancer in community hospitals. J Gerontol 1987;42:185–190.

47. Greenfield S, Blanco DM, Elashoff RM, Ganz PA. Patterns of care related to age of breast cancer patients. JAMA 1987;257:2766–2770.

48. Mann B, Samet J, Key C, Goodwin JM, Goodwin JS. Changing treatment of breast cancer in New Mexico from 1969 through 1985. JAMA 1988;259:3413–3417.

49. Silliman RA, Guadagnoli E, Weitberg AB, Mor V. Age as a predictor of diagnostic and initial treatment intensity in newly diagnosed breast cancer patients. J Gerontol: Med Sci 1989;44:M46–50.

50. Bergman L, Dekker G, van Leeuwen FE, Huisman SJ, van Dam FSAM, van Dongen JA. The effect of age on treatment choice and survival in elderly breast cancer patients. Cancer 1991;67:2227–2234.

51. Nicolucci A, Mainini F, Penna A, et al. The influence of patient characteristics on the appropriateness of surgical treatment for breast cancer patients. Ann Oncol 1993;4:133–140.

30/ Musculoskeletal and Rheumatic Diseases Common to the Elderly

John A. Flynn, Fredrick M. Wigley

GENERAL APPROACH TO MUSCULOSKELETAL PROBLEMS IN THE ELDERLY

Pain and dysfunction of the musculoskeletal system are a common and challenging clinical problem in the elderly patient. Loss of muscle and joint function is second only to cardiovascular disease as a cause for disability in the elderly. Elderly patients frequently have muscular disease of the lower extremity or arthritis of weight-bearing joints that restricts their ability to ambulate; while articular disease of the small joints of the hands impairs fine motor function and the capacity to do many simple tasks. At the same time, degenerative changes in the articulations of the spine and loss of normal vertebral disk physiology are almost universal in the elderly, often leading to pain, deformity, or loss of function.

The evaluation of the musculoskeletal system in the elderly is complicated by many factors. The aging process itself, in the absence of a specific disease process, is associated with a loss of muscle mass and strength. The loss of muscle function may affect the elderly patient's ability to perform normal daily activities. Often the elderly patient has other health problems that mimic musculoskeletal disease, impair the normal functional capacity, or prevent the use of helpful medications and/or various forms of physical therapy. Medications can also either cause conditions that may mimic rheumatic illness or lead to a drug-induced myopathy. In addition, some helpful diagnostic tests, such as the sedimentation rate, the rheumatoid factor, and the antinuclear antibody, are often abnormal in the elderly because of the aging process itself. Radiological evidence of osteoarthritis is present in almost all elderly patients but may not be the cause of their musculoskeletal complaint. In fact, there is often a disparity between the pain a patient expresses and the radiological evidence of joint abnormalities. The physician must have a keen sensitivity to these many complicating factors and must use a systematic approach to the evaluation of the elderly patient.

Epidemiologic studies have demonstrated that age, sex, and the genetic matrix of the patient influence disease expression. Therefore, the approach to any patient with arthritis begins by appreciating the differential diagnosis based on the prevalence of disease defined by age, sex, and ethnic background (Table 30.1). For example, while osteoarthritis is almost universal, nodular osteoarthritis is uncommon in blacks and erosive osteoarthritis is more common in women than men. Polymyalgia rheumatica is more common in Caucasians than in other racial groups. Gout is usually seen in middle-aged men but is equally common in both sexes in the elderly population.

Other factors that influence the disease expression include the patient's occupation, habits, drug usage, and medical history. Hypertrophic pulmonary osteoarthropathy is associated with lung cancer, and therefore, this type of arthritis is usually seen in the smoker. Carpal tunnel syndrome frequently occurs in the diabetic or in the patient who worked in a occupation with repetitive injury to the hands and wrists. Secondary osteoarthritis of the knees has been associated with frequent stress or trauma to joints such as that seen in professional dancers, athletes, or workers required to do repeated knee bending. Drug-induced lupus is associated with the use of hydralazine or procainamide, while myopathy may develop in patients with renal insufficiency taking colchicine. An appreciation of these environmental factors and other characteristics of the host with a musculoskeletal complaint sets the scene for the rest of the evaluation.

To make a definite diagnosis, it is important to systematically characterize the pattern, the num-

Table 30.1
Differential Diagnosis of Arthritis in the Older Adult

	Middle years: ages 30–60
Predominant gender	
Male:	Gout
Female:	Rheumatoid arthritis (RA)
	Polymyositis/dermatomyositis
	Erosive osteoarthritis
	Sjögren's syndrome
	Scleroderma
Both:	Seronegative RA
	Vasculitic syndromes
	Elderly: ages 60+
Predominant gender	
Male:	Diffuse idiopathic skeletal hyperostosis (DISH)
	Hypertrophic pulmonary osteoarthropathy (HPO)
Female:	Primary generalized osteoarthritis
	Polymyalgia rheumatica
	Giant cell arteritis
	Late-onset SLE
Both:	Secondary osteoarthritis
	Metabolic disorders
	Crystal arthritis
	Tumor-related syndromes
	Soft tissue syndromes

ber of abnormal joints, the intensity of the joint pain, and the course of the joint problem. For example, gout typically is an episodic, intense monarthritis; rheumatoid arthritis is an additive symmetrical polyarthritis that causes dull pain and stiffness within the joints. In this review we have characterized the pattern of the musculoskeletal involvement in the context of reviewing each specific disorder.

A careful assessment of any extraarticular manifestations of disease is also important. For example, in a chronic inflammatory process such as polymyalgia rheumatica or rheumatoid arthritis, fatigue is a common extraarticular complaint; in a noninflammatory arthritis such as osteoarthritis, the patient generally feels well. Fatigue is usually associated with a sense of weakness. Definite loss of muscle power can result from either primary muscle disease or disuse atrophy secondary to pain or prolonged limitations in limb motion. The presence of subcutaneous nodules is a helpful clue in the diagnosis of rheumatoid arthritis, but similar lesions can be seen with metastatic skin lesions, tophaceous gout, or vasculitis. Every patient with arthritis must have a comprehensive physical examination so that ex-

traarticular features of the disease are appreciated.

The laboratory testing necessary to confirm the diagnosis is best determined by the findings of the history and physical examination. A test such as a positive rheumatoid factor has more clinical importance if the history and physical findings suggest a diagnosis of rheumatoid arthritis. Radiological evidence of osteoarthritis should correlate with the history of pain on motion of the joint before a cause and effect is confirmed.

Despite a careful assessment at the bedside and appropriate laboratory testing, the diagnosis may still be unresolved. Added information can then be obtained by characterizing the course of the arthritis, including the response to a therapeutic trial. It is often necessary and important to define all dimensions of the clinical and laboratory presentation before confirming the diagnosis and deciding the treatment program.

OSTEOARTHRITIS (1)

Osteoarthritis is second only to cardiovascular disease as a major cause of disability among the elderly. It has been estimated that 2 to 6 of 1000 individuals in the general population are incapacitated by osteoarthritis and 5% of persons between the ages of 55 to 64 lose 3 or more months of employment because of osteoarthritis. Studies have shown a striking influence of age on the expression of osteoarthritis, with severe disease being more common in the elderly and radiologically defined disease increasing exponentially after the age of 50.

Although osteoarthritis is the most common joint disease in the elderly, it is generally overlooked as a significant clinical problem until its late stages, at which time the patient begins to have incapacitating symptoms. Early symptoms of osteoarthritis, such as the loss of hand dexterity or stiffness in the knees, are often not mentioned by the patient because of the concept that these symptoms are expected as one gets older. Many physicians tell patients that osteoarthritis is caused by aging or that the joint surface (cartilage) wears down, the "wear and tear" theory. In fact, osteoarthritis is not just a cartilage disease or simply a normal process of aging. It is a disease that involves the entire joint, including the muscles, tendons, ligaments, and nervous and vascular supply. Osteoarthritis results from a complex process that is clearly associated with aging, but it is also influenced by several other important factors including the patient's genetic makeup, the state of the subchondral bone, inflammation, the presence or absence of joint injury or laxity, gender, hormones, and a variety of mechanical factors such as overuse of a particular joint or the presence of obesity (1, 2). Appreciation that osteoarthritis is not simply the result of an aged, worn cartilage will help in the design of an effective therapeutic approach.

SYMPTOMS OF OSTEOARTHRITIS

The usual complaints of osteoarthritis are pain and stiffness. The pain is usually dull (occasionally sharp) and of moderate intensity. It is aggravated by stress to the involved joint (e.g., prolonged walking, stair climbing). Stiffness is usually present after a period of rest (gelling). In contrast to the patient with rheumatoid arthritis who has morning stiffness that lasts for several hours, the stiffness of osteoarthritis disappears in seconds or minutes following gentle movement of the joint. However, prolonged joint movement will often lead to pain; particularly if a weight-bearing activity is stressful to the joint.

Stiffness and pain may be associated with a lack of normal joint function; patients may be unstable or have a sense of weakness when they begin joint motion. Patients often give up activities that they enjoyed during their younger years, such as knitting, typing, or other such hobbies that require fine motor movement or a strong grip. Osteoarthritis involving the hip or knee joint is commonly associated with discomfort and alterations in the patient's ability to perform daily activities and simple exercises. As a consequence of inactivity, muscle atrophy with weakness and/or clumsiness in gait may develop. Osteoarthritis involving the axial skeleton is often associated with degenerative disk disease. Stiffness and decreased range of motion is common in the cervical or lumbar regions of the spine.

While radiological changes of osteoarthritis can be seen in multiple joints, the patient usually has clinical symptoms in only one or two joints: the knee, the neck, the back, and/or occasionally the hip. Less commonly involved joints are the first MP joint of the foot or the first carpal-metacarpal joint of the hand (base of the thumb). Occasionally, the patient will complain of discomfort in the midfoot area, particularly the diabetic patient. Osteoarthritis of the interphalangeal joints of the fingers is more likely to be a cosmetic problem than one of pain or significant loss of function (3), while osteoarthritis of the knee or hip is one of the leading causes of disability in the elderly population (4). Physical and radiological findings of osteoarthritis in the wrist, elbow, shoulder, or ankles usually indicate a form of osteoarthritis that is secondary to some other process.

SIGNS OF OSTEOARTHRITIS

The most common physical finding in osteoarthritis is enlargement of a peripheral joint in the absence of inflammatory signs. This is coupled with loss of normal range of motion. The enlargement of the joint is secondary to bone remodeling and osteophyte formation. Heberden's and Bouchard's nodes of the interphalangeal joints (Fig. 30.1) are examples of the joint enlargement seen in primary osteoarthritis. The joints of the spine and the hips manifest osteoarthritis by a decrease in range of motion. Crepitation during movement may also be felt over major joints such as the knees. In the late stages of osteoarthritis, malalignment of the joint and atrophy of adjacent muscle groups are seen.

In patients with osteoarthritis, inflammatory signs of the involved joints (soft tissue swelling or joint warmth) are usually either absent or very subtle. When intense inflammatory signs are

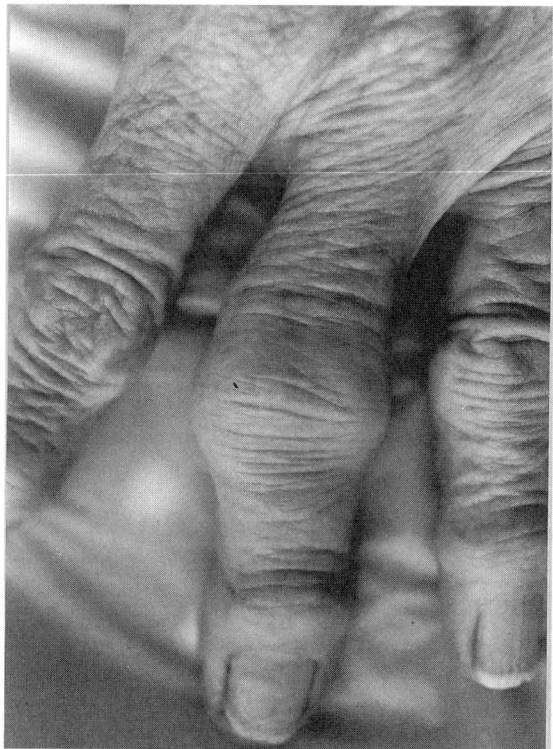

Figure 30.1 Clinical features of osteoarthritis. Photograph of finger demonstrating Heberden's nodes and distal interphalangeal joint and Bouchard's nodes of proximal interphalangeal joint.

present, one needs to consider another process such as crystal-induced arthritis or infection. Arthrocentesis of the involved joint should be done whenever there are impressive inflammatory signs. The joint fluid should be examined and sent for culture and crystal analysis in this situation.

CLINICAL STAGES OF OSTEOARTHRITIS

Osteoarthritis has different clinical stages. First, there is an asymptomatic stage in which the patient has no complaints, but if tested, biochemical abnormalities of the articular cartilage can be demonstrated. Although measurements of these biochemical events are not presently available to the clinician, it is estimated that this process begins in the 4th decade. The first symptoms of osteoarthritis are often associated with signs of soft tissue swelling secondary to mild synovitis. This inflammatory stage is usually subtle and short in duration. The most common clinical situation is the late "mechanical" phase. In this stage, the patient presents with various degrees of pain and stiffness. The physical examination demonstrates loss of joint function and/or malalignment, and the radiograph demonstrates loss of joint space. The mechanical problems that result in joint dysfunction are the predominant cause of pain and disability in the elderly patient. In this late stage of disease a comprehensive management program must be designed.

DIAGNOSTIC TESTING IN OSTEOARTHRITIS

Osteoarthritis is defined radiologically by joint space narrowing that is accompanied by osteophyte formation (5, 6) (Fig. 30.2). Bony eburnation and subchondral cysts can also be seen. Although the presence of an osteophyte is considered necessary to make a definite radiological diagnosis of osteoarthritis, longitudinal studies have suggested that joint space narrowing occurs prior to osteophyte formation. Radiological evidence of osteoarthritis is almost uniformly present in the elderly. However, it is common that radiological abnormalities do not correlate with the clinical complaint of musculoskeletal pain. Frequently, osteoarthritis is inappropriately blamed for pain in the elderly only because radiological changes are seen of the joints in the region of the pain. It is most important that a careful clinical assessment of the patient first be done to determine if the radiological findings correlate with the signs and symptoms.

On occasion, magnetic resonance imaging (MRI) and computed tomography (CT) scanning are helpful diagnostic procedures, particularly of

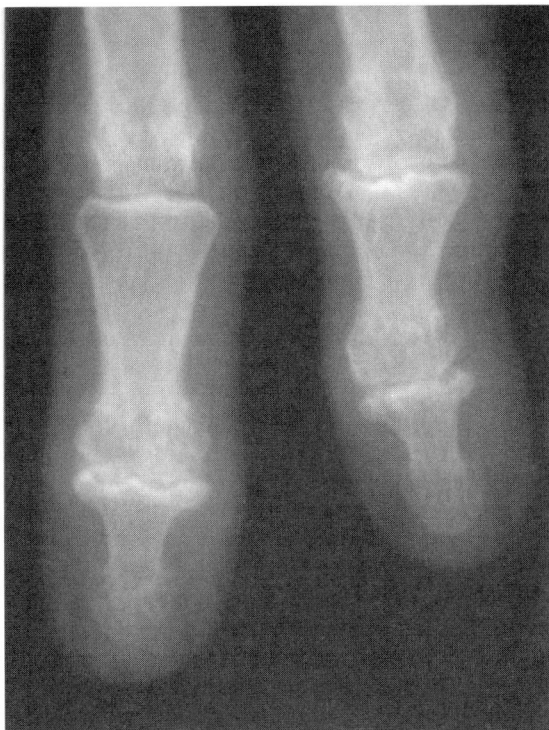

Figure 30.2 Radiological features of osteoarthritis. Radiograph of distal and proximal interphalangeal joints of the fingers demonstrating loss of joint space, osteophyte formation, bony eburnation, and subchondral cyst.

the spine, to rule out spinal stenosis, or of the knee to evaluate for soft tissue lesions or internal knee derangements involving the cartilage, ligaments, or menisci.

SUBSETS OF OSTEOARTHRITIS

Osteoarthritis can also present as different subsets of disorders. In general, osteoarthritis is usually classified as either primary or secondary disease. Primary osteoarthritis is defined not only by its clinical expression but also by the fact that the underlying cause is not completely understood. This is the most common situation in the elderly. Secondary osteoarthritis is associated with a defined underlying condition that is thought to contribute to or cause the articular changes.

Primary osteoarthritis usually involves either the peripheral joints and/or the axial skeleton in a specific pattern: distal interphalangeal joints (Heberden's nodes), proximal interphalangeal joints (Bouchard's nodes), the first carpal-metacarpal joint, the cervical and lumbar spine, the hips, knees, midfoot, and the first metatarsal joint. The presence of osteophyte formation on the interphalangeal joints defines the nodular pattern of primary osteoarthritis. Most patients have an isolated symptomatic joint; the minority have painful osteoarthritis involving many joints. Generalized nodular (Heberden's and/or Bouchard's nodes) osteoarthritis is thought to be genetically determined and has a age of onset between 40 and 60 years. It is more common in Caucasian females.

Erosive inflammatory osteoarthritis is another subset of osteoarthritis that is characterized by relatively intense inflammatory changes in the small joints of the hands, particularly the distal and proximal interphalangeal joints. Mild to moderate synovitis is present in the early stages of this subset of osteoarthritis. Eventually joint deformity can occur, including instability and then ankylosis. Radiological evidence of erosive changes is seen. Erosive osteoarthritis is more common in women than men and has a relatively younger age of onset (typically occurring soon after menopause) than primary localized osteoarthritis. Acute flares and periods of increased discomfort can wax and wane over years. This pattern of inflammatory changes sometimes mimics late-onset rheumatoid arthritis. Nonsteroidal antiinflammatory drugs are often necessary to control the inflammatory process, but these drugs do not seem to change the natural course of the disease.

Secondary causes of osteoarthritis can occur at any age. One particular secondary form that has been associated with the elderly patient is calcium crystal deposition disease. Radiological evidence of osteoarthritis can occur from many joint disorders: inflammation, hypermobility, injury, metabolic disorders, infection, or neuropathic processes.

MANAGEMENT OF OSTEOARTHRITIS

The key to the successful management of patients with osteoarthritis is to establish realistic goals and expectations. The patient needs to understand that symptomatic osteoarthritis is likely associated with a failing joint that has significant mechanical problems. A medication alone will not solve the situation; a comprehensive program including an altered life style may be necessary to reduce symptoms. The physician should understand the overall health status, general capacity, and goals of the patient. For example, a patient who is able to comfortably live on one floor at home and is either not capable or does not desire

vigorous activity, may do quite well with a conservative medical program. On the other hand, patients who are still participating in athletic activity (shopping, golfing, etc.) and are in general good health may choose surgical intervention to reach their goals. Treatment starts with education about the problem and a careful assessment of all dimensions of the patient's health and functional capabilities.

Reduction of joint stress is one key principle to follow when treating symptomatic osteoarthritis. Avoiding prolonged walking, stair climbing, or repetitive knee bending may reduce symptoms. Consultation with a physical therapist early in the course of treatment is recommended to help the patient learn methods to reduce joint stress, as well as to devise an exercise program and ways to assist the patient with activities of daily living.

Exercise is important not only because it maintains strength and stability but also because it may reduce pain. Studies have shown that patients with osteoarthritis become generally deconditioned as a consequence of immobility. Regular exercise, which does not stress the joint but conditions the patient, will improve the aerobic condition of the patient. Aquatic exercise and group exercise programs have been used successfully in the elderly population to achieve these goals. Exercise aimed at muscle strengthening (isometric or dynamic isotonic exercise) is important to maintain stability and reduce joint pain. If the mechanical component of the joint disease is so severe that exercise causes increased joint pain, surgical repair may be the only method to reduce pain and improve function.

Antiinflammatory medication should be used with caution in the elderly (7, 8). In fact, inflammation is generally not the cause of pain in osteoarthritis. The pain in osteoarthritis is thought to be secondary to joint failure; a process that involves all the components of the joint including the loss of articular cartilage, poor muscle tone, malalignment of the joint, and instability. Analgesic medication may adequately control the symptoms of osteoarthritis. A recent study demonstrated that acetaminophen was as effective as a nonsteroidal antiinflammatory drug (NSAID) in controlling the pain of moderate knee osteoarthritis. Intermittent use of a NSAID alone or in combination with acetaminophen is also helpful. Narcotics should be avoided.

Chronic use of a NSAID may be necessary in patients with severe osteoarthritis, particularly when inflammatory signs are present. No one NSAID has been shown to be more efficacious than any other in the treatment of osteoarthritis, although there may be individual patient preferences both in terms of effectiveness and tolerance. A reasonable trial of a given NSAID is 1 to 4 weeks, starting with a low dose and adjusting to an effective dose. Every effort should be made to use a low-dose schedule of the NSAID.

Intraarticular corticosteroids can be used as an adjunct to the medical regimen. In general, intraarticular corticosteroids are less effective in osteoarthritis, compared with the dramatic responses in an inflammatory arthritis like rheumatoid arthritis. Repetitive injections of corticosteroids should be avoided. In fact, if a joint requires multiple injections, it probably means this is an inappropriate method of therapy and that a significant mechanical component is present. There is no role for systemic corticosteroids in the treatment of osteoarthritis.

Consultation with an orthopaedic surgeon is appropriate when the patient is failing medical therapy. The decision to move to surgical intervention is complex, but patients should not be denied surgery solely on the basis of age. One must consider the patient's general medical condition, response to a comprehensive medical program, and goals and expectations. The goal of surgery should be to decrease pain and to improve independent function. Arthroscopic surgery has been used to remove joint debris and to repair degenerative and torn meniscus. An arthroscopic approach is a reasonable intermediate procedure to consider in the patient whose symptoms suggest an internal knee derangement.

Arthroplasty remains the primary option for many patients with end-stage osteoarthritis. Total joint reconstruction of the hip and knee are almost universally successful and have a reasonably low morbidity. In the elderly patient, long-term failure of the prosthesis from wear is of less concern than it is in the younger more active individual. However, in the elderly it is particularly important that the bone and supporting muscles are strong enough to predict a good surgical outcome.

REGIONAL MUSCULOSKELETAL DISORDERS

THE PAINFUL BACK (9, 10)

In the general population, low back pain is the most common localized musculoskeletal complaint that confronts the physician. This is not different in the elderly population; however, the causes of axial skeletal and low back discomfort in the elderly are different than in other age groups (Table 30.2). Acute low back strain occurs less commonly in the elderly than in the younger

Table 30.2
Common Causes of Low Back Pain in the Elderly Patient

Mechanical
Muscular strain
Osteoarthritis
Degenerative disk disease
Spinal stenosis
Metabolic bone disease
Osteoporosis
Osteomalacia
Neoplastic
Myeloma
Leukemia
Metastatic disease
Paget's disease
Diffuse idiopathic skeletal hyperostosis (DISH)

populations. Therefore, the elderly patient who presents with acute onset of back pain without obvious cause should have a radiograph done of the symptomatic area to rule out a bony lesion. Simple muscular backache can occur, but in the elderly there is usually associated evidence of structural problems of the axial apophyseal (facet) joints and/or degenerative disk disease. In any age group, poor posture, weak abdominal muscles, inappropriate stress to the muscles of the lumbar region, or acute trauma may lead to back discomfort. The simple "muscular strain" can be treated conservatively with rest, local measures such as massage and heat, and the use of an analgesic such as acetaminophen or low doses of a nonsteroidal antiinflammatory medication. Recovery should occur in 2 to 4 weeks; if not, further evaluation and diagnostic tests should be considered.

Probably the most common cause of back pain and limitation of motion is osteoarthritis and degenerative disk disease. Complaints are usually located in the lumbar and/or cervical areas. Thoracic back discomfort is distinctly unusual and should make one consider another etiology. The pain is generally insidious in onset, often present since younger years (30 to 40 years of age), dull in nature, sharp on extreme range of motion and, in the low back, aggravated by forward flexion. Pain in the neck that is aggravated by extension and relieved by flexion suggests osteoarthritis of the facet joints of the cervical vertebral bodies. Approximately 70% of patients over the age of 70 will have radiographic evidence of cervical degenerative disk disease, most frequently in C5-C6 or C6-C7. Stiffness after periods of inactivity is typical of osteoarthritis and/or degenerative disk disease.

If the pain radiates into the legs or arms, then a radiculopathy secondary to nerve root compression may be present. A sciatica secondary to impingement of L-4–5 or L-5, S-1 is the most common type of nerve root entrapment syndrome.

Conservative medical management is appropriate unless the pain is not reasonably controlled or a progressive neurologic syndrome emerges. Medical management follows the same principles that are detailed in the section on osteoarthritis.

Spinal Stenosis

Spinal stenosis is an important cause of low back pain and dysfunction in the elderly (11, 12). It can be caused by compression of the spinal canal because of extensive bony enlargement secondary to osteoarthritis of the vertebral body facets and soft tissue changes secondary to degenerative disk disease. It can also occur in the cervical area. Spinal stenosis in the lumbar region is usually preceded by a history of previous back problems including scoliosis, intervertebral disk disease, spondylolisthesis, enlarged ligamentum flavum, or enlarged posterior longitudinal ligament. It may also occur as a result of other acquired bony diseases such as Paget's disease, acromegaly, renal osteodystrophy, or late-stage ankylosing spondylitis or secondary to malignant mass or bony collapse from tumor invasion.

Typically the discomfort of spinal stenosis is dull and moderate, aggravated by moving into extension (lying down, stretching backward), and improved with stooping forward by flexing the hips and knees. The pain may radiate into the posterior legs or buttock, causing a discomfort that is often aggravated by ambulation (pseudoclaudication). Leg numbness or muscle weakness as well as other neurologic impairment can occur, including an upper motor lesion and/or bowel or bladder dysfunction. In lumbar spinal stenosis there are relatively few physical findings. Specifically, demonstrable sensory or muscular deficits are seen in the minority of patients. The straight leg test is negative. In approximately 40% of patients there is a decreased or absent ankle reflex.

The neurogenic claudication of spinal stenosis must be differentiated from vascular claudication. Patients with vascular claudication will have relief with standing and lying flat, and will have diminished peripheral pulses; patients with spinal stenosis will have worsened pain when standing upright in the extended position.

Plain radiographs are of little value in making the diagnosis of lumbar spinal stenosis. Electromyelography studies, however, are abnormal in about 80% of patients. The abnormalities are frequently seen in multiple levels in a bilateral distribution. The traditional gold standard for diagnosis is CT myelography. This allows evaluation of the bony and soft tissue causes of spinal stenosis as well as evaluating for concomitant nerve root entrapment. Recently, MRI has been used by many to diagnosis spinal stenosis, but there have been no controlled studies yet published to demonstrate superiority over CT myelography.

Conservative treatment is appropriate in the absence of significant pain or neurologic deficit. There is, however, no evidence to suggest that this offers any improvement in symptoms. Surgical decompressive laminectomy is the treatment of choice for relief of pain, functional limitation, or neurologic deficit. It is important to fully appreciate the entire extent of spinal cord compression prior to undergoing surgical therapy. There have been some recent anecdotal reports of the use of intrathecal corticosteroids for the relief of spinal stenosis. This therapy, however, has not been subjected to a randomized control trial to determine its efficacy.

Diffuse Idiopathic Skeletal Hyperostosis (DISH)

By age 50 years, approximately 60% of women and 80% of men will form anterior and lateral osteophytes of the vertebral column (spondylosis deformans). Diffuse idiopathic skeletal hyperostosis (DISH) is a disorder characterized by calcification and ossification of the anterior longitudinal ligament that occurs in the absence of degenerative disk disease or inflammatory back disease (13). The ossification may extend over several vertebral bodies and is associated with moderate to marked limitations of movement of the thorax and low back. DISH is often an asymptomatic radiological finding. However, it may be an important cause of complaints of decreased range of motion and stiffness with discomfort. Bony "spurs" may occur at other sites including the tip of the elbow or the heel. This process rarely causes nerve root entrapment and generally can be managed with conservative measures of education and physical therapy.

THE PAINFUL SHOULDER (14)

The painful shoulder is a common musculoskeletal complaint in the elderly, usually presenting as either unilateral or bilateral pain that radiates into the upper arm or deltoid muscle groups on elevation of the arm(s) laterally or over the head. Abduction of the arm to 45° involves the muscles of the rotator cuff. These muscles insert onto the humeral head and are located beneath the acromion of the scapula. The insertion of these muscles has a limited blood supply and because of its location is subject to chronic impingement, injury, and microtears. Subsequently, inflammation and deposition of calcium-containing crystals (hydroxyapatite) takes place in these tissues. Patients present with a painful arch of motion of the arm from 0 to 45° of abduction or they may have decreased motion of the arm (the frozen shoulder syndrome). They may also present with an acutely painful shoulder girdle with signs of inflammation. The acute inflammatory events are secondary to bursitis/tendinitis as a reaction to the local release of calcium-containing crystals from the soft tissue into the bursae, tendons, or joint.

The acute inflammatory event is best treated with rest and a NSAID. Alternatively, corticosteroids can be instilled into the subdeltoid region of the shoulder girdle. In the indolent phase of this process, protection of the shoulder and regular physical therapy to prevent limited motion is the preferred treatment.

A painful shoulder can also be caused by osteoarthritis of the acromioclavicular (AC) joint. In this situation patients present with pain at the AC joint as they elevate the arm beyond 45° of abduction, such as raising the arm over the head. Rarely, surgical resection of the end of the clavicle is necessary to relieve pain.

Biceps tendinitis can present as anterior shoulder girdle pain and swelling. This condition is aggravated by pronation of the forearm, flexion-extension of the forearm, or compression over the biceps tendon. Rest and short-term use of a NSAID almost always results in successful treatment.

True glenohumeral joint arthritis (the true shoulder joint) is uncommon in the elderly patient, probably because this joint is spared from osteoarthritis. Limitation of shoulder movement is almost always secondary to bursitis, rotator cuff disease, or the restriction from the chronic impingement syndrome. Arthritis of the glenohumeral joint leads to restriction of the shoulder movement during flexion-extension or external-internal motion.

BURSITIS

Bursitis is inflammation in a bursal sac(s) that normally lines and lubricates movement between bones, tendons, ligaments and/or muscles. The bursae may become inflamed because of trauma (microbleeding or tears), infection, systemic inflammation (e.g., rheumatoid arthritis), microcrystalline deposition, or for no well-defined reason. The patient presents with pain that is localized and aggravated with motion. If the bursa is superficially located (e.g., the olecranon bursae), then swelling, heat, or redness may be present. Fever is usually absent.

Sites of daily trauma, such as the olecranon bursa over the elbow and the prepatellar bursa of the knee, are the areas where bursitis is more likely to occur. Other sites include the trochanteric bursa (lateral upper thigh), anserine bursa (tibia at the anterior medial knee), ischial bursa (over the ischial tuberosity), and semimembranosus-gastrocnemius bursa (Baker's cyst).

The Baker's cyst is of special importance because it can rupture and result in severe pain and swelling in the involved knee and leg. This typically occurs in people with some underlying arthritic knee condition. The patients will typically complain of acute onset of calf pain and calf swelling that occurs when the popliteal cyst dissects down into the calf muscle. This event may mimic thrombophlebitis and has been coined the pseudothrombophlebitis syndrome (15). In anyone with acute leg pain and swelling, this diagnosis should be considered and not mistaken for deep venous thrombosis. Traditionally, diagnosis was established with an arthrogram; however, now ultrasonography can detect a ruptured cyst. Therapy requires rest for the joint and intraarticular injection of corticosteroids. This should provide prompt relief within a matter of hours.

Whenever possible an acutely inflamed bursae should be aspirated to obtain bursal fluid for examination (including polarization microscopy for crystals) and culture. Crystal-induced bursitis and infection have high leukocyte counts (25,000 to 50,000 cells per mm^3), while in other etiologies the white count is usually low. Olecranon bursitis is a common site for septic bursitis, usually secondary to *Staphylococcus aureus* infection (16). Infectious bursitis will require both appropriate antibiotics and drainage. In the elderly patient, it is recommended that the patient be hospitalized for management of septic bursitis.

Noninfectious bursitis can best be treated with rest and a short course of a NSAID. If this fails to resolve the situation, then a local injection of corticosteroids may be helpful.

TENOSYNOVITIS

Tenosynovitis or tendinitis can occur at any age; either secondary to overuse (exercise) or trauma or associated with a generalized inflammatory arthritis (e.g., rheumatoid arthritis). Common sites for tendinitis include the flexor tendons of the fingers (the trigger finger), the abductor or extensor tendons of the thumb (De Quervain's syndrome), dorsal extensor tendons of the wrist, or insertion of muscles at the elbow (tennis elbow). However any tendon can be involved. Tendinitis can be distinguished from ganglions (cystic swelling of the synovial sheath) and a Dupuytren's contracture (hyperplasia of the palmar fascia) because tendinitis tends to have an acute onset and a short course compared with the chronic noninflammatory nature of ganglions and contractures. Diffuse palmar fascia thickening has been associated with ovarian carcinoma and longstanding diabetes. Tenosynovitis is best managed by splinting the involved area (rest) and using a NSAID for a short time.

MICROCRYSTALLINE DISEASE

The most common cause of acute monarticular arthritis in the elderly patient is a crystal-induced arthritis. The main forms of microcrystalline arthritis are triggered by monosodium urate crystals (gout) and calcium pyrophosphate dihydrate crystals (pseudogout) (17). Pseudogout clinically mimics gout, but the treatment approach for each microcrystalline-induced arthritis is different (see below). It is, therefore, important to perform an arthrocentesis to identify the exact crystal and distinguish crystal-induced arthritis from other causes of acute monarthritis, in particular, a septic arthritis. Recent studies have shown that a variety of other crystals can cause acute arthritis, bursitis, or tendinitis. These include basic calcium phosphate (BCP) crystals and calcium oxalate crystals (18).

GOUT (19)

Hyperuricemia leads to the deposition of monosodium urate crystals in soft tissue (the tophi) and in the structures of the joint. The urate crystals are proinflammatory and provoke an acute arthritis that is usually monarticular and intense. In the absence of defined secondary factors (e.g., renal failure, diuretic use), young and middle-aged men are more likely to have an elevated serum uric acid level and gout than are premenopausal women. In fact, in men over the age of 30 years, gout is the most common cause of an inflammatory arthritis. In the elderly population, hyperuricemia becomes equally prevalent in both men and women.

Symptoms of Gout

Gout classically presents as an acute intense monarticular arthritis that mimics a septic arthritis, a soft tissue infection (cellulitis), or thrombophlebitis. The most frequently involved joints are those of the lower extremity including the metatarsal phalangeal joint of the great toe (podagra) as well as the ankle and knee. Typically, an attack begins abruptly for no apparent reason; the joint rapidly swells and becomes warm, erythematous, and so exquisitely painful that the patient will not move the joint or allow it to be touched. Gouty arthritis is episodic and will spontaneously resolve in 3 to 10 days without treatment. Patients can have "mini" attacks that are less intense and are difficult to diagnosis. Occasionally, the gout attacks occur in the upper extremity, particularly in the olecranon bursae. A polyarticular presentation is uncommon as an initial presentation, but multiple joint involvement is typical of untreated tophaceous gout (20). Tophaceous deposits around the joints of the fingers can be mistaken for the nodules of osteoarthritis or even rheumatoid arthritis in the elderly patient (Fig. 30.3). Recurrent untreated gout attacks and local deposition of urate will cause bone and joint destruction leading to joint deformities and remarkable disability. The other major sequela of hyperuricemia is nephrolithiasis from uric acid stones.

Laboratory Diagnosis

During an acute gout attack the patient may have a remarkable leukocytosis associated with fever, thus making a major concern. The serum uric acid level is influenced by several factors and, therefore, is of limited value during an acute attack. Arthrocentesis of the involved joint and synovial fluid analysis are important procedures to establish the diagnosis of gout. In gout, the joint fluid is inflammatory with decreased viscosity, high protein level, and elevated polymorphonuclear leukocytes. The synovial fluid leukocyte count is generally above 50,000 cells per mm³, levels also seen in septic arthritis. Gram staining of the fluid sample and culture should be negative for bacteria. Monosodium urate crystals are easily identified in the joint fluid by using a polarizing microscope; they are needle-shaped crystals and bright yellow when the crystal's long axis is parallel to the axis of light from the polarizer (negatively birefringent).

Management of Gout

Patients who have asymptomatic elevations of the serum uric acid (no history of either renal

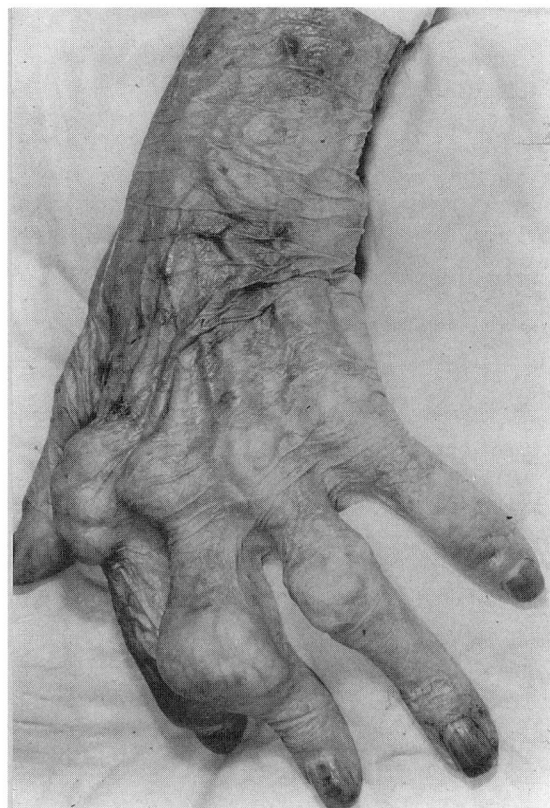

Figure 30.3 Clinical features of tophaceous gout. Photograph of hand demonstrating large tophi secondary to recurrent gouty arthritis and hyperuricemia.

stones or gouty arthritis) do not need any specific treatment. Treatment of the acute gout attack and prevention of recurrent attacks are the main problems to be addressed in the gouty patient. After diagnosing acute gouty arthritis, the principal aim of therapy is solely to suppress inflammation and relieve pain. Treatment of hyperuricemia should not be undertaken until the acute attack is suppressed. In the elderly, it is important to carefully review other medical problems and the physiologic condition of the patient before starting any drug treatment.

NSAIDs are effective in rapidly reducing inflammation and pain in gouty arthritis. No one NSAID has been shown to be more efficacious than another in the treatment of gout. The NSAID should be started at full dose and continued until the attack resolves (usually with 24 to 48 hours). Critical contraindications to NSAIDs are evidence of renal or hepatic insufficiency or active gastric lesions. Elderly patients are at a greater risk for NSAID-related toxic reactions, particularly gastritis, peptic ulceration, or gastrointestinal bleed-

ing. Acute effects of NSAID on renal function are also more common in the elderly patient. Caution should be exercised by documenting normal renal function before using a NSAID and by using the NSAID for the shortest period necessary to control the attack. The NSAID should be stopped in the asymptomatic intercritical period.

Colchicine has been used successfully for over 100 years for the treatment of acute gouty arthritis (21). Colchicine is thought to work by suppressing leukocytes from ingesting the urate crystal and by reducing the production of locally produced chemoattractants. It can be given orally in small frequent doses; however, oral colchicine usually causes significant gastrointestinal distress including abdominal cramps, diarrhea, or nausea and vomiting. These gastrointestinal side effects can be avoided by giving colchicine by a slow i.v. infusion. The i.v. route of administration, however, has been complicated by a significant risk of severe toxic reactions. Patients with renal and hepatic insufficiency and/or elderly patients have been shown to have a higher risk of these toxicities. Colchicine is not recommended as the initial drug treatment of acute gouty arthritis in the elderly.

Corticosteroids are also very effective for suppressing the inflammation of acute gout. These drugs should be considered when a NSAID or colchicine are contraindicated (50). The steroids can be administered either orally or intravenously in moderate doses to suppress inflammation (20 to 30 mg p.o. daily for several days). Intramuscular injections of ACTH or corticosteroids are not recommended. Preferably, intraarticular injection of corticosteroids following joint aspiration can be done. Intraarticular injection of corticosteroids is extremely effective when acute gout affects one joint.

After the acute attack has subsided, the physician should address any risk factors for hyperuricemia that can be corrected. For example, a myelodysplastic disorder (e.g., polycythemia vera) can cause excess uric acid production and hyperuricemia; excess alcohol intake can both increase urate production and decrease its renal excretion; thiazide diuretics will decrease renal uric acid secretion and increase serum uric acid. If hyperuricemia persists after addressing potentially reversible causes of hyperuricemia, then a drug that lowers serum uric acid should be considered. If the patient has had only one gout episode and if there is a low or normal excretion of urate (low risk for renal stone), then colchicine alone can be used in low doses (0.6 mg orally once or twice daily) for prophylaxis against new attacks. Patients with renal insufficiency are at risk for developing colchicine-induced myopathy.

Recurrent acute gout can also be prevented by normalizing the serum uric acid level, decreasing the total body urate content. This is accomplished by reducing uric acid formation or by increasing the rate of uric acid excretion. Therapy to lower serum uric acid should be reserved for patients who have recurrent gouty attacks, a renal stone, or tophaceous gout. Uricosuric medications (probenecid) can be used in patients without renal insufficiency, low or normal uric acid excretion, and no history of uric acid nephrolithiasis. The xanthine oxidase inhibitor allopurinol lowers the production of urate and is the more practical drug to use in the elderly patient to normalize the serum uric acid. It is recommended that allopurinol be started at 100 mg p.o. daily and increased by 100 mg every 2 weeks until the serum uric acid is normalized. The average dose needed is usually 300 mg daily. Low-dose oral colchicine (0.6 mg p.o. q.d. or b.i.d.) should be started before allopurinol treatment to prevent a new gout attack, which may occur as tissue uric acid shifts rapidly during decreases in serum uric acid.

PSEUDOGOUT

The acute inflammatory monarthritis that occurs secondary to calcium pyrophosphate dihydrate (CPPD) crystals mimics gout and, therefore, is called pseudogout (22). Deposition of CPPD crystals in the articular cartilage (chrondrocalcinosis) is very common in the elderly. Chrondrocalcinosis is usually an asymptomatic finding that is more common in men than in women.

Symptoms of Pseudogout

Like gouty arthritis, pseudogout presents as an episodic, acute, intense arthritis that can involve one or several joints. The attacks are typically self-limited and most usually affect the knee or the radiocarpal joint in the wrist. A minority of patients present with a symmetric polyarthritis that mimics rheumatoid arthritis, including the constitutional symptoms of fatigue, morning stiffness, and low-grade fever. Pseudogout may have also present as "mini" attacks or "pseudo-osteoarthritis." Arthrocentesis of the involved joint should be done when possible so that the crystal can be identified and joint fluid can be sent for culture. The CPPD crystals are the rod-shaped crystals that are blue when viewed with parallel light on the polarizing microscope (positively birefringent).

Management of Pseudogout

Chondrocalcinosis and attacks of pseudogout have been associated with a number of diseases, including hypothyroidism, hyperparathyroidism, and hemochromatosis (48). These disorders should be considered, particularly in the younger patient. Treatment of pseudogout revolves around the appropriate use of a NSAID or, if necessary, corticosteroids to suppress acute inflammation. There are no drugs to alter the tissue level of CPPD crystals. Fortunately, unlike with gout, recurrent attacks of pseudogout are infrequent.

DIFFUSE SOFT TISSUE PAIN SYNDROMES (23)

Diffuse pain syndromes are not unique to any age group. They fall into two major categories: noninflammatory and inflammatory (Table 30.3). Noninflammatory pain occurs more frequently, falling into one of five major causes: musculoskeletal pain associated with psychiatric illness, chronic pain syndrome, metabolic disorders, fibromyalgia, and malingering. Some neurologic disorders can mimic diffuse pain syndromes because they are associated with a loss of normal musculoskeletal function and a sense of muscular stiffness (e.g., Parkinson's disease).

Patients with psychiatric disorders, particularly depression, can have symptoms of musculoskeletal pain. The pain is often bizarre, poorly characterized by the patient, not well localized, and usually free of any associated physical find-

Table 30.3
Differential Diagnosis of Diffuse Pain in the Elderly

Noninflammatory
    Depression
    Chronic pain syndrome
    Metabolic disorder
    Hyperthyroidism
    Hypothyroidism
    Hyperparathyroidism
    Vitamin D deficiency
    Fibromyalgia (fibrositis)
    Malingering
Inflammatory
    Rheumatic diseases with late-age onset
        Polymyositis
        Rheumatoid arthritis
        Sjögren's syndrome
    Systemic lupus erythematosus
    Chronic infections
    Systemic vasculitis
        Giant cell arteritis
    Malignant neoplasms

ings. The psychiatric disorder is evidenced by a careful history including consultation with family members. Management of the pain syndrome will not be successful without a comprehensive program for the psychiatric illness. Chronic diffuse pain can occur in the absence of a defined psychiatric disorder, usually following a persistent local source of pain such as a severe injury to a joint. Metabolic disorders, particularly thyroid disease, may be associated with myalgia, arthralgia, muscle weakness, and diffuse or localized pain. Recognition of a metabolic disorder in the elderly patient is most important. Correction of the imbalance usually improves the soft tissue pain.

Fibromyalgia (fibrositis) is characterized by noninflammatory aches, pain, and stiffness in many muscle groups, primarily around the neck and shoulder girdle, low back area, and upper legs and knees (24, 25). Patients typically state that they "hurt all over" and that they have a poor sleep pattern. During the day, they feel fatigued, anxious, and/or depressed. The examination is normal with the exception of trigger points of subjective tenderness that can be found at multiple specific sites. Laboratory data are normal in primary fibromyalgia, and often the patient has seen several physicians, seeking help for the pain. Although the typical patient is a younger female, one should not forget that fibromyalgia can occur in any age group and may be overlooked in the older patient. Management for fibromyalgia includes education, counseling, physical therapy (especially exercise), analgesic medication (either acetaminophen or low doses of a NSAID), and consideration for a low nighttime dose of a tricyclic antidepressant medication. Narcotics should be avoided. Fibromyalgia tends to be a chronic relapsing disorder despite a comprehensive program.

POLYMYALGIA RHEUMATICA (PMR) (26–28)

Polymyalgia rheumatica is a clinical syndrome that is seen almost exclusively in patients over the age of 50 years (mean age of onset 70; range 50 to 90). It is more common in women and Caucasians, particularly individuals of Scandinavian descent. The incidence of PMR increases with each decade over the age 50 but varies depending on the ethnic background of the population studied. It has been estimated that in Olmstead County, Minnesota, USA, the incidence is 19.8 per 100,000 in persons 50 to 59 years of age and 112 per 100,000 in persons 70 to 79 years of age.

Symptoms of PMR

PMR is manifested by an aching discomfort and stiffness involving symmetrically the neck, shoulders, and hips. It commonly begins acutely over a 2-week period but may also have an insidious onset and course. Pain and stiffness are usually significantly worse at night and in the morning hours or after periods of rest (gelling). The pain generally improves as the patient moves the involved muscles and joints, but debilitating pain in the shoulder and hip girdle usually progresses during simple daytime activities. In fact, the patient's ability to provide self-care may become impaired. Although muscle weakness is uncommon, the patient may be unstable and subject to falls due to pain and stiffness.

PMR often involves the joints of the fingers and the wrist in a pattern similar to that of rheumatoid arthritis. Less commonly, the patient has swelling of the sternoclavicular joint(s). Other clinical signs and symptoms supporting the presence of an inflammatory illness are usually prominent. These include a low-grade fever, weight loss, fatigue, mood changes, and lethargy. The symptoms of PMR may cause patients to withdraw from their usual social activity or to develop a profound depression.

Signs and Laboratory Parameters in PMR

On physical examination the patient may appear chronically ill and may have a depressed affect. There is usually no objective evidence of muscle weakness. Range of motion of the shoulders and hips is frequently limited by pain and stiffness. The presence of joint effusions, especially within the fingers, wrists, and knees, is not uncommon. Carpal tunnel entrapment may occur secondary to wrist synovitis. Laboratory studies will often show evidence of a systemic inflammatory reaction: a remarkably elevated erythrocyte sedimentation rate (ESR), mild leukocytosis, and a normochromic, normocytic anemia of "chronic disease." An elevated serum alkaline phosphatase is found in 20 to 60% of patients secondary to a nonspecific granulomatous process in the liver. The analysis of synovial fluid, when present, shows only moderate inflammation with typically fewer than 15,000 synovial WBCs/mm^3. Muscle enzyme levels are normal as are electromyelograms.

PMR is a clinical syndrome that requires the exclusion of other specific diseases. Several disorders may mimic PMR. The arthritis of PMR is similar to rheumatoid arthritis. In fact, the onset of rheumatoid arthritis in the elderly patient may present with months of muscular aches and stiffness before the onset of inflammatory joint changes. Some have suggested that late onset of seronegative rheumatoid arthritis is, in fact, the articular manifestation of PMR. Polymyositis has been confused with PMR, but patients with polymyositis usually present with weakness and minimal muscular pain. Endocrine disorders such as hypothyroidism may have muscular pains and/or a myopathy with weakness. Malignancy and chronic infection may also present as a PMR-like syndrome. One also needs to consider soft tissue pain syndromes such as fibrositis or the muscular manifestations of true depression in an elderly patient. Finally, giant cell arteritis may present as a PMR syndrome.

Management of PMR

PMR has no known etiology, and therefore, treatment is directed at the inflammatory process. It is reasonable to use a NSAID as an initial mode of treatment in patients without signs or symptoms of associated giant cell arteritis. However, a NSAID generally provides only mild to moderate relief of symptoms. PMR is dramatically responsive to relatively low doses of oral corticosteroids. In fact, the rapid resolution of symptoms within 24 hours following a oral dose of 10 to 20 mg of prednisone is so characteristic and unique to PMR that this dramatic response to corticosteroids is helpful in confirming the diagnosis. The toxicity of corticosteroid usage in the elderly patient must always be given careful consideration. The signs and symptoms of active disease resolve rapidly, thus in most patients the prednisone dosage can be tapered to a low dose of 5 mg daily within a few weeks. Corticosteroids can generally be discontinued after a 1- to 2-year period. Patients who are resistant to corticosteroid therapy are so uncommon that the diagnosis of PMR should be questioned. If the patient is intolerant or not responsive to corticosteroids, then consideration can be given to immunosuppressive therapy.

GIANT CELL ARTERITIS (29–31)

Giant cell arteritis (GCA) is also referred to as cranial or temporal arteritis because the signs and symptoms occur as a result of inflammatory lesions of the vessels extending off the aortic arch into the temporal and cranial arteries (excluding intercerebral blood vessels). Like PMR, GCA presents almost exclusively in Caucasian patients over the age of 50 years. Approximately 10 to 20% of patients who have PMR will have occult GCA detected by biopsy of an asymptomatic temporal artery.

Patients with GCA may present in a variety of ways, the most common being new and persistent headache. While temporal headache is characteristic, any location of headache may occur. In addition, most patients are profoundly ill with constitutional symptoms including fatigue, mood changes, weight loss, anorexia, and myalgia. Fever is usually low grade, but occasionally GCA can present with fever of unknown origin. Visual disturbances including diplopia, blurred vision, and unilateral or bilateral transient loss of vision are common symptoms of GCA. These symptoms may precede one of the most devastating complication of this condition, permanent loss of vision secondary to occlusion of the ophthalmic artery. Other symptoms that affect the head and neck include the sensation of nodules over the scalp, pain in the jaws on chewing (jaw claudication), tongue pain, throat pain, and unexplained cough. GCA is a generalized process, so that ischemic injury can occur in the distribution of any major muscular artery including the coronary circulation.

Laboratory studies typically show a markedly elevated sedimentation rate, leukocytosis, and a normocytic, normochromic anemia. Frequently, the serum alkaline phosphatase level will be mildly elevated. A definitive diagnosis requires a temporal artery biopsy with pathology demonstrating arterial wall necrosis and multinucleated giant cells within the medial portion of the vessel. Investigations have suggested that a unilateral temporal artery biopsy will miss the diagnosis in up to 15% of cases, while bilateral biopsies that are negative for arteritis would exclude GCA 95% of the time.

Management of GCA

When there is a high clinical suspicion for active GCA, the patient should be started promptly on prednisone at a dosage of 1 mg per kilogram per day (prednisone 60 to 80 mg p.o. daily). Prompt treatment with corticosteroids may prevent the occurrence of blindness or other vascular events. Within a period of several days after initiating corticosteroids the patient should undergo a diagnostic temporal artery biopsy to confirm the clinical diagnosis. Whenever possible, the biopsy specimen should first be obtained from a symptomatic side. Because the inflammatory changes are not uniformly present in the temporal artery, the biopsy specimen should be at least 3 cm in length. This generous biopsy specimen allows careful pathological sectioning and thorough evaluation of the vessel wall. Biopsy of the other temporal artery should be considered if the first biopsy specimen is negative and the diagnosis is unclear. After clinical signs and symptoms have resolved, prednisone taper can begin slowly and cautiously. The sedimentation rate and other laboratory parameters should have dramatically improved. The corticosteroids can be tapered by lowering the dose by 5 mg every 5 to 7 days. Relapses of disease activity uncommonly occur as the dosage of corticosteroids reaches approximately 5 to 15 mg of daily prednisone. It has been reported that most patients can have corticosteroids stopped after a 2-year period of treatment, but in the authors' experience, a low maintenance dose of 5 mg daily is needed in some cases.

MUSCLE WEAKNESS IN THE ELDERLY PATIENT

The elderly patient often complains of muscle weakness, clumsiness, or instability in the absence of significant pain. This is a challenging clinical problem because the differential diagnosis of muscle weakness in the elderly patient is extensive (Table 30.4). A systematic approach needs to be established that considers not only the effect of aging on the muscle but also a superimposed process that may either directly or indirectly cause muscle injury or dysfunction (49).

Amyotrophic lateral sclerosis (ALS) is a degenerative disease of the nervous system that presents with progressive weakness of the muscles of the limbs, trunk, neck, tongue, and respiration (32). ALS has an increased risk with age, with the average age of onset in the early 60s. Although easy to diagnose, ALS is most often misdiagnosed and confused with cervical and lumbar spondylitic myelopathy. ALS is a clinical diagnosis based on the presence of insidious but progressive muscle weakness with muscle fasciculations in the absence of sensory loss, bowel or bladder incontinence, or ocular muscle weakness.

Cervical spondylosis generally presents with sharp pain on movement of the head and neck and progressive loss of range of motion. This may progress to a myelopathy manifest as painless weakness in the arms, muscle fasciculations, and muscle atrophy. In the lower extremity, a spastic paralysis with sensory loss helps distinguish cervical spondylosis from ALS. CT scanning or MRI will make the diagnosis of cervical spondylosis. Treatment can be conservative in the absence of progressive neurologic deficits. Lumbar spondylosis may also lead to numbness and weakness in the lower extremities (see Spinal Stenosis).

Polymyositis is an inflammatory process involving striated muscle (33). It has a mean age of onset in the 3rd to 4th decade, with a female predominance in all age groups. The patient presents with the insidious onset of proximal limb/girdle muscle weakness. Muscle pain and stiffness are minimal. Typically, the weakness is first experienced in the lower extremities, causing difficulty rising from a low chair or climbing steps. Later the weakness is sensed in the arms; patients complain of difficulty combing their hair or working with their hands above their head. In severe cases, all striated muscle groups are involved with profound weakness, inability to rise from a supine position, compromised swallowing, and even respiratory distress secondary to impaired diaphragmatic function. Other systems can be involved including a cardiomyopathy, pulmonary fibrosis, inflammatory rashes (dermatomyositis), or a systemic vasculitis.

The etiology of polymyositis is unknown, but tumor-related myositis emerges as a problem in the elderly patient. In the absence of autoantibodies (a positive antinuclear antibody) and if the age of onset is greater than 50, one must be concerned about an associated malignancy. Cutaneous vasculitis, an aggressive course, and unresponsiveness to corticosteroids have also been associated with tumor-related myositis.

The diagnostic workup for polymyositis should include evidence of symmetrical proximal muscle weakness, elevated serum muscle enzymes (creatine kinase, aldolase, alanine aminotransaminase, and/or aspartate aminotransaminase), typical electomyographic changes, and a positive muscle biopsy. Dermatomyositis has characteristic inflammatory skin changes including a viola-

Table 30.4
Age-related Neuromuscular Problems

Amyotrophic lateral sclerosis
Myasthenia gravis
Polymyositis
    Adult polymyositis
    Dermatomyositis
    Myositis associated with malignancy
    Inclusion body myositis
Drug-induced myopathies
    Colchicine
    Lovastatin
    Corticosteroids
    Alcohol
Oculopharyngeal muscular dystrophy
Other myopathies in the elderly
    Thyrotoxic myopathy
    Compressive myelopathy due to cervical spondylosis
    Tumor-related syndromes

ceous discoloration of the eyelids (heliotrope), a scaly erythematous rash over the knuckles (Gottron's sign), inflammatory erythematous skin on the face and chest, and sometimes photosensitivity. Management includes careful assessment for an underlying tumor. The mainstay of therapy is corticosteroids in moderate to high dosages. In resistant cases immunosuppressant medications may be necessary.

Inclusion body myositis is most often seen in males over the age of 50. This disease progresses slowly, with initial complaints of proximal muscle weakness of both the arms and legs and later distal muscle weakness. The creatine kinase level is only mildly elevated or it can be normal. There is no evidence of an autoimmune process, and at the stage at which patients present, they are generally not responsive to corticosteroids or other immunosuppressive therapy. Muscle biopsy is diagnostic of inclusion body myositis, demonstrating a myopathy with eosinophilic intranuclear and cytoplasmic inclusions in muscle fibers.

Myasthenia gravis is an autoimmune disorder that affects muscle motor end-plate function (34). Myasthenia gravis of late onset (age 50 to 70 years) more often affects men than women. Both ocular and voluntary muscle groups are involved in most cases. Easy fatigability of the limbs, manifest by the inability to do repetitive tasks, is typical of myasthenia gravis. Ptosis, diplopia, difficulty with swallowing, a forward stooping of the head, a nasal voice, and regurgitation of food or liquids into the nasal passages are also typical. The weakness waxes and wanes and seems to be aggravated by exertion, stress, infections, and warm temperatures. Older patients often respond more readily than younger patients to immunosuppressive therapy.

Drug-induced myopathies are particularly important to consider in the differential diagnosis of muscle weakness in the elderly. Like drug use in general, drug-induced myopathy is more common in the elderly population. Drug-induced myopathies are often mistaken for polymyositis because they may present with proximal muscle weakness, moderate to mild muscle pain, and elevated muscle enzyme levels. Colchicine myopathy may develop in the gout patient taking daily colchicine, particularly if there is renal dysfunction, a common combination in the elderly (35). Lovastatin myopathy occurs in older patients being treated for hypercholesterolemia and in transplant patients. Corticosteroid-related myopathy often begins in proximal muscles of the lower extremity as painless muscle weakness that can then progress to other muscle groups. The muscle enzymes

are normal in steroid myopathy, and muscle biopsy demonstrates type 2 muscle fiber atrophy. Alcohol abuse and associated alcoholic myopathy should not be forgotten in the elderly patient. Alcoholic myopathy generally presents as painless weakness of the pelvic and thigh muscles, often in association with a peripheral neuropathy.

Oculopharyngeal muscular dystrophy is the only muscular dystrophy that presents more commonly in the elderly population. Ptosis and dysphagia are more prevalent than is limb muscle weakness. Muscle biopsy is distinctive in this disorder.

AUTOIMMUNE DISEASES IN THE ELDERLY

Systemic Lupus Erythematosus

Systemic lupus erythematosus (SLE) is typically a disorder of young women, with a peak incidence in the second through fourth decades. Patients over the age of 50 represent 6 to 20% of patients with SLE (37, 38). Several studies have characterized "late onset" SLE and determined the presence of specific clinical features suggesting that SLE in the elderly patient may be a distinct subset of this disease.

Female predominance is seen in late-onset SLE; however, in the older population, there is a proportionally greater number of males than in younger-age SLE. Frequently, the symptoms of active SLE are misdiagnosed; the interval from the onset of symptoms to the diagnosis can be many months. The symptoms of late-onset SLE differ from those of disease in the younger age group. Arthritis is less common in the elderly patient. Serositis, presenting as pleuritis and/or pericarditis, occurs more frequently in late-onset disease than in younger patients. Rashes, photosensitivity, lymphadenopathy, Raynaud's phenomenon, and renal and central nervous system involvement are uncommon in the elderly patient, while pulmonary disease, the sicca complex (dry mouth and eye), and neuropathy are common. When glomerulonephritis is present it rarely progresses to renal failure.

Patients with late-onset SLE will have antinuclear antibodies, commonly anti-Ro (SSA); antibody to double-stranded DNA is rarely seen. In all age groups a normochromic, normocytic anemia, lymphopenia, and an elevated sedimentation rate are typical of active disease.

Long-term follow-up of patients with late-onset SLE demonstrates a relatively benign course with a good prognosis. Conservative medical therapy is appropriate. Serositis or arthritis may be treated with a NSAID, while skin rashes can be managed with topical corticosteroids. Hydroxychloroquine is useful in controlling the disease and preventing flares. Low-dose corticosteroids may be necessary in some patients. Immunosuppressive drugs are rarely used.

DRUG-INDUCED LUPUS

The syndrome of drug-induced lupus includes clinical symptoms that are quite similar to those of late-onset SLE (39). The drugs that have been most strongly associated with this syndrome include hydralazine, procainamide, isoniazid, chlorpromazine, and methyldopa. However, over 50 drugs have been implicated in causing a lupuslike illness. This syndrome typically occurs in older males because they are more likely to have a medical condition that requires the drugs that induce lupus.

Fever, arthritis, or inflammation of serous membranes (pleural/pericardial) are the usual features of drug-induced lupus. Unlike idiopathic SLE, it is distinctly unusual for neurologic, hematologic, rashes, lymphadenopathy, and renal disease to occur in drug-induced lupus.

The symptoms of drug-induced lupus often are mild and usually begin several months after starting the causative medication. Antinuclear antibodies are present in 100% of patients with this condition and are predominantly directed toward nuclear histones (40). Anti-double-stranded DNA, anti-SM, hypocomplementia, and Coombs-positive hemolytic anemia are less likely to occur in drug-induced lupus than in spontaneous SLE. Therefore, these laboratory differences are helpful in distinguishing idiopathic from drug-induced lupus.

The prognosis of drug-induced lupus is excellent because the illness is reversible with cessation of the offending medication. NSAIDs or, on occasion, low-dose corticosteroids may be necessary to control the inflammatory response. All symptoms should resolve within several weeks, and further medical therapy should not be required.

Sjögren's Syndrome

Sjögren's syndrome is an autoimmune disorder that involves certain exocrine glands and presents with a variety of clinical problems (41). While most patients have only the sicca complex (dry eye, xerophthalmia; and dry mouth, xerostomia), Sjögren's syndrome may be a systemic disorder commonly associated with musculoskeletal complaints. Sjögren's syndrome may exist alone (primary Sjögren's syndrome) or it may be associated with another disease (secondary Sjögren's syndrome), usually a rheumatic disease like rheumatoid arthritis or SLE. Primary Sjögren's syndrome is found primarily in older women (mean age at onset 50 to 60).

Patients with primary Sjögren's syndrome often have chronic upper airway dryness and bronchitis, difficultly swallowing, inability to chew dry foods, difficulty with speech, increased problems with dental caries, trouble with dentures, diffuse dry skin, and sicca vaginitis. A nondeforming, nonerosive polyarthritis that mimics rheumatoid arthritis has been reported in 50 to 60% of patients. Polymyositis may present as proximal muscle weakness. Extraglandular lymphocytic infiltration of viscera and a systemic vasculitis may occur, particularly in patients over the age of 50. Chronic pulmonary disease, renal abnormalities (e.g., glomerulonephritis, renal tubular acidosis), and focal or diffuse central nervous system disease can also be seen in patients with primary Sjögren's syndrome. Although most patients have a benign sicca syndrome, there is an increased risk of developing a lymphoma or pseudolymphoma syndrome (42).

Physicians should be aware that primary Sjögren's syndrome can cause both systemic and musculoskeletal disease in the elderly. Laboratory assessment will demonstrate hypergammaglobulinemia, a positive rheumatoid factor, and the presence of autoantibodies, particularly antinuclear antibody, and anti-Ro and anti-La antibodies. When suspicious of Sjögren's syndrome, an ophthalmologic workup should include testing for dry eyes by both Schirmer's test and rose bengal staining for corneal lesions. When there is a diagnostic dilemma, a lip biopsy is indicated to examine the minor salivary glands for the characteristic lymphocytic infiltration. Management of patients with Sjögren's syndrome is primarily focused on reduction of dryness to eye and other mucous membranes with topical wetting agents. Antiinflammatory and immunosuppressive drugs are reserved for patients with active systemic disease.

LATE-ONSET RHEUMATOID ARTHRITIS (RA) (43)

Rheumatoid arthritis is an inflammatory systemic disease that affects predominantly women in the 3rd to 4th decade of life (44). Its pivotal clinical problem is chronic symmetrical polyarthritis that causes erosive changes of the structures of diarthrodial joints. Deformity of the joints, loss of function, and disability are common outcomes despite current therapy for RA.

When RA begins in the elderly patient (after the age of 60 years), there characteristically is a long period of arthralgias and myalgias before the onset of frank arthritis. Stiffness and pain in the limb girdles and synovitis limited to the fingers and wrist are typical of late-onset RA. The diagnosis of PMR is often entertained in patients with late-onset RA because of the similarity of clinical features of both of these conditions. In fact, some have suggested that late-onset RA is not a distinct disease but actually is the arthritis of PMR. In general, the course of the arthritis of late-onset RA is less aggressive than RA of young-onset disease; rheumatoid nodules are less common, and rheumatoid factor is frequently not present. Patients who do have high-titer rheumatoid factor are more likely to have a destructive polyarthritis similar to the younger age onset disease.

In managing patients with late-onset RA one should consider PMR in the differential diagnosis. Patients with late-onset RA have a good response to low-dose corticosteroids (10 to 15 mg p.o. daily), but they are less likely to have the dramatic overnight response seen in patients with PMR. NSAIDs are often helpful. In the absence of retinal disease, hydroxychloroquine is often used first as a slow-acting remitting agent. Other remitting agents (e.g., gold, D-penicillamine, methotrexate) can be used but are generally not necessary because of the benign course of late-onset RA.

MALIGNANCY

In the elderly population one must always consider malignancies as a source of musculoskeletal symptoms (45). The associated malignancy may be either overt or occult. One such condition is hypertrophic osteoarthropathy (HPO) (46). This is typically caused by a pulmonary neoplasia and results in clubbing of the extremities, painful periostitis of the long bones, and polyarthritis. Usually the tumor is obvious at the time of onset of articular symptoms. The acute periostitis is manifested by paresthesia and severe discomfort, predominately of the long bones of the lower extremities, worsened when the extremities are in the dependent position. In addition, the patients may have a symmetric polyarthritis involving the small joints of the hands and feet, similar to that seen in rheumatoid arthritis. NSAIDs may provide symptomatic relief, but therapy should be directed toward reducing the tumor burden.

In the elderly patient, dermatomyositis and polymyositis are also known to occur in association with malignancies (47). In a recently published series of 788 patients, approximately 12% were diagnosed with an associated malignancy. Malignant tumors may also cause muscle weakness as a consequence of muscle wasting or an associated carcinomatous myopathy or secondary to neurologic sequelae such as Lambert-Eaton syndrome.

There are a number of other less common musculoskeletal syndromes that have been described in association with malignancies. Carcinomatous polyarthritis is a term used to describe the symmetrical polyarthritis that occurs in close temporal relationship to the development of malignancy. This arthritis typically has an explosive onset, is symmetric, and is predominantly a lower extremity arthritis, sparing the joints of the upper extremity. The articular symptoms of carcinomatous polyarthritis will improve with successful treatment of the underlying malignancy and may relapse as the tumor recurs. Ovarian tumors have been described to be associated with a palmar fascitis presenting as the abrupt onset of thickening and contractions within the palmar fascia. Rheumatic manifestations have also been reported in approximately 10% of patients with hematologic myelodysplastic syndromes. The manifestations include cutaneous vasculitis, peripheral neuropathy, and a clinical "lupuslike" syndrome.

REFERENCES

1. Moskowitz RW, Howell DS, Goldberg VM, Mankin HJ, eds. Osteoarthritis: diagnosis and medical/surgical management. 2nd ed. Philadelphia: WB Saunders, 1992.
2. Hamerman D. The biology of osteoarthritis. N Engl J Med 1989;320(20):1322–1330.
3. Kallman DA, Wigley FM, Scott WW Jr, Hochberg MC, Tobin JD. The longitudinal course of hand osteoarthritis in a male population. Arthritis Rheum 1990;33:1323–1332.
4. Felson DT, Naimark A, Anderson J, Kazis L, Castelli W, Meenan RF. The prevalence of knee osteoarthritis in the elderly. The Framinghan Osteoarthritis Study. Arthritis Rheum 1987;30:914–918.
5. Kellgren JH, Lawrence JS. Radiological assessment of osteoarthritis. Ann Rheum Dis 1957;16:494–501.
6. Scott WW, Lethbridge-Ceiku M, Richle R, Wigley FM, Tobin JD, Hochberg MC. Reliability of grading scales for individual radiological features of osteoarthritis of the knee. Invest Radiology 1993;28:497–501.
7. Clements PJ, Paulus HE. Nonsteroidal anti-inflammatory drugs (NSAIDs). In: Kelley WN, Harris ED Jr, ed. Textbook of rheumatology. Philadelphia: WB Saunders, 1993:700–730.
8. Weinblatt ME. Nonsteroidal anti-inflammatory drug toxicity: increased risk for the elderly. Scand J Rheumatol Suppl 1991;91:9–17.
9. Frymoyer JW. Back pain and sciatica. N Engl J Med 1988;318:291–300.
10. Bornstein DG, Wiesel SW, eds. Low back pain: medical dagnosis and comprehensive management. 1st ed. Philadelphia: WB Saunders, 1989.

11. Hall S, Bartleson JD, Onofrio BM, Baker HL, Oka-zaki H, O'Duffy JD. Lumbar spinal stenosis: clinical features, diagnostic procedures, and results of surgical treatment in 68 patients. Ann Intern Med 1985;103:271–275.

12. Moreland LW, Lopez-Mendez A, Alarcon GS. Spinal stenosis: a comprehensive review of the literature. Semin Arthritis Rheum 1989;19:127–149.

13. Resnick D, Shapiro RF, Wiesner KB, et al. Diffuse idiopathic hyperostosis (DISH) (ankylosing hyperostosis of Forestier and Notes-Querol). Semin Arthritis Rheum 1978;7:153–187.

14. Thornhill TS. Shoulder pain. In: Kelley WN, Harris ED Jr, Ruddy S, Sledge CB, eds. Textbook of rheumatology. Philadelphia: WB Saunders, 1993:417–440.

15. Katz RS, Zizic TM, Arnold WP, Stevens MB. The pseudothrombophlebitis syndrome. Medicine 1991; 56(2):151–164.

16. Ho G Jr, Tice AD, Kaplan SR. Septic bursitis in the prepatellar and olecranon bursae. Ann Intern Med 1978;89:21–27.

17. Doherty M, Dieppe P. Crystal deposition disease in the elderly. Clin Rheum Dis 1986;12:97–116.

18. McCarty D, ed. Crystalline deposition diseases. Clinical rheumatic diseases. Philadelphia: WB Saunders, 1988:14.

19. Kelley WN, Schumacher R Jr. Gout. In: Kelly WN, Harris ED Jr, Ruddy S, Sledge CB, eds. Textbook of rheumatology. Philadelphia: WB Saunders, 1993:1291–1336.

20. Hadler MM, Franck A, Bress M, Robinson R. Acute polyarticular gout. Am J Med 1974;56:715–719.

21. Roberts WN, Liang MH, Stern SH. Colchicine in acute gout. JAMA 1987;257:1920–1922.

22. McCarty DJ. Arthropathies associated with calcium-containing crystals. Hosp Pract 1986;21(10): 109–120.

23. Sheon RP, Moskowitz RW, Goldberg VM, eds. Soft tissue rheumatic pain: recognition, management, prevention. 2nd ed. Philadelphia: Lea & Febiger, 1987.

24. Goldebenberg DL. Fibromyalgia, chronic fatigue, and myofascial pain syndromes. Curr Opin Rheumatol 1992;4:247–257.

25. Bennett RM, Goldenberg DZ, eds. The fibromyalgia syndrome. Rheumatic disease clinics. Philadelphia: WB Saunders, 1989:15.

26. Chaung T, Hunder GG, Ilstrup PM, Kurland LT. Polymyalgia rheumatica. Ann Intern Med 1982; 97:672–680.

27. Cohen MD, Ginsburg WW. Polymyalgia rheumatica. Rheum Dis Clin North Am 1990;16:325–339.

28. Ayoub WT, Franklin CM, Torretti D. Polymyalgia rheumatica. Duration of therapy and long-term outcome. Am J Med 1985;79:309–315.

29. Huston KA, Hunder GG, Lie JT, Kennedy RH, Elveback LR. Temporal arteritis: a 25-year epidemiologic, clinical, and pathologic study. Ann Intern Med 1978;88:162–167.

30. Chmelewski WL, McKnight KM, Agudelo CA, Wise CM. Presenting features and outcomes in patients undergoing temporal artery biopsy. Arch Intern Med 1992;152:1690–1695.

31. Hamilton CR, Shelley WM, Tumulty PA. Giant cell arteritis: including temporal arteritis and polymyalgia rheumatica. Medicine 1971;50:1–27.

32. Swash M, Schwartz MS. What do we really know about amyotrophic lateral sclerosis? J Neurol Sci 1992;113:4–16.

33. Dalakas MC. Polymyositis, dermatomyositis and inclusion-body myositis. N Engl J Med 1991; 325(21):1487–1498.

34. Phillips LH, Melnick PA. Diagnosis of myasthenia gravis the 1990's. Semin Neurol 1990;10:62–69.

35. Kuncl RW, Duncan G, Watson D, Alderson K, Rogawski MA, Peper M. Colchicine myopathy and neuropathy. N Engl J Med 1987;316:1562–1568.

36. Stevens MB. Connective tissue disease in the elderly. Clin Rheum Dis 1986;12:11–32.

37. Urowitz MB, Stevens MB, Shulman LE. The influence of age on the clinical pattern of SLE. Arthritis Rheum 1967;10:319–.

38. Baker SB, Rovira JR, Campion EW, Mills JA. Late onset systemic lupus erythematosus. Am J Med 1979;66:727–736.

39. Fritzler MJ, Rubin RL. Drug induced lupus. In: Wallace DJ, Hahn BH, eds. Dubois' lupus erythematosus. 4th ed. Philadelphia: Lea & Febiger, 1993; 442–453.

40. Totoritis MC, Tan EM, McNally EM, Rubin RL. Association of antibody to histone complex H2A-H2B with symptomatic procainamide-induced lupus. N Engl J Med 1988;318:1431–1436.

41. Talal N. Sjögren's syndrome: historical overreview and clinical spectrum of disease. Rheum Dis Clin North Am 1992;18:507–515.

42. Kassaw SS, Thomas TL, Moutsopoulos HM, Hoover R, Kimberly RP, et al. Increased risk of lymphoma in sicca syndrome. Ann Intern Med 1978;89:888–892.

43. Deal CL, Meenan RF, Goldenberg DL, Anderson JJ, Sack Burton S, et al. The clinical features of elderly-onset rheumatoid arthritis. Arthritis Rheum 1985; 28:987–998.

44. Wigley FM. Rheumatoid arthritis. In: Barker LR, Burton JR, Zieve PD, eds. Principles of ambulatory medicine. Baltimore: Williams & Williams, 1991: 880–990.

45. Caldwell DS, McCallum RM. Rheumatologic manifestations of cancer. Med Clin N Am 1986;70:385–417.

46. Vogh A, Blumenfeld S, Gritner LB. Diagnostic significance of pulmonary hypertrophic osteoarthropathy. Am J Med 1955;18:51.

47. Sigurgeirsson B, Lindelöf B, Edhag O, Allander E. Risk of cancer in patients with dermatomyositis or polymyositis. N Engl J Med 1992;326:363–367.

48. Jones AC, Chuck AJ, Arie EA, Green DJ, Doherty M. Diseases associated with calcium pyrophosphate deposition disease. Sem Arthritis Rheum 1992; 22:188–202.

49. Lacomis D, Chad DA, Smith TW. Myopathy in the elderly. Neurology 1993;43:825–828.

50. Groff GD, Franck WA, Raddatz DA. Systemic steroid therapy for acute gout: a clinical trial and review of the literature. Sem Arthritis Rheum 1990; 19:329–336.

31/ Osteoporosis and Other Metabolic Disorders of the Skeleton in Aging

Michele Frances Bellantoni

Table 31.1 lists the metabolic bone diseases that may first present in older adulthood. For all of these disorders, the goal of patient care is to prevent bony fractures. This chapter focuses on the management and, where possible, the prevention of the most common of the bone disorders of the elderly: osteoporosis, osteomalacia, hyperparathyroidism, and Paget's disease.

OSTEOPOROSIS

PATHOPHYSIOLOGY OF OSTEOPOROSIS

Adult bone is a metabolically active body tissue. At the cellular level, bone remodeling occurs at discrete foci in the skeleton, called bone-remodeling units. Each cycle begins with activated osteoclasts lining the bone surface. Over a period of about 2 weeks, the osteoclasts excavate a lacuna on the surface of cancellous bone or a cavity within cortical bone. Bone formation then occurs as osteoblasts secrete matrix proteins that are calcified. The impact of bone remodeling at the tissue level is determined by both the rate of bone turnover and the balance of the amount of bone resorbed and formed at each unit (1). During times when bone mass is maintained, resorption is coupled to formation.

Osteoporosis is defined as low bone mass resulting from an excess of bone resorption over bone formation, with resultant bone fragility and increased risk of fracture. A population-based data model has estimated that 54% of 50-year-old women will sustain osteoporosis-related fractures during their remaining lifetime (2). Significant morbidity, mortality, and medical expense result from osteoporosis-related fractures. Spinal fractures, which occur in 25% of white women by age 65 years, cause pain, deformity, and disability. Hip fractures result in at least short-term institutionalization in over 50% of patients, and are associated with a mortality rate of 5 to 20% within

the first year of fracture (3). Moreover, it is estimated that over 10% of women who sustain hip fractures become dependent in functional status, while many more never regain their full prefracture level of activity. The financial cost of osteoporosis in the United States each year exceeds 10 billion dollars (4).

RISK FACTORS FOR OSTEOPOROSIS

Bone mineral density in the elderly is the result of a peak bone mass that occurs in late adolescence, the maintenance of bone mass during young adulthood, and the subsequent bone loss that occurs over time. Based on family and twin studies, a low peak bone mass can result from as yet unrecognized genetic defects (5), with other factors such as malnutrition, chronic disease states, and exogenous glucocorticoid use contributing to reductions in peak bone mass. The maintenance of bone mass during young adulthood depends upon the maintenance of normal endocrine function including ovarian, adrenal, and testicular function; adequate calcium intake; and weight-bearing exercise. Frequent conditions that result in the loss of bone mass in young adults include menstrual irregularities resulting from severe weight loss or excessive exercise, gonadal dysfunction in women or men related to chronic disease, and the use of exogenous corticosteroids, cigarettes, or alcohol.

Estrogen deficiency results in accelerated bone loss at the time of menopause. It is likely that bone loss begins before the cessation of menses (6, 7). The time course and magnitude of the perimenopausal bone loss appear to be variable, and the factors other than the loss of ovarian estrogen production that contribute to and modulate the bone loss during this period are not completely understood. For example, the menopause is associated with a significant reduction in ovarian testosterone and adrenal androgen production.

326

Rates of bone loss during the menopausal transition can be up to 4% per year and may last 10 to 15 years (8). It is estimated that a third to a half of all bone loss in women may be attributable to the menopause (1). While men do not experience an easily identifiable menopause, hypogonadism in men is associated with accelerated bone loss (9).

Cross-sectional data suggest that bone loss continues in older women and men but that the degree of bone loss varies from site to site. In one study, decrements in bone density between women age 65 to 69 years and women 85 years and older exceeded 16% in the distal and proximal radius, the calcaneus, and the proximal femur; the difference in bone mineral density of the lumbar spine between the two groups was 6% (10). The primary causes for bone loss in older adults are unknown; however, dietary interventions including calcium (11) and vitamin D (12) and weight-bearing exercise (13) have been shown to reduce the rate of bone loss and may to a small degree reverse bone loss in older adults. It is thought that estrogen deficiency plays little part in the continued bone loss in women over age 65 years; however, transdermal estrogen replacement therapy has been shown to reduce bone turnover at least short-term in some older women (14). Secondary osteoporosis can be caused by excessive exposure to endogenous or exogenous glucocorticoids and thyroid hormone as well as hyperparathyroidism and multiple myeloma. It is also possible that deficiencies in growth hormone and insulinlike growth factor I can contribute to bone loss in older men and women (15).

SCREENING FOR OSTEOPOROSIS

While osteopenia can be diagnosed with standard radiography, this technique requires the loss of as much as 30% of bone mineral density. Thus, standard radiography is not an acceptable method to determine early or mild bone loss. Bone mineral densitometry is a useful technique for predicting the risk of fracture based on comparisons with age-matched controls. Single-photon absorptiometry, the first commercially available technique for the noninvasive measurement of bone mineral density, passes a beam of highly collimated monoenergetic photons from a radionuclide source through the area to be measured. The observed attenuation of the beam is a function of the density of the tissues through which the beam is passed.

Unlike single-photon absorptiometry, which requires a constant soft tissue path length, thereby limiting the technique to measurements of the peripheral skeleton, dual-energy absorptiometry uses two photon energies to allow the separation of bone and soft tissue mass attenuation. Dual-energy absorptiometry is used to measure bone mineral density of the lumbar spine and proximal femur. More recently, the radiation spectrum of gadolinium-153 has been simulated by x-ray techniques. Dual-energy x-ray absorptiometry scans now provide the most precise measurements of bone mineral density with 1% precision for spine, and 1 to 2% for femur scans, and with lowest radiation exposure, at doses per scan of less than 0.03% of the natural yearly radiation.

One criticism of bone densitometry is that the technique does not distinguish vertebral bone mass from fatty infiltrate. Also, degenerative changes that are common in the spinal column with aging, like fatty infiltrate, result in falsely elevated bone mineral density measurements with absorptiometry techniques. In contrast, quantitative computed tomography (CT) allows the direct measurement of trabecular or total bone density; however, this technique is costly and also has greater radiation exposure than dual-energy x-ray absorptiometry. While studies have shown that single-photon absorptiometry of the appendicular skeleton equally predicts non-spine fracture risks, as compared with dual-energy x-ray absorptiometry (16), it has been suggested that imaging of the trabecular component of the proximal femur using dual-energy techniques may better predict femoral fracture (17).

One study has documented that the results of bone densitometry substantially influence women's decisions about preventive measures for osteoporosis (18). There is considerable controversy about the appropriate use of bone densitometry as a screening test for osteoporosis. However, it is generally accepted that women who are at increased risk for osteoporosis should be screened with bone densitometry at yearly to biyearly intervals. Decreases in bone mineral density of more than 1% per year are considered clinically significant changes, which may be corrected by the interventions described below. Examples of patients who might benefit from such screening include a postmenopausal woman who has a strong family history of osteoporosis and who is not receiving estrogen replacement therapy, men and women who require long-term exogenous steroid therapy, and premenopausal women with menstrual irregularities. A single densitometry screen may be useful to a woman who is unwilling

Table 31.1
Metabolic Bone Disorders of the Elderly

Disorder	Metabolic Bone Defects	Common Risk Factors
Osteoporosis	Bone resorption predominates over formation	Postmenopausal women; hypogonadal men; chronic steroid, tobacco, or alcohol use
Osteomalacia	Mineralization defect associated with impaired or insufficient vitamin D metabolism	Home-bound or institutionalized elderly; inadequate intake of dairy products; gastric surgery
Hyperparathyroidism	PTH-induced accelerated bone resorption	Postmenopausal women
Renal osteodystrophy	Secondary hyperparathyroidism that results in accelerated bone resorption; osteomalacia related to impairment of vitamin D metabolism in the kidney; aluminum toxicity from phosphate buffers	Moderate to severe renal insufficiency; renal tubular defect; heavy metal exposures
Paget's disease	Increase in both bone resorption and formation	Late manifestation of paramyxoviral infection such as measles or respiratory syncytial virus
Malignant disorders	Bone resorption related to ectopic hormonal production (lung and kidney); direct invasion of tumor causing either increased resorption (breast, thyroid, myeloma) or increased osteoblastic function (prostate)	Underlying malignancy
Infectious disorders	Accelerated bone resorption resulting from infection of bone (tuberculosis, osteomyelitis)	Diabetes mellitus, chronic wound overlying bone, vascular insufficiency
Genetic disorders that may present in later life		Genetic predisposition
Hypophosphatasia	Disorders of alkaline phosphatase activity	
Osteogenesis imperfecta	Type I collagen defects causing brittle bones	
Osteopetrosis	Impairment of bone resorption	
Pyknodysostosis	Sclerosing bone dysplasia	

to take estrogen therapy without evidence of low bone mass.

Although densitometry provides an accurate assessment of bone mass, it does not provide information on the present rate of bone turnover. Bone-specific proteins and their metabolites can be measured in blood and urine specimens to estimate the current rates of bone formation and resorption (19). Serum procollagen peptide and osteocalcin measurements reflect bone formation, while urine pyridinoline cross-links measure collagen breakdown products that reflect bone resorption. These biochemical markers combined with bone densitometry are useful in determining which patients are at risk for osteoporosis-related fractures, such as a postmenopausal woman who

has a low baseline bone mineral density and evidence of accelerated bone turnover.

DIAGNOSTIC EVALUATION FOR OSTEOPOROSIS

Serum calcium and alkaline phosphatase levels are expected to be normal in osteoporosis but may be abnormal in other metabolic bone diseases such as hyperparathyroidism and osteopenia caused by vitamin D deficiency (20, 21). A patient who presents with osteoporosis and elevated serum calcium and alkaline phosphatase levels should be further evaluated with a serum measurement of intact molecule parathyroid hormone. The presentation of elevated alkaline phosphatase, muscle weakness, and osteoporosis in the setting of inadequate dietary intake of vitamin D or a predisposition to malabsorption should prompt an evaluation for vitamin D deficiency. It is suggested that a serum 25 vitamin D level be measured to assess the adequacy of vitamin D stores (22). Serum procollagen peptide and osteocalcin combined with the measurement of pyridinoline cross-links in a 2-hour timed urine sample provide current evidence of the rate of bone turnover.

Further diagnostic studies are recommended on the basis of the clinical presentation. For example, patients receiving thyroid supplements should be assessed for bone loss related to supraphysiologic thyroxine replacement. In this setting, a serum measurement of thyroid stimulating hormone utilizing a supersensitive assay technique is suggested. The finding of a suppressed hormone level indicates excessive replacement. Serum protein electrophoresis is appropriate in patients with elevated total protein in whom multiple myeloma is suspected. While the measurement of calcium excretion in a 24 hour collection of urine is useful, the practicality of the test often precludes its use in a geriatric patient population.

PREVENTION AND TREATMENT OF OSTEOPOROSIS

Table 31.2 summarizes preventive strategies for various patients at risk of osteoporosis. There is well-documented evidence that estrogen replacement therapy results in prevention of the accelerated bone loss attributed to the menopause. The minimum fully effective dose of oral estrogens is either 0.625 mg of conjugated equine estrogen or 1 mg 17β-estradiol per day. Alternatively, a transdermal patch may be worn continuously that administers 50 to 100 μg of 17β-estradiol per day. One study of daily low-dose estrogen, 0.3 mg conjugated equine estrogen, combined with 2 g of calcium supplementation showed efficacy of this regimen to prevent short-term bone loss (23); however, this has not been confirmed in long-term studies. In contrast, the 0.625-mg dose has been studied longitudinally with 20-year published data to support its efficacy as well as studies documenting the prevention of hip fractures (24).

Given the well-documented efficacy of estrogen in the prevention of osteoporosis, the routine use of perimenopausal hormone replacement is becoming commonplace. Controversy exists about the maximum age or length of menopausal duration at which the initiation of estrogen is of benefit. The beneficial effects of estrogens on bone have been demonstrated on patients up to age 70 years and in women with established osteoporosis (14); however, it appears that to achieve maximum benefit, estrogen replacement must begin at least at the time of cessation of menses.

Frequent side effects of estrogens in older women include breast tenderness and bloating, both of which tend to peak by 6 weeks of therapy (25). The effects of postmenopausal estrogen replacement therapy on clotting factors are not clinically significant, unlike those of oral contraceptive treatments (26). A poorly studied potential side effect of long-term estrogens is biliary stone formation associated with the changes in cholesterol metabolism resulting from the relatively high levels of estrogens achieved in the portal circulation following oral estrogen therapy. The most controversial aspect of estrogen replacement remains the potential increase in breast cancer resulting from prolonged estrogen use. To date, most studies support no significant increase in breast cancer risk in women receiving postmenopausal estrogen therapy (27).

The duration of estrogen treatment is difficult to determine, although several factors must be considered in the decision to stop estrogen treatment. First, accelerated bone loss occurs immediately following estrogen withdrawal (28). Data obtained from the Framingham Study suggest that for the long-term preservation of bone mineral density, women should take estrogen for at least 7 years after the menopause and that even this duration of therapy may have little residual effect on bone density in women 75 years of age and older (29). A further consideration for the initiation and the maintenance of long-term estrogen replacement therapy is the potential protection against cardiovascular disease in postmenopausal women (30). A practical approach is to begin hormonal therapy during the menopausal transition and to maintain therapy until long-term prevention of osteoporosis is no longer an important aspect of health care for an individual woman or a significant adverse event related to the therapy is experienced.

Progestins appear to enhance the effect of estrogen on bone (31); at the same time, the progestins appear to antagonize the effects of estrogen on the endometrium to prevent endometrial hyperplasia. Recent studies suggest that low-dose daily progestin, such as medroxyprogesterone acetate 2.5 to 5 mg daily added to daily estrogen, may improve compliance by preventing monthly vaginal bleeding. However, a significant portion of women experience unpredictable bleeding in the first 6 months of this treatment (32). An al-

Table 31.2
Patient-oriented Prevention and Treatment Strategies for Osteoporosis

Common Clinical Presentations	Suggested frequency of Diagnostic Evaluation[a]	Pharmacologic Interventions	Nonpharmacologic Interventions
Any perimenopausal woman Special emphasis if thin, smoker, sedentary, family history of fracture, early natural or surgical menopause	Yearly to biyearly if estrogn therapy is not taken	Daily estrogen combined with cycled progestin[b] (low-dose contraceptives in nonsmoker until menopausal transition is complete)	Dietary calcium and vitamin D[c] Weight bearing exercise Smoking cessation Modest alcohol and caffeine intake
Postmenopausal woman Age up to 70 years	Yearly to biyearly if estrogen therapy is not taken	Individual risk/benefit-profile of daily combined estrogen and progestin[b]	As above
Postmenopausal woman History of breast or endometrial cancer	Yearly to biyearly if tamoxifen therapy is not taken	Individual risk/benefit-profile of daily tamoxifen; antiresorptive therapies in high-risk patients[d]	As above
Symptomatic hypogonadism in an older man	Yearly to biyearly if testosterone therapy is not taken	Individual risk/benefit profile of parenteral testosterone; antiresorptive therapies in high-risk patients[d]	As above
Chronic steroid use	Yearly to biyearly to monitor bone loss	Antiresorptive therapy prophylactically[d]	As above
Osteoporosis-related fracture	Initial evaluation and yearly to monitor therapy	Antiresorptive therapy[d]	As above; physical therapy to strengthen abdominal and paraspinal muscles; fall prevention

[a]Diagnostic evaluation includes bone mineral density scan of spine and hip, routine chemistries to exclude other metabolic bone disorders, and serum/urine markers of bone turnover.
[b]Hysterectomy negates the need for progestin cotherapy.
[c]Total daily intake of calcium 1000–1500 mg/day and vitamin D 400–800 IU.
[d]FDA-approved therapy includes calcitonin; potential benefit of cyclical bisphosphonate therapy.

ternative therapy that results in predictable monthly vaginal bleeding is sequential progestin, medroxyprogesterone acetate 10 mg daily for 10 to 14 days at the beginning of each calendar month combined with daily estrogen.

In the past, progestins were added to estrogen therapy even for women who had undergone hysterectomy, under the assumption that progestins counterbalanced the effects of estrogen on breast tissue, analogous to the uterine effects. It is now known that both estrogens and progestins stimulate breast tissue growth. This effect on the breast, combined with the dose-related adverse effect on cholesterol profiles, precludes the use of progestins in women who are no longer at risk of endometrial cancer because of hysterectomy.

For women who have proven breast cancer, estrogen and progestin therapy are contraindicated. The nonsteroidal antiestrogen, tamoxifen, which is used in the treatment of breast cancer, has been shown in vitro to inhibit bone resorption and in a small clinical trial, to increase bone density (33). Tamoxifen also improves the lipid profile, yet there are potential adverse effects of therapy such as thromboembolic disease and hepatic and endometrial tumors (34). Large-scale clinical trials are under way to assess the benefits and risks of this therapy for women who have contraindications to estrogen treatment.

Anabolic steroids increase bone mass in osteoporotic women; however, their adverse effects on lipid profiles and their potential to cause hepatic dysfunction make them inadequate substitutes for estrogen therapy. Testosterone replacement increases bone loss in hypogonadal men (35); however, the benefits of this therapy may be offset in elderly men by exacerbating both prostatic hypertrophy and cardiac risk factors such as lipoprotein profiles. Studies are ongoing to establish a method of testosterone replacement that provides an overall health benefit to hypogonadal men.

In addition to gender-appropriate sex hormone replacement therapy, calcium intake is important in maintaining bone mass. It is suggested that postmenopausal women should receive between 1000 and 1500 mg of elemental calcium daily. This is roughly equivalent to four 8-ounce glasses of milk daily. As most older American women do not consume a sufficient quantity of dairy products to meet their calcium needs, calcium supplementation is recommended. The most common side effect of calcium therapy is constipation. In women with normal renal function, no monitoring of electrolytes is needed to prevent hypercalcemia. In newly postmenopausal women, high calcium intake does not confer the same degree of osteoporosis prevention as estrogen replacement therapy (36). In contrast, bone loss in elderly women whose dietary calcium intake is below 400 mg daily is retarded when calcium supplementation is provided to the level of 1000 mg daily (11).

For the treatment of established osteoporosis, calcitonin was the first drug approved by the Food and Drug Administration (FDA). While calcitonin deficiency is thought to have little impact on the development of osteoporosis, antiresorptive effects of exogenous calcitonin have been documented in patients with osteoporosis. However, the studies of calcitonin in osteoporotic patients are short-term, 1 to 2 years duration. In addition, there are no studies demonstrating the efficacy of calcitonin in preventing fractures, the current standard of efficacy for osteoporosis treatments.

The usual dose of calcitonin is 100 international units (IU) of the salmon preparation or 0.50 mg of the recombinant human form subcutaneously three times weekly. Nocturnal injections are suggested to minimize the effects of nausea and facial flushing that may be experienced as a result of either the salmon or the recombinant human preparations. An intradermal test dose of salmon calcitonin 10 IU is recommended to test for allergic response before therapy. The cost and inconvenience of subcutaneous injections are the major drawbacks to calcitonin therapy (37). Intranasal preparations are under investigation. Other more recent studies have combined calcitonin in a cyclical fashion with parathyroid hormone therapy,

to test the hypothesis that the combined therapy would stimulate bone formation and reduce resorption (38). In previous studies, calcitonin has been studied in the setting of acute vertebral compression fracture and has been shown to be more effective than placebo in the short-term management of bone pain (39).

Bisphosphonates are a class of synthetic pyrophosphate analogues that bind strongly to hydroxyapatite crystals. They are adsorbed onto newly synthesized bone matrix and prevent bone resorption through inhibition of osteoclastic activity. Bisphosphonates also inhibit bone formation, but more recent compounds inhibit bone resorption more than bone formation. Currently available drugs in this class are poorly absorbed and may cause gastrointestinal symptoms. To date, these drugs have been studied for efficacy in both the prevention of bone loss and the treatment of established osteoporosis. Short-term prevention of bone loss has been established for early postmenopausal women (40) and for patients receiving corticosteroid therapy (41).

For the treatment of established osteoporosis, pulse therapy with etidronate has been tested in placebo controlled studies. At least two studies have shown a 50% reduction in the incidence of vertebral deformity (42, 43). Based on these studies, the commonly prescribed dosage of etidronate is 400 mg daily for 14 days every three months, which is taken in place of the usual daily calcium supplementation of at least 1000 mg. It must be noted, however, that to date this therapy has not been approved by the FDA because of concerns about inadequate bone formation with extended or prolonged therapy. Newer agents in this class of drugs are being tested, which have been shown in vitro to have less deleterious effects on bone formation.

Other antiresorptive agents include calcitriol, the active metabolite of vitamin D, and thiazide diuretics. Both agents improve calcium balance; calcitriol increases gastrointestinal absorption of calcium, while thiazides decrease renal excretion of calcium. Vitamin D replacement in deficient elders reverses secondary hyperparathyroidism (44). However, the therapeutic efficacy of calcitriol or synthetic analogues of calcitriol in the treatment of osteoporosis without vitamin D deficiency is unclear. Initial therapy with low-dose calcitriol can prevent hypercalcemia and renal stones, yet inactive metabolites of vitamin D may be associated with fewer adverse effects for patients who have dietary vitamin deficiency without metabolic defects caused by renal insufficiency. Thiazide diuretic use has been associated with reduced risk of fracture (45); however, this is not a consistent observation. A randomized, placebo-controlled study is needed before thiazides can be recommended as antiresorptive therapy.

None of the above therapies stimulate bone formation, but rather they prevent bone resorption. Fluoride has been shown to stimulate osteoblast function. However, some studies of fluoride therapy have resulted in increased fracture incidence that was likely related to the dose-dependent effect of fluoride to impair mineralization of newly formed bone. Dosages of fluoride below 45 to 75 mg daily combined with 1000 mg calcium per day may offset the mineralization defects seen with higher-dose therapy (46). Other adverse effects include gastrointestinal side effects (nausea, dyspepsia, and hemorrhage) and rheumatic complaints such as tendinitis and arthralgia, including lower extremity pain syndrome caused by incomplete fractures. These have been decreased by the use of extended-release formulations and by reducing the daily dose (47).

However, one study of postmenopausal women with osteoporotic vertebral compression fractures, which used a maximum daily dose of 60 mg of enteric-coated tablets with dose reductions for adverse symptoms and serum fluoride levels above 15 μmol/L, reported that almost 40% of the subjects were intolerant of the drug within the first 18 months of treatment (48). Yet, those patients who tolerated the therapy experienced a mean increase in vertebral bone mineral density of 8.4% per year, one of the highest achievable increases in bone density documented by therapeutic agents. Similar increases in lumbar density have been achieved in a second cohort of postmenopausal osteoporotic women, accompanied by 4% per year increases in proximal femur, but 2% decreases in radial cortical bone (49). Of note, these changes persisted throughout 4 years of study. However, the most controversial aspect of fluoride treatment is the effect on fracture rates.

In summary, while fluoride has the potential to increase bone density, the potential abnormal structure and fragility of bone with excess fluoride content and the clinical side effects of fluoride preclude its use routinely in the current management of patients with osteoporosis. However, ongoing studies of fluoride may determine safe and efficacious uses for this therapy in the future.

The effect of parathyroid hormone on bone metabolism is dose-dependent. While sustained elevated circulating levels of parathyroid hormone result in osteoclast-mediated bone resorption, intermittent low-dose therapy, designed to mimic the endogenous pulsatile secretion of parathyroid hormone, has been shown to stimulate bone formation. In small groups of osteoporotic patients, sequential therapy with parathyroid hormone and calcitonin over 14 months increased trabecular vertebral bone by 12% (50). Combined therapy with calcitriol gave a similar result, but a plateau effect was reached after 12 months, followed by a decrease in mean bone mineral density. In addition, there was a concomitant decrease in cortical bone of the radius, raising concerns that prolonged therapy may result in increased fractures in appendicular bone. Current research is under way to determine the mechanism for the different responses of trabecular and cortical bone to parathyroid hormone therapy.

Other potential stimulators of bone formation include the hormones of the somatotrophic axis: growth hormone–releasing hormone, growth hormone, and insulinlike growth factor I. To date in small clinical trials, growth hormone replacement in deficient young adults increased cortical and trabecular bone density, and in healthy older men, increased lumbar bone density by 1.6% over 6 months (51). Bone-derived growth factors may prove useful to activate bone. Potential therapeutic agents include transforming growth factor β, platelet-derived growth factor, fibroblast growth factors, and bone morphogenetic proteins.

Weight-bearing exercise is important in the maintenance of bone mass (52). Immobility including bed rest or systemic illnesses can cause rapid bone loss. Exercise prescriptions for elderly patients must minimize adverse events resulting from comorbid conditions such as cardiovascular disease and degenerative joint disease. Extension and isometric exercises minimize vertebral compression in patients with severe vertebral osteopenia (53). Fall prevention is paramount in patients at risk for fractures because of severe osteoporosis. Other important behavioral interventions include smoking cessation and judicious alcohol and caffeine intake. Pain management of muscle spasms and the mechanical deformities of severe kyphosis include heat, massage, physical therapies, and analgesics.

In summary, osteoporosis is a common bone disorder, particularly of older women, with significant morbidity and mortality resulting from spinal deformity and hip fractures. Preventive strategies include adequate lifetime calcium intake and exercise, and postmenopausal hormone replacement. Treatment for osteoporosis is less well established, with each therapy posing potential difficulties including cost, side effects, and lack of long-term efficacy.

OSTEOMALACIA

Vitamin D deficiency in the elderly can result in deep bone and muscle pain, muscle weakness, hyperesthesia, and fractures related to osteopenia and osteoporosis. The elderly are susceptible to vitamin D deficiency for several reasons. Less vitamin D is manufactured through the skin because aged skin has less precursor and converts these precursors more slowly. In addition, lotions and creams are applied topically to prevent skin cancer. These lotions effectively filter out the UV light needed for the conversion of vitamin D precursors in the skin. Frail elderly are often physically unable to venture outdoors, and window glass effectively filters out the UV light. Restrictions of high-cholesterol foods, including dairy products and organ meats, result in insufficient dietary sources of vitamin D precursors. In addition, medications such as phenytoin may interfere with vitamin D metabolism. Studies of homebound elderly suggest that the RDA for vitamin D of 200 IU may be insufficient to prevent osteomalacia and that vitamin D supplementation of 400 IU per day of ergocalciferol is needed in this population (22).

HYPERPARATHYROIDISM

Primary hyperparathyroidism is characterized by excessive production of parathyroid hormone, which leads to hypercalcemia via two mechanisms: (a) osteoclast-mediated bone resorption and (b) calcium conservation at the level of the renal glomerulus. The recognized prevalence of mild forms of this condition has increased since the automation of serum chemistry analyzers and the routine use of blood work in medical evaluations. The incidence of hyperparathyroidism in men over the age of 60 years is one new case per 1000 of population per year, with twice this frequency for women of similar age (54). Thus, this is a condition that primarily affects postmenopausal women. The disease course can vary in severity from the benign presentation of asymptomatic abnormal serum chemistries to a constellation of clinically relevant adverse events including constipation, hypertension, accelerated bone loss, peptic ulcer disease, pancreatitis, nephrocalcinosis, nephrolithiasis, and renal insufficiency. Added to this list are varied psychiatric symptoms including anxiety, depression, and cognitive impairment.

The diagnosis of hyperparathyroidism is considered when an elevation in serum calcium level is accompanied by a decreased or low normal serum phosphate level. Serum alkaline phosphatase may be either minimally or more strikingly elevated. Urinary calcium excretion is less than 250 mg/g Cr, while urinary cyclic AMP is typically elevated.

There are multiple radioimmunoassays for the measurement of serum parathyroid hormone levels. Assays that measure intact molecule, aminoterminal fragments, or midmolecule are recommended to confirm the diagnosis; measurements of carboxy-terminal fragments can give false elevations in the setting of renal insufficiency. Hypercalcemia accompanied by suppressed parathyroid hormone levels suggests either a malignancy or sarcoidosis, depending on the associated clinical findings. The measurement of parathyroid hormone–related protein may be clinically useful when an underlying malignancy is not identifiable, although currently this assay is not widely available.

The radiographic findings, like the severity of the condition, are varied in hyperparathyroidism, ranging from diffuse osteopenia to more specific radiographic signs. The latter include extensive cortical bone resorption such as subperiosteal resorption of the radial aspect of the second and third phalanges, the distal clavicles, and the skull, which gives a salt and pepper appearance. In both cortical and trabecular bone, deep burrows resulting from resorption may be filled by fibrous tissue, giving a cystic appearance to the bone, termed osteitis fibrosa cystica. Bone tissue replaced by highly vascularized fibrous tissue, called brown tumors, may be misinterpreted as giant cell tumors of bone. Bone densitometry typically reflects more extensive involvement of cortical bone over trabecular bone, resulting in greater reductions in bone mineral density of the radius and hip than of the lumbar spine.

Definitive therapy for hyperparathyroidism is surgical resection of the adenoma; however the indications for surgery in older patients are controversial. Probable indications for surgery include low bone mass (greater than 2 to 2.5 standard deviations below mean for age as assessed by densitometry), recurrent renal calculi, and pancreatitis (20). Hypercalcemia greater than 12 mg/dL, osteitis fibrosa, reduced and falling bone mass, and refractory ulcer disease are also targeted for surgical correction. Based on this strategy for surgical referrals, the appropriate evaluation should include a bone mineral density scan to assess for osteopenia. Hypertension, hypercalcemia less than 12 mg/dL, and psychiatric symptoms are thought not to be indications for surgical resection. It must be noted, however, that others have reported that the psychiatric symptoms may be amenable to surgical correction. Also in question is the issue of a surgically correctable improvement in renal function in a patient with reduced creatinine clearance but with no prior history of renal calculi. The overall health status of the patient must be assessed in the decision for surgery, including the relative impact of the consequences of hyperparathyroidism on function as compared with comorbid conditions.

Mild forms of the disease can be managed with estrogen replacement therapy in postmenopausal women. Daily doses of conjugated equine estrogen of 1.25 mg and ethinyl estradiol 50 μg have been shown to arrest accelerated bone turnover in postmenopausal women with hyperparathyroidism.

PAGET'S DISEASE

Osteitis deformans was well described by Sir James Paget in 1877. The condition is common in older adults; studies have shown prevalence data ranging from 1 to 3% in areas of the United States to 10 to 15% of elderly Europeans, with a male to female ratio of 3 to 2. The condition is characterized by focal areas of active bone turnover, which include both increased osteoclast-mediated resorption and excessive bone formation. The diseased bone is deformed, with thickened cortices and coarse trabeculations resulting in painful skeletal deformity, fragility, and fractures (55). The most commonly affected sites include the femur, spine, pelvis, humerus, tibia, cranium, and sternum. Clinical symptoms range from bone pain, skeletal deformity, changes in skin temperature overlying areas of active bony involvement, pathologic fractures, and nerve compression syndromes, particularly of the thoracic and lumbar spine.

Degenerative joint disease is common in the joints adjoining affected weight-bearing bones. Complications include cranial nerve compression syndromes from basilar invagination, hearing loss related to alterations in the acoustical properties of bone, and alterations in blood flow related to metabolically active areas of bony involvement. Osteosarcomas, fibrosarcomas, and benign giant cell tumors develop in 2 to 4% of patients with symptomatic Paget's disease. The pathogenesis of Paget's disease is unknown, but it is hypothesized that the condition is a late manifestation of an earlier paramyxoviral infection such as measles, respiratory syncytial, or canine distemper viruses. However, the viral-type inclusions identified on an ultrastructural level are not specific to Paget's disease.

It is estimated that perhaps 10 to 20% of patients with Paget's disease are asymptomatic and are diagnosed as a result of abnormal serum chemistries and radiographs performed for unrelated problems (56). Serum levels of alkaline phosphatase and osteocalcin levels are abnormal, particularly when bone formation is markedly increased. A second voided urine sample obtained following overnight fast should yield an elevation in the ratio of hydroxyproline to creatinine, particularly when bone resorption is markedly increased. Radiographic findings include cortical thickening and a mixture of lytic and sclerotic changes, although either presentation may predominate. Lytic areas of the skull are referred to as osteoporosis circumscripta. Transverse lucencies of long bones, called pseudofractures, may progress to frank fractures. Nuclear bone scans using technetium-labeled polyphosphonate or diphosphonate scanning often reveal additional areas of asymptomatic or radiographically undetectable involvement.

Clinically, the radiographic changes of Paget's disease can be difficult to distinguish from those seen in metastatic prostate or breast cancer. The advent of serum markers such as prostate-specific antigen may help in the diagnosis; however, as both metastatic malignancy and Paget's are relatively common conditions in the elderly, they may coexist. Computerized tomography may be helpful, with pagetoid lesions demonstrating bony expansion adjacent to areas of resorption. At times, a therapeutic trial is performed as a first line of treatment, as biopsy confirmation of questionable lesions can be technically difficult and may require an open biopsy technique rather than a less invasive percutaneous approach.

The treatment of the asymptomatic patient is controversial. Treatment strategies range from no treatment other than baseline assessment of the extent of skeletal involvement with nuclear imaging to the treatment of asymptomatic patients with either active metabolic disease, as suggested by elevations of alkaline phosphatase levels to more than twice normal, or with involvement of the weight-bearing joints of the legs and spine to prevent bowing deformities. Pain syndromes must be carefully evaluated for potential nerve entrapment and joint manifestations, which may require management in addition to the treatment of the bone pain of Paget's disease.

Calcitonin therapy is effective in reducing osteoclast-mediated bone resorption in Paget's disease. It is recommended that an initial daily dose of 25 to 50 IU of salmon or 0.25 mg human calcitonin be given nightly with an incremental increase in dose every 1 to 2 weeks until a clinical response is observed, with usual maintenance doses of 100 IU salmon and 0.50 mg human calcitonin (55). In the treatment of a pseudofracture, this dose is maintained until there is radiographic evidence of fracture healing and a reduction in the serum alkaline phosphatase level, at which time a dose reduction to 50 IU units per day then three times weekly is suggested (56).

Bisphosphonates are effective in reducing bone resorption and have the advantage of oral therapy. Etidronate dosing is 5 to 10 mg per kilogram per day. However, etidronate therapy should be limited to 6 months at a time because of adverse effects on bone mineralization. For this reason, bisphosphonates are not recommended in the setting of acute fracture or immediately following orthopaedic surgery. Calcium supplementation is suggested to improve mineralization. Combination calcitonin therapy for 6 weeks, followed by low-dose daily etidronate, 5 mg per kilogram for 6 months, has been suggested (56). Relapses are treated in a similar fashion. Alternatively, pulse therapy with high-dose etidronate 20 mg per kilogram per day may be beneficial when given monthly every 4 months. The more recently developed bisphosphonates such as pamidronate appear to have no clinically significant effects on bone mineralization and may prove with further testing to be viable options for long-term therapy.

It should be noted that 15% of patients experience an exacerbation in pain during the first 1 to 3 months, with marked increases in alkaline phosphatase levels and osteolytic progression noted on radiography. In this setting, calcitonin should be substituted for bisphosphonate therapy. The chemotherapeutic agent mithramycin, while providing a rapid response, is reserved for the patient with impending paraplegia or one whose disease no longer responds to the standard therapies. Gallium nitrate is being tested for its effects on osteoclast activity.

Regardless of the therapy, monitoring serum alkaline phosphatase levels and clinical symptoms is useful. Assessments are recommended monthly for the first 3 months, with serial testing determined by the clinical response and treatment plan. Serial radiographs of areas of active disease targeted for treatment are also useful. Bone scanning is not useful during bisphosphonate therapy.

REFERENCES

1. Riggs BL, Melton LJ III. The prevention and treatment of osteoporosis. N Engl J Med 1992;327:620–627.
2. Chrischilles EA, Butler D, Davis CS. A model of lifetime osteoporosis impact. Arch Intern Med 1991; 151:2026–2032.
3. Cummings SR, Kelsey JL, Nevitt, et al. Epidemiology of osteoporosis and osteoporotic fractures. Epidemiol Rev 1985;7:178–208.
4. Christiansen C. Consensus development conference: prophylaxis and treatment of osteoporosis. Am J Med 1991;90:107–110.
5. Matkovic V, Fontana D, Tominac C, et al. Factors that influence peak bone formation: a study of calcium balance and the heritance of bone mass in adolescent females. Am J Clin Nutr 1990;52:878–888.
6. Sowers MR, Clark MK, Hollis B, et al. Radial bone mineral density in pre- and perimenopausal women: a prospective study of rates and risk factors for loss. J Bone Miner Res 1992;7:647–657.
7. Johnston CC, Hui SL, Witt RM, et al. Early menopausal changes in bone mass and sex steroids. J Clin Endocrinol Metab 1985;61:905–911.
8. Geusens P, Dequeker J, Verstraeten A, et al. Age-, sex-, and menopause-related changes of vertebral and peripheral bone: population study using dual and single photon absorptiometry and radiogrammetry. J Nucl Med 1986;27:1540–1549.
9. Seeman E, Melton II LJ, O'Fallon WM, Riggs BL. Risk factors for spinal osteoporosis in men. Am J Med 1983;75:977–983.
10. Seiger P, Cummings ST, Black DM, et al. Age-related decrements in bone mineral density in women over 65. J Bone Miner Res 1992;7:625–632.
11. Dawson-Hughes B, Dallal GE, Kall EA, et al. A controlled trial of the effect of calcium supplementation on bone density in postmenopausal women. N Engl J Med 1990;323:878–883.
12. Tilyard MW, Spars GFS, Thomson J, Dovey S. Treatment of postmenopausal osteoporosis with calcitriol or calcium. N Engl J Med 1992;326:357–362.
13. Pocock NA, Eisman JA, Gwinn TH, et al. Muscle strength, physical fitness and weight but not age predict femoral neck bone mass. J Bone Miner Res 1989;4:441–447.
14. Lufkin EG, Wahner HW, O'Fallon WM, et al. Treatment of postmenopausal osteoporosis with transdermal estrogen. Ann Intern Med 1992;117:1–9.
15. Corpas E, Harman SM, Blackman MR. Human growth hormone and human aging. Endocr Rev 14:20–39.
16. Black DM, Cummings SR, Genant HK, et al. Axial and appendicular bone density predict fractures in older women. J Bone Miner Res 1992;7:633–638.
17. Mazess RB, Barden H, Ettinger M, Schultz E. Bone density of the radius, spine, and proximal femur in osteoporosis. J Bone Miner Res 1988;3:13–17.
18. Rubin SM, Cummings SR. Results of bone densitometry affect women's decisions about taking measures to prevent fractures. Ann Intern Med 1992;116:990–995.
19. Gunberg CM, Lian JB, Gallop PM, et al. Urinary γ-carboxyglutamic acid and serum osteocalcin as bone markers; studies in osteoporosis and Paget's disease. J Clin Endocrinol Metab 1983;57:1221–1225.
20. Potts JT. Management of asymptomatic hyperparathyroidism. J Clin Endocrinol Metab 1990;70:1489–1493.
21. Demaux BB, Arlot ME, Chapuy MC. Serum osteocalcin is increased in patients with osteomalacia: correlations with biochemical and histomorphometric findings. J Clin Endocrinol Metab 1992;74:1146–1151.

22. Gloth FM, Tobin JD, Sherman SS, et al. Is the recommended daily allowance for vitamin D too low for the homebound elderly? J Am Geriatr Soc 1991; 39:137–141.

23. Ettinger B, Genant H, et al. Postmenopausal bone loss is prevented by treatment with low-dosage estrogen with calcium. Ann Intern Med 1987;106:40–45.

24. Nachtigall LE, Nachtigall MJ. Hormone replacement therapy. Obstet Gynecol 1992;4(6):907–913.

25. Bellantoni MF, Harman SM, Cullins VE, et al. Transdermal estradiol with oral progestin: biological and clinical effects in younger and older postmenopausal women. J Gerontol 1991;46:M216–222.

26. Chetkowski RJ, Meldrum DR, Steingold KA, et al. Biologic effects of transdermal estradiol. N Engl J Med 1986;314:1615–1620.

27. Henrich JB. The postmenopausal estrogen/breast cancer controversy. JAMA 1992;268:1900–1902.

28. Christiansen C, Christiansen MS, Transbol I. Bone mass in postmenopausal women after withdrawal of oestrogen/gestagen replacement therapy. Lancet 1981;1:459–461.

29. Felson DT, Zhang Y, Hannan MT. The effect of postmenopausal estrogen therapy on bone density in elderly women. N Engl J Med 1993;329:1141–1146.

30. Barrett-Connor E, Bush TL. Estrogen and coronary heart disese in women. JAMA 1991;265:1861–1867.

31. Gallagher JC, Kable WT, Goldgar D. Effect of progestin therapy on cortical and trabecular bone: comparison with estrogen. Am J Med 1991;90:171–178.

32. Weinstein L, Bewtra C, Gallagher JC. Evaluation of a continuous combined low-dose regimen of estrogen-progestin for treatment of the menopausal patient. Am J Obstet Gynecol 1990;162(6):1534–1542.

33. Fornander T, Rutqvist LE, Sjoberg, et al. Long-term adjuvant tamoxifen in early breast cancer: effect on bone mineral density in postmenopausal women. J Clin Oncol 1990;8:1019–1024.

34. DeGregoriao MW. Is tamoxifen chemoprevention worth the risk in healthy women? J NIH Res 1992; 4:84–87.

35. Finkelstein JS, Klibanski A, Neer RM, et al. Increases in bone density during treatment of men with idiopathic hypogonadotropic hypogonadism. J Clin Endocrinol Metab 1989;69:776–783.

36. Riis B, Thomsen K, Christiansen C. Does calcium supplementation prevent postmenopausal bone loss? A double-blind, controlled clinical study. N Engl J Med 1987;316:173–177.

37. McDermott MT, Kidd GS. The role of calcitonin in the development and treatment of osteoporosis. Endocr Rev 1987;8:377–390.

38. Hodsman AB, Fraher LJ, Ostbye T, et al. An evaluation of several biochemical markers for bone formation and resorption in a protocol utilizing cyclical parathyroid hormone and calcitonin therapy for osteoporosis. J Clin Invest 1993;91:1138–1148.

39. Lyritis GP, Tsakalakos N, Magiasis B, et al. Analgesic effect of salmon calcitonin in osteoporotic vertebral fractures: a double-blind placebo-controlled clinical study. Calcif Tissue Int 1991;49:369–372.

40. Reginster JY, Lecart MP, Deroisy R, et al. Prevention of postmenopausal bone loss by tiludronate. Lancet 1989;2:1469–1471.

41. Reid IR, King AR, Alexander CJ, Ibbertson HK. Prevention of steroid-induced osteoporosis with (3-amino-1-hydroxyroprylidene)-1,1-bisphosphonate (APD). Lancet 1988;1:143–146.

42. Watts NB, Harris ST, Genant HK, et al. Intermittent cyclical etidronate treatment of postmenopausal osteoporosis. N Engl J Med 1990;323:73–79.

43. Storm T, Thamsborg G, Steiniche T, et al. Effect of intermittent cyclical etidronate therapy on bone mass and fracture rate in women with postmenopausal osteoporosis. N Engl J Med 1990;322:1265–1271.

44. Perry HM, Miiler DK, Morley JE, et al. A preliminary report of vitamin D and calcium metabolism in older African Americans. J Am Geriatr Soc 1993;41:612–616.

45. LaCroix AZ, Wienpahl J, White LR, et al. Thiazide diuretic agents and the incidence of hip fracture. N Engl J Med 1990;322:286–290.

46. Kleerekoper M, Balena R. Fluorides and osteoporosis. Annu Rev Nutr 1991;11:309–324.

47. Pak CYC, Sakhaee K, Zerwekh JE, et al. Safe and effective treatment of osteoporosis with intermittent slow release sodium fluoride: augmentation of vertebral bone mass and inhibition of fractures. J Clin Endocrinol Metab 1989;68:150–159.

48. Hodsman AB, Drost DJ. The response of vertebral bone mineral density during the treatment of osteoporosis with sodium fluoride. J Clin Endocrinol Metab 1989;69:932–938.

49. Riggs BL, Hodgson SF, O'Fallon WM, et al. Effect of fluoride treatment on the fracture rate in postmenopausal women with osteoporosis. N Engl J Med 1990;322:802–809.

50. Hesch RD, Rittinghaus EF, Harms HM, Delling G. Die fruhtherapie der osteoporose mit (1–38) parathormon und calcitonin-nasal spray. Med Klin 1989;84:488–498.

51. Rudman D, Feller AG, Nagraj HS, et al. Effects of human growth hormone in men over 60 years old. N Engl J Med 1990;323(1):1–5.

52. Prince RL, Smith M, Dick IM, et al. Prevention of postmenopausal osteoporosis: a comparative study of exercise, calcium supplementation, and hormone replacement therapy. N Engl J Med 1991;325:1189–1195.

53. Sinaki M, Mikkelsen BA. Postmenopausal spinal osteoporosis: flexion versus extension exercises. Arch Phys Med Rehabil 1983;65:593–596.

54. Heath H, Hodgson SF, Kennedy MA. Primary hyperparathyroidism, incidence, morbidity, and potential economic impact in a community. N Engl J Med 1980;302:189–193.

55. Bone HG, Kleerekoper M. Paget's disease of bone. J Clin Endocrinol Metab 1992;75:1179–1185.

56. Merkow RL, Lane JM. Paget's disease of the bone. Endocrinol Metab Clin North Am 1990;19:177–203.

32/ Musculoskeletal Injuries in the Elderly

John C. Gordon

Discussion of musculoskeletal injuries in elderly persons is not an isolated listing of cause, effect, and treatment. Such injuries evoke different responses in different age groups. The location and severity of injury, the quality of bone and soft tissues, and the healing process combine to dictate the recovery rate of an individual patient. Conditions such as deafness, blindness, impaired mental status, cardiovascular abnormalities, and use of multiple medications may significantly affect treatment and rehabilitation. Progress and prognosis of orthopaedic injury in the older patient is very different from that in the younger individual.

Aging itself makes the elderly patient different. As adults grow older, there are physical and psychological alterations that affect function. Muscle fibers decrease in number and become atrophic. Slight flexion contractures of joints occur. Density of bone is decreased by demineralization, resulting in osteoporosis. Collagen, which comprises 40% of the body's protein, thickens and becomes less elastic and mobile, which, in turn, affects the mobility and recovery capability of the skin, bone, cartilage, muscle, and joint surfaces. Changes in bone density and blood supply also affect the healing response in an elderly patient.

Effects of injury on attitude and independence of the elderly patient must be assessed and treated, when possible, as must any disability from other medical and physical causes. Skeletal injury complicates and upsets an elderly person's already delicate balance of living and may worsen medical problems already present (1, 2). Injury may force patients into health care systems they have avoided. Patients may equate hospitalization with dying, and injury with loss of independence. They may try to recover that independence by minimizing problems and trying to avoid or shorten hospitalization. A practitioner must provide straightforward explanation, a positive yet realistic attitude, and much reassurance.

Ideal goals of orthopaedic treatment are restoration of preinjury function and prevention of further injury. Even these modest goals may be elusive in the elderly, and extensive counseling for the patient and the family is necessary. One should not promise a restoration of normal function after injury if it was initially compromised by arthritis or other disease. Bones are thin, tissues are stiff, and recovery is slow in the elderly. Early rehabilitation is extremely important, both for restoring and for maintaining the patient's physical independence. Prevention of further injury involves more than just "fixing" a fracture. Hospital discharge and postinjury planning is crucial. Home health aids, Meals on Wheels, visiting nurses, home therapists, and others are used to ease the transition and to speed acclimation at home. Home evaluation surveys to prevent recurrent or aggravating injuries are helpful, noting the need for wheelchairs, canes, bedside commodes, bathroom and stairway railings, and removal of scatter rugs (3, 5).

INTERVIEW

When an elderly patient is seen in the office setting, the chief complaint is often pain, but may also include deformity, spasm, or joint stiffness. Reduction of function may cause frustration and resentment of a process over which the individual has little or no control. Resentment and/or the fear of lost independence may make an older person nervous and difficult to treat.

Extra gentleness and reassurance must be a part of every interview. The physician must not rush in or out, or leave the patient alone in the examination room for a long time. A hurried interview will make any patient more agitated and apprehensive. During history-taking, gently turning, touching, or massaging the injured area will often put the patient at ease and facilitate physical examination. It is necessary to explain the problems and proposed treatment in layman's terms. Patients do not remember all that the physician says and will remember even less if explanations are in complicated medical terms. Written instructions coupled with practical demonstrations are necessary to enable the older patient to carry out the recommended exercises. Instructions from a staff member or practical teaching by a physical therapist are helpful. In prescribing exercises, therapy, or medication for a certain injury, the physician must remain aware of the person as a whole, including previous injuries, past and present medical history, present medication, economic issues, psychosocial factors, and nutritional status.

The emergency room setting only exacerbates the anxiety and agitation patients may feel. Often, they have been waiting for hours before the x-rays are taken, the diagnosis is made, and the specialist has arrived. A few extra minutes to reassure the patient and allay anxieties is time well spent and may facilitate the examination.

REHABILITATION

Rehabilitation attempts to return the patient to a preinjury level of functioning. Careful assessment must be made of the nature of injury or surgery and the potential of each patient. Rehabilitation programs must begin immediately and be directed toward the whole patient. A hip fracture may necessitate nonweightbearing for 1 to 3 months, during which time independent mobility may be lost because of lack of upper body strength, instability of Parkinsonism, fear of falling, etc. Special problems affecting rehabilitation potential must be addressed preoperatively, if possible. Exercise programs and walker instructions are very beneficial before elective lower extremity surgery.

Rehabilitation goals must be reassessed periodically while the patient is healing. It is important when treating the elderly to tailor a rehabilitation program to the individual patient and not order cookbook programs applicable to a younger patient. Reassurance, periodic evaluations, home visits by physical therapists and social service workers, and assessment of family or friend support systems are necessary. Fear, uncertainty, and even hostility may prevent a patient from following any rehabilitation program. Impaired mental status, deafness, and blindness may hamper a patient's progress, as may pulmonary or cardiovascular diseases.

HEALING FACTORS

Bone density and strength decrease with age. Osteoporosis and osteomalacia are common in the elderly and seem to be a function of increased bone resorption rather than of decreased bone for-

mation (6). Calcium and protein intake and absorption are being studied as potential causes of loss of bone density, as well as effects of estrogens, exercise, and dieting in weight control. It is certain that the loss of mineral bone density in the elderly has multiple causes. With decreased density and strength, bones are more easily fractured by falls and minor trauma. This fact, combined with the decreased mobility and stability of the elderly, partially explains the high incidence of fractures and deformities in this age group. However, the elderly are quite capable of healing their fractures and do so with rapidity and voluminous callus. Unfortunately, the elderly are often osteoporotic before fracture and have bones already at risk. Immobilization and reduced activity secondary to fracture cause more osteoporosis and increase subsequent risk. Pain in the fracture area may increase both elements. Therefore, while the elderly may heal the fracture well, the underlying weak bone may require longer protection and more graduated rehabilitation than in a younger person.

TOTAL JOINT REPLACEMENT

As the older population increases, the effects of trauma, medical conditions, and normal wear and tear on joints are more pronounced. Many older persons are candidates for the pain relief and functional improvement afforded by total joint replacement (Fig. 32.1, A and B).

Total joint replacements traditionally last 5 to 15 years before needing replacement, depending on the joint replaced, the activity and weight of the patient, and the strength of the bone-cement-metal fixation. The patient is cautioned against having unrealistic expectations, such as complete restoration of former activity levels and lifestyle. Pain is the major reason for replacement, not the restoration of normal movements nor the ability to play a certain sport or, for example, to jog. Middle-aged to elderly patients with restricted motion but no pain are better advised to wait until pain is a significant factor and interferes with their lifestyle and well-being before considering total joint replacement, other medical factors being equal.

While total hip replacement is an appropriate treatment for some acute femoral neck fractures, a cemented endoprosthesis is preferable in most cases. It provides good stability, less postoperative pain, and easy conversion to a total hip replacement if necessary. Endoprosthetic replacement entails considerably less surgery and reduces the incidence of the complications of em-

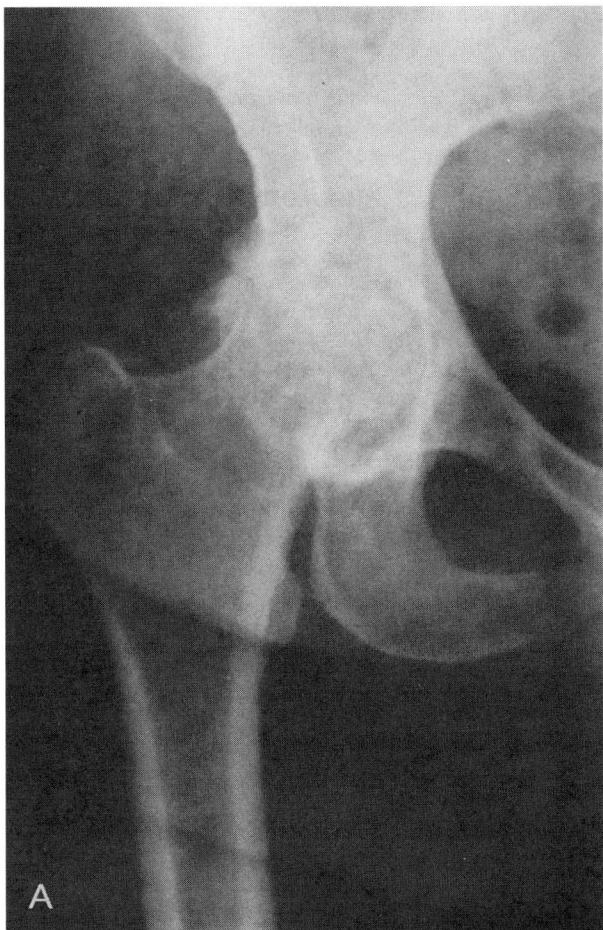
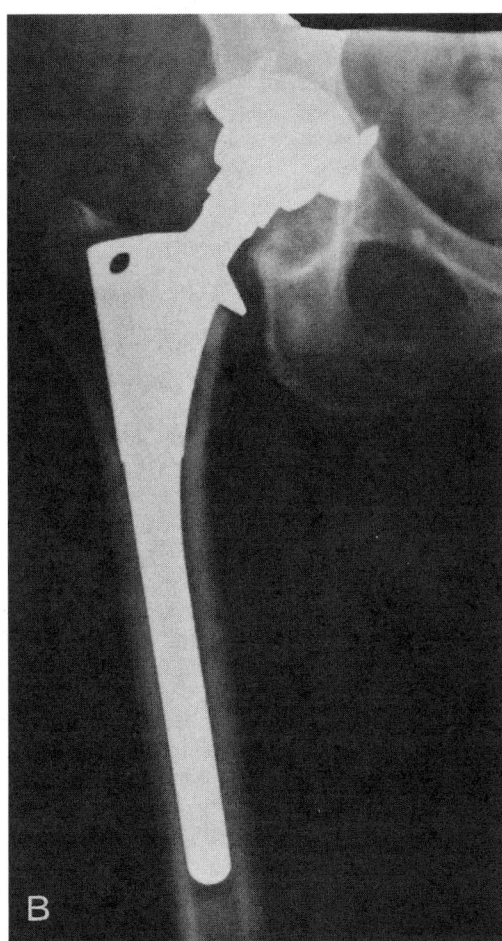

Figure 32.1. **A**, Severe degenerative joint disease of hip; cartilage has been eroded, joint is nearly ankylosed, and pain is severe. **B**, Postoperative total hip replacement; function and length have been restored and patient now walks without pain.

bolism, infection, and heterotopic bone formation. The morbidity and mortality rates of total hip replacements were twice as great as in endoprosthetic replacements in the acute fracture. With better techniques, anesthesia, and equipment, this ratio has been reduced, but a statistical difference still exists.

Today's state-of-the-art in joint replacement is quite good in total hips and good in total knees. Total shoulder replacement will relieve pain but all types compromise motion and strength to some degree. Total elbows, ankles, and wrists are salvage procedures at present and have been disappointing in long-term follow-ups. Finger joint replacement for rheumatoid arthritis and other medical and traumatic joint diseases has been quite good. The strength is less, the range of motion is moderate, but pain is relieved. Technical

advancements continue to improve motion, pain relief, and compatibility of joint replacements.

UPPER EXTREMITY INJURIES

The principal purpose of the upper extremity is functional placement of the hand. Impaired mobility of the shoulder, elbow, or wrist can be compensated by the remaining two joints. Proper positioning and/or maintenance of a functional range of motion of the wrist, elbow, or shoulder after injury will prevent disability of the hand. Sufficient strength and range of motion are usually regained, allowing satisfactory function, but special attention to the adjacent uninjured joints is important in preventing stiffness, such as frozen shoulder. Reflex sympathetic dystrophy (persistent vascular spasm) can occur and require aggressive physical therapy, nonsteroidal antiinflammatory drugs (NSAIDs), and sometimes sympathetic nerve blocks. Constant motion of the extremity, elevation and compression to reduce edema, and the use of appropriate analgesics and NSAIDs can generally relieve these conditions. The physical function of the elderly may be restricted before the injury. Previous injury, arthritic deformity of the fingers, flexion contractures of the elbow and decreased strength of the arm and hand, etc. must all be assessed by history and compared with the present evaluation. This will give a general direction to the goals of rehabilitation.

SHOULDER PAIN

Shoulder pain (Fig. 32.2) can be confusing to the examiner. Potential causes in the elderly include minor or major trauma, strains or overuse syndromes, arthritic changes, and degenerative changes secondary to medical disease. Soft tissue pain must be differentiated from degenerative joint pain and those from metastatic disease by the history and physical, x-rays, bone scan, etc. Subacromial bursitis, biceps tendinitis, adhesive capsulitis, and rotator cuff tears can mimic one another, cause significant pain and disability, and may be refractory to treatment.

Subacromial bursitis is caused by pinching and recurrent compression of the bursa between the edge of the acromion on one side and the rotator cuff and humeral head on the other. The patient has pain on attempted abduction of the arm against resistance and on direct palpation of the bursa.

Biceps tendinitis results from an irritation of the long head of the biceps tendon in the bicipital groove from trauma or degenerative disease. It causes significant pain in the region of the insertion of the pectoralis major, especially when the patient is trying to do overhead work. The patient avoids lifting heavy objects and tries to keep the arm by the side with the elbow flexed. Abduction is painful, and other movements of the shoulder are limited. To test for biceps tendinitis, have the patient pronate the forearm and flex the elbow to 90°. Grasp the patient's wrist and ask the patient to supinate against resistance. When pain is localized to the anteromedial aspect of the shoulder, Yergason's sign for biceps tendinitis is positive.

Selective injection of Xylocaine into the bursa or along the tendon with resultant relief of pain will often distinguish one from the other. Ice, rest, NSAIDs, physical therapy, and a sling for support while the irritation subsides are helpful. Physical therapy usually includes heat and phonophoresis (ultrasound with steroid cream). Recurrences are not uncommon but may respond well to steroid injection and/or the above therapies.

Adhesive capsulitis is a progressive and painful tightening of the shoulder joint that restricts motion in all directions. Fifty percent of cases have a traumatic history, whereas the rest have no specific inciting incident. As motion becomes more painful, patients self-limit their movement, setting up a vicious circle of pain and decreased motion. Eventually the process will completely reverse, but this takes 2 to 3 years. The diagnosis is made by history and restricted movement in all directions. Treatment is aggressive physical therapy, NSAIDs, and reassurance for 1 to 6 months. Shoulders that are not responding to treatment within 4 to 10 weeks and are constantly painful may require closed manipulation under general anesthesia to break up the adhesions. This will usually start the patient on the road to recovery over 1 to 3 months.

Recent research divides adhesive capsulitis into types 1, 2, and 3. Types 1 and 2 seem to respond well to arthroscopic synovectomy.

Type 1: restricted motion abnormal but not grossly inflamed or boggy synovium
Type 2: restricted with inflamed synovium
Type 3: restricted but synovium has burned-out look (5)

Rotator cuff tears in the older population are usually extensive, happen with minimal trauma, and result from chronic irritation and thinning of the avascular area of the supraspinatus tendon under the acromion. The size of the tear and the activities of the patient will dictate how much disability ensues. Common problems are inability to work overhead and to abduct the arm with any strength. Pain is variable and located just below the acromion process. In a complete rupture, active abduction above 40° is impossible, passive abduction is full and usually painless, and once positioned, the arm can be held in a vertical position by deltoid contraction (abduction paradox). In partial ruptures of the supraspinatus, active and passive abduction are usually abandoned because of pain located at the insertion of the deltoid muscle that often radiates down the lateral aspect of the arm. It occasionally travels down the dorsal forearm as far as the wrist.

Many older patients are able to adapt their lifestyles and activities to limited motion and strength below shoulder level. Those with chronic pain and significant loss of motion may require

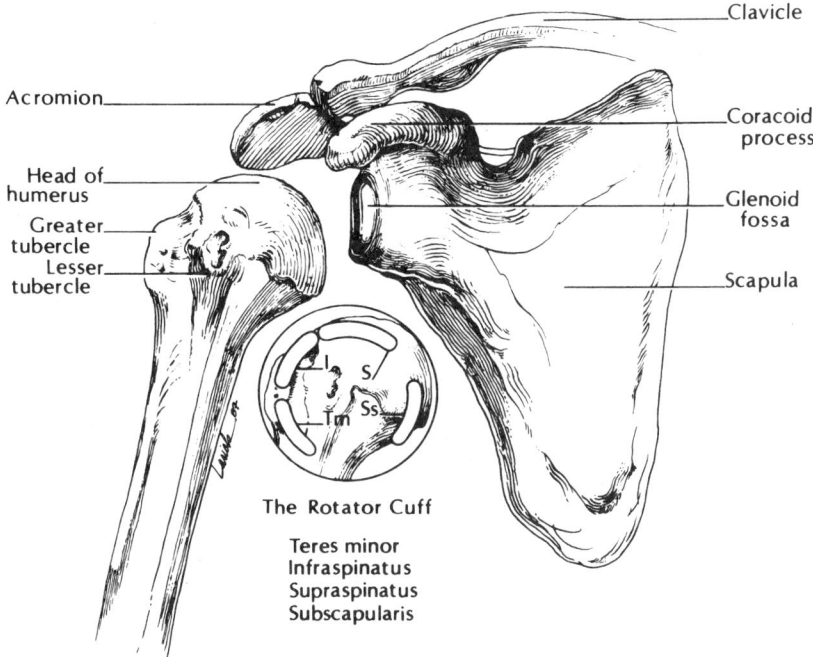

Figure 32.2. Bony anatomy of the shoulder joint, anterior view.

decompressive acromioplasty and/or a rotator cuff repair. The results vary with the size of the tear and the quality of the tissues used in the repair. Full function is usually not regained in the older patient, but a painless and moderately functioning shoulder is possible.

Occurring primarily in middle-aged and older men, "Popeye" muscle deformities are caused by rupture of the long head of the biceps tendon just below the humeral head or at the radial attachment (Fig. 32.3). They are accompanied by a sharp pain in the upper arm and result in mild-to-moderate edema and ecchymosis. It is common for the elderly patient to appear at the doctor's office weeks or months after injury, wondering about the "bump" in the arm, but without complaining of any functional loss. Operative repair is rarely warranted and is only indicated in the first 2 to 3 weeks, after which scarring precludes an acceptable result. Even without surgical repair, the patient usually regains 90% of strength and a full functional range of motion with only a minor cosmetic deformity.

Thoracic outlet syndromes must be considered in the differential diagnosis of shoulder pain. Subclavian vessel and brachial plexus compression with certain positions of the upper extremity may cause weakness and aching. It is more common in middle-aged patients. Frequent causes of compression are scalene muscles, cervical ribs, and di-

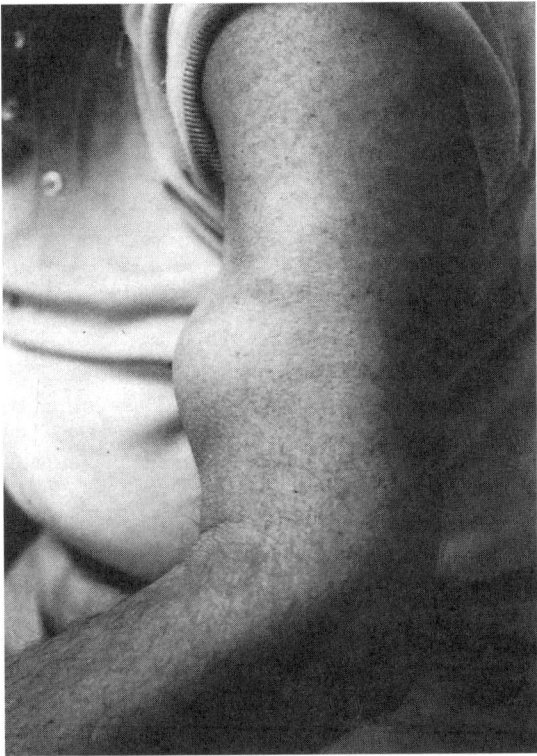

Figure 32.3. "Popeye" muscle. The tendon of the long head of the biceps is ruptured at the shoulder. Attempts at flexing the biceps caused the muscle to contract into a ball.

rect trauma to the base of the neck. Various degrees of sensory and/or vascular abnormalities can occur in the affected extremity. Treatment is directed at relieving the offending pressure.

Differential diagnosis of shoulder pain must rule out neoplastic disease such as an apical lung neoplasm with either pain from the tumor itself extending to the arm or metastatic lesions from breast or prostate. Pain and/or swelling and the absence of trauma must raise the suspicion of neoplasm. X-rays revealing pathologic fracture or bone-destroying lesions confirm this suspicion. Definitive diagnosis is established on biopsy. Internal fixation to prevent pathologic fractures or to stabilize an existing fracture provides good palliation and comfort.

HUMERAL HEAD AND NECK FRACTURES

Humeral head and neck fractures are common in the elderly (Fig. 32.4). Bone in these areas lacks strength and is unable to withstand a fall on the outstretched arm. Impacted fractures are usually stable, are minimally displaced, and may not be comminuted. Pain is not prolonged. Exercises are begun early, and the overall result is good. Nonimpacted fractures are less stable, are moderately

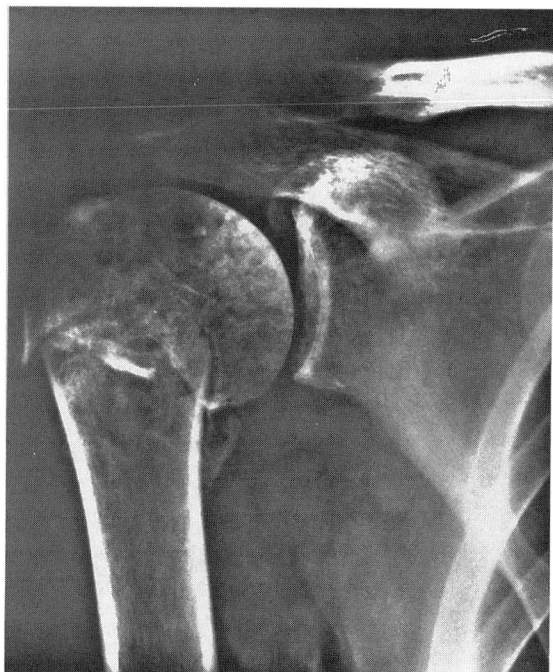

Figure 32.4.   Comminuted, impacted, slightly angulated fracture of the humeral head. The articular surface is intact, and the overall functional result should be good.

displaced, and can be comminuted or noncomminuted. Pain is prolonged, exercises are delayed, and the fracture may require closed or open reduction. The end result is less satisfactory.

With some fractures, mild deformity and no operative treatment are acceptable. Disimpaction of the fracture to achieve exact anatomic realignment rarely improves the functional result. Even malaligned but impacted fractures will be stable enough to begin careful range of motion exercises within 7 to 10 days. Careful instruction and counseling regarding the injury, the method of treatment, and the expected results are important. Generally, treatment is nonoperative, emphasizing protection and support in a Velpeau sling with early guarded mobilization. Pendulum (Codman) exercises (described in the next paragraph) should begin at 1 to 5 days, depending upon the degree of pain and the status of the fracture. Overhead strength and mobility will be partially lost varying with the patient's age, type of fracture, and response to rehabilitation. However, ordinary activities of daily living, such as eating, dressing, hair combing, and others below 90° or shoulder level are almost always recovered.

Home exercises must be carefully taught and demonstrated to the patient and family or friends who will be with the patient. Long-term physical therapy is seldom necessary, but repeated instruction and encouragement by physical therapists early in the course of treatment are beneficial. The physician should inform the patient that edema and ecchymosis of the upper arm and even of the forearm and hand often occur with this injury. Range of motion exercises of the elbow and wrist are as necessary as those for the shoulder to prevent stiffness. The usual progression of home shoulder exercises begins with pendulum (Codman) exercises, advancing to pulley exercises, walking up walls with the fingers to improve abduction, and combing the hair and scratching the small of the back repeatedly to improve rotation.

Pendulum (Codman) exercises are designed to negate gravity and are done by bending over 90° at the hip, putting the good arm on a table for support, and swinging the affected arm in gentle and increasingly larger circles for 1 to 5 minutes, 5 to 10 times per day. These exercises should start with the arm in a sling and then progress out of the sling as the range of motion increases and the arm feels better.

Rope or pulley exercises are designed to allow the good arm to help elevate the injured one, thereby facilitating gradual protected range of motion exercises for the injured arm, joint, muscles, and bone. A rope or towel is placed over a hook or a door, both sides of the towel are grasped as high as possible, and each arm is alternately raised and lowered. As with many postfracture courses, improvement begins slowly, then progresses rapidly, and the last 15% of improvement can take up to a year. It is important for the practitioner to maintain an optimistic but realistic attitude during this time and to encourage the patient to do the same.

FRACTURE/DISLOCATION OF THE HUMERAL HEAD

Fracture/dislocation of the humeral head poses special problems in the elderly. Preexisting arthritic changes and comminution of the humeral head may compromise any treatment that is carried out. Open reduction of the dislocation is often necessary because no leverage can be applied directly when the humeral head is comminuted and the shaft is broken at the surgical neck. Severe edema of the shoulder and comminution of the humeral head also frustrate reduction and alignment. Open reduction and internal fixation with wires, screws, or plates is difficult unless the fragments are of respectable size and the bone quality is sufficient. The underlying osteoporosis may thwart even this effort. Placing the fragments in good position, with the articular surface turned toward the glenoid, and treating the injury as an unimpacted, comminuted humeral head fracture may be all that is possible. Long-term prognosis remains guarded. When the comminution and displacement preclude a satisfactory result, early prosthetic replacement is worthy of consideration.

Dislocated shoulders with avulsion of the greater tuberosity occur equally in the elderly and young, but again, special difficulties occur in the elderly when the joint is arthritic and the head or the greater tuberosity is also fragmented because of the underlying osteoporosis. Treatment falls into two categories: those needing closed reduction and those needing open reduction and internal fixation. Fragments not displaced into the joint space usually will go back into close proximity to the original fracture site when the shoulder joint is reduced. This shoulder will function well when healed, although abduction may be limited by the position of the fragments under the acromion. If the avulsed greater tuberosity remains displaced inside the joint after closed reduction, open reduction and internal fixation is required.

Both of these injuries are then treated with a Velpeau sling followed by careful pendulum ex-

ercises in 7 to 10 days. Attention is again paid to elbow and wrist motion while the shoulder is healing. The prognosis depends upon the preinjury status of the glenohumeral joint, the degree of injury, and the response to rehabilitation. Partial loss of motion, especially above shoulder level, is not unusual.

DISLOCATIONS OF THE SHOULDER

More than 95% of all shoulder dislocations are anterior (Fig. 32.5) and occur when the person falls on the outstretched arm, forcing the shoulder into abduction and external rotation, and levering the humeral head anteriorly out of the joint. The patient with an anterior dislocation typically presents after a fall with loss of the normal rounded contour, a prominent acromion, the arm held in internal rotation and pressed to the side, and all attempts at movement painful. Neurovascular integrity must be determined by checking pulses and testing sensory and motor distributions of the median, ulnar, and radial nerves. The most common complication is axillary nerve injury with loss of sensation near the insertion of the deltoid muscle and absence of deltoid and teres minor muscle contraction. Anteroposterior (A/P) and lateral or transthoracic x-rays should be obtained. An axillary view will also help identify the position of the dislocated humeral head.

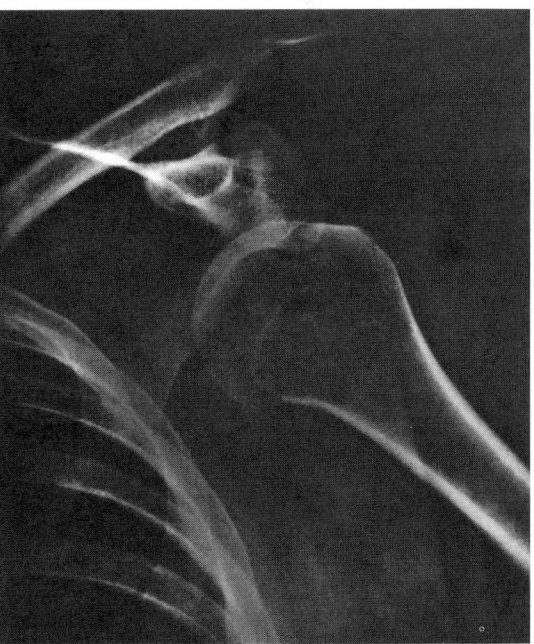

Figure 32.5. Anterior and inferior dislocation of the shoulder.

Closed reduction uses three methods, all preceded by steady traction on the arm in abduction to reduce muscle spasm before any reduction is attempted. The method favored by the author is that described by Stimson. The Stimson, Kocher, and Hippocratic methods are well described in standard orthopaedic texts.

In the postreduction period, the shoulder is immobilized in a Velpeau sling for 1 to 2 weeks, then taken out of the sling and used actively for all motions below shoulder level and inside of shoulder width for the next 6 weeks. For the entire 6 weeks, the patient should sleep in the Velpeau sling to prevent redislocation at night. Strengthening exercises for the biceps, pectoralis major, and anterior deltoid muscles are instituted early. Pendulum exercises are begun within 1 week to prevent stiffness, but range of motion exercises for the wrist and elbow are started immediately. The patient should refrain from abduction and external rotation movements as much as possible for 3 to 4 months to maximize the chances of preventing dislocation.

The frequency of recurrent dislocation in the elderly depends upon the severity of the dislocation and associated injuries around the shoulder, but is much less common than in the young. Ninety percent of those 20 years of age may experience recurrent dislocation, but less than 20% of those 50 years of age will redislocate. Recurrence in those older than 50 years is even less common. Complicating factors, such as a tearing of the anterior glenoid labrum (Bankhart lesion) or a compression fracture of the posteromedial portion of the humeral head (Hill-Sachs lesion) may lead to chronic instability requiring operative repair. Short- and long-term care, including operative treatment, is designed to restrict abduction and external rotation for a specified period of time. Operations include combinations of muscle/tendon shortening, bone blocks, and tendon transfers. Surgery is successful in preventing redislocations in over 93% of the patients, but range of motion and endurance of the shoulder is often decreased for over-the-head work.

Posterior dislocations of the shoulder in the elderly do occur, but are uncommon. The major problem of a posteriorly dislocated shoulder is that of misdiagnosis, because the A/P x-ray of a posterior dislocation can appear normal. Axillary or tangential views are used to verify the dislocation. Reduction of a posterior dislocation can be difficult and should be referred to the orthopaedic surgeon. After reduction, the shoulder must be immobilized in a sling and swathe. Chronic instability may necessitate operative repair.

An occurrence unique in the elderly is the long-term, dislocated shoulder, which may be unnoticed by nursing home personnel or family at home. It may not be reported by the patient, who is either unable to communicate the problem or considers it a minor disability or a sprain that eventually will get better. The humeral head is lodged beneath the coracoid, and the patient has relatively little pain. The range of motion is surprisingly good, lacking primarily abduction beyond 60° and external rotation beyond 50°. There is an obvious defect in the shoulder where the humeral head should be. Edema may be present, but it is usually minimal in the chronic dislocations.

Closed reduction without general anesthesia is difficult and sometimes impossible. Reduction often accomplishes very little. The range of motion may improve slightly, but the joint may become painful or begin to dislocate repeatedly. If the range of motion is moderate and painless, the dislocation has been present for more than 2 weeks, and the patient can do most activities below shoulder level without difficulty, then aggressive efforts to reduce the dislocation by closed or open means are seldom warranted. If the patient has continuous pain and restricted motion to the point of disability, closed or open reduction under general anesthesia may be considered.

ACROMIOCLAVICULAR SEPARATIONS AND FRACTURED CLAVICLES

"Separated shoulders" are uncommon in the elderly and are often confused historically with shoulder dislocations. Questioning the patient regarding the method of injury usually will differentiate the two conditions. A separated shoulder refers to disruption of the acromioclavicular (AC) joint, involves the AC ligament and the coracoclavicular (CC) ligament, and occurs by falling directly on the acromion or point of the shoulder and forcing it downward. Three grades of injury thus occur:

Grade I: only the AC ligament is stretched
Grade II: the AC ligament is torn, the CC ligament is stretched, and the tip of the clavicle may be slightly elevated
Grade III: the AC ligament and CC ligament are ruptured and the tip of the clavicle is elevated, giving a prominent bump to the shoulder

Treatment is almost always nonoperative. Strength recovery is good, and pain is usually minimal. If the AC joint becomes chronically painful and measures such as NSAIDs or local steroid injections give no relief, distal resection (Mumford procedure) of the clavicle can be effective.

A fracture through an osteoporotic clavicle is a common occurrence in the elderly from a fall striking the posterolateral surface of the shoulder, pushing the shoulder forward and snapping the clavicle that acts as a strut for the shoulder. Treatment with a figure-of-eight clavicle brace results in good healing in 3 to 8 weeks, though recent reports state a brace is often not needed. Several simple tactics will make the patient more comfortable. A clavicle brace should be tightened periodically by the family over the first 4 to 5 days. It does not have to be tightened immediately and is much more comfortable if tightened gradually as the swelling and spasm decrease. Mark the clavicle straps to gauge the advancement of about 1 inch on each side per day until the brace is moderately tight or "comfortably uncomfortable."

Have the patient sleep in a semi-sitting (semi-Fowler's) position either in a recliner chair or on a reading pillow for the first week for comfort. Place a folded sheet or narrow pillow between the shoulder blades to support the center of the back up to the occiput and prevent the bed from pushing the shoulders forward against the brace. Encourage patients to put their thumbs under the brace, like thumbs under suspenders, to (a) push the shoulders back for comfort and healing; (b) relieve pressure on the neurovascular structures in the axilla; and (c) air out the axilla to prevent chafing from the brace. For the first 5 to 7 days, no motion will be comfortable; for the next 5 to 7 days, pain will occur with sudden and major movements; after that, patients will be relatively comfortable. The clavicle brace should be worn full-time for 3 weeks but may be removed for bathing and replaced. Clavicle fractures routinely heal in all age groups, but may take slightly longer in older patients and should be protected until healing is complete.

HUMERAL SHAFT FRACTURES

Fractures of the humeral shaft occur in the elderly with direct trauma or a fall, with or without twisting, resulting in various combinations and degrees of comminution and angulation. Splintering of osteoporotic bone is common. Appropriate immobilization allows union to occur rapidly within 3 to 6 weeks. A hanging cast is the traditional treatment for humeral shaft fractures and, while cumbersome for some, is an effective and proven modality. Hanging casts are only applicable for patients who can adjust to sitting up much

of the time, allowing the cast to hang, thus pulling the fracture fragments into longitudinal alignment. Lying down causes loss of traction, and the usefulness of the cast is negated. Repeated angulation of the fracture leads to a fibrous nonunion. A Velpeau cast or dressing is a useful alternative. A Velpeau cast is used to splint and secure the arm to the side of the body, with pads and rolls of gauze around the arm and the torso. While effective and comfortable, it does require once-a-week changing to prevent skin breakdown under the arm and in the axilla. It is a less effective treatment for the overriding and shortened fractures that lengthen with hanging cast treatment.

Intramedullary pin fixation is an effective method in a few displaced and noncomminuted mid and lower shaft fractures. This is most appropriately used in relatively nonosteoporotic bone when there is unstable displacement of horizontally fractured ends. Therefore, its use in the elderly patient is limited. This can achieve early alignment, early motion, good healing, and increased comfort. The pin is electively removed under local or general anesthesia after several weeks or months.

Another very effective treatment modality is the fracture brace, a form-fitted, heat-molded plastic brace that conforms to and supports the humerus. This can be used as a primary treatment or after any of the above operative treatments in the mid and lower shaft fractures, allowing early protected motion and healing.

Complications of humeral shaft fractures are radial nerve injury, malunions, and delayed or fibrous nonunions. The radial nerve, which wraps around the humeral shaft, must be evaluated for injury, especially in displaced proximal one-third fractures of the humerus. Injury to this nerve is the most common nerve complication of humeral shaft fractures, causing wrist drop and the inability to extend thumb and finger metacarpophalangeal joints fully. Spontaneous recovery of the radial nerve is the rule, and the wrist, thumb, and fingers may be splinted until that recovery occurs. The humerus can tolerate malunions with shortening and angulation very well. Rotational deformities may cause problems and require derotational osteotomies because of the inability to get the hand toward the mouth or in certain directions. Delayed or fibrous nonunions are the most common complications of humeral fractures and may require operative fixation with bone grafting to heal the fractures. Fracture braces may be especially valuable in long-term nonoperative care.

SUPRACONDYLAR FRACTURES

Treatment methods for supracondylar fractures of the humerus depend upon the integrity of the elbow joint, i.e., the humeral/ulnar joint. If the distal humerus is split in a "T" fashion, open reduction and internal fixation are indicated. Evaluation of neurovascular status is critical before and repeatedly during treatment. Manipulation, reduction, and posterior splinting or casting will suffice for most pure supracondylar fractures. Use of olecranon pin traction for difficult fractures or those with moderately severe perielbow edema is an effective alternative. In the elderly, however, this type of treatment should not be used routinely. It requires a patient to be in bed too long, and osteoporosis, stiffening of joints, and exacerbation of medical problems may result.

ELBOW DISLOCATIONS

Elbow dislocations are not uncommon in the older patient. They occur as the patient falls backward on the outstretched hand, hyperextending and dislocating the elbow posterolaterally. The olecranon is prominent posteriorly and the arm is held in semiflexion. The elbow should be packed in ice in a comfortable position until reduction is attempted. In uncertain cases, feel the points of the olecranon and the medial and lateral condyles. If the elbow is extended, these three points will be in a straight line. If the elbow is flexed to 90°, they should form an equilateral triangle. If not, then the elbow is dislocated. The dislocation and the reduction are confirmed with A/P, lateral, and oblique radiographs. Draw a straight line on the x-ray through the radial shaft and head and extend it through the center of the capitulum. If this line does not go through the center of the capitulum on all views and at any angle, then the elbow remains dislocated.

The complications of elbow injury in the elderly depend upon the status of the underlying tissues. Fragments of osteoporotic bone in the joint may require removal. Already delicate skin may tear or slough after elbow injury. Preexisting arthritic changes and muscle stiffness may compromise the result. Although permanent neurovascular impairment is rare, the status of the arm should be assessed before treatment is instituted, after reduction, and during the first several days. The five "P's" of neurovascular compression (pain, pallor, pulselessness, paralysis, and paresthesia) should be recognized. However, the best indicator of an impending compartment syndrome, secondary to a fracture, is the sixth "P", painful passive extension of the fingers. If this occurs, compartment syndrome must be suspected until disproven. Immediately remove all splints and compressive dressings and extend the elbow to 10 or 15° of flexion. Elevate the arm. If there is no improvement, fasciotomy is necessary before irreversible muscle and nerve damage occurs. Volkmann's ischemic contracture is a disastrous and preventable sequel of unrecognized neurovascular compromise.

Early motion is essential in the treatment of dislocated elbows. Without it, the elbow will be stable but restricted. Within 7 to 10 days, the patient is taught active range of motion exercises in the sling, to better extend and flex the elbow and rotate the forearm. Avoid passive stretching, as it irritates elbow structures and actually decreases the range of motion regained. Loss of full extension is common, but this is rarely a functional disability.

OLECRANON INJURIES

Olecranon fractures occur from a direct fall or blow to the flexed elbow. Undisplaced olecranon fractures are treated with casting and early motion in 1 to 3 weeks, avoiding a long immobilization. A palpable "gap" in the bone indicates the more common displaced fracture, which requires open reduction and internal fixation. Internal fixation allows early active range of motion within 3 to 7 days and nets excellent results. Minimal loss of full extension is a frequent but minor complication. Other complications, such as stiffness and pain, often depend upon the amount of comminution and the status of the reduction.

Traumatic olecranon bursitis is rare in the elderly. It is a contusion of the point of the elbow causing enlargement and fluid formation in the bursa. It may appear dramatically edematous and infected looking with induration and redness, but a culture of the aspirate is negative. The problem will resolve in several days to weeks when treated with ice, NSAIDs, time, and avoidance of further contusion. Rheumatoid arthritis and other medical diseases may inflame bursas. Treatment is directed to the underlying disease process. Chronically inflamed and enlarged bursas may be excised.

RADIAL HEAD AND NECK FRACTURES

Radial head and neck fractures occur when the patient falls directly on the hand, and force is transmitted through the forearm to the radial head. Pain and edema occur over the radial head, accompanied by decreased flexion and extension and decreased pronation and supination because of pain or displaced fragments. Impacted radial head and neck fractures are treated with a short immobilization period and early active range of motion exercises. Displaced fractures require open reduction, excision, or prosthetic replacement if they physically restrict rotation of the forearm. A loss of some pronation is easily compensated, but loss of supination poses a larger problem and requires more aggressive treatment. Some mild loss of extension and full rotation is to be expected. If arthritic changes develop, later excision of the radial head will be helpful with relief of pain, although recovery of full motion is rare.

When the patient falls directly on the flexed forearm, the ulna may fracture and displace the radial head anteriorly. The treatment of this "Monteggia" fracture is by open reduction and internal fixation of the ulna and reduction of the radial head. Radial head reduction is again confirmed on x-ray by drawing a line through the radial shaft and the head that must pass through the capitulum.

FOREARM FRACTURES

Forearm fractures result from falls on the hand or direct trauma to the forearm. Edema and deformity may be clinically present at the fracture site, or the deformity may be much more subtle. In the elderly, nondisplaced distal and midshaft forearm fractures are treated with a long-arm cast, giving careful attention to the neurovascular status. Repeat the x-rays each week to detect any collapsing of the radius and ulna toward one another because this causes significant loss of forearm rotation. Displaced fractures require open reduction and internal fixation. Even then, some pronation-supination ability may be lost. Exact fracture management is described in several authoritative texts, for example, Rockwood and Green (7).

Rehabilitation for forearm and elbow fractures requires active and passive exercises, such as holding the wrist in a pronated position for 10 seconds with slight tension, then in supination, and repeating. This will gain rotation if it is carried out on a routine basis. Range of motion exercises for the wrist and shoulder should also be carried out.

WRIST

Wrist fractures from falls onto the outstretched hand are extremely common in the elderly. The distal radius and ulna are the weakest points of the upper extremity and have thin cortices with mostly cancellous bone. Colles' or posteriorly displaced fractures of the distal radius are the dinner-fork deformity fractures, so-called because the side view contour of the broken wrist resembles a dinner fork. Anteriorly displaced (Smith's) fractures and intraarticular (Barton's) fractures of the distal radius are less common, but not rare. Often associated with a fracture of the ulnar styloid, Colles' fractures are noted for a moderate degree of postreduction loss of position because the posterior cortex is often comminuted and provides little postreduction support.

Fortunately, the wrist tolerates mild-to-moderate angulation while retaining a good functional result. In most cases, closed manipulation and reduction under local or general anesthesia will restore alignment. A short- or long-arm cast is applied with the wrist in flexion and ulnar deviation and then trimmed to allow metacarpophalangeal joint motion. The fracture is immobilized 5 to 6 weeks, after which intensive range of motion exercises are started. In the more comminuted, unstable fractures, internal fixation or an external fixator is used.

Physical therapy is helpful. Finger exercises, which are started immediately and continued during and after the immobilization period, are important for strengthening. Squeezing a rubber ball will increase gross hand strength and rough motion, but the patient must also squeeze a cloth or something very small while making a fist and get the fingers into the palm for closer grip strength and fine motion. "Silly Putty" works very well for this. The immediate and major postreduction problem is edema distal to the fracture site. Gordon's sling, a stockinet taped to the cast, will keep the hand elevated above the elbow at night, the time when postreduction edema most often develops. The stockinet is attached to a hook on the wall with the elbow resting on the bed and the hand elevated at right angles to the bed. Other techniques for preventing edema and post-immobilization stiffness include placing the hand on top of the head, reaching for the sky several times a day, and actively moving the fingers as if waving. Passive finger exercises are also important. Range of motion exercises for the elbow and the shoulder are included in the patient's instructions.

Besides stiffness of wrist and fingers and angular deformity of the wrist, a major complication is median nerve compression causing a carpal tunnel syndrome. If the patient has unremitting pain and numbness into the median nerve distribution of the hand, edema or a fracture fragment may be compressing the nerve in the carpal tunnel canal. Cast change, positional change, or a formal carpal tunnel release may be required early in the course of treatment. Late releases may also be required.

HAND INJURIES

Fractures of the metacarpals and phalanges are not common in the elderly and are usually minimally displaced when they do occur. Stiffness and functional loss often arise because the injury is superimposed upon a preexisting deformity or arthritic change. Protected motion as early as possible reduces these problems. Treatment for extraarticular fractures of the metacarpals is short-term, hand-cast immobilization with active exercises in a buddy splint for the fingers (one finger taped to the other in two areas) for 2 to 3 weeks, followed by a circumferential strapping for the metacarpals. Phalangeal fractures are treated with a finger traction hand cast for 2 to 3 weeks, followed by active motion in a buddy splint. Buddy splinting for both injuries should be done in as much flexion as possible, for it is the grip that needs to be restored. Extension of the fingers will return and slight loss does not cause a functional disability. Loss of finger flexion, and therefore, grip strength, does cause functional loss. Intraarticular fractures require reduction with nearly anatomic alignment and/or open reduction with fixation. The postoperative course is the same as for a closed injury.

Fractures of the thumb are divided into impacted nondisplaced fractures and displaced fractures. Impacted, nondisplaced, or relatively nondisplaced, fractures of the thumb can be treated with thumb spica immobilization for 2 to 3 weeks. The thumb has good mobility and compensates well for minor angulation and/or stiffness. Displaced thumb fractures require pin fixation by closed or open means, especially for the displaced intraarticular fracture of the first metacarpal base (Bennett's fracture). This fracture is inherently unstable and will migrate proximally without fixation.

Proximal interphalangeal (PIP) joint dislocations are almost always posterior and should be reduced and held in a flexion splint for 5 to 10 days and then begun on flexion exercises with a buddy splint. Again, extension will be regained over time, but flexion needs to be actively pursued. Permanent residual swelling around the PIP and the distal interphalangeal (DIP) joints is a rule, but usually does not interfere with function, only with the wearing of rings on that finger.

Mallet fingers, or baseball fingers, are avulsion fractures or ruptures of the extensor tendon at the base of dorsum of the distal phalanx, allowing un-opposed flexion of the DIP joint. The DIP joint is splinted in extension for 3 to 6 weeks. The principal complications of treatment are stiffness and pain, especially in the already arthritic finger. Functional loss, with or without treatment, is minimal.

TRUNK INJURIES

Rib fractures are common in the older population, partly because of osteoporosis and partly because of increased frequency of falls in the older age group. Direct palpation over the fracture site will cause pain, but remote palpation on the fractured rib will move the fracture and also cause pain at the fracture site. This will help distinguish a fractured rib from a contusion of the chest wall. Strapping may be used to support the rib cage, but should not mechanically impair respiratory excursion. When two or more ribs are fractured, admission to the hospital is advised for observation and stabilization. Treatment is usually symptomatic. Intercostal nerve blocks may be needed for severe pain. The physician must be aware of the adjacent internal structures. For example, an injury to the lungs or liver or spleen may lead to pneumonia and/or pneumothorax or internal bleeding. If there is any suspicion of internal injury, chest x-rays or serial hematocrits are obtained, as well as liver and spleen scans. Splinting of the rib cage from a fracture not uncommonly causes pneumonia. Incentive spirometry, deep breathing exercises, and mild analgesics may be required.

Falls and automobile accidents cause most of the pelvic fractures in this age group. Evaluation of the supporting columns, i.e., a weightbearing line drawn through the hip joint, the ilium, the sacroiliac joint and up through the spine, dictates weightbearing stability and mobilization factors. Most pelvic fractures are only mildly displaced. Bed rest from several days to 2 or 3 weeks and then gradual mobilization is usual. Major traumatic injuries to the pelvis are life-threatening, with a 10 to 50% mortality rate from blood loss, cardiovascular failure, and local complications such as infection. Immediate care in a major trauma center is mandatory.

Complications of pelvic fracture include prolonged pain from ligament disruption and fragmentation of bone—especially around the symphysis pubis and sacroiliac joints. A walker or a cane, medication, and reassurance over time is tried at first. Treatment of these complications after prolonged local care may be operative, but is beyond the scope of this chapter.

SPINE FRACTURES

Acute onset of back pain in the elderly is vertebral compression fracture until proven otherwise. Osteoporotic bone in the vertebral column is particularly susceptible to this injury. A sudden blow or fall on the buttock may cause a compression fracture, but the cause may be far more subtle, such as a sudden twist of the body or a missed step. Typically, the pain of a vertebral compression fracture is acute, but gradually improves over 5 to 20 days. Often patients may not even seek medical help, and old compression fractures are picked up on an x-ray done for some other reason.

An appropriate period of bed rest, followed by stabilization with a brace or body cast, mild analgesics, and protected mobilization with a walker or cane, is the usual sequence in treatment. If appropriate, early resumption of activities will lessen the increase of osteoporosis. Treatment of compression fractures necessitates the awareness of complications. Paralytic ileus, secondary to spine injury, occurs frequently, and is manifested by loss of bowel sounds, bloating, nausea, and vomiting. A nasogastric tube or rectal tube for decompression and keeping the patient without food until the bowel sounds recur are usually all that are necessary to treat this complication. Neurologic deficits must be detected and treated. X-ray evaluation of the neural canal must be correlated with clinical evaluation of the patient to assess neurologic compromise. Any questionable compromise of the spinal canal may require tomograms, CAT scans, or magnetic resonance imaging (MRI) for definitive diagnosis and treatment.

A new and accurate method of gauging a patient's vertebral bone density is dual photon absorptiometry (DPA). DPA compares patients against an age-matched population and computes the relative risk of fracture. DPA provides a reliable and reproducible serial comparison and is the test of choice in evaluating the progress of any planned or ongoing treatment for osteoporosis.

COCCYDYNIA

Coccydynia represents pain from a fracture or contusion resulting from a fall directly on the coccyx. With either diagnosis, treatment is nonoperative and often prolonged. The patient should sit on a pillow or a rubber ring at all times, use a high soft chair, do stretching exercises, take NSAIDs, and have patience. Because several months to a year or more may be necessary for the discomfort to resolve, these patients need constant reassurance of eventual relief. Coccygectomy is a salvage procedure, and its results are equivocal.

FRACTURES OF THE ACETABULUM

Fractures of the acetabulum involve the posterior, medial, and superior surfaces and must be suspected after hip trauma without a fracture of the proximal femur. When there is direct horizontal trauma to the flexed knee while sitting or falling, the femoral head is driven posteriorly and punches out the posterior wall of the acetabulum. This is a common, so-called dashboard injury. The femoral head is typically displaced posteriorly to the acetabulum, so the patient presents with a thigh that is flexed, shortened, internally rotated, and virtually "locked" in that position. All attempts at movement are painful and meet with resistance.

Pre- and postreduction x-ray evaluation of this injury is very crucial and sometimes difficult to achieve. The patient must lie on the affected side on the x-ray table. The patient is then turned approximately 45° anteriorly so that a tangential view of the posterolateral surface of the affected acetabulum can be taken. Reduction may require general anesthesia. Nondisplaced fractures can be treated closed and immobilized for several weeks with a Bermuda shorts walking cast that keeps the leg and hip straight and stable. If the posterior fragment is unstable, the femur will be unstable and dislocate posteriorly while sitting or bending over. This injury will require open reduction and internal fixation of the posterior fragment.

Medial wall fractures are the result of direct trauma to the greater trochanter or the lateral side of the femur, driving the femoral head medially into the acetabulum. Pain and restricted motion are present in all attempts at movement. Distal skeletal traction is the treatment of choice. If the nondisplaced fracture is not recognized and treated, the femoral head will migrate medially and protrude into the pelvis. Operative reduction may be necessary in these fractures or when the femoral head is locked inside the pelvis or the medial wall remains displaced after reduction of the femoral head.

Forces transmitted directly upward through the femur to the acetabulum, such as from jumping from a height, result in superior dome fractures that compromise the weightbearing capability of the hip joint. Full motion may be present, although painful. The treatment is nonweightbearing for 8 to 12 weeks and may include open reduction and internal fixation to restore the integrity of the dome. Inability of many elderly patients to comply with the nonweightbearing regimen compromises many long-term results because of displacement of the fracture fragments. Stiffness may ensue, and some will develop arthritic changes within a short time. Periodic x-rays are necessary to identify any collapse or displacement because displacement of medial and superior surface fractures can necessitate difficult reconstructive total hip replacements.

LOWER EXTREMITY INJURIES

Lower extremity injuries involve more than just treatment of the affected area. In the elderly, a fracture or serious injury to the hip or leg may mark the end of independence or significantly decrease a patient's mobility. Upper body strength may not be sufficient for the use of crutches or a walker. The ability to drive, go up and down stairs, go to the toilet, or make one's dinner, and even the ability to answer the phone may be compromised. Evaluation of the home and family support situations, use of Visiting Nurses Association or nurses aides, physical therapy, strengthening exercises for the upper extremities, Meals on Wheels, or temporary placement in a nursing home are among the many supports to consider when treating lower extremity injuries in this age group. In a significant number, acute disability will last 6 to 20 weeks. This must be foreseen, and appropriate home and social services planning and referrals provided.

All of the problems and complications that occur in lower extremity injuries can be found in the treatment of hip fractures. Among these are shortening, rotation, infection, fibrous nonunion and nonweightbearing for several weeks or months. The strength of the arms and of the good leg is tested as well as balance, motor coordination and sensation, stamina, and judgment. Rehabilitation potential is also tested. Many studies have been done to try to develop preoperative rehabilitation predictors. Several preoperative factors have been shown to be of significance and were rated on a scale of 1 to 100 (3). Some of these are

1. Mental awareness (status)
2. Independent ambulation
3. Social interaction inside the home
4. Social interaction outside the home
5. Age

In general, those who were mentally alert preoperatively were alert postoperatively. These patients better understood the nature of the injury and the demands for rehabilitation. Those who were independent ambulators before surgery most often achieved a comparable level of ambu-

lation postoperatively. Those who had participated in outside activities and were active at home preoperatively, most often returned to preoperative activity levels after the surgery. Evaluation by age discerned a natural division between "young old" and "old old." Old old begins at 80 to 85 years and is characterized as less healthy, less productive, and less independent than the young old. They have greater needs in all areas and require more time to improve their level of functioning. The old old tend to have lower preoperative assessment and lower postoperative recovery scores. By evaluating these and other parameters, an estimate of the level of functional return can be given to the family and social worker to facilitate posthospital planning (9–12).

Immediate postoperative mortality is a concern in elderly patients with hip fractures. Six-month mortality estimates of 15 to 50% have been reported. In a 10-year Minnesota study of 456 persons over age 60 years (13), 32% of the women and 17% of the men sustained a hip fracture before age 90 years. The 4-month postoperative fracture mortality rate was 12% higher than that of an age-matched population without hip fractures. After 4 months, the mortality rate of both groups was the same. Other studies have verified that age is directly related to mortality rate (2). These mortality rates after hip surgery persist, even though aggressive operative treatment has definitely decreased the mortality rate over nonoperative treatment.

Historically, many patients with hip fractures treated nonoperatively would succumb to complications of pneumonia, emboli, pressure sores, and infections. Among those treated operatively, the mortality rate was less but still substantial, especially in the first 6 months after surgery (10). Advances in anesthesia, fixation devices, and joint replacement metallurgy have helped reverse this statistic, giving the patient a 60 to 90% chance of long-term, postoperative survival. The importance of preoperative and postoperative medical stability in keeping the mortality rate and morbidity rate down cannot be overemphasized. A significant number of the elderly admitted for hip fractures have medical problems that are untreated or require updated evaluation before they can tolerate the trauma of surgery (1). A recent study has even correlated lower serum albumin with fixation failures in hip fractures. While the stability of the fracture and the position of the hip screw were the direct causes of fixation failure, the high correlation of low serum albumin with those that did fail suggests that nutritional supplementation may reduce the failure rate. Surgical fixation or hip replacement in the first 24 to 48 hours, followed by early mobilization, lessens the complications and allows easier nursing care, faster recovery, and rehabilitation. The present attitude is more surgically aggressive toward these fractures, thus decreasing the mortality and morbidity inherent in long-term, nonoperative treatment.

HIP FRACTURES (PROXIMAL FEMUR FRACTURES)

Hip fracture is the "fracture of the elderly." It is the most common injury and reason for hospitalization in the elderly and causes more long-term disability than any other injury. Definitive treatment of hip fracture within the first 24 to 72 hours, early ambulation, and physical therapy have combined to reduce the morbidity, hospitalization time, and recovery time, but the problem is still significant (14).

Hip fractures usually result from falls. The patient has pain and inability to bear weight on the affected limb, and all attempts at movement are painful. The leg is characteristically shortened, slightly flexed, and externally rotated.

Hip fractures are divided into three categories: subcapital, intertrochanteric, and subtrochanteric fractures (Fig. 32.6). Subcapital fractures involve the area of the femoral neck and are stable or unstable. Stable fractures are impacted in slight valgus and heal well, and internal fixation with threaded pins gives an excellent result. Unstable fractures are displaced in a varus position, roll posteriorly and shorten, and do not heal well. Unstable subcapital fractures are best treated by replacement with endoprostheses, that is, prosthetic hip joints without an acetabular replacement. Endoprostheses last for 2 to 10 years without the need for conversion to total hips to alleviate pain, depending upon the bone stock and the activity of the patient.

Theoretically, ambulation can begin immediately. In practice, partial weightbearing for 4 to 6 weeks is advised. Painless, but somewhat decreased, motion is usual in these patients. Femoral neck fracture in the elderly has its own special complication—aseptic necrosis of the femoral head. The blood supply to the femoral head is already reduced and is then further compromised by the fracture. Reasonable efforts should be made in younger (55 to 70 years old) patients toward retaining their own hips, even with slight displacement and the increased chance of aseptic necrosis and further surgery. In a patient over 70 years of age with a displaced fracture, an endo-

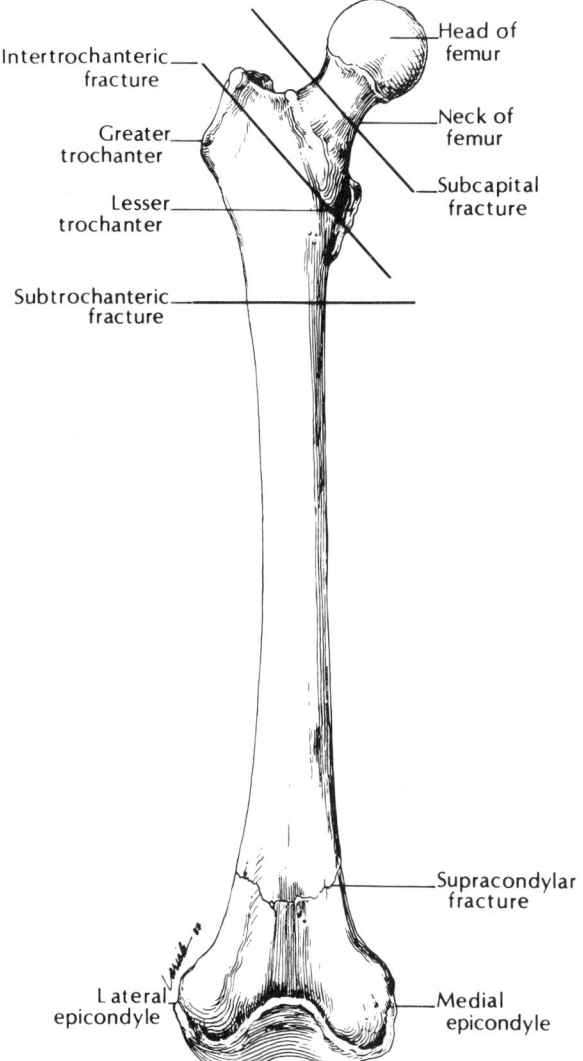

Figure 32.6.   Anterior view of right femur showing anatomic designation and levels of hip fractures.

prosthesis is the treatment of choice. Any patient who, for mental or physical reasons, would be unable to tolerate a nonweightbearing status and/or later surgery is also an excellent candidate for an endoprosthesis (15).

Intertrochanteric fractures involve the area along a general line between the greater and lesser trochanters of the femur (Fig. 32.7A). They are usually displaced and require open reduction and internal fixation, most often by a sliding hip compression screw and plate, which allows mechanical and functional impaction and fixation (Fig. 32.7B). Healing is prompt over 2 to 3 months,

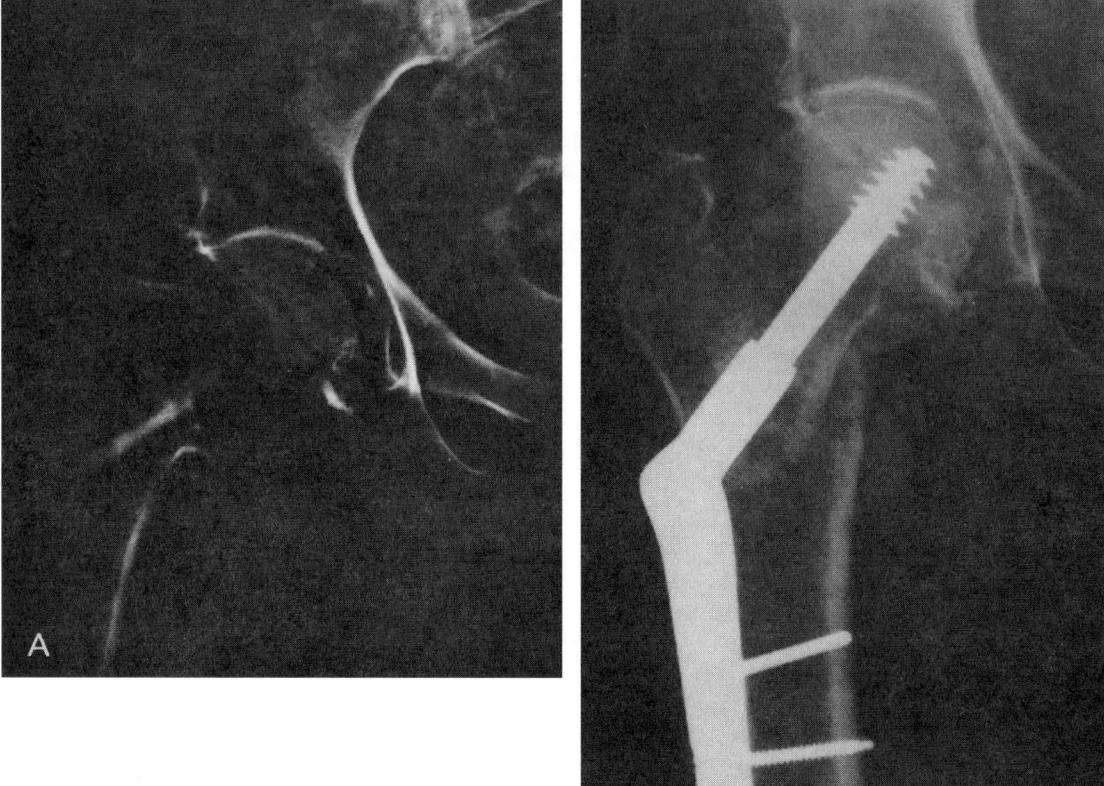

Figure 32.7.   A and B, Comminuted and displaced intertrochanteric fracture of the femur. Fracture fixed with sliding hip compression screw. Alignment has been restored.

and fixation devices are of such quality as to protect most fractures from displacement. The patient remains nonweightbearing for 8 to 10 weeks, during which time range of motion exercises of the hip are encouraged. Partial weightbearing with a walker and/or crutches then commences and should progress to full weightbearing by 12 to 16 weeks. Complications are uncommon, but include delayed union, malrotation, and stiffness.

Subtrochanteric fractures, those below the lesser trochanter, are mechanically unstable and require either intermedullary fixation or a long side-plate fixation. These fractures need a longer healing time, closer follow-up, and extended weightbearing protection and have a risk of refracture in the early stages. Delayed union is not uncommon in these fractures and may require later bone grafting.

FEMORAL SHAFT FRACTURES

Femoral shaft fractures usually result from significant direct trauma, for example, an auto-

mobile accident or a fall from a height. The leg is edematous, is shortened, and lies in external rotation. Femoral shaft fractures respond well to skeletal traction, followed by hip spica cast or a cast brace to give a solid and satisfactory union. This enforced immobilization, however, increases morbidity in the elderly. Internal fixation with intermedullary rods or compression plates, though preferable, has to be weighed against the condition of the patient and quality of the bone. Osteoporotic femurs may splinter from attempts at internal fixation, complicating an already difficult situation. The application of a cast brace, with or without surgical fixation, will allow earlier mobilization and reduced morbidity. Nonweightbearing and partial weightbearing continue for 4 to 9 months, depending upon the fracture, the fixation, and the quality of the bone.

Delayed union occurs occasionally, but loss of hip and knee motion is more frequent. The most acute concern is blood loss. A femoral fracture allows the escape of 2 units of blood into the thigh at once. Vital signs must be monitored, fluid replaced, and blood pressure stabilized as needed.

SUPRACONDYLAR FRACTURES OF THE FEMUR

Supracondylar fractures of the femur (Fig. 32.6) occur as a result of direct trauma or a fall with a twisting motion. Deformity and malalignment just above the knee are usually evident. Minimally displaced fractures can be treated with traction and cast bracing. Surgical treatment is preferred if alignment and displacement are a problem and after the usual factors of age, medical and physical condition, and bone stock are considered. Cast bracing after closed or open reduction enables earlier ambulation.

Complications include malalignment and entrapment of the quadriceps in the healed fracture site. A displaced, intraarticular fracture must be internally fixed for the knee to be functional. Malalignment of a supracondylar fracture changes the normal tracking of the extensor mechanism and alters the weightbearing forces through the knee. The possible results are painful catching of the patella against the femoral condyle, early patellofemoral and/or knee compartment arthrosis, and decreased extensor strength. When the muscle is caught in the fracture site, there is inability to actively or passively flex the knee fully or to actively extend the knee fully (extensor lag). Extensor lag causes instability with walking on levels or declines, difficulty in ascending or descending stairs, and problems rising from a sitting position. Inability to flex the knee at least 90° impairs the ability to walk up the stairs or to sit easily. Patients have to step over the stair when climbing or kick the leg out in front to sit down, literally dropping into the chair.

These impairments can be devastating to the individual who was functioning independently before the injury. Early protected mobilization is helpful to reduce this complication, but closed manipulation may have to be considered when a significant loss of the range of motion is present at the 4- to 8-week level.

PATELLAR INJURIES

Patellar injuries in the elderly are usually the result of direct trauma from a fall or automobile accident. The knee area becomes very edematous, and the patient is unable to extend the knee against gravity or any weight. There is often a palpable transverse defect in the middle of the pa-

tella. X-rays confirm a patellar fracture, ranging from nondisplaced to wide open and shattered.

Nondisplaced patellar fractures with good quadriceps function can be treated with a long-leg cast and knee immobilizer for 3 weeks, followed by gradual knee flexion exercises for 4 weeks. The knee immobilizer is used for comfort during that time. Walking is encouraged during the first week after the fracture.

Displaced fractures require open reduction and internal fixation to restore strength and stability. Loose, comminuted fragments should be excised. If large fragments are present and provide a stable articular surface, they should be preserved and the extensor mechanism repaired. The inferior pole can be discarded, but if more than two-thirds of the patella is severely fragmented, a patellectomy may be necessary.

In an older person, forceful contraction of the quadriceps mechanism to prevent a fall may rupture the quadriceps just proximal to the patella. Inability to extend the knee and a palpable defect in the muscle just above the patella confirm the diagnosis and indicate a need for operative repair. Postoperatively, a knee immobilizer is used for 4 to 6 weeks. Graduated knee flexion exercises and quadriceps-setting exercises are begun at 2 to 3 weeks. Rehabilitation often takes 6 months or more, but the results are usually quite good.

TIBIAL PLATEAU FRACTURES

Tibial plateau fractures are compression injuries that depress the central portion of the medial or lateral tibial plateau. These fractures occur when a sudden force is directed upward through the foot and the leg, compressing the knee joint at an angle, as with falling from a height and landing directly on the foot. The lateral tibial plateau is more often affected than the medial plateau. X-rays may show an obvious fracture, but in some cases, the findings may be much more subtle. A lateral x-ray of the knee may show a double density where the plateau on the affected side is below the plateau on the noninvolved side instead of overlapping and indicates a tibial plateau fracture.

Open reduction and internal fixation are considered if the depression is more than 8 mm, the resulting angulation is greater than 5° of valgus and 10° of varus, or widening of the fracture line and displacement of the tibial plateau indicates fragment instability. The entire corticocancellous bone complex of the tibial plateau is elevated and fixed with a plate or a long-lag screw and washer. After a closed or open reduction, the extremity is kept in a long-leg, bent-knee cast for 3 weeks, followed by 3 to 5 weeks of range of motion exercises, before any partial weightbearing is allowed. Graduated weightbearing then progresses over the next 4 to 8 weeks. Exercises for the muscles of the upper arms and both legs are instituted immediately to prevent stiffening and loss of strength due to disuse atrophy. Valgus and varus deformities may result, compromising ambulation in the older person. Bracing, canes, proximal tibial osteotomies, or partial or total knee replacement may then be required to restore satisfactory ambulation.

TIBIAL SHAFT FRACTURES

Direct trauma to the tibia from falls or accidents causes most tibial shaft fractures in the elderly. X-rays will reveal nondisplaced fractures or confirm obvious deformities. Treatment of tibial shaft fractures depends upon the degree of displacement and whether they are compound or simple. Casting, especially with the newer synthetic or fiberglass casting materials, can provide excellent and lightweight stabilization during the healing process. Open reduction and internal fixation can be used in difficult, unstable, or displaced fractures. Off-center or bayonet alignment and some shortening can be tolerated, but proper rotational or angular alignment is critical to allow the elderly patient continued ambulatory independence. In the elderly, careful assessment of the neurovascular status, the condition of the skin, and the quality of the bone is necessary. Delayed or fibrous nonunions of the tibia are present at any age, but the added complications of pressure ulcers, diabetic or vascular skin breakdown, and osteoporotic bone are far greater in the elderly.

ANKLE AND FOOT FRACTURES

Ankle and foot fractures are very common in the elderly. A stone, a slippery walk, or a rug may cause a misstep and a broken ankle or foot. Deformity and edema are usually present. X-ray will confirm the clinical opinion and note the extent of the fracture. If the ankle joint or mortise is disrupted (the talus is displaced from under the tibia), then the bony integrity and the ligamentous attachments of the medial malleolus, the lateral malleolus, and the posterior malleolus must be evaluated. If both bone and ligament are intact with the mortise disrupted, then a fracture more proximal in the leg must be suspected, almost always of the proximal fibula. Good alignment is mandatory, especially of the fibular malleolus

that supports the ankle mortise. Closed manipulation is usually very successful in the older patient, but marginal reduction or displaced articular fragments require internal fixation. Delayed union can occur, and ankle stiffness is frequent. Early protected weightbearing can help reduce these problems.

Os calcis fractures occur from a direct blow to the calcaneus, usually from a fall, or as in jumping from a height. Os calcis fractures are usually impacted, comminuted, and often disrupt the subtalar joint. X-rays will outline the extent of the fracture and the displacement. Closed or open reductions are infrequent and have inconsistent results. Postfracture edema may be striking, and long-term disability from pain may result. If long-term disability pain is present, a subtalar fusion or triple arthrodesis may be required to restore ambulation and independence.

Fifth metatarsal base fractures are one of the most common fractures in the foot and also are one of the more common of all fractures in the elderly. This is an avulsion fracture, resulting from a sudden contraction of the peroneus brevis tendon attachment to the base of the fifth metatarsal when trying to straighten the foot, when the foot is suddenly inverted. Displacement is usually minimal, and this fracture responds well to a short-leg walking cast for 3 to 4 weeks. Delayed or painful nonunion is a complication that may require surgical correction.

Fractures at the metatarsal shafts usually occur from direct trauma or twisting. Good alignment must be maintained, and the tendency of the metatarsal shaft to collapse realized. Special attention to supporting the arch in the cast will prevent this complication. It may also be necessary to delay weightbearing in the more unstable metatarsal shaft fractures. Painful and persistent soft tissue edema on the dorsum of the foot after a fracture, dislocation, or serious soft tissue injury may lead to the devastating complication of reflex sympathetic dystrophy. In the author's experience, more than one-half of patients with reflex sympathetic dystrophy of the foot had no fracture present.

Toe phalangeal fractures and dislocations result from direct trauma or "catching" the toe on a furniture corner or a rug. Both injuries should be reduced into good alignment and treated with buddy-splint taping and with attention to circulation. When the taping becomes more of a nuisance than the toe injury, it is discontinued. Edema usually persists for a lengthy period and may never fully resolve. Rarely, the fracture or dislocation is nonreducible and requires operative treatment.

SUMMARY

Treatment of musculoskeletal system injuries in the elderly differs from that of the young in that the practitioner must be acutely aware of the effect of preexisting medical problems, psychosocial impact of injury, and potential complications on the morbidity and mortality of this patient population. The practitioner must consider physiologic aspects of aging, drug metabolism in the elderly, and problems of healing with age and realize that the precarious homeostatic balance of elderly patients is easily upset. While concentrating on specific treatment and rehabilitation, the practitioner must draw on both medical and ancillary hospital and community-based support systems to care for the total person.

Acknowledgment. I wish to acknowledge the contributions of James Hitzrot, M.D., whose tireless editing and encouragement made this chapter possible. I am also indebted to Ms. Hunt Gressitt for her technical and editorial assistance.

REFERENCES

1. Furey JG. Complications following hip fractures. J Chronic Dis 1967;20:103–113.
2. Kenzora JE, McCarthy RE, Lowell JD, Sledge CB. Hip fracture mortality. Clin Orthop 1984;186:45–56.
3. Moss N. The psychology of the aging athlete. In: Kerlan RK, ed. Clinics in sports medicine. Philadelphia: WB Saunders, 1991:431–444.
4. Brown M. Special considerations during rehabilitation of the aged athlete. In: Lehman RC, Delitto A, eds. Clinics in sports medicine. Philadelphia: WB Saunders, 1989:893–901.
5. Hannafin JA. Pathophysiology of the frozen shoulder. Sports Medicine Conference. Greater Baltimore Medical Center, Baltimore, 1993.
6. Adams P, Davies T, Sweetman P. Osteoporosis and the effects of aging on bone mass in men and women. Q J Med 1970;39:601–615.
7. Rockwood CA, Green DP. Fractures. Philadelphia: JB Lippincott, 1975.
8. Carey RG, Posabac EJ. Manual for the level of rehabilitation scale (LORS). Park Ridge, IL: Office of Evaluation and Research, Lutheran General Hospital, 1977.
9. Rowe CR. The management of fracture in elderly patients is different. J Bone Joint Surg 1965; 47:1043–1059.
10. Lukens L. Six months after hip fracture. Geriatr Nurs 1986;7:202–206.
11. Katz S. Jackson BA, Jaffee MW, Littell AS, Turk CE. Multidisciplinary studies of illness in aged persons. VI. Comparison study of rehabilitated and nonrehabilitated patients with fractures of the hip. J Chronic Dis 1962;15:979–984.
12. Miller CW. Survival and ambulation following hip fracture. J Bone Joint Surg [Am] 1978;60:930–934.
13. Gallagher TC, Melton LJ, Riggs BL, Bergstrath E. Epidemiology of fractures of the proximal femur in Rochester, Minnesota. Clin Orthop 1980;150:163–171.
14. Villar RN, Allen SM, Barnes SJ. Hip fractures in healthy patients. Operative delay versus prognosis. Br Med J 1986;293:1203–1204.
15. Boyd HB, Salvatore JE. Acute fracture of the femoral neck: internal fixation or prosthesis? J Bone Joint Surg 1964;46:1066–1068.

33/ Foot Health for the Elderly Patient

Geoffrey M. Habershaw, Thomas E. Lyons

Most everyone desires to live a long and fulfilling life, and indeed we encourage our society to find new ways to improve quality and duration of life. The incidence of chronic disease increases as people age (1). Among the chronic diseases are foot problems, which are very common in the aged. Often these alterations in health, including those affecting the foot, affect the functional ability of the elderly patient. The podiatrist plays a major role in promoting the overall health of the elderly by providing comfort, optimizing functional ability, and limiting disability.

Optimal foot health adds to the ease with which the elderly may be cared for. Preventative care of the foot avoids deterioration, and the onset of problems may be delayed or eliminated. Proper foot care can decrease morbidity, and ultimately mortality, in patients with diabetes and peripheral vascular disease (2). Minor foot problems, including painful calluses and toe and nail deformities, may be an underappreciated cause of instability and falls (3).

Foot care in the elderly is important in maintaining mobility and independence (4). The active, mobile geriatric enhances quality of life and medical well-being. The lack of mobility can result in many forms of physiologic deconditioning in the elderly. The tragedy of immobilization and the negative effect it has on normal physiology should never be due to ineffectual management of lower extremity dysfunction.

CHANGES IN THE FOOT WITH AGING

With the aging process, there are a number of degenerative changes that simultaneously affect the various components of the foot. Many patients develop peripheral vascular disease. Manifestations of arterial insufficiency are common. The posterior tibial and dorsalis pedis pulses are often diminished or absent. The foot is cooler, especially distally, near the toes. Thinning of the skin with a shiny appearance may be present. Loss of hair growth over the lower leg and dorsum of the foot is common. The nails become thick and brittle. Dependent rubor and pallor with elevation are seen frequently with more severe forms of arterial insufficiency. In light of this decreased perfusion, it is easier for patients to develop ulcerations.

Peripheral nervous system dysfunction occurs in the elderly, especially those over 70 years of age. One or more disease entities associated with peripheral neuropathy may be present, and the distinction between the various entities may be difficult. Symptoms may or may not be present but can include numbness, a feeling of tightness around the feet, and burning sensations. Shooting pains and paresthesias may also be present. Physical examination findings include absent or diminished patellar and Achilles tendon reflexes and altered light touch, vibratory, and pain sensation. A reduction in strength with distal muscular atrophy may be present (6). Elderly patients frequently have a decreased sensitivity to pain and pressure. Although this may not be pronounced, they are at risk for skin injury and ulceration.

A number of changes occur in the pedal skin with age. The stratum corneum contains less moisture and thus is more brittle, contributing to dry skin. Turnover time for the stratum corneum is increased significantly, necessitating a longer treatment period for superficial fungal infections (7). The epidermal rete ridges flatten, resulting in a decreased area of contact between the dermis and epidermis. This is significant, as the removal of an adhesive corn pad or friction between the skin and a poorly fitting shoe can easily result in tearing of the epidermis. The dermis, too, become thinner with age and is more easily damaged. The cutaneous circulation decreases with age and may delay wound healing. It also results in delayed clearance of the substances that come in contact with the skin and may result in prolonged cases of contact dermatitis. Furthermore, the signs of inflammation may not be as striking, make the diagnosis of such entities as cellulitis more difficult. Decreased sweating is also common and adds to dryness of the skin.

The subcutaneous tissue tends to resorb with age. As it does, there is less protection for those areas of the foot that come in contact with the shoe, especially bony prominences. The subcutaneous fat of the heel is composed of dense adipose tissue contained within fibrous septa. Its thickness is normally approximately 2.0 cm. On the ball of the foot, vertical fibers connect the dermis to the plantar aponeurosis (8). Essentially this arrangement provides for columns of retained adipose tissue, designed to bear weight, absorb shock, and provide a cushion. Resorption of some of this fat invariably occurs with age. Also, the retaining fibers in the ball of the foot and heel may rupture, resulting in displacement of the fat, leading to less cushion and a cause of plantar foot pain that can be quite disabling.

Musculoskeletal changes with age are also seen. There is a loss of muscle mass secondary to a reduction in muscle cells, connective tissue, and muscle tissue fluids (1). This helps to explain the thinning of the calves and atrophy of the intrinsic muscles of the foot, leading to a prominence of the ball and heel. Also, as people age, a progressive pronation, or flattening, of the arch occurs. Other clinical entities that tend to become progressive over the years include bunion and hammertoe deformities, which tend to become more rigid and fixed with time. Bony spurs may be noted on the inferior and posterior aspect of the calcaneus and may or may not be symptomatic. Arthritic changes with dorsal spur formation are common in the midfoot. Rearfoot osteoarthritis is not frequently seen, even though significant involvement may be present in the hips and knees.

The cumulative effect of these changes often results in a painful foot. Compensation for this foot pain often consists of an antalgic gait. The antalgic gait, which consists of twists and rotations of the lower extremities, alters normal knee, hip, and pelvic position, and this may lead to pain at these sites.

NAIL DISORDERS

Nail problems are very common in the elderly. Sixty to 70% of patients presenting to podiatrists have one or more nail disorders (9). These frequently result from a number of conditions, including acute and chronic trauma and virtually any systemic disease affecting the skin and its appendages, with fungal infection being the most common.

Onychomycosis is due to the invasion of the nail plate caused by the penetration of hyphae either along the surface or sides of the nail plate. The prolonged turnover of the stratum corneum and an altered immune response add to the chronicity of the disease (7). Mycotic nails may serve as a reservoir for reinfection of local skin structures, specifically the interdigital areas and the sole of the foot.

The altered growth pattern of the nails often predisposes them to fungal infection. Insidious trauma caused by shoe gear and progressive digital and forefoot deformities contributes to distortion of the nails and increases the likelihood of mycotic infection. The color of the nail changes in the involved area and can be white, yellow, or brown. As the condition progresses, the nail can become very thick with an abundance of subungual debris. The nail plate becomes distorted with ridges and pitting, and a foul odor may be present. Frequently pressure on the thick nail plate from shoe gear will cause minute hemorrhage under the nail, giving it a black discoloration. The nail plate often becomes detached distally from the underlying nail bed. Partial or total nail loss may occur.

Although the fungal invasion of the nail plate itself does not cause pain, the thickened nails are often a source of problems. Pain may result from pressure of the shoe pressing the nail down into the toe. With this, calloused tissue frequently develops in the nail grooves, resulting in discomfort and pain. In addition, the rough irregular nail may catch on hose, resulting in traumatic partial or total avulsion of the nail. Patients with arterial insufficiency may develop subungual abscesses. Ulcers may form in the nail bed or grooves, with resulting tissue loss. Osteomyelitis is a potential complication because of the close proximity of the distal phalanx and should be suspected when ulcerations are present for extended periods.

Dermatophytes, including *Trichophyton, Microsporum*, and *Epidermophyton* species, are typically the causative agents. Frequently, the clinical appearance of one species is indistinguishable from that of another species (10).

The diagnosis of onychomycosis is confirmed via KOH preparation and culture. Thin shavings of nail are placed in a drop of potassium hydroxide solution on a glass slide and gently heated. Evidence of fungal hyphae is noted under microscopic examination. The thin shavings may also be placed in fungal culture media.

The simplest mode of therapy for mycotic nails consists of debriding the nail and keeping the nail plate as thin as possible. For motivated patients, the topical application of an antifungal liquid such as clotrimazole or miconozole may be considered. The success of this therapy is directly proportional to the zeal with which it is approached by the patient. The nail must be kept as thin as possible, and the medication must be applied at least twice daily for several months. Success with this therapy is 50–50 at best. Oral therapy is also available with griseofulvin, ketoconazole, and fluconazole and is far more successful for onychomycosis of fingernails. The cure rate for mycotic infection of toenails with oral agents is low, and recurrence is high. Surgical avulsion and treatment of the nail bed as the nail plate grows back is largely ineffective. Avulsion of the nail plate and matrixectomy are acceptable forms of treatment in the case of chronically painful nails or those associated with recurrent bacterial infections. Most cases of onychomycosis can be managed with local debridement of the nail plate on a regular basis.

Onychocryptosis, or an ingrown toenail, is a condition in which the medial and lateral borders of the nail plate are curved into the skin. Its expression is largely hereditary. Occasionally, a subungual exostosis exerts pressure on the underside of the nail plate, forcing the sides into the soft tissue. Shoe pressure or incidental trauma may drive the nail into the soft tissues, puncturing the skin, resulting in pain and often infection. Improper cutting of the corners too far proximally may also result in pain and infection as the nail grows out into the soft tissue.

For pain and infection localized to the distal corner of the nail, removal of the leading edge is performed, often without local anesthesia. If the nail edge cannot be reached or the entire border of the nail is painful and infected, a partial nail avulsion should be performed. With infection involving a large part of the nail with purulence noted under the nail plate, the condition should be treated with a total nail avulsion. The procedure for nail avulsion is as follows:

1. Anesthetize the toe, using a digital block at the base of the toe. Never inject in and around the nail, as it is extremely painful. Lidocaine 2% plain is an appropriate local anesthetic.
2. The area should be prepared with a local antiseptic, such as povidone iodine.
3. A tourniquet may be used at the base of the toe, using a Penrose drain secured with a hemostat. It is easy to forget to remove a tourniquet that has been secured to itself without an instrument to serve as a reminder.
4. Using an elevator, carefully detach the soft tissue from the section of nail to be removed.
5. Split the nail plate with nail nippers, and gently remove the nail section with a hemostat. A partial nail avulsion frequently necessitates removal of the outer

third of the nail plate. When performing a total nail avulsion, splitting a nail down the middle facilitates removal.
6. Loose debris and granulation tissue should be debrided accordingly.
7. Povidone iodine 1/4 strength is then applied, followed with a sterile gauze dressing.

Patients are then instructed to change the dressing twice daily thereafter, instilling povidone iodine 1/4 strength into the affected area. Antibiotics should be prescribed with severe infection or for patients with significant peripheral vascular disease.

For recurrent episodes of infection or pain, a chemical matrixectomy can be performed only when the pedal pulses are palpable and never in patients with peripheral vascular disease or neuropathy (11). For those with diminished pulses but adequate perfusion documented with noninvasive vascular studies, nail procedures such as the Frost or Suppan can be performed, in which the nail and matrix are excised by sharp dissection as a procedure in the operating room. Patients should be placed on antibiotics, as the postoperative infection rate can be as high as 10%.

Onychauxis is a hypertrophy or thickening of the nail plate. This condition is seen with trauma, peripheral vascular disease, infection, and certain dermatologic diseases (12). Pain occurs with onychauxis when a tight shoe with a low toe box hits the thickened nail. Treatment includes debridement of the thickened nail to keep it as thin as possible. Permanent removal is a possibility in appropriate cases.

Onychogryphosis, or ram's horn nail, is the term for a nail associated with onychauxis or onychomycosis that has not been cut and grows out to a long, curved, thick nail. The nail may grow to a length of 3 or 4 inches and may curve and press on other structures of the foot, causing pain, especially in shoe gear. Treatment involves simple debridement of the nail.

Another nail disorder is a subungual hematoma, which occurs with acute trauma to the toe, resulting in bleeding beneath the nail plate. The accumulation of blood under the nail results in increased pressure and pain. After obtaining radiographs to rule out a fracture or dislocation, the fluid is then drained through a small hole made in the nail plate with the use of a drill, hot paper clip, or Concept cautery device. Pain is usually relieved immediately.

With chronic trauma, small areas of hemorrhage appear under the nail plate, giving part or all of the nail a black discoloration. This is usually seen when the nail is very thick and tight shoes are worn. Debridement to decrease the thickness of the nail plate and advising patients to wear shoes with adequate room should be sufficient. Chronic subungual hematomas can be confused with subungual melanomas. Many times the distinction can be made with debridement of the nail plate and the underlying subungual hematoma with the use of an electric burr. While the subungual hematoma can be debrided away, this is clearly not the case with a subungual melanoma.

COMMON DERMATOLOGIC FOOT PROBLEMS

Tinea pedis is a common pedal manifestation in the elderly. As in onychomycosis, a slower turnover of the stratum corneum, a depressed inflammatory response, and a decreased cellular immunity contribute to the chronicity of the problem. If there is involvement of the toenails, a cure without relapse is nearly impossible. Many elderly patients have some form of the disease without realizing it.

The two most common organisms involved are *Trichophyton rubrum*, followed by *T. mentagrophytes*, often associated with an acute inflammatory form of the disease (13). There are four basic forms of tinea pedis. The first is a chronic intertriginous form with involvement of the web spaces, especially of the lesser digits. The involved areas often have macerated, peeling skin with fissuring. These fissures can serve as a portal of entry for bacteria, resulting in a secondary cellulitis. The second form is a chronic scaly form, usually caused by *T. rubrum*. It is characterized by chronic papulosquamous hyperkeratotic lesions associated with the sole of the foot in what is often termed a moccasin distribution. The involved area may be a small patch or it may involve the entire sole. It tends to be bilateral. The third type is an acute vesicular form and is often caused by *T. mentagrophytes*. A fourth presentation is an acute ulcerative, vesiculopustular form that is often associated with secondary bacterial infection (14).

An attempt should be made to identify the causative agent via KOH preparation and fungal culture. Bacterial cultures should be performed when secondary bacterial involvement is suspected.

Treatment consists of debriding vesiculobullous lesions and prescribing astringent soaks and antifungal medication. Oral medications are rarely used to treat tinea pedis. They are expensive and rarely successful long-term, with recurrences common, even after prolonged therapy. Most patients are happy to keep the condition in check with topical therapy.

Xerosis, or dry skin, is very common in the elderly. It is due to an inadequate water content of the stratum corneum. The elderly are predisposed to it because of the changes that occur in the skin with aging. Certain disease states may also be implicated, including peripheral vascular disease, hypothyroidism, and dehydration. Weather conditions play a role, as it tends to worsen during the winter or in climates with a low relative humidity (15). It is not a life-threatening condition, but it is often annoying and uncomfortable because of itching, scaling, inflammation, and painful fissures that may develop.

Treatment consists of limiting soaking and the use of harsh soaps. Prolonged exposure to water can actually dry the skin. Bath oils are of some help but should not be recommended to frail elderly patients because with their use, the bathtub can become slippery, putting these patients at risk for falls. Occlusive agents, such as a lanolin or Eucerin are recommended, and their application is generally twice daily. Occlusive agents are especially effective when applied just after bathing. Generally the more effective occlusive agents are more greasy and less pleasing to patients. Keratin-softening agents are also very useful and quite effective preparations, containing urea and lactic acid. Lac-Hydrin (ammonium lactate 12%) is highly effective and readily available (10).

Heel fissures are common problems in the elderly. They are often seen in patients with xerosis, chronic tinea pedis, peripheral vascular disease, and keratosis palmaris et plantaris. They can be very painful and a source of significant morbidity, especially in those with peripheral vascular disease. Long-standing fissures can become secondarily infected with tissue loss. Treatment consists of debridement of the hyperkeratoses and rehydration of the skin with topical therapy. An antifungal agent with an occlusive vehicle would be ideal in those patients with an underlying component of tinea pedis. Difficult cases are managed with the use of moisturizing agents under occlusion with Saran wrap. Patients are instructed to apply a generous amount of the moisturizing agent to the affected area, wrap the foot in Saran wrap, and cover with a sock overnight. Excellent results are often obtained, although this treatment may need to be repeated up to three times weekly.

DISORDERS OF THE FOREFOOT

Hallux abducto valgus with bunion deformity is common in the elderly. The deformity is the result of a deviation of the great toe toward the lesser digits, with a prominence or bunion noted medial to the 1st metatarsophalangeal joint. The deformity may be mild to severe. Severe deformities may be associated with subluxation of the 1st metatarsophalangeal joint. Pain often results from pressure against the prominence from shoe gear and may lead to the formation of a painful bursa. Patients with peripheral vascular disease or neuropathy are at risk for ulceration. Treatment for painful bunion deformities includes rest, ice (for those without peripheral vascular disease and neuropathy), and a short course of a nonsteroidal antiinflammatory agent, provided there are no contraindications. Comfort can be obtained with padding and bunion shields. An attempt should be made to wear shoes wide enough to accommodate the deformity, and shoe stretching is often of great help. Finally, if all else fails, surgery should be considered.

Hallux limitus and hallux rigidus are conditions also frequently associated with a bunion. In this deformity, the motion of the great toe is limited in dorsiflexion. It frequently results in cartilage degeneration and osteophyte production. In this case, the bunion is primarily dorsal or dorsomedial, and little deviation of the great toe exists. To compensate for this lack of motion, the great toe interphalangeal joint hyperextends. Treatment consists of modifications in shoe gear to accommodate the bunion and wearing a shoe with a low heel. A rocker-bottom sole may be beneficial. Surgical procedures are available and should be considered when other treatments are unsuccessful.

Tailor's bunion, or bunionette, deformity is another deformity associated with the lateral aspect of the 5th metatarsophalangeal joint. An associated medial deviation of the 5th toe is often present. Treatment includes padding and wearing appropriate shoe gear, wide enough to accommodate the deformity. Stretching the shoe to accommodate the prominence is helpful, and surgery, when indicated, is often very successful.

Hammertoes, or contractures of the lesser digits, are a very common pedal deformity. A hammertoe is associated with hyperextension of the metatarsophalangeal joint and hyperflexion of the proximal interphalangeal joint. A mallet toe is similar in that there is hyperflexion only at the distal interphalangeal joint. A claw toe is a combination of a hammer toe and a mallet toe. Pain often results from shoe gear rubbing against the skin over the dorsal aspect of the interphalangeal joints, with corns frequently developing. Corns are thickening of the stratum corneum. Frequently a corn develops with inflammation of the underlying structures. Not infrequently, because of the contracture, a retrograde force will push the metatarsal head plantarly, and a painful callus may develop on the ball of the foot. As patients age, hammertoe deformities that were once flexible often become more and more rigid. Treatment involves debridement of the hyperkeratotic lesions, padding, and wearing appropriate shoe gear to provide sufficient room. Should this not provide adequate relief, surgical procedures to correct the deformities can be considered, if desired.

Morton's neuroma is a common source of discomfort in the forefoot. Also referred to as an interdigital neuroma, it is most frequently seen in the distal 3rd intermetatarsal space, and to a lesser extent, in the distal 2nd intermetatarsal space. It is a neuritic condition involving fibrous enlargement of the common digital nerve and seems to occur secondary to chronic, repetitive microtrauma of the nerve against the distal edge of the intermetatarsal ligament. Symptoms include burning sensations, sharp pain that radiates to the toes or proximally up the leg, numbness, tingling sensations, and a dull ache on the ball of the foot. These symptoms are worse with tight or narrow shoes, and relief may be obtained by removing the shoe and massaging the infected area. Treatment includes counseling patients on proper shoe gear with an adequate width. In addition, padding placed just proximal to the metatarsophalangeal joints may produce relief. Nonsteroidal medications may be helpful, and a trial for up to 2 weeks may be necessary. An injection of a corticosteroid can produce relief, but it is often temporary. If all else fails, surgical resection of the neuroma can be performed with generally good results.

Plantar calluses are often seen in the elderly. They are often present under one or more metatarsophalangeal joints, as well as the rim of the heel. Their formation is the result of repetitive moderate stress of musculoskeletal elements moving in relation to the skin. The pressures involved in the formation of calluses are not sufficient to cause ulceration in the sensate patient. They are very common in the elderly population, especially in those with fat pad atrophy of the ball of the foot. The calluses are a thickening of the stratum corneum. The callus may be diffuse or discrete, with a core of hyperkeratotic tissue that extends deep. With weightbearing, the hyperkeratotic tissue is pushed into the deeper structures, resulting in pain that can be severe and can limit ambulation. Treatment consists of debridement of the hyperkeratotic tissue and often results in immediate relief. Keratin-softening products containing urea or aluminum lactate 12% (Lac-Hydrin) are also beneficial in keeping these lesions soft.

MIDFOOT DISORDERS

It is common to see manifestations of osteoarthritis in the midfoot. Although significant spurring may be noted over the dorsal aspect of the midfoot, it is rare to see noticeable joint pain in this region. Still, the dorsal spurs may cause discomfort due to irritation of the overlying structures. Dorsal tendinitis, tenosynovitis, and bursitis are seen when shoe gear presses the dorsal midfoot soft tissue structures into the osteophytes. Local nerve irritation can occur, specifically to the medial dorsocutaneous nerve and to the deep peroneal nerve as they course over this region. Symptoms such as burning, tingling, and paresthesias may exist. All of the complaints frequently respond to icing, a short course of nonsteroidal antiinflammatory medications, and shoe gear modifications. Shoes that are open over the dorsum of the foot and those with padded tongues are helpful. Shoe laces should also be kept loosely tied.

REARFOOT DISORDERS

Heel pain is a term that includes several clinical entities. Among the most common is plantar fasciitis, which is common among all podiatric patients, including the elderly. Pain develops at the plantar medial aspect of the heel near the insertion of the plantar fascia. The discomfort frequently is worse in the morning and subsides with ambulation, although the first few steps may be quite painful. The pain typically returns with prolonged ambulation toward the end of the day. The condition is worse with flat shoes or walking barefoot. Radiographs may reveal a spur at the inferior aspect of the calcaneus, historically thought to cause the pain by irritating the adjacent soft tissues. However, many active people with very large infracalcaneal spurs never have heel pain. Rather, the pain appears to be secondary to inflammation at the insertion of the plantar fascia into the inferior calcaneus. Factors predisposing to plantar fasciitis include pronation, obesity, and recent onset of new activity. Pronation, where the arch flattens somewhat with weightbearing, stresses the plantar fascia at its attachment to the medial calcaneal tubercle, with inflammation developing. The elderly may be particularly predisposed to plantar fasciitis, as weight gain into the eighth decade and a progressive flattening of the arch are common. Many patients will have just begun a walking program as part of weight loss or cardiac rehabilitation.

Conservative therapy is very successful, and arch support is the mainstay of therapy. A foot strapping and an over-the-counter arch support with nonsteroidal inflammatory medication may be sufficient. Cortisone injections are helpful in very painful cases. Care must be taken to avoid injecting cortisone into the fat pad, to avoid fat pad atrophy. It is important to realize that injection therapy and medication are beneficial short-term and that arch support is often necessary to maintain long-term relief. A custom-made foot orthosis may be needed if simpler, inexpensive, over-the-counter inserts are inadequate. Surgery is indicated in intractable cases, but this is very rare.

Infracalanceal bursitis is also sometimes seen, often in conjunction with fat pad atrophy and/or rupture of the fibrous retaining system of the fat pad. The pain is due to the inflammation of the infracalcaneal bursa, located between the calcaneus and fat pad. Unlike plantar fasciitis, pain is not usually seen upon arising in the morning but rather with continued weightbearing throughout the course of the day. Pain is noted with palpation directly plantar to the heel, and the plantar contour of the calcaneus may be palpable as well. Treatment is limited and consists of wearing shoes with a soft sole with inserts that provide additional cushioning. Cortisone injections into the painful bursa may produce relief, but caution should be exercised in cases of significant fat pad atrophy.

Posterior heel pain may occur due to retrocalcaneal bursitis, in inflammation of the bursa, located between the calcaneus and the Achilles tendon, just superior to its insertion. The Achilles tendon inserts into the lower two-thirds of the calcaneus, and a bursa is present between the Achilles tendon and the upper one-third of the bone. The pain is frequently secondary to shoe gear impinging on the area. Treatment involves shoe gear modifications, heel lifts, and a short course of nonsteroidal therapy. For persistent cases, physical therapy may be indicated. Cortisone injection into this bursa is often avoided, as it may predispose to rupture of the Achilles tendon.

An inflamed bursa may also be present between the skin and the Achilles tendon, just superior to its insertion. It is usually due to pressure from shoe gear. A bulla may be present as well. Treatment consists of icing, nonsteroidal antiinflammatory medications, padding, and modification of shoe gear to relieve pressure on this area.

Posterior tibial tendinitis is a common source of pain that is often misdiagnosed. The tendon courses posterior to the tibia and medial malleolus. At the tip of the medial malleolus, it courses inferiorly and anteriorly, inserting onto the medial and plantar structures of the midfoot. Inflammation of the posterior tibial tendon is prone to develop in many elderly patients, since weight gain and a progressive flattening of the arch tend to occur. The tendon is in close proximity to the tibial nerve, and pain in this area is often attributed to a tarsal tunnel or a neuritic condition. Uncomfortable nerve studies are sometimes ordered and usually are normal, and the pain is attributed to "arthritis." The diagnosis of posterior tibial tendinitis is simple and merely requires palpating the tendon with the foot plantarflexed and inverted. Localized edema along the course of the tendon is common. Treatment consists of icing, nonsteroidal antiinflammatory medication, strapping of the foot, and physical therapy. A custom foot orthosis is usually indicated to provide support and long-term relief. The response to therapy with these simple measures is often excellent. Cortisone injections are never indicated, as they increase the risk of rupture of the posterior tibial tendon, which is very debilitating.

Achilles tendinitis in the elderly is relatively uncommon. However, pain may be noted at the insertion of the Achilles tendon, and radiographs may reveal spurs or calcifications on the posterior calcaneus. Treatment consists of heel lifts, nonsteroidal antiinflammatory medication, and physical therapy. Relief may require removal of the posterior spur and calcifications, provided the patient is a good surgical candidate.

THE ARTHRITIC FOOT

The arthritic foot, caused by either degenerative joint disease or rheumatoid arthritis in the geriatric patient, can be an incapacitating condition that warrants aggressive management to help maintain mobility. The contiguous joint structures including bone, hyaline cartilage, ligaments, synovium, joint capsule, tendon and sheaths, and muscles are all subject to degenerative changes with advancing age. Bone becomes osteopenic and cartilage thins and fragments. Adjacent molecules of collagen and the soft tissue elements become cross-linked and thereby stiffen and lose resiliency. Fluidity of motion and decreased support follow lessening muscular strength. The degenerative process ensues, leading to compromise.

The foot is particularly susceptible to these changes because of the tremendous forces generated by locomotion. The vaulted arch structure of the foot places the midfoot at particular risk of degenerative joint disease. Breakdown here is due to the "keystone" function of the bases of the metatarsals and cuneiform bones. Failure of optimal joint function at this level causes swelling and pain. Lacing shoes over this area may be very uncomfortable.

The subtalar and ankle joints are not as commonly involved in osteoarthritis. Degenerative joint disease of these areas is usually related to history of prior trauma or inflammatory joint disease. Destruction at these areas can cause severe pain and disability. Ankle-foot orthoses, special shoeing, and nonsteroidal antiinflammatory drugs are usually necessary to delay the need for surgical arthrodesis of these joints.

The most clinically significant area for degenerative changes is the forefoot. Deformity, which develops slowly over the years, may accelerate the process of joint and soft tissue breakdown. Degenerative changes are usually seen at the most dynamic structure of the forefoot, the first ray, hallux, first metatarsal, and first cuneiform. Hallux valgus with bunion deformity or hallux rigidus (degenerative joint disease of the first metatarsal phalangeal joint) causes the great toe to play less of a role in the dissipation of forces during gait. Other forefoot structures will be under greater stress because of the compensation for less than optimal first metatarsal phalangeal joint function. The lesser metatarsal phalangeal joints are also sites for degenerative changes. Subluxation and dislocation of the metatarsal phalangeal joints places tremendous stress below the ball of the foot. Thinning of the plantar fat pad and formation of thick calluses adds to disability.

Treatment includes concentration on providing cushioning, support, and accommodation of deformity. Orthotics that combine soft and firm materials are preferred. Combinations of plastazote and Spenco or PPT are very useful. Supporting the foot to control intrinsic foot motion will lessen joint inflammation. Walking and running shoes may be used if there is not excess deformity. An orthotic that ends at the ball of the foot can usually be used. Excess deformity such as hallux valgus, hammertoes, and subluxed or dislocated metatarsal phalangeal joints require the use of extra-depth shoes. They are useful because they allow the insertion of a cushioned orthotic while leaving room for the foot.

Custom molded shoes are only necessary when there is such severe deformity that conventional shoe wear is not possible. Molded shoes should be fabricated with resilient leathers and flat soles including the arch area of the shoe. The molded orthotic should provide all the cushioning and support and thereby can be replaced regularly. They should be laced to the toe and of rigid construction.

Regular visits are important to keep nails appropriately trimmed and corns and calluses thinned. Blisters may occur at these sites that allow infection and ulceration. Pads medicated with salicylic acid should not be used in a geriatric patient because of the potential for chemical burn.

Surgical therapy should be considered when nonsurgical care fails to provide sufficient comfort, deformity is severe enough to prevent wearing shoes, or there is chronically recurrent infection caused by deformity. Postoperative planning is essential for this patient population. The use of a walker or crutches after foot surgery may be necessary for weeks. It may be impossible for the geriatric patient with arthritis to use these devices effectively. Rehabilitation or nursing facility may be necessary after foot and ankle surgery.

THE DIABETIC FOOT

Care of the foot of a patient with diabetes mellitus begins before there are any complications of the disease. Good habits should begin at the time the diabetes is diagnosed. The elderly diabetic has the same risk factors as the younger diabetic, but in addition, is subject to the risks of the geriatric years.

All diabetic patients must be encouraged to maintain good hygiene, with daily bathing, including the foot. Soaking of the feet is not necessary and indeed not recommended. It will contribute to drying of the skin. It also may delay healing of any open wound by spreading existing infection and slowing development of granulation tissue. Daily inspection of the feet by the patient, family, or health care worker is very important. The diabetic should be encouraged never to go barefoot. Many geriatric patients give their own insulin injections. Broken insulin needles are the most common foreign body encountered in the feet of diabetics. All diabetics should be taught not to break the needle off the syringe. The syringe and needle should be disposed of intact, in a proper receptacle.

Diabetes, in and of itself, does not preclude self-care of the feet. When complications of peripheral neuropathy or peripheral vascular disease begin to occur, self-care of the nails and calluses must stop. This is also true for the diabetic with poor eyesight, joint disease, or inability to reach the feet. The geriatric physician must pay close attention to the feet, making sure to inspect the skin for any breaks, especially interdigitally on the plantar surface and the heels. Peripheral pulses, when palpable, are the only circulation test necessary. Nonpalpable pulses need not be tested further as long as the patient is active and the skin is intact.

Shoes should be shaken out before putting them on. All diabetics with complications should change their shoes and socks every 3 to 4 hours. This allows for brief inspection, changes pressure points, and causes friction to be minimized. Any break in the skin can then be caught early, and treatment can begin before infection has a chance. The modern walking shoes are good, because they have desirable qualities. The upper materials are soft leather or man-made material. The soles are cushioned, and the heel counters firm. They are laced, and the tongue and collar of the shoe are cushioned. Extra-depth shoes should be used if there is digital or other forefoot deformity. Molded shoes are necessary only if the foot has changed shape because of disease; for example, Charcot foot. Soft custom-molded orthotics such as plastazote may be used with all of these shoes.

Neuropathic ulceration develops because of a combination of faulty dynamic and static deformities of the musculoskeletal system and peripheral neuropathy. Repetitive moderate stress, that responsible for plantar callus formation, is also the chief cause of the neuropathic ulceration. When preventive efforts have failed, concentration on four factors will achieve healing of neuropathic ulceration. First, there must be adequate arterial blood flow, preferably palpable pedal pulses. Second, spreading sepsis must be absent. Incision and drainage is sometimes necessary to drain infection and remove necrotic tissue. Exposed bone should be removed. Third, the blood sugar level should be controlled as close to normal as possible. Fourth, weight should be removed from the involved site. There is no substitute for total nonweightbearing with a walker or crutches. Weight dispersion pads should be used for an outpatient. Failure of the ulcer to heal in a reasonable period of time (4 to 6 weeks) should cause the clinician to recheck the four major elements necessary for healing. Hospitalization is necessary if the ulcer fails to close.

Application of topical agents to help close ulcerations is only secondary to the primary factors previously mentioned. Antiseptics, such as povodone iodine, should be diluted to 1/4 strength. The use of normal saline in a wet-to-dry dressing appears to be sufficient. Application of topical growth factors has still to prove its benefit versus cost. It is, however, an area of great potential, and research should continue as to its efficacy.

REFERENCES

1. Blocker WP. Maintaining functional independence by mobilizing the aged. Geriatrics 1992;1:42–56.
2. Jekel JF. A public health perspective on podiatric medicine. J Am Podiatr Med Assoc 1990;80:158–160.
3. Tinnetti M, Speechley M. Prevention of falls among the elderly. N Engl J Med 1989;320:1055–1062.
4. Hsu JD. Foot problems in the elderly patient. J Am Geriatr Soc 1971;19:880–886.
5. Levine R. Social implications of immobility. Clin Podiatr 1984;1:255–259.
6. Taylor R, Bradley WG. Peripheral neuropathies. In: Hazzard WR, Andres R, Bierman E, Blass JP, eds. Principles of geriatric medicine and gerontology. New York: McGraw-Hill, 1990:977–982.
7. Balin AK. Aging of human skin. In: Hazzard WR, Andres R, Bierman E, Blass JP, eds. Principles of geriatric medicine and gerontology. New York: McGraw-Hill, 1990:383–412.
8. Sarrafian SK. Anatomy of the foot and ankle. 1st ed. Philadelphia: JB Lippincott, 1983:350–356.
9. Krantz CE. A nail survey of 4,600 patients. J Natl Assoc Chirop 1950;40:5–11.
10. Arnold HL, Odom RB, James WD. Andrew's diseases of the skin. 8th ed. Philadelphia: WB Saunders, 1990:81.
11. Yale JP. Podiatric medicine, 3rd ed. Baltimore: Williams & Wilkins, 1987:221–223.
12. Helfand AE. Onychial disorders in the older patient. Clin Podiatr Med Surg 1993;10:59–68.
13. Arnold HL, Odom RB, James WD. Andrew's diseases of the skin. 8th ed. Philadelphia: WB Saunders, 1990:331–333.
14. Abramson C. A new look at dermatophytosis and atopy. In: McCarthy DJ, ed. Podiatric dermatology. Baltimore: Williams & Wilkins 1986:133–145.
15. Robinson JR. Dermatitis, dry skin, dandruff, seborrheic dermatitis, and psoriasis products. In: Feldman EG, ed. Handbook of non-prescription drugs. Washington, DC: American Pharmaceutical Association, 1991:819–824.

34/ Endocrinology and Aging

Steven R. Gambert

For years, gerontologists and endocrinologists alike have been intrigued by a possible relationship between some alteration in the endocrine system and the aging process itself. In fact, the "father" of both fields is considered to be the same individual, Brown-Séquard, a noted French scientist who claimed in 1889 that a water-soluble extract of dog testes gave him an "astonishing degree of rejuvenation" and improved his longstanding problem of impotence. Despite the fact that we now know that there is no testosterone or for that matter any other sex steroid or hormone in this water-soluble extract, the link between hormones and aging was set forward.

Over the years, one or another hormone received some degree of notoriety amid claims that it was the "key" to the aging process. Diabetes mellitus was thought to be an excellent model for aging because of the common features of thickened basement membranes, atherosclerotic changes, and cataracts, among other findings. Needless to say, diabetes mellitus is currently considered to be a disease and not a part of the aging process. An insensitivity to thyroid hormone action was also theorized as a possible explanation for the aging process or at least some of the manifestations seen more commonly during later life.

What exact role the sex steroids play in the aging process is also a topic of great concern. It is well known that the female reproductive system undergoes changes as part of the normal aging process. Menopause not only leads to changes in the genitourinary tract but also accelerates the loss of minerals from bone and leads to an alteration in the lipid composition of the mature woman. Male hormones have been linked to preservation of muscle mass as well as to an increased tendency toward developing certain diseases during later life.

Recently, growth hormone has been resurrected as a potentially significant factor in how well we preserve our muscle mass, general well-being, and appetite (1). Growth hormone, however, is not new to the field of aging and in fact was first postulated in 1914 by Simmonds to be a vital determinant of the aging process (2). In 1959, Groen postulated that the hypothalamus provided a central control of aging, a theory further propagated by Dilman in 1971 (3) and Frolkis in 1972 (4). About the same time, Denkler reported that he had identified a peptide within the pituitary that he called DECO, for decreasing oxygen consumption hormone, that presumably "programmed" the aging process. Rats that had their pituitaries removed and were given supplements of all known pituitary hormones other than this peptide reportedly no longer demonstrated many of the otherwise "normal" aging changes, including a preservation of the ability to reject foreign substances injected under the skin, protein synthesis as measured by new hair growth, and sensitivity of the β-adrenergic nervous system as based on aortic strip response to isoproterenol. Unfortunately, these studies were abruptly discontinued and have not been reproduced.

While the endocrine system remains a likely target for additional research regarding the normal process of aging, it is certain that aging is associated with a higher incidence of disorders or diseases of the endocrine system, including diabetes mellitus, hypothyroidism, apathetic thyrotoxicosis, among others, and that there is an often atypical presentation to endocrine diseases during later life. This chapter discusses the diagnosis and management of several disorders of the endocrine system that appear commonly during later life.

PITUITARY

ANATOMIC CHANGES WITH AGING

Both anatomic and histologic changes in the pituitary gland have been described with aging. By age 80, the weight of the adenohypophysis is approximately 25% from its peak of 400 mg during young adulthood. With age, there is a reduction in blood supply, a higher percentage of cells that are chromophobic and basophilic, and a relative decrease in acidophilic cells. A higher number of adenomas and colloid-filled cysts have also been described during later life.

HORMONAL CHANGES WITH AGING

Although there have been reports of altered secretion of various neuropeptides by the aging pituitary gland, no significant findings have been agreed upon, and clearly age should not be used to explain an abnormality of pituitary function. While the half-life of ACTH, adrenocorticotropin hormone, was reported by Friedman et al. (5) to increase slightly with age, there is no increase in circulating levels or response of ACTH to stimulation as demonstrated by the metyrapone stimulation test. The ability to secrete growth hormone in response to arginine stimulation or postsurgical stress also appears to be preserved throughout life as a function of normal aging.

Circulating levels of growth hormone have been reported to be lower or without difference in older persons, compared with younger ones; it remains uncertain whether this represents a deficiency state in need of correction or some necessary adaptation or response to age. Studies measuring blood sugar and free fatty acids following infusions of growth hormone fail to demonstrate differences with increasing age. Growth hormone is elevated without regard to age following infusions of arginine or postoperatively (6). Although Hontela (7) and Kaiser (8) reported a diminished response of TSH (thyroid-stimulating hormone) to TRH (thyroid-releasing hormone) stimulation in older subjects, compared with younger ones, there is no consensus about the physiologic effect of this finding. Prolactin release has not been shown to be affected by age, and the pituitary continues to respond to stimulation with L-dopa and 2-bromo-ergocryptine (9). Peptides related to female reproduction demonstrate principles of normal physiology. As the primary endorgan fails, in this case the ovary, the pituitary responds with higher levels of stimulating peptides, e.g. LH and FSH. Although the failure of a gland in certain circumstances is considered to be a disease and not a normal consequence of aging, in this case, failure of ovarian function is considered to be an inevitable consequence of growing old.

Studies of old male Wistar rats report a diminished secretion of antidiuretic hormone (ADH) by the neurohypophysis (10). This is associated with an increased excretion of water and fluid and electrolyte changes. Miller found that the quantity of ADH excreted in urine paralleled very closely the changes in ADH content of the neurohypophysis (11). While young rats had a prompt fall in urine output when water was withheld, older rats continued to excrete water despite the lack of fluid intake. In other words, there was a difference in the pattern of the response to dehydration in aging rats, perhaps related to a change in the sensitivity of the osmoreceptors. This has also been shown to occur in human subjects. When infused with hypertonic solutions, elderly individuals report less thirst than younger individuals and drink significantly less free water when presented with the option to drink ad libitum.

While everyone agrees that hypopituitarism is a disease and not a normal accompaniment of the aging process, elderly persons demonstrate a loss of body hair and changes in the skin compatible with an endocrinopathy. There is a general reduction in the skin's collagen content and thickness. Because normal aging and growth hormone deficiency are both associated with an increase in percentage body fat, a decrease in lean body mass, and a decrease in bone mass and protein synthesis, there is a possibility that reduced growth hormone secretion could account for some of these effects (12).

Recent data suggest a role for growth hormone administration in a subset of elderly men who exhibit significant muscle wasting (13). While there has been an increase in muscle mass and a reduction in body fat compatible with a more youthful state reported following growth hormone injection in a select group of elderly men, additional studies are needed before making any definitive conclusions regarding growth hormone replacement therapy. Fears of prostatic hypertrophy, stimulation of malignant cells, and development of carpal tunnel syndrome among other problems need to be weighed against any potential desired outcome. Prospective clinical trials of replacement of growth hormone in both elderly men and women are now in progress.

THYROID

CHANGES WITH AGE

The thyroid gland becomes relatively smaller, lower lying, and retrosternal with age. There is an increase in interfollicular fibrotic tissue and the development of both macronodules and micronodules. Follicles appear distended and are lined by flattened follicular cells. Large vacuolated thyrotrophs, a decrease in blood supply, and fibrolymphocytic infiltration are also more commonly noted.

HORMONAL CHANGES WITH AGING

Studies that can distinguish between healthy individuals and those who have age-prevalent illness are essential if one is to differentiate between the effects of normal aging and diseases that occur more frequently in the aged. Serum levels of free L-thyroxine (T_4) remain constant throughout life, as do levels of free triiodothyronine (T_3). However, the half-life of serum T_4 increases with age from an approximate value of 4 days during youth to 7 days during young adulthood to 9.3 days during later life. Since less T_4 is produced by the thyroid gland with age, serum levels remain constant.

Nevertheless, this change in half-life has clinical significance in that the time to reach a steady-state level on any given dose of thyroid hormone replacement is related to the half-life. It takes approximately five half-lives to reach a steady state, thus mandating a longer time between dosing intervals with increasing age. In addition, this change results in a lower target dose for thyroid hormone replacement in older persons than in younger ones. While the average T_4 replacement dose for young hypothyroid adults is 0.15 mg, the dose is approximately 0.1125 mg for older hypothyroid persons. As with any medication, individual titration is essential.

Serum TSH does not change with normal aging. Despite this, many more older persons will have elevated serum TSH levels because of a higher incidence of primary failure of the thyroid gland, resulting in hypothyroidism or subclinical hypothyroidism. In a study using the Framingham population, it was noted that of those persons over the age of 60 who had normal levels of serum T_4, approximately 14% had slight elevations of serum TSH, and 5.9% had serum TSH levels clearly within the hypothyroid range (14). Studies have confirmed these data and report that of those who have clear elevations of serum TSH despite a normal level of serum T_4, the likelihood of developing hypothyroidism is great, with over 80% becoming hypothyroid within 4 years. In addition, the presence of antimicrosomal antibodies is also associated with a high risk of progression to hypothyroidism. For this reason, most clinicians advocate starting these individuals on thyroid hormone replacement. The presence of subclinical hypothyroidism may not be as benign as was once thought. Studies have confirmed an increased systolic time interval associated with subclinical hypothyroidism and improvement as measured by quality of life scales following thyroid hormone replacement, compared with placebo (15).

Hypothyroidism is an age-prevalent disease that occurs most frequently during later life. Although the most common cause is thought to be immunologic, past radiation therapy or surgery to the thyroid gland should be considered. While hypothyroidism presents with the same signs and symptoms regardless of one's age, elderly persons may not be readily diagnosed because so many other problems that occur during later life may confuse the situation. Paresthesias, weakness, constipation, memory disturbances, dry atrophic skin, and cardiomegaly are just a few of the presenting problems that may be confused with normal aging or age-prevalent disease. For this reason, it is currently recommended that all persons over the age of 50 be screened for thyroid abnormalities and that screening be repeated periodically thereafter. Hypothyroidism most commonly results from a primary failure of the thyroid gland and can be confirmed by detecting low circulating levels of serum T_4 and an elevated serum TSH level. Low levels of both circulating thyroid hormone and serum TSH suggest pituitary dysfunction.

Once a decision is made to treat a person with either frank hypothyroidism or subclinical hypothyroidism, thyroid hormone replacement should be initiated with T_4. Due to the "burst" effect of T_3 on the myocardium and the short half-life of this hormone, T_3 should not be used to treat hypothyroidism, especially in elderly persons. The dose of T_4 should initially be small, 0.0125 or 0.025 mg, and increased gradually, allowing a steady state to be reached between dosage adjustments. This may require a wait of 4 to 6 weeks, given the age-related change in half-life for T_4 that is further prolonged by hypothyroidism. Serum levels of T_4 should be monitored; the final dose is that which reduces serum TSH to within normal levels without causing unwanted side effects. In general, elderly persons require approximately 0.1125 mg of T_4 to maintain a euthyroid state.

Of all persons with *hyperthyroidism*, approximately 15% are over the age of 60. While the most common cause of hyperthyroidism at any age is Graves' disease, a toxic nodule is most common in elderly individuals. Men and women appear to be affected equally during later life, contrasted with a predominate female distribution during youth. Elderly persons classically present with few of the more traditional signs and symptoms; cardiovascular changes, muscle wasting, and weight loss are most common. Congestive heart failure is noted in over half, atrial fibrillation in 40%, and new or worse angina in 20%. Anorexia is a common finding leading to malnutrition, weight loss, and eventually muscle wasting and weakness. This is in contrast to an increase in appetite in younger adults who are hyperthyroid. Data from animal studies suggest an age-related change in neuropeptide response to thyroid stimulation in areas of the brain that control appetite (16). While few elderly who become hyperthyroid complain of frequent bowel movements, a correction of a pre-existing constipation is not uncommon.

While most young persons who have hyperthyroidism have elevated levels of both T_4 and T_3, older persons may have isolated elevations of either T_4 or T_3 alone. This likely results from years of a failing thyroid gland being stimulated by TSH, resulting in nodule formation and in certain cases, autonomy. If clinical data suggest hyperthyroidism and T_4 levels are not elevated, the clinician should obtain a serum T_3 level before dismissing hyperthyroidism as a possibility. Although the serum TSH level may be suppressed with age, a suppressed TSH based on the newer ultrasensitive assay is compatible with a diagnosis of hyperthyroidism.

Elderly persons may also present with an almost compete absence of symptoms and signs in what has been referred to as apathetic thyrotoxicosis (17). In this disorder, elderly persons appear to be extremely depressed, with apathetic-appearing facies, blunted affect, and significant anorexia and weight loss. Muscle wasting is pronounced, and proximal muscle weakness results in an inability to transfer and remain independent. Once again, thyroid glands are commonly nonpalpable, eye findings nonexistent, and cardiovascular findings often confused with preexisting disease. Unfortunately, many persons with apathetic thyrotoxicosis are evaluated for, and even unnecessarily treated for, major depression and/or presumed malignancy.

Treatment of hyperthyroidism mandates reduction in circulating levels of thyroid hormone. Antithyroid medications take several weeks to work and therefore should be given promptly to reduce circulating levels of thyroid hormone before definitive therapy. In most cases, definitive therapy will require radioactive iodine; antithyroid medications should be continued and individually titrated while the former treatment continues to work over the next weeks to months. While many clinicians fail to initiate the antithyroid medications before radioactive iodine therapy, this increases the risk of a radiation-induced thy-

roiditis. When the clinical condition mandates more immediate action than possible through the above mechanism, the addition of iodine (Lugol's solution) to the antithyroid medications will accelerate the decline in circulating levels of thyroid hormone. The use of β-blockers can also help reduce cardiovascular effects from increased levels of thyroid hormone, though caution is advised because of the relatively high risk of unwanted cardiovascular side effects.

PARATHYROID

Although there are pathological changes that occur in parathyroid gland tissue with advancing age, such as an increase in the number of oxyphilic cells, there appears to be no major change in parathyroid hormone (PTH) levels. There is an increase in interstitial fat within the parathyroid gland, and colloid vesicles and microcysts are frequently noted on pathological review. There is an increase in nodule formation, especially in women over the age of 50. Many of the studies that have reported an increase in PTH with age unfortunately measured PTH using an antibody that recognizes only the C-terminal portion of the hormone. Since this inactive fragment is cleared by the kidney and renal function declines with increasing age, an increase in this fragment should be expected and has no clinical consequence. While other studies have reported an increase in PTH with age using other antibodies, there is not universal agreement, and any increase must be evaluated in relation to calcium levels to rule out an underlying hyperparathyroidism.

HYPERPARATHYROIDISM

Clinically, the main problem to consider in relation to the parathyroid gland is hyperparathyroidism. While this may result from a diffuse hyperplasia of all four parathyroid glands, it may be due to a tumor. Approximately two-thirds of the cases of primary hyperparathyroidism occur in persons over 50 years of age, with a preponderance being women. Most result from single or multiple adenomas, with a small number associated with parathyroid growth outside the neck region.

The advent of automated mass screening for serum chemistries has led to an increase in the number of persons identified with elevated serum calcium levels. Immobility is a risk factor for hypercalcemia, and individuals who have borderline high levels of serum calcium may develop seriously elevated levels when left immobile. This is a particular problem in elderly individuals who have had borderline hyperparathyroidism for many years and now require greater intervention. Although sodium is coupled to calcium in the kidney and increased sodium intake can help reduce calcium levels by increasing a mechanism of excretion, elderly persons may not tolerate this therapy because of cardiovascular compromise. Particular attention should be given to fluid and electrolyte status; diuretic therapy (Lasix) can increase sodium and thus calcium excretion but must be used only with careful monitoring. Hydrochlorothiazide uncouples the sodium-calcium unit and can actually increase calcium levels in this setting.

Clinical

Approximately two-thirds of persons with hyperparathyroidism have clinical evidence of renal calculi or osteitis fibrocystica. There may also be symptoms of decreased excitability of neuromuscular structures, muscular weakness, constipation, anorexia, nausea, abdominal cramps, dryness of mucous membranes, fatigue, apathy, and confusion. Some individuals also complain of a generalized bone pain, and pathological fractures may occur. Nephrocalcinosis may be noted on radiographs, and renal colic and/or hematuria should alert the clinician to a possible problem. The electrocardiogram may show a shortened QT interval.

Treatment

Treatment of hyperparathyroidism rests on removing the cause, be it an adenoma or gland hyperplasia. Depending on the level of the hypercalcemia and the underlying health status of the patient, surgical intervention may be delayed while medical management is attempted. As mentioned previously, delaying surgical therapy when the patient is able to tolerate it may result in an even more difficult situation later on if the aged patient becomes more frail, immobile, and a greater surgical risk.

Medical management rests on fluids, sodium intake as tolerated, diuretic therapy with Lasix, and oral ingestion of phosphate. Phosphates increase the risk of renal calcification and GI disturbance, however, with the potential for diarrhea and electrolyte abnormalities. In some cases, phosphates may need to be given intravenously. While this is a potent way to reduce calcium levels, diffuse calcifications may result, with a particular problem if the kidneys are affected. Newer therapy also includes subcutaneous injections of calcitonin. While this is also a potent treatment,

it generally is short-lived because of the development of antibodies and does nothing to correct the underlying problem. Other causes of hypercalcemia should be ruled out, especially malignancy at this time in life.

HYPOPARATHYROIDISM

Hypoparathyroidism in the elderly is rare and almost always results from prior neck surgery for thyroid disease. Transient hypoparathyroidism is common following thyroid or parathyroid surgery. This presumably results from damage to the glands themselves or to their blood supply. In addition, both hyperthyroidism and hyperparathyroidism may suppress normal parathyroid gland activity and thus the need for reequilibration following surgery. Mild hypocalcemia may be asymptomatic or be accompanied by nonspecific changes involving the CNS. Chronic hypocalcemia is associated with cataract formation, calcification of the basal ganglia, and symptoms involving the CNS, including depression, dementia, or even a frank psychosis. When hypocalcemia becomes severe, a neuromuscular irritability, or tetany, may occur. Tetany is characterized by paresthesias, particularly around the mouth, and muscle spasms, most notably affecting the hands, feet, and face. This rarely occurs with calcium levels above 7 mg/dL (ionized levels of calcium above 3 mg/dL) unless there is concurrent alkalosis. Clinically, hypocalcemia may be associated with clinical signs of latent neuromuscular irritability even before tetany is noted. The Chvostek sign, or a contraction of the facial muscles elicited by tapping the facial nerve and Trousseau sign, a carpopedal spasm caused by a reduction of the blood supply to the hand when a tourniquet, most commonly an inflated blood pressure cuff, is applied to the arm for 3 to 5 minutes, should be looked for. The ECG may show a prolongation of the QT interval. Administration of calcium and vitamin D should successfully manage low levels of calcium resulting from hypoparathyroidism.

ADRENAL

The adrenal glands have more fibrous tissue with aging. Although there is a decrease in the secretion of cortisol by the zona fasciculata, there is no change in the circulating levels of corticosteroids because of reduced clearance. The adrenal glands maintain their ability to respond to ACTH by increasing levels of cortisol. The circadian rhythmic pattern of adrenal cortical activity reportedly remains unchanged by age, with plasma cortisol levels normally peaking in the AM hours and reaching a minimum in late afternoon. Aldosterone secretion has been reported to decrease with age, though the clinical significance of this report remains unknown.

Perhaps the most common cause of hypercortisolism is the iatrogenic use of corticosteroids for a variety of medical conditions. Since steroid use can suppress the pituitary-adrenal axis, adrenal insufficiency is also a risk following discontinuation of therapy. Cushing's disease, although most common during middle life, may occur at any age and is due to hyperstimulation of the adrenal glands by a pituitary-hypothalmic abnormality. Cushing's syndrome results from overproduction of cortisol by an adenoma of the adrenal gland itself. There are rare cases of nonendocrine tumors that produce either an ACTH-like substance or a substance that acts on the hypothalamus to stimulate the ACTH-releasing factor. In general, these factors are suppressed by relatively high doses of steroids. Individuals with Cushing's disease loose the normal diurnal plasma cortisol variation and early on may be detected by failure to see a "lower" level of PM cortisol. Cushing's disease is commonly associated with a hypokalemic alkalosis, "moon"-shaped or round facies, hirsutism, purplish abdominal striae, buffalo hump, and new appearance of acneiform lesions. Signs of virilization suggest adrenal tumors that secrete elevated levels of androgen.

Treatment of hypercortisolism depends upon the cause of the problem. Iatrogenically caused hypercortisolism can be treated by reducing exogenous steroid therapy. In most cases, this must be done in a manner that does not exacerbate the underlying condition that led to the use of steroids in the first place. Do not stop the therapy abruptly, as the adrenal glands will need time to return to normal function following a period of suppression. Cushing's disease may be treated by performing adrenalectomy or treatment of the pituitary itself with radiation. Adrenal adenomas are excised in most cases. Following surgery, replacement therapy with a cortisol equivalent should be instituted promptly. Because the adrenal can increase corticosteroid output to a maximum of 300 mg/day hydrocortisone equivalent under stress, normal replacement dosages may not be sufficient during episodes of acute medical conditions including infections, burns, and surgery. Under these circumstances, the patient is best treated with continual intravenous steroid coverage because the half-life of circulating cortisol given intravenously as a one-time injection is approximately 15 minutes.

Addison's disease may occur at any age and is most commonly due to an autoimmune phenomenon. It is important to rule out other causes such as tuberculosis and metastatic involvement of the adrenal glands, as these appear to be more common in elderly persons. While chronic use of corticosteroids may suppress the adrenal's production of cortisol, the production of mineralocorticoids usually remains intact because of the preservation of stimulation from ACTH and the renin-angiotensin-aldosterone system. In cases in which an autoimmune or infiltrative process destroys the adrenal glands themselves, both corticosteroid and mineralocorticoid production is affected, and thus therapy is directed at replacement of both. The adrenal gland may also develop a problem with the zona glomerulosa that produces mineralocorticoid activity. Conn syndrome has been used to characterize primary hyperaldosteronism resulting from a small benign adenoma of the adrenal cortex that produces an excess of aldosterone. Although this problem is due to an adenoma in 95% of cases, the disorder may also result from a bilateral hyperplasia, nodular hyperplasia, or carcinoma of the gland. Elderly persons more commonly develop a problem with aldosterone excess due to a secondary factor such as cirrhosis or other hepatic diseases, nephrosis, cardiomyopathies, or malignant hypertension. Aldosteronism is characterized by hypertension and hypokalemic alkalosis. Since these findings may also be noted in cases of Cushing's disease, a complete workup will be needed to determine the actual cause of the problem. Primary aldosteronism is confirmed by an elevated urinary aldosterone level, alkaline urine, and low or absent renin activity. In most cases, surgery is the treatment of choice. Underlying causes of this problem should be treated as identified.

OVARY

Perhaps one of the best-studied changes accompanying the aging process is the decline in ovarian function that accompanies aging. This change has clearly been shown to have physiologic effects, most notably on the cardiovascular system and the skeleton. This topic is discussed elsewhere in this book.

TESTIS

As mentioned earlier in this chapter, there has long been an interest in male hormones and their possible relationship to aging. This interest has been fueled by research touting the "benefits" of testosterone administration to elderly men. While it is clear that replacement of testosterone for men with suboptimal levels improves libido, sexual potency, and muscle mass, treatment for men with normal levels is not advised. There is a general decline in the mass and weight of the testicles with age. The tubules undergo some atrophy, and the intertubular spaces become more fibrous. Leydig cells decline, and there is an increase in tubular wall size, compromising the ability of the tubules to conduct spermatogenesis.

The testes have a dual function: production of spermatozoa and secretion of sex steroids, mainly testosterone. Whereas spermatogenesis is under the control of testosterone and the pituitary hormone follicle-stimulating hormone (FSH), testosterone secretion is regulated by another pituitary hormone, luteinizing hormone (LH). LH and FSH are collectively referred to as gonadotropins and are under the control of a hypothalamic hormone, luteinizing hormone–releasing hormone (LHRH). LHRH release is regulated by circulating testosterone levels through a negative feedback system. It now appears that testosterone is converted to estrogen within the hypothalamus before it exerts its action on the neurons responsible for LHRH secretion (18).

Although mean levels of circulating serum testosterone decline in men over 50 years of age, levels for most men remain within the range of normal for men of any age (19). Because of an increase in the binding of testosterone to plasma testosterone-binding globulin (TeBG), levels of free testosterone are lower than would be expected on the basis of total testosterone measurements. Testosterone secretion is probably reduced with age; data show increased gonadotropin levels with age, diminished response to exogenous human chorionic gonadotropin (hCG), and reduced Leydig cell mass. Vermeulen et al. reported a decrease in the overall rate of metabolism of testosterone with age (20).

Dihydrotestosterone (DHT) has been reported to decrease, remain unchanged, or increase with age, similar to what has been reported regarding estradiol in men. Serum LH and FSH progressively increase with age, regardless of the presence or absence of decreased testosterone levels. The increased LH level, despite the maintenance of testosterone levels, is compatible with a Leydig cell defect that is compensated by enhanced gonadotropic stimulation. This is compatible with the decrease with age in peak testosterone response following hCG stimulation. A decreased hypothalamic sensitivity to feedback inhibition by sex steroids with age is another possible mechanism for the gonadotropin rise noted. Age-related decreases in gonadotropin responses to LHRH have been reported.

IMPOTENCE

There is no relationship between sexual potency and serum testosterone levels as long as levels are within normal range. Levels below 200 ng/dL at any age are considered suboptimal and deserve further evaluation. More commonly, impotence is due to a variety of psychological and medical conditions, including the health of the patient and his partner, or medication side effects. Organic causes of impotence can usually be detected by measuring nocturnal penile tumescence. The use of testosterone in the elderly should presently be restricted to the overtly hypogonadal, as long-term risks of testosterone are yet unknown; there is an increased risk of prostatic hypertrophy, with some investigators questioning a higher risk of prostatic cancer.

Male sexual physiologic response has been well described by Masters and Johnson (21). Regardless of age, sexual response can be divided into four phases: (a) the excitement phase, during which, in response to various sexual stimuli, the heart rate and blood pressure increase; increased blood flow to the pelvis leads to penile erection and some increase in testicular size; other changes occur including erection of the nipples, skin flushing, and increased muscular tension; (b) the plateau phase, during which the excitement state is maintained for variable lengths of time; (c) the orgasmic phase, during which muscular tension reaches its peak and contractions of various pelvic muscles occur leading to ejaculation; and (d) the resolution phase, during which physiologic parameters return gradually to preexcitement levels. The last phase includes a refractory period during which new sexual stimuli elicit no response.

There is a decline in libido and sexual performance with age, though many feel that the former is not "normal" but rather a result of a variety of physical, social, and psychological factors. Sexual activity, as determined by Kinsey, peaks in the mid to late teens and starts declining in the 20s and early 30s, reaching almost zero by the ninth decade of life. This was later confirmed in a study of upper-middle-class men in the Baltimore Longitudinal Study of Aging (22). Impotence, while relatively rare under the age of 40, increases with age and affects up to 8% of all men by age 55, 25% by age 65, and over 50% by age 75.

There are age-related alterations in the physiology of sexual response. Studies of nocturnal penile tumescence show a rapid decline in total duration as a percentage of total REM sleep time during the 20s and 30s, with a relatively small decline thereafter (23). There is a reduction in the excitatory phase, with increased stimulation required for erection. Multiorgasmic capacity declines throughout life after the mid teens, and refractory periods increase, with some elderly men reporting refractory periods of up to 24 hours or longer.

CONCLUSION

This chapter discusses only a few of the endocrine problems that are more common during later life. While the problem of diabetes mellitus is discussed elsewhere (Chapter 35), diabetes mellitus is perhaps the most common endocrine problem affecting the elderly, with 40% of all diabetic individuals being over the age of 65. With the change in demography that is occurring, this problem will most certainly grow; approximately 8% of persons of 65 and 22% of persons over 80 years of age currently have diabetes mellitus, on the basis of National Diabetes Data Group criteria.

When considering any endocrinological problem in an older person, it is imperative to remember that many of the signs and symptoms that are usually associated with the illness are often dismissed as being due to "aging" or some other age-prevalent problem. Because hypothyroidism and diabetes mellitus are common at this time in life, screening for these illnesses with blood testing is deemed appropriate and cost-effective. For other problems, a high index of suspicion, often based on a change in usual routine or some nonspecific finding, should lead to further testing. Early recognition and treatment can do a great deal to promote maximal functioning among the elderly and maintain quality life for as long as possible.

REFERENCES

1. Rudman D, Feller AG, Nagraj HS, et al. Effects of human growth hormone in men over 60 years old. N Engl J Med 1990;323:1–6.
2. Simmonds, M. Uber Hypophysenschwund mit todlichem Ausgang. Dtsch Med Wochenschr 1914;7:94–99.
3. Dilman VM. Age-associated elevation of hypothalamic threshold to feedback control, and its role in development, ageing, and disease. Lancet 1971; 11:1211–1219.
4. Frolkis VV, Bezrukov V, Duplenko YK, Genis ED. The hypothalamus in aging. Exp Gerontol 1972; 7:169–184.
5. Friedman M, Green MF, Sharland DE. Assessment of hypothalamic-pituitary-adrenal function in the geriatric age group. J Gerontol 1969;24:292–297.
6. Blichert-Toft M. Secretion of corticotrophin and somatotrophin by the senescent adenohypophysis in man. Acta Endocr Suppl 1975;195:1–157.
7. Hontela S. Triiodothyronine turnover in hospitalized psychogeriatric patients. J Am Geriatr Soc 1975;23:241–247.
8. Kaiser FE. Variability of response to thyroid-releasing hormone in normal elderly. Age Ageing 1987; 16:345–354.
9. Rozencweig M, Heuson JC, Bila S, et al. Effects of 2-Br-a-ergocryptine, L-dopa and cyclic imides on serum prolactin in postmenopausal women. Eur J Cancer 1973;9:657–664.
10. Dunihue FW. Reduced juxtaglomerular cell granularity, pituitary neurosecretory material, and width of the zona glomerulosa in aging rats. Endocrinology 1965;77:948–951.
11. Miller M, Moses AM. Radioimmunoassay of urinary antidiuretic hormone with application to study of the Brattleboro rat. Endocrinology 1971;88:1389–1396.
12. Corpas E, Harman SM, Blackman MR. Human growth hormone and aging. Endocr Rev 1993;14:20–39.
13. Kaiser FE, Silver AJ, Morley JE. The effect of recombinant human growth hormone on malnourished older individuals. J Am Geriatr Soc 1991; 39:235–240.
14. Sawin CT, Chopra D, Azizi F, et al. The aging thyroid: increased prevalence of elevated serum thyrotropin levels in the elderly. J Am Med Soc 1979; 242:247–250.
15. Ridgway EC, Cooper DS, Walker H, et al. Peripheral responses to thyroid hormone before and after L-thyroxine therapy in patients with subclinical hypothyroidism. J Clin Endocrinol Metab 1981; 53:1238–1242.
16. Gambert SR. Interaction of age and thyroid hormone status on beta-endorphin content in rat corpus striatum and hypothalamus. Neuroendocrinology 1981;32:114–117.
17. Lahey FH. Non-activated (apathetic) type of hyperthyroidism. N Engl J Med 1931;204:747–748.
18. Kastin AJ, Schally AV. Release of LH and FSH after administration of synthetic LHRH. J Clin Endocrinol Metab 1972;34:753–757.
19. Hjorton R, Hsieh P, Barberia J, et al. Altered blood androgens in elderly men with prostate hyperplasia. J Clin Endocrinol Metab 1975;41:793–796.
20. Vermeulen A, Rubens R, Verdonck L. Testosterone secretion and metabolism in male senescence. J Clin Endocrinol Metab 1972;34:730–735.
21. Kinsey AC, Pomeroy WB, Martin CE. Sexual behavior in the human male. Philadelphia: WB Saunders, 1948.
22. Martin CE. Factors affecting sexual functioning in 60–79 year old married males. Arch Sex Behav 1981;5:399–420 .
23. Karacan I, Williams RL, Thronby JI, et al. Sleep related penile tumescence as a function of age. Am J Psychiatry 1975;132:932–937.

35/ Diabetes Mellitus in the Elderly Patient

Rebecca A. Silliman

Diabetes mellitus is common in old age, afflicting 2.7 million people 65 years of age and older, most of whom have type II disease (1). The personal and economic costs are great, with $5.16 billion dollars being spent each year on medical care for these patients. Most of this expense is for inpatient costs, with most being attributed to the care of cardiovascular complications (2). Indeed, in old age the challenges to clinicians are to prevent microvascular and macrovascular complications insofar as possible, and when they do occur, to minimize their effects on patients' functioning.

EPIDEMIOLOGY

Almost half of all diabetics are 65 years of age or older, with an approximately even split between men and women. The absolute number of older persons with diabetes will continue to rise for the foreseeable future for at least two reasons: (a) the rate of diagnosed diabetes in persons 65 to 74 years of age and ≥ 75 years has increased about 2.5 times in the past 30 years and (b) the number of older persons at risk is growing. Since about half of all cases in older persons are undiagnosed, if methods of detection improve, the numbers of clinically recognized cases could rise even further (1).

DIAGNOSIS

Although the "poly" symptoms (polydipsia, polyuria, and polyphagia) are considered by many to be pathognomonic of diabetes, this is often not true in older persons for several reasons. First, these symptoms are nonspecific and may be due to other conditions. Second, they may not be present because of age-related or disease-related changes in organ function. Third, they may be masked by other conditions. Thus, relying on them alone will result in both false positives and false negatives. The challenge to the clinician is to maintain a high level of suspicion, yet be prudent with glucose testing.

The accepted criteria for diagnosing diabetes in adults include (a) an elevation in plasma glucose to ≥ 200 mg/dL, accompanied by symptoms such as polydipsia, polyuria, polyphagia, and weight loss, or (b) a fasting plasma glucose of ≥ 140 mg/dL on at least two occasions. In the unusual circumstance in which diabetes is suspected and plasma glucose criteria are not met, two oral glucose tolerance tests with the 2-hour plasma glucose being ≥ 200 mg/dL with one intervening value (between 0 and 2 hours) being ≥ 200 mg/dL are required to make the diagnosis (3).

SCREENING

As with other conditions, screening for diabetes would be indicated if the treatment of asymptomatic patients resulted in better outcomes, if the burden of suffering associated with it were high, and if the screening test were sensitive and specific, simple and inexpensive, safe, and acceptable for both patients and practitioners (4). Although no one would argue that the burdens associated with diabetes are great, a simple screening test is lacking, and there is no good evidence that early detection and treatment improve outcomes for patients with type II disease (5, 6). The U.S. Preventive Services Task Force, however, recommends that among persons aged 65 and over consideration be given to screening those at high risk: the markedly obese, women with a history of gestational diabetes, and those persons with a family history of diabetes (5).

Once diabetes has been detected clinically, screening for complications, specifically for retinopathy and foot lesions, can be effective in reducing morbidity, as discussed below.

MANAGEMENT

DIET AND WEIGHT LOSS

Most type II diabetics are overweight, although a subset of older patients are either of normal weight or underweight (7). Although what constitutes an optimal diabetic diet for older persons is unknown, weight loss, even if modest, in obese older persons can improve metabolic control, thereby reducing symptoms of hyperglycemia. Indeed, a primary reason for attempting to achieve metabolic control in old age is to make patients feel better by (a) reducing polyuria and incontinence and (b) improving vision and a general sense of well-being.

Recently reported findings of two randomized controlled trials of intensive therapy in type I patients indicate that such therapy results in better glycemic control and a reduced incidence of complications, particularly microvascular complications (8, 9). Although generalizing these results to type II patients, particularly older type II patients, is problematic, it is probably reasonable to try to achieve the best metabolic control possible, being careful to balance the potential benefits of glycemic control (e.g., decreased symptoms associated with hyperglycemia, prevention of the hyperosmolar state, and the possible reduction of risk for microvascular and macrovascular complications) against the costs (e.g., dollar costs of medications, monitoring supplies, provider visits, and food; effects on lifestyle; and risk of hypoglycemia).

Achieving weight loss and metabolic control is not easy. Lifelong dietary habits are difficult to change, as are notions of what constitutes a "healthy" diet. This may be compounded by the fact that older patients frequently must rely on someone else for food acquisition and preparation. In addition, they may live in households where food preferences are disparate. Furthermore, financial considerations may interfere with patients' procuring appropriate foods, such as fresh fruits and vegetables.

Although weight loss in obese persons should be attempted, for many this will not be possible. For this group as well as those who are either underweight or of normal weight, the best strategy should be to help them achieve a balanced diet that includes fruit and legume sources of carbohydrate, restricts the amount of animal fat while maintaining the intake of protein at 0.8 to 1 gm/kg of body weight, and incorporates fiber in moderate amounts (7). Adequate fluid intake of nonsucrose-containing beverages is also important. This alone may help to reduce glucose levels and will correct mild volume contraction related to osmotic diuresis.

DRUG THERAPY

Drug therapy is probably warranted if metabolic control cannot be achieved by the combination of diet, exercise, and weight loss. In choosing between sulfonylurea drugs and insulin, risks and benefits and patient preferences must be taken into account.

The sulfonylurea drugs (tolbutamide, acetohexamide, tolazamide, chlorpropamide, glipizide, and glyburide) are the most frequently prescribed agents for treating hyperglycemia. Yet they rarely are able to achieve euglycemia. Furthermore, there are few data that support either their short- or long-term efficacy (10), and in the University Group Diabetes Program (UGDP) trial, tolbutamide-treated patients died more frequently from cardiovascular disease than did patients treated with diet alone, or diet and insulin (11). Finally, over time the effectiveness of these drugs diminishes, probably because of a combination of patients' difficulty with dietary restrictions and a diminution of beta cell function over time.

Nonetheless, oral agents are easy to use and are frequently preferred by patients. The choice of agent should take into account the following considerations. First, since all are metabolized at least in part by the liver, they should be used with care in patients with severe liver disease. Second, renal insufficiency will prolong the half-lives of tolbutamide, glyburide, and glipizide. Third, because of its long half-life, a risk factor for hypoglycemia, and its propensity to cause hyponatremia, chlorpropamide should be avoided in older persons (10). Fourth, since glyburide can also cause hypoglycemia in older persons, it also should be used with caution. Glipizide, the other second-generation agent, may be preferable because it does not have any active metabolites. The advantage that both of these newer agents have over the older ones is that they are less likely to interact with other drugs; a disadvantage is that they cost more, since generic forms are not yet available.

Insulin therapy may be needed to achieve metabolic control and may be preferable to oral agents, given their risks. The decision to treat with insulin must include an assessment of patients' beliefs about insulin and the potential for its safe use. For example, since most older patients have type II disease, they are likely to have had experiences with other family members with diabetes. Insulin therapy is frequently instituted after several years of diagnosed disease duration, at a time when disease complications may be manifest. Thus, the development of worsening complications may be falsely attributed to the insulin itself. This and other fears should be explored with patients. In addition, visual and cognitive function and manual dexterity require careful evaluation if patients will be administering the insulin themselves. If not, the adequacy of informal or formal supports to consistently and safely manage insulin therapy must be evaluated.

Insulin therapy is frequently instituted in the hospital setting, when a diagnosis of diabetes is first made in conjunction with an admission for an acute infectious illness or for a complication, or when a patient is admitted for complicated hyperglycemia (e.g., for the diabetic hyperosmolar state or ketoacidosis). Given the differences in diet, physical activity, and stress levels that exist in the hospital and the home setting, particular attention should be paid to monitoring the transition from hospital to home. This is a time when serious hyperglycemia or hypoglycemia is likely to occur, either because of changes in these factors or because of misunderstandings about dosing and the technical aspects of insulin administration.

Although in recent years the addition of insulin to an established oral agent regimen has been advocated, a recent meta-analysis of trials comparing insulin plus sulfonylurea agents with insulin alone has failed to demonstrate a significant improvement in glycemic control. Furthermore, the one study reviewed that studied diabetics with a mean age of 70 or above only involved nine patients (12). Given the complexities of such a regimen and the potential for complications, it is difficult to advocate such a regimen in most older persons.

MONITORING

Although self-monitoring of blood glucose is safe and relatively easy for most patients to manage, its use has not been studied systematically in older persons. The main reasons to consider glucose monitoring in older patients are (a) to prevent the development of hypoglycemia in patients treated with hypoglycemic medications, particularly during times of illness or when medication changes are planned, and (b) to guide adjustments of hypoglycemic therapy in conjunction with glycosylated hemoglobin levels. The glycosylated hemoglobin (hemoglobin A_{1C}) reflects glucose levels over the previous 8 to 12 weeks and is therefore useful in monitoring glycemic control over time.

CARDIOVASCULAR RISK FACTORS

Findings from the San Luis Valley Diabetes Study that compared cardiovascular risk factor patterns in patients with diabetes with those in patients with impaired glucose tolerance suggest that the adverse risk factor profile seen so frequently in diabetics may develop either before or concomitantly with the development of diabetes (13). Regardless of when risk factors develop, diabetics are more likely to be hypertensive, to have elevated lipid levels, and to be obese (13, 14). These are equally strong risk factors for coronary disease in diabetics and in nondiabetics. Furthermore, diabetes itself is a risk factor for coronary heart disease (14, 15), and its presence not only negates the protective effect of female gender but also confers a worse prognosis in women who develop myocardial infarctions and congestive heart failure (14).

While there is no evidence that treating these risk factors confers the same or greater benefit as in nondiabetics, given the two- to threefold increased risk of myocardial infarction and stroke in diabetics, it is prudent to try to modify cardiovascular risk factors, particularly in older persons, in whom additional comorbidities may cause important decrements in already compromised physical, social, and emotional function. Targeting obesity would theoretically have the greatest impact on clinical outcomes, since it is a coronary heart disease risk factor and contributes to adverse lipid profiles and hypertension. However, the difficulties associated with its modification, as outlined above, will likely blunt the effectiveness of this approach in many older persons.

Although attempts at weight loss should not be discounted or neglected, an equally important strategy for risk factor reduction is the treatment of existing hypertension. Accumulating evidence suggests that treatment with angiotensin converting enzyme (ACE) inhibitors can decrease proteinuria and preserve the glomerular filtration rate in patients with type II diabetes, whether or not they have hypertension (16, 17). This is an important observation, since at least 20% of type II patients will develop nephropathy.

Although older persons have generally been excluded from these studies, since many older diabetics have cardiac conditions that warrant the use of an ACE inhibitor, this class of antihypertensives should be the class of choice for treating hypertension in these patients. Careful attention should be paid to potassium levels when beginning therapy, since hyperkalemia may develop in those with even mild renal insufficiency. While cost and dry cough are other side effects of concern, the additional advantage of these agents is that they do not cause or exacerbate urinary incontinence, constipation, lipid abnormalities, or hyperglycemia.

The treatment of lipid abnormalities in old age is controversial, regardless of whether patients have diabetes or not (see Chapter 24). Once dietary manipulations have been made and hyperlipidemia persists, consideration should be given to drug therapy if LDL levels remain markedly elevated and other risk factors are present. Niacin should be avoided, since it can worsen glycemic control.

Finally, although rates of cigarette smoking decline with age, an important subset of smokers survive to old age. Recent evidence suggests that the hazards of cigarette smoking for men and women, particularly with respect to cardiovascular mortality, extend into later life. Furthermore, the risk of death from cardiovascular disease for former smokers is similar to that of "never smokers," independent of the age at which people quit (18). Taken together, these data should compel clinicians to work with their older diabetic smokers to help them to quit.

EYE DISEASE

Data from the 1976–80 National Health and Nutrition Survey indicate that among diabetics aged 65 to 74, one-quarter have serious trouble seeing, even with glasses (1). This is because of both the ravages of diabetic retinopathy and the fact that older diabetics are likely to have comorbid eye conditions, namely cataracts and glaucoma. While 22% report that they have cataracts and 6% report that they have glaucoma (1), data from the Wisconsin Epidemiologic Study of Diabetic Retinopathy (WESDR) indicate that the prevalence of these conditions is actually much higher on the basis of physical examination. In that study of 1370 patients 30 years and older, over 95% of diabetics $\geqslant$ 65 years of age had evidence of cataracts; 7.5% had glaucoma. By comparison, between 35 and 40% in this age group who were not taking insulin had diabetic retinopathy; this rose to 50 to 70% in insulin users; about 8% had macular edema (19). Clearly, older diabetics experience a considerable burden of eye disease. Given the critical importance of visual function to overall functional independence, eye disease in older diabetics deserves critical attention by clinicians.

The risk of developing diabetic retinopathy increases with duration of disease. Because patients with type II disease frequently have had their disease for some time before diagnosis, they may already have retinopathy by the time they are diagnosed. It may be manifested by early nonproliferative changes or by more severe proliferative changes. Because of the likelihood of prevalent retinopathy, all newly diagnosed diabetics should be referred for ophthalmologic evaluation, not only for the presence of retinopathy but also for the presence of cataracts and glaucoma.

Ideally this evaluation should include stereoscopic fundus photography, since even in the best hands dilated ophthalmoscopy only has a sensitivity of about 80% for detecting proliferative retinopathy (20). The American College of Physicians, in conjunction with the American Diabetes Association and the American Academy of Ophthalmology, has recently published guidelines stating that if initial stereoscopic screening is negative, further screening need not occur until 4 years later, when annual screening with stereoscopic photographs or dilated ophthalmoscopy should begin. This strategy, of course, demands that careful attention be given to ensuring that patients are followed carefully to avoid missing the 4-year anniversary. If stereoscopic photographic screening is not available, dilated ophthalmoscopy should be performed annually (21).

The reasons for being compulsive about ophthalmologic screening are that (a) one-third of the cases of blindness in diabetics are due to retinopathy, (b) laser photocoagulation therapy has been shown to reduce that rate of vision loss in patients with proliferative retinopathy and macular edema, and (c) treatment of comorbid eye disease may also help to preserve visual function. In spite of these compelling reasons, in a study of community care of diabetics in Michigan in the mid-1980s, only about half of patients with type II disease reported ever having seen an ophthalmologist (22). Furthermore, only 58% of eyes of older patients identified as having high-risk characteristics for visual loss in the WESDR study had received photocoagulation treatment by the time of follow-up, in spite of letters to patients that outlined the importance and need for this intervention (19).

FOOT CARE

Sixty-four percent of amputations in diabetics occur in patients 65 years of age and older; the rate of lower extremity amputations in this age group is 101/10,000 (26). In addition to the monetary costs of amputations, they obviously have a profound effect on patients' mobility and may precipitate institutionalization.

Peripheral vascular disease and sensory neuropathy are risk factors for lower extremity trauma and falls, as well as for amputation. A recent case-control study has demonstrated that lack of patient education is an additional important risk factor for amputation (24). Patients do not engage in preventive care of their feet, and physicians infrequently examine diabetics' feet. Improved self-care and physician attention to foot abnormalities, however, can be achieved relatively easily and inexpensively, with resulting improvement in patient outcomes (25). Patients should be instructed in self-examination methods, nail and callus care, washing techniques, and what constitutes appropriate footwear. Since many older persons have fungal infections of their nails and may not be able to safely cut them, referral to a podiatrist is a prudent strategy. For their part, physicians should examine diabetic feet at each patient visit. This examination can be used to reinforce important patient foot care behaviors. Although there is still much to learn about the prevention and treatment of diabetic foot lesions, successful implementation of these strategies is a place to start.

COGNITIVE FUNCTION

Compared with age-matched nondiabetic controls, older diabetic patients are likely to perform more poorly on cognitive tests that require long-term memory processes, specifically reasoning, learning (recall), and visuospatial processing (26). These changes are similar to those associated with normal aging, but whether they are manifestations of an accelerated aging process or occur via other mechanisms is not clear. Older diabetics are also more likely to have strokes and may experience adverse effects on cognition from hyperglycemia and hypoglycemia and hyperosmolar and hypoosmolar states. These are additional reasons for maintaining metabolic stability and for treating hypertension. Indeed, recent studies suggest that improved glycemic control improves some aspects of cognitive function in older patients with type II disease (27).

Because of diabetes-related changes in cognitive function, the increased likelihood of vascular dementia (both age- and diabetes-related), and the increased incidence of primary degenerative dementia with age, periodic assessment of cognitive function in older diabetics is essential. This can serve to reassure the "worried well," who may have concerns about memory problems, and to identify early those beginning to experience subtle difficulties. Careful attention to these issues may uncover adverse drug effects and other metabolic derangements (e.g. hypothyroidism) and will identify those who may need additional help from clinicians and family or friends in adhering to complex treatment regimens.

COMORBIDITY

By virtue of their having diabetes and having manifestations of the complications described above, as well as by virtue of being older, older type II diabetics are likely to have considerable coexisting disease. The fact that these patients take several medications, and the likelihood that they may have diminished organ function (especially renal function) and decreased physiologic reserve together mean that they are at an increased risk of adverse drug effects. Careful attention therefore needs to be paid to avoiding drug-drug interactions. In addition, since compliance with medications is known to diminish as the number of medications and the complexity of the regimen increases, thought needs to be given to ways of decreasing the total number of medications (e.g. using one medication for multiple indications). This may also help with cost, which is frequently an issue for older persons on fixed incomes.

FAMILY CONSIDERATIONS

In addition to being a family disease because of inheritance, diabetes is a family disease because of its effects on patients' lives. Not only are complications devastating, but following complex dietary, medication, and monitoring regimens may be overwhelming. When patients are biomedically and/or functionally frail, help from family and others is essential. Until recently, little attention has been given to the central role that families play in the management of older persons with chronic disease (28, 29), in spite of the well-known role that they play in the community care of frail older persons (30). Although there is some evidence from studies involving younger patients with type II disease that regimen-specific family support is correlated with higher rates of regimen adherence, no such studies have been done with older patients. If patients are having difficulty adhering to treatment regimens, if they rely on family members for certain activities (e.g., food preparation, managing medications), or if they have functional disabilities, their family members or other informal care providers need to be educated about diabetes and receive instruction and support in methods of management.

SUMMARY AND CONCLUSIONS

Diabetes is a common condition in older persons and is associated with considerable economic and personal costs. Attention to the prevention and management of cardiovascular, eye, and foot disease is therefore critical. Whether this can be achieved by maintaining tight glycemic control is not known. Although reducing blood glucose levels to values that eliminate hyperglycemic symptoms while minimizing the potential for hypoglycemic reactions should be attempted and cardiovascular risk factors treated, equal attention should be given to preventing eye and foot complications, where screening and treatment interventions have known efficacy.

REFERENCES

1. Harris MI. Epidemiology of diabetes mellitus among the elderly in the United States. Clin Geriatr Med 1990;6:703–719.
2. Weinberger M, Cowper PA, Kirkman MS, Vinicor F. Economic impact of diabetes mellitus in the elderly. Clin Geriatr Med 1990;6:959–970.
3. Anonymous. Position statement: office guide to diagnosis and classification of diabetes mellitus and other categories of glucose intolerance. Diabetes Care 1991;14(suppl 2):3–4.
4. Fletcher RH, Fletcher SW, Wagner EH. Clinical epidemiology—the essentials. Baltimore: Williams & Wilkins, 1982:59–74.
5. U.S. Preventive Services Task Force. Screening for diabetes mellitus. In: Fisher M, ed. Guide to clinical preventive services: an assessment of the effectiveness of 169 interventions. Report of the U.S. preventive services task force. Baltimore: Williams & Wilkins, 1989:95–103.
6. Singer DE, Samet JH, Coley CM, Nathan DM. Screening for diabetes mellitus. Ann Intern Med 1988;109:639–649.
7. Reed RL, Mooradian AD. Nutritional status and dietary management of elderly diabetic patients. Clin Geriatr Med 1990;6:883–901.
8. Reichard P, Nilsson B-Y, Rosenqvist U. The effect of long-term intensified insulin treatment on the development of microvascular complications of diabetes mellitus. N Engl J Med 1993;329:304–309.
9. American Diabetes Association Position Statement. Implications of the Diabetes Control and Complications Trial, June 1993.
10. Halter JB, Morrow LA. Use of sulfonylurea drugs in the elderly. Diabetes Care 1990;13(suppl 2):86–92.
11. University Group Diabetes Program. A study of the effects of hypoglycemic agents on vascular complications in patients with adult-onset diabetes. II. Mortality results. Diabetes 1970;19(suppl 2):789–815.
12. Peters AL, Davidson MB. Insulin plus a sulfonylurea agent for treating type 2 diabetes. Ann Intern Med 1991;115:45–53.
13. Burchfiel CM, Hamman RF, Marshall JA, Baxter J, Kahn LB, Amirani JJ. Cardiovascular risk factors and impaired glucose tolerance: the San Luis Valley Diabetes Study. Am J Epidemiol 1990;131:57–70.
14. Kannel WB. Lipids, diabetes, and coronary heart disease: insights from the Framingham Study. Am Heart J 1985;110:1100–1107.
15. Koskinen P, Manttari M, Manninen V, Huttunen JK, Heinonen OP, Frick MH. Coronary heart disease incidence in NIDDM patients in the Helsinki Heart Study. Diabetes Care 1992;15:820–825.
16. Kasiske BL, Kalil RSN, Ma JZ, Liao M, Keane WF. Effect of antihypertensive therapy on the kidney in patients with diabetes: a meta-regression analysis. Ann Intern Med 1993;118:129–138.
17. Ravid M, Savin H, Jutrin I, Bental T, Katz B, Lishner M. Long-term stabilizing effect of angiotension-converting enzyme inhibition on plasma creatinine and on proteinuria in normotensive type II diabetes patients. Ann Intern Med 1993;118:577–581.
18. LaCroix AZ, Lang J, Scherr P, Wallace RB, Cornoni-Huntley J, Berkman L, et al. Smoking and mortality among older men and women in three communities. N Engl J Med 1991;324:1619–1625.
19. Klein BEK, Klein R. Ocular problems in older Americans with diabetes. Clin Geriatr Med 1990; 6:827–837.
20. Singer DE, Nathan DM, Fogel HA, Schachat AP. Screening for diabetic retinopathy. Ann Intern Med 1992;116:660–671.
21. American College of Physicians, American Diabetes Association, and American Academy of Ophthalmology. Screening guidelines for diabetic retinopathy. Ann Intern Med 1992;116:683–685.
22. Anderson RM, Hess GE, Davis WK, Hiss RG. Community diabetes care in the 1980s. Diabetes Care 1988;11:519–526.
23. Morley JE, Kaiser FE. Unique aspects of diabetes mellitus in the elderly. Clin Geriatr Med 1990; 6:693–702.
24. Reiber GE, Pecoraro RE, Koepsell TD. Risk factors for amputation in patients with diabetes mellitus: a case-control study. Ann Intern Med 1992;117:97–105.
25. Litzelman DK, Slemenda CW, Langefeld CD, et al. Reduction of lower extremity clinical abnormalities in patients with non-insulin-dependent diabetes mellitus: a randomized, controlled trial. Ann Intern Med 1993:119:36–41.
26. Tun PA, Nathan DM, Perlmuter LC. Cognitive and affective disorders in elderly diabetics. Clin Geriatr Med 1990;6:731–745.
27. Meneilly GS, Cheung E, Tessier D, Yakura C, Tuokko H. The effect of improved glycemic control on cognitive functions in the elderly patient with diabetes. J Gerontol:Med Sci 1993;48:M117–M121.
28. Adelman RD, Greene MG, Charon R. The physician-elderly patient-companion triad in the medical encounter: the development of a conceptual framework and research agenda. Gerontologist 1987; 27:729–734.
29. Silliman RA. Caring for the frail older patient: the doctor-patient-family caregiver relationship. J Gen Intern Med 1989;4:237–241.
30. Stone R, Cafferata GL, Sangl J. Caregivers of the frail elderly: a national profile. Gerontologist 1987; 27:616–626.

Syndrome X

In 1988 Reaven hypothesized the existence of syndrome X, a syndrome characterized by insulin resistance, with glucose intolerance, hyperinsulinemia, increased VLDL triglyceride, decreased

HDL cholesterol, and hypertension resulting as a consequence (1). Since all of these are risk factors for the development of coronary artery disease, Reaven postulated that insulin resistance might be an important underlying defect.

In spite of considerable evidence from animal and human studies, a major limitation of these studies has been that they have been cross-sectional. A recent report based on longitudinal data from the San Antonio Heart Study has documented that fasting insulin levels precede the development of low HDL cholesterol, increased triglycerides, and type II diabetes mellitus. Furthermore, higher baseline insulin concentrations were associated with the development of multiple metabolic disorders, even with controlling for changes in adiposity (2).

At present the clinical implications of these findings remain to be fully elucidated, particularly in relation to older persons. Nonetheless, an elevated insulin level is a strong risk factor for the development of type II diabetes, and in patients with hypertension who are at risk for developing type II diabetes, it is probably prudent to avoid drugs that may worsen insulin resistance (e.g., thiazides and β-blockers) unless there are other compelling reasons to use them (2).

REFERENCES

1. Reaven GM. Role of insulin resistance in human disease. Diabetes 1988;37:1595–1607.
2. Haffner SM, Valdez RA, Hazuda HP, Mitchell BD, Morales PA, Stern MP. Prospective analysis of the insulin-resistance syndrome (syndrome X). Diabetes 1992;41:715–722.

36/ Geriatric Dermatology

Bruce E. Beacham

Clinical aspects of aging skin are familiar to anyone who can picture the appearance of an elderly person. The skin becomes wrinkled on the face and is often variable in pigmentation. These changes merely reflect dehydration and decreases in elasticity, vascularity, and subcutaneous fat in the dermis, as well as the melanocytic inability to spread out melanin granules in an orderly fashion. These most common clinical changes of the aged skin are highly variable and may be garnished with many other changes, all of which depend on genetic factors and the environment, especially the cumulative effects of ultraviolet radiation.

Several informative studies have characterized the most prevalent disorders of the skin of the elderly (1–3). This chapter provides a discussion of many well-known problems of aging skin and an update on therapies and diagnostic strategies when appropriate. The general categories for discussion include pruritus, common dermatoses, infections, bullous diseases, and tumors of the skin.

PRURITUS AND XEROSIS

Pruritus is probably the most common presenting symptom in dermatology and includes both localized and generalized itching, with or without an accompanying eruption. It may also be described as stinging, crawling, or burning and is really a modified form of pain, with impulses being transmitted through slow afferent fibers.

In the elderly, pruritus is a common problem that has a number of causes (4). Xerosis and asteatotic eczema are regularly seen in the elderly, especially in the winter. Alkaline soaps, too frequent bathing, low humidity, rough clothing, alcohol, poor nutrition, and cholesterol-lowering drugs aggravate the above conditions and pruritus. Dry skin (most commonly seen over the lower legs) may fissure, appear shiny, and crack, with subsequent inflammatory changes. On the back, such skin looks pale and dry and has attached irregular small scale. Pruritus associated with xerosis is best controlled by restricting the amount of bathing, lubrication with an α-hydroxy acid lotion or ointment, and the avoidance of soap. It may be necessary to use a mild-to-moderate topical corticosteroid and a systemic antihistamine to control pruritus. Antihistamines blocking H1, H2, or both types of receptors, as well as nonsedating types such as terfenadine, may be used.

Aquagenic pruritus is a symptom complex consisting of itching, burning, or prickling at the sites of contact with any type of water (5). Polycythemia vera must be ruled out. An important subset of aquagenic pruritus exists in the elderly, associated with dry skin and several other conditions. This form often occurs in women, worsens in the winter, and, unlike other varieties of aquagenic pruritus, responds to emollient therapy (6).

Pruritus may also be associated with numerous other skin diseases besides asteatotic eczema and xerosis. These include scabies, insect bite reactions, drug sensitivity, dermatitis herpetiformis, and urticaria. If no skin disease is evident, the pruritus may be associated with an underlying systemic disorder. Pruritus may be associated with malignancy, especially myeloproliferative disorders. Other systemic diseases associated with pruritus include chronic renal failure, cholestatic liver disease, iron deficiency anemia, diabetes, thyrotoxicosis, and psychiatric and neurologic disorders.

GERIATRIC NAIL DISORDERS

Age-associated nail changes are common in the elderly. Nails appear yellow and opaque, more brittle, with longitudinal ridging, and become rougher and irregular, especially at the distal nail plate. These changes are associated with a variety of exogenous and endogenous influences, including trauma, infections, concurrent dermatologic or systemic disorders, as well as those changes normally associated with aging (7). Common onychodystrophies of the elderly are hypertrophy of

380

the nail, subungual corn, ingrown nail, enlargement of nail, splinter hemorrhages, subungual hematomas, and hyperkeratotic tissue in nail folds. Fungal and bacteria cultures, systemic workup, and x-rays may be necessary before therapy is considered for any of the above conditions. Treatment for these disorders includes local measures such as rehydration of the nail, correction of faulty biomechanics and trauma, proper nutrition, antibiotics, antifungals, or surgical correction of the defect.

COMMON DERMATOSES

CONTACT DERMATITIS

Contact dermatitis may be due to a true allergic reaction most commonly found on exposed skin in an asymmetric distribution associated with itching and burning sensations. Erythematous macules, papules, and vesicles appear, and affected sites are often hot and swollen. Later, exudation, crusting, and secondary infection may occur. The pattern of the eruption is often diagnostic of the dermatitis, e.g., linear streaked vesicles on the extremities or swelling of the genitals in the case of poison ivy contact dermatitis. The location of the eruption will often suggest the cause and should direct questioning about possible allergens or irritants. Chronic allergic or irritant contact dermatitis may appear less red, scaled, dry, and fissured, but nonetheless it is still secondary to repeated exposure to an irritant or allergen.

Although the elderly individual may present with typical clinical features of allergic contact dermatitis, several features of contact dermatitis in the elderly should be noted. Older individuals generally show relatively little vesiculation or inflammation and have scaling as a prominent feature of eruption. Hyperpigmentation and lichenification are present early in the eruption, and itching is usually severe. Contact dermatitis tends to persist and is generally more resistant to therapy than in the younger age groups. These differences in clinical reactions may be related to the decreased ability to mount a delayed hypersensitivity reaction (8) and to the reduced reactions to standardized skin tests observed in the elderly (9). When the etiology of contact dermatitis remains obscure, patch testing can be performed to determine whether the patient has a true allergy. In cases of intractable contact dermatitis of unexplained origin, the possibility of underlying systematic disease or internal malignancy must be considered. Elderly patients with persistent eczematous dermatosis resembling contact dermatitis may in reality have a form of mycosis fungoides.

The most common causes of allergic dermatitis in the elderly are topical medications such as neomycin, nitrofurazone, paraben preservatives, vitamin E cream, lanolin, and ethylenediamine hydrochloride applied to stasis ulcers. These sensitizing agents may produce widespread and even generalized eruptions and play a central role in the production of the autosensitization often associated with eruptions. Many elderly individuals have developed allergic contact dermatitis in response to medications or adhesives used in transdermal drug delivery systems (10), the most common of which include nitroglycerine, scopolamine, and clonidine.

Several other contact dermatitis problems that appear to be more common in the elderly include hair dye dermatitis secondary to paraphenylene diamine present in older dyeing solutions, ragweed dermatitis, photodermatitis, and systemic eczematous contact dermatitis (11).

Therapy for contact dermatitis consists of removal of the offending agent, coupled with the application of moderate- to high-potency topical corticosteroid cream or ointment. Oral antihistamines and aluminum acetate compresses may also provide some symptomatic relief. Severe or widespread contact dermatitis usually requires a 2-week course of systemic corticosteroid therapy using a tapering dosage schedule.

DERMATITIS MEDICAMENTOSA

Dermatitis medicamentosa is an acute or chronic inflammatory reaction to a drug. Almost any drug, whether ingested, injected, inhaled, or absorbed, may cause any type of skin eruption in any individual at any time. The eruption usually recurs on reexposure to the same or related drug and may be quite life-threatening, requiring emergency treatment.

Drug eruptions have been estimated to occur in 18 to 30% of all hospitalized patients and to account for 3 to 5% of hospital admissions (12). Furthermore, approximately one-third of these patients hospitalized for a drug eruption developed a second drug reaction in the hospital. The latter phenomenon reflects the so-called broadening of the base of hypersensitivity to drugs once one has developed a drug reaction. The elderly take multiple medications and demonstrate a variety of pathologic states that may predispose to certain drug eruptions. In fact, one study found that almost 23% of cutaneous eruptions caused by drug ingestion occurred in patients over 60 years of age (13).

Drug eruptions may have a variety of clinical appearances, depending upon the type of drug, environmental factors, and pathologic state of the patient. These eruptions can be classified as erythematous, eczematoid, lichenoid, acneiform, urticarial, bullous, fixed drug, exfoliative, nodose, exanthematous, photosensitive, and purpuric. Each of these eruption patterns is associated with certain drug groups; this knowledge is often helpful in determining which drug may be responsible for certain types of eruptions (Table 36.1).

Treatment of these various eruptions includes discontinuation of the offending medications, antihistamines, topical menthol, and steroid lotions. More severe drug eruptions, such as toxic epidermal necrolysis and erythema multiforme, may require hospitalization and the use of systemic corticosteroids.

URTICARIA

Urticaria (hives) secondary to drugs is quite common, and the offending drug may be easily identified and discontinued in straightforward cases. However, in the elderly, management is often a problem because the patient may be on many essential medications that are difficult to discontinue or replace. In these instances, the urticaria may continue beyond 6 weeks and be classified as a chronic type. Even after the suspected drugs are discontinued, the eruption may continue and its etiology become more and more obscure. At this juncture, not only drugs should be considered as the cause of urticaria but also unusual types of infection, gallstones, and sinusitis.

A careful history, physical examination, and judicious use of laboratory studies is essential and may be helpful. Extensive laboratory testing, however, has a very low yield and is not cost-effective (14).

Hives are characterized by edema and erythema (wheals), which last as individual lesions from 1 to 5 hours, with complete resolution to normal skin. There are often multiple lesions, which can form a variety of shapes including arcuate, circular, or serpiginous configurations. Severe pruritus usually accompanies these lesions, and rarely, angioedema involving the mouth, the eyelids, or larynx may occur. A common component accompanying urticaria is dermatographism. This condition reflects histamine release with subsequent urticaria after light stroking or pressure on the skin, leaving patterns conforming to the shape of the pressure.

When no obvious cause has been uncovered to explain urticaria, it is appropriate to treat empirically with antihistamines such as hydroxyzine, an H1-receptor blocker, and cimetidine, an H2-receptor blocker, if necessary. More recently, the nonsedating antihistamine terfenadine has been very useful in the elderly with urticaria or pruritus. The use of doxepin, which reportedly blocks both H1 and H2 receptors, has also been quite helpful but has significant anticholinergic effects not well tolerated by the elderly.

STASIS DERMATITIS AND ULCERATION

Stasis dermatitis is an eczematous, red, edematous, sometimes oozing eruption, with or without

Table 36.1
Classification of Drug Eruptions According to Morphology[a]

Morphology	Medications Associated with Rash
Erythematous	Bismuth, barbiturates, sulfonamides, antihistamines, penicillins
Lichenoid or eczematous	Gold, quinidine, methyldopa (Aldomet, Amodopa), antituberculous, antiarrhythmic, and anticonvulsant agents
Acneiform	Corticosteroids, bromides, iodides
Urticarial	Penicillins, antibiotics, reactions to sera
Bullous	Iodides, penicillamine, bleomycin (Blenoxane)
Fixed drug	Phenolphthalein, tetracycline, nalidixic acid (NegGram), barbiturates
Exfoliative	Gold
Nodular	Sulfathiazole, salicylates, oral contraceptives
Exanthematous photodistribution	Phenothiazines, chlorothiazide (Diachlor, Diuril), dimeclocycline, griseofulvin (Fulvicin, Grisactin), oral hypoglycemics
Erythema multiforme target lesions	Allopurinol (Zyloprim), barbiturates, dapsone, digitalis, phenytoin (Dilantin), gold, hydralazine (Alazine, Apresoline), salicylates, sulfonamides, tetracycline, trimethoprim-sulfamethoxazole (Bactrim, Septra, etc.)

[a]From Beacham BE. Common Dermatoses in the Elderly. Am Fam Physician 1993;47:1445–1450. With permission.

ulceration, on the lower legs, which invariably demonstrate venous insufficiency. The condition may be acute, as described above, or chronic, with lichenification and fibrotic and atrophic pigmented skin with scars over previously healed ulcer sites. The condition may be associated with any other medical condition that may cause edema of the lower extremities. Stasis dermatitis may be difficult to differentiate from tinea infection, and potassium hydroxide preparation testing may be helpful.

Therapy is directed at removal of edema, along with lubrication and mild topical steroid preparations. Occasionally, systemic antibiotics are necessary for secondary bacterial infection, after bacterial cultures for antibiotic sensitivity have been performed. Ulceration is best treated with aluminum acetate solution soaks, debridement using topical medications, or surgical intervention. If it is certain that no infection or diabetes exists, the use of Unna paste boots or biologic dressings is quite helpful (15).

Another important factor when treating ulceration with topical medication is the relative ease of sensitization to these agents. A recent study demonstrated a high incidence of allergy to lanolin, topical antibiotics, and cetearyl alcohol in patients with venous stasis ulcers (16). Incomplete healing responses may necessitate patch testing those patients to rule out contact sensitivity.

Finally, it is imperative that once the acute phase of this disorder has been controlled, some form of compression therapy is instituted after excluding coexisting arterial insufficiency. This will undoubtedly delay a worsening of this chronic condition, although the progress depends in great part upon the improvement of the circulation in the affected limb. This may require consultation with a vascular surgeon.

ACNE ROSACEA

Acne rosacea is a chronic inflammatory condition that occurs primarily in middle-aged and elderly individuals. Women are more frequently affected than men. It is usually localized to the central facial region and is always associated with erythema. The erythema is often associated with small telangiectatic vessels, and there may be a varying degree of papules and pustules. Severe nasal involvement may lead to scarring and papularity known as rhinophyma, which is most often seen in males. Eye involvement, including conjunctivitis, iritis, and blepharitis, may also be seen.

The etiology of acne rosacea is still poorly understood. Dietary factors such as alcohol and caffeine, which have been reported to increase erythema, are sometimes implicated. In addition, fluorinated steroids and heat also appear to make acne rosacea worse. Increased vascular lability, increased production of sebum, and reactions to the follicular mite, *Demodex folliculorum*, have been suggested as having a role in the pathogenesis.

Acne rosacea must be differentiated from lupus erythematosus, seborrheic dermatitis, acne vulgaris, and polymorphous light eruption.

Therapy of mild acne rosacea consists of 1% hydrocortisone cream and the cessation of precipitating factors, and perhaps the use of a 1 to 2% precipitated sulfur preparation applied twice daily. If these measures fail or if the acne rosacea is particularly inflammatory or extensive, the use of systemic tetracycline, 250 to 1000 mg daily, usually controls the disease. In recalcitrant cases, the use of metronidazole both orally and topically (17) as well as oral retinoids, has been suggested to be helpful (18).

BULLOUS DISEASES

Bullous diseases of the elderly may be life-threatening. The most important encountered in this age group include bullous pemphigoid, benign mucous membrane pemphigoid, linear IgA bullous disease, epidermolysis bullosa acquista, and pemphigus vulgaris. In the first four conditions, blisters develop at the junction between the dermis and epidermis, with some differences in each case in the exact location of the lysis.

The clinical differential diagnosis of bullous diseases may be difficult but can be clarified by considering such factors as the age of the patient at onset, the pattern and distribution of the blisters, presence of the Nikolsky sign, and the drug history (19).

Bullous pemphigoid is the most common blistering disorder of the elderly and occurs equally in both sexes. The mean age of onset is 72 years, and 85% of the cases begin in patients over 60 years of age (20, 21). Bullous pemphigoid is a chronic, nonscarring, vesicular bullous disease in which nongrouped bullae occur on normal to urticarial skin. The bullae are most commonly seen over the flexural areas but may be localized. They may be pear-shaped and quite dense and may contain clear or hemorrhagic fluid (Fig. 36.1). The oral mucosa is involved in approximately one-third of the patients and has a negative Nikolsky's sign reflecting an inability to dislodge peripheral uninvolved epidermis. The typical course of this disease may last a year, with a variable number of flares.

Benign mucous membrane pemphigoid, epidermolysis bullosa acquista, linear IgA bullous disease, and pemphigus vulgaris are less commonly seen in the elderly. The diagnosis and therapy of these conditions have been reviewed in detail elsewhere (22–25). Therapy for the bullous pemphigoid includes the use of prednisone and azathioprine. In the neutrophil-predominant bullous pemphigoid, dapsone appears to be quite beneficial. For localized bullous pemphigoid, the treatment of choice is still topical steroids and perhaps the addition of erythromycin.

Association between bullous pemphigoid and internal malignant neoplasms is not clear. Accumulated evidence points to a lack of relationship at this time. Extensive studies for cancer appear unwarranted (26, 27). There does appear to be a bullous pemphigoid/bullous erythema multiforme–like eruption associated with internal malignancy (28). There also exists a possible association between malignancy and linear IgA disease (29).

INFECTIONS OF THE SKIN

SUPERFICIAL FUNGAL AND BACTERIAL INFECTIONS

Superficial and dermatophytic (tinea) fungus infections are common in the elderly person but are often not symptomatic. Several series have demonstrated incidences of tinea pedis with onychomycosis of 50% and tinea versicolor of 17% in the elderly considered in the specific studies (30). Erythrasma, a low-grade bacterial infection caused by *Corynebacterium tenuens*, involves the intertriginous and moist areas of the body and has been reported to occur in 10% of elderly women (31). The use of Wood's light makes the diagnosis of tinea versicolor easier and is specific in the diagnosis of erythrasma, which fluoresces a coral red. Intertrigo, a mechanical frictional problem in flexural regions of the body with frequent secondary infection with monilial organisms, involves the axilla, groin, and inframammary regions, especially in diabetic individuals. More recently, tinea capitis in the elderly has been reported to be caused by *Trichophyton tonsurans* and clinically may mimic seborrheic dermatitis or discoid lupus erythematosus (32).

Seborrheic dermatitis is a chronic eczematous disorder of the scalp, face, chest, and intertriginous zones that affects 20% of the elderly population (33). The cause of seborrheic dermatitis is unknown, but the yeast *Pityrosporum* has been suggested as being involved in the pathogenesis,

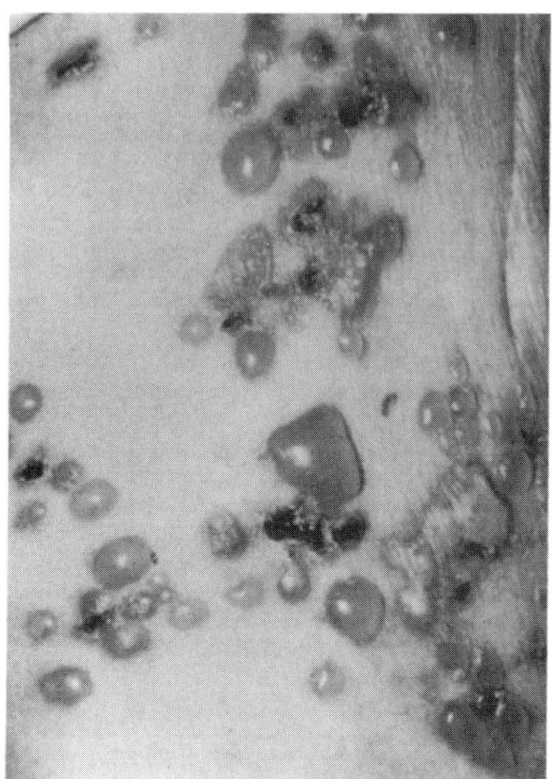

Figure 36.1   Bullous pemphigoid.

and topical antifungals appear to improve the condition (34).

Treatment of these superficial infections ranges from topical antifungal agents, such as miconazole or clotrimazole, for tinea infections to oral griseofulvin for tinea capitis and onychomycosis.

Resistant onychomycosis and certain dermatophyte infections may necessitate the use of newer broad-spectrum antifungals such as terbinafine. This allylamine rapidly penetrates the distal nail and quickly reaches fungicidal levels, requiring a shorter course of therapy than that with griseofulvin. Tinea versicolor can be treated with topical selenium sulfide preparations applied to the entire integument for 10 minutes each day for 10 days and/or a short course of ketoconazole if the case has been refractory and is extensive. Erythrasma is effectively treated with Safeguard soap, topical erythromycin, or clindamycin. Intertrigo should be managed with meticulous cleaning of the involved area and proper ventilation, as well as the application of clotrimazole or miconazole topical creams.

Superficial infections present a significant problem for elderly diabetic, immunocompromised, or vascular-incompetent elderly persons. A low-grade infection often allows other bacteria an excellent portal of entry. These superficial infections require treatment in such individuals to avoid more serious complications. Proper foot and leg care are essential. The use of proper orthotics to avoid the formation of large corns and removal of any onychographytic nails by nonsurgical means such as concentrated urea ointment, are often indicated (35). Again, topical antifungals are useful in any tinea infection, but the use of griseofulvin may be indicated for the more serious type of dermatophytic infections. Topical antibiotics such as mipuracin are extremely helpful in the control of superficial staphylococcal infections. More serious and/or resistant yeast infections may require ketoconazole for an extended period of time, necessitating proper monitoring of the blood count and liver profile.

DEEP BACTERIAL INFECTIONS

Cellulitis and erysipelas present as acute problems and can be life-threatening in the elderly. Systemic antibiotics such as penicillin and erythromycin are helpful and should be used against β-hemolytic streptococcal infections for at least 10 days. In addition, the use of heat in the case of cellulitis and cool soaks in the case of erysipelas is beneficial. For recurrent attacks of cellulitis and erysipelas, it is often necessary to keep the elderly patient on continuous antibiotics at a lower dosage after adequate treatment of the initial infection has been accomplished.

VIRAL INFECTIONS

Herpes zoster and herpes simplex are viral infections that may cause significant morbidity in the elderly. Herpes zoster usually occurs in the fifth to seventh decade of life. The offending agent, varicella-zoster virus, is the same virus that causes chicken pox or varicella in children. After the primary infection, the virus remains dormant in the ganglion of the sensory nerve roots. Precipitating factors such as trauma, radiotherapy, immunosuppression, and stress have been identified as reactivating the virus and causing the clinical condition of herpes zoster. Nevertheless, the exact pathogenesis of herpes zoster remains unclear. In most cases, it seems to occur in healthy individuals, but it may also be seen in individuals with internal malignancies, especially in the lymphoma and leukemia group.

The condition usually begins with pain and burning and is followed by the appearance of grouped vesicles in a dermatomal distribution.

Occasionally there is associated headache, malaise, or low-grade fever. Any of the nerves can be involved, in the following order of frequency: thoracic, trigeminal, cervical, lumbar, and sacral regions. Involvement of the ophthalmic branch of the trigeminal nerve may affect the eye and result in a serious conjunctivitis, iritis, or uveitis. Involvement of the facial nerve can lead to facial palsy and ear pain known as Ramsey Hunt's syndrome.

A few vesicles outside the main distribution of the eruption are not uncommon. However, if there are more than a dozen such lesions outside the dermatomal distribution of the initial eruption, dissemination has occurred. This is more commonly seen in immunosuppressed individuals and those with lymphoreticulate disorders. A presumptive diagnosis can usually be made with the use of a Tzanck smear. Cells scraped from the base of an early vesicle with a #15 scalpel blade are smeared on a microscope slide, then stained with Wright's or Giemsa solution. Multinucleated giant cells, balloon cells, and occasionally intranuclear viral inclusion bodies are seen on microscopic examination. This test will not differentiate zoster from herpes simplex, and false positives and false negatives can occur. The use of tissue culture or monoclonal antibodies may then be necessary for precise identification of the virus.

Therapy for the acute phase of herpes zoster is largely aimed toward symptomatic relief and control of secondary infection. Analgesia and open compresses with aluminum subacetate solution applied four times a day for 15 to 20 minutes are helpful. Secondary infection is best controlled with erythromycin, 250 mg orally four times daily for 10 days. The use of oral acyclovir in doses of 800 to 1200 mg five times a day for 10 days has also been reported to be effective (36). With the advent of newer analogues of acyclovir that provide better absorption, this treatment of the acute phase with acyclovir orally has become more feasible.

The incidence of postherpetic neuralgia (PHN) increases rapidly with age. The percentage of elderly patients with PHN roughly correlates with the age of the patient. For example, 60% of patients that are approximately 60 years of age will develop PHN following typical herpes zoster infection. In addition, recurrence of herpes zoster infection is seen most commonly in patients more than 60 years of age. PHN resolves within 2 months in 50% of patients and within 1 year in 70 to 80% but may last 5 to 20 years (37). The pain experienced from PHN may be so debilitating and disturbing that it rules the patient's life and can even lead to suicide.

In view of the morbidity caused by PHN, many therapeutic modalities have been suggested and tried to control or prevent the discomfort experienced by the patient. Some of the therapeutic regimens that have been tried include antiviral agents such as acyclovir (37, 38) and famciclovir (39), which have demonstrated a significant pain benefit in PHN. The use of systemic corticosteroids early in the course of herpes zoster to prevent PHN is controversial (40–42). Psychoactive agents such as levodopa (43) and amitriptyline (44) have been reported to have some success in controlling the symptoms. More recently, the use of capsaicin topically four times daily for 1 month often helps to decrease PHN, theoretically by decreasing substance P (45).

Herpes simplex infection of the recurrent type occurs in 20 to 45% of the general population in the United States. Lesions of herpes simplex appear as grouped vesicles on an erythematous base. A tingling, burning sensation often precedes the clinical eruption by a few hours to days. The vesicles usually last 2 to 3 days before rupture, resulting in shallow erosions or crusts. Herpes simplex virus type I infection usually occurs around the mouth and in the oral cavity, but may occur at any body site where a superficial break in the stratum corneum has allowed the herpes simplex virus to enter. Herpes genitalis, usually caused by herpes simplex virus type II, is rarely seen in the elderly. Recurrent herpes simplex infection of the buttocks region, especially in elderly females, is not uncommon (46).

Diagnosis of herpes simplex virus infection can be presumptively made with a Tzanck preparation, as with herpes zoster infection. The virus may also be grown in tissue culture or identified by a micro-ELISA technique using a monoclonal antibody.

Therapy consists of drying agents such as ether, camphor, or 4% thymol in alcohol. Additionally, topical acyclovir ointment applied every 3 hours for 48 to 72 hours may slightly shorten the course of the infection. Intraocular lesions can be very effectively treated with idoxuridine, 0.1%, and arabinoside. The most effective systemic therapy is acyclovir, 200 mg orally five times a day for 10 days. This also may be used to prevent recurrent episodes after the initial 10 days of therapy for the acute disease, at a dose of 40 mg twice daily for 4 months or longer, if necessary. Unfortunately, recurrence after cessation of acyclovir is the rule.

Warts of all types can occur in the elderly person (47–49), but filiform and pedunculated warts of the face and neck are perhaps the most common. Occasionally, warts may develop cutaneous horns or become irritated and must be differentiated by biopsy from actinic keratosis and squamous cell carcinoma.

Effective therapy for warts includes the destruction of the lesion by a variety of measures including not only physical but immunologic means. The most common form of therapy is cryosurgery, but this should not be used on eyelids or on the lower extremities. Topical caustic agents may also be used, but only with great caution.

BIOLOGIC EFFECTS OF ULTRAVIOLET RADIATION

Many of the changes commonly referred to as skin aging, such as fine wrinkles, irregular pigmentation, and patchy roughness, are not the result of intrinsic aging but the consequences of solar damage or photoaging. The blue-eyed, sandy-complexioned person is more prone to develop actinic changes than dark-skinned individuals with natural pigment that provides some degree of photoprotection. Every decade beginning at the age of 30, the number of melanocytes per unit area is reduced by approximately 10%, which increases the penetration of ultraviolet light and resultant sun damage (50).

Years of overexposure to the sun result in leathery, atrophic, pebbly, yellowish, textured, wrinkled, and sagging skin (Fig. 36.2). Despite a decreased number of melanocytes in the skin with aging, it is quite clear that the aged still get hyperpigmented or variably pigmented skin in sun-exposed areas. Experimental and clinical evidence demonstrates that nonspecific immune suppression results in cancer formation in animals (51–54).

There is a direct relationship between chronic sun exposure and the development of precancerous and cancerous growths in the skin. Early and continual solar protection can help prevent premature aging of the skin and such changes as atrophy, sebaceous hyperplasia, and life-threatening skin cancers. The best protection, perhaps, is clothing, avoidance of sunlight between the hours of 10 AM and 3 PM, and sunscreens. The daily use of tretinoin on sun-damaged skin may prevent the development of new actinic keratoses and alter involutional structural changes in the skin. Tretinoin has recently been used successfully in the treatment of photoaged skin (55) and non-sun-exposed skin of the elderly (56).

TUMORS OF THE SKIN

The elderly frequently present with a variety of benign, premalignant, and malignant skin tumors. These skin tumors arise from one of three basic tissues in the skin: epidermal, melanocytic, or mesodermal (Table 36.2). Epidermal tumors usually demonstrate the loss of surface lines, scaling, and hyperkeratosis and may occasionally be pigmented. Melanocytic lesions are usually pigmented with a brown to black color. Mesodermal tumors are papulonodular in appearance and may have a red or yellow color. The various lesions may be either malignant or benign. Generally, malignant lesions have a rapid rate of growth, are irregular in contour, vary in pigment, and have a tendency to ulcerate or bleed. Finally, skin tumors may arise from internal malignancy and may be the first sign of this occult disease.

BENIGN TUMORS OF THE EPIDERMIS

Solar lentigo, or age spots, are benign lesions seen in more than 90% of Caucasians over 70 years of age and occur in areas of highest sun exposure, especially the face and dorsal aspects of

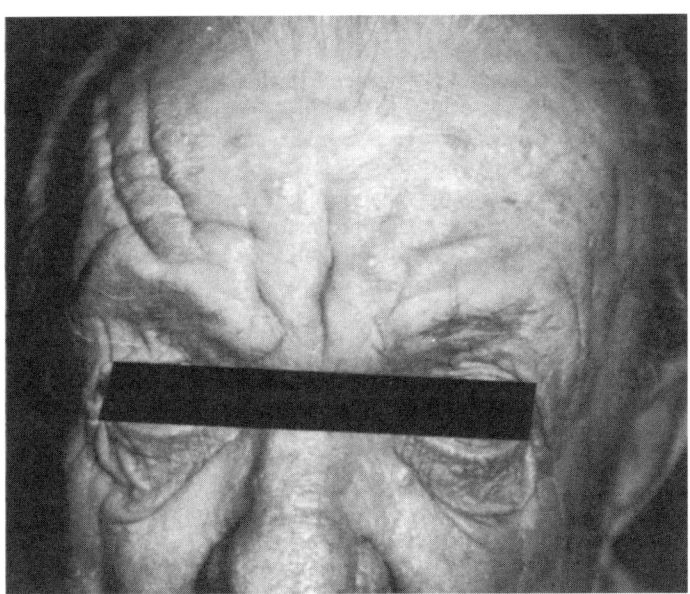

Figure 36.2 Actinic changes of the skin.

Table 36.2
Benign and Malignant Tumors of the Skin According to Tissue of Origin

Tissue of Origin	Benign	Premalignant and Malignant
Epidermal	Solar lentigo Seborrheic keratosis Keratoacanthoma Epidermal cyst Sebaceous hyperplasia	Basal cell carcinoma Squamous cell carcinoma
Melanocytic	Lentigo Pigmented nevi Blue nevus	Lentigo maligna Lentigo maligna melanoma Acral lentiginous melanoma Superficial spreading melanoma Nodular melanoma
Mesodermal	Dermatofibroma Angioma Angiokeratoma Fibroepithelioma	Angiosarcoma Kaposi's sarcoma

the hands (58). They are without question induced by solar radiation and are now being seen in younger populations because of our society's penchant for suntanning. Clinically, these lesions appear as macular, uniform, dark brown lesions that vary in size from pinpoint to more than 1 cm and often coalesce. Histologically, the rete ridges are elongated with small bud-like extensions. The number of melanocytes has been reported to be increased by approximately 10%, and they appear to have increased capacity for melanin production. Treatment of this condition with bleaching creams such as hydroquinone usually is not successful, primarily because the solar lentigo represents an epidermal proliferation. Cryotherapy or trichloracetic acid is often necessary to lighten or remove these lesions. Sunscreens undoubtedly help to decrease the rate of appearance and darkening of these lesions.

Seborrheic keratoses or seborrheic warts are also among the most common skin lesions of the elderly and are found in up to 88% of persons over 65, half of whom had 10 or more lesions (57). They may often be confused with solar lentigo. Seborrheic keratoses, however, appear to be more variable in color, have a more hyperkeratotic and verrucous appearance, and tend to occur over the seborrheic areas. Lesions may number into the hundreds and appear primarily on the back, chest, and face, with a familial predisposition (Fig. 36.3). Seborrheic keratoses often appear as greasy brown to black papules and look as if they are stuck on the skin. The lesion slowly enlarges over the years and may reach several centimeters in diameter. Individual lesions are variable in

color, shape, and adherence and may be mistaken for a malignant melanoma, junctional nevus, or pigmented basal cell carcinoma. Occasionally, the lesion may become irritated and quite tender or may develop into a cutaneous horn.

Eruptive seborrheic keratoses associated with internal malignancy are known as the sign of Leser-Trelat, first described in 1890. Lesions appear clinically as inflamed or even pigmented seborrheic keratoses. Historically, only 50% were typical seborrheic keratoses; the other half resembled acanthosis nigricans (58–60). Most commonly, eruptive keratoses are found on the trunk, and 65% of cases occurred before or concurrent with the diagnosis of internal malignancy. Forty percent of the cases were associated with adenocarcinoma of the stomach. Lymphoma and leukemia were associated with 25% of the cases. The prognosis of this condition is extremely poor; 25% of the patients with the sign of Leser-Trelat die in 1 to 38 months (58–60).

Therapy is not required for seborrheic keratoses unless the lesions are cosmetically unacceptable, inflamed or atypical in appearance. Removal may be achieved simply by curettage or with cryosurgery. In the case of a truly atypical appearing keratosis, complete excision may be necessary. In patients with numerous seborrheic keratoses, the use of topical α-hydroxy acids has been reported as an effective but slow method of removal of these lesions. A more recent report evaluated ammonium lactate in the treatment of seborrheic keratoses. It failed to support other reports of significant beneficial effects of α-hydroxy acid lotions on seborrheic keratoses (61).

Figure 36.3   Multiple seborrheic keratoses.

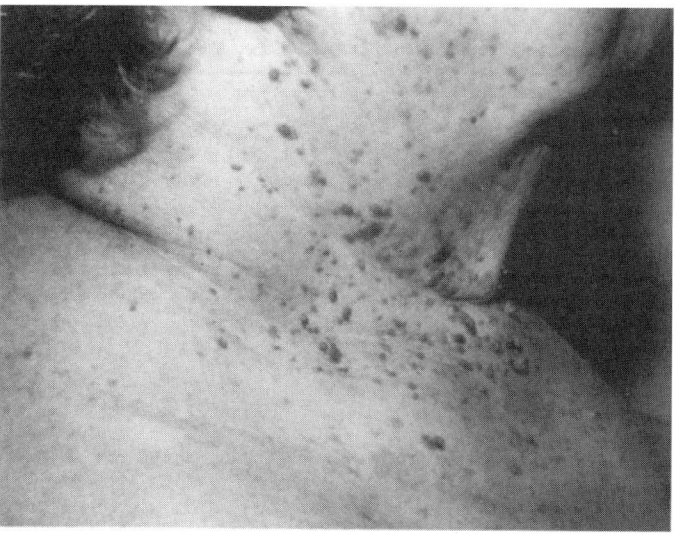

Keratoacanthoma is a benign tumor occurring most commonly on sun-exposed skin in elderly individuals. The tumor most commonly is seen on the face and dorsum of the hands. It is usually solitary and dome-shaped with a central crater of keratinaceous plug (Fig. 36.4). It characteristically arises within a period of approximately 2 to 8 weeks, reaching a size of 1 to 2 cm in diameter, and may be quite destructive. It remains constant in size for another 2 to 8 weeks, then often involutes over several weeks, becoming a depressed, hypopigmented scar. Rarely, a keratoacanthoma may transform into a squamous cell carcinoma. When this occurs, it is often controversial whether the initial lesion was not that of a squamous cell carcinoma (62). Two variants of multiple keratoacanthomas exist and are termed multiple self-healing and eruptive (63–65).

Solitary keratoacanthoma must be differentiated from squamous cell carcinoma, which grows much more slowly, occurs in sun-exposed areas, and has an irregular shape with a tendency to ulcerate and not involute. Frequently, the diagnosis rests on histologic evaluation of the completely excised tumor, and even then differentiation from squamous cell carcinoma may be difficult (66). The patient must always be followed up carefully as if the tumor is a true carcinoma. Other disorders to rule out include basal cell carcinoma, giant molluscum contagiosum, warts, irritated seborrheic keratoses, and inverted follicular keratosis, all of which warrant a biopsy to help differentiation.

Most keratoacanthomas undergo a benign self-healing course but may leave a large, unsightly scar. For cosmetic reasons and the rare case of malignant transformation, treatment is almost always preferred. Surgical excision of the solitary type is the treatment of choice for both cosmetic concerns and accurate histologic study. Curettage and electrodesiccation can also be effective in tumor removal. Others have reported the use of intralesional injection of 5-fluorouracil (5-FU) to be quite effective, especially for large mutilating types of keratoacanthoma or in lesions occurring on the nose and lips (66). Treatment for multiple keratoacanthomas is not effective, but some investigators advocate the use of systemic immunosuppressives or etretinate (67, 68).

PREMALIGNANT TUMORS OF THE EPIDERMIS

Premalignant lesions of the epidermis include actinic keratosis and Bowen's disease, both of which are predominantly seen in the elderly. Actinic keratoses appear as a keratotic papule or a red, scaling macule that may be surrounded by an erythematous halo (Fig. 36.5). They are often multiple and are more easily felt than seen since they have a rough quality. They are most prevalent in areas that receive heaviest solar exposure, such as the alopecic scalp, ears, cheeks, lower lip, nose, dorsum of the hands, and arms. Left alone, actinic keratoses gradually progress to basal cell carcinoma or squamous cell carcinoma over a period of years. At times, the scale may become quite thick, especially in lesions over the dorsal aspects of the hand, and should be viewed with suspicion. When these lesions become infiltrated or elevated or become tender, malignant change may have occurred (69). Approximately 15 to 20% of actinic keratoses are said to evolve into squamous cell carcinomas that have an extremely low potential for metastases (70).

Solitary or multiple hypertrophic actinic keratoses may be treated with cryosurgery. For numerous poorly defined actinic keratoses on the face, scalp, and ears, topical treatment with 5-FU is preferable. It should be noted, however, that 5-FU works poorly on lesions over the dorsal aspects of the hand and forearms, recurrent actinic keratoses, or lesions classified as cutaneous horns. Cryosurgery and surgical excision may be necessary for these resistant lesions.

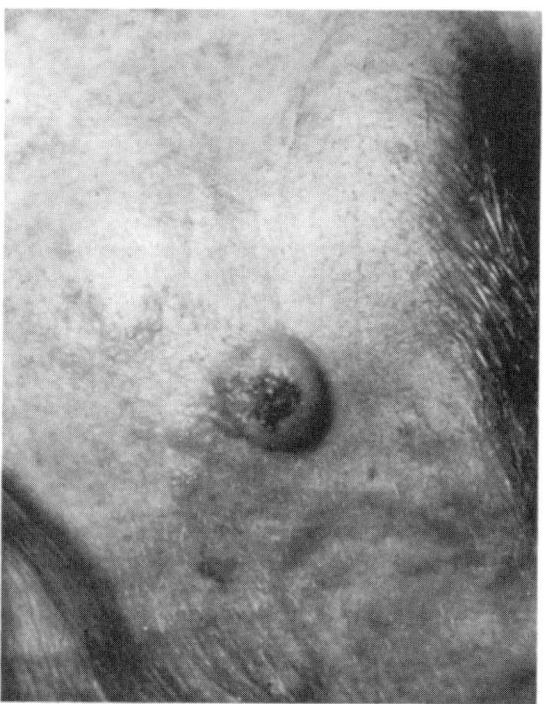

Figure 36.4 Solitary keratoacanthoma.

Figure 36.5   Multiple actinic keratoses.

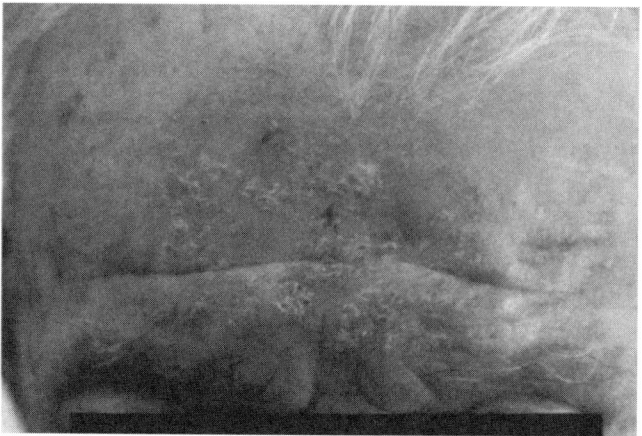

Another newer method used in the treatment of multiple actinic keratoses has been the topical use of tretinoin before 5-FU or cryosurgery or as a primary therapy (71). Short-term exposure to 5% 5-FU cream applied twice daily for 5 to 7 days, followed by immediate treatment with pyruvic acid, appears to be another effective treatment for actinic keratoses, with rapid healing (72). Actinic cheilitis of the lower lip has been treated by 5-FU, tretinoin, cryosurgery, partial lipectomy, and Moh's chemosurgery.

Bowen's disease is an intraepidermal-epidermoid cell carcinoma in situ. The lesion is usually seen as a well-circumscribed, scaly, indurated red plaque that may occur anywhere on the body. The lesion is often mistaken for psoriasis or eczema, which may delay biopsy. When Bowen's disease occurs on non-sun-exposed areas it may be associated with an increased prevalence of internal malignancy. The lesions may slowly enlarge over many years to nodular, invasive squamous cell carcinoma with a potential for metastasis. The lesion characteristically resists topical steroid application, which should suggest the need for a skin biopsy. A variant of Bowen's disease, so-called erythroplasia of Queyrat, occurs in the glans penis in uncircumcised men and may appear as a red, velvety, well-circumscribed plaque (73). In addition, Bowen's disease has been reported as a pigmented lesion resembling a melanoma or a pigmented basal cell carcinoma (74). In both these variants, it is absolutely necessary to perform a biopsy to establish the correct diagnosis.

Treatment of Bowen's disease has included electrodesiccation and curettage, 5-FU application, cryosurgery, excision, and Moh's chemosurgery. Regardless of the type of therapy used, it is exceedingly important for these patients to have close follow-up examinations.

MALIGNANT TUMORS OF THE EPIDERMIS

In the elderly, the most common malignant tumor arising from the epidermal basal cells or cutaneous appendages is the basal cell carcinoma. This particular carcinoma is highly variable in appearance and may be flat, nodular, flesh-colored, black, scar-like, or ulcerative. They are usually found in sun-exposed areas, especially on the face and neck in light-skinned individuals. Ninety-three percent of basal cell carcinoma occur on the head and neck, 60% alone above a line drawn from the ear to the corner of the mouth, and 7% on the trunk (62). They are slow-growing and rarely metastasize.

Nodular ulcerative basal cell carcinoma, the most common form, presents as a waxy or pearly nodule with central ulceration and telangiectatic vessels threading across translucent, rolled, sloping borders (Fig. 36.6). Superficial basal cell carcinoma often presents as multiple lesions and appears as superficial, sharply marginated plaques, with pearly, thread-like borders with a central crust. They occasionally appear like psoriasis and are often on the trunk (Fig. 36.7). Basal cell carcinoma may be deeply pigmented, looking much like a melanoma. Pigmented basal cell carcinoma does not differ in malignant potential from non-pigmented basal cell carcinoma but does seem to be more common in brown-eyed individuals. The most subtle form of basal cell carcinoma is the morpheaform or sclerosing type. It is also the most difficult to cure because of its nondistinct borders. It appears as a flatter, depressed, scarred patch that slowly enlarges to form a plaque. Telangiectasias are present, and there is a shiny, waxy quality to the lesion.

Squamous cell carcinoma has a much greater propensity to metastasize than basal cell carci-

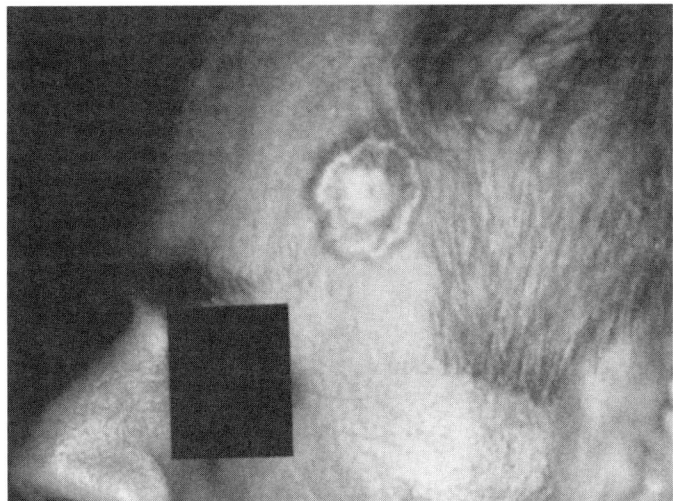

Figure 36.6 Nodular ulcerative basal cell carcinoma.

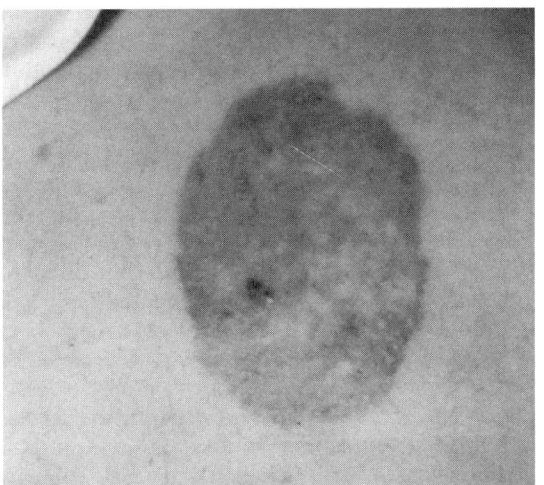

Figure 36.7 Superficial basal cell carcinoma.

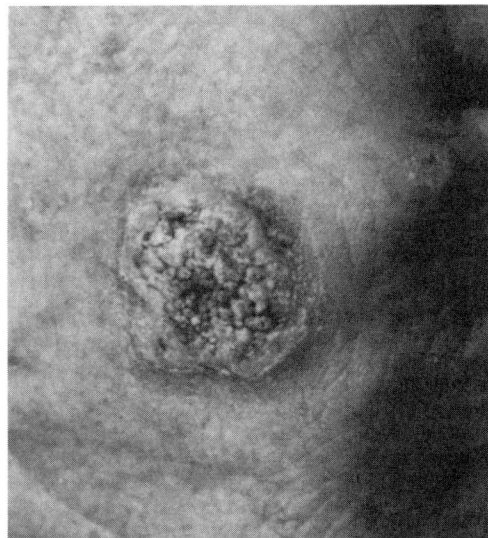

Figure 36.8 Squamous cell carcinoma.

noma but is far less frequent. It is most commonly seen on the face and the dorsal aspects of the hands but may occur on any sun-exposed surface or chronically irritated or damaged area. The clinical appearance of squamous cell carcinoma is also quite variable and may be scaled, ulcerative, nodular, and fungating. Most squamous cell carcinomas appear as solitary keratotic nodules with an erythematous base and nondistinct borders (Fig. 36.8). These often develop into a shallow ulcer that is covered by scale and has a cribriform floor.

Squamous cell carcinoma is usually preceded by intraepidermal carcinoma or a premalignant lesion such as an actinic keratosis, actinic cheilitis, or leukoplakia of the lower lip or buccal mucosa. Verrucous carcinoma, a special form of squa-

mous cell carcinoma, has a warty condylomatous appearance and may be seen most commonly on the penis and foot; it is often misdiagnosed as a wart (75). Squamous cell carcinoma has the potential for rapid growth, but it is unpredictable how long it will remain localized to the epidermis before involving the underlying dermis or metastasizing. Invasive squamous cell carcinoma arising in actinic keratoses is less likely to metastasize than carcinoma arising from Bowen's disease, previously irradiated tissue, or scars resulting from chronic infection or trauma. Squamous cell carcinoma arising in areas of no sun exposure such as the penis, anus, or vermillion border is much more rapidly invasive than squamous cell carcinoma occurring in sun-exposed areas (76).

Therapy for either basal cell carcinoma or squamous cell carcinoma must be tailored for the individual lesion on the basis of many factors (77). These include cell type, tumor size, ease of defining margins clinically, and depth of invasion as indicated by biopsy. In addition, the age and general health of the patient, previous treatment of recurrent cancers, postoperative patient disability, length of time treatment takes, and cosmetic factors all must be taken into account before selecting the best method of therapy for each specific skin cancer. Although the most satisfactory treatment is surgical excision with normal skin margins, it might be more appropriate to use cryosurgery, radiotherapy, or electrodesiccation and curettage. In unusually large, deep, or recurrent lesions, especially around the nose, the use of Moh's histographic chemosurgery may be necessary. Regardless of the procedure, the malignant tissue must be removed in its entirety. The area must then be observed at regular 3-month intervals to assess whether recurrences have occurred.

MELANOCYTIC TUMORS

Many variations occur in benign nevocellular nevi, which first appear in persons from birth to adolescence. Throughout their existence, they may change in color, shape, and size. Often these changes are normal changes associated with aging, irritation, or pregnancy. When suspicious changes occur in any type of nevocellular lesion, lesions should be removed, and histologic evaluation is mandatory.

The benign types of nevocellular tumors of the skin are junctional nevi, dermal nevi, compound nevi, halo nevi, and blue nevi. Junctional nevi are macular and have a uniform brown or black color that does not diffuse into normal skin. The margins are regular. Dermal nevi usually have little or no pigment and are elevated, skin-colored soft papules or nodules with regular margins. They grow slowly with age and may become irritated by friction and thus necessitate removal. Compound nevi combine the characteristics of dermal nevi and junctional nevi and appear as an elevated nodule with uniform brown color and contour. The halo nevus is a junctional nevus with an area of hypopigmentation surrounding the lesion, with a resulting white macule. Blue nevi are not common, and consist of small dark blue to blue-black smooth firm nodules that may occur on any surface of the body. Because of its color, the blue nevus is often excised for histologic differentiation from melanoma.

The number of nevocellular nevi increases up to the fourth decade and then begins to diminish. New nevocellular nevi after the age of 40 should be viewed with suspicion and dictate close follow-up or biopsy to rule out malignancy. Those that do occur after the age of 40 are histologically junctional nevi, but 25% of those originally read as junctional nevi in this older age category were reevaluated and thought to be atypical in appearance.

Lentigines are lesions caused by a slight increase in the melanocyte number and definite increase in melanocyte pigmentation and have been discussed earlier (Benign Tumors of the Epidermis).

Lentigo maligna, a lesion of the head and neck of the elderly, is premalignant and may develop into lentigo maligna melanoma. Lesions are irregularly pigmented and are often noted by the patient to have changed in size, shape, and contour (Fig. 36.9). The lesion histologically is essentially a melanoma in situ. There is a tendency for this tumor to extend down through hair follicles and adnexal structures into the dermis. It has been estimated that 50% of these lesions will become invasive malignant melanoma if not adequately treated, and a further 10% will metastasize (78, 79). It is also clear that lentigo malignant melanoma behaves biologically like other malignant

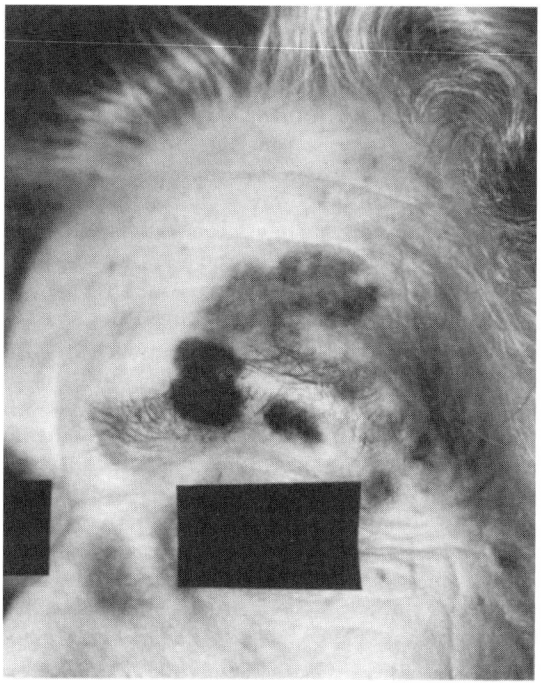

Figure 36.9   Lentigo maligna melanoma.

melanomas. It is absolutely essential that lesions with these characteristics undergo biopsy in several different locations for histologic evaluation and correct diagnosis.

Therapy for lentigo maligna revolves around complete surgical excision with 0.5- to 1.0-cm margins and has been reported to have a 90% cure rate (80). When treating lentigo maligna or lentigo maligna melanoma, one must consider the age as well as cosmetic appearance following such a surgical procedure. Other methods that are available include cryosurgery with a double freeze-thaw cycle, which results in a full-thickness destruction of the dermis (81). This type of procedure should be avoided in areas such as the scalp, eyelids, alae nasi, and nasolabial folds. If the patient is not a good candidate for surgical procedures, conventional radiation or ortho-voltage has also been reported to have a 90% cure rate (82).

Malignant melanoma is the most malignant of all skin cancers. Prognosis varies with the depth of invasion of the tumor. Melanoma varies from macular to nodular forms, with colors ranging from flesh-tint to pitch black. The border tends to be irregular, and growth may be rapid. It tends to be seen on the upper back of 50- to 60-year-old men as the nodular form.

The lentigo maligna melanoma, as discussed above, occurs in the elderly individual and develops from a preexisting lentigo maligna. These lesions expand in the horizontal plane within the dermis for years before entering the vertical growth phase. This is also the case with acral lentiginous melanoma. Acral lentiginous melanoma is also a type of superficial melanoma, with pigmented lesions occurring on the palms and soles, especially in blacks and elderly individuals. These lesions tend to grow slowly, and after years exhibit variations in color such as blacks, blues, and reds. They may also become papular and nodular, signaling overt melanoma.

Nodular melanoma lesions often appear as dark, blue-black to reddish brown nodules without surrounding hyperpigmented macular areas. The surface may be smooth or ulcerated. Nodular melanoma has the poorest prognosis because it has an early vertical growth phase, and often metastases are present at the time of initial presentation.

Differential diagnosis in the case of malignant melanoma may be difficult when dealing with other pigmented lesions and almost always necessitates an excisional biopsy with histologic evaluation whenever a lesion is suspicious. The definitive diagnosis of suspicious pigmented lesions is best confirmed by a total excisional biopsy. When the lesion is too large to excise easily, an adequate representative incisional biopsy may be performed. This must provide enough tissue to evaluate depth of invasion for prognostic and therapeutic purposes. When the tumor thickness, measured from the stratum corneum to the deepest dermal melanoma cells, is less than 0.76 mm, metastasis to local lymph nodes is unlikely, and prognosis is very favorable. If this depth is greater than 1.5 mm, prognosis is poor, because the likelihood of lymph node involvement is not easily predictable.

Wide excisional surgery is the preferred method of initial treatment of melanomas. On an extremity, a melanoma with a tumor depth of 0.76 mm or greater also seems best treated with wide excision plus local chemoperfusion of the limb. The value of node dissection is unclear, but when necessary, continuous node dissection is best. Treatment of disseminated malignant melanoma is chemotherapy or immunotherapy. These are experimental therapies that require well-organized surgical-oncologic-immunologic faculty working in concert.

MESODERMAL TUMORS

Mesodermal tumors of the elderly include both benign and malignant lesions. The most common benign tumors include hemangiomas, venous lakes, angiokeratomas, dermatofibromas, fibroepitheliomas, and sebaceous hyperplasia. Malignant mesodermal tumors include dermatofibroma sarcoma protuberans, Kaposi's hemorrhagic sarcoma, and angiosarcoma. These lesions are dermal or subcutaneous in position and are often papulonodular. They do not usually alter the surface texture of the epidermis, and their color is usually a variation of red, blue, or yellow.

Angiomatous lesions of the skin in the elderly are quite common, easily identified by their red to blue color and the ability to force blood out of the lesion with light pressure. Cherry angiomas are bright red papular lesions seen on the trunk and are very common in the elderly. Venous lakes on the face, especially the lips, are also common in the elderly and appear as blue papular or nodular lesions. Angiokeratomas of Fordyce are small red to bluish black papular tumors on the scrotum that begin in middle age and become quite numerous and common in the elderly. The angiomatous lesions persist indefinitely and usually require no therapy other than reassuring the patient of its benign nature.

Dermatofibromas may occur anywhere but are most common on the arms and legs. They appear as firm brown to pink papules or nodules. They dimple when palpated and have a very hard consistency. Lesions are generally asymptomatic but may become irritated from shaving, especially over the legs in women, and necessitate excision. Fibroepitheliomas or skin tags are papillomatous lesions usually occurring over the neck, axillae, groin, and inframammary regions and are thought to be familial. They begin in persons of middle age and progress in size and number. They may easily be removed by electrodesiccation and curettage, scissor excision followed by hemostasis, or cryosurgery. The occurrence of the fibroepitheliomas and their association with adenomatous colonic polyps has recently been reported, but its significance needs further study (83).

MALIGNANT MESODERMAL TUMORS

Two important malignant tumors of mesodermal origin are Kaposi's hemorrhagic sarcoma and angiosarcoma. Kaposi's sarcoma is relatively uncommon and is usually seen in elderly patients, unless immunosuppression occurs, as in the case of renal transplants or if acquired immune deficiency syndrome is present (84). Classic Kaposi's sarcoma lesions begin on the lower legs, usually as blue papules or plaques. Elderly men are more commonly affected than women, and lesions occur much more commonly in persons of Mediterranean descent and in Africans. Cutaneous lesions may exist alone or in conjunction with systemic lesions, particularly in the gastrointestinal and lymphoreticular systems. Therapy consists of local radiation, vinblastine, or cyclophosphamide, all with variable but generally good results, largely dependent upon the extent of disease or immunologic status of the patient.

Angiosarcoma is an aggressive tumor, usually seen in the scalp of elderly patients. Lesions may appear as reddish purple nodules that may bleed but are generally asymptomatic. Nodular components are often only the tip of the tumor mass, which may infiltrate deeply into the scalp and underlying tissue. Any unexplained angiomatous-appearing nodular tumor of the scalp in the elderly should alert the physician to consider the diagnosis of angiosarcoma. Treatment of this tumor requires wide excision, usually with grafting, and the prognosis is generally poor because the diagnosis is made late in the course of this malignancy.

SUMMARY

Cutaneous problems encountered when treating the elderly patient are often common to all age groups. However, changes in the skin resulting from metabolic alterations, sun exposure, occupational hazards, and underlying diseases create a milieu that allows many disorders to occur with greater frequency and severity in the elderly than in younger individuals. The physician must be able to recognize these pathologic changes and decide on appropriate therapy.

REFERENCES

1. Tindall JP, Smith JG. Skin lesions of the aged and their association with internal changes. JAMA 1963;186:1039–1042.
2. Weismann K, Krakaver R, Wancher B. Prevalence of skin diseases in old age. Acta Derm Venereol 1981;66:352–353.
3. Welton DG, Greenberg BG. Trends in office practice of dermatology, part III. Arch Dermatol 1964;90:296–304.
4. Rajka G. Investigation of patients suffering from generalized pruritus, with special reference to systemic disease. Acta Derm Venereol (Stockh) 1966;49:190–194.
5. Steinman H, Greaves MW. Aquagenic pruritus: an analysis of 36 patients. J Am Acad Dermatol 1985;13:91–96.
6. Kligman AM, Greaves MW, Steinman H. Water-induced itching without cutaneous signs. Arch Dermatol 1986;122:183–186.
7. Cohen PR, Sher RK. Nail changes in the elderly. J Geriatr Dermatol 1993;1(1):45–53.
8. Waldorf DS, Willkens RD, Decker JD. Impaired delayed hypersensitivity in an aging population: association with antinuclear activity and rheumatoid factors. JAMA 1968;203:831–834.
9. Roberts-Thompson ID, Whittingham S, Youngchaiyerd U, et al. Aging, immune response and mortality. Lancet 1974;2:368–370.
10. Fisher AA. Dermatitis due to transdermal therapeutic systems. Cutis 1984;34:526–527.
11. Fisher AA. Contact dermatitis in elderly patients. In: Contact dermatitis. Philadelphia: Lea & Febiger, 1986:58–61.
12. Melmon KL. Preventable drug reactions—causes and cures. N Engl J Med 1971;284:1361–1368.
13. Kauppinen K. Cutaneous reactions to drugs. Acta Derm (suppl) 1972;68:1–89.
14. Jacobson KW, Branch LB, Nelson HS. Laboratory tests in chronic urticaria. JAMA 1980;243:1644–1646.
15. Apelqvist J, Larsson J, Stenstrom A. Topical treatment of necrotic foot ulcers in diabetic patients: a comparative trial of Duoderm and Mezinc. Br J Dermatol 1990;123:787–792.
16. Wilson CL, Cameron J, Powell SM, Cherry G, Ryan TJ. High incidence of contact dermatitis in leg ulcer patients; implications for management. Clin Exp Dermatol 1991;16:250–253.
17. Pyer J, Burton JL. A double blind trial of metronidazole. Lance 1976;1:1211–1212.
18. Plewig G, Wikolowiski J, Wolff HH. Action of isotretinoin in acne rosacea and gram-negative folliculitis. J Am Acad Dermatol 1982;6:766–785.
19. Goldbert SH, Bronson D. Blistering diseases. Diagnostic help for primary care physicians. Postgrad Med 1991;89(2):159–62.

20. Gammon WR. Chronic acquired bullous diseases in the elderly—diagnosis and treatment. Presented at the Westwood Carolina Conference on Clinical Dermatology, Oct 8–10, 1986.

21. Hamm G, Wozniak KD. Bullous pemphigoid antigen concentration in normal human skin in relation to body area and age. Arch Dermatol Res 1988; 280:416–419.

22. Gammon WR, Briggamon RA, Woodley DT, et al. Epidermolysis bullosa acquisita—pemphigoid-like disease. J Am Acad Dermatol 1984;11:820–832.

23. Pearson JR, Rogers RS III. Bullous and cicatricial pemphigoid. Mayo Clin Proc 1977;52:54–56.

24. Shelley WB, Shelley ED. Advanced dermatologic therapy. Philadelphia: WB Sanders, 1987:172–173.

25. Wilson BO. Linear IgA bullous dermatosis: an immunologically defined disease. Int J Dermatol 1985;24:569–574.

26. Lindelof B, Islam N, Eklund G, Arfors L. Pemphigoid and cancer. Arch Dermatol 1990;126:66–68.

27. Venning VA, Wojnarowska F. The association of bullous pemphigoid and malignant disease: a case control study. Br J Dermatol 1990;123:439–445.

28. Anhalt GO, Kim S, Stanley JR, et al. Paraneoplastic pemphigus: an autoimmune mucocutaneous disease associated with neoplasia. N Engl J Med 1990;323:1729–1735.

29. McEvoy MM, Connolly SM. Linear IgA dermatosis: association with malignancy. J Am Acad Dermatol 1990;22:59–63.

30. Michalowski R, Rodziewicz H. Pityriasis versicolor in the aged. Br J Dermatol 1965;77:388–390.

31. Michalowski R, Rodziewicz H. Incidence of erythrasma in elderly women. Arch Dermatol 1965; 92:396–397.

32. Moberg S. Tinea capitis in the elderly. A report on two cases caused by *Trichophyton tonsurans*. Dermatologica 1984;169(1):36–40.

33. Young AW, Jr. Seborrhea in the geriatric patient: incidence, implication, management. Geriatrics 1969;24:144–150.

34. Farr PM, Shuster S. Treatment of seborrheic dermatitis with topical ketoconazole. Lancet 1984; 2:1271–1272.

35. Farber EM, South DA. Urea ointment in the nonsurgical avulsion of nail dystrophies. Cutis 1978;22:689–692.

36. Bean B, Brava C, Balfour HH. Acyclovir therapy for acute herpes zoster. Lancet 1982;2:118–121.

37. Straus SE, Moderator. Varicella-zoster virus infections: biology, natural history, treatment and prevention. Ann Intern Med 1988;108:221–227.

38. Wood MJ, Johnson RW, McKendrick MW, Taylor J, Mandal BK, Crooks J. A randomized trial of acyclovir for 7 days or 21 days with and without prednisone for treatment of acute herpes zoster. N Engl J Med 1994;330:896–900.

39. Beutner K. Antivirals in the treatment of pain. J Geriatr Dermatol 1994; 2(Suppl A)(6):23A–28A.

40. Keczkes K, Basheer AM. Do corticosteroids prevent postherpetic neuralgia? Br J Dermatol 1980; 102:551–555.

41. Esmann V, Kroon S, Peterslund NA, et al. Prednisolone does not prevent post-herpetic neuralgia. Lancet 1987;2:126–129.

42. Elliott FA. Treatment of herpes zoster with high doses of Prednisone. Lancet 1964;2:610–611.

43. Kernbaum S, Hauchecorne J. Administration of levodopa, for relief of herpes zoster pain. JAMA 1981;246:132–134.

44. Weis D, Sriwatana KUK, Weintraub M. Treatment of postherpetic neuralgia and acute herpetic pain with amitriptyline and perphenazine. S Afr Med J 1982;62(9):274–275.

45. Bernstein JE, Korman NJ, Bickers DR, et al. Treatment of chronic post-herpetic neuralgia with topical capsaicin. J Am Acad Dermatol 1989;21:265–270.

46. Raimer SS, Pursley TV. Office management of viral skin infections in the elderly. Geriatrics 1981; 36:53–63.

47. Adler A, Safa B. Immunity in wart resolution. J Am Acad Dermatol 1979;1:305–309.

48. Briggaman RA, Wheeler JCE. Immunology of human warts. J Am Acad Dermatol 1979;1:297–303.

49. Pass F. Warts: biology and current therapy. Minn Med 1974;57:844–847.

50. Gilchrest BA, Glog FB, Szabo G. Effects of aging and chronic sun exposure on melanocytes in human skin. J Invest Dermatol 1979;73:141–143.

51. Koranda FC, Dehmel FM, Kahn G, et al. I. Cutaneous complications in immunosuppressed renal homograft recipients. JAMA 1974;229:419–424.

52. Fisher M, Kripke M. Suppressor T lymphocytes control the development of primary skin cancers in ultraviolet irradiated mice. Science 1982;216:1133–1134.

53. Walder BR, Robertson MR, Jeremy D. Skin cancer and immunosuppression. Lancet 1971;2:1281–1283.

54. Westburg SP, Stone OJ. Multiple cutaneous squamous cell carcinomas during immunosuppressive therapy. Arch Dermatol 1973;107:893–895.

55. Weiss JS, Ellis CN, Headington JT, Tincoff T, Hamilton TA, Voorhees JJ. Topical tretinoin improves photoaged skin: a double-blind vehicle controlled study. JAMA 1988;259:527–532.

56. Kligman AM, Dogadkina MS, Lavker RM. Effects of topical tretinoin on non-sun-exposed protected skin of the elderly. J Am Acad Dermatol 1993;29:25–33.

57. Droller H. Dermatologic findings in a random sample of old persons. Geriatrics 1953;10:421–424.

58. Elewski BE, Gilgor RS. Eruptive lesions and malignancy. Int J Dermatol 1985;24:617–629.

59. Halery S, Feverman EJ. The sign of Leser-Trelat: a cutaneous marker for internal malignancy. Int J Dermatol 1985;24:359–361.

60. Venencie PY, Perry HO. Sign of Leser-Trelat: report of two cases and review of the literature. J Am Acad Dermatol 1984;10:83–88.

61. Kalus MV, Wehr RF, Rogers RS III, Russell TJ, Krochmal L. Evaluation of ammonium lactate in the treatment of seborrheic keratoses. J Am Acad Dermatol 1990;22:199–203.

62. Lynch PJ. Common malignant and premalignant tumors of the skin. Ariz Med 1977;34:90–91.

63. Ghadially FW. Keratoacanthoma. In: Fitzpatrick RB, Eisen AZ, Wolfe K, Freedberg IM, Austen KF, eds. Dermatology in general medicine: textbook and atlas. 2nd ed. New York: McGraw Hill, 1979:383–389.

64. Sommerville J, Milne JA. Familial primary self-healing squamous epithelioma of the skin (Ferguson Smith type). Br J Dermatol 1950;62:485–490.

65. Winkleman RK, Brown J. Generalized eruptive keratoacanthoma: report of cases. Arch Dermatol 1968;87:615–623.

66. Odom RB, Goette DK. Treatment of keratoacanthomas with intralesional 5-fluorouracil. Arch Dermatol 1978;114:1779–1783.

67. Cristofolini M, Piscioli F, Zumiani G, et al. The role of etretinate in the management of keratoacanthoma. J Am Acad Dermatol 1985;12:633–638.

68. Goette DK, Odom RB, Arrott JW, et al. Treatment of keratoacanthoma with topical application of fluorouracil. Arch Dermatol 1982;118:309–311.

69. Yu RCH, Pryce DW, MacFarlane AW, Stewart TW. A histopathological study of 643 cutaneous horns. Br J Dermatol 1991;124:449–452.

70. Parler F. Skin tumors: malignant and premalignant. Geriatrics 1983;38(10):79–114.

71. Bercovitch L. Topical chemotherapy of actinic keratosis of the upper extremity with tretinoin and 5-fluorouracil: a double blind controlled study. Br J Dermatol 1987;116:549–552.

72. Griffin TD, Van Scott EJ. Use of pyruvic acid in the treatment of actinic keratoses: a clinical and histopathologic study. Cutis 1991;47:325–329.

73. Goette DK. Review of erythroplasia of Queyrat and its treatment. Urology 1976;8:311–315.

74. Fisher GB, Greer KE, Walker AN. Bowen's disease mimicking melanoma. Arch Dermatol 1982; 118:444–445.

75. Swanson NA, Taylor WB. Plantar verrucous carcinoma. Arch Dermatol 1980;116:794–797.

76. Robinson JK. Skin problems of aging. Geriatrics 1983;38:57–65.

77. Spencer AD. Treatment of skin cancer using multiple modalities. J Am Acad Dermatol 1982;7:143–171.

78. Jackson R, Williamson GS, Beattie WG. Lentigo maligna and malignant melanoma. Can Med Assoc J 1966;95:846–851.

79. Koh HK, Michalik E, Sober AJ, et al. Lentigo maligna melanoma has no better prognosis than other types of melanoma. J Clin Oncol 1984;2:994–1001.

80. Maize JC. Pigmented lesions in the elderly. Presented at the Westwood Carolina Conference on Clinical Dermatology. Oct 8–10, 1986.

81. Zacharian SA. Cryosurgical treatment of lentigo maligna. Arch Dermatol 1982;118:89–92.

82. Dancuart F, Harwood AR, Fitzpatrick PJ. The radiotherapy of lentigo maligna and lentigo maligna melanoma of the head and neck. Cancer 1980; 45:2279–2283.

83. Chobanian J, Van Ness MM, Winters C Jr, et al. Skin tags as a marker for adenomatous polyps of the colon. Ann Intern Med 1985;103:892–893.

84. Harwood AR, Osoba D, Hofstader SL, et al. Kaposi's sarcoma in recipients of renal transplants. Am J Med 1979;67:759–765.

37/ Hematologic Problems of the Elderly

John K. Erban

Hematologic abnormalities in elderly patients should be recognized early, for they often are the earliest indicators of failing health. Disorders are no different than those for the population at large, however the frequencies of diseases such as cancer and renal insufficiency, which lead to secondary effects on the hematopoietic system, do increase with age. This chapter focuses on factors that effect changes in blood counts or blood viscosity, leading to clinical disease in the elderly.

THE HEMATOPOIETIC SYSTEM

Normal hematopoiesis produces red cells with an average life span of 120 days, platelets with an average life span of approximately 7 to 10 days, and neutrophils with a half-life of approximately 10 hours. Levels of the white blood cell count, platelets, and hematocrit are determined by balances in production and consumption. Erythropoietin (EPO), granulocyte colony-stimulating factor (G-CSF), granulocyte/monocyte stimulating factor (GM-CSF), interleukin 3 (IL-3), as well as stem cell factor and factors stimulating megakaryocyte growth and platelet production are produced by stromal cells within the bone marrow, and many have been purified, cloned, and produced for pharmacologic use. Increased production of growth factors in response to infectious stresses leads to increased production of neutrophils, monocytes, and platelets when required by the host. Production of some but not all cytokines may decrease with age, but there is no evidence for stem cell exhaustion within the normal life span of humans (1, 2). Cytogenetic analysis of bone marrow may also show loss of the Y chromosome in aging men, but this is unassociated with disease (3).

DISORDERS OF THE RED CELLS

The assumptions that age is an independent risk factor for anemia and that older persons become anemic as they age are hazardous and lead to the false conclusion that anemia is the inevitable consequence of aging. The normal reference ranges of hemoglobin and hematocrit should be considered similar for elderly and nonelderly patients. Freedman and Marcus (4) have concluded that standard hematologic levels for the population include roughly 80% of the unselected elderly population, a substantial minority of whom may have an underlying medical illness leading to anemia. While minor variations in red blood cell indices and values may exist, one comparison of patients over the age of 60 with those aged 20 to 39 yielded hemoglobin levels only 0.3 g/dL higher and 0.3 g/dL lower in elderly men and women, respectively, than in the younger cohorts of patients (5). A significant overlap therefore exists between the normal red blood cell levels in elderly patients and their younger counterparts. Anemia of senescence, if it exists, should be considered an extremely rare entity and a diagnosis of exclusion. Elevation of the hemoglobin and hematocrit should always be considered abnormal, although in most cases secondary causes will be found (see below).

ANEMIA

Evaluation of causes for anemia should begin with an evaluation of the peripheral blood smear and a determination of the mean red cell volume (MCV), mean corpuscular hemoglobin (MCH), mean corpuscular hemoglobin concentration (MCHC), and the reticulocyte count. Practically, once a diagnosis of anemia has been made, the MCV is the most important parameter for discerning the underlying cause. Table 37.1 lists causes of anemia classified by the MCV.

Anemia with Microcytic Red Blood Cells

A low MCV implies decreased hemoglobinization of the red cells, which when new is most commonly the result of iron deficiency. Occasional patients of Mediterranean or Asian heritage will be unaware of an inherited thalassemic trait until evaluation during the older years. A low serum ferritin level will help to distinguish iron deficiency from thalassemia. Diagnosis of iron deficiency is usually straightforward after examination of the blood smear and measurement of the serum ferritin, in the absence of underlying chronic illness or inflammation. Normal levels of circulating ferritin can be seen with coexistent iron deficiency if there is ongoing hepatitis or if the patient has an occult infection or carcinoma (6). In this situation, evaluation of the bone marrow by bone marrow aspiration and biopsy under local anesthesia provides invaluable information on the total marrow iron stores, the "gold standard" for the diagnosis of iron deficiency.

Iron deficiency is pathologic and in the absence of a significantly altered diet should prompt an exhaustive evaluation for the cause. The most common causes in the older male population are colonic neoplasms including asymptomatic cancers and polyps, peptic ulcer disease, gastritis, and arteriovenous malformations, which may be found throughout the gastrointestinal tract. In older women, the same causes should be considered, and the reproductive organs should be thoroughly evaluated for occult blood loss from uterine carcinoma or fibroid tumors.

Table 37.1
Causes of Anemia Classified by Mean Cell Volume (MCV)

Group I: microcytic anemias (low MCV)
　Iron deficiency
　Thalassemias
　Lead poisoning
　Sideroblastic anemia
　Anemia of chronic disease (less commonly)

Group II: macrocytic anemias (high MCV)
　B_{12} deficiency
　Folate deficiency
　Hypothyroidism
　Ethanol abuse
　Hemolysis with reticulocytosis
　Myelodysplasia or preleukemia
　Liver disease
　Drug effects

Group III: normocytic anemias (normal MCV)
　Nephropathy with uremia
　Infiltration of the bone marrow
　Anemia of chronic disease (more commonly)
　Hypothyroidism

An occasional patient will present with microcytic indices as a manifestation of sideroblastic anemia. Iron studies are normal, yet the patient has microcytosis and anemia of unclear etiology. The peripheral smear demonstrates basophilic stippling of the red blood cells. Bone marrow aspirate and biopsy with iron stains will reveal the presence of iron in the marrow and ringed sideroblasts in the red blood cell precursors. Identification of sideroblastic anemia may prompt consideration of pyridoxine deficiency or chronic isoniazid use in the treatment of tuberculosis or its prophylaxis. In the absence of either of the above, a likely diagnosis is refractory anemia with ringed sideroblasts, which is considered in the diagnosis of the myelodysplasias (Table 37.2).

Anemia with Macrocytic Red Blood Cells

Anemias associated with macrocytic indices are another group that in the aged population have many reversible causes and should be thoroughly investigated. Initial history includes a comprehensive list of medications because some, such as hydroxyurea and diphenylhydantoin, induce macrocytosis. Dietary history is critical to rule out excessive ethanol use, which raises the MCV, or to determine risk for B_{12} or folate deficiency in the diet. Anemia with associated macrocytosis is a cardinal manifestation of vitamin B_{12} deficiency and can occur with minimal or no other associated neurologic symptoms. Fatigue is common.

Identification of the patient with B_{12} deficiency often begins with the discovery of macrocytosis with mild anemia; however associated hematologic findings include leukopenia with hypersegmentation of the neutrophils, thrombocytopenia, or, in severe cases, pancytopenia. The bilirubin and LDH are often mildly elevated. Evaluation of the marrow can show severe changes and a predominance of megaloblastic and immature precursors, which has rarely led in the past to erroneous diagnoses of leukemia. While the he-

Table 37.2
Myelodysplastic Syndromes (MDS)[a]

Refractory anemia
Refractory anemia with ringed sideroblasts
Refractory anemia with excess blasts
Chronic myelomonocytic anemia
Refractory anemia with blasts in transformation

[a]Adapted from Bennett J, Catovsky D, Daniel M, et al. Proposals for the classification of the myelodysplastic syndromes. Br J Haematol 1982;51:189–199.

matologic manifestations of the disorder are completely reversible with B_{12} administration, neurologic complications, including combined systems disease and dementia are irreversible when present for long duration. Hematologic manifestations of B_{12} deficiency can be corrected with supplemental folic acid replacement, while the neurologic manifestations cannot. Supplemental folate will mask the early hematologic signs of vitamin B_{12} deficiency and is never prescribed unless an evaluation reveals normal levels of vitamin B_{12}.

Causes of B_{12} deficiency include nutritional deficiency, a history of partial or complete gastrectomy, diseases of the terminal ileum, fish tapeworm infestation or resection of the terminal ileum, or pernicious anemia. Diets devoid of red meat are most likely to lead to lower levels of vitamin B_{12} over time. Anti–parietal cell antibodies and anti–intrinsic factor antibodies are present in serum in a large percentage of patients with pernicious anemia (7, 8). Associated autoimmune disorders include such entities as Hashimoto's thyroiditis, Addison's disease, or vitiligo. Most patients found to have decreased B_{12} levels without a dietary cause will have associated atrophic gastritis and achlorhydria (9). Therefore, the standard three-part Shilling test, which identifies the mechanism of inadequate absorption, is not necessary in most cases. Only the occasional patient will have a history that suggests an intestinal process such as bacterial overgrowth/blind loop syndrome, terminal ileitis, or infection with the fish tapeworm *Diphyllobothrium latum.*

Further evaluation of the patient with documented B_{12} deficiency is controversial. The finding of atrophic gastritis has led to concern about the subsequent development of gastric cancer. The incidence of atrophic gastritis in patients with documented gastric carcinoma is as high as 85 to 90%, although the total population at risk for atrophic gastritis also increases significantly with age (10). Most investigators do recognize a slightly increased risk of gastric cancer with pernicious anemia, yet the optimal screening for gastric cancer in patients with pernicious anemia has not been determined. At a minimum, frequent history, physical examination, and stool analysis for occult blood should be performed.

Treatment of vitamin B_{12} deficiency involves monthly injection of 100 µg vitamin B_{12} for life, unless dietary inadequacies have been identified as the cause. Oral B_{12} repletion has no place in the management of nondietary B_{12} deficiency.

Folate deficiency is usually dietary and due to a lack of fresh green vegetables in the diet. In ad-

dition, patients with a significantly increased red blood cell turnover associated with chronic hemolytic anemias can become folate deficient if not supplemented, and patients on dihydrofolate reductase inhibitors or medications that inhibit the generation of tetrahydrofolates, such as trimethoprim/sulfamethoxazole or methotrexate, do become functionally deficient in folic acid. The evaluation consists of measurement of serum folate levels or red blood cell folate if the patient has recently taken folate supplementation and is still suspected of being folate deficient. A single healthy meal can raise serum folate levels to normal. Red blood cell folate levels are insensitive to recent dietary intake and will identify deficiency in these cases. Folic acid (1 mg daily) supplementation is well tolerated orally and will reverse the deficiency. As noted above, folate should never be used to correct the hematologic abnormalities of B_{12} deficiency because it will delay the diagnosis and not prevent the development of neurologic complications.

Reticulocytosis in the setting of anemia causes elevation of the MCV, and in the absence of bleeding should prompt an evaluation for hemolysis. The MCV is elevated because of the increased size of reticulocytes. A detailed drug history should always be sought when confronted with hemolytic anemia, as medications such as α-methyldopa, penicillins, and many other drugs have been implicated in the development of hemolytic anemia. Nonimmune hemolysis suggests an intrinsic red cell defect, which is usually hereditary and diagnosed earlier in life; however its importance should be considered when hemolysis without an immune cause is identified. Particular consideration of glucose-6-phosphate dehydrogenase deficiency is important, as oxidant stress upon the red cells from medications or infection can lead to fluctuations in the hemoglobin level and acute hemolytic reactions. The direct Coombs test, which identifies immunoglobulin or complement bound to the red cell, confirms the diagnosis of immune hemolytic anemia. Immune hemolysis is often accompanied by increased lactic dehydrogenase (LDH) and mild indirect hyperbilirubinemia. Certain drugs may cause the Coombs test to be positive in the absence of hemolysis. Autoimmune hemolysis can be a presenting sign of hematologic malignancy, especially lymphoma and chronic lymphocytic leukemia (CLL), where it suggests progressive disease and a poorer prognosis. Other causes of immune hemolytic anemia include systemic lupus erythematosus and cold agglutinin disease. Fifty percent of newly diagnosed immune hemolytic anemias will be associated with B cell lymphoproliferative diseases.

Mild macrocytosis and the presence of target cells in the smear point to liver disease as the cause, because of redundancy of the cell membrane and increased cell surface area and volume. A most important cause of anemia in the elderly population, associated with macrocytosis and increased MCV, is hypothyroidism. Often the onset of symptoms is gradual, and the complete blood count is remarkable for macrocytosis in the absence of target cells or reticulocytosis. The anemia responds promptly to normalization of the thyroxine and TSH levels. Myelodysplasia in the elderly is rarely associated with isolated anemia; however macrocytosis is commonly found in patients with myelodysplastic syndromes. Most often, other abnormalities in the white blood cells and platelets lead to consideration of myelodysplasia. Bone marrow aspirate and biopsy are diagnostic.

Anemia with Normocytic Indices

Most anemias are normocytic and may be categorized as primary, originating in the bone marrow, or secondary, due to underlying illness. Primary marrow disorders associated with normocytic anemias include refractory anemias with or without sideroblasts associated with myelodysplasia. Multiple myeloma, a malignant disorder of plasma cells associated most often with monoclonal gammopathy, osteolytic lesions on bone survey, a markedly elevated sedimentation rate, and (in late stages) renal failure and hypercalcemia, may present in many ways including isolated normochromic, normocytic anemia. Rouleaux alignment of the red blood cells on peripheral smear is a key to consideration of the diagnosis.

Secondary causes of normocytic anemias include the anemia of chronic disease, endocrinopathies including hypothyroidism, and renal failure with decreased erythropoietin production. Malignancy and chronic inflammation deserve special mention. The definition of chronic disease should not include limited, early-stage malignancy, but rather, signifies a systemic process. Iron studies in anemia of chronic disease usually demonstrate increased ferritin and decreased serum iron levels with decreased total iron binding capacity. The diagnosis of anemia of chronic disease should be made with caution. A documented chronic illness is a sine qua non, and age alone is not a sufficient criterion to make the diagnosis. The sedimentation rate is most often elevated in

anemia of chronic disease; for example, in the case of temporal arteritis, a diagnosis most commonly found in patients over the age of 60 (11).

Occasionally, combined deficiencies such as concurrent iron and folate deficiency will produce an averaged, normal MCV by automated analysis. The RDW, which is an index of the distribution of red cell size, will be increased in this case. As always, examination of the peripheral blood smear is crucial to determine whether two populations of red cells exist, suggesting combined disorders.

POLYCYTHEMIA

Polycythemia vera is most commonly associated with leukocytosis and/or thrombocytosis, often with splenomegaly (see below). When found as a secondary disorder, polycythemia is most likely secondary to hypoxia as a result of pulmonary emphysema or chronic cardiac disease and congestive heart failure. Polycythemia may be relative, due to hemoconcentration, or absolute, due to true increase in the red blood cell mass as determined by an isotopic red cell mass determination. The consequence of an hematocrit over 50 includes increased whole blood viscosity, which rises dramatically as the hematocrit approaches 60. Increased hematocrit and viscosity induce increased afterload on the heart, hypertension, and decreased perfusion to cerebral, coronary, or peripheral circulation.

Evaluation, after confirmation of an absolute increase in the red cell mass, should include an arterial oxygen saturation, a carboxyhemoglobin concentration in smokers, and a serum erythropoietin level to distinguish primary from secondary polycythemia. Secondary polycythemia is associated with elevated erythropoietin levels, unlike polycythemia vera. In the absence of a disorder of oxygen delivery, the older patient should be investigated for disorders associated with increased erythropoietin production such as renal cell carcinoma, cystic kidneys, hepatic lesions including hepatoma, and cerebellar and other rarer tumors (12). In an elderly patient, polycythemia commonly leads to ischemic symptoms, especially when associated with cerebrovascular, cardiovascular, or peripheral vascular disease. When symptoms of hypoperfusion are present, consideration should be given to emergent treatment with phlebotomy and crystalloid repletion until the hematocrit drops below 50.

DISORDERS OF WHITE BLOOD CELLS

Isolated deficiency of white blood cells infrequently occurs except in the setting of drug-induced neutropenia and agranulocytosis (13). Occasionally patients with autoimmune disorders may present with neutropenia in the absence of other hematologic findings. Drugs that are commonly encountered and which may cause neutropenia include antibiotics such as sulfonamides and prolonged use of penicillins, as well as analgesics. Antiseizure medications and antiarrhythmics may also induce neutropenia. The deficiency is corrected within 7 to 10 days after withdrawal of the drug. Certain medications such as tamoxifen may induce mild decreases in the white blood cell count that can be followed without need to discontinue the drug in most cases.

Leukocytosis in the elderly patient should prompt a careful examination of the blood smear for morphologic changes. In the absence of acute infection, neutrophilia suggests an underlying chronic inflammatory condition or a response to malignancy. The white blood cell differential should be examined carefully. Increases in the eosinophil or basophil count may suggest allergic reaction or vasculitis in the setting of eosinophilia, or chronic myeloproliferative disorder in the case of basophilia. Lymphocytosis with atypia in the setting of a flulike illness, when severe, may indicate cytomegalovirus infection, toxoplasmosis, or infectious mononucleosis, which should not be ruled out solely because of the age of the patient (14). Early chronic lymphocytic leukemia is associated only with an absolute increase in the number of lymphocytes in the blood, mainly mature in appearance, and is usually discovered after a complete blood count has been performed for other reasons.

The identification of new defects in leukocyte function at an older age is rare and associated mainly with other hematologic disorders in the setting of myelodysplasia or acute or chronic leukemia. A decrease in the absolute lymphocyte count may occur with age, which may be a manifestation of illness and immunosuppression. Decreasing lymphocyte counts may predict decreased survival over the next 3 years (15).

DISORDERS OF PLATELETS

The platelet count does not change with age, nor does platelet function change. Platelet counts may decrease in response to medications commonly prescribed in elderly patients, such as histamine-receptor blockers and antiarrhythmics. Quinidine-induced thrombocytopenia can lead to severe, life-threatening bleeding and profound thrombocytopenia. The major mechanism is thought to be a response to antibody binding to platelets in the presence of drug (16). The treatment is withdrawal of the drug and, if clinically indicated by bleeding or profound thrombocytopenia, administration of platelets. Heparin induces a mild decrease in the platelet count in all patients, and an idiosyncratic severe thrombocytopenia in as many as 5% of patients who are on daily doses. Thrombocytopenia associated with acute arterial thromboembolic disease is characteristic of heparin-induced thrombocytopenia and requires immediate cessation of the anticoagulant.

Thrombocytopenia due to peripheral destruction of platelets can be distinguished from drug suppression of the marrow by examination of the blood smear and bone marrow aspirate. Peripheral destruction is accompanied by decreased but large platelets on peripheral smear. The response to platelet transfusion in the setting of peripheral destruction is poor, unlike the case of marrow suppression. The distinction can be made easily by aspiration of the bone marrow and assessment of megakaryocyte numbers. If there is no significant splenomegaly or other cause for thrombocytopenia, immune thrombocytopenic purpura should be considered and can be treated either with corticosteroids or more rapidly but at greater cost by infusion of intravenous gamma globulin at high dose over 2 to 4 days (17).

Elevations of the platelet count can be seen as a response to chronic infection or occult malignancy. In combination with microcytic anemia, thrombocytosis should suggest iron deficiency. In all of the secondary causes for thrombocytosis, elevations above 1,000,000/μL are uncommon and suggest a primary myeloproliferative disorder. Essential thrombocythemia usually presents in the later years and may be manifest by an isolated platelet count elevation. The distinction between essential thrombocythemia or other marrow disorders leading to platelet elevations and secondary causes for platelet elevations can sometimes be difficult, although most often platelet counts over 1,000,000/μL are associated with primary disorders of the marrow.

MYELOPROLIFERATIVE DISORDERS

Bi- or trilineage abnormalities in the peripheral blood should prompt consideration of primary diseases of the bone marrow. It is virtually certain that simultaneous identification of changes in the red cell, white cell, and platelet series together will identify many patients who have primary diseases of the bone marrow, with other causes being much less likely.

Myeloproliferative disorders, described and characterized by William Damashek at Tufts-New England Medical Center in the 1950s, are an interesting group of diseases that are more likely to occur in the older population (18). The myeloproliferative diseases include agnogenic myeloid metaplasia (or myelofibrosis with myeloid metaplasia), polycythemia vera, essential thrombocythemia, and chronic myelogenous leukemia. Each is associated with varying degrees of fibrosis in the marrow, splenomegaly, and specific abnormalities in the blood counts; however, significant overlap exists among these entities, and ancillary tests are often needed to define the disorder.

The leukocyte alkaline phosphatase level is usually elevated or normal in all of the disorders except chronic myelogenous leukemia, in which it is abnormally low. Myelofibrosis is associated with prominent tear-drop-shape changes in the peripheral blood red cell series, massive splenomegaly, and variably elevated white cell and platelet counts. The course is usually indolent, although acute myelofibrosis as a manifestation of megakaryocytic leukemia has been described. The appearance of fevers in a patient with myelofibrosis, in the absence of infection, suggests a transformation in the disease and a poorer prognosis (19).

Nonhematologic causes of severe myelofibrosis include disseminated tuberculosis and metastatic carcinoma to the bone marrow. Polycythemia vera can be distinguished by the profound increase in the red cell mass out of proportion to increases in the other cell lines, although secondary elevations of both white blood cells and platelets are common.

Occasionally, the patient with polycythemia will present with a *normal or low* hematocrit, microcytic indices, and an elevation in the platelet count more typical of essential thrombocythemia. In this case the decreased MCV should alert the physician to concurrent iron deficiency due to loss of blood from the gastrointestinal tract. Iron replacement therapy is contraindicated because it would result in a dramatic and symptomatic rise in the hematocrit. Gastrointestinal blood loss as a manifestation of abnormal platelet function in the myeloproliferative syndrome does occur; however an evaluation for lesions accounting for blood loss is indicated.

The myeloproliferative diseases are not associated with specific chromosomal abnormalities with the exception of chronic myelogenous leukemia, in which 95% of cases are associated with a 9:22 chromosome translocation, the Philadelphia chromosome. Identified in 1960 by Nowell

and Hungerford, this abnormality has proven to be a specific marker of chronic myelogenous leukemia (20). Five percent of CML cases are not associated with the Philadelphia chromosome; molecular probes will confirm the diagnosis in these cases.

Patients may have lassitude, sweats, and weight loss or may present without symptoms after routine blood work discovers an elevated white cell count. Older age has been identified as an independent marker of poorer prognosis, with a shorter median survival for patients over the age of 60 than for those younger (21).

Proper diagnosis of chronic myelogenous leukemia is essential, because the prognosis is significantly different than that with myeloproliferative disorders in general. Fifteen percent of patients diagnosed with CML will transform each year to acute myelogenous leukemia (60%) or acute lymphoblastic leukemia (25 to 30%), which are highly refractory to further therapy (22); clinical transformation of polycythemia vera or essential thrombocythemia to a more acute disease is rare in the absence of alkylator therapy or ^{32}P treatment.

The management of chronic myelogenous leukemia in the elderly patient involves regulation of the white blood cell count and platelet count, although patients as old as 60 have been considered for allogeneic bone marrow transplantation if a suitable donor can be found. Hydroxyurea, busulfan, and α-interferon have all been used to control the white blood cell and platelet counts. The use of α-interferon in CML has increased, and a recently reported randomized trial comparing α-interferon and hydroxyurea with hydroxyurea alone has demonstrated increased survival in patients who received interferon (23). Busulfan has recently been shown to be inferior to hydroxyurea in the management of chronic-phase CML (24).

Management of the myeloproliferative disorders other than CML is specific to the abnormality. Phlebotomy for polycythemia is benign and should be done weekly until the patient is iron deficient and the hematocrit stabilizes. If platelet count elevations are problematic, hydroxyurea can be prescribed to lower the count. The use of ^{32}P, which is highly effective, should be avoided because an increased risk of late-onset leukemia has been identified in patients who have been so treated. Patients with essential thrombocythemia should be monitored carefully for signs of bruising, bleeding, or thrombosis. Many patients have associated atherosclerosis and are at risk for coronary or cerebrovascular events. The platelet count should be lowered aggressively if the patient has been symptomatic. The occasional patient who presents with platelet counts between 1,000,000 and 3,000,000/μL and who is symptomatic should be treated with immediate platelet pheresis and initiation of hydroxyurea. Aspirin should not be used empirically in asymptomatic patients because some will manifest bleeding and not vascular insufficiency as their hemostatic defect.

Patients with agnogenic myeloid metaplasia should be managed conservatively. Occasionally, severe and progressive pancytopenia, painful splenomegaly, or cachexia due to splenic compression of the stomach suggests the need for splenectomy; however this should be considered only in extreme circumstances as prior series on splenectomy in this disorder have demonstrated a high 30-day postsurgical mortality. Irradiation of the spleen is an alternative method of decreasing its size.

HODGKIN'S DISEASE AND NON-HODGKIN'S LYMPHOMA

Hodgkin's disease may present with protean manifestations, especially in the elderly patient. Lassitude, fever, anorexia, or night sweats may be the only symptoms. The disease has a bimodal frequency, with the second peak incidence in the sixth decade. Prognosis is heavily determined by staging at the time of diagnosis, which in turn depends upon the number of nodal groups involved and presence or absence of fever, night sweats, or 10% or more weight loss (B symptoms). Isolated involvement of the bone marrow is rare. The treatment of Hodgkin's disease is highly successful, even in advanced-stage disease, if full-dose therapy can be administered; however combination chemotherapy is demanding and is often not tolerated by the patient. For this reason, survival may be compromised in the older population (25).

Non-Hodgkin's lymphoma (NHL) depends much more upon histologic subtype than upon staging to identify prognosis and need for therapy. Unlike Hodgkin's disease, NHL is more likely to be diffuse at presentation. Several classification schema have attempted to stratify tumor types based on histology in an attempt to define prognostic factors; the Working Formulation is one commonly applied classification schema (26). Paradoxically, high-grade lymphomas have a more aggressive course but a higher chance of overall cure with chemotherapy than do low-grade tumors.

LYMPHOPROLIFERATIVE DISEASES AND PLASMA CELL DYSCRASIAS

Clonal expansion of lymphocytes or plasma cells can give rise to a number of syndromes that are much more common in elderly patients than in a younger population.

Chronic lymphocytic leukemia (CLL) is usually a disorder of B cell, rarely T cell, origin. The long-term survival depends upon the stage of disease at diagnosis, with patients with asymptomatic lymphocytosis (stage O) demonstrating 10- to 15-year median survivals. Staging depends upon the presence of adenopathy (stage I), hepatic or splenic enlargement (stage II), anemia (stage III), or thrombocytopenia (stage IV) (27). Associated hypogammaglobulinemia is common, and patients often present with recurrent sinopulmonary infections, prompting a complete blood count and discovery of the characteristic changes on smear. Treatment should be reserved for those with progressive cytopenia, symptomatic organomegaly or lymphadenopathy, or immune thrombocytopenia or anemia.

Waldenstrom's macroglobulinemia is a malignant proliferation of B lymphocytes with plasmacytoid features that secrete monoclonal IgM, causing hyperviscosity with extreme elevations. Circulatory disturbances and changes in retinal vasculature ("box-car" venous configurations) may result. Patients tend to be older and male (28). The marrow shows infiltration with B lymphocytes, and the patient often manifests anemia and rarely thrombocytopenia. Treatment with alkylating agents and prednisone to lower the IgM improves hyperviscosity, although plasmapheresis is occasionally needed to control symptoms.

The incidence of multiple myeloma has increased over the past decade and is more frequent with age, commonly appearing in the seventh decade (29). The disease is characterized by a clonal expansion of plasma cells that in most circumstances secrete immunoglobulin. Background levels of normal immunoglobulins are depressed, and the patient often experiences anemia, recurrent infection, and bone pain. Infrequently renal failure is the initial manifestation, and all patients with newly diagnosed renal insufficiency should have a serum and urine evaluation for monoclonal immunoglobulin or light chains. The patient may experience significant bone pain from osteolytic lesions in the skeleton that are not seen on bone scan. Hypercalcemia is found in advanced disease and can be managed with hydration and diphosphonate and steroid administration initially. The diagnosis of myeloma is usually not difficult when monoclonal immunoglobulin or light chain is identified in association with anemia and bone lesions. The blood smear will show normochromic, normocytic anemia, with rouleaux alignment of the red cells. Analysis of the bone marrow will show increased numbers of clonal plasma cells with cytologic atypia. Untreated, median survival of patients with myeloma is 6 to 9 months. Treatment has extended survival to 2 to 3 years.

The identification of a monoclonal immunoglobulin spike on serum electrophoresis is not sufficient to make a diagnosis of myeloma. In the absence of bone lesions and with minor increases only in the percentage of plasma cells in the marrow, monoclonal gammopathy of uncertain significance (MGUS) should be considered. The background level of immunoglobulins is normal in this entity, and there is no evidence of renal failure, bone disease, or anemia. In long-term study, one-quarter to one-third of patients with MGUS will progress to overt myeloma or a related disorder over the next 10 to 20 years (28); therefore, careful evaluation over time is necessary and should include serial complete blood counts and quantitation of the monoclonal spike, in addition to immunoelectrophoresis of serum and urine.

Isolated plasmacytoma may be found by plain x-ray in elderly patients with site-specific bone pain. The associated monoclonal gammopathy resolves with resection or radiation of the lesion. Despite the focal nature of the process, most patients diagnosed with isolated plasmacytoma will go on to develop disseminated disease (30).

Treatment of multiple myeloma involves the use of alkylating agents such as melphalan in combination with prednisone, or vincristine, adriamycin, and dexamethasone, with corticosteroid being an important part of any initial therapy. Pulse dexamethasone alone has been used to decrease tumor burden. More aggressive regimens have yet to be proven to show advantage over the easily administered alkylator and steroid combination for most cases.

The diagnosis of marked splenomegaly and pancytopenia should prompt consideration of hairy cell leukemia because of the dramatically successful therapies for this disease. Patients may have recurrent bacterial infections but more commonly present with significant pancytopenia and marked splenomegaly. Often the diagnosis is elusive and may be found only after splenectomy or after several bone marrow biopsies. This diagnosis is important because remissions and cures are possible with the use of 2-chlorodeoxyadenosine, pentostatin, or interferon. Each has a role;

however, 70% of patients enter complete durable remissions with 2-CDA, and up to 95% of patients remit after 2 courses (31). The medical therapy for hairy cell leukemia is one of the most remarkable evolutions of medical therapy for any malignant disease. The role of splenectomy in the modern era of medical therapy for hairy cell disease is unclear, though durable long term remissions have clearly been demonstrated with splenectomy alone.

MYELODYSPLASIA

The myelodysplastic syndromes (MDS) are more common in the aging population. Finding trilineage abnormalities on blood smear and the combination of anemia, thrombocytopenia, and leukopenia should always alert to the possibility of disease within the marrow. The myelodysplastic conditions (listed in Table 37.2) include an orderly progression from refractory anemia to refractory leukemia with excess blasts in transformation. Many are associated with chromosomal disorders such as deletion of the long arms of chromosomes 5 or 7 or trisomy 8. The presence of cytogenetic abnormalities may predict a poorer outcome (32).

Treatment is supportive, although occasional patients respond to androgen therapy. G-CSF and GM-CSF have no chronic role in the disorder. Left untreated, peripheral blood counts may fall to severely depressed levels or the disease may transform to acute leukemia. The therapy of acute leukemia arising out of myelodysplasia is disappointing, with prolonged and profound pancytopenia a possibility. Aggressive chemotherapy and bone marrow transplantation for myelodysplasia should be reserved for younger patients. Finding pancytopenia warrants performance of a bone marrow aspirate and biopsy, with attention to chromosomal analysis. Treatment of myelodysplastic patients requires frequent counseling and attention to the problems of anemia, thrombocytopenia, and infection. Patients may require frequent blood transfusions and commonly develop iron overload from transfusion. Easy brusibility, mucosal bleeding, and retinal bleeding, fatigue, and infection all occur frequently in elderly patients.

The median survival with myelodysplastic syndromes varies with the number of blasts and the degree of cytopenia; however, overall survival is approximately 50% at 1 year (33). Transfusions of platelets and packed red blood cells is for symptomatic relief and not to maintain arbitrary levels. Infections should be aggressively treated without delay, as host defenses against bacteria are decreased. Particularly common are dental and perirectal infections, and preventative care in the mouth and removal of carious teeth are critical, as is attention to proper bowel function and avoidance of rectal fissures or hemorrhoidal inflammation. Vaccination of patients against pneumococcal pneumonia and influenza is recommended.

The incidence of myelodysplasia and acute leukemia after prior treatment for another malignancy is of increasing interest. The increased incidence of leukemia following chemotherapy for breast cancer, for example is extremely low but real (34). Patients with Hodgkin's disease have increased incidences of leukemia and solid tumors when followed long-term. The peak incidence of leukemia and MDS occurs about 7 years after chemotherapy, and the incidence of secondary tumors is approximately 7 to 15%, although follow-up continues (35, 36).

ACUTE LEUKEMIA

A diagnosis of leukemia provokes profound fear in all patients, especially those who are older, since therapeutic options are more limited than for the patient who is 20 to 40. Acute leukemia can present de novo or can arise from a myelodysplastic condition over months. The acute leukemias are defined by either myeloid or lymphoid features (37, 38) using the French-American-British classification system. Several important specific features are worth noting.

Promyelocytic leukemia associated with a translocation of chromosomes 15 and 17 may have a better prognosis and can be treated with oral *trans*-retinoic acid rather than with standard cytotoxic drugs as initial inductive therapy. This disease is associated with disseminated intravascular coagulation more commonly than are the other acute leukemias.

Identification of acute lymphoblastic leukemia (ALL) in the older patient usually is not associated with a prior myelodysplastic condition; however, approximately 15 to 17% are associated with the Philadelphia chromosome. Therapy for ALL is usually associated with eventual relapse in the adult, unlike in children, where 70% or more are cured.

Therapy for acute myelogenous leukemia (AML) in the elderly population is controversial. Standard therapy for AML in patients less than 60 years of age includes an anthracycline for 3 days and cytosine arabinoside infusion for 7 days, or newer regimens that combine anthracycline, cytosine arabinoside, and etoposide. Mucositis and infectious complications occur with frequency and are associated with a higher mortality and morbidity in older patients. Cardiac function must be sufficient to allow use of anthracyclines, which are associated with a dose-dependent cardiotoxicity. Attempts to control morbidity and mortality by decreasing the anthracycline and cytosine arabinoside doses have been proposed as the most appropriate form of therapy. Alternatively, a 21-day infusion of cytosine arabinoside at low doses has been recommended. The decision to treat with standard induction therapy or cytosine arabinoside is controversial and depends upon the overall health of the patient and the experience of the hematologist. Often, supportive care alone is the most appropriate therapy for the patient.

OTHER CAUSES OF PANCYTOPENIA

Pancytopenia in an otherwise healthy older patient should prompt consideration of several other entities in addition to those mentioned above. Hypoplastic or aplastic anemia presents with lassitude, bruising or bleeding, or infection. Other than low blood counts, the blood smear is normal. Drug-induced suppression of the marrow should be considered, which may be reversible upon cessation of the drug. Chloramphenicol and phenylbutazone may be associated with irreversible marrow aplasia. Since marrow transplantation is not generally a consideration in patients over age 60, therapies are limited to those that include immunosuppression, such as antithymocyte globulin or cyclosporine and corticosteroid therapy.

Paroxysmal nocturnal hemoglobinuria (PNH) should be considered whenever the combination of iron deficiency and pancytopenia is seen. PNH is a clonal stem cell disorder that leads to pancytopenia and increased susceptibility of red blood cells to hemolysis. Hemosiderin in the urine is increased, and ongoing hemolysis leads to loss of iron. Patients may present with hypercoaguability and rare thrombotic complications such as Budd-Chiari syndrome. The molecular defect in PNH responsible for increased hemolytic sensitivity to complement has recently been identified (39).

SUMMARY

Approaching the patient to establish a hematologic diagnosis requires broad consideration, as many hematologic abnormalities are explained by systemic illnesses or caused by other disorders. The importance of establishing the hematologic diagnosis is clear, since certain abnormalities will lead to discovery of significant disease that may be easily treated, such as hypothyroidism or pernicious anemia. Hematologic abnormalities yield a wealth of information about the general condition of the patient. Evaluation of the blood counts and review of the peripheral blood smear, coupled with a detailed history and physical examination will provide a cost-effective and elegant basis upon which to formulate a diagnosis.

REFERENCES

1. Shank WA Jr, Balducci L. Recombinant hemopoietic growth factors: comparative hemopoietic response in younger and older subjects. J Am Geriatr Soc 1992;40:151–154.
2. Rothstein G. Hematopoiesis in the aged: a model of hematopoietic dysregulation. Blood 1993;82:2601–2604.
3. Sandberg AA. The chromosomes in human cancer and leukemia. North Holland, NY: Elsevier, 1980.
4. Freedman ML, Marcus DL. Anemia and the elderly: is it physiology or pathology? Am J Med Sci 1980; 280:81–85.
5. Garry PJ, Goodwin JS, Hunt WC. Iron status and anemia in the elderly: new findings and a review of previous studies. J Am Geriatr Soc 1983;31:389–399.
6. Lipschitz DA, Cook JD, Finch CA. A clinical evaluation of serum ferritin as an index of iron stores. N Engl J Med 1974;290:1213–1216.
7. Irvine WJ, Davies SH, Teitelbaum S, Delamore I, Williams A. The clinical and pathological significance of gastric parietal cell antibody. Ann NY Acad Sci 1965;124:657–691.
8. Schade SG, Abels J, Schilling RF. Studies on antibody to intrinsic factor. J Clin Invest 1967;46:615–620.
9. Nilsson-Ehle H, Landahl S, Lindstedt G, et al. Low serum cobalamin levels in a population study of 70- and 75-year old subjects: gastrointestinal causes and hematological effects. Dig Dis Sci 1989;34:716–723.
10. Hoffman NR. The relationship between pernicious anemia and cancer of the stomach. Geriatrics 1970; 25:90–102.
11. Bethlenfalvay NC, Nusynowitz ML. Temporal arteritis: a rarity in the young adult. Arch Intern Med 1964;114:487–489.
12. Thorling EB. Paraneoplastic erythrocytosis and inappropriate erythropoietin production. Scand J Haematol 1972;17(S):13–85.
13. Bottiger LE, Bottiger B. Incidence and cause of aplastic anemia, hemolytic anemia, agranulocytosis and thrombocytopenia. Acta Med Scand 1981; 210:474–479.
14. Schnader KE, van der Horst CM, Klotman ME. Epstein-Barr virus and the elderly host. Rev Infect Dis 1989;11:64–73.
15. Bender BS, Nagel JE, Adler WH, Andres R. Absolute peripheral blood lymphocyte count and subsequent mortality of elderly men. The Baltimore Longitudinal Study of Aging. J Am Geriatr Soc 1986; 34:649–654.
16. Christie DJ, Mullen PC, Aster RH. Fab-mediated binding of drug-dependent antibodies to platelets in quinidine- and quinine-induced thrombocytopenia. J Clin Invest 1985;75:310–314.
17. Bussel JB, Pham LC, Aledort L, Nachman R. Maintenance treatment of adults with chronic refractory immune thrombocytopenic purpura using repeated intravenous infusions of gammaglobulin. Blood 1988;72:121–127.
18. Damashek W. Some speculations on the myeloproliferative syndromes. Blood 1951;6:372–375.
19. Varki A, Lottenberg R, Griffin R, Reinhard E. The syndrome of idiopathic myelofibrosis: clinicopathologic review with emphasis on the prognostic variables predicting survival. Medicine (Baltimore) 1983;62:353–371.
20. Nowell PC, Hungerford DA. A minute chromosome in human chronic granulocytic leukemia. Science 1960;132:1197.
21. Kantarjian H, Keating M, McCredie K, et al. Old age: a sign of poor prognosis in patients with chronic myelogenous leukemia. South Med J 1987;80:1228–1232.
22. Rosenthal D, Canellos G, de Vita V, Gralnick H. Characteristics of blast crisis in chronic granulocytic leukemia. Cancer 1975;35:199–207.
23. Giles FJ, Aitchison R, Syndercombe CD, Schey S, Newland AC. Recombinant alpha 2B interferon in combination with oral chemotherapy in late chronic phase chronic myeloid leukemia. Leuk-Lymphoma 1992;7:99–102.
24. Hehlmann R, Heimpel H, Hasford J, et al. Randomized comparison of busulfan and hydroxyurea in chronic myelogenous leukemia: prolongation of survival by hydroxyurea. Blood 1993;82:398–407.
25. Erdkamp FL, Breed WP, Bosch LJ, Wijnen JT, Blijham GB. Hodgkin's disease in the elderly. A registry-based analysis. Cancer 1992;70:830–834.
26. The Non-Hodgkin's Lymphoma Pathologic Classification Project: National Cancer Institute sponsored study of classifications of non-Hodgkin's lymphomas. Summary and description of a working formulation for clinical usage. Cancer 1982; 49:2112–2135.
27. Rai KR, Sawitsky A, Cronkite EP, et al. Clinical staging of chronic lymphocytyic leukemia. Blood 1975;46:219–234.
28. Kyle RA, Garton JP. The spectrum of IgM monoclonal gammopathy in 430 cases. Mayo Clin Proc 1987; 62:719–731.
29. Kyle RA. Plasmas cell proliferative disorders. In: Hoffman R, Benz EJ Jr, Shattil SJ, Furie B, Cohen HJ, eds. Hematology: basic principles and practice. New York: Churchill Livingstone, 1991:1026.
30. Batille R, Sany J. Solitary myeloma: clinical and prognostic features in a review of 114 cases. Cancer 1981;48:845–851.
31. Estey EH, Kurzrock R, Kantarjian HM, et al. Treatment of hairy cell leukemia with 2-chlorodeoxyadenosine (2-CDA). Blood 1992;79:882–887.
32. Nowell PC. Cytogenetics in preleukemia. Cancer Genet Cytogenet 1982;5:265–278.
33. Tricot G, Vlietinck R, and Boogaerts MA, et al. Prognostic factors in the myelodysplastic syndromes: importance of initial data on peripheral blood counts, bone marrow cytology, trephine biopsy and chromosomal analysis. Br J Haematol 1985;60:19–32.
34. Curtis R, Boice J, Stovall M, et al. Risk of leukemia after chemotherapy and radiation treatment for breast cancer. N Engl J Med 1992;326:1745–1751.

35. Tester WJ, Kinsella TJ, Waller B, et al. Second malignant neoplasms complicating Hodgkin's disease: the National Cancer Institute experience. J Clin Oncol 1984;2:762–769.

36. Tucker MA, Coleman CN, Cox RS, et al. Risk of second cancers after treatment for Hodgkin's disease. N Engl J Med 1988;318:76–81.

37. Bennett J, Catovsky D, Daniel M, et al. Proposed revised criteria for the classification of myeloid leukemia. A report of the French-American-British Cooperative Group. Ann Intern Med 1985;103:620–625.

38. Bennet J, Catovsky D, Daniel M, et al. French-American-British (FAB) Cooperative Group: the morphological classification of lymphoblastic leukaemia-concordance among observers and clinical correlations. Br J Haematol 1981;47:553–562.

39. Takeda J, Miyata T, Kawagoe K, et al. Deficiency of the GPI anchor caused by a somatic mutation of the PIG-A gene in paroxysmal nocturnal hemoglobinuria. Cell 1993;73:703–711.

40. Bennett J, Catovsky D, Daniel M, et al. Proposals for the classification of the myelodysplastic syndromes. Br J Haematol 1982;51:189–199.

38/ Surgical Principles for the Aged

Alan W. Hackford

It is obvious that the nature of surgical practice is changing as a result of changing population demographics. The median age on most general surgical services now exceeds what was once considered a contraindication to operate. These facts obligate surgeons to be better able to assess risk in the context of multiple comorbid conditions. They must thoroughly understand the natural history of the diseases of the elderly, particularly malignancy, so that they can balance the possibilities for cure, the benefits of palliation, and the life expectancy of the patient. Finally, surgeons must be aware of the physiologic impact of aging and its effect on clinical presentations and the incidence, type, and severity of postoperative complications.

RISK ASSESSMENT

The variable rate of age-related physiologic change and the impact of comorbid conditions require that each surgical patient be individually assessed for risk. The bulk of morbidity and mortality related to surgery in the elderly derives from the cardiorespiratory systems. Fifty percent of mortality alone results from cardiovascular complications. The best and most cost-effective screening tools remain the history and physical. Scoring systems have emerged that allow reasonably accurate risk projection. The most generic of these is the classification system used by the American Society of Anesthesiologists (ASA). Patients older than 80 by definition are at least ASA class 2. In a series of over 500 patients, less than 1% of class 2 patients died. Patients with severe systems disturbances that were not life threatening (class 3) have a 4% mortality. By contrast, 25% of ASA class 4 (with life-threatening physiologic derangement) patients died. Emergent operations double the risk (1).

Twenty percent of potentially avoidable mortality is attributed to cardiac causes (2). History, physical examination, and ECG are the cornerstones of cardiac risk assessment. The historical

factors of age above 70 years, diabetes, and previous myocardial infarction (MI) within 6 months are important. In addition, physical features of congestive heart failure, systolic murmurs, and irregular rhythms and ECG findings of arrhythmia are significant risk factors.

In the 1970s, multivariant analysis led to the development of the Cardiac Risk Index by Goldman et al. (3). This has become the "gold standard" for risk assessment and a straightforward method for stratifying patients by cardiac status. High-risk (class III and IV) patients should be evaluated by an exercise tolerance test to further stratify risk (4).

Significant advances in anesthetic techniques and perioperative monitoring have somewhat clouded the utility of more extensive screening evaluations, with the exception of systolic murmurs. Post-MI reinfarction rates of 30% for surgery within 3 months and 15% between 3 and 6 months reported in the 1970s have been reduced to 6 and 2%, respectively (5). Dipyridamole myocardial scintigraphy is of particular benefit in patients who are unable to perform or who have an abnormal exercise tolerance test. The negative predictive value of scintigraphy is 100% for normal examinations and 88.5% for fixed perfusion defects (6). The positive predictive value of identifying myocardium at risk defined by reversible perfusion defects, however, is 12% for a single defect in the absence of congestive heart failure and 36.7% for multiple defects. The cardiac mortality was 1.3% for the former and 5.9% for the latter (6). In contemporary studies using limited screening or clinicians blinded to the scintigraphy results, the rates of MI or cardiac death have been comparable to those in series reporting routine screening of all patients (7, 8). Given current morbidity and mortality of cardiac revascularization, coronary catherization is recommended only for patients with single reversible defects associated with congestive heart failure or multiple reversible defects. Patients with abnormal rhythms on

ECG should undergo 24-hour ambulatory monitoring and identified disturbances be treated preoperatively (9). Congestive heart failure needs aggressive medical management, and angina should be stabilized. Any discontinuation of β-blockade, calcium channel blockers, and/or nitrates increases risk. Antihypertension medications should be continued right up to the day of the procedure.

Pulmonary complications account for 40% of postoperative morbidity and 20% of mortality in the elderly (2). In addition to physiologic change related to age, coexisting chronic obstructive pulmonary disease can increase the risk by a factor of 20 (10). Functional deficits are further compounded by any significant malnutrition. History taking in these patients should always elicit the patient's level of activity, dyspnea, cough, smoking, or previous thromboembolic events. Based on historical or physical findings, if problems are suspected, spirometry should be done. FEV_1 and maximum voluntary ventilation combine a variety of variables such as physiologic function with motivation and stamina and reliably predict the risk of a postoperative cardiopulmonary event (11). Abnormal spirometry should trigger a full set of pulmonary function studies, including response to bronchodilators and arterial blood gases. High-risk patients defined by pulmonary function tests (PFTs) can decrease risk by more than 60% with a preoperative regimen involving cessation of smoking, breathing exercises, the use of bronchodilators for reversible elements, and antibiotics for patients with productive cough (12). The use of deep breathing exercises and incentive spirometry has been found to be equally effective and alone has reduced pulmonary complication rates by 50% (12). Evidence of CO_2 retention ($pCO_2 > 45$ mm Hg) is an indication of severe impairment, and elective interventions should be abandoned. Additional findings indicating high risk are maximum breathing capacity of less than 50% of expected and an FEV_1 below 2 L (11). Should surgery still be necessary in identified high-risk patients, a prolonged period of postoperative ventilatory support can be anticipated. On the other hand, patients identified as low risk by normal history and physical and/or spirometry can anticipate a 3% pulmonary complication rate (12).

All elderly patients should be considered at risk for thromboembolic events, and prophylactic measures such as low-dose heparin or intermittent venous compression should be used.

The impact of other organ system dysfunction on surgical outcome is important but much less so than the cardiopulmonary systems. History taking should identify patients at risk for liver disease or those who may have obstructive uropathy. All patients undergoing surgery should have prothrombin time measured, which is a good indicator of hepatic synthetic function, and a creatinine determination, which, within the limits of normal physiologic decline in glomerular filtration rate (GFR), will identify patients with poor renal function.

The presence of significant protein energy malnutrition, defined as sufficient protein loss to impair physiologic function, needs to be screened for. In one study of elderly patients awaiting major gastrointestinal resection 43% had less than 10% weight loss, 17% had more than 10% loss, and 40% had more than 10% weight loss with associated measurable impairment. The latter group suffered from a significant increase in postoperative complications and length of hospitalization (13). This effect is largely mediated through impairment of respiratory muscle function. Both vital capacity and peak expiratory flow rates are significantly decreased when protein depletion exceeds 20% (14). Comorbid conditions, however, may confuse the interpretation of static lung volumes, in which case hand grip dynamometry is easily obtained and correlates well with protein loss (15).

The value of identifying patients at risk lies in the demonstrable reversibility of this effect within a matter of 3 to 4 days of nutritional repletion, either parenterally (16) or enterally (17). Using plasma transferrin level as a biochemical marker, repletion inducing a 10% increase in value was associated with a fivefold decrease in operative mortality for malignant disease (18). Clinical assessment, incorporating history of recent weight change and dietary intake, the presence of gastrointestinal symptoms, the level of physiologic stress, and overall functional capacity, is at least as effective in predicting hospital infections as anthropometric and biochemical measures (19). While it is difficult to specifically isolate the contribution of malnutrition, in cases of more than 10% weight loss with demonstrable physiologic impairment, a few days of enteral caloric supplementation, if possible, or parenterally, if not, will have a positive effect in reducing morbidity and mortality.

The ability to maintain functional well-being is an additional and fundamental determinant in decision making in the elderly. At the heart of independent function is mental status. Varying degrees of dementia may develop in the elderly as a component of aging, and this represents an important risk for the development of postoperative confusion, which occurs in 7 to 15% of patients (2, 10). It can be distinguished from underlying dementia by its acute onset, waxing and waning character, and the accompaniment of psychomotor changes. The "sun-downing" agitated patient will, in 50% of cases, have an acute underlying physiologic cause readily detected by evaluation of electrolytes, BUN, glucose, blood gases, and volume status (20). Dementia is also associated with analgesic use and decreased mobility postoperatively and with multiple medical problems and polypharmacy preoperatively.

Preoperative screening beyond typical blood work and chest x-ray should include an assessment of mental status. The Folstein Mini-Mental State Examination tests orientation, short-term recall, memory loss, and attention. It requires only about 10 minutes to administer and has been well validated (21). Once a baseline has been established, periodic perioperative review is very helpful in the early detection of postoperative confusion.

The preservation of mental capacity is pivotal in achieving optimal functional outcomes in the elderly. A technically successful surgical intervention that results in the patient moving from an independent living situation to a nursing home is very costly in terms of health care resources and may not have been in the patient's best interests. In fact, health and illness status must be assessed to develop the goals of the intervention. Such assessment can also measure the existence, extent, and impact of preexisting chronic conditions and define the preoperative quality of life. Dozens if not hundreds of functional assessment tools have been developed, although many are unvalidated, and most are adapted for administrative assessments in formulating health care policy rather than for clinical assessment of individual patients (22).

Five basic areas should be evaluated. In addition to physical health and mental function, the performance of activities of daily living (ADLs) and the status of social supports and economic resources assume significant importance in the elderly. In patients disabled with regard to ADLs, recovery also occurs through three stages: the return of independence in feeding and continence, followed by recovery in transfer and toileting, and finally, recovery in bathing and dressing (23). There are no good data available on the impact of surgery on independence in ADLs. The optimal data tool needs to be quick, easily administered in a variety of circumstances, and reliable.

The Katz index, in conjunction with instrumental ADLs and the mini-mental status evaluation, provides a comprehensive description of the patient's sociobiologic function. Postoperative monitoring in these areas provides data on recovery and deterioration, often signals the development of complications, and should trigger a systematic evaluation for an underlying pathologic process. Deficits identified preoperatively may warrant a period of rehabilitative or physical therapy to maximize function. In fact, if such therapies are anticipated postoperatively, their preoperative introduction will allay anxiety and help ensure maximum benefit.

PREOPERATIVE MANAGEMENT

Preparation for a planned operative procedure should begin in the office. Anxiety plays a significant role in perioperative stress and may be associated with significant myocardial ischemia (24). Preoperative familiarity with the procedures and supportive therapies reduces the fear of the unknown and improves performance. Reminiscence interviewing, with its focus on positive past experiences for the patient, is effective in reducing state anxiety scores and enhancing self-efficacy scores (25) and yields benefits beyond the provision of emotional support. Special training is not required, and in fact, peer-administered interviews are most effective. Most hospital settings have retired seniors who could provide volunteer counseling work.

In the current medical-economic climate of the 1990s, convalescence planning needs to begin preoperatively. Medical and personal requirements can be anticipated for which arrangements need to be made. This should be done in conjunction with supporting family members. Hospital social services can provide a comprehensive inventory of available community services and help identify economic and personnel resources. Families need to recognize that there may be a period of several weeks in which functional lapses can be anticipated.

Any aids that the patient uses (e.g. hearing aids, glasses, canes) should be brought to the hospital, as every effort to avoid sensory deprivation should be made. Familiar objects such as pictures or other objects also help reduce stress, anxiety, and depression. The patient should bring some extra, loose clothing and anticipate an active postoperative period.

PRESENTATION

Elective surgical procedures can be performed in the elderly safely and with very acceptable mortality. In patients over 90 years of age, mortality for elective procedures is 2.3% (26). On the other hand, in urgent procedures mortality rises to 16% and further to 45% for emergent procedures. Thus, conditions that can be anticipated to cause an urgent or emergent situation should be addressed in as elective a setting as possible.

Often intervention is delayed because of atypical presentations. Comorbid conditions may mask signs and symptoms, and nonspecific features such as lethargy, confusion, or agitation may predominate. Pain thresholds are higher in the elderly and, when present, are more likely to be associated with surgical pathology than in younger patients. Localization of pain is also less precise. In fact, the elderly patient with significant sepsis is more likely to present with hypothermia and/or evidence of bone marrow suppression. Conversely, fever and elevated white blood cell counts are more likely to be absent in acute abdominal disease such as appendicitis or diverticulitis. Accordingly, a higher index of suspicion for surgical illness should exist when dealing with the elderly. The decline in physiologic reserve makes these patients much less tolerant of a delay in diagnosis.

The goals of surgery should be clearly defined. Up to 50% of procedures are in the context of malignant disease. This fact highlights the issues of surgical objectives and quality of life and, in particular, the role of palliation. The value of prophylactic or screening procedures must also be placed in the context of anticipated life expectancy. Finally, the surgical procedure contemplated should be consistent with the patient's functional status.

PERIOPERATIVE MANAGEMENT

Once the decision to operate, based on a consideration of the relative risks and benefits, has been made, the issues of type of anesthesia and perioperative cardiovascular monitoring need to be considered. It has been argued that all patients over 65 undergoing a major surgical procedure should be managed with right heart catheterization (27). This recommendation is based on the finding that only 13.5% of such patients had normal measured hemodynamic, respiratory, and oxygen transport function. However, the ASA classification of physical status alone was reasonably accurate in predicting functional impairment, although it could not predict the specific physiologic defect. It would seem most cost-effective therefore to combine the risk factors identified with cardiac and pulmonary screening with overall physical status and use right heart catheterization in those

patients with moderate or severe cardiorespiratory impairment.

Time should be anticipated between Swan-Ganz catheter placement and surgery to allow optimization of derived physiologic variables. Such monitoring is also of great value in minimizing the physiologic perturbations that occur around an operation consequent to the stress response, fluid shifts, and changes in vasomotor tone as a result of anesthetic agents. In patients where frequent arterial blood gas determinations are anticipated or noninvasive blood pressure monitoring methods are inadequate, a radial artery cannula should be considered as well.

The choice of anesthetic is a significant variable and should take into account the impact on postoperative mental function and respiratory function. It should further minimize hemodynamic instability, particularly at induction and intubation, and optimize the oxygen supply to demand ratio. Tachycardia and hypotension have been associated with a significant increase in cardiac morbidity and mortality (28). General anesthesia, while allowing the surgeon to perform prolonged procedures with a controlled airway, may be complicated by extreme swings in blood pressure. "Cardiac" anesthesia, using high doses of various opiates, has been shown to decrease the peaks in circulating stress hormones, glucose levels, energy expenditures, and cardiac pulse rates (29). There are also significant changes in pulmonary functional residual capacity, FEV_1, and vital capacity that exacerbate the normal decline in physiologic reserve associated with aging. Manipulation of the airway may precipitate bronchospasm and certainly diminishes the patient's ability to clear airway secretions. Mental functions may also be adversely affected.

Spinal (subarachnoid) or epidural anesthesia provides an alternative modality, which, as the patient is awake with preservation of cough reflexes, eliminates the respiratory problems associated with general anesthesia. Further, depending on the amount of sedatives and narcotics used in conjunction with regional anesthesia, there may be less postoperative confusion (30). It does require some degree of patient cooperation and may have more limited value in prolonged upper abdominal procedures.

Hypotension may occur following the establishment of regional anesthesia, as a result of its sympatholytic effect. This is particularly pronounced in hypovolemic patients. Bradycardia may occur with higher levels because of unopposed vagal tone. The blunted cardioregulatory responses in the elderly exacerbate these effects.

If a catheter is left in the epidural space, postoperative analgesia can be continued. This is particularly useful in preventing the airway collapse that results from upper abdominal splinting secondary to incisional pain. The combination of light general anesthesia with continuous epidural analgesia appears to be an optimal modality for managing the high-risk elderly patient. The cardiovascular effects tend to balance one another, and an epidural analgesic can be continued for 24 to 48 hours postoperatively. The complication rate may be significantly lower with this combination of anesthetic techniques (31).

Whatever anesthetic modality is used, particular attention needs to be paid in the elderly to the issue of hypothermia. Thermoregulatory responses are blunted, and this worsens with age (32). Shivering dramatically increases oxygen demand and metabolic stress. A variety of intraoperative warming devices are available and should be used during the procedure, particularly if it is anticipated to be lengthy with significant visceral exposure.

POSTOPERATIVE MANAGEMENT

The postoperative course in the elderly presents some fairly unique problems. Mental and functional status play significant roles. Cardiorespiratory complications predominate in this age group, and aggressive measures are needed to prevent atelectatic changes and increases in metabolic stress. High-risk patients identified preoperatively may well benefit from 24 to 48 hours of mechanical ventilation before extubation. In "at-risk" patients, preventative measures have been shown to reduce complications by up to 50% (12). Intermittent positive-pressure breathing (IPPB) was introduced in the 1960s, but more recent studies looking at airway closure reversal have shown that voluntary maximum inhalation is as effective (33). This provides the basis for the use of bedside incentive spirometry. The supine position alone contributes to morbidity by exacerbating the ventilation perfusion mismatch resulting from the postoperative loss of diaphragmatic function. Early mobilization, therefore, is also important. The extent of cardiac monitoring is determined by the preoperative assessment. Patients with Swan-Ganz catheters are going to be in an intensive monitoring environment, with continuous ECG monitoring. Most major postoperative fluid shifts occur within 96 hours. Effort needs to be made to reduce perioperative stress by controlling CNS confusional states. Pain control is essential to reduce atelectasis and metabolic stress, but responses to narcotics can be paradoxical, and smaller doses should be used (34). Supplemental oxygen will also improve the myocardial oxygen supply to demand ratio.

The use of intensive care modalities in the elderly has raised some moral and economic issues, particularly in an era of soaring health care costs (35). Several studies have shown that age alone is not an adequate predictor of long-term survival and quality of life (36). In looking at all patients over 65 years of age, acuity of illness on admission and at 48 hours, as defined by the medisgroup algorithm, is 10 times more likely to predict length of stay than age (37). Further, the length of non-traumatic surgical intensive care unit (ICU) stays did not correlate with postdischarge quality of life as measured by the sickness impact profile (22, 38). Even in the aged population (over 75 years of age), there do not appear to be significant differences in quality of life as assessed by ADLs and patient-based assessment following intensive care. Most of the patients studied would undergo intensive care again (36). However, in both groups, 30% of patients moved from living at home to a nursing home environment following their hospitalization. This is not, however, significantly different from the percentage of patients discharged to nursing homes from general acute care beds (39). Thus an ICU-specific negative impact on outcome in the elderly has not as yet been demonstrated.

In general, the postoperative management of the elderly presents the clinician with a different set of priorities than used with younger patients, specifically regarding the maintenance of functional levels. A significant number of patients are discharged from an acute hospital episode with diminished functional capacity as measured by the various tools previously discussed. While in the hospital, every effort should be made to maintain the patient's orientation and daily routine. Any and all sensory aids used by the patient, such as hearing aids, should be at the bedside. Mobilization should be as rapid as possible, and if necessary, aggressive physical rehabilitation can be instituted. The benefit of such a program outweighs the risk of increased injuries that may result.

Patients should be allowed to wear comfortable clothing from home that doesn't interfere with nursing requirements. They should be encouraged to maintain their own basic ADLs commensurate with their preoperative capability. Primary nursing provides important continuity for the patient; the primary nurse should begin teaching early and encourage self-maintenance frequently. The loss of independence is a severe psychological blow to the patient, and lost ground is difficult to regain. Behavioral modification with some form of incentive may restimulate motivation. Medical devices that confine patients to their beds, such as Foley catheters or intravenous tubes should be eliminated as soon as is medically feasible.

Postoperative confusional states are common, and it is unfortunate that sedation and restraints are frequently used. If such behavior is a regression, then it is incumbent on the physician to rule out any underlying infectious or metabolic cause. While restraints have the obvious benefit of an immediate impact on behavior, their use seriously degrades the maintenance of functional capacity. In addition, the use of restraints is associated with higher in-hospital mortality, nosocomial infection rates, and pressure sore rates (40). Communication between members of the health care team is vital. The decision to restrain is made most often by nursing staff for perceived safety or liability issues. In up to 15% of instances, the physician is unaware that restraints are in use (41).

The use of pharmacologic restraints (e.g., neuroleptic, anxiolytic, or sedative/hypnotic agents) may also help control agitated behavior, but the incidence of falls and fractures may increase. Major tranquilizers are preferred because they are less likely to worsen confusion, increase agitation or cognitive dysfunction, or aggravate depression (42).

Environmental modalities may be helpful, such as increased lighting or getting the patient out of the room and near a nurses station. Actually leaving bed rails down will decrease the risk of falls. Diversionary activities such as radio, television, or visits by the occupational therapist are helpful. Psychosocial intervention dealing with anxiety, depression, and stress management will help allay any underlying emotional disturbances (40). Reminiscence interviewing from peer volunteers can help reestablish a patient's sense of dignity and self-worth.

A multidisciplinary team approach to the elderly is essential in optimizing functional outcomes. In addition to physician-nursing-psychiatric liaison, physical therapy, occupational therapy, and social work services can provide invaluable assistance in discharge planning and arranging support systems for the home. This alone may help allay the fear and depression an elderly patient feels in the hospital. Unfortunately, such multidisciplinary teams or units increase hospital costs; however, global costs in elderly care can be substantially reduced.

In a prospective trial involving 120 medical and surgical patients randomized to either routine postoperative care on an acute care ward or to a geriatric evaluation unit (GEU), the number of discharges back to home increased by 20%, and the number to nursing homes decreased by 17.3% using the GEU (39). Subsequent rehospitalizations were reduced, and fewer days were spent in an institutionalized setting. In the first year of follow-up, there was a greater than 50% reduction in mortality and a significant improvement in basic and instrumental ADLs and morale scores in GEU patients. After adjustment for mortality, the global cost of care was reduced by over 20% at 1 year, and using 1982 census statistics, annual nursing home admissions could be reduced by as many as 200,000 (39).

CONCLUSION

In considering surgery, a whole new set of values must emerge that focuses on quality of life and functional outcomes. We must be able to assess the biologic not the chronologic age of patients and their capacity for independent function. We must be able to measure or predict the impact of an intervention on the patient's quality of life and, therefore, its value. Most difficult of all is withholding an intervention. We must avoid treating the family and ourselves and stay focused on the patient. In the current climate of cost containment, we must also critically assess physician practice patterns, not simply in terms of yield but in terms of incremental benefit.

Finally, health care policy must take a more global view of cost. The current directives of managed health care are driving patients from the hospital sooner and are not willing to underwrite the cost of the geriatric evaluation team concept. These efforts at reducing expenses will significantly increase the cost burden to society in increased utilization of outpatient services and nursing home beds. Remember that the price for the loss of independent function as a result of an acute surgical illness may be incalculable to the elderly individual. Every effort should be made in surgical and nursing practice to preserve these values.

REFERENCES

1. Djokovic JL, Hedley-Whyte J. Prediction of outcome of surgery and anesthesia in patients over 80. JAMA 1979;242:2301–2306.
2. Seymour DG, Pringle, R. Postoperative complications in the elderly surgical patient. Gerontology 1983;29:262–270.

3. Goldman L, Caldera DL, Nussbaum SR, et al. Multifactorial index of cardiac risk in noncardiac surgical procedures. N Engl J Med 1977;297:845–850.

4. Gerson MC, Hurst JM, Hertzberg VS, Baughman R, Rouan GW, Ellis K. Prediction of cardiac and pulmonary complications related to elective abdominal and non-cardiac thoracic surgery in geriatric patients. Am J Med 1990;88:101–107.

5. Rao TLK, Jacobs KH, El-Etr AA. Reinfarction following anesthesia in patients with myocardial infarction. Anesthesiology 1983;59:499–505.

6. Bry JDL, Belkin M, O'Donnell TF, et al. An assessment of the positive predictive value on cost effectiveness of dipyridamole myocardial scintigraphy in vascular surgery patients. J Vasc Surg, 1994;19:112–124.

7. Kresowik TF, Bower TR, Garner SA, et al. Dipyridamole thallium imaging in patients being considered for vascular procedures. Arch Surg 1993;128:299–302.

8. Mangano DT, London MJ, Tubau JF, et al. Dipyridamole thallium-201 scintigraphy as a preoperative screening test. A reexamination of its predictive potential. Circulation 1991;84:493–502.

9. Fleg JL, Kennedy HL. Cardiac arrhythmias in a healthy elderly population: detection by 24-hour ambulatory electrocardiography. Chest 1982;81:302–326.

10. Seymour DG, Vaz FG. A prospective study of elderly general surgical patients: post-operative complications. Age Ageing 1989;18:316–326.

11. Tisi GM. Perioperative evaluation of pulmonary function. Validity, indications, and benefits. Am Rev Respir Dis 1979;119:293–310.

12. Stein M, Cassara EL. Preoperative pulmonary evaluation and therapy for surgery patients. JAMA 1970;211:787–790.

13. Windsor JA, Hill GL. Weight loss with physiologic impairment—a basic indicator of surgical risk. Ann Surg 1988;207:290–296.

14. Windsor JA, Hill GL. Risk factors for postoperative pneumonia: the importance of protein depletion. Ann Surg 1988;208:209–214.

15. Windsor JA, Hill GL. Grip strength: a measure of the extent of protein loss in surgical patients. Br J Surg 1988;75:880–882.

16. Christie PM, Hill GL. Effect of intravenous nutrition on nutrition and function in acute attacks of inflammatory bowel disease. Gastroenterology 1990;99:730–736.

17. Stokes MA, Hill GL. Improvement in physiological function with enteral nutrition. Br J Surg 1991;78:758–759.

18. Buzby GP, Foster J, Rosato EF. Transferrin dynamics in total parenteral nutrition. J Parenter Enteral Nutr 1979;3:34–39.

19. Detsky AS, Baker JP, Mendelson RA, Wolman SL, Wesson DE, Jeejeebhoy KN. Evaluating the accuracy of nutritional assessment techniques applied in hospitalized patients: methodology and comparisons. J Parenter Enteral Nutr 1984;8:153–159.

20. Millar HR. Psychiatric morbidity in elderly surgical patients. Br J Psychiatry 1982;138:17–20.

21. Folstein MF, Folstein SE, McHugh PR. "Mini-Mental State": a practical method for grading the cognitive state of patients for the clinician. J Psychiatr Res 1975;12:189–198.

22. Fillenbaum GG. The wellbeing of the elderly. Approaches to multidimensional assessment. WHO Offset Publication 84. Geneva, Switzerland: WHO, 1985.

23. Katz S, Akpom CA. A measure of primary sociobiological functions. Int J Health Serv 1979;6:493–507.

24. Rozanski A, Bairey CN, Krantz DS, et al. Mental stress and the induction of silent myocardial ischemia in patients with coronary artery disease. N Engl J Med 1988;318:1005–1012.

25. Rybarczyk BD, Auerbach SM. Reminiscence interviews as stress management interventions for older patients undergoing surgery. Gerontologist 1990;30:522–528.

26. Adkins RB, Scott HW. Surgical procedures in patients aged 90 years and older. South Med J 1984;77:1357–1364.

27. DelGuercio LRM, Cohn JD. Monitoring operative risk in the elderly. JAMA 1980;243:1350–1355.

28. Mangano DT. Perioperative cardiac morbidity. Anesthesiology 1990;72:153–184.

29. Campbell BC, Parikh RK, Naismith A, Reid JL. Comparison of fentanyl and halothane supplementation to general anesthesia on the stress response to upper abdominal surgery. Br J Anesth 1984;56:257–261.

30. Riis J, Lomholt B, Haxholdt O, et al. Immediate and long-term mental recovery from general versus epidural anesthesia in elderly patients. Acta Anaesthesiol Scand 1983;27:44–49.

31. Yeager MP, Glass DD, Neff RK, Brinck-Johnsen T. Epidural anesthesia and analgesia in high-risk surgical patients. Anesthesiology 1987;66:729–736.

32. Vaughan MS, Vaughn RW, Cork RC. Postoperative hypothermia in adults: relationship of age, anesthesia and shivering to rewarming. Anesth Analg 1981;60:746–751.

33. Bartlett RH, Gazzaniga AG, Geraghty T. Respiratory maneuvers to prevent postoperative pulmonary complications: a critical review. JAMA 1973;224:1017–1021.

34. Thompson TL, Moran MG, Nies AS. Psychotropic drug use in the elderly. N Engl J Med 1983;308:134–138.

35. Levinsky NG. Age as a criterion for rationing health care. N Engl J Med 1990;322:1813–1816.

36. Chelluri L, Pinsky MR, Donahoe MP, Grenvik A. Long-term outcome of critically ill elderly patients requiring intensive care. JAMA 1993;269:3119–3123.

37. Dunlop WE, Rosenblood L, Lawrason L, Birdsall L, Rusnak CH. Effects of age and severity of illness on outcome and length of stay in geriatric surgical patients. Am J Surg 1993;165:577–580.

38. Iafrati M, Cherr G, Carey D, Schwaitzberg SD. Survival and quality of life after long term non-traumatic SICU stays. Crit Care Med 1993;21 (supp): S213.

39. Rubenstein LZ, Josephson KR, Wieland GD, English PA, Sayre JA, Kane RL. Effectiveness of a ger-

iatric evaluation unit. N Engl J Med 1984;311:1664–1670.

40. Cefalu CA. Hospital restraint use in the elderly: a review of the literature and practical guidelines for use. Hosp Physician 1993;June:25–35.

41. MacPherson DS, Lofgren RP, Granieri R. Deciding to restrain medical patients. J Am Geriatr Soc 1990;38:516–520.

42. Savoy J, Lazarus LW, Jarvik LF. Comprehensive review of psychiatry. Washington, DC: American Psychiatric Press, 1991:292–293,315,320,460,553–554.

39/ Pressure Ulcers

Practical Considerations in Their Prevention and Treatment

Elise M. Coletta

A pressure ulcer is defined as a "lesion caused by unrelieved pressure resulting in damage of underlying tissue" (1). Elders are particularly prone to pressure sores because of the predispositions of physiologic aging changes and common diseases. Although many areas of medicine have advanced over the last several decades, the prevention and treatment of pressure ulcers remains a significant area of medical ignorance. At present, there are few good scientific data on the most effective preventive and therapeutic regimens for pressure sores, and many anecdotal treatments are in common practice. A recent, retrospective, 5-year (1983 to 1988) review in a long-term care setting found that 72 different pressure ulcer treatments were used in this one facility, thereby highlighting the lack of a uniform standard of practice (2).

Pressure ulcers are a concern for anyone involved in the treatment of elders because of the consequent patient morbidity and suffering as well as the cost of care (3). Although development of a pressure sore in a high-risk patient is not necessarily associated with poor quality care, this is often assumed to be the case (3). There are over 17,000 lawsuits a year related to pressure ulcers, with settlements as high as 4 million dollars (3).

EPIDEMIOLOGY

Approximately 3 million persons are presently affected by pressure sores in the United States (3). Over 50% of all pressure ulcers occur in patients age 70 years or older (3, 4). More than 60% of all pressure ulcers develop in the acute care setting (3). Actual occurrence rates for pressure sores have been difficult to determine because of methodological problems with the present data (1). In-hospital incidence rates vary from 2.7 to 29.5%, while prevalence rates range from 3 to 30% (5).

The best estimate of hospital prevalence rate is 9.2% (1).

Pressure ulcers are a frequent reason for nursing home placement and remain a common problem in that setting. In long-term care, the 1-year incidence rate is 13%, while the prevalence rate varies from 2 to 25% (6–8). Pressure ulcers are more frequent with increased length of nursing home stay (1). Twenty to 22% of patients will develop pressure ulcers within 2 years of admission to a long-term care facility (5, 7). The focus of care in a nursing home often makes this setting preferable for healing pressure sores, and in general, long-term care facility staff are quite skilled in application of preventive skin care protocols. However, the serious coexisting illnesses of nursing home residents can make the occurrence of skin breakdown almost inevitable at times.

Little is known about occurrence rates in the home care setting and more research is needed in this area. Pressure sores are also common with certain illnesses. There is a 60% prevalence in quadriplegic patients and a 66% incidence in elderly patients with femoral fracture (1).

The development of a pressure ulcer is a bad prognostic sign and is associated with a fourfold increase in in-hospital mortality (7–9). Nonhealing sores are associated with a sixfold increase in mortality (8). Twenty-three to 37% of patients with pressure ulcers die during hospitalization; most of these deaths are the result of severe underlying illnesses (4).

Pressure ulcers are very costly. In 1984, the treatment cost for a stage IV pressure sore was 40 thousand dollars (10, 11). In the United States, annual expenditures for the prevention and treatment of pressure ulcers exceeds 5 billion dollars (3).

PATHOGENESIS

It is thought that pressure ulcers can develop when the skin is subjected to four mechanical forces: pressure, shearing force, friction, and maceration (7, 12, 13). Of these four forces, pressure must be present for skin breakdown (13, 14), although the intensity and duration of pressure that is damaging varies, depending on multiple intrinsic and extrinsic factors (14–16). Skin does not respond well to pressure forces; the only skin area capable of withstanding substantial pressure for long periods of time is the soles of the feet. The epidermis is more resistant to pressure damage than is muscle (7, 14).

Pressure effects on skin and muscle have been well studied in animal models (15, 17). The studies done with pigskin are most relevant, as porcine skin is very similar to the human integument (17). When skin is compressed between a contact surface and a bony prominence, pressure effects become concentrated over the bone. In comparison to the skin surface, pressure effects are more widely dispersed at the level of the bone, thereby producing a cone-shaped area of tissue damage (7, 13). As capillary pressure (32 mm Hg) is exceeded, local tissue ischemia develops. Two hours of pressure greater than 32 mm Hg theoretically should damage skin and muscle; however, clinical evidence is of much greater skin tolerance (14). In porcine studies, no skin breakdown developed with 200 mm Hg of pressure for 15 hours (14); 200 mm Hg pressure for 16 hours or 600 mm Hg pressure for 11 hours was needed for full thickness skin breakdown (4). As a point of reference, a 70-kg person produces approximately 150 mm Hg of pressure over the greater trochanter when lying on their side on a regular mattress (17). Seated pressure over the ischium is 500 mm Hg (17).

The pressure threshold for ulcer development is decreased by the soft tissue changes seen with paraplegia (muscle atrophy), local infection (tissue necrosis), repetitive trauma (muscle scarring), and the presence of any additional adverse mechanical factors (4, 14). Along with the absolute amount of pressure, its duration is of significance (15). Muscle tolerates pressure applied intermittently (relieved every 5 minutes) better than the same amount of pressure applied continuously (15).

The cycle of pressure-induced skin damage is the following: when capillary pressure is exceeded, capillaries and lymphatics occlude, thereby producing ischemia. These blood vessels leak, leading to interstitial edema and hemorrhage. Because of the lack of circulation, metabolic wastes accumulate, causing bacterial deposition and tissue necrosis (8, 12–14).

Shearing force can be defined as "the sliding of adjacent surfaces of laminar elements providing a progressive relative displacement" (13). This mechanical force is especially relevant to the sacral area. The sitting patient on a reclining chair, or a semirecumbent patient in bed can slide forward, during which the sacral skin remains stationary while the deeper tissues shift. These forces undermine dermal tissues and stretch and angulate dermal blood vessels, causing thrombosis and occlusion (13, 17). In older persons, sacral shearing forces can reduce blood flow in the sacral vessels by two-thirds (4).

Whereas shearing force effects occur more at the dermal level, frictional forces are most important in the development of superficial lesions (4). Strong abrasive forces are placed on the epidermis when patients are pulled across bed linens or reposition themselves by using elbows and heels (17). These frictional forces remove the stratum corneum and cause epidermal blistering (4, 13). At pressures below 500 mm Hg, frictional forces increase the incidence of pressure ulcers (17). As a further example of the additive effect of these mechanical forces to pressure damage, friction and repetitive pressure of as little as 45 mm Hg will lead to pressure ulcers (17). Such minimal pressures are easily exceeded in the at-risk elderly patient.

The final factor in skin breakdown is maceration. As with frictional forces, maceration is most important in the development of shallow lesions (4). Maceration leads to epidermal injury (1). In addition, moderate moisture or the other extreme, excessive dryness, both lead to an increase in frictional forces (18). Dry skin is further associated with fissuring of the stratum corneum, which reduces its effectiveness as a barrier to mechanical injury (1).

RISK FACTORS

Pressure ulcers occur because of a combination of extrinsic (adverse mechanical forces) and intrinsic (patient susceptibility) factors (16). Each elderly individual has a different risk for skin breakdown necessitating an individualized approach to prevention.

Over 100 risk factors have been associated with the development of pressure ulcers (19); the most common ones are listed in Table 39.1. Immobility is the most important factor in the development of skin breakdown (4). One study revealed that hospital patients who made 50 or more spontaneous movements a night developed no pressure sores, whereas 90% of patients who moved 20 or less times per night developed skin breakdown (19). The risk of pressure ulcer development may be highest in the newly immobile patient. Ten to 25% of elders who develop pressure sores do so in the first 2 weeks of their hospital stay (4, 11, 20). Age is also a significant risk factor for pressure ulcers because of age-related skin changes. These changes include epidermal thinning; an increase in skin permeability; decreases in dermal vessel number, skin elasticity, wound repair rate, and dermal and subcutaneous tissue mass; and a flattening of rete pegs, which then predisposes to friction and shear force injury (4, 12).

One cross-sectional study found that only three of the factors listed in Table 39.1 are independently associated with the development of pressure ulcers in a bedridden patient. These factors are low serum albumin, fecal incontinence, and fracture (21). In a separate analysis with a cohort design, a history of stroke, bed- or chair-bound status, and impaired nutritional status were independent predictors of new pressure sore development (22).

PRESENTATION AND COURSE

Although the typical pressure sore is difficult to mistake for anything else, the clinician should think of other possible etiologies when presented with an ulcerative lesion. This differential diagnosis includes stasis ulcer, ischemic ulcer, vasculitides, cancer, radiation injury, early ischial-rectal abscess, deep mycotic infection, pyoderma gangrenosum, and other ulcerative, dermatologic conditions (4, 13). Location is also helpful in differential diagnosis; pressure sores are commonly distributed over bony pressure points (13). Eighty percent of all pressure ulcers occur over the sacrum, ischia, greater trochanters, heels, and lateral malleoli (4).

Once a pressure ulcer is diagnosed, staging of the lesion is imperative. Staging is helpful in the selection of appropriate therapy and also allows generalization of research data. A commonly accepted pressure ulcer staging system was developed at a consensus conference of the National Pressure Ulcer Advisory Panel in March 1989. This system, an adaptation of an original model by Shea, is presented in Table 39.2 (23). Stage I ulcers (nonblanching erythema) involve no epidermal breakdown and may be difficult to diagnose in a dark-skinned individual (1). Nonblanching erythema develops as pressure-damaged vessels allow plasma to leak into the surrounding tissues (4).

Reactive, or blanching, erythema is produced by the restoration of blood flow to an area previ-

Table 39.1
Risk Factors for Pressure Ulcers[a]

Advanced age	Fracture
Anemia	Immobility
Corticosteroid therapy	Increased or decreased skin temperature
Decreased level of consciousness	Insensate skin
Dehydration	Low serum albumin
Dementia	Major surgery
Edema	Malnutrition
Extremes of weight (high or low)	Paralysis
Fecal incontinence	Peripheral vascular disease
Foley catheter use	Urinary incontinence

[a]Adapted from Olson B. Effects of massage for prevention of pressure ulcers. Decubitus 1989;2(4):32–37; Inman KJ, Sibbald WJ, Rutledge SS, Clark BJ. Clinical utility and cost-effectiveness of air suspension bed in the prevention of pressure ulcers. JAMA 1993;269(9):1139–1143; Allman RM, LaPrade CA, Noel LB, et al. Pressure sores among hospitalized patients. Ann Intern Med 1986;105:337–342; and Robson MC, Phillips LG, Lawrence WT, et al. The safety and effect of topically applied recombinant basic fibroblast growth factor on the healing of chronic pressure sores. Ann Surg 1992;216(4):401–408.

Table 39.2
Staging System for Pressure Ulcers[a]

Stage	Description
I	Nonblanching erythema of intact skin
II	Partial-thickness skin loss involving the epidermis and/or dermis; these lesions present clinically as an abrasion, blister, or shallow crater
III	Full-thickness skin loss down to, but not through, underlying fascia; these lesions present clinically as a deep crater that may be undermined
IV	Full-thickness skin loss with extensive tissue destruction and necrosis that may include damage to muscle, bone, or supporting structures; these lesions may be undermined and have sinus tracts

[a]Adapted from Panel for the Prediction and Prevention of Pressure Ulcers in Adults. Pressure ulcer in adults: prediction and prevention. Clinical practice guideline, no. 3. AHCPR Publ no 92-0047. Rockville, MD: Agency for Health Care Policy and Research, Public Health Service, U.S. Department of Health and Human Services, May 1992; and Goode PS, Allman RM. The prevention and management of pressure ulcers. Med Clin North Am 1989;73(6):1511–1524.

ously under pressure and is different from, and of less concern than, nonblanching erythema. The presence of blanching erythema should be used to identify skin areas at particular risk for breakdown. Lesions cannot be staged unless eschar and all necrotic debris are removed (7). A dark eschar often signifies a full-thickness skin lesion (4, 7). Deep lesions may look deceptively benign because of undermining that occurs secondary to the previously mentioned cone-shaped pattern of pressure damage (see Pathogenesis section) (13).

The healing process also differs by ulcer stage. The more superficial stage I and II lesions heal by epithelial cell migration from the ulcer edges. With appropriate treatment this healing process should occur in a matter of days to weeks (4, 12). Stage III and IV lesions heal from the buildup of granulation tissue at the wound base. This process typically requires many months to occur (4, 12).

PREVENTION

Prevention of pressure ulcers is possible and is both time- and cost-effective (3, 24). Several studies have shown that instituting preventive measures for high-risk patients in an acute care setting can decrease the rate of pressure sore development by more than 50% (3, 4). Prevention of pressure ulcers begins with a risk factor assessment of the patient. Those individuals at highest risk should receive the most substantial preventive interventions. Indiscriminate use of resources just serves to increase cost. Upon admission to a health care facility or home care agency, a patient should be assessed for skin breakdown potential using a standardized scale (1). Assessment should then recur at a frequency determined by the patient's risk status (1).

Two well-tested, standardized scales have been developed to assist in identification of patients at high risk for skin breakdown. Although these scales are somewhat lacking in specificity (5, 7, 25), their use does promote systematic patient evaluation. The Norton scale assesses five factors: physical condition, mental state, activity, mobility, and incontinence, each graded from 1 to 4, with 4 reflecting the highest functioning (8, 26). Low scores (≤12) are associated with higher risk of pressure ulcer development. The Norton scale has been tested in the acute care setting.

The Braden scale contains six subscales: sensory perception, skin moisture, activity level, mobility, nutritional status, and friction and shear (25, 27). Each subscale is scored 1 to 4, except friction and shear, which is scored 1 to 3. Again, the highest subscale score indicates the most intact state (25, 27). A low score (≤16) predicts pressure sore development, with a reported sensitivity of 100% and specificity ranging from 64 to 90% (7, 25). The Braden scale has good interrater reliability and has been used in the acute hospital and long-term care settings (25).

Preventive interventions should address the four mechanical forces causal in pressure ulcer development (see Pathophysiology section). Treatable risk factors (Table 39.1) should be sought and remedied, as possible. The Agency for Health Care Policy and Research sponsored an interdisciplinary, non-Federal panel of health care providers and a consumer representative to develop recommendations for the prevention of pressure ulcers in the adult patient. Table 39.3 contains a summary of their recommendations that was published as a Clinical Practice Guideline in May 1992 (1). Panel participants reviewed all available research data to produce the guideline. Note that only two of the recommended interventions are based on good research data. Twenty recommendations are based on expert opinion or panel consensus (5). This highlights the lack of valid, scientifically derived data on the subject of pressure ulcer prevention.

At-risk patients should most appropriately be placed on a standardized protocol for skin care. All of the recommended preventive interventions may not be appropriate for each individual patient. Certainly, in some elders, the goal of medical treatment may be comfort and not cure, and in this situation, more limited intervention may be appropriate.

The following discussion explains and augments the guidelines presented in Table 39.3. Initial recommendations improve skin tolerance to pressure and prevent other forms of skin injury. The skin should be kept well hydrated and treated gently in all therapeutic interventions. It should be patted dry after cleansing (13). Skin massage has been recommended for years to promote blood flow; however, recent evidence suggests that massage is damaging, as it causes tearing of dermal tissues (5, 10). Extrinsic factors like catheter tubing, food particles, and wrinkled sheets can be a source of skin irritation and subsequent breakdown (28). A well-padded footboard will prevent sliding and shear force injury, especially if the head of the bed is elevated less than 20° (or more than 70°) (19).

Pressure-relieving overlays for a standard mattress are appropriate, but the use of these and other gadgets will never supplant the need for good basic skin care. All at-risk patients should

Table 39.3
Guidelines for Pressure Ulcer Prevention

1. A structured, comprehensive, educational program should be developed for all health care providers (doctors, nurses, and therapists), patients, and caregivers. The program should be evaluated for effectiveness.[a]
2. While the patient is in bed, use a written, systemic turning schedule to reposition the at-risk patient approximately every 2 hours, if consistent with overall patient treatment goals.[b]
3. Any at-risk patient should be placed on a pressure-relieving surface (foam, static-air or alternating-air mattress, gel or water mattress).[b]
4. Do not massage the skin over bony prominences.[b]
5. Document and perform daily, comprehensive, skin inspection.[c]
6. Keep skin clean using mild soap and water. Minimize the application of pressure and frictional forces during cleansing.[c]
7. Avoid ambient low humidity (less than 40%) and cold. Use moisturizers on dry skin.[c]
8. Minimize skin exposure to moisture. Assess and manage any urinary or fecal incontinence. Use absorbent underpants, when necessary, to help keep skin dry. Topical agents that produce a moisture barrier can be used.[c]
9. Lessen frictional and shearing-force injury through proper positioning, transferring, and turning.[c]
10. Friction may be decreased through the use of lubricants (cornstarch, creams), protective films (transparent film dressings, skin sealants), protective dressings (e.g., hydrocolloids), and protective padding.[c]
11. Use foam/pillows for bed positioning. Keep bony prominences from contact with each other.[c]
12. The bed-bound patient requires positioning to provide complete heel pressure relief.[c]
13. Avoid the use of doughnut cushions.[c]
14. Avoid positioning directly on the greater trochanter.[c]
15. Use lifting devices (sheets, bed trapeze) to alleviate frictional forces.[c]
16. Maintain the head of the bed as flat as possible, consistent with medical restrictions. The head of the bed should be elevated for as little time as possible.[c]
17. A patient in a chair should reposition q. 1 hour and weight shift q. 15 minutes.[c]
18. Positioning of chair-bound patients should include consideration of the following factors: pressure relief, postural alignment, weight distribution, and balance. Use a pressure-relieving seat cushion.[c]
19. Provide appropriate nutritional assessment and support.[c]
20. Maintain/improve mobility as possible.[c]
21. A written skin care plan should be used to document patient risk assessment and preventive interventions. The patient's response to preventive interventions should be monitored and documented. The skin care plan should be adjusted to the patient's response to treatment.[c]

[a]Based on good research-based evidence.
[b]Based on fair research-based evidence.
[c]Based on expert opinion and panel consensus.

be placed on a pressure-relieving mattress surface. There are many different pressure-relieving devices on the market. For prevention of pressure ulcers, there is no evidence that one device is better than another (1). Regular 2-inch "egg crate" foam pads do not substantially decrease local pressure but can increase comfort and may help prevent pressure sores (29). Other differently constructed foam pads are inexpensive and will decrease local pressure below capillary pressure (29). Sheets should be left somewhat loose over foam mattresses so as not to detract from their pressure-distributing characteristics.

Air mattresses are more expensive but also effective (11). Doughnut devices should not be used, as they may decrease circulation to the central area and promote venous congestion and edema (4). Sheepskin is not a pressure-relieving device but is somewhat compressible, so it may distribute pressure more evenly. The main purpose of

sheepskin is to reduce friction between surfaces and absorb moisture (30). The heels are very susceptible to pressure-induced skin damage and must be well protected in the bed-bound individual. There are several prefabricated products that elevate the heel off the bed (31), but an effective and less expensive alternative is placing a thick pillow lengthwise under the calf.

On a more systemic level, the patient's nutritional needs should be quickly assessed, and appropriate nutritional support provided, with special attention to the intake of protein, calories, vitamin C, and zinc (1).

The Clinical Practice Guideline puts a strong emphasis on structured, educational interventions that teach the multidisciplinary health care team, the patient, and any other caretakers about appropriate skin care (1). In addition, formal introduction of facility-wide protocols for skin care is promoted. There is good research evidence that such protocols are effective in decreasing the incidence of pressure ulcers (5, 12).

TREATMENT

Treatment of a pressure ulcer depends on wound characteristics. Suggested therapy by ulcer stage is summarized in Table 39.4. In general, any new therapy should be used for at least 2 to 4 weeks before therapeutic effectiveness is judged (5). The use of any therapeutic agent should be reassessed after the intended goal of treatment is accomplished. For any ulcer, the first part of treatment should be to review all aspects of the preventive skin care protocol (Table 39.3) to determine potential areas for improvement. The characteristics of the pressure ulcer should be documented, including location, dimension, signs of infection, and the presence or absence of undermining, sinus tracts, necrotic tissue, and exudate (32).

PRESSURE-RELIEVING MATTRESSES AND OVERLAYS

If a patient is not on a pressure-relieving mattress, development of a sore should indicate the need for such a surface (12). If an "egg crate", for example, is in use, perhaps a surface with greater pressure-relieving capacity should be substituted. Pressure relief can be provided by a variety of devices at varying cost. Deep-cut foam cube mattress overlays improve healing time of pressure

Table 39.4
Treatment of Pressure Ulcers

Stage	Treatment
I	Review preventive skin care protocol and improve its application, as much as possible
II	Review preventive skin care protocol and improve its application, as possible Hydrocolloid or moisture vapor–permeable dressing
III & IV	Review preventive skin care protocol and improve its application, as possible Consider low-air-loss or air-fluidized bed[a] Surgical debridement, as necessary Antiseptic/antibacterial treatment if wound is locally infected Wet to dry saline dressings if necrotic tissue is present Change to saline or Ringer's lactate moist dressing when wound is clean

[a]See text for explanation.

ulcers (20). Low-air-loss and air-fluidized beds are effective but costly (6, 9) and should be reserved for the patient who has not responded to less aggressive treatment. In one prospective, controlled, randomized trial comparing an air-fluidized bed with an alternating air mattress covered by foam, the air-fluidized bed improved the healing rate of large pressure ulcers, but there was no difference in median length of hospital stay or in-hospital death rates (9).

The air-fluidized bed consists of a woven fabric sheet covering ceramic beads through which warm, pressurized air is circulated. Air-fluidized beds do decrease local pressure below capillary pressure. They also provide a clearly movable contact surface for the skin, which may decrease friction and shearing force (9). However, these beds have drawbacks, including the promotion of insensible fluid loss and ineffective cough. Poor cough can occur because of the absence of firm back support on this type of bed surface (9). Patient repositioning and transfers are also difficult on an air-fluidized bed. The combination of limited positioning options and impaired cough mechanism may increase the risk of aspiration pneumonia (9). These problems do not occur on a low-air-loss bed system, which consists of multiple, inflatable, fabric pillows attached to a modified hospital bed frame (6).

No pressure-relieving mattress surface replaces the need for regular turning and repositioning of the patient. No randomized controlled trials on optimal turning frequency have been conducted in humans; therefore, no hard-and-fast rules can be made regarding turning frequency (12). Although the "turn every 2 hour rule" is generally recommended, this may be insufficient or excessive, based on the particular skin tolerance and risk factor profile of the individual patient (4).

WOUND DRESSINGS

Almost every concoction known has been placed on or into pressure ulcers in an attempt to heal them. Few data are available to support the efficacy of most of these therapies. With a stage II, III, or IV ulcer, some form of wound dressing is appropriate. The clean stage II lesion may be best treated by a moisture-vapor-permeable dressing or hydrocolloid dressing (5, 7, 33, 34). Moisture-vapor-permeable dressings are sterile, transparent, polyurethane sheets that are impermeable to water and bacteria but permeable to moisture vapor and oxygen. This dressing should be changed when it becomes nonadherent, usually in 1 to 3 days.

Dressing adherence may be a problem in lesions with extensive exudate (34). The contact surface of hydrocolloid dressings mixes with wound fluid to form a gel on the ulcer surface. This gel allows migration of epithelial cells onto the ulcer surface (5, 12). Hydrocolloid dressings should also be changed when nonadherent, typically every 3 to 4 days. Neither dressing should be used on an infected pressure ulcer. Both are, overall, less costly than the alternative of wet-to-dry saline dressings because of improved healing time and decreased nursing time for treatment (5, 33, 34).

For a stage II lesion with copious exudate, dextranomer, a system of hydrophilic microspherical polymer beads, may be used to absorb exudate and necrotic material (12, 28). However, this substance may be hard to remove from wounds (12). Stage III and IV pressure ulcers are more of a challenge to heal. After any necessary debridement is accomplished, granulation and reepithelialization occur most quickly in a moist environment (12, 19, 35). Moist saline or Ringer's lactate solution dressings (changed or remoistened with 3 mL of solution every 4 hours) can be used in this setting (12, 19). Unfortunately, this dressing procedure is quite labor intensive.

ANTISEPTIC/ANTIBACTERIAL AGENTS

The reduction of bacterial counts to less than 10^5/g of tissue and the removal of necrotic material, including eschar, are two key points in successful healing of pressure ulcers (4, 36). Numerous antiseptic agents are in common use. However, although bactericidal, several of these products are cytotoxic in certain concentrations and may, therefore, delay wound healing (37). In fibroblast studies, 1% povidone-iodine, 0.25% acetic acid, 3% hydrogen peroxide, and 0.5% sodium hypochlorite (Dakin's solution) were all 100% cytotoxic to fibroblasts, and in animal models, all but hydrogen peroxide delayed wound healing (37). Hydrogen peroxide was found to be minimally bactericidal (36). Dilute povidone-iodine (0.001%) and sodium hypochlorite (0.005%) are bactericidal, but noncytotoxic, concentrations of these solutions. Povidone-iodine can be systemically absorbed and will inactivate chemical debriding agents (12).

Antibacterial agents appear to be noncytotoxic (37) but may select for resistant organisms (38). Pressure ulcers can then serve as a reservoir of antibiotic-resistant bacteria and nosocomial infection (4, 9). There is also the potential for contact dermatitis or a hypersensitivity reaction with topical antibacterial agents. One percent sulfadiazine cream reduces bacterial counts quickly and is 100% effective in lowering counts below 10^5/g of tissue after 3 weeks of use (36). In this same study, cleansing with sterile 0.9% normal saline was 78.6% effective in reducing bacterial colony counts below 10^5/g of tissue within 3 weeks (36). Therefore, the role of topical antibiotics is not entirely clear. Use of these agents should probably be reserved for the locally infected wound. Topical antibiotics should be discontinued when signs of infection (purulence, odor) have abated (28, 36).

DEBRIDEMENT

Surgical debridement is often necessary when necrotic tissue can be seen. The presence of necrotic tissue is associated with high bacterial counts, so successful debridement also promotes wound disinfection. The bacteremia rate during debridement is 50%, necessitating antibiotic prophylaxis for patients at risk for endocarditis (7). Wet-to-dry saline dressings (changed every 8 hours) and whirlpool baths can also be used for debridement, but both are rather nonselective treatments (12, 19, 33). New granulation tissue may be removed along with necrotic debris. Chemical agents for debridement are available, but there are no good studies on the utility of these agents, and their continued use may damage healthy tissue (13).

Surgical closure is rarely considered for older persons but may be appropriate in the medically stable, more vigorous patient, in whom rapid healing would positively affect functional status and quality of life (39). Aggressive local debridement and disinfection must precede definitive surgery (40). Four surgical options are available: simple secondary closure, skin graft, local rotation skin graft, and fascial or muscle flap (40). Muscle flap closure is especially good for large wounds. Because of the retained vascular supply, healing time is often improved with muscle flap procedures (40). Surgery is not a panacea however. Sixty-one percent of those patients who initially healed after surgery subsequently had breakdown of their surgical sites within 9.3 months (41). The breakdown rate after a flap procedure can be as high as 79% (42).

NUTRITION

Adequate nutrition is imperative to healing of all pressure ulcers (19, 33). One randomized, placebo-controlled trial suggested that vitamin C supplementation (500 mg b.i.d.) is helpful (4). There are presently insufficient data on the role, if any, of zinc supplementation in the patient who is not zinc deficient (12). In addition, treatment of anemia and control of hyperglycemia may be helpful (13).

Future pressure ulcer treatments may include some new directions of care. Both platelet-derived growth factor and recombinant basic fibroblast growth factor are under study, with some preliminary evidence of success (41, 42).

COMPLICATIONS

Sixty thousand people per year die of pressure ulcer–related complications (19). Two basic types of complication can occur. The first is caused by direct extension of the ulcer into neighboring tissues and includes erosion into the bowel or bladder and joint disarticulation and infection. The second type of complication is infectious, including cellulitis, generalized sepsis, osteomyelitis, and tetanus.

Cellulitis is suggested by the presence of fever and wound erythema, purulent drainage, and odor (4, 7). Because of surface contamination with many organisms, surface wound cultures correlate poorly with the actual infecting bacteria. Tissue culture is more appropriate for identification of these organisms (8). Stage III and IV ulcers are likely to be infected with polymicrobial flora (Gram-positive, Gram-negative, and anaerobic organisms). A foul-smelling ulcer suggests anaerobic infection (4). In nursing homes, especially, methicillin-resistant *Staphylococcus aureus* may be a problem. Treatment of cellulitis should include local antiseptic/antibacterial agents as well as systemic antibiotics. Pressure ulcers almost by definition have poor circulation, so some antibiotics (e.g., first-generation cephalosporins) may not penetrate well into the tissues (4, 36). Appropriate presumptive antibiotic therapy, pending culture results, would include cefoxitin with an antipseudomonal aminoglycoside or imipenem cilastin.

Sepsis (bacteremia) related to pressure ulcers has a greater than 50% in-hospital mortality rate among patients 60 years of age or older (12). Pressure ulcer–related sepsis occurs at a rate of 1.7 cases per 10,000 hospital discharges (33). Twenty to 38% of patients with pressure sore–related bacteremia have polymicrobial (including anerobic) sepsis (4) necessitating broad antibiotic coverage. Wound debridement is imperative to remove the necrotic tissue that is often the source of the bacteremia (4).

Osteomyelitis is not a particularly common complication of pressure ulcers but can be a difficult problem to diagnose. Osteomyelitis is seen in approximately 33% of stage IV ulcers (39) and 26% of nonhealing sores (3, 4). Usual organisms are Gram-negative rods or anaerobes. These bacteria are frequently multidrug resistant (43). The diagnosis of osteomyelitis should be considered when a pressure ulcer does not heal well or there is surgical breakdown after a repair procedure (43).

No radiologic test is particularly specific for the diagnosis of osteomyelitis. The "gold standard" for diagnosis remains histologic changes seen on bone biopsy (43). Plain radiographs are often abnormal in osteomyelitis, but it can be difficult to differentiate actual osteomyelitis from pressure-induced bone changes (43). X-rays may be helpful in identifying appropriate areas for biopsy (43). Gallium scans are sensitive but not specific for the detection of osteomyelitis. They are typically positive in stage IV lesions (43). Bone scans are sensitive (65 to 100%) but, again, not specific for the diagnosis for osteomyelitis (43). Specificity rates have ranged from 30 to 57% (43). Therefore, a negative bone scan makes the diagnosis of osteomyelitis very unlikely (43). CT scans will detect areas of bone destruction and provide the opportunity for CT-guided bone biopsy. MRI can detect marrow edema, but this procedure has not found a clinical place in the diagnosis of osteomyelitis as yet.

Bone cultures are usually done at the time of biopsy and can be helpful if the wound is prepared appropriately. Preceding debridement and disinfection of the ulcer will decrease the chance of a false-positive culture (43). One study has suggested that at least one positive response from a specific combination of laboratory tests has a sensitivity of 89% and a specificity of 88% for the diagnosis of osteomyelitis (44). The positive results are a white blood cell count of 15,000/mm^3 or above, an abnormal plain radiograph, and an erythrocyte sedimentation rate of 120 mm/hr or above (44).

An uncommon, but important, complication of pressure ulcers is tetanus infection. Deep indolent sores can lead to heterotopic calcifications that may be associated with the development of tetanus (13). Elders as a group have low immunization rates against tetanus (45). In the surveillance year 1989 to 1990, several of the 117 diagnosed cases of tetanus were associated with pressure ulcers (45). It is recommended that elderly patients without evidence of up-to-date tetanus immunization receive appropriate wound prophylaxis and immunization.

Pressure sores are an important and common problem among elders. Although much is yet to be known about the prevention and treatment of these lesions, we do presently have sufficient knowledge to prevent or heal most pressure ulcers.

REFERENCES

1. Panel for the Prediction and Prevention of Pressure Ulcers in Adults. Pressure ulcer in adults: prediction and prevention. Clinical practice guideline, no. 3. AHCPR Publ no 92–0047. Rockville, MD: Agency for Health Care Policy and Research, Public Health Service, U.S. Department of Health and Human Services, May 1992.
2. Frantz RA, Gardner S, Harvey P, Specht J. The cost of treating pressure ulcers in a long-term care facility. Decubitus 1991;4(3):37–38,40,42.
3. Moss RJ, LaPuma J. The ethics of pressure sore prevention and treatment in the elderly: a practical approach. J Am Geriatr Soc 1991;39(9):905–908.
4. Allman RM. Pressure ulcers among the elderly. N Engl J Med 1989;320:850–853.
5. Xakellis GC. Guidelines for the prediction and prevention of pressure ulcers. J Am Board Fam Pract 1993;6(3):269–278.
6. Ferrell BA, Osterweil D, Christenson P. A randomized trial of low-air-loss beds for treatment of pressure ulcers. JAMA 1993;269(4):494–497.
7. Spoelhof GD, Ide K. Pressure ulcers in nursing home patients. Am Fam Physician 1993;47(5):1207–1215.
8. Emanuele JA, Katz T, Levien DH. Pressure sores. How to prevent and treat them. Postgrad Med 1992; 91(7):113–118,120.
9. Allman RM, Walker JM, Hart MK, Laprade CA, Noel LB, Smith CR. Air-fluidized beds or conventional therapy for pressure sores. Ann Intern Med 1987;107:641–648.
10. Olson B. Effects of massage for prevention of pressure ulcers. Decubitus 1989;2(4):32–37.
11. Inman KJ, Sibbald WJ, Rutledge SS, Clark BJ. Clinical utility and cost-effectiveness of air suspension bed in the prevention of pressure ulcers. JAMA 1993;269(9):1139–1143.
12. Goode PS, Allman RM. The prevention and management of pressure ulcers. Med Clin North Am 1989;73(6):1511–1524.
13. Reuler JB, Cooney TG. The pressure sore: pathophysiology and principles of management. Ann Intern Med 1981;94:661–666.
14. Daniel RK, Priest DL, Wheatley DC. Etiologic factors in pressure sores: an experimental model. Arch Phys Med Rehabil 1981;62:492–498.
15. Kosiak M. Etiology of decubitus ulcers. Arch Phys Med Rehabil 1961;42:19–29.
16. Versluysen M. Pressure sores in elderly patients. The epidemiology related to hip operations. J Bone Joint Surg [Br] 1985;67(1):10–13.
17. Dinsdale SM. Decubitus ulcers: role of pressure and friction in causation. Arch Phys Med Rehabil 1974; 55:147–152.
18. Sultzberger MB. Studies on blisters produced by friction: I. Results of linear rubbing and twisting techniques. J Invest Dermatol 1966;47:456–465.
19. Perez ED. Pressure ulcers: updated guidelines for treatment and prevention. Geriatrics 1993; 48(1):39–41,43–44.
20. Andrews J, Balai R. The prevention and treatment of pressure sores by use of pressure distributing mattresses. Decubitus 1988;1(4):14–21.
21. Allman RM, LaPrade CA, Noel LB, et al. Pressure sores among hospitalized patients. Ann Intern Med 1986;105:337–342.
22. Berlowitz DR, Wilking SVB. Risk factors for pressure sores. A comparison of cross-sectional and cohort-derived data. J Am Geriatr Soc 1989;37:1043–1050.
23. Shea JD. Pressure sores. Classification and management. Clin Orthop 1975;112:89–100.
24. Oot-Giromini B, Bidwell FC, Heller NB, Park ML, Prebish EM, Wicks P, Williams PM. Pressure ulcer prevention versus treatment, comparative product cost study. Decubitus 1989;2(3):52–54.
25. Bergstrom N, Braden BJ, Laguzza A, Holman V. The Braden scale for predicting pressure sore risk. Nurs Res 1987;36(4):205–210.
26. Norton D. Calculating the risk: reflections on the Norton scale. Decubitus 1989;2(3):24–31. Published erratum in Decubitus 1989;2(4):10.
27. Braden BJ. Clinical utility of the Braden scale for predicting pressure sore risk. Decubitus 1989; 2(3):44–46,50–51.
28. Guggisberg E, Terumalai K, Karron JM, Rapin CH. New perspectives in the treatment of decubitus ulcers. J Palliat Care 1992;8(2):5–10.
29. Anonymous. Treatment of pressure ulcers. Med Lett Drug Ther 1990;32:17–18.
30. Denne WA. An objective assessment of the sheepskins used for decubitus sore prophylaxis. Rheumatol Rehabil 1979;18:23–29.
31. Pinzur MS, Schumacher D, Reddy N, Osterman H, Havey R, Patwardin A. Preventing heel ulcers: a comparison of prophylactic body-support systems. Arch Phys Med Rehabil 1991;72(7):508–510.
32. Pieper B, Mikols C, Mance B, Adams W. Nurses' documentation about pressure ulcers. Decubitus 1990;3(1):32–34.
33. Gorse GT, Messner RL. Improved pressure sore healing with hydrocolloid dressings. Arch Dermatol 1987;123:766–771.
34. Sebern MD. Pressure ulcer management in home health care: efficacy and cost effectiveness of moisture vapor permeable dressing. Arch Phys Med Rehabil 1986;67:726–729.
35. Xakellis GC, Chrischilles EA. Hydrocolloid versus saline-gauze dressings in treating pressure ulcers: a cost-effectiveness analysis. Arch Phys Med Rehabil 1992;73(5):463–469.
36. Kucan JO, Robson MC, Heggers JP, Ko F. Comparison of silver sulfadiazine, povidone-iodine and physiologic saline in the treatment of chronic pressure ulcers. J Am Geriatr Soc 1981;29:232–235.
37. Lineaweaver W, Howard R, Soucy D, et al. Topical antimicrobial toxicity. Arch Surg 1985;120:267–270.
38. Hirschmann JV. Topical antibiotics in dermatology. Arch Dermatol 1988;124:1691–1700.
39. Siegler EL, Lavizzo-Mourey R. Management of stage III pressure ulcers in moderately demented nursing home residents. J Gen Intern Med 1991; 6:507–513.

40. Anthony JP, Huntsman WT, Mathes SJ. Changing trends in the management of pelvic pressure ulcers: a twelve-year review. Decubitus 1992;5(3):44–47,50–51.

41. Robson MC, Phillips LG, Lawrence WT, et al. The safety and effect of topically applied recombinant basic fibroblast growth factor on the healing of chronic pressure sores. Ann Surg 1992;216(4):401–408.

42. Robson MC, Phillips LG, Thomason A, et al. Recombinant human platelet-derived growth factor-BB for the treatment of chronic pressure ulcers. Ann Plast Surg 1992;29(3):193–201.

43. Sugarman B. Pressure sores and underlying bone infection. Arch Intern Med 1987;147:553–555.

44. Lewis VL, Bailey MH, Pulawski G, Kind G, Bashiom RW, Hendrix RW. The diagnosis of osteomyelitides in patients with pressure sores. Plast Reconstr Surg 1988;81:229–232.

45. Prevots R, Sutter RW, Strebel PM, Cochi SL, Hadler S. Tetanus surveillance—United States, 1989–1990. MMWR 1992;41(#SS-8):1–9.

40/ Ocular Disorders of the Aged Eye

Cynthia Mattox, Helen K. Wu, Joel S. Schuman

Eighty million Americans have a medical or surgical disease of the eye and visual system (1, 2). Over 1 million Americans are legally blind, and Americans over the age of 65 represent 50% of the U.S. blind population (2). Thirteen percent of Americans over the age of 85 are blind (3, 4). Many more Americans, nearly 3 million, are visually impaired. In a population-based study, the rate of visual impairment in subjects 80 years and older was 15 to 30 times greater than that in subjects aged 40 to 50 (3). In addition, many individuals are unaware of their eye disease.

A thorough ophthalmologic evaluation will allow diagnosis and possible treatment of many common and uncommon eye diseases. Individuals 65 and older, in the absence of symptoms or other indications, should have a comprehensive eye examination every 1 to 2 years (5). Ophthalmologists are in the unique position of being able to provide not only primary eye care for the elderly, but also comprehensive medical and surgical eye care, as well as having an understanding of the other medical conditions that afflict the older population.

EYELIDS AND LACRIMAL SYSTEM

The function of the eyelids is to provide protection and lubrication for the surface of the globe. The eyelids are composed of an anterior lamella consisting of the cilia, the dermis, the orbicularis oculi muscle, and the lid retractors (Fig. 40.1, A). The tarsal plate, which is composed of dense connective tissue, and the palpebral conjunctiva constitute the posterior lamella (Fig. 40.1, B).

The meibomian glands, as well as the sebaceous glands of Zeis and the apocrine glands of Moll, contribute to the lipid layer of the tear film. The lacrimal and accessory lacrimal glands supply the aqueous portion of the tears, while the conjunctival goblet cells produce the mucinous layer of the tear film, which adheres to the superficial conjunctival and corneal surfaces. The tears drain through the upper and lower lid puncta, located

nasally, through the canaliculi, and into the nasolacrimal sac. The nasolacrimal duct extends from the sac and opens into the nose inferior and lateral to the inferior turbinate.

STRUCTURAL CHANGES ASSOCIATED WITH AGING

Dermatochalasis is the progressive laxity of the delicate eyelid skin, which may cause visual impairment by obstructing the superior visual field. This may be associated with *blepharoptosis*, the drooping of the upper lid because of levator aponeurotic dehiscence; less commonly, myogenic disorders such as myasthenia gravis may be associated with ptosis.

The lids may develop horizontal laxity, with subsequent *lagophthalmos*, or inability to completely close the lids. *Entropion*, the inward rotation of the eyelid margins, may be due to involutional changes or cicatrizing processes involving the posterior lamella, such as Stevens-Johnson syndrome or ocular cicatricial pemphigoid. *Trichiasis* (malpositioned eyelashes) may be present alone or in conjunction with entropion. *Ectropion*, the outward rotation of the lid margin, may be a consequence of involutional, cicatricial, or inflammatory processes of the anterior lamella, as well as paralytic sequelae of seventh nerve palsies. These eyelid malpositions may produce tearing and ocular discomfort secondary to mechanical irritation or exposure keratopathy. The treatment of these structural changes is generally surgical.

Obstruction of any portion of the lacrimal tract may lead to abnormal tearing. The most common reasons for tearing, however, are aqueous hyposecretion or tear film abnormalities. The proper workup for tearing should thus include examination of the lids and tear film for dry eyes, blepharitis, and possible mechanical irritation from trichiatic lashes or lid malpositions. Stenotic puncta or lacrimal sac obstruction should be evident with inspection and palpation. Involutional stenosis of the nasolacrimal duct is the most common form of

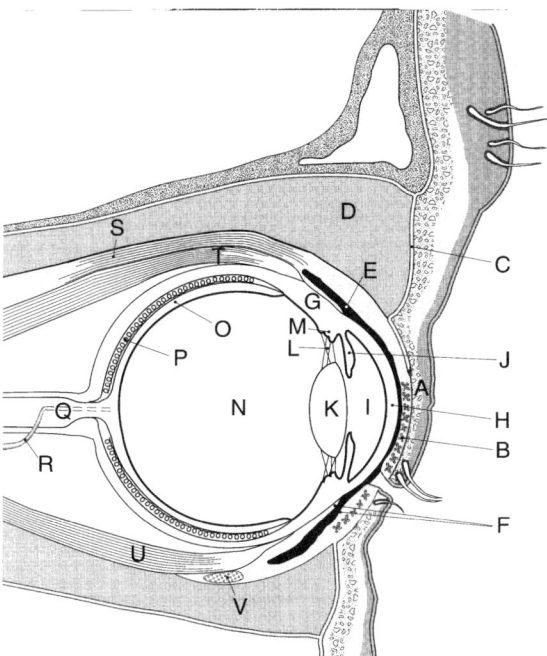

Figure 40.1. Cross section anatomy of the eye, orbit, and eyelids. *A*, Anterior lamellae of the eyelid; *B*, posterior lamellae of the eyelid; *C*, orbital septum; *D*, orbital fat; *E*, tear film; *F*, conjunctiva; *G*, sclera; *H*, cornea; *I*, anterior chamber; *J*, iris; *K*, lens; *L*, zonules; *M*, ciliary body; *N*, vitreous; *O*, retina; *P*, choroid; *Q*, optic nerve; *R*, ophthalmic artery; *S*, levator muscle; *T*, superior rectus muscle; *U*, inferior rectus muscle; *V*, inferior oblique muscle.

nasolacrimal duct obstruction in elderly individuals and is more common in women (6). The treatment for lacrimal tract obstruction depends upon its anatomic location. Stenotic puncta may be enlarged with a simple snip procedure, while lacrimal sac and nasolacrimal duct obstructions usually require silicone intubation and dacryocystorhinostomy, in which a bony ostium is created between the sac and the nasal cavity.

EYELID NEOPLASMS

Basal cell carcinoma is the most common malignancy of the eyelid skin, accounting for over 90% of tumors (7). It is most likely associated with ultraviolet exposure and occurs with increased frequency in southern climates and in individuals with fair skin. It occurs with the greatest frequency on the upper lids and medial canthus and has the worst prognosis in the medial canthal area. Typically, the lesion is painless, grows slowly, and has the appearance of a nodular ulcer with raised rolled edges ("rodent ulcer"). It ranges

from light to dark brown in color. It may also appear as a diffuse, indurated, tan, plaquelike lesion (morpheaform) with ulcerated areas or nodules interspersed throughout. The diagnosis is made with an excisional biopsy.

The treatment of basal cell carcinoma is generally surgical. The technique of Mohs' micrographic surgery, with careful stepwise excision and microscopic monitoring of the surgical margins, has a lower recurrence rate than other methods (8). Chemotherapy may be used in unresectable tumors.

Squamous cell carcinoma of the eyelid is much less common than basal cell carcinoma and accounts for less than 5% of malignant eyelid tumors. It too occurs in areas of actinic exposure, most commonly in the lower lid. Squamous cell tumors grow more rapidly than basal cell carcinomas and are locally destructive, with extension into surrounding structures. They may arise in areas of actinic keratosis and may resemble other benign lid lesions or basal cell carcinomas. Metastasis occurs in only 0.5% of squamous cell carcinomas that arise from sun-damaged skin, although metastasis may occur more frequently in tumors from chronically inflamed areas (9). Clinically the tumor is flat and mildly erythematous, with overlying telangiectasias and scaling. As the tumor grows, it often develops an ulcer with surrounding induration and loss of the eyelashes. Surgical excision with frozen section examination of the margins is the treatment of choice for squamous cell carcinomas of the eyelid.

Sebaceous cell carcinoma, like the superficial variant of basal cell carcinoma, is felt to be multicentric in origin and exhibits pagetoid, or horizontal, spread. It is found most frequently in elderly people and has a variable clinical presentation. It may present as a chronic unilateral blepharitis, and a high degree of clinical suspicion is necessary. It arises from the meibomian glands, glands of Zeis, and the sebaceous glands in the caruncle. It is diagnosed with a full-thickness lid biopsy. The prognosis for sebaceous cell carcinoma is worse than that for basal or squamous cell carcinoma, with a mortality rate of 20% or more because of metastasis (10). The treatment includes surgical excision, including possible orbital exenteration, and radiation therapy.

Nonmalignant tumors of the eyelids include seborrheic and actinic keratosis and keratoacanthoma, among others. Seborrheic keratosis is quite common and appears as an elevated, light brown, greasy plaque on the skin. The tendency to develop these lesions is inherited as a dominant trait. Actinic keratosis, on the other hand, is considered a premalignant lesion and develops in individuals who have had excessive sun exposure. It is associated with surrounding inflammatory changes in the skin and may progress to squamous cell carcinoma (11). Keratoacanthoma develops rapidly over several weeks and may be mistaken for a squamous cell carcinoma. It is a large, round, elevated lesion with a central depressed core of keratin. These lesions are treated with simple excision and should always be examined histopathologically.

Blepharitis is a common condition characterized by inflammation of the anterior eyelid margin or by meibomian gland dysfunction in the posterior lids. It is frequently associated with *dry eye syndrome*, which is defined as aqueous hyposecretion and/or tear film dysfunction leading to ocular surface irritation. Both entities occur more commonly in elderly patients, and dry eye syndrome is more common in women. Patients with blepharitis and dry eyes complain of burning, foreign body sensation, redness, mild itching, and tearing. These symptoms are worse in the evening and exacerbated by prolonged reading or wind if dry eye is present. Patients with keratoconjunctivitis sicca associated with autoimmune processes such as Sjögren's syndrome may experience more severe pain, photophobia, and blurry vision.

Blepharitis may be secondary to staphylococcal infection, but noninfectious blepharitis is equally common. Infectious organisms that inhabit the eyelids may produce infections or inflammation of the lids and cornea or even lead to endophthalmitis after intraocular surgery. It is therefore important to recognize and treat significant blepharitis.

The signs of **anterior staphylococcal blepharitis** include collarettes, or material deposited at the base of the eyelashes, as well as broken or absent cilia (madarosis). A mucopurulent discharge, hordeolum and chronic conjunctivitis, and sometimes corneal changes, are associated clinical signs. The clinical course of blepharitis waxes and wanes. The treatment for staphylococcal blepharitis includes lid hygiene and topical antibiotics. Patients should be instructed to scrub the eyelid margins with dilute baby shampoo or a commercial preparation, using the fingers or a washcloth to loosen the crusts from the lashes, followed by a thorough rinsing with warm water. Warm compresses may be applied to the lids with a clean washcloth. Lid hygiene measures should be performed each morning as part of the patient's daily routine. Antibiotic ointments, such as erythromycin or bacitracin, may be applied to the lids before bedtime for at least 6 weeks. Eyelid cultures are usually unnecessary unless the condition is severe.

Noninfectious types of blepharitis include seborrheic blepharitis or meibomitis. Patients with seborrheic blepharitis may exhibit oily lid margins, crusting of the lashes, conjunctivitis, and an associated seborrheic dermatitis. Meibomitis involves the posterior eyelid surface and is characterized by thickened irregular lid margins with inflammation around the orifices of the glands. The material within the glands, when expressed, may have a thickened consistency. Chalazion formation can also be associated. Many patients with meibomitis have acne rosacea. The treatment for noninfectious blepharitis includes lid hygiene measures, warm compresses, and systemic tetracycline or its derivatives for 6 to 8 weeks, or longer if necessary.

Patients with **dry eye syndrome** may have mild conjunctival injection, a low tear meniscus, and an abnormal tear breakup time, which is the interval between the blink and the separation of the tear film. In patients with keratoconjunctivitis sicca, rose bengal stains the desiccated conjunctival and corneal surfaces and mucus strands in the tear film. The Schirmer test quantifies tear production by measuring the millimeters of wetting of a strip of filter paper inserted into the inferior fornix. Topical anesthesia is used to measure basic tear secretion; less than 10 mm of wetting is considered abnormal. Treatment includes artificial tear preparations, lubricating ointment at bedtime, punctal occlusion, and the use of humidifiers and side shields on glasses. A tarsorrhaphy can minimize exposure in patients with severe disease.

CONJUNCTIVA AND CORNEA

Conjunctivitis is a common condition in all age groups; it may be classified as acute or chronic and may be due to infectious or noninfectious causes. It generally does not cause structural damage to the eye, but certain organisms, such as *Neisseria gonorrhoeae*, may invade the cornea and cause blindness if untreated. The symptoms are usually nonspecific and include irritation, discharge, photophobia, and itching. The conjunctiva is typically diffusely erythematous, and a follicular or papillary response may be discernible in the palpebral conjunctiva by slit lamp examination.

Patients with **bacterial conjunctivitis** have a mucopurulent discharge. Although the disease is generally self-limited, cultures should be obtained if a bacterial infection is suspected. Treatment includes topical broad-spectrum antibiotic agents, such as erythromycin or bacitracin ointments, for 5 to 7 days. The antibiotic regimen may be modified on the basis of results from culture and sensitivity testing. Any patient with gonococcal or meningococcal infection, however, should be hospitalized and treated systemically with intravenous antibiotic therapy, because of the rapid and destructive clinical course of these infections.

Patients with **adenoviral conjunctivitis**, which is the most common of the viral infections, may have associated upper respiratory tract flulike symptoms. The discharge is more watery than that associated with bacterial infections. The disease is self-limited and typically lasts up to a week. The presence of preauricular lymphadenopathy, as well as rapid progression with bilateral spread, is characteristic of epidemic keratoconjunctivitis, caused by adenovirus types 8 and 19. This condition affects the corneal epithelium, with subsequent photophobia and blurry vision. It is highly contagious and may be contracted in health care environments, such as physicians' offices. Viral conjunctivitis does not require therapy except lubricants and topical vasoconstricting agents for symptomatic relief.

Allergic conjunctivitis is characterized by itching, which may be severe, and a stringy white mucous discharge. In addition, these patients frequently experience concurrent seasonal allergic symptoms. Cold compresses and topical nonsteroidal agents or antihistamine preparations help to relieve itching. Environmental control of the offending allergen is the most effective therapy; in addition, systemic antihistamines, topical sodium cromolyn and topical steroid medication may be required. Topical steroids are a last resort and should always be administered by an ophthalmologist, as these agents may induce glaucoma and cataract formation.

The differential diagnosis of conjunctivitis includes primary conjunctival conditions as discussed above; in addition, patients with systemic diseases such as Stevens-Johnson syndrome or ocular cicatricial pemphigoid may exhibit chronic conjunctival inflammation. Other causes of chronic conjunctivitis include occult neoplasm (squamous or sebaceous cell carcinoma), retained foreign body, eyelid abnormalities, chronic dacryocystitis or orbital processes such as arteriovenous shunt or thyroid disease. Topical medications, such as antiglaucoma agents, may also cause chronic irritation. If a neoplastic or cicatricial systemic process is suspected, a conjunctival biopsy should always be performed.

The cornea is the major refracting surface of the eye (Fig. 40.1, *H*). Its transparency allows transmission of light to the retina, and it provides structural integrity to the globe. The cornea consists of five layers: epithelium, Bowman's membrane, stroma, Descemet's membrane, and endothelium. The endothelium functions as a metabolic pump that transports fluid across its surface, thus keeping the cornea dehydrated and clear. The number of endothelial cells and the pumping action of the endothelium decrease with age. Corneal edema may occur secondary to the loss of endothelial cells. The normal decrease in endothelial cells caused by aging is usually insufficient to cause corneal edema, unless there is an underlying dystrophy or trauma from intraocular surgery.

Fuchs' dystrophy, first described in 1910, is characterized by corneal epithelial and stromal edema, associated with endothelial changes called guttata, which are warty excrescences of Descemet's membrane. The endothelial cells are abnormal or absent overlying the guttata and produce a thickened basement membrane. It is more common in women and is bilateral, although it may be asymmetric. Initially, these individuals are asymptomatic. Symptoms of early stromal edema include blurry vision in the morning, which clears throughout the day as the evaporation from the ocular surface leads to stromal dehydration. As the endothelial function decreases over time, the visual acuity decreases, and epithelial edema or bullae may occur, with subsequent pain and tearing. The treatment of Fuchs' endothelial dystrophy consists of topical hyperosmotic agents for morning stromal edema and may progress to therapeutic contact lens use for pain relief from corneal epithelial edema and ruptured bullae. If further corneal decompensation occurs and visual rehabilitation is required, corneal transplantation may be very successful.

Individuals who have had cataract extraction with intraocular lens implantation may develop progressive corneal stromal edema with subsequent epithelial swelling similar to the changes seen in Fuchs' dystrophy. This condition, known as **pseudophakic bullous keratopathy**, may also be seen in aphakic individuals and requires corneal transplantation for improvement of vision. The development of improved cataract surgical techniques and intraocular lens implants has decreased the incidence of pseudophakic bullous keratopathy in recent years (12).

Infectious diseases of the cornea are another cause of decreased vision and pain and should always be suspected in individuals who complain of a sudden onset of red eye, photophobia, and tearing. Contact lens wearers, in particular, are more susceptible to microbial keratitis, including *Pseudomonas* and *Acanthamoeba* infections. Staphylococcal infections may lead to peripheral corneal infiltrates that progress slowly, while Gram-negative bacterial infections progress rapidly and may lead to corneal perforation. *Acanthamoeba* is a ubiquitous protozoan found in soil, swimming pools, hot tubs, and lake water. It is also associated with homemade saline solution. Fungal keratitis is more common in southern climates and in immunocompromised individuals. Herpes simplex and varicella zoster infections may cause corneal anesthesia and scarring. Varicella zoster infections also produce pain and vesicular skin lesions in a dermatomal distribution and may involve all the structures of the eye and surrounding orbit.

The management of most corneal infections includes Gram and Giemsa staining of material obtained by scraping the bed of the ulcer, as well as culture and sensitivity testing. Fortified broad-spectrum antibiotics that are normally used for intravenous therapy may be applied topically up to every 15 minutes initially. Modification of the treatment regimen is based on culture results and clinical response. Corneal biopsy may be necessary to diagnose fungal or *Acanthamoeba* infections. Prolonged topical therapy is usually successful, but surgical treatment may be necessary in severe cases. Herpes simplex keratitis is treated with topical antiviral agents. Oral acyclovir may be helpful in treating and preventing recurrent keratitis. Acute varicella zoster infections are treated for 10 days with 800 mg of acyclovir orally five times daily to minimize ocular complications (13).

Indications for **corneal transplantation** include corneal scarring due to trauma or herpetic infections, severe keratoconus, and corneal dystrophies involving the deeper layers of the stroma. Corneal grafts have a success rate approaching 90%. The success rate decreases markedly, however, if the underlying pathology includes inflammatory or infectious diseases, such as herpes simplex keratitis, which may induce corneal neovascularization (14). Superficial corneal scarring or anterior basement membrane corneal dystrophies may be an indication for superficial keratectomy or partial-thickness lamellar corneal transplantation.

Presbyopia is the most ubiquitous condition affecting the aging population. Presbyopia develops in the aging eye when accommodation for near focusing becomes so weak that visual aids (bifocals) are required. This usually begins in the mid-40s and progresses with aging. Accommodation of the normal eye is produced by the ciliary muscle, which contracts and causes a change in the shape and therefore the power of the crystalline lens (Fig. 40.2, *A*). A more rigid lens from metabolic aging may play a part in the decreased ability to accommodate with aging. However, in recent years, experimental evidence in aged monkeys has suggested that a loss of ciliary muscle contractility and/or innervation may play a large role in the development of presbyopia (15). As yet, there is no chemical or surgical remedy for the loss of accommodation.

The lens is located behind the iris and is supported by zonular fibers that arise from the internal layers of the eye (Fig. 40.1, *K, L*). By adulthood, the lens measures 9 mm in equatorial diameter, and 5 mm in anterior-posterior thickness. The lens consists of several layers and becomes thicker with age.

Cataract is defined as an opacity in the lens. Epidemiologically, cataract is age-related. At the present time, there is no medical therapy to prevent the formation or progression of cataract in an otherwise healthy eye. The production of cataractous changes is a multifaceted progressive process, and the precise sequence of events has yet to be elucidated. Two fundamental processes seem to occur in the lens to produce cataract. The lens cortex may become overhydrated and the lens nucleus proteins become aggregated. The resulting changes cause a deterioration in the highly organized structure of the lens, and opacification results. Oxidative damage and photooxidation over decades of chronic exposure may contribute to the development of cataract (16). The lens has high concentrations of the antioxidants glutathione and ascorbic acid that decrease with age. However, there is a lack of concrete evidence in humans that supplemental antioxidants will slow the progression of cataract formation. Poor nutrition producing deficiencies of trace minerals and certain vitamins has also been found to cause experimental cataract in animals, but the role in human cataractogenesis is uncertain.

Other than aging, there are some specific entities that may cause cataract in the older patient. Blunt trauma, electrical shock, or ionizing radiation may cause cataract to develop acutely or with a delayed onset. Large osmotic shifts in a patient's fluid balance may produce reversible or irreversible cataract changes due to swelling of the lens fibers.

Systemic conditions may predispose to the development of cataract. Diabetes mellitus is associated with the earlier onset and a higher incidence of cataract. Many drugs have been reported to cause cataract. Corticosteroids given long-term often produce posterior subcapsular cataract changes. Chlorpromazine, naphthalene, dinitrophenol, p-dichlorobenzene, and others have been implicated in cataract formation.

Most patients with cataract changes have a combination of opacities in the nuclear and cortical layers. Nuclear sclerosis occurs as the increase in number and density of lens fibers accrues, and produces a gradual decline in visual acuity. Initially the change may manifest as an increase in myopia, in which patients will find that they are able to read without glasses or a change in the eyeglass prescription is necessary. The progressive yellowing of the lens will cause poor hue discrimination. Cortical cataract changes often appear as spoke-shaped opacities and will result in varying amounts of decreased vision. Posterior subcapsular cataract tends to be more prevalent in a somewhat younger population and in patients on chronic corticosteroids. Visual difficulty is found in bright light because of severe glare once the central axis of the pupil is affected.

CATARACT SURGERY

The prevalence of cataract in Americans between age 65 and 74 is about 50% (17, 18). The prevalence increases to 70% in Americans over the age of 75. In 1988, about 1.25 million cataract extractions were performed in the U.S., while the visual disability associated with cataract accounts for over 8 million office visits per year (17, 19).

Nonsurgical management of cataract involves accurate refraction and changes of spectacle correction. Eventually, the vision will not improve significantly with a change in lens prescription. Once the optical modalities no longer meet the patient's needs, the patient may be offered cataract surgery based on the ophthalmologist's full evaluation.

The technological advances in cataract surgery over the past two decades have been enormous. Extracapsular cataract extraction and phacoemulsification are microsurgical techniques that remove the cataract and leave the posterior lens capsule intact so that an intraocular lens implant may be placed. Intraocular lens implants are small disk-shaped pieces of polymethylmethacrylate (or more recently, silicone or hydrogels) that are manufactured with differing powers. The power of the implant is determined by the optical properties of the patient's eye, measured with sophisticated instrumentation. The vast majority of cataract surgery is done on an outpatient basis with local anesthesia and mild intravenous sedation. Adequate wound healing and stabilization

occur by 4 to 8 weeks, and the patient is then prescribed new eyeglasses, if necessary.

Visual acuity after cataract surgery is 20/40 or better in 97% of patients without coexisting ocular pathology. Patients experience significant improvement in their quality of life functions such as nighttime and daytime driving, community and home activities, and mental health and life satisfaction, along with the improvement in their visual function (20). In addition, patients who undergo necessary cataract surgery in both eyes report greater subjective improvement than patients who undergo surgery in one eye alone (21).

Complications following cataract surgery do occur, however. The lifetime incidence of retinal detachment increases after cataract surgery and may be as high as 3% (22). Opacification of the remaining posterior capsule of the lens is fairly common and may necessitate opening with a laser months to years later. Cystoid macular edema following cataract surgery may cause temporary and sometimes permanent visual impairment. Less common but sight-threatening complications include secondary glaucoma, hyphema, intraocular lens dislocation, endophthalmitis, and expulsive glaucoma choroidal hemorrhage.

GLAUCOMA

Glaucoma is the second most common cause of blindness in the United States. Among black Americans, it is the leading cause of blindness. Of the 2 million people who have glaucoma, nearly half are unaware of their disease (23, 24). Up to 15 million people have characteristics that put them at risk for developing glaucoma (25). Glaucoma increases markedly in prevalence with age. One in 10 elderly blacks and one in 50 elderly whites have glaucoma in the U.S. (24).

Glaucoma is not a single disease, but rather a group of diseases that have common findings. Glaucoma refers to a condition that has an intraocular pressure that is too high for the health of the optic nerve, which goes on to develop a characteristic optic atrophy and pattern of visual field loss. The damage, once it occurs, is irreversible. The goal, therefore, is early identification and treatment to prevent further loss of visual function.

Intraocular pressure is the function of three features of the eye: the rate of aqueous fluid production by the ciliary body (Fig. 40.1, *M*), the resistance to aqueous outflow through the trabecular meshwork in the anterior chamber angle (Fig. 40.2A), and the venous pressure of the episcleral veins. In most eyes with elevated intraocular pressure, increased resistance to outflow through

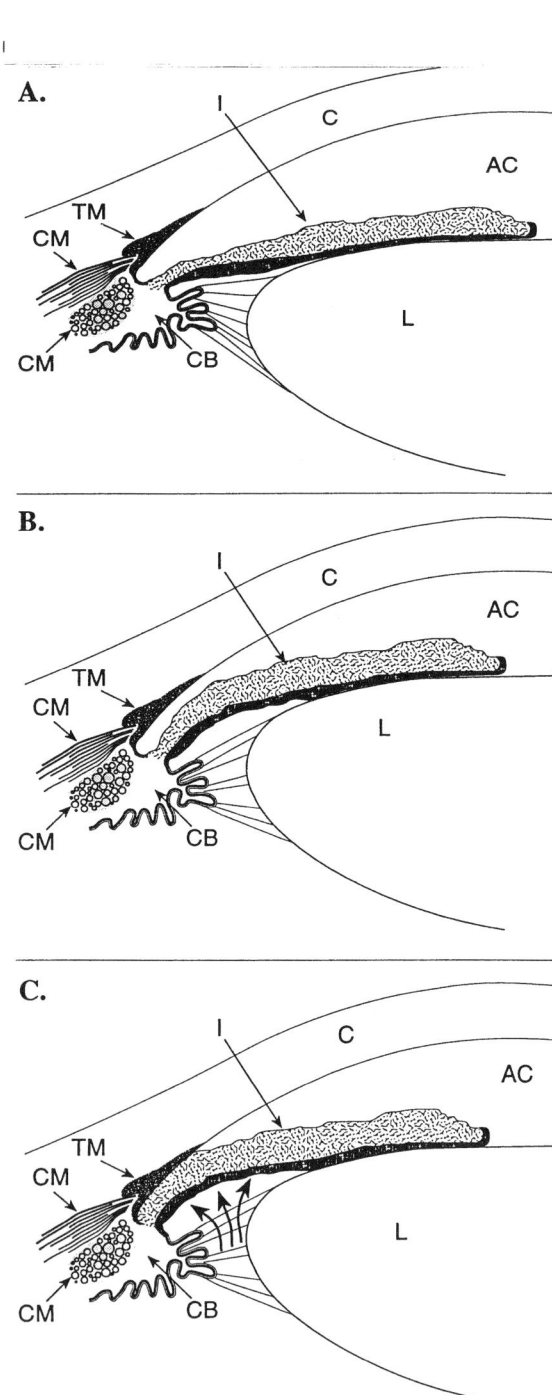

Figure 40.2.   Detail of the anterior chamber angle. **A,** Open angle. **B,** Narrow angle. **C,** Angle closure. (Cornea (*C*), anterior chamber (*AC*), iris (*I*), lens (*L*), ciliary body (*CB*), trabecular meshwork (*TM*), ciliary muscle (*CM*).)

the trabecular meshwork is at fault. The intraocular pressure is not the only cause of the disease, however. Some patients are predisposed to develop glaucoma for reasons that are not fully elucidated. It is likely a multifactorial genetic tendency that makes an individual susceptible to glaucoma. The known risk factors for glaucoma are high intraocular pressure, black race, old age, family history, myopia, high hyperopia, diabetes, and vascular disease.

Routine direct ophthalmoscopy of the optic disk in all adult patients by the primary care physician will identify possible glaucoma. Although the cup-to-disk ratio varies, usually a cup-to-disk ratio of 0.3 in whites and 0.5 in blacks is considered normal. The optic disks should be symmetric. Larger cups, especially vertically oval ones that have a cup-to-disk ratio greater than 0.6, are suspicious (Fig. 40.3). The disk rim should be of uniform thickness throughout its temporal portion, without notches, localized atrophy, or splinterlike hemorrhages. Intraocular pressure measurements should be a part of a routine physical examination of adults over 40. The population "normal" level of intraocular pressure is 21 mm Hg or less. However, glaucoma may develop with levels of intraocular pressure in the "normal" range. Primary care physicians should become facile in the use of a Schiotz tonometer for routine examinations, as well as for eye emergencies that may present to the office. Other hand-held devices are available, but usually at higher cost and with less accuracy. If the primary care physician does not include measurement of intraocular pressure in practice, the patient should be referred to an ophthalmologist.

During routine comprehensive examinations, the ophthalmologist will take a medical and family history and perform an examination that includes several tests to screen for glaucoma. These include Goldmann applanation tonometry, gonioscopy (a mirrored-lens examination of the anterior chamber angle), and dilated fundus examination, with detailed evaluation of the optic disks and nerve fiber layer. Patients who have risk factors for glaucoma may undergo visual field testing by automated or manual methods.

Open-angle glaucomas have no obvious macroscopic mechanical restriction to outflow; angle-closure glaucomas have an impediment to outflow from mechanical blockage by the peripheral iris (Fig. 40.2). Open-angle glaucomas account for most glaucomas in the United States, and primary open-angle glaucoma constitutes 70% of glaucoma in adults.

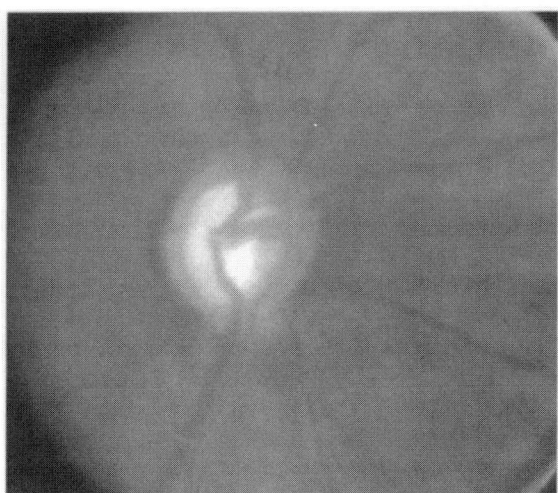

Figure 40.3. Clinical photograph of a glaucomatous optic disk with characteristic enlargement of the optic disk cup. Note the thin optic disk rim, especially inferiorly.

Primary open-angle glaucoma does not cause any symptoms until late in the course of the disease, when near total loss of the visual field becomes obvious to the patient. The elevated intraocular pressure often found is a chronic condition and does not produce any sensation of fullness or pain. The early visual field loss develops slowly and affects the peripheral and paracentral fields without affecting the central visual acuity, so the patient may not detect any visual change until the disease is far advanced. The diagnosis is made by finding characteristic optic disk cupping and typical visual field changes in the presence of an open, normal-appearing angle. The intraocular pressure may or may not be elevated beyond what is considered the population "normal" of 21 mm Hg.

Pigmentary glaucoma, pseudoexfoliation glaucoma, and steroid-induced glaucoma are other types of open-angle glaucoma. Patients who are on systemic or topical steroids for any condition may develop steroid-induced intraocular pressure elevation and glaucoma. Even skin creams containing steroids that are used near the eye may cause steroid-induced glaucoma if used on a continuing basis. The steroids modify the intracellular structure of the trabecular meshwork cells and increase the resistance to outflow. The effect may or may not be reversible.

Although it is uncommon and occurs in only 0.1% of people over the age of 40 in the U.S., **acute angle-closure glaucoma** is a true emergency. A patient who develops acute angle-closure glaucoma is already predisposed by an anatomically narrowed anterior chamber angle depth (Fig. 40.2B). Very often a narrow angle exists in patients who are moderately to highly hyperopic. Acute angle closure occurs more frequently in females than in males, and in whites than in blacks, with an intermediate occurrence in Asians. The peak prevalence is between ages 55 and 70 (26).

The anterior chamber depth decreases normally with age because of the increasing size of the lens. In patients who already have a narrowness to the chamber angle, the iris becomes apposed to the anterior surface of the lens. This impedes the normal flow of aqueous fluid from its production site behind the iris to the drainage site in the trabecular meshwork. The pressure builds up behind the iris, causing the peripheral iris to bow forward, further obstructing aqueous outflow (Fig. 40.2C). The fluid production continues, and an acute rise in pressure ensues. It is this rapid rise in intraocular pressure that is responsible for the severe pain that accompanies this condition.

The unilateral presentation of pain and redness is sudden, can be excruciating, and may be attributed to sinus pain or headache. It is not uncommon for nausea and vomiting to occur. Less than 5% of cases present with bilateral attacks, although the narrow angle is a bilateral condition. The vision becomes blurred as the cornea becomes swollen and edematous. Corneal edema is responsible for patient complaints of halos or rainbows around lights. The anterior chamber may appear shallow, and the pupil is mid-dilated and nonreactive.

The attack often occurs in the evening, during periods of dim illumination, or during physical or emotional stress or excitement when the pupil becomes mid-dilated and has the greatest surface contact with the anterior lens. Rarely, a dense, swollen neglected cataract will precipitate an angle-closure glaucoma. Patients who have narrow angles and have undergone pharmacologic dilation may develop angle-closure glaucoma as the dilation slowly wanes and the iris becomes arrested in mid dilation. Certain common medications may predispose patients with narrow angles to angle closure, including any with anticholinergic side effects such as decongestants, tricyclic antidepressants, and antispasmodics.

The diagnosis is made by the clinical appearance of the eye and a usually severely elevated intraocular pressure. The ophthalmologist will use gonioscopy to confirm the closed angle in the involved eye and the narrow angle in the fellow eye. Treatment should be started immediately. The goals of treatment are to first lower the intraocular pressure as rapidly as possible with medical treatment and then to relieve the angle

Table 40.1
Systemic Side Effects of Glaucoma Medications

Topical β-blockers	Exacerbate COPD or asthma
Timoptic (timolol)	Exacerbate congestive heart failure
Betagan (levobunolol)	Bradycardia
Betoptic-S (betaxolol)	CNS disturbances and depression
OptiPranolol (metipranolol)	Impotence
Ocupress (carteolol)	Worsening of myasthenia gravis
Adrenergic agonists	Hypertension
(epinephrine)	Dysrhythmias
Adrenergic α-2 agonists	None
(apraclonidine)	
Cholinergic agents (miotics)	Acute poisoning by overdosage of anticholinesterases: sweating, GI disturbances, defecation, bradycardia, respiratory paralysis
Anticholinesterases: (echothiophate iodide, demecarium bromide, physostigmine)	
Direct-acting: (pilocarpine, carbachol)	Acute poisoning by overdosage of direct-acting agents: sweating, salivation, nausea, tremor, hypotension
Carbonic anhydrase inhibitors	Lethargy
Diamox (acetazolamide)	Anorexia
Neptazane (methazolamide)	Paresthesias
	Metabolic acidosis
	Hypokalemia
	Renal lithiasis
	Blood dyscrasias: aplastic anemia, agranulocytosis, thrombocytopenia

obstruction definitively with a laser iridectomy. The hole in the iris provides a channel for aqueous to flow to the anterior chamber, and the iris settles back, relieving the outflow obstruction. It provides protection against further attacks of angle-closure glaucoma and should be performed in the fellow eye as well.

Chronic angle-closure glaucoma may develop in patients who have chronic apposition of the iris against the trabecular meshwork, for anatomic reasons, or in patients who are chronically treated with the medications mentioned above. Asians and blacks seem to be at higher risk for this type of glaucoma. Laser iridectomies may be successful in relieving the iris apposition, but damage to the delicate trabecular meshwork cells may have occurred, producing a "mixed" open- and closed-angle form of glaucoma.

The goal of glaucoma treatment is to lower intraocular pressure to a safe level and prevent further damage to the optic nerve and visual field. Medical therapy is usually the initial treatment in the U.S. Topical glaucoma medications all have the potential for systemic side effects, because they are drained through the nasolacrimal duct system and absorbed by the nasal mucosa. Patients, however, often do not attribute systemic symptoms to their eyedrops. Patients presenting to their primary care physician should be questioned about ophthalmic medications.

β-Adrenergic antagonists are usually the first line of therapy (Table 40.1). The β-blockers lower intraocular pressure by reducing aqueous fluid production. They can be given once or twice a day and are usually well tolerated.

An adrenergic agonist, epinephrine, enhances outflow from the eye, but local side effects limit its use. Dipivefrin (Propine) is an agent that is cleaved into epinephrine once inside the eye. It tends to have fewer local side effects, although it is usually not as effective as other agents.

Miotics have been used for decades to treat glaucoma by increasing the outflow of aqueous. They have few systemic side effects but many ocular side effects. They cause miosis and may produce eye and brow ache from ciliary spasm, induce some myopia, and may cause unacceptable dimness in the presence of cataract. Pilocarpine has the mildest of these discomforts but requires administration four times a day in its drop form. A gel and an extended-release device preparation are available, but older patients often experience difficulty with their administration.

An adrenergic α-2 agonist is currently approved for use perioperatively during laser surgery. Apraclonidine has no known systemic side effects and is a potent inhibitor of aqueous fluid production. It has greatly increased the safety of ocular laser procedures by reducing the risk of postoperative pressure elevations. Studies on the efficacy of aproclonidine and similar agents for chronic use are in progress.

Oral carbonic anhydrase inhibitors, acetazolamide (Diamox) and methazolamide (Neptazane), lower intraocular pressure by reducing aqueous fluid production up to 50%. Their systemic side effects often limit their use, especially in older patients. Topical preparations of these drugs are in their final phases of investigation and await FDA approval.

Laser trabeculoplasty is applied with an argon or diode laser by directing small, focused spots of light energy at the trabecular meshwork. The desired results are an improvement in outflow facility and a lowered intraocular pressure. Studies in patients with primary open-angle glaucoma have shown laser trabeculoplasty to be safe and effective, although approximately 50% of patients will show a loss of effect by 5 years (27). Current practice in the U.S. is to offer laser trabeculoplasty before glaucoma filtration surgery.

Glaucoma filtration surgery is usually offered after medical and laser therapies have failed to provide adequate control of the glaucoma. The surgery involves the creation of a fistula from the anterior chamber of the eye to the subconjunctival space. Eyes that have failed multiple surgeries may undergo cyclodestructive procedures or the implantation of an artificial aqueous drainage device.

REFERENCES

1. Sommer A. Disabling visual disorders. In: Last JM, ed. Maxcy-Rosenau public health and preventive medicine. 12th ed. East Norwalk, CT: Appleton-Century-Crofts, 1986.
2. American Academy of Ophthalmology. Eye care for the American people. San Francisco: American Academy of Ophthalmology, 1987.
3. Tielsch JM, Sommer A, Witt K , Katz J. Blindness and visual impairment in the urban population: the Baltimore Eye Survey. Arch Ophthalmol 1990; 108:286–290.
4. Klein R, Klein BEK, Linton KLP, DeMets DL. The Beaver Dam Eye Study: visual acuity. Ophthalmology 1991;98:1310–1315.
5. American Academy of Ophthalmology. Comprehensive adult eye examination. San Francisco: American Academy of Ophthalmology, 1992.
6. McCord CD. The lacrimal drainage system. In: Tasman W, Jaeger EA, eds. Duane's clinical ophthalmology. Philadelphia: JB Lippincott, 1989;4:1–33.
7. Ferry A. The eyelids. In: Sorsby A, ed. Modern ophthalmology. Philadelphia: JB Lippincott, 1972; 4:833–853.
8. Margo CE, Waltz K. Basal cell carcinoma of the eyelid and periocular skin. Surv Ophthalmol 1993; 38:169–192.
9. Dryden RM, Wilkes TD. Periocular squamous cell carcinoma. In: Fraunfelder F, Roy F, eds. Current

10. Jacobiec FA. Sebaceous tumors of the ocular adnexa. In: Albert DA, Jacobiec FA, eds. Principles and practice of ophthalmology. Philadelphia: WB Saunders, 1994;3:1745–1770.
11. Doxana MT, Iliff WJ, Iliff NT, Green WR. Squamous cell carcinoma of the eyelids. Ophthalmology 1987; 94:538–541.
12. Mamalis N, Anderson CW, Kreisler KR, Lundergan MK, Olson RJ. Changing trends in the indications for penetrating keratoplasty. Arch Ophthalmol 1992;110:1409–1411.
13. Hoang-Xuan T, Buchi ER, Herbort CP, et al. Oral acyclovir for herpes zoster ophthalmicus. Ophthalmology 1992;99:1062–1071.
14. Vail A, Gore SM, Bradley BA, Easty DL, Rogers CA. Corneal graft survival and visual outcome. Ophthalmology 1994;101:120–127.
15. Bito LZ, DeRousseau CJ, Kaufman PL, Bito LZ. Age-dependent loss of accommodative amplitude in rhesus monkeys: an animal model for presbyopia. Invest Ophthalmol Vis Sci 1982;23:23–31.
16. Datiles MB, Kinoshita JH. Pathogenesis of cataracts. In: Tasman W, Jaeger EA, eds. Duane's clinical ophthalmology, vol 1. Philadelphia: JB Lippincott, 1991;chap 72B:1–8.
17. National Advisory Eye Council. Vision research; a national plan: 1983–1987. Washington, DC: U.S. Department of Health and Human Services, 1987:87–2755.
18. Leibowitz HM, Krueger DE, Maunder LR, et al. The Framingham Eye Study monograph: an ophthalmological and epidemiological study of cataract, glaucoma. diabetic retinopathy, macular degeneration, and visual acuity in a general population of 2631 adults, 1973–1975. Surv Ophthalmol (suppl) 1980;24:335–610.
19. Office of the Inspector General. Medicare cataract implant surgery. Washington, DC: U.S. Department of Health and Human Services, 1986.
20. Brenner MH, Curbow B, Javitt JC, Legro MW, Sommer A. Vision change and quality of life in the elderly. Arch Ophthalmol 1993;111:680–685.
21. Javitt JC, Brenner H, Curbow B, Legro MW, Street DA. Outcomes of cataract surgery: improvement in visual acuity and subjective visual function after surgery in the first, second, and both eyes. Arch Ophthalmol 1993;111:686–691.
22. Wetzig PC, Thatcher DB, Christiansen JM. The intracapsular versus the extracapsular cataract technique in relationship to retinal problems. Trans Am Ophthalmol Soc 1979;77:339.
23. Bankes JL, Perkins ES, Tsolakis S, Wright JE. The Bedford Glaucoma Survey. Br Med J 1968;1:791–796.
24. American Academy of Ophthalmology. Primary open angle glaucoma. San Francisco: American Academy of Ophthalmology, 1992.
25. Tielsch JM, Sommer A, Katz J, Royall RM, Quigley HA, Javitt J. Racial variations in the prevalence of primary open angle glaucoma: the Baltimore Eye Survey. JAMA 1991;266:369–374.
26. Lowe RF, Ritch R. Angle closure glaucoma. In: Ritch R, Shields MB, Krupin T, eds. The glaucomas. St. Louis: CV Mosby, 1989;825–853.
27. Shingleton BJ, Richter CU, Bellows AR, et al. Long-term efficacy of argon laser trabeculoplasty. Ophthalmology 1987;94:1513–1518.

41/ Retinal Disorders of the Aged Eye

Elias Reichel, Jay S. Duker, Carmen A. Puliafito

As the eye ages, a host of conditions can affect the vitreoretinal interface, the retinal circulation, the retinal pigment epithelial-choroidal complex, and the optic nerve. Most of these conditions may result in moderate to severe visual loss. The rapid identification of retinal emergencies (Table 41.1) and the early recognition of conditions that may be amenable to laser photocoagulation (Table 41.2) can result in the prevention of severe visual loss. All of the conditions described in this chapter are typically evaluated and treated by a retina specialist who performs laser photocoagulation, scleral buckling procedures, and vitrectomies. Many general ophthalmologists evaluate patients with diabetic retinopathy and perform laser photocoagulation when indicated, but typically do not perform vitreoretinal surgery.

Preventing blindness is an important factor in improving the elderly's ability to function autonomously and lead productive lives. The individual, familial, and societal burdens that are the result of retinal blinding disorders are not insignificant and can be profound.

VITREORETINAL DISORDERS

RHEGMATOGENOUS RETINAL DETACHMENT

Retinal detachment secondary to a tear or hole (rhegma) of the retina is typically seen in individuals over the age of 50. The incidence of occurrence is higher in patients who have had antecedent cataract extraction or myopia. Some 25,000 people in the United States will suffer from retinal detachment each year. The mechanism of hole or tear formation is detachment of the posterior vitreous from the surface of the retina, which is a common occurrence in individuals over the age of 55.

Symptoms of posterior vitreous detachment include floaters and flashing lights. Floaters may be found with retinal hole or retinal tear formation or vitreous hemorrhage secondary to avulsion of a retinal blood vessel. Symptoms of retinal de-

tachment include a decline in central vision if the macula is involved; more commonly, a peripheral visual field defect is detected by the patient. Examination of the retina by binocular indirect ophthalmoscopy and including scleral depression is the most important way to identifying retinal tears and detachment. Techniques for repair of retinal detachments include photocoagulation, pneumatic retinopexy, scleral buckling, and pars plana vitrectomy (removal of the vitreous gel). Rapid referral to an ophthalmologist is indicated if retinal detachment is suspected, so that intervention may improve the chances for saving central and peripheral vision.

MACULAR HOLE

Idiopathic macular holes result in loss of central vision to the 20/60 to 20/400 range. A partial or complete hole in the neurosensory retina located in the fovea is observed clinically. This condition typically occurs in the sixth to eighth decades of life. The prevalence of this condition is 1 in 3000. Formation of macular holes may be due to vitreoretinal traction caused by the separation of the posterior vitreous. The chances for bilaterality of this condition are 5 to 10%. Vitrectomy surgery may play a role in improving central visual acuity in patients affected with this disorder (1).

IDIOPATHIC EPIRETINAL MEMBRANE

Epiretinal membranes ("cellophane maculopathy") are typically seen in patients over the age of 50. Bilaterality occurs 20% of the time. Posterior vitreous detachment is thought to result in small dehiscences of the internal limiting membrane of the retina, causing glial cells to proliferate on the surface of the retina. Retinal distortion may result from contraction of the epiretinal membrane. Cystoid macular edema may also occur, secondary to loss of normal retinal capillary integrity. In general, when visual acuity

Table 41.1
Retinal Emergencies

Bacterial endophthalmitis
Central retinal artery occlusion
Choroidal neovascularization
Retinal detachment
Giant cell arteritis

Table 41.2
Retinal Disorders Amenable to Laser Treatment

Choroidal neovascularization
Macular edema secondary to branch retinal vein
   occlusion or diabetes
Proliferative diabetic retinopathy or severe
   nonproliferative diabetic retinopathy
Retinal neovascularization associated with branch or
   central retinal vein occlusion
Retinal tears or holes

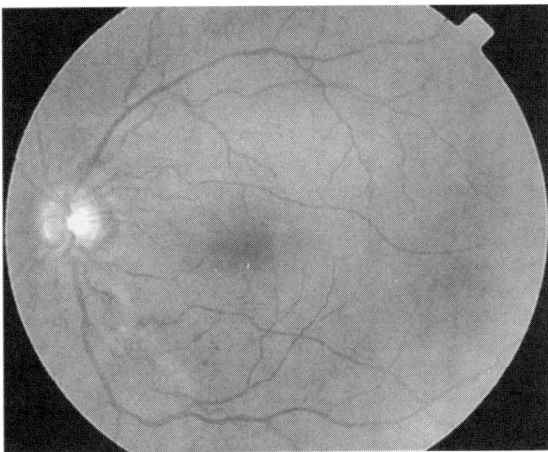

Figure 41.1 Dot hemorrhages, microaneurysms, and exudate in a patient with background diabetic retinopathy.

drops to the 20/100 level or less, surgical removal of the epiretinal membrane can be performed by pars plana vitrectomy in an attempt to improve vision (2).

RETINAL VASCULAR DISORDERS

DIABETIC RETINOPATHY

Individuals who have been diagnosed with type II diabetes mellitus have a significant risk of diabetic retinopathy or diabetic maculopathy after a 15-year duration of diabetes. Type II diabetes is typically diagnosed in middle age; therefore, retinopathy is usually a problem in individuals over the age of 50. Individuals diagnosed with diabetes should be examined on a yearly basis for evidence of retinopathy by an ophthalmologist or expert in retinal diseases. Background changes represent the earliest signs of diabetic retinopathy and include microaneurysms, "dot and blot" hemorrhages, cotton-wool spots, and venous beading (Fig. 41.1). Proliferative diabetic retinopathy is evidenced by the formation of new retinal blood vessels on the surface of the retina and into the vitreous cavity. These abnormal blood vessels can hemorrhage within the vitreous cavity and create traction on the retina, resulting in retinal detachment.

Diabetes can affect central visual acuity as well. Abnormal retinal capillaries can form microaneurysms. These microaneurysms leak serous or lipid exudate into the retina, and this can result in macular edema. Diabetic macular edema is the most common cause of loss of vision in type II di-

abetics. Fluorescein angiography aids in the diagnosis and in the treatment strategy for individuals who have macular edema.

The prompt identification of proliferative diabetic retinopathy or maculopathy is critical to the visual well-being of the diabetic patient because both of these problems have proven to be treatable by laser photocoagulation (3, 4). The goal of laser photocoagulation in proliferative diabetic retinopathy is to halt the progression of new blood vessels that can result in vitreous hemorrhage and provide a scaffold for retinal detachment. Pars plana vitrectomy is an important technique for clearing the vitreous cavity of blood and removing the fibrovascular scaffold that allows the development of tractional retinal detachment (5).

BRANCH RETINAL VEIN OCCLUSION

Branch retinal vein occlusion (BRVO) typically occurs in individuals over the age of 60. Symptoms include loss of central vision and visual field defects. Associated systemic conditions include hypertension (approximately 75% of the time), diabetes (10%), and arteriosclerosis. Acute changes on fundus examination show superficial hemorrhages, retinal edema, and cotton-wool spots in a sector of the retina. An obstructed vein can be seen which is dilated and tortuous. Fluorescein angiography typically shows slow filling of the obstructed vein. Invariably the site of occlusion is an arteriovenous crossing site. Loss of vision is typically due to macular edema. Retinal neovascularization also occurs, with the possibility of subsequent vitreous hemorrhage. Laser photocoagulation is of proven benefit for the two major complications, macular edema and retinal neo-vascularization (6, 7).

CENTRAL RETINAL VEIN OCCLUSION

Some 90% of patients with occlusion of the central retinal vein are older than 50 years of age. Systemic associations include cardiovascular disease (75%), systemic hypertension (60%), and diabetes (35%). Blood dyscrasias, dysproteinemias, and vasculitides all may result in central retinal vein occlusion (CRVO). CRVO is characterized on fundus examination as displaying tortuous retinal veins, retinal edema, intraretinal hemorrhage, and cotton-wool spots throughout the entire retina. It is important to remember that the retinopathy of carotid occlusive disease has some characteristics similar to those of CRVO.

CRVO may present in two forms: nonischemic or ischemic. Capillary perfusion in the nonischemic group is normal or near-normal as determined by fluorescein angiography. Subsequent retinal or anterior segment neovascularization is unusual in this group of patients. Ischemic CRVO is characterized by widespread capillary nonperfusion on fluorescein angiography. The visual prognosis is poor in this group of patients, and only 10% of eyes with ischemia end up with better than 20/400 visual acuity. Anterior segment neovascularization is a frequent complication, and retinal neovascularization may be seen as well. Management of patients with this disorder includes diagnosing and treating any underlying medical condition that may predispose to CRVO. Laser photocoagulation plays a role in the treatment of retinal and anterior segment neovascularization.

BRANCH RETINAL ARTERY OCCLUSION

Acute branch retinal artery occlusion (BRAO) results in an edematous white retina caused by infarction of the inner retina at a branch retinal arteriole secondary to an embolus. Patients typically present with visual field defects and/or loss of central vision. Cholesterol emboli arise from the carotid arteries, platelet-fibrin emboli are associated with large vessel arteriosclerosis, and calcific emboli originate from cardiac valves. Evaluation and management of patients is geared toward determining the specific systemic etiology of the emboli. Therefore, carotid noninvasive testing and cardiac echography are important tests in determining the etiology of this condition. There is no specific treatment for BRAO.

CENTRAL RETINAL ARTERY OCCLUSION

Central retinal artery occlusion (CRAO) is characterized by a sudden, severe, painless loss of vision. Acuity is typically worse than 20/400. CRAO is generally caused by emboli or intraluminal thrombosis of the central retinal artery. A cherry spot can be seen with mild to severe degrees of retinal whitening. Systemic etiologies of CRAO are similar to those of BRAO. Giant cell arteritis is another possible cause of central retinal artery occlusion and a very rare cause of branch retinal artery occlusion. Therefore a sedimentation rate should be obtained in patients with CRAO and BRAO. Signs of embolic disease affecting other organ systems (e.g., stroke) should be sought if retinal emboli are suspected as causing the retinal infarct. Carotid noninvasive studies and color Doppler imaging are useful in assessing flow through the carotid, ophthalmic, and retinal circulations.

CRAO is recognized as an ophthalmic emergency, and therapy should be instituted promptly, including measures to reduce intraocular pressure and to dilate the arterial bed by inhalation of 95% oxygen/5% carbon dioxide. There may also be a role for thrombolytic agents. Even with immediate treatment, the prognosis for good visual acuity is poor. Long-term complications of central retinal artery occlusion include anterior and posterior segment neovascularization (8).

CHOROIDAL DISORDERS

AGE-RELATED MACULAR DEGENERATION

Age-related macular degeneration is the leading cause of blindness in the United States. Affected individuals are typically over the age of 60; the prevalence of this disorder rises with increasing age. Approximately 2% of patients over the age of 65 have severe loss of vision (<20/200) due to this disorder. The hallmark of this condition is the sudden loss of central vision, which is typically associated with the "wet" or exudative form of this disease. Choroidal neovascularization results in hemorrhage, lipid exudate, or serous exudate that is typically observed in the macula (Fig. 41.2). Prompt referral to an ophthalmologist for fluorescein angiography is necessary to define the location and extent of the abnormal choroidal blood vessels that result in visual loss. Indocyanine green angiography is a new technique that may also help to determine the extent and location of the abnormal blood vessels underneath the retina (9). Early signs of age-related macular degeneration include drusen. Only a minority of pa-

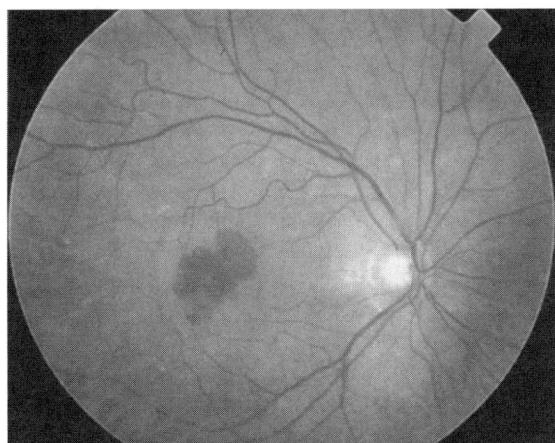

Figure 41.2 Retinal hemorrhage associated with age-related macular degeneration.

tients who have drusen will experience loss of vision secondary to the exudative changes of age-related macular degeneration.

Laser photocoagulation is the only treatment proven to be of benefit for the choroidal neovascular sequelae of this disorder (10). Low-vision aids, particularly magnifiers, telescopes, and computers have proven useful for individuals with loss of central vision.

VITREORETINAL COMPLICATIONS OF CATARACT SURGERY

Cataract surgery is typically performed in elderly individuals. Two important vision-threatening complications include acute bacterial endophthalmitis and cystoid macular edema. Identification of these problems and referral to an ophthalmologist is extremely important to preserve vision threatened by these complications.

BACTERIAL ENDOPHTHALMITIS

Bacterial endophthalmitis is a true emergency and one of the most feared complications of intraocular surgery (11). The most common setting is after cataract surgery, and typically it occurs within 2 weeks after surgery. Approximately 1 in 1000 surgeries will be complicated by acute bacterial endophthalmitis (12). The most common causative organism is *Staphylococcus epidermidis*. Less commonly, *Staphylococcus aureus*, streptococcal species, and Gram-negative bacteria may be identified. In most cases, the bacteria come from the patients' own conjunctival flora.

Patients typically present with eye pain and loss of vision. Anterior chamber inflammation

may be associated with a hypopyon (layered leukocytes). The vitreous is cloudy, and there is a poor view of the retina. Immediate referral to an ophthalmologist is necessary if this condition is suspected. Pars plana vitrectomy with installation of intravitreal antibiotics and steroids has been successful in treating this condition.

CYSTOID MACULAR EDEMA

Cystoid macular edema (CME) is characterized by intraretinal edema. A decline in central vision is the hallmark of this condition. The most common setting for CME is following cataract surgery (13). The incidence of visually symptomatic CME is approximately 5%. Cystoid spaces within the retina can be seen within the perifoveal area of the macula. Typically CME occurs 6 to 10 weeks after cataract surgery, and this condition may spontaneously improve approximately 75% of the time. Fluorescein angiography is used to diagnose this condition. Steroid drops, nonsteroidal anti-inflammatory drops, and periocular steroids may be useful in cases that do not spontaneously improve.

OPTIC NERVE DISORDERS

GIANT CELL ARTERITIS

Giant cell arteritis has a multitude of systemic complications. The primary vision-threatening disorder is one that affects the optic nerve and causes an anterior (arteritic) optic neuropathy. Visual loss is rapid. There may be concomitant systemic complaints that include headache, weight loss, malaise, jaw claudication, and proximal muscle weakness. Preauricular tenderness or an enlarged temporal artery may be signs of temporal arteritis. A "stat" erythrocyte sedimentation rate (ESR) should be performed on any patient suspected to have this condition. The general rule is that any patient who is suspected to have giant cell arteritis who is over the age of 50 with an ESR greater than 50 should have immediate biopsy of a temporal artery (14). Biopsy should also be performed if the diagnosis of giant cell arteritis is entertained, even if the sedimentation rate is normal, as 10% of patients with this condition will have a normal ESR.

If the diagnosis is suspected, high-dose steroids should be administered immediately. The role of steroids is to protect the individual from the sequelae of other organ disease (e.g., prevent loss of vision in the unaffected eye). Temporal artery biopsy should be performed within 3 days of initiating steroid treatment, because steroid treatment will reverse the pathological signs of this condition when administered for longer periods of time. High-dose intravenous steroids are preferred over steroids administered by mouth.

ANTERIOR (NONARTERITIC) ISCHEMIC OPTIC NEUROPATHY

Infarction of the optic nerve usually occurs in patients over the age of 50. This condition is associated with hypertension and diabetes mellitus. There is an acute loss of vision unassociated with pain. Vision may vary from being normal to having no light perception. Altitudinal or arcuate visual field defects are seen. On ophthalmoscopy, the optic disk is partially swollen, and there may be hemorrhages within the nerve fiber layer. Vision is rarely recovered. No proven treatments exist for this condition. The role of optic nerve sheath fenestration is controversial in the treatment of this disorder.

REFERENCES

1. Kelly NE, Wendel RT. Vitreous surgery for idiopathic macular holes: results of a pilot study. Arch Ophthalmol 1991;109:654–659.
2. Michels RG. Vitrectomy for macular pucker. Ophthalmology 1984;91:1384–1388.
3. The Diabetic Retinopathy Study Research Group. Photocoagulation treatment of proliferative diabetic retinopathy: the second report of Diabetic Retinopathy Study findings. Ophthalmology 1978;85:82–106.
4. The Early Treatment of Diabetic Retinopathy Study Research Group. Photocoagulation for diabetic macular edema. Arch Ophthalmol 1985;103:1796–1805.
5. The Diabetic Retinopathy Vitrectomy Study Research Group. Early vitrectomy for severe vitreous hemorrhage in diabetic retinopathy. Arch Ophthalmol 1985;103:1644–1651.
6. The Branch Vein Occlusion Study Group. Argon laser photocoagulation for macular edema in branch vein occlusion. Am J Ophthalmol 1984;98:271–282.
7. The Branch Vein Occlusion Study Group. Argon laser scatter photocoagulation for prevention of neovascularization and vitreous hemorrhage in branch vein occlusion. Arch Ophthalmol 1986;104:34–41.
8. Duker JS, Sivalingam A, Brown GC, Reber R. A prospective study of acute central retinal artery obstruction. Arch Ophthalmol 1991;109:339–343.
9. Reichel E, Puliafito CA. ICG-enhanced diagnosis and treatment of choroidal neovascularization in age-related macular degeneration. In: Lewis H, Ryan SJ, eds. Medical and surgical retina. Philadelphia: Mosby Year Book, 1993.
10. Macular Photocoagulation Study Group. Argon laser photocoagulation for senile macular degeneration: results of a randomized clinical trial. Arch Ophthalmol 1982;100:912–918.
11. Puliafito CA, Baker AS, Haaf J, Foster CS. Infectious endophthalmitis: a review of 36 cases. Ophthalmology 1982;89:921–929.
12. Javitt JC, Vitale S, Canner JK, et al. National outcomes of cataract extraction. Endophthalmitis following outpatient surgery. Arch Ophthalmol 1991;109:1085–1089.
13. Gass JDM, Norton EWD. Cystoid macular edema and papilledema following cataract extraction: a fluorescein, funduscopic and angiographic study. Arch Ophthalmol 1966;76:646–653.
14. Hedges TR, Gieger GL, Albert DM. The clinical value of negative temporal artery biopsy specimens. Arch Ophthalmol 1983;101:1251–1254.

42/ Geriatric Ear, Nose, and Throat Problems

Milton G. Yoder

Ear, nose, and throat problems, ranging from impacted cerumen and postnasal drip to malignancies and epistaxis, are often neglected by older people. They deny their existence, and sometimes these symptoms are dismissed by older people because they assume that discomfort, loss of function, and changes in structure are obvious consequences of aging. Sometimes these problems are totally ignored for reasons associated with the stigma surrounding old age: fears of complaining too much, of beginning to fail, or of becoming senile. The same ear, nose, and throat problems that can affect the young patient also can affect the elderly patient. However, the emotional, mental, and physical needs of an elderly patient may be quite different from those of a younger person. Accordingly, the prescribed course of treatment should be developed with an understanding of the special needs for this age group (1, 2).

The sequelae of otorhinolaryngologic diseases are especially serious because they disrupt an important human function—verbal communication. The inability to hear others and/or to speak to others may be the most devastating handicap of old age. This handicap isolates a person who otherwise would have the physical and mental capacity to lead a happy and useful life. Communicatively handicapped persons will withdraw from both the environment and social stimulation, increasing their debilitation, depression, and lack of motivation for living (3).

To assist the otolaryngologist in the diagnosis and treatment of communicative disorders, an audiologist and/or speech therapist or speech pathologist may be needed. The audiologist is a nonmedical professionally trained person who specializes in the measurement of hearing loss, in the nonmedical rehabilitation aspects of the hearing impaired, and in the diagnosis of vestibular or balance disorders. The audiologist has either a Master's or a Ph.D. degree and must meet certi-

fication or licensure requirement. The speech therapist or pathologist meets the same academic and certification/licensure requirement as the audiologist and is concerned with the diagnosis and treatment of speech and language disorders.

EAR

Hearing impairment is classified as conductive, sensorineural, or mixed. Conductive hearing loss may be caused by anything that precludes the normal transmission of sound through the external auditory canal, tympanic membrane, or middle ear ossicles. Various conditions frequently result in conductive hearing loss including impacted cerumen, tympanic membrane perforation, otitis media, and discontinuity or fixation of the middle ear ossicles. Sensorineural hearing loss occurs when the inner ear, auditory nerve (cranial nerve eight), brainstem, or cortical auditory pathways are not functioning properly. Mixed hearing loss is a combination of a conductive hearing loss superimposed on a sensorineural hearing loss (4).

EXTERNAL AUDITORY CANAL

The aging process affects all portions of the otologic mechanism (external auditory canal, middle ear ossicles, cochlear apparatus, and vestibular system). The external auditory canal is affected by virtue of a decrease in both the number and the activity of ceruminal glands. These glands are located only in the outer one-half of the external auditory canal. Cerumen is never present in the inner half or osseous portion of the external auditory canal unless it is pushed there or accumulates as a result of pressure from the use of headphones or telephones. The cerumen can be intimately adherent to the skin of the external canal in elderly patients. The hearing loss from impacted cerumen is insidious and can result in difficulty with communication. Careful, slow,

441

time-consuming efforts are necessary to separate the cerumen from the intact skin without causing otalgia (pain) or bloody otorrhea. These efforts include curettage, suctioning, and irrigation with room temperature water. Irrigation should not be performed if the tympanic membrane has not been examined before or if there is a history of perforation of the tympanic membrane (5).

The skin of the external auditory canal may become atrophic and dry as a result of atrophy of the epithelium and the sebaceous glands. In elderly individuals, itching of the skin can be attributed to the dryness, but pruritus sometimes is a major complaint even when no apparent clinically significant abnormality is discovered by the examining physician. This itching is a frequent but unwelcome symptom associated with senile skin. This problem can be exacerbated by vigorous efforts to remove accumulated dry cerumen with cotton-tipped applicators and other foreign instruments. This self-induced trauma further increases the problem. Bathing with hot water, especially in the winter when the air is dry, removes moisture from the skin. Drying the external canal with rubbing alcohol or alcohol-acetic acid mixture may help prevent otitis externa; however, it removes fat and increases the dryness, leading to further irritation and itching of the external auditory canal. Efforts must be directed toward breaking the cycle by avoiding moisture, trauma, and defatting agents in the external auditory canal. Emollients, such as glycerin, act as an epidermal seal to slow the loss of moisture from the skin.

There is not an increased incidence of infections in the external auditory canal. However, there does seem to be an increased amount of otalgia and tenderness in the ear canal when there is a disease process. One aggressive external ear disease is malignant otitis externa, which is a *Pseudomonas* osteitis and osteomyelitis of the temporal bone. This life-threatening disease process is usually seen in elderly diabetic patients.

Mild dermatoses, furunculosis, and occasional infected sebaceous cysts sometimes involve the outer one-half of the external auditory canal. These infections should be treated early with topical medication in a cream vehicle. These may contain an antibiotic or steroid compound, depending upon the disease process. Adjunctive oral antibiotics may be needed (6).

Benign bony growths that narrow the external auditory canal can also predispose patients to impacted cerumen. These bony growths consist of either benign osteophytes, which may narrow the canal medially, or benign lateral osteomas. Although malignant changes occur infrequently in the external auditory canal, persistent bloody otorrhea or an increased amount of granulation-appearing tissue should arouse suspicion of a neoplastic process. It is imperative to obtain a biopsy early to establish the correct diagnosis. The vast majority of carcinomas of the external auditory canal are squamous cell carcinomas. Basal cell carcinomas and ceruminomas (including adenomas, pleomorphic adenomas, adenoid cystic carcinomas, and adenocarcinomas) occur. These processes should be considered in all patients who complain of chronic otalgia with or without otorrhea, hearing loss, vertigo, or facial nerve paralysis (7).

MIDDLE EAR

In 1974, Etholm and Belal (8) reported that arthritic changes of the ossicular articulations within the middle ear do occur. There is a hyalinization of the joint capsules, calcification of the articular cartilage, and calcification of the joint capsule itself. These changes are strictly age related with no sexual predilection. Surprisingly, there is almost no associated conductive hearing loss with these changes.

Atrophic or sclerotic changes of the tympanic membrane are common in the aged, but these changes do not usually cause appreciable losses of hearing. If there is marked retraction of the tympanic membrane or malfunction of the ossicular chain, there is accompanying moderate to severe conductive hearing loss. If there is a serous middle ear effusion, eustachian tube inflation with proper medication usually effectively treats it. Occasionally myringotomy with aspiration of the fluid and possible placement of a tympanostomy tube is required to restore eustachian tube function.

Perforations of the tympanic membrane can occur in various locations and are of various sizes. These may be due to direct injury from a foreign object, such as cotton-tipped applicators, pencils, or pens. These perforations also may be sustained from a blow to the ear from a fall or a hand slap to the side of the head. The pressure changes in the middle or external ear result as a barotraumatic change. Bleeding, vertigo, and secondary infection may accompany these. Otologic examination and audiologic evaluation are necessary in these perforated tympanic membranes. When there is a small perforation in the tympanic membrane without middle ear complications, simple patching with tissue paper, temporalis fascia, or sclera (banked) may be effective in closing the perforation to restore the hearing. The larger tympanic membrane perforation may require tympanoplasty or a myringoplasty, depending upon the status of the middle ear ossicles.

Otosclerosis is a bony disease causing conductive hearing loss as a result of fixation of the footplate of the stapes. Otosclerosis also may affect other parts of the labyrinth and otic capsule, causing a sensorineural hearing loss. It affects approximately 10% of the population and is usually bilateral. Otosclerosis most commonly starts in early adult life; however, it may not be recognized until secondary presbycusis sets in. The aging sensorineural hearing loss added to a previously unrecognized borderline conductive hearing loss then becomes evident. The diagnosis of otosclerosis is made by the patient's medical history, otologic examination, and audiologic evaluation.

There are three possible approaches to treatment. The patient may choose surgical correction, a hearing aid, or a combination of these two. The latter may be the most desirable with severe hearing loss, as the surgery may improve it to the point that a hearing aid can be used to greater advantage. In older medical literature, arguments have been made against ear surgery for the elderly patient. However, there is no age limitation as long as the general condition of the patient is good. As with younger patients, each candidate for surgery must be evaluated on an individual basis. Klotz (9) reported postoperative results of stapedectomies in elderly patients after 2 years of observation. He found that elderly patients did just as well as younger patients. Goodhill (10) reported excellent results from stapedectomy, averaging a 34.6-decibel gain for patients over 70 years of age with profound mixed-type hearing loss.

In older patients with larger perforations, cotton should be worn in the ear canal during exposure to cold temperatures or cold wind to avoid vertigo. Middle ear and mastoid tumors do occur in the aged population. These malignancies must be considered when there is a chronic draining ear and an abundance of granulation tissue. However, the most common tumor in the middle ear and mastoid area has to be cholesteatoma. After thorough audiologic, otologic, and radiologic evaluation and medical therapy failure, chronic otorrhea may require mastoid and/or tympanic membrane surgery (11).

INNER EAR

Presbycusis

In the United States, hearing loss constitutes one of the most common physical disabilities. Twenty-five percent of people between 65 and 74 years of age and 50% of people 75 years of age or older experience hearing difficulties. For older adults, the major auditory dysfunction is the result of presbycusis. By taking a complete history of the patient and by having a thorough audiologic, otologic, and, if necessary, radiologic evaluation, presbycusis is a diagnosis made by exclusion. Variables associated with presbycusis include metabolism, arteriosclerosis, smoking, noise exposure, genetic factors, diet, and stress. According to Schuknecht (12), there are four categories of presbycusis: (a) sensory, (b) metabolic or strial, (c) neural, and (d) mechanical or cochlear conductive.

As a result of the imbalance in hearing for low and high frequencies, speech may be heard in a distorted or even unintelligible manner. Presbycusis patients usually know when they are being spoken to, but they may not always understand what is said. The words are distorted by the patient's imperfect auditory system. When the distortion problem is compounded by a difficult listening situation, such as several people talking at once, patients with presbycusis will have an especially difficult time. More reliance on visual cues, such as reading lips, is important. The presbycusis patient who has difficulty with vision has an even worse problem.

There is no known prevention for presbycusis. However, the amount of hearing loss in the geriatric patient is usually the end result of a combination of multiple factors. The most serious complicating factor for most male patients is that they have spent a lifetime in a noisy working environment. The effects of prolonged exposure to high-intensity noise are similar to the effects of presbycusis in that the hearing for higher frequencies is usually affected first. There is no effective, after-the-fact treatment for noise-induced hearing loss. It can be prevented by avoiding excessively noisy environments and by wearing ear protective devices when exposed to high noise levels above 80 decibels.

Treatment of presbycusis with vasodilators, vitamins, diuretics, steroids, hormones, etc. has been attempted with little evidence of success. Because the possibility of improving presbycusis by medical therapy is limited, other approaches are often needed to assist the geriatric patient. The primary source of help is auditory rehabilitation. This includes the use of hearing aids, auditory training, assistive listening devices, and training in lip-reading. The task of the otorhinolaryngologist and audiologist is to thoroughly examine patients, evaluate their auditory function, assess their ability to benefit from amplification, and counsel them and their families.

Although a relatively large number of geriatric patients wear hearing aids, many elderly individuals deny a hearing loss, refuse to get their hearing evaluated, and refuse to consider wearing a hearing aid. The decision to evaluate the hearing and to consider wearing a hearing aid must be made by the patient, but awareness and encouragement by family and friends should be made if there is a possibility of a hearing loss and/or lost communicative skills. If a hearing aid can help the elderly individual, the family and close friends should be counseled about the hearing aid itself, assistive listening devices, training in lip-reading, and auditory training.

The hearing aid is a small, personalized, loudspeaker system consisting of a battery-operated microphone, amplifier, and speaker. The net effect of passing a sound through a hearing aid is to make the sound louder through amplification. The hearing aid cannot correct discrimination or differentiation of words as the hearing aid can only make sounds louder. Therefore, the hearing aid is most useful in face-to-face conversation as lip-reading can aid in discriminating or differentiating the word. When the distance from the source of the desired sound increases, ambient noise and reverberant sound interfere more with what the individual wants to hear.

Many elderly patients purchase and wear a hearing aid for a period of time, then they have complaints concerning the hearing aids and even may stop using them. The most common complaints of hearing aid users are squealing of the aid, excessive background noise, uncomfortable loudness at certain pitches, and less effectiveness in group conversations. Adjustments to the earmold or hearing aid usually can correct these complaints.

The elderly hearing-impaired individual whose vision is also impaired is doubly handicapped because of decreased ability to lip-read. As blind individuals are more dependent on their sense of hearing, hearing-impaired individuals are more dependent on their sense of sight. Light-flashing door bells, telephones, and fire alarm systems are used by many hearing-impaired individuals.

Home assistive listening devices include special telephone devices and television and radio earpiece receivers. It is important for the hearing-impaired individual to be aware of the assistive listening devices that are available in the community. These include the infrared and loop systems that may be found in places of worship, movie theaters, or other places of public entertainment.

Patients may find that they may gain 15 decibels in hearing by the use of ear cupping, placing a hand directly behind the auricle and deflecting the sound. Patients may find that they prefer the hearing aid in the ear canal itself or behind the ear, whatever their individual situation is. If for cosmetic reasons a patient does not want a hearing aid that can be seen, then an implantable hearing aid would be a solution to this problem. Implantable hearing aids give better sound, appear more natural and cosmetic, and require an operative procedure to implant the hearing aid in proximity to the mastoid bone.

Rules and regulations regarding the evaluation and issuance of hearing aids vary from state to state as they have resulted from certain problems and policies in those states. Most areas now require a complete audiogram by an audiologist or certified hearing aid dealer, medical evaluation by an otolaryngologist, and the opportunity for the individual to try the hearing aid before purchasing it.

Although there are many auditory function tests, the audiogram is the basic test to evaluate hearing loss. Pure-tone levels at individual frequencies can be tested as well as discrimination of words. In general, there are three types of hearing loss: neurosensory, conductive, and mixed (combination of neurosensory and conductive). Figure 42.1 shows these three types of hearing loss.

Hearing impairment presents in many different ways. The patient may be aware of a sudden, gradual, or questionable hearing loss. Sometimes individuals are not aware of a hearing loss and they actually deny the existence of such a problem, while their family and friends are aware of the problem. When oral communication decreases between two individuals, there is a possibility of hearing loss, and an audiogram should be considered. Because of the increased incidence of hearing loss in the elderly, screening of elderly people has been encouraged.

Tinnitus

Tinnitus is a major problem for the geriatric patient. Tinnitus is a buzzing, ringing, hissing, or similar type of sound that usually is related to hearing loss in the higher frequencies. This may be related to presbycusis or prolonged noise exposure. Aspirin and other medications may cause hearing loss and tinnitus. Tinnitus is a bothersome and troubling symptom that may or may not be of ear origin. Sometimes there can be objective cause, and sometimes the cause cannot be found. Subjective tinnitus occurs when the patient is aware of the ringing, buzzing, humming, whistling, roaring, or clicking sound; however, the examiner cannot hear it. Objective tinnitus is a

AUDIOGRAM

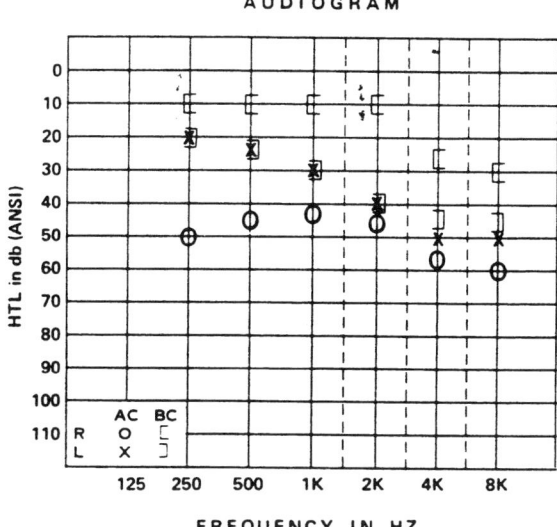

	RT EAR	LT EAR
SPEECH RECEPTION THRESHOLD (SRT)	45db	30db
DISCRIMINATION	100%	96%

Left ear (X, ⅂) demonstrates neurosensory loss. Right ear (Ꝺ, ⊏) demonstrates conductive loss with a mixed loss at 4K and 8K.

Figure 42.1. Audiogram of elderly individual demonstrating both neurosensory and conductive hearing losses.

bruit that can be heard by the examining physician. There are two types; one is the ear tinnitus (tinnitus aurium) and head tinnitus (tinnitus cranii). Cochlear and retrocochlear lesions can produce unilateral tinnitus. Ménière's disease is frequently accompanied by an ipsilateral tinnitus on the side with the hearing loss and vertigo. Acoustic neuroma and cerebellar pontine angle tumors also are characterized by an ipsilateral tinnitus. Unilateral tinnitus is a bothersome symptom that requires a thorough diagnostic evaluation.

There is no specific treatment for tinnitus aurium. Tinnitus is difficult to treat, and the patient needs to understand that it may persist forever. Treatment of tinnitus may include therapy for the underlying condition, such as a psychosomatic problem. Elimination of aspirin or similar medication may reduce the tinnitus. There is hope of converting the decompensated tinnitus into a compensated state. Acoustic sedation is helpful, as patients usually are most bothered at quiet times, such as when they are trying to fall asleep at night. The use of a bedside radio or tape recorder frequently helps provide an artificial

source of ambient noise to mask out this objective tinnitus. Some people require the use of tinnitus maskers that give them a sound constantly throughout the day. As there is no specific medical therapy for ear tinnitus, there is no effective surgery for tinnitus per se at this time. If the tinnitus becomes a major factor and is a unilateral process, then only as a last resort would a unilateral obliterative operation be considered.

Sudden Hearing Loss

Sudden hearing loss is a topic unto its own. Vascular changes can occur involving branches of the internal auditory artery. This type of loss is due to constriction or occlusion of the blood vessels or hemorrhage within the organ of Corti. Multiple medical regimens have been tried; however, there is not one form of therapy that has been proven to be most effective.

VESTIBULAR SYSTEM

Vestibular complaints have been recorded in over 50% of elderly patients living alone. *Vertigo* is a specific term used to describe the symptoms of the vestibular system including the peripheral labyrinthine, retrolabyrinthine, and central nervous system vestibular components. *Dizziness* is a vague term that may include giddiness, imbalance, faintness, "wooziness," and passing out. Dizziness may be used to describe cortical or visual disorientation, altered states of consciousness, and limb incoordinations. Balance depends on the input and proper functioning from the vestibular, visual, and proprioceptive pathways. Impaired function in any one of these three components may yield symptoms of dizziness (11). In the vestibular system, the disease process is usually in the sensory epithelium, the primary afferent fibers, and the vestibular apparatus.

Histopathology of the aged vestibule reveals a decrease of up to 40% in myelinated nerve fibers (with myelinated fibers of the cristae being affected most often). The otoconia of the saccule degenerate progressively from the posterior to the anterior end, and the saccular membranes have been shown to rupture more frequently in the elderly. Tissue between the endolymphatic duct and the bony vestibular aqueduct becomes fibrotic (13). Finally, postural vertigo (cupulolithiasis) is associated with dense deposits of insoluble particles in the pars superior at the ampule of the posterior semicircular canal (2). In addition to the general decrease of vestibular sensitivity, Schuknecht (14) has described four age-related conditions of dysequilibrium: (*a*) cupulolithiasis, (*b*) ampullary dysequilibrium, (c) macular dysequilibrium, and (d) vestibular ataxia.

NYSTAGMUS

Nystagmus is an objective finding that accompanies vertigo. It is characterized by a slow movement to one side with a corrective fast return movement to the other side. By convention, nystagmus is identified by the direction of the quick component. Thus, a nystagmus to the left means a nystagmus that has a slow movement to the right and a quick corrective component to the left.

The direction of the nystagmus may be horizontal, vertical, diagonal, or rotary. Manifest nystagmus can be observed with the naked eye under ordinary conditions. Occult nystagmus can be observed by using a +20 Freznel lens to abolish fixation or by electronystagmography. Electronystagmography is a diagnostic test that allows us to differentiate central nervous disorders from peripheral disorders within the labyrinth.

Vertical nystagmus can be produced either by peripheral labyrinth or by central nervous system disorders. Peripheral vertical nystagmus can originate from the semicircular canals, utricle, and saccule of the labyrinth. The symptoms of vertigo may be accompanied by nausea, vomiting, and generalized malaise. Common causes of peripheral vertigo include labyrinthitis, Ménière's disease, and labyrinthine fistula. Central vertical nystagmus may be caused by tumor in the temporal lobe (transverse gyrus of Heschl), by cerebral arteriosclerosis, and by lesions of the midbrain, pons, cerebellum, and brainstem. Lesions of the posterior inferior cerebellar artery will involve vestibular nuclei and their connections to the medial longitudinal fasciculus. Peripheral and central pathways can interact also.

NOSE

In aging, the nose loses its internal moisture and capability as there is decreased mucus production. The mucus is thicker, and the patient may complain of a thickness in the nose. Aging also brings on an absorption of the adipose tissue and atrophy of muscle within the nose itself. The most significant nasal finding in the aged patient is the increased fragility and sclerosis of blood vessels, contributing to epistaxis.

Cartilaginous changes show that the elderly person's nasal dorsum is convex with a retracted columella and a downward rotation of the lobule. These nasal changes are accentuated by loss of muscle mass of the orbiculus oris, absorption of facial adipose tissue, loss of teeth, and absorption of the maxilla and the mandible, causing a loss in the vertical dimension of the lower one-third of the face. The patient's nasal airway is decreased as the tip droops and the columella becomes retracted. There can be some fragmentation between the upper lateral cartilage and the lower lateral cartilage, causing collapse in the nasal valve area. Sometimes septoplasty and a tip rhinoplasty are done for elevation of the nasal tip to improve the airway. A resection of 2 to 4 mm of the lower lateral cartilage rotates the tip upward to improve the nasal airway.

In the elderly, the most distressing nasal condition is epistaxis. A nosebleed can be severe enough to threaten the life of the patient; furthermore, epistaxis can be challenging to treat because elderly patients have a higher percentage of posterior nasal bleeding than other patients. Typically, posterior epistaxis occurs in the middle of the night, causing the patient to wake up gagging on a mouthful of blood, which requires emergent treatment. Epistaxis can be caused by multiple factors, but certainly, the aging process with increased fragility and sclerosis of the blood vessels is the most important factor. Hypertension and sicca (dryness) condition that is accentuated by the loss of internal moisture contribute to epistaxis among the elderly. Other causes of epistaxis in the elderly are trauma, septal perforation, blood dyscrasias, use of medications (aspirin, Coumadin, etc.), benign tumors of the nose and sinuses, malignant tumors of the nose and sinus, atrophic rhinitis, Wegener's granulomatosis, and mucormycosis.

Atrophic rhinitis is a progressive chronic disease in which the nasal fossae are greatly enlarged as a result of atrophic changes in the mucosa and underlying bone. Thick, smelly, adherent crusts are formed in the nasal passages. Atrophic rhinitis is also known as ozena, derived from the Greek word meaning "stench." The infecting organisms of mucormycosis are species of *Absidia*, *Mucor*, or *Rhizopus*. It is associated with facial cellulitis, acute rhinosinusitis and gangrenous mucosal changes. It occurs in diabetic patients or in patients who have received immunosuppressive therapy for lymphomas, leukemias, or connective tissue disorders. Intranasal examination is diagnostic with the finding of a black inferior turbinate resulting from necrosis of the inferior turbinate. The disease process can progress rapidly and may cause death by extension into the intracranial area.

Acne rosacea is a pustular dermatologic condition that may affect the nose. If it becomes advanced, it develops into a rhinophyma, which is hypertrophy of the underlying sebaceous glands in the affected area, giving rise to a very bulbous nasal tip. Acne rosacea can be controlled by the application of mild steroid cream to the affected areas. If the lesion advances to rhinophyma, then surgical removal should be done by dermabrasion or carbon dioxide laser resection (15).

Postnasal drip is one of the more frequent symptoms in the elderly patient. Postnasal drip usually is accompanied by a sinusitis and, of course, has to do with thickening of the mucus. The key to this diagnosis is to elicit a history of the color and type of drainage, to do a thorough nasopharyngeal and nasal examination, to document with sinus x-rays or computerized axial tomography scans, and to consider diagnostic nasal and/or sinus endoscopy. Furthermore, the postnasal drip may cause a chronic cough, clearing of the throat, a catch-in-the-throat, and/or hoarseness. If the medical treatment of chronic sinusitis is unsuccessful, then surgical sinus endoscopy will be needed to correct the osteomeatal complex blockage causing the maxillary, ethmoid, frontal, and/or sphenoid sinusitis. The techniques of endoscopic sinus surgery continue to be refined and expanded to relieve chronic sinusitis and its pulmonary sequelae (16, 17).

Taste and smell are related chemical senses. It is possible to have malfunction of one or both of them. However, more complaints center around the loss of olfaction. An acute loss of sense of smell (anosmia) can be related to an upper respiratory infection. Because of the short-term effect, the patient is rarely seen for this condition. Chronic anosmia occurs after blockage of the air currents through the nose. This may be due to nasal polyps, benign tumors, malignant tumors, influenzalike viral infections, surgery, or radiation, and high doses of aspirin or similar drugs can also cause this effect. Closed head trauma and diseases such as cancer, hyperthyroidism, hepatitis, and liver disease can also alter the sense of smell and taste (15).

ORAL CAVITY

Aging significantly alters the dentition, oral cavity mucosa, and salivary glands. The mucosa has thinner epithelium (especially tunica propria), blunted rete pegs, decreased collagen, fewer functioning capillaries, and decreased water content. Arteriosclerosis delays and reduces healing, plus the tissue is more prone to injury. Salivary gland production is diminished 25% by loss of secretory parenchymal volume, acinar hyalinization, and salivary ductal adhesions. As a result,

there is an increase in dental caries, mucosal atrophy, and mucosal burning, with a decreased taste bud sensitivity.

Glossodynia (burning pain in the tongue) may be caused by anemia (folic acid, iron, or B_{12} deficiency), candidiasis, denture irritation, lichen planus, xerostomia, neuropathy of diabetes mellitus, postviral neuropathy, or carcinoma. Sometimes it incorporates the entire mouth to cause a burning mouth syndrome. Usually the patient does not demonstrate any lesion. If no cause can be found and psychosomatic conversion can be eliminated, then the patient may require a lemon and glycerin mouthwash and possibly a tranquilizer.

Geographic tongue is also known as migratory glossitis. This can be secondary to a minor viral infection; however, it usually is of no consequence. Some people in their normal state have geographic tongue.

Fordyce granules, which are the fourth most common oral lesions in the elderly, are ectopic sebaceous glands that are benign, raised, yellow-to-white areas on the buccal or lip mucosa. No treatment is required.

Angular cheilitis is most evident at the oral commissures that are fissured, macerated, erythematous, and tender. Loss of connective tissue support causing redundant skin folds allows pooling of saliva and resulting candidiasis. Application of nystatin cream to the oral commissure usually corrects angular cheilitis; however, correction of ill-fitting dentures and management of iron or vitamin B deficiency may be required.

Candidiasis appears to be more common in the elderly than in other age groups. It occurs after prolonged and/or intensive antibiotic therapy and also in debilitated individuals. A typical clinical picture consists of white patches on the throat and hypopharynx, with mild inflammatory reaction to the underlying tissue. Mycostatin mouthwash suspension is usually effective. For advanced cases, the patient may need systemic treatment with intravenous amphotericin B.

Lichen planus is a benign chronic disease usually caused by emotional or physical stress. Nonerosive lichen planus has a roughened, asymptomatic, hyperkeratotic leukoplakia on the mucosa; the painful erosive type has vesicles and bullae. There is no definite correlation between lichen planus and oral cavity carcinoma.

Temporomandibular joint syndrome (TMJ), or Costen's syndrome, is defined as a dysfunction of the temporomandibular joint with severe pain in the joint itself, the ear, or adjacent structures. Causes can be dental malocclusion, acute trauma to the mandible, clenching of the teeth with muscular contraction, arthritis, or tumors in the area. TMJ can cause vertigo, a ringing type tinnitus, or a clicking or popping sensation when the jaw is opened. Nonsurgical treatment includes use of topical heat, soft diet, physical therapy, analgesics, steroids, dental splints, bite blocks, biofeedback, and psychotherapy. In the event that these are unsatisfactory, then exploratory surgery of the temporomandibular joint should be considered (18).

SPEECH ALTERATIONS

Hoarseness, difficulty swallowing, and painful swallowing increase with the patient's age. If any of these symptoms persist, the patient must have an indirect laryngoscopy mirror examination. If a thorough mirror examination cannot be done, then fiberoptic laryngoscopy can be carried out. Sometimes a barium swallow is also needed for aid in diagnosis. Causes range from benign vocal cord nodules and diverticulum to aggressive malignant tumors. Gastroesophageal reflux is one of the more common disorders causing hoarseness, catch-in-throat, or dysphagia.

Vocal strain occurs more frequently in the geriatric patient. The aging process affects the voice pitch, quality, and volume and the rate of speech to varying degrees in different individuals. The voice intermittently changes to what is described as a tired, failing, and faltering type of voice. A wavering tone and decreased volume result in a lessened ability to communicate. Articulation also may be significantly distorted by missing teeth, dentures, or stroke. Chronic vocal strain can result from voice misuse.

The elderly voice has a change in pitch after age 50 years. According to data obtained by Honjo and Isshiki (19), men have a vocal fold atrophy causing an increase in fundamental frequency, whereas women have a vocal fold edema causing decreased fundamental frequency. The muscles of the larynx, especially the thyroarytenoid muscle, become atrophic. The voice becomes drier as the false vocal cords have a reduction in mucous glandular production and may actually show some squamous metaplasia. The cricoarytenoid joint and the cricothyroid joint may develop a relaxation of the joint capsule or partially become fixed.

As a result of some of the preceding changes, the patient may develop a spastic dysphonia type of voice. The patient develops a tight and squeezed voice sound with extreme tension and a strained, creaking, choking type of vocal attack. The patient complains of reduction in clarity and volume with no pathologic findings evident on indirect or direct laryngoscopy. Speech therapy is most helpful. For true documented spastic dysphonia, recurrent laryngeal nerve sectioning should be considered only after intensive speech therapy has been deemed a failure.

Laryngeal dysfunction secondary to vocal cord paralysis entails special problems. Unilateral vocal cord paralysis can be due to many different etiologic factors ranging from laryngeal carcinoma to left chest disease to central nervous system disorders. Of patients developing unilateral vocal cord paralysis, 30% never have the cause determined. After allowing about 6 months for spontaneous resolution of the paralysis, it may be desirable to eliminate aspiration of liquids and foods and to attempt to improve the voice and the effectiveness of the cough reflex by injecting Teflon (polytetrafluoroethylene), placed lateral to the paralyzed cord.

Bilateral abductive vocal cord paralysis does not affect the voice quality as much. However, it affects the inspiratory function of the larynx, requiring corrective surgery. The patient would benefit from a lateralizing procedure of the vocal cord, such as arytenoidectomy, or perhaps a valved tracheostomy tube.

Dysphonia secondary to gastroesophageal reflux is usually found in obese patients who have a chronic sore throat and a globus sensation with possible pain over the thyrohyoid membrane. Physical examination reveals erythema of the arytenoid mucosa. If the problem is advanced enough, contact granuloma or hyperkeratosis of the true vocal cords can be seen. Treatment includes diet, elevation of the head of the bed, antacids, and H_2-receptor blocking agents (1, 2).

Senile bowing of the vocal cords is secondary to muscle atrophy and loss of connective tissue. Dryness of the laryngeal mucosa (laryngitis sicca) results from atrophy of the mucous glands. Voice tremor can be associated with other tremors in the head and neck area and may be a solitary finding. The voice will quiver with sudden abrupt changes, similar to those found in spastic dysphonia.

Dysarthria also may cause inarticulation or problems in communication. Dysarthria may be found in patients suffering from cerebral vascular accidents, trauma, Parkinson's disease, Huntington's chorea, or lower or upper motor neuron disease.

TRACHEOSTOMY

If a short-term or long-term tracheostomy is necessary, the patient and the family should have proper preoperative counseling. It is necessary to explain the purpose of the procedure and that the patient will probably be without a voice until the tracheostomy tube can be effectively occluded. Humidification of the patient's immediate environment is very important. Suctioning and cleaning of the airway with saline solution is also very important in limiting crusting and thinning the secretions. Suctioning should be reduced to a minimum as soon as possible, so as not to remove any more cilia from the trachea than is absolutely necessary.

FACIAL NERVE PALSY

Facial nerve palsies are usually of idiopathic origin. Bell's palsy is a diagnosis by exclusion of all other causes of the facial nerve palsy. Herpes zoster oticus (Ramsay Hunt syndrome), cholesteatoma in a chronic suppurative otitis media, carcinoma of the middle ear, and parotid tumor are a few of the causes of a facial palsy. The most important step in the initial assessment of facial palsy is exclusion of any middle ear pathology or tumors along the distribution of the facial nerve.

OTALGIA

Otalgia may originate within the ear itself or may be referred from numerous structures in the head and neck. Pain originating within the ear is usually due to an acute inflammation within the outer or middle ear. Referred pain is a common important phenomenon. A number of cranial nerve sensory components to the external and middle ear also are sensory components to the pharynx, hypopharynx, and larynx; a lesion elsewhere in the head and neck area may be manifest as otalgia. Otalgia may be a symptom of a carcinoma on the base of the tongue, pharynx, or larynx. Furthermore, ordinary common causes of such referred pain include cervical osteoarthrosis and TMJ dysfunction. In both, pain may be centered on the ear, but they usually show differing radiations, with the former having a cervical root distribution and the latter having a preauricular, maxillary, and mandibular pattern.

HEAD AND NECK CANCERS

Head and neck cancers comprise 5% of all malignancies in the body. They occur more frequently in the elderly than in the younger population. Because of the possible pronounced functional and cosmetic deformities from ablative surgery, early diagnosis to allow the least destructive therapy is important. Poor oral hygiene, alcohol, and smoking are prime factors in the formation of these head and neck tumors.

Common geriatric complaints that should be investigated for possible malignancy include neck masses, hoarseness, dysphagia, dyspnea, hearing alterations, painful teeth, swollen face, bad breath, otalgia, and hemoptysis. Common presenting symptoms include proptosis due to tumors of the orbit or ethmoid, frontal, or maxillary sinuses; epistaxis associated with cancer of the paranasal sinuses or nose; ulceration of the mouth; hoarseness associated with laryngeal carcinoma; and dysphagia resulting from laryngeal and esophageal tumors. Facial swelling also can result from tumors of the parotid gland, floor of the mouth, maxillary sinus, palate, or mandible.

The most common malignancy in the head and neck area is epidermoid squamous cell carcinoma. If the laryngeal lesions are found early, a cure rate greater than 95% can be achieved. The early lesions are treated with radiation, carbon dioxide laser resection, or partial laryngectomy. While still providing a possible cure rate, advances in surgical techniques of partial laryngectomy can preserve the voice and deglutition to many moderately advanced cases. Total laryngectomy is still required in advanced tumors, and this sometimes is done in combination with radiation (1, 2).

Carcinoma of the oral cavity occurs most commonly in the older age groups. Age itself is not a contraindication to surgery, as extensive head and neck surgery is generally well tolerated by the elderly patient. Johnson et al. (20) reported that in 27 cases of composite resection in patients over 65 years of age, the surgical complications were equivalent to or less than those of an equally paired younger age group. There was an increase in associated medical complications for the elderly population; however, the head and neck complications were fewer. Rehabilitation time for oral alimentation and for discharge of the patient was essentially the same in both age groups. Age also is no contraindication to partial laryngeal surgery, as it seems to be tolerated relatively well in the elderly patient. Tucker (21) viewed 27 cases of conservation laryngeal surgery in the elderly age group. He found his 11% complication rate with no deaths compared favorably with the rates for total laryngectomy and radiotherapy alone. McGuirt et al. (22) reported no increased incidents of surgical complications in the group above 70 years of age. His series also had a slight increase in medical complication; however, the head and neck complications were equal.

Thyroid malignancies act more aggressively in the elderly because more anaplastic or undifferentiated carcinomas occur. Hoarseness, dysphagia, dyspnea, and enlarging neck mass are symptoms of thyroid cancer. The most useful diagnostic techniques are fine-needle aspiration and radioactive imaging. Surgical resection is the initial treatment of choice for thyroid malignancies. For follicular or papillary carcinoma, radioactive iodine ablation and thyroid supplementation are recommended after total or near-total thyroidectomy (with a modified neck dissection for positive lymphatic involvement). For medullary carcinoma, external radiation to the neck and mediastinum and thyroid supplementation should be given after total thyroidectomy and regional lymphatic resection. For anaplastic carcinoma, external radiation, possible chemotherapy, and thyroid supplementation should be given after total thyroidectomy and regional lymphatic resection (23).

The geriatric population has skin changes that are of significance to the otolaryngologist. Basal cell carcinoma, squamous cell carcinoma, malignant melanoma, and the numerous premalignant skin lesions are discussed elsewhere in this textbook.

In summary, it would appear that age alone is not a criterion for withholding curative surgery from an elderly patient. Instead, postponing an operative procedure is unwise. Consequently, the head and neck surgeon should evaluate each patient on the basis of preexisting medical problems, the preexisting psychologic and mental condition, the type of surgery required with possible reconstructive procedure, probable postoperative functional state, and the support facilities available where the operation will be done. Only after weighing all of these considerations should the surgeon make recommendations regarding major head and neck surgery.

There has been significant improvement in rehabilitation of the laryngectomee after total laryngectomy. In addition to an electrolarynx and esophageal speech, there are now multiple approaches to the surgical reconstruction of the speaking mechanism.

Cosmetic and reconstructive facial surgery is of growing importance to the aging population. The physician must pay careful attention to the patient's desires, needs, and physical capabilities. Reconstructive surgery is very crucial in the rehabilitation of a cancer patient. The postsurgical defect following removal of a malignancy may require both functional and cosmetic surgery. Recent developments with microsurgery, regional flaps, free flaps, and myocutaneous flaps have improved reconstructive surgery significantly (24, 25).

REFERENCES

1. Cummings CW, Fredrickson JM, Harker LA, Krause CJ, Schuller DE, eds. Otolaryngology—head and neck surgery. 2nd ed. Baltimore: Williams & Wilkins, 1993.
2. Paparella MM, Shumrick DA, eds. Otolaryngology. 3rd ed. Philadelphia: WB Saunders, 1991.
3. Boone DR, Bayles KA, Koopmann CF. Communicative aspects of aging. Otolaryngol Clin North Am 1982;15:313–327.
4. English GM, ed. Otolaryngology. 2nd ed. Philadelphia: Harper & Row, 1986.
5. Anderson RG, Meyerhoff WL. Otologic manifestations of aging. Otolaryngol Clin North Am 1982; 15:353–370.
6. Gates G, ed. Current therapy in otolaryngology—head and neck surgery. 5th ed. St. Louis: CV Mosby, 1994.
7. Senturia BH. Diseases of the external ear. New York: Grune & Stratton, 1980.
8. Etholm B, Belal A. Senile changes in the middle ear joints. Ann Otol Rhinol Laryngol 1974;83:49–54.
9. Klotz RE, Kilbane M. Hearing in an aging population, preliminary report. N Engl J Med 1962; 266:277–280.
10. Goodhill V. Diseases, deafness, and dizziness. New York: Harper & Row, 1979.
11. Ballenger JJ. Diseases of the nose, throat, ear, head, and neck. 13th ed. Philadelphia: Lea & Febiger, 1985.
12. Schuknecht HF. Further observations on the pathology of presbycusis. Arch Otolaryngol 1964; 80:369–382.
13. Johnsson LG. Degenerative changes and anomalies of the vestibular system. Laryngoscope 1971;81: 1682–1693.
14. Schuknecht HF. Pathology of the ear. Cambridge: Harvard University Press, 1974.
15. Patterson CN. The aging nose: characteristics and correction. Otolaryngol Clin North Am 1980;13: 275–278.
16. Lamear WR, Davis WE, Templer JW, et al. Partial endoscopic middle turbinectomy augmenting functional endoscopic sinus surgery. Otolaryngol Head Neck Surg 1992;107:79–84.
17. Metson R. Endoscopic treatment of frontal sinusitis. Laryngoscope 1992;102:712–716.
18. Koopman CF, Coulthard SW. The oral cavity and aging. Otolaryngol Clin North Am 1982;15:293–312.
19. Honjo I, Isshiki N. Laryngoscopic and voice characteristics of aged persons. Arch Otolaryngol 1980; 106:149–150.
20. Johnson JT, Rabuzzi DD, Tucker HM. Composite resection in the elderly: a well tolerated procedure. Laryngoscope 1977;87:1509–1515.
21. Tucker HM. Conservation laryngeal surgery in the elderly patient. Laryngoscope 1977;87:1995–1999.
22. McGuirt WF, Loevy S, McCabe BF, Krause CJ. The risks of major head and neck surgery in the aged population. Laryngoscope 1977;87:1378–1382.
23. Holt GR, Mattox DE. Decision making in otolaryngology. St. Louis: CV Mosby, 1984.
24. Chavpil M, Koopman CF. Age and other factors regulating wound healing. Otolaryngol Clin North Am 1982;15:259–268.
25. Koopman CF. Special considerations in managing geriatric patients. In: Otolaryngology—head and neck surgery. St. Louis: CV Mosby, 1987.

43/ Geriatric Dentistry

R. I. Garcia

The scope of geriatric dental practice has changed dramatically over the past decade as a result of demographic trends, secular changes in oral disease prevalence, and the growing awareness that aging per se does not appear to be a major risk factor for oral diseases. The focus of geriatric dentistry has in turn shifted from predominant attention to the needs of elders in long-term care settings and the replacement of missing teeth in the edentulous patient. Increasingly, there is growing emphasis on providing the benefits of comprehensive oral health care, encompassing all the dental specialties where appropriate, to the growing population of community-dwelling elders. In addition, the need for such comprehensive care is projected to grow into the future as more and more elders are maintaining their dentition throughout their life span. Because persons over 65 typically see physicians more regularly and more often than they see a dentist, there is also an important need for non-dentist health care providers to identify oral problems early, undertake appropriate interventions, and make timely referrals for further evaluation and treatment. In particular, those elders who are seen by physicians more frequently are typically those with a greater burden of comorbidities of aging and who are in turn at highest risk for developing oral problems.

The recent changes in geriatric dental practice have come about in great part because new research findings have debunked a number of old myths about the oral health of elders. The seemingly simple question, "What are the effects of aging on oral health?" has proven to be quite complex and difficult to answer. The formulation of testable hypotheses has often been complicated by the large number of confounders for which the available data are often inadequate. Furthermore, needed information pertaining to the medical and psychosocial factors that can affect specific outcome measures of oral health status frequently is unavailable.

The two major longitudinal studies of aging and oral health in the U. S., the oral physiology component of the Baltimore Longitudinal Study of Aging and the VA Dental Longitudinal Study–Normative Aging Study in Boston, aim to identify the precursors and risk factors associated with age-related changes in oral health (1). These studies have made important contributions in this regard, showing that any disproportionate levels of oral disease or dysfunction found in elders appear to be related more to the presence of comorbid conditions than to any normative age-related changes in the oral cavity. For example, salivary gland function remains fundamentally unchanged with aging (2). Subjective reports of dry mouth symptoms ("xerostomia") and objective measures of decreased salivary flow in certain elders are not due to age but rather are associated with certain systemic conditions (3) or specific medication usage (4). Similarly, the clinical appearance and condition of oral mucosa do not significantly change with age in otherwise healthy elders (5). The ability of elders to chew is also unaffected by age (6). Rather, tooth loss and the presence or absence of adequate tooth replacements are the major factors affecting mastication. In turn, food selection and diet are not significantly related to age but rather to dentition status (7).

AGING AND CHANGES IN ORAL STRUCTURES AND FUNCTION

DENTAL CARIES, PERIODONTAL DISEASES, AND TOOTH LOSS

Tooth loss is not an inevitable consequence of aging. Rather, it represents an endpoint to a complex interaction among dental diseases (caries and periodontitis) and behavioral and attitudinal factors toward tooth retention and treatment preferences on the part of both the patient and provider. Perhaps the most significant oral health–related change taking place in the population is the decline in tooth loss. In the U. S., there are now more elders with teeth than without (8). Comparison of national data over the past four decades clearly shows declines over time in the number of missing teeth per person. The trends for the prevalence of complete edentulism are similar (Table 43.1). In the most recent U. S. national survey, only one-third of those 65 and older were completely edentulous, a reverse of the situation 30 to 40 years earlier. Even in the Northeast region of the U. S., an area historically known for its high prevalence of dental disease and tooth loss, secular trends toward better oral health and tooth retention are evident. In a 1991 random sample of elders, the New England Elders Dental Study found that over two-thirds had teeth. More importantly, of those elders with teeth, over 80% had kept most of their teeth.

This decreasing rate of edentulism is expected to continue into the future, as current younger-age cohorts in the population demonstrate a similar trend regarding tooth retention. Important factors involved in this trend include a decline in dental caries incidence, related in large part to widespread availability of fluoride (9), a change in professional philosophy concerning retention of the natural dentition, and a concomitant change in the public's expectations about keeping their teeth for a lifetime (10). In addition, the acceptance of preventive dentistry and the improvement in oral hygiene behaviors by adults have also led to declines in the prevalence of periodontal diseases in elders (8).

Periodontal disease, manifested as gingival inflammation and loss of tooth-supporting alveolar bone, has been traditionally viewed as the predominant cause of tooth loss in adults. However, more recent data from longitudinal epidemiologic studies have not confirmed this long-held belief. Results from the Rand Health Insurance Experiment (11) showed that less than 4% of tooth extractions could be ascribed to periodontal disease in a sample of 1210 young and middle-aged

adults. Similarly, the presence of root caries and coronal caries was found to be a significantly more important predictor of tooth loss than was periodontal condition in a community-based sample of elders in rural Iowa (12). Longitudinal results from the VA Normative Aging Study also show that the presence of dental caries is a more important predictor of tooth loss than periodontal disease (13). A repeated observation from many studies has been the major contribution to tooth loss of provider decisions to remove otherwise healthy teeth to facilitate a prosthetic treatment plan (14). Clearly, factors other than caries and periodontitis are important to understanding tooth loss, including sociocultural and economic factors, access to and availability of care, and provider treatment preferences.

Dental caries, both coronal and root decay, remain major problems in elders (8), with the annual incidence in elders being equivalent to that seen in high-risk populations of children and adolescents, when incidence rates are adjusted for the number of tooth surfaces at risk for decay. As with tooth loss, multiple risk factors are at play. Specific groups of elders may also be identified who are at dramatically higher risk for caries, including those with Alzheimer's disease (15) and those with salivary gland dysfunction (16).

Gradual changes do occur over time in the adult dentition. There is a tendency toward mesial, or forward, drift of the teeth over time, which may result in anterior crowding. Tooth enamel typically exhibits attrition in later years on the occlusal and incisal surfaces of the teeth. The severity of such attrition is highly variable and due to masticatory forces, coarseness of the diet, and oral habits such as bruxism or grinding. Fracture lines may also develop in the enamel over time. Internal to the enamel is the dentin layer, with a mineral density like that of bone. Dentin continues to be formed throughout life by an odontoblastic cell layer within the dental pulp. With age, the dentin layer thickens while the pulp narrows. Abrasion of the tooth root at the cementoenamel junction may result from mechanical processes such as excessive tooth brushing or from erosion. Gingival recession, a common finding in elders, results in increased exposure of root surfaces. Because cementum, the mineral layer that covers tooth roots, is less dense than enamel, it is much more susceptible to decay, leading to the increased risk for root surface caries noted in elders.

Periodontal changes typical of aging include not only gingival recession with root exposure but also loss of the attachment apparatus, including the tooth-supporting alveolar bone (17). However,

Table 43.1
Prevalence of Tooth Loss in the United States

Survey Year	Type	Ages Sampled	Edentulous (%) Overall Population	Edentulous (%) Ages 65–74
1957–58	NHIS-I	All ages	13	55
1960–62	NHES-I	18–74	17	50
1971	NHIS-II	All ages	11	45
1971–74	NHANES-I	18–74	15	46
1985–86	NIDR	All ages	4	37

changes in bone appear to be minimal in systemically healthy elders, with severe and extensive periodontal destruction limited to a small proportion of the population. The rate of periodontal attachment loss and alveolar bone loss can be particularly great in those elders with specific risk factors (17, 18). Cigarette smoking has been identified as a major risk factor for attachment loss and alveolar bone loss (18, 19), as well as for other oral problems in elders (20). The effects of smoking appear to go beyond simply local effects in the oral cavity and involve inhaled tobacco smoke, as men who are exclusively pipe and cigar smokers are at much lower risk than those who smoke cigarettes (18). Cigarette smokers have also been shown to have lower bone mineral density at various skeletal sites and are at higher risk for osteoporosis (21). Oral bone changes may also reflect systemic bone metabolism (22). In turn, persons with lower bone mineral at various skeletal sites (e. g., hip, spine, radius) are also at higher risk for tooth loss (23).

In addition to osteoporosis, the other major comorbidity of aging with important oral consequences is non-insulin-dependent diabetes mellitus (NIDDM). With over 10% of elders affected by NIDDM and an equivalent number having impaired glucose tolerance, the impact of these conditions as risk factors for oral disease is quite large. Both the prevalence and the severity of periodontal disease have been found to be greater in persons with NIDDM, and they are at higher risk for tooth loss (24, 25). Adult diabetics report xerostomia symptoms at high rates (26), although subjective reports do not appear to correlate well with measured stimulated or unstimulated salivary flow rates (27). Changes in the composition of saliva in diabetics, rather than changes in the flow rates, have been hypothesized to account for the xerostomia symptoms and may also explain in part the increased incidence of oral mucosal candidal infections noted in diabetics (28).

SALIVARY GLAND FUNCTION, XEROSTOMIA, AND ORAL CANDIDIASIS

Salivary gland function, as measured by salivary flow rates, remains essentially unchanged with age in the absence of systemic disease or certain medication usage (2–4, 26–29). Minor changes in the electrolyte composition of parotid saliva have been noted with age (30). Decreases in saliva secretion are well correlated with a number of specific medical disorders (31, 32) and have also been related to the use of certain common medications (4, 28). Interestingly, most studies

have shown poor correlations between patient-reported symptoms of xerostomia and objective measures of salivary flow rates (33). Elders with diminished salivary flow, but not those with subjective complaints, have been found to have higher salivary yeast counts and to be at higher risk for oral candidiasis (34). Yeasts are normal commensals in the oral cavity but may result in oral lesions under certain conditions, including use of antibiotics, presence of salivary dysfunction, presence of inadequate prostheses, and more rarely with the use of inhaled corticosteroids in asthmatics (35). Such infections may present in various forms (36), including acute pseudomembranous candidiasis (thrush) with raised whitish plaques that may be scraped off leaving an erythematous and often ulcerated base; chronic hyperplastic candidiasis; and chronic atrophic candidiasis. The latter is often accompanied by angular cheilitis, linear ulcerated fissures at the corners of the mouth that may be superinfected with bacteria.

NUTRITION, ORAL HEALTH, AND MASTICATION

Longitudinal research findings have clearly demonstrated that masticatory function and food selection do not change as a direct result of aging (6, 7). A stable dentition and the absence of medical problems or medication usage affecting salivary function or taste result in the maintenance of normal function and diet over time. However, the worse one's dental status, the more compromised is one's ability to adequately chew and swallow food. Poor oral health, missing teeth, and inadequate prosthetic replacements may lead to severe compromises in nutrition (37). This may in turn have a significant negative impact on general health and well-being. For example, one recent study found that the best predictor of involuntary weight loss among frail elderly was the number of oral problems present (38). Given the remaining high prevalence in elders of missing teeth, ill-fitting dentures, and their associated problems, improvements in oral health could make a significant impact on the nutritional status of elders.

Dietary preferences of elders do not tend to change progressively with age, but rather will change as masticatory function decreases with progressive tooth loss or is compromised by inadequate replacement of missing teeth. Under such conditions, patients may prefer softer and more easily chewed foods, including a shift to packaged, processed foods, and may also select foods that are sweeter, saltier, or overly seasoned, because the gustatory sensation is diminished by poorer oral health status. In turn, such shifts in food selection may have systemic health consequences and may affect the medical management of comorbid conditions, such as hypertension and diabetes.

In parallel to the apparent stability of masticatory function with aging, there appear to be only minor changes in taste perception with aging (39). When alterations in taste and smell are noted in elders, they are related to underlying disease rather than to normative age changes in chemosensation (40). In contrast, evidence exists that alterations in swallowing ability may occur with aging and be related to altered oropharyngeal proprioception.

ORAL CANCER

The incidence of oral cancer is higher in older patients and is more common in males than females. Similar to other aspects of oral health in elders, oral cancer is not an inevitable consequence of aging but is rather very significantly associated with specific preventable risk factors, primarily alcohol and tobacco use. Approximately 4 to 5% of all cancers occur in the oral cavity and adjacent tissues. Oral carcinomas are typically squamous cell type and occur at different intraoral sites with varying frequency (Table 43.2).

Carcinoma of the lip is chiefly associated with pipe smoking and exposure to sunlight. Carcinoma of the tongue may present as ulceration, leukoplakia, or an erythematous patch (erythroplakia), often with a hyperkeratotic periphery. The lateral borders of the tongue are the most common sites of dysplastic and neoplastic lesions. On the buccal mucosa and gingiva, lesions may have a highly variable appearance including ulcerated, indurated mass with leukoplakia. Adenocarcinomas may arise from the minor salivary glands, where they may appear as a painless, firm, or fluctuant masses, most frequently occurring near the juncture of the hard and soft palate.

Table 43.2
Frequency of Primary Occurrence of Oral Cancer by Intraoral Site

Location	Occurrence (%)
Tongue	50
Floor of the mouth	15
Gingiva and alveolar mucosa	12
Lip	9
Palate	9
Buccal mucosa	3

Patients who receive head and neck radiation therapy should receive a comprehensive oral evaluation before treatment begins. Elimination of oral infection, maintenance of ideal oral hygiene, and a daily topical fluoride regimen must be established to prevent rampant dental caries and oral mucositis, which can be important sequelae to salivary gland dysfunction resulting from radiation treatment. All necessary dental extractions should be performed before therapy, to avoid the risk of osteoradionecrosis following extractions.

ORAL HEALTH ASSESSMENT IN ELDERS

SELF-ASSESSMENT AND THE DENTAL SCREENING INITIATIVE

Oral problems, like other health problems, are best managed if identified early. However, neither patients nor nondental health care professionals are often comfortable with their abilities to diagnose oral conditions, and such problems thus go unrecognized until they progress significantly. The DENTAL screening initiative (Table 43.3) is being developed to provide a simple self-administered questionnaire for patients' self-assessment of their oral health status and to facilitate their obtaining needed consultation and follow-up care. This simple instrument also helps physicians, nurses, dietitians, and other health care providers to easily identify oral problems in their elder patients. The goals of this screening process are to identify and treat sources of potential oral infection, to improve the ability to eat a balanced diet comfortably, and to facilitate social interactions by improving appearance and self-esteem and permitting ease of eating and speaking.

CLINICAL EXAMINATION

A visual and digital oral examination should primarily be a simple and targeted attempt to identify the presence of, or potential for, oral infection. Teeth should be noted and the number in each jaw counted. The level of hygiene of remaining teeth, and of dentures if present, should also be noted. Problems needing immediate attention include grossly decayed or fractured teeth, teeth that move laterally or vertically with finger pressure, purulence from the gingiva or other soft tissue structures, and areas of ulceration or desquamation. In addition, areas of leukoplakia and erythroplakia may be noted for subsequent oral cancer evaluation.

Oral hygiene is also a major concern in the edentulous patient. Even the best-fitting dentures

Table 43.3
The DENTAL Screening Initiative

Determine Your Oral Health

Warning signs of poor oral health are often overlooked. You can use the answers to the following six statements to evaluate your own oral health. Read each statement below. If you answer YES to one or more statements, you should contact your dental or medical provider and ask for assistance.

D	I have a **D**ry mouth.
E	I have **E**ating or swallowing problems, or my **E**ating habits have changed in the past year as a result of problems with my teeth or mouth.
N	I have **N**ot had a dental exam in the past year.
T	I have frequent **T**ooth or mouth pain, or **T**ender, bleeding gums.
A	Problems with my teeth or gums have **A**ffected my **A**ppearance or my social interactions with family, friends, or coworkers.
L	I have **L**esions or sores in my mouth.

You should realize that these warning signs do not represent the diagnosis of any condition. Instead they suggest that you may be at risk of poor oral health and that you should visit a professional who can help you determine the best course of action to enhance your dental health.

may cause mucosal irritation in areas of constant contact and may harbor oral yeasts and bacteria. In patients with chronic candidiasis, dentures must be treated to eliminate an important source of reinfection. All dentures should be removed from the mouth at bedtime and should not be worn when asleep. Dentures need to be brushed daily for proper plaque removal. An appropriate oral hygiene regimen should be adhered to routinely on a daily basis to promote optimal cleansing of oral tissues and dental prostheses. Cleansing aids can be modified to make patients with physical limitations more self-reliant and responsible for their own care. Providers for patients unable to self-care as well as for those under long-term care should set a simple goal that every day their patients will go to sleep with clean mouths. Daily brushing with topical fluoride gels may prevent dental decay and also may prevent progression of gingivitis and periodontal disease. A variety of other highly effective products, including oral rinses, are readily available as adjuncts to routine oral hygiene procedures (41).

The basic clinical screening that should be performed on all patients is a simple oral and soft tissue examination of the head and neck:

1. Observe face and neck for any swelling, asymmetry, lesions, or unusual pigmentation, and palpate lymph nodes and glands of the face and neck.
2. Observe and palpate buccal mucosa, floor of the mouth, palate, and tongue. When observing the tongue, grasp the tip with a gauze pad, gently extend, and view both of the lateral borders of the tongue.
3. Check salivary duct patency for any signs of blockage or inflammation.
4. Check the teeth for decay, mobility, and level of oral hygiene.
5. Check the gingiva ("gum") for inflammation, purulence, and bleeding.

MANAGEMENT OF COMMON ORAL PROBLEMS IN ELDERS

As elders often see physicians and other health care providers more frequently than they see dentists, the recognition of oral problems by the non-dentist plays a key role in providing comprehensive care by facilitating early intervention and appropriate referrals for more definitive treatment. In this regard, the diagnosis of dysplastic and neoplastic lesions (leukoplakia, erythroplakia) and the identification and treatment of caries and periodontal infections are of primary importance. Prompt referral to a dentist is indicated.

Xerostomia is often reported by elders and may be managed by the use of various commercially available saliva substitutes and oral lubricants. Severe xerostomia has been treated with some success with secretagogues, including pilocarpine and carbacholine, in those patients with some residual salivary gland function (42, 43). Such patients can also benefit from the use of oral rinses containing fluoride or chlorhexidine (41).

"Burning mouth" (stomatodynia) and "burning tongue" (glossodynia) are other common complaints and may be reported together with dry mouth symptoms. Pain can be mild to severe. Vitamin deficiencies, especially vitamin B complex, may be implicated, and other conditions such as anemias and Sjögren, Mikulicz, and Plummer-

Vinson syndromes may also be associated with xerostomia and "burning" or "itching" sensations and may also be brought about by side effects of medications used to manage psychologic and psychiatric problems. Treatment may consist of drug substitution, modification of dosage of the implicated medication, use of vitamin supplements when a deficiency is identified, or use of salivary gland stimulants or saliva substitutes. In addition, subclinical oral candidiasis must be ruled out as a cause of the "burning mouth" symptoms. A course of treatment with an oral antifungal agent may be appropriate.

Denture sores (denture stomatitis) are commonly seen in elderly patients who wear dentures. Denture stomatitis may appear as reddened, inflamed areas, frequently seen on the palate corresponding with the denture base. Denture sore mouth typically results from poor oral hygiene and failure to cleanse dentures properly.

Candida albicans, normally resident in healthy persons, may proliferate in certain patients as the result of (*a*) malnutrition, (*b*) antibiotic therapy, (*c*) steroid therapy, (*d*) diabetes, or (*e*) xerostomia. Antifungal oral rinse and swallow suspensions used for a 2-week period, such as Mycostatin, are usually the treatment of first choice in uncomplicated cases. Also appropriate are clotrimazole troches, and ketoconazole and fluconazole tablets used systemically for 14 days.

Angular cheilitis is an inflammatory fissuring and ulceration at the commissures (corners) of the lips and may occur either unilaterally or bilaterally. Causes include loss of vertical dimension due to overclosure of the jaws in edentulous persons, vitamin deficiencies, and xerostomia. Infection with *C. albicans* may also be present. Treatment may include fabrication of appropriately fitting dentures, as well as use of antifungal ointments such as Mycostatin, when a diagnosis of *C. albicans* is made.

Papillary hyperplasia is often seen in patients wearing dentures for extended periods of time without removal. This condition appears as a raised papular lesion in the mucosa or gingiva under or alongside the edge of complete dentures.

Ulcerations occasionally may appear on any mucosa in older adults because of trauma or inadequate dentures. The ulceration caused by an overextended denture will, on examination, be consistent with the margin of the denture or site of irritation. If left unadjusted, the area of the ulceration may eventually lead to a reactive hypertrophy of epithelial tissue, known as an epulis fissuratum.

Fibroepithelial polyps, or irritation "fibromas," are frequently observed lesions in the buccal mucosa of the tongue, the vestibular mucosa, or the lips. They may be either sessile or pedunculated and are generally smooth-surfaced and firm upon palpation. Causes include ill-fitting dentures, irritation from fractured dental restorations or teeth, or oral habits such as cheek or lip biting. They are remarkable only if they are a source of discomfort or interfere with function.

Temporomandibular (TM) joint disorders are articulation dysfunctions of the TM joint, between the glenoid fossa of the skull and the condylar process of the mandible. Studies have generally been inconclusive in correlating physical changes such as internal derangements of the TM joint with symptomatology. Patients may experience pain, tenderness, swelling, limited movement, and clicking in the area of the joint. Pain may also be referred to the ears or temporal region and may lead to earaches or temporal headaches. Initial treatment usually is symptomatic with the use of analgesic and antiinflammatory medications. More detailed radiographic evaluation is indicated in patients with persistent or progressive symptoms.

Idiosyncratic oral manifestations of pharmacologic therapy, particularly with psychotropic drugs, are a common reason for dental consultation in the medical management of elders. In particular, polypharmacy in older persons may lead to a variety of side effects that have oral manifestations, including xerostomia, mucositis, glossodynia, stomatodynia, desquamation of the oral mucosa, and gingival bleeding.

ETHICAL ISSUES IN ORAL HEALTH CARE FOR ELDERS

Oral health care may be viewed as a value in its own right, but it must also be viewed as an integral part of comprehensive patient care. Critical as it is to the nutritional, psychologic, and physical well-being of elders, oral health care plays a key role in geriatric health assessment and treatment. Under ideal circumstances, where social, economic, and medical contraindications do not present significant barriers to treatment options, health care providers are able to reach clinical decisions about appropriate levels of care with some confidence about the long-term outcomes of the chosen interventions. Such decisions become more difficult in certain categories of older patients (15, 44, 45), particularly those with a high burden of comorbidities, those with dementia, and those with especially limited life expectancies. Ethical considerations also come into play regarding issues of informed consent to treatment in patients with certain conditions, while at the same time the dentist wishes to carry out "ideal" treatment in all patients. In geriatric dentistry we must accept a basic premise that age per se should not determine treatment. As we have learned that aging is not a major risk factor for oral diseases, we have also learned that comprehensive dental care, including implant dentistry, is highly appropriate in certain elders and even beneficial to their feelings of general well-being. Nevertheless, treatment decisions in most elders require consideration of a multiplicity of factors, medical, dental, psychological, social, and economic, to determine the most appropriate level of care to be provided. Appropriate care may be viewed as that level of intervention that considers the patient's physical and mental ability to tolerate or accept treatment, with the goal of restoration and maintenance of function, which also corresponds to the patient's own perception of need and quality of life (46–48).

The management of the oral health care needs of residents in long-term nursing care facilities presents particular dilemmas regarding how to provide comprehensive and appropriate dental care to elders who may be severely compromised. Concern for the oral health status of the patient is often not a priority in the geriatric evaluation process. While the medical and nursing staff may be aware of oral problems, there may not be a clear understanding of how such problems can be resolved nor how oral problems can play a major role in the overall well-being of the patient.

One simple triage scheme for approaching the issue of appropriateness could involve an initial level of minimal care of patients, including the elimination of sources of infection and relief of pain through an appropriate intervention (extraction, cleaning, antibiotic therapy, etc.). The subsequent restoration of teeth to establish adequate oral function would constitute intermediate care. Advanced care would comprise the full range of dental services, including endodontic and periodontal surgical care and comprehensive prosthetic dentistry. A basic set of preventive interventions, such as daily oral hygiene (self-care or assisted), topical fluorides, and oral rinses, could be made available to all patients to prevent the recurrence and progression of oral diseases. A similar program of preventive and comprehensive care would be appropriate for the ambulatory, community-dwelling elder. However, financial concerns often present a major barrier to the provision of appropriate oral health care for elders.

All can be potentially faced with significant financial burdens when different dental treatments are recommended. Few elders, either employed or retired, have insurance coverage for their oral health needs. Federal and state programs do not typically provide comprehensive, nor in many cases even minimal, oral health care benefits to elders.

Difficult judgments must be made about what level of care is to be considered "appropriate" for a particular patient. For example, should extensive dental restorative and prosthetic care be provided to patients with dementia? Should decayed teeth be extracted or aggressively treated with restorative, endodontic ("root canal"), and periodontal therapy in the patient with a short life expectancy because of an underlying medical condition? Should dentures be provided to long-term nursing care residents who did not have them before admission? Is there any circumstance in which no treatment, or "watchful waiting," is an appropriate option in geriatric dentistry? Can one specify the goals of oral health care for particular categories of patients to better determine appropriateness of care? Which elders are more likely to benefit from specific types of interventions and how can we best identify such patients?

CONCLUSION

With the ability to better identify those elders at highest risk for oral problems, we can better target our preventive and therapeutic interventions. We have learned much regarding the prevalence and severity of oral diseases, such as dental caries and periodontal diseases, in elders. In addition, the essential relationship of systemic disease development and medication usage to oral health status is now better understood, with observed age-related changes in gustation, mastication, swallowing capability, and salivary gland function evaluated in that context. In contrast, much less is known about the impact of oral conditions on general well-being. A number of other important issues remain unresolved regarding the relationship of aging and oral health status. We have made great progress in the biomedical domain but less in the psychosocial domain. What are the relationships between health behaviors and attitudes and specific oral health outcomes? Do attitudes about oral health and preventive health behaviors change with aging? How do self-assessments of elders' oral health affect their behavioral functioning, social interactions, and sense of well-being? What interventions are most effective in increasing elders' oral health-promoting behaviors and in turn their oral health and function? How do we determine appropriateness of oral health care for different groups of elders? How can the financial barriers to access to appropriate dental care, which affect the vast majority of elders, be eliminated? Finally, we need to learn to what extent improving access to, and use of, comprehensive dental care services by elders can significantly affect their oral health status and their quality of life.

REFERENCES

1. Garcia RI, Chauncey HH. Longitudinal studies of aging and oral health. J Dent Res 1991;70:865–866.
2. Ship JA, Baum BJ. Is reduced salivary flow normal in old people? Lancet 1990;336:1507.
3. Sreebny L, Valdini A. Xerostomia. Part I: relationship to other symptoms and salivary gland hypofunction. Oral Surg Oral Med Oral Pathol 1988; 66:451–458.
4. Sreebny LM, Schwartz SS. A reference guide to drugs and dry mouth. Gerodontology 1986;5:75–80.
5. Wolff A, Ship JA, Tylenda CA, Fox PC, Baum BJ. Oral mucosal appearance is unchanged in healthy, different aged individuals. Oral Surg Oral Med Oral Pathol 1991;71:569–572.
6. Feldman RS, Kapur KK, Alman JE, Chauncey HH. Aging and mastication: changes in performance and swallowing threshold with the natural dentition. J Am Geriatr Soc 1980;28:97–103.
7. Garcia RI, Perlmuter LE, Chauncey HH. Effects of dentition status and personality on masticatory performance and food acceptability. Dysphagia 1989; 4:121–126.
8. National Institute of Dental Research. Oral health of United States adults: the National Survey of Oral Health in U.S. Employed Adults and Seniors: 1985–86, national findings. National Institutes of Health NIH publ no 87–2868. Hyattsville, MD: U.S. Dept. of Health and Human Services, Public Health Service, 1987.
9. Ripa L. A half-century of community water fluoridation in the U.S.: review and commentary. J Public Health Dent 1993;53:17–44.
10. Branch BR, Antczak AA, Stason WB. Toward understanding the use of dental services by the elderly. Spec Care Dent 1986;6:38–41.
11. Bailit HL, Braun R, Maryniuk GA, Camp P. Is periodontal disease the primary cause of tooth extraction in adults? J Am Dent Assoc 1987;14:40–44.
12. Hand JS, Hunt RJ, Kohout FJ. Five-year incidence of tooth loss in Iowans aged 65 and older. Community Dent Oral Epidemiol 1991;19:48–51.
13. Chauncey HH, Glass RL, Alman JE. Dental caries. Principal cause of tooth extraction in a sample of U.S. male adults. Caries Res 1989;23:200–205.
14. Niessen LC, Weyant RJ. Cause of tooth loss in a veteran population. J Public Health Dent 1989; 49:19–23.
15. Jones JA, Lavalee N, Sinclair C, Garcia RI. Caries incidence in patients with dementia. Gerodontology 1993;10:76–82.
16. Fox PC, van der Ven P, Sonies BC, Weiffenbach JM, Baum BJ. Xerostomia: evaluation of a symptom

with increasing significance. J Am Dent Assoc 1985; 110:519–525.
17. Brown LJ, Oliver RC, Loe H. Periodontal dieases in the US in 1981: prevalence, severity, extent and role in tooth mortality. J Periodontol 1989;60:363–370.
18. Feldman RS, Bravacos JS, Rose CL. Association between smoking different tobacco products and periodontal disease indexes. J Periodontol 1983; 54:481–487.
19. Ahlqwist M, Bengtsson C, Hollender L, Lapidus L, Osterberg T. Smoking habits and tooth loss in Swedish women. Community Dent Oral Epidemiol 1989;17:144–147.
20. National Cancer Institute and National Institute of Dental Research. Tobacco effects in the mouth. Washington, DC: Government Printing Office, 1992:25–26. NIH publ. no. 92–3330.
21. Krall EA, Dawson-Hughes B. Smoking and bone loss among postmenopausal women. J Bone Miner Res 1991;6:331–337.
22. Jeffcoat MK, Chestnut CH. Systemic osteoporosis and oral bone loss. J Am Dent Assoc 1993;124:49–56.
23. Krall EA, Dawson-Hughes B, Papas A, Garcia RI. Tooth loss and skeletal bone density in healthy postmenopausal women. Osteoporosis Int 1994;4:104–109.
24. Schlossman M, Knowler WC, Pettit DJ, Genco RJ. Type II diabetes and periodontal disease. J Am Dent Assoc 1990;121:532–536.
25. Nelson RG, Schlossman M, Budding LM, et al. Periodontal disease and glucose tolerance in Pima Indians. Diabetes Care 1990;13:836–840.
26. Sreebny LM, Yu A, Green A, Valdini A. Xerostomia in diabetes mellitus. Diabetes Care 1992;15:900–904.
27. Cherry-Peppers G, Sorkin J, Andres R, Baum BJ, Ship JA. Salivary gland function and glucose metabolic status. J Gerontol 1992;47:M130–M134.
28. Sreebny LM, Valdini A, Yu A. Xerostomia part II: Relationship to nonoral symptoms, drugs and diseases. Oral Surg Oral Med Oral Pathol 1989; 68:419–427.
29. Baum BJ. Salivary gland fluid secretion during aging. J Am Geriatr Soc 1989;37:453–458.
30. Chauncey HH, Feller RP, Kapur KK. Longitudinal age-related changes in human parotid saliva composition. J Dent Res 1987;66:599–602.
31. Atkinson JC, Travis WD, Pillemer SR, et al. Major salivary gland function in primary Sjögren's syndrome and its relation to clinical features. J Rheumatol 1990;17:318–322.
32. Ship JA, DeCarli C, Friedland RP, Baum BJ. Diminished submandibular salivary flow in dementia of the Alzheimer type. J Gerontol Med Soc 1990; 45:M61–M66.
33. Fox PC, Busch KA, Baum BJ. Subjective reports of xerostomia and objective measures of salivary gland performance. J Am Dent Assoc 1987;115:581–584.
34. Narhi TO, Ainamo A, Meurman JH. Salivary yeasts, saliva, and oral mucosa in the elderly. J Dent Res 1993;72:1009–1014.
35. Stead RJ, Cooke NJ. Adverse effects of inhaled corticosteroids. Br Med J 1989;298:403–404.
36. Holmstrup P, Axell T. Classification and clinical manifestations of oral yeast infections. Acta Odontol Scand 1990;48:57–59.

37. Wayler AH, Muench ME, Kapur KK, Chauncey HH. Masticatory performance and food acceptability in persons with removable partial dentures, full dentures and intact natural dentition. J Gerontol 1984; 39:284–289.

38. Sullivan DH, Martin W, Flaxman N, Hagen JE. Oral health problems and involuntary weight loss in a population of frail elderly. J Am Geriatr Soc 1993;41:725–731.

39. Weiffenbach JM, Cowart BJ, Baum BJ. Taste intensity perception in aging. J Gerontol 1986;41:460–464.

40. Kadi J, Greer RO Jr, Jafek BW. Oral evaluation of patients with chemosensory disorders. Ear Nose Throat J 1989;63:373–380.

41. Cianco SG. Agents for the management of plaque and gingivitis. J Dent Res 1992;71:1450–1454.

42. Johnson JT, Ferretti GA, Nethery WJ, et al. Oral pilocarpine for post-irradiation xerostomia in patients with head and neck cancer. N Engl J Med 1993;329:390–395.

43. Joensuu H, Bostrom P, Makkonen T. Pilocarpine and carbacholine in treatment of radiation-induced xerostomia. Radiother Oncol 1993;26:33–37.

44. Friedlander AH, Solomon DH. Dental management of the geriatric alcoholic patient. Gerodontics 1988; 4:23–27.

45. Weyant RJ, Jones JA, Hobbins MJ, et al. Oral health status in VA nursing home residents. Community Dent Oral Epidemiol 1993;21:227–233.

46. Atchison KA, Dolan TA. Development of the Geriatric Oral Health Assessment Index. J Dent Educ 1990;54(11)680–687.

47. Gift HC, Redford M. Oral health and the quality of life. Clin Geriatr Med 1992;8(3):673–683.

48. Kressin NR, Spiro A, Bosse R, Garcia RI. Assessing oral health related quality of life: findings from the Normative Aging Study. Med Care 1994, in press.

SECTION II

Care of the Elderly Patient
Other Considerations

44/ Successful Aging

Psychosocial Factors and Implications for Primary Care Geriatrics

William Rakowski, Deborah N. Pearlman, John B. Murphy

Geriatrics is not restricted to dealing with the burdens of coping with and treating illness, impairment, and disease. In this century we have seen significant increases in life expectancy and remarkable declines in mortality at all ages. Especially in the past 10 years, major additions have been made to the gerontologic literature which emphasize the potential for sustained good health. In a longer-term historical view, it can be argued that over the past 20 years, the age period of 65 to 75 has gradually become a time of life that the large majority of older persons can hope to enjoy in good health and functional status. We are now working to bring these benefits to the oldest elderly. However, as life expectancy has increased, the importance of maintaining quality of life into old age has become clear. An important question being asked with increasing frequency is, "How can older persons achieve a truly successful aging?" With a focus on quality as well as quantity of life, the terms productive (1), healthy (2), successful (3) and effective (4) aging have attracted a great deal of interest.

This chapter reviews the literature in the area of what is commonly referred to as "psychosocial epidemiology." Generally speaking, topics in psychosocial epidemiology include a person's self-ratings of health, along with social support and social involvement. This review explores how this research may provide clinicians with insights into what may help their older patients to achieve the goal of "successful aging." Chapter 3, Health Maintenance for Older Persons, addresses lifestyle practices demonstrated to be risks for disease (e.g., smoking and heart disease) and completes the picture of psychosocial and behavioral influences on health.

The reason for dealing with successful aging as a general objective, and with these psychosocial topics specifically, is grounded in the day-to-day demands of primary care. As the chapter on the Demography of Aging illustrates, the older population is heterogeneous. A challenge facing primary care physicians is knowing which information reported by or solicited from patients is most important to act upon. Where should the physician's time be directed to benefit the patient? Studies now in the literature showing that subjective reports of how good one's health is perceived to be, of how connected the person is to social groups, and of certain lifestyle habits can be "flags" for identifying persons who are at risk of adverse health outcomes. Careful listening by the physician, along with timely follow-up questions when risks are suspected, may provide a key to early intervention that can promote a patient's successful aging.

SUCCESSFUL AGING

There is no single agreed-upon standard against which to measure successful aging—and there is no reason to expect that there ever will be such a universal consensus. Primary care physicians will adopt personal definitions to apply to their patients. Therefore, careful choice of the elements that can go into the definition is important.

ELEMENTS OF A DEFINITION

"Successful aging" conveys decidedly positive connotations about a person's status. However, several different criteria may be used as the standard for defining successful aging. These include some combination of (*a*) avoiding premature mortality; (*b*) maintaining functional health status compared with others who are declining; (*c*) improving functional status compared with one's own previous levels; (d) remaining independent despite the onset of illness and functional losses; (e) remaining productive and contributing to society through channels such as part-time work or volunteering; (f) retaining one's material and economic resources for as long as possible; (g) maintaining one's intellectual, cognitive, and creative skills; (h) adjusting psychologically to the losses that can be encountered during later adulthood; (i) maintaining positive outlooks along broad dimensions such as life satisfaction, self-concept, and future orientation; and (j) achieving an especially well-integrated life perspective and personal quality that is often called "wisdom."

These options differ in specific versus general focus, but regardless of which one is chosen, they indicate that "successful aging" is defined by much more than the function of a single organ or the absence of individual illnesses. Successful aging is a composite concept. In a 12-year longitudinal study (1971–1983), Roos and Havens (5) defined successful aging as meeting the following criteria: being alive and not in a nursing home in 1983, not more than 59 days of home care in 1983, independent in activities of daily living (ADLs), not in a wheelchair, no help needed going outdoors or walking outdoors, excellent to fair self-rated health, and seven or more correct answers on a mental status test. This definition is complex because it includes several domains; yet, 20% of their sample met these criteria after 12 years.

Guralnik and Kaplan (6) defined "healthy aging" as the top 20% of their sample on a composite index that was based on reports of functional health and exercise. Similarly, both Mor et al. (7) and Harris et al. (8) used functional status criteria (ADLs, instrumental ADLs [IADL], and higher level functional items) to create subgroups of "well elderly" and "physically able" elderly. Rowe and Kahn (3) distinguished "usual" from successful aging, with usual aging denoting normative trends that occur in the nondiseased older population.

Clearly, the Roos and Havens (5) definition is the most comprehensive of the four studies cited. In fact, it is the only one that explicitly used the term successful aging. However all four studies demonstrate the use of composite indicators rather than reliance on individual elements.

A DEFINITION FOR PRIMARY CARE PHYSICIANS

These definitional considerations are very important, but primary care geriatrics also operates under several constraints that may affect which criterion is seen as the most realistic and achievable. The amount of contact between physician and patient is extremely limited relative to the time that the individual spends alone, with family, with friends, and in other settings. In addition, physician-patient contact is often initiated by new illnesses or exacerbations of existing problems. These health issues tend to dominate appointment time. It is therefore reasonable to ask whether primary care physicians can be expected to have a heavy influence over outcomes of successful aging that are expansive or very broad, such as improved life satisfaction, enhanced productivity, maintaining intellectual and cognitive skills, or promoting creativity and contributions to society. The potential impacts of primary care physicians for successful aging are most likely (and realistically with most patients) going to be observed in health-related arenas. Influence over broader domains is a great bonus.

In any definition of successful aging, deciding whether to use the individual or the group as the reference point for comparison is an important decision. In other words, should "success" be defined idiographically (i.e., relative to the person's own prior level) or should it be defined nomothetically (i.e., relative to a group-based criterion)? The idiographic approach allows "success" to be defined in personally salient ways and makes individuals accountable only to themselves. The idiographic approach emphasizes the question, "What is my personal aging trajectory, and how can it be improved upon?" On the other hand, one individual's progress may not seem especially significant in the bigger picture of what occurs in the larger population. Small personal gains relative to a disadvantaged starting point often do not seem that important. This is the classic issue faced by clinicians in the care of chronically ill persons for whom progress often comes only in small steps achieved by hard work by both the patient and the clinician, with no highly visible reward beyond the satisfaction of having made a small but positive contribution.

In contrast, the nomothetic approach provides a population-based standard against which successful aging can be defined. Because it is population-based, this standard is likely to have greater acceptability by some professionals and government. Individuals or groups who are outperforming a reference population almost automatically gain attention, praise, and perhaps more resources to continue their efforts. This type of comparative approach is consistent with how success is culturally defined in competitive circumstances such as athletic events or professionally by the researcher's continuing quest to secure federal grant dollars and to publish papers.

However, this similarity to competition is also the root of a potential difficulty with the nomothetic approach. In particular, although outperforming a large group is hard to deny as a criterion for ascribing success, there is also the risk that an increasingly stringent criterion will be applied over time to define what constitutes success. While we have no intention of dampening the goals and performance of the truly exceptional older person or the especially influential physician, it is also important to maintain a critical eye on what should define success for individuals who are engaged in meeting the demands of daily life, often with nagging chronic conditions.

Therefore, an appropriate and modest definition of successful aging that might be considered as a goal by physicians in primary care geriatrics would be for the patient to remain in good functional health for as long as possible. In essence, this means optimizing what is commonly referred to as "active life expectancy"—years of life that are free of limitations on performing regular daily activities because of illnesses or other conditions. Active life expectancy emphasizes the quality of years alive, not simply extending the number of those years.

This definition is especially useful because it can be used in two ways. On one hand, it can be used nomothetically, by contrasting a patient's status with a normative, population-level database. On the other hand, it can be used idiographically, by comparing individuals with their own previous status, i.e., taking their own aging trajectory as the reference point.

In sum, the criteria for defining successful aging set the goals toward which persons are encouraged to strive. Our position is that successful aging should not be defined by criteria that require "heroic efforts" to be achieved. From the standpoint of the physician in clinical practice, it would seem prudent to adopt a position that allows as many persons as possible to believe that they can experience "successful aging" in some way. If an older individual either has the potential to outperform, or is in fact outperforming, the nomothetic reference group, that information can be legitimately conveyed and the goal can be pursued. However, the physician should be equally ready to adopt an idiographic approach for patients whose success in aging is most likely going to be based on maintaining or exceeding their own prior status. For those patients, successfully influencing the course of their own aging is an appro-

priate, justified, and valuable reward. The challenge, of course, lies in finding clues during medical visits that give insights into an older person's individual aging process and then devising intervention strategies to help that older person age as successfully as possible. Self-reports of health status and of social involvements are two sources of such clues.

SELF-ASSESSMENTS OF HEALTH

The potential relationships between personal state-of-mind and effects on physical health have been discussed and researched for decades. In research on aging, one of the intriguing questions has been whether individuals' subjective assessments of their health could somehow influence subsequent physical health status for better or worse—perhaps even at the level of mortality rates. The intuitive hypothesis is that favorable assessments would be reflected in a longevity advantage and that mortality rates would increase as subjective ratings become more negative. In large part, that hypothesis has been confirmed in several studies, although there are exceptions (9).

GLOBAL RATINGS OF HEALTH

Investigations of subjective health assessments and mortality have used simple questions, amenable to the design of large surveys. These questions are also very amenable to colloquial discussion during a patient visit. Most investigations have used a single question asked at a baseline interview to predict subsequent health status. One type of question is, "Would you say your health in general is excellent, very good, good, fair, or poor?" (10). This question implies no comparison with other persons, such as age peers. A second type of question asks for a subjective assessment relative to age peers or even to chronological age (e.g., "For your age would you say, in general, your health is excellent, good, fair, poor, or bad," [11]; "Compared to other people your own age, would you say that your general health is excellent, good, fair, poor, or very poor" [12]).

Several reports now show that older persons who rate their health "fair" or "poor" have a higher risk of mortality than persons who rate it "excellent" (1, 8, 10–16). In some of these reports, even persons who rate their health "good" rather than "excellent" show a higher risk of death during the follow-up period.

This consistency is impressive for several reasons. First, subjective health has been routinely assessed with a single question that has a simple four- or five-category set of responses. The fact that such a basic assessment repeatedly shows a relationship to mortality suggests that a reliable relationship exists. This relationship between subjective ratings and mortality appears to hold for women and for men (10, 16). Secondly, relationships between subjective ratings at a baseline interview and later mortality have been found over periods covering up to 12 years. Predictive associations over such a range of time attest to a phenomenon that should not be ignored. Third, these predictive relationships have been found despite the use of procedures that statistically correct for numerous other variables such as age, gender, social support, medical conditions, and functional health status, which might effect mortality.

The fact that two versions of a general self-rating are used (i.e., without and with comparison to a reference group) raises the question of whether they are interchangeable or whether each one contributes unique information. Recent data support the latter, showing that both versions of the general health rating made a contribution to predicting mortality over 6 years when they were used simultaneously in a statistical analysis (14). The information the answers provide is therefore not entirely redundant, which suggests that the primary care physician should seriously consider comments by patients that they perceive themselves as being less healthy or active than age peers.

OTHER RATINGS AND OUTCOMES

Some studies have used ratings other than the global self-assessment, and some have used self-ratings to predict outcomes other than mortality. Perceiving a lack of projects for the future was related to mortality over 4 years in a rural French sample (17). Other analyses showed that persons with poorer self-rated health, with a lack of future projects, and who felt useless had greater loss of functional status over 4 years (18). Feeling useless was most robustly associated with mortality in analyses that controlled for age, sex, and several other variables. In addition, the risk of mortality is higher for older persons with at least one impairment in ADLs who also gave "old age" as the main cause of that impairment (19).

COMMENTS ON SELF-RATED HEALTH

The epidemiologic data cited above have come from secondary analyses of surveys that were not designed specifically to study self-rated health or successful aging. Furthermore, findings to date have also been constrained by the content of those surveys. For example, there are no studies yet that have obtained self-rated health information at two points in time, such as a year apart, to investigate whether changes in self-assessment are associated with longer-term health-related outcomes. Deliberately incorporating more self-assessment questions in baseline and follow-up surveys will permit analyses to address more complex issues relevant for patient care.

At the present time there is no solid evidence that shows why the association between baseline self-assessments and subsequent health status exists. As noted above, controlling for health status explains some of the association, but not completely. One possibility is that more sophisticated physical and functional status assessment measures will account for even more of the association. If so, then the effects for self-rated health would only be a marker for the effects of physical status. However, this extreme outcome is not likely, since self-rated health and objective health appear to be different phenomena. That is, although physical health and self-rated health are correlated, the association between them is not perfect.

It is also possible that favorable self-assessments influence health status through physiologic mediators. If self-assessments reflect other day-to-day psychological affective states, such as depression, then such general life outlooks may have physical sequelae. For example, the social support literature poses the hypothesis that psychological status can influence susceptibility to illness through effects on neuroendocrine or immune system function (20). Review of this possibility is beyond the scope of this chapter, but it is an intriguing area of study.

Finally, self-assessments may affect health status because of an intermediate association with health-related practices. Persons with more favorable self-ratings may act on symptoms of illness in a more timely fashion than persons who already believe that their health is poor. The important point is that although both groups act on a symptom, the difference may lie in such aspects of the action as timeliness and persistence after symptom perception. To the extent that persons with unfavorable self-ratings tend to have less timely or consistent preventive and symptom-related actions, they are giving over control of long-term health outcomes to the fundamental soundness of their biology. If their fundamental biology is strong, their long-term health status will be adequate. However, if their fundamental biology or the function of key organs is frail, then decline will be rapid and reflected in morbidity and mortality outcomes. Persons with poorer evaluations of their health may also take a longer time to label something as a "symptom" that needs to have action taken. The implication is that even though the time from "symptom labeling" until "taking action" would be the same for persons with better and those with poorer self-rated health, those perceiving poorer health may have inadvertently delayed contacting a physician by having a longer time pass before labeling something as a problem in the first place.

SOCIAL INVOLVEMENTS AND SUPPORT

In recent decades a great deal of research has demonstrated the positive effects of social support. The evidence suggests that being integrated into a network of family and friends reduces the risk of morbidity and mortality (3, 21–23). Mortality has been significantly related to outside-home activities, social activities (the higher the activity the lower the mortality), and the number of persons per household (the more persons the lower the mortality) even when controlling for age, health status, and coronary heart disease risk factors (24). For example, unmarried and socially isolated people are more likely to become ill or die than persons who are socially integrated (e.g., married, involved with extended family, friends, and organizations).

There are still areas of debate and uncertainty regarding whether the preferred concept should be "social support," "social network," "social involvement," or "social integration." These discussions are important in theoretical formulations and research development because the choice of definition affects the way questions are asked in a survey or in the clinical setting. Differences in definition, however, should not obscure the fact that social context is important for health and that indications of a patient's social support need to be attended to by primary care providers. We use the term social support in this chapter knowing that some imprecision still exists; but we prefer to emphasize issues and findings that have widespread endorsement and clinical relevance.

Although there is broad acceptance that social support influences health and mortality, there is still debate about how social support prevents illness and/or enhances health. At least two explanations have been offered. The "main effects" hypothesis states that social support has an independent and positive effect on individual well-being even when other potential explanatory variables are included in an analysis (21). This means that the presence or absence of social support influences health to a comparable degree—for better or worse—across persons with a wide variety of personal characteristics (this is referred to as a "main effect" in statistical terminology). This benefit could occur through the transmission of health beliefs and values in the social network or through the active encouragement of health-promoting behaviors (25, 26).

The second view, the "buffering effect" hypothesis, states that social support is effective primarily in circumstances of stress rather than in general (27, 28). There are three ways in which support may promote health when stressors exist: the perception that others are willing to help may bolster the ability to cope with a stressful situation; social support might influence biologic responses to a stressful situation (e.g., blood pressure) so that individuals are less reactive to stress; or, social support might affect physical health and mortality indirectly through its effect on high-risk coping behaviors such as drinking and smoking (20, 25, 26). House et al. (23) boldly claim that the absence of social support is a risk factor for morbidity and mortality which rivals the effects of many well-established health risk factors such as smoking, obesity, and high blood pressure.

AGE DIFFERENCES

Among the elderly, the role of social support in maintaining health and promoting recovery from illness is important because aging is associated with increased health and social problems and thus greater need for help. The benefits of social support may be less available to the elderly than to younger adults, in that aging is often accompanied by a constriction of social relationships frequently associated with the death of relatives and friends (29–31). In addition, problems with physical mobility may make it more difficult to maintain relationships later in life (32). Thus, to the extent that social support influences recovery from or adaptation to health problems, elderly persons can be at a disadvantage (30).

On a more optimistic note, however, older people's support networks are not necessarily devastated by aging. The elderly have smaller networks than younger people do, as people in the older person's support network die and are not replaced. Yet the elderly live closer to, and have more frequent contact with, persons in their support network than younger persons do, and older persons also have known their network members longer (21, 29, 32, 33).

Because the need for health-related support increases with age, age-related losses in the size of the social network could result in diminished access to social support at a time of critical need. A wide social network, however, does not necessarily ensure adequate social support. Individuals who depend on a small intimate core of family members or friends generally cope better with serious health problems than those who have a wider support network but lack intimate relationships (27). Thus it seems prudent for clinicians to ask specific questions about who provides the support (e.g., spouse, adult child, friend, neighbor), how well the patient knows the support provider, and the type of support provided for specific problems. In addition, support should be recognized as a two-way street. Reciprocity is an important feature of social interaction. Few persons truly enjoy always being "supported." Even persons with a family caregiver because of health problems want to feel that they can still contribute or give something meaningful in return.

GENDER DIFFERENCES

Many researchers have noted that the nature of social ties is different for women and men. Women appear to have larger networks and a greater variety of people in those networks, providing many kinds of support (32, 34). In addition, women are more likely than men to keep in touch with kin, to be more involved in kin-related activities (35), and to mention their friends as confidants (34). Women's extensive social support resources have important implications in later life. Older women are more likely than older men to be living with family members or to be living closer to children and to have more contact with close friends and neighbors (21, 31, 32, 36–38). In addition to having a wider range of supportive relationships, older women are more likely than their male counterparts to have interpersonal relationships that are characterized by intimacy, advice, guidance, and emotional support (31, 32).

Gender differences also occur in the exchange of social support. Older women are more likely than older men to receive emotional and social support from children (32, 34, 36, 38) and to think that elderly persons, if unable to care for themselves, should be cared for by children and other close family members (39).

In contrast, the social supports of older men are more limited. Men rely more heavily for instrumental and emotional support on a single person, their wives (34, 37, 40). Men's paucity of close relationships has led to widespread concern that older men who outlive their spouses easily become isolated (40). As noted, the loss of health leading to physical or mental impairment is a major stressor, and the lack of supportive social relationships is a risk factor for morbidity and mortality (23, 40). It can be argued that the greater diversity in older women's relationships—both in range and type of social resources—may give women a "support advantage," balancing the effects of aging on health (32).

Findings from the bereavement literature offer some additional insights into successful aging. Widowhood affects physical health and mortality, but the effect is greater for men than for women (21, 25). For men, the situation may be characterized more by a continuing state of low levels of social support and integration. It may be important for physicians to deliberately encourage the activation of an older man's network, rather than assume it is operating and conveying benefits.

IMPLICATIONS FOR CLINICAL PRACTICE

Risk factor identification in clinical settings (both medical and psychosocial risks) needs to take into consideration the exigencies of the clinical practice of primary care geriatrics and thus must be practical. There is only sufficient time to gather the most important information and to do so in an efficient manner. The precious little time available in clinical encounters should not be spent on activities that are unlikely to produce tangible results. Since the relationships between self-rated health and social support with health outcomes are correlational and not necessarily causal, one might contend that pursuing these psychosocial variables as part of a clinical encounter is not justified. However, unlike many medical assessments, these domains can be assessed without expensive and invasive methods. Furthermore, in addition to identifying powerful predictors of subsequent health outcomes, the process of gathering this information shows the patient interest and caring on the part of the clinician. Finally, much of the necessary data can be gathered reliably and efficiently.

In the domain of self-perceived health, two brief questions are likely to be the very effective markers: "Would you say that your health is excellent, very good, good, fair, or poor?" and "Compared with others your age, would you say that your health is excellent, very good, good, fair, or poor?" Persons willing to answer only fair or poor certainly merit follow-up, but even a "good" response might be alerting, depending on the patient's tone of voice and overall demeanor.

Social support is more difficult to assess briefly. However, tools exist that allow reliable and efficient data collection (41). The "family genogram" (42) and the "family circle" (43) are two such tools, which graphically represent family structure and social support in the medical record. Epidemiologic investigations have often obtained results by asking relatively straightforward questions about regularity of contact with family and friends and activities usually done outside of one's residence such as membership in clubs, going to spectator events such as movies, and even doing volunteer work. It is important to note that the objective is not to convince persons to be involved in all of these activities—having at least a few is sufficient. Instead, attention is directed at those persons who seem to be the least involved, to try and determine whether increasing their social connectedness will be a benefit. And, being alert for the reciprocity of the patient's social interactions is advised.

Well-established strategies for interventions to remedy continually poor self-perceived health status and sustained, limited social support are currently lacking. As noted earlier, poor self-perceived health in the patient who lacks objective evidence of poor health for such an extreme view may just be the result of inaccuracies that undoubtedly can accompany one-question, global impressions (e.g., a transient mood, the recent death of a close friend). However, encountering such a discrepancy should still clue the clinician to look for an as yet undiagnosed illness or to try harder to remedy a patient's harmful health-related behaviors. An argument can be made for monitoring self-rated health and social support just as one monitors physical and cognitive function (see Chapter 2), and the lack of tested interventions should not preclude such monitoring.

A CAUTION ON EMPLOYING THE CONCEPT OF SUCCESSFUL AGING

Using the label of "successful aging" in geriatrics and applying it to older persons with certain characteristics begs the issue of what constitutes "unsuccessful aging." This question arises most immediately in two contexts. First, are individuals who are not labeled as aging successfully automatically designated as aging unsuccessfully? And secondly, are older persons initially designated as aging successfully now suddenly considered unsuccessful if their status falls below the criterion point?

These are significant questions not only for the self-concept of the older person but also for the primary care physician who must interpret health status changes to a patient. It is all well and good to hold up lofty and intellectually gratifying standards for a goal such as successful aging, but it is also necessary to keep a perspective on how persons are labeled and treated when they do not meet those standards.

Another consideration is the implication that successful aging is under the individual's personal control. On one hand, the label of aging successfully would denote positive evaluations of the individual's skills and certainly be a boost to one's ego. On the other hand, to imply that someone is not aging successfully could just as easily be taken as a judgment that the individual had somehow failed and therefore become a severe blow to one's self-concept. This situation would be unfair, since the course of one's aging is not completely under personal control.

In short, the concept of successful aging is a double-edged sword, and our good intentions to use it as a standard for giving praise and stimulating motivation should not blind us to the possibility of doing a disservice to other older persons. Some older persons may, in fact, age unsuccessfully. However, trying to arrive at that definition would require a separate chapter, probably much more complex than the present one.

CONCLUSION

As a popular saying goes, "If it were easy to do, it would have been done already." Creating a definition of successful aging, as well as integrating the concept into primary care geriatrics, falls squarely into that category. The big picture can indeed be complex and will take years of research and practice to refine—if it can ever truly be accomplished to anyone's ultimate satisfaction. The approach taken and recommendations made in this chapter have purposely adopted a modest view of the definition of success. The reader is encouraged to review more empirically detailed, disciplinarily diverse, and perhaps more interesting discussions of successful aging than the one here (e.g., 44).

However, primary care physicians can take actions to promote successful aging among their patients. Psychosocial and behavioral factors are important, and indications of a patient's status are not difficult to obtain. Everyone needs a reason to get out of bed in the morning, and these social, psychological, and behavioral elements of life seem to be second to none in providing such reasons. Remember that successful aging need not follow a lock-step model or formula for everyone. Just as the older population itself is diverse, different paths can be followed. In the experience of personal aging and the process of one's life review, it would be among the most horrifying of thoughts that there was no longer a way to reap a measure of success from the final years of one's life. Primary care physicians who can help to leave this opportunity open, if only in the domain of physical health and functioning, will be performing a truly useful service beyond medical care per se.

REFERENCES

1. Butler RN, Gleason HP, eds. Productive aging: enhancing vitality in later life. New York: Springer, 1985.
2. Benfante R, Reed D, Brody J. Biologic and social predictors of health in an aging cohort. J Chronic Dis 1985;38:385–389.
3. Rowe JW, Kahn RL. Human aging: usual and successful. Science 1987;237:143–149.
4. Curb JD, Guralnik JM, LaCroix AZ, et al. Effective aging: meeting the challenge of growing older. J Am Geriatr Soc 1990;38:827–828.
5. Roos NP, Havens B. Predictors of successful aging: a twelve-year study of Manitoba elderly. Am J Public Health 1991;81:63–68.
6. Guralnik JM, Kaplan GA. Predictors of healthy aging: prospective evidence from the Alameda County study. Am J Public Health 1989;79:703–708.
7. Mor V, Murphy J, Masterson-Allen S, et al. Risk of functional decline among well elders. J Clin Epidemiol 1989;42:895–904.
8. Harris T, Kovar MG, Suzman R, Klienman JC, Feldman JJ. Longitudinal study of physical ability in the oldest old. Am J Public Health 1989;79:698–702.
9. Idler EL, Angel RJ. Self-rated health and mortality in the NHANES-I Epidemiologic Follow-up Study. Am J Public Health 1990;80:446–452.
10. Idler EL, Kasl SV. Health perceptions and survival: do global evaluations of health status really predict mortality? J Gerontol 1990;46:S55–65.
11. Mossey JM, Shapiro E. Self-rated health: a predictor of mortality among the elderly. Am J Public Health 1982;72:800–808.
12. Idler EL, Kasl SV, Lemke JH. Self-evaluated health and mortality among the elderly in New Haven, Connecticut and Iowa and Washington Counties, Iowa, 1982–1986. Am J Epidemiol 1990;131:91–103.
13. Rakowski W, Mor V, Hiris J. The association of self-rated health with two-year mortality in a sample of well-elderly from the Longitudinal Study of Aging. J Aging Health 1991;3:527–545.
14. Rakowski W, Fleishman J, Mor V, Bryant S. Self-assessments of health and mortality among older persons: do questions other than global self-rated health predict mortality? Res Aging 1993;1:92–116.
15. Jagger C, Clarke M. Mortality risks in the elderly: five year follow-up of a total population. Int J Epidemiol 1988;17:111–114.
16. Wolinsky FD, Johnson RJ. Perceived health status and mortality among older men and women. J Gerontol 1992;47:S304–312.
17. Grand A, Grosclaude P, Bocquet H, Pous J, Albarede JL. Disability, psychosocial factors and mortality among the elderly in a rural French population. J Clin Epidemiol 1990;43:773–782.
18. Grand A, Grosclaude P, Bocquet H, Pous J, Albarede HL. Predictive value of life events, psychosocial factors and self-rated health on disability in an elderly rural French population. Soc Sci Med 1988; 12:1337–1342.
19. Rakowski W, Hickey T. Mortality and the attribution of health problems to aging among older adults. Am J Public Health 1992;8:1139–1141.
20. Cohen S, Syme SL. Issues in the study and application of social support. In: Cohen S, Syme SL, eds. Social support and health. New York: Academic Press, 1985:3–22.
21. Antonucci TC. Personal characteristics, social support, and social behavior. In: Shanas E, Binstock RH, eds. Handbook of aging and social sciences. 2nd ed. New York: Van Nostrand, 1985:94–128.
22. Antonucci TC, Jackson JJ. Social support, interpersonal efficacy, and health: a life course perspective. In: Carstensen L, Edelstein BA, eds. Handbook of clinical gerontology. New York: Pergamon, 1987: 291–311.
23. House JS, Landis KR, Umberson D. Social relationships and health. Science 1988;241:540–549.
24. Welin L, Tibblin G, Svardsudd K, Ander-Peciva S, et al. Prospective study of social influences on mortality: the study of men born in 1913 and 1923. Lancet 1985;1(8434):915–918.
25. Berkman LF. The relationship of social networks and social support to morbidity and mortality. In: Cohen S, Syme SL, eds. Social support and health. New York: Academic Press, 1985:241–262.
26. Umberson D. Family status and health behaviors: social control as a dimension of social integration. J Health Soc Behav 1987;28:306–319.
27. Arling G. Strain, social support and distress in old age. J Gerontol 1987;42:107–113.
28. Cohen S, Wills TA. Stress, social support, and the buffering hypothesis. Psychol Bull 1985;98:310–357.
29. Antonucci TC, Akiyama H. Social networks in adult life and a preliminary examination of the convoy model. J Gerontol 1987;42:519–527.
30. Minkler M. Social support and health of the elderly. In: Cohen S, Syme SL, eds. Social support and health. New York: Academic Press, 1985:199–213.
31. Vaux A. Variations in social support associated with gender, ethnicity, and age. J Soc Issues 1985;41:89–110.
32. Depner CE, Ingersoll-Dayton B. Supportive relationships in later life. Psychol Aging 1988;3:348–357.
33. Antonucci TC, Depner CE. Social support and informal helping relationships. In: Wills TA, ed. Basic processes in helping relationships. New York: Academic Press, 1982:233–254.
34. Antonucci TC, Akiyama H. An examination of sex differences in social support among older men and women. Sex Roles 1987;17:737–749.
35. Chappell N. Health and helping among the elderly: gender differences. J Aging Health 1989;1:102–120.
36. Hess B. Sex roles, friendship and the life course. Res Aging 1979;1:494–515.
37. Powers EA, Bultena GL. Sex differences in intimate friendships of old age. J Marriage Fam 1976; 38:739–747.
38. Spitze G, Logan J. Gender differences in family support: is there a payoff? Gerontologist 1989;29:108–113.

39. Seelbach WC. Gender differences in expectations for filial responsibility. Gerontologist 1977;17:421–425.
40. Levitt MJ, Antonucci TC, Clark MC, Rotton J, Gordon EF. Social support and well-being: preliminary indicators based on two samples of the elderly. Int J Aging Hum Dev 1985–86;21:61–77.
41. Saultz JW. Family-centered health care. In: Taylor RB, ed. Family medicine: principles and practice. 3rd ed. New York: Springer, 1988.
42. Jolly W, Froom J, Rosen MG. The genogram. J Fam Pract 1980;10:251–255.
43. Thrower SM, Bruce WE, Walton RF. The family circle method for integrating family systems concepts in family medicine. J Fam Pract 1982;15:451–457.
44. Baltes PB, Baltes MM, eds. Successful aging: perspectives from the behavioral sciences. Cambridge: Cambridge University Press, 1990.

45/ Cell Biology and Physiology of Aging

John J. Brink, William Reichel

Aging in humans is a universal biologic and psychological phenomenon that is associated with positive and negative connotations determined by the cultural environment. In physical terms, normal aging may be considered as the time-related differential decline in biologic functions of both the whole organism and its parts, ultimately resulting in death. In psychological terms, normal aging may be considered as the development of the individual accompanied by age-specific culturally determined roles and expectations.

A distinction should be made between loss of function because of aging and loss of function because of disease. Normal aging may be accompanied by a decline in the number or capacity of cells needed for optimal functioning of the individual. Disease states of individual components, while often age-related, imply a potential for prevention or reversibility of pathology. An example of normal aging is the age-related loss of neurons in the brain, while disease states include severe memory impairment, malignancy, cataracts, presbycusis, and marked skin wrinkling.

The dual processes of the loss of cells and gradual decline in function are associated with aging, which combined with the accumulation of abnormal changes associated with disease, promote a distorted view of aging. The functional decline of a critical organ such as the brain because of Alzheimer's disease or Parkinson's disease is often misconstrued as the result of an aging process, even though other organs may still be normal. The frequency of pathology with age beyond 30 years is unfortunately common. Thus "old age" becomes synonymous with diseases such as osteoporosis, atherosclerosis, and cancer. The inability to distinguish between nonpathological aging and pathology-related aging is a result of medical advances that make prevention and treatment of disease increasingly possible.

To more clearly define the biologic and molecular changes known to occur, aging can be divided into two domains comprised of intrinsic and extrinsic factors (Table 45.1). Intrinsic factors include the individual's genetic constitution, which determines maximum longevity, while extrinsic factors are environmental exposures that impinge on the individual's survival in the environment. Both overfeeding and starvation contribute to shorter than average life spans in many animal species, and the ability of these and other extrinsic factors to influence expression of genetic potential has been studied extensively in the past decade, although not specifically in humans. A distinction has to be made between a substantial deprivation of food intake (starvation) and partial reduction (i.e., 30% to 60%) in daily food consumption. In the former case, deterioration of survival capacity is accelerated, whereas in the latter case, biologic adaptation to diminished oxygen demands (lower metabolic rate) slows deterioration in laboratory animals. Whether such dietary reduction will retard aging in humans remains to be seen (1).

GENETIC FACTORS

The existence of genes associated with the aging process is indicated by the wide variation in maximal survival times among different organisms (2). These times can vary from 4600 years for the bristlecone pine to 4 to 6 weeks for the fruit fly. Among mammals the average longevity ranges from a low of 12 months for the shrew to between 70 and 80 years in humans. Studies on longevity in fruit flies have shown that their average life span can be extended by inbreeding of long-lived individuals. The health and activity of these long-lived progeny also seems to be more youthful than age-matched normals (3). Similar inbreeding experiments with mice gave the same result of extended life span. Moreover, it is known that human longevity is enhanced in people with long-lived parents who lived under similar lifestyle and economic conditions (4).

Early studies by Hayflick (5) on the mitotic capacity of isolated human fibroblasts to reproduce

Table 45.1
Biologic Factors in Human Aging

Factors	Biologic Role
Intrinsic	
Genetics	Genes specifically acquired to retard aging effects of endogenous metabolic toxins and genes to suppress the tendency toward unlimited cell proliferation
Basal metabolism	Maintenance of energy-generating capacity by mitochondrial DNA and its decline by damage to it from oxygen radicals
Endocrine system	Progressive decline in reproductive and homeostatic functions beyond age 30
Immune system	Gradual functional loss of immune responses needed for protection against extrinsic pathogens
Extrinsic	
Exercise	Protection against chronological decline of organ systems
Diet	Retardation of functional loss by balanced food intake
	Excessive or unbalanced dietary intake leading to cardiovascular disease
Mutagens	Enhanced decline of normal and orderly function of genes
Radiation	Destruction of genetic control of tissue functions

in cell culture have shown that such cells can reproduce only a limited number of times. When skin fibroblasts from individuals of different ages were cultured, a calculation of the maximum number of mitoses that remained in these cells showed a net decline of mitotic capacity with age. Starting with a maximum of 61 mitoses remaining for cells from newborns, the numbers decline by three mitotic divisions per subsequent decade of life (3, 6). Extrapolation of this value to an age for zero remaining divisions suggests a maximal reproductive life for fibroblasts from normal humans of somewhat more than 200 years. This restricted mitotic potential has been confirmed for similar cells derived from many other species and has a unique value for each species (6).

The existence of a finite number of cell doublings in differentiated cells is accounted for by a molecular mechanism in chromosomes that pre-vents terminal ends of the chromosomes (telomeres) from being completely replicated in each mitotic cycle (7). Each successive cell division causes a progressive shortening of a repeating nucleotide sequence (TTAGGG) in the telomere until a point is reached at which DNA replication is no longer possible (8). Malignant cells, sperm, and ova express a gene, not active in cells with limited mitotic potential, that produces the enzyme telomerase to *correct* the mitotic shortening of telomeres and thus confer immortality on these and other cells. The HeLa cell line is an example of an immortal human cell line that expresses this gene (7).

Immortalization or malignant transformation of cells can arise from other genetic mechanisms as well, such as through the action of genes that control cell proliferation in normal growth. Cells produce protective enzymes that counteract metabolic toxins that otherwise might lead to genetic and cellular damage and induce malignant transformation. These protective components, derived from both internal and external sources, are listed in Table 45.2. If these protective mechanisms fail, cell transformation may result.

BASAL METABOLISM

The cellular locus of energy production from oxygen resides in the mitochondria. As a result of normal metabolic activity, reactive free radical derivatives of oxygen such as superoxide anion (O_2^-) and hydrogen peroxide (H_2O_2) are generated

Table 45.2
Aging Resistance Factors in Cells

Endogenous protection (cellular origins)	
Enzymes that degrade free radicals and peroxides	Superoxide dismutase
	Catalase
	Glutathione peroxidase
Enzymes that facilitate replacement of damaged cellular components	Peptidases (proteins)
	Phospholipases (membranes)
	Nucleases (DNA)
Exogenous protection (dietary origins)	
Compounds that act as free radical scavengers	Vitamin E (tocopherol)
	Vitamin A (retinol)
	Vitamin C (ascorbate)
	BHT (butylated hydroxytoluene)
Factors that reduce free radical production	Diminished food consumption by 30–60% of optimal caloric intake

and produce destructive oxidation of membranes, proteins, and DNA. The major defenses against such destruction are the protective enzymes superoxide dismutase and catalase, which remove the reactive free radicals derived from O_2^- and H_2O_2, as well as regenerative systems such as the enzymes associated with the removal, repair, and replacement of cell constituents. Components that turn over slowly or not at all, such as proteins and DNA, will accumulate damage over time. This damage eventually leads to the cell's demise or impairment of cellular function. The lipofuscin pigment found in aged neurons as a result of their high metabolic activity is typical of the oxidative debris found in cells. DNA in neuronal mitochondria is particularly vulnerable to oxidative damage because these cells do not multiply after birth. Oxidative debris is also seen in other tissues where a common measure for metabolic loss is the decline in VO_2max, the maximum oxygen extraction capacity of the lungs (9–11).

Cross-sectional studies of the aging population have shown that several physiologic parameters such as body weight, basal metabolism, renal clearance, and cardiovascular function decline with age (12, 13). Longitudinal studies on the other hand, suggest that specific individuals show gains rather than losses with age (13). Buskirk and Hodgson found that the VO_2max in some older exercising individuals was elevated relative to generally sedentary peers, even though the slopes for decline for both groups were parallel (10). Aging, as measured by loss of physiologic function, thus needs to be defined in more precise terms that distinguish between "usual," "normal," and "ideal" changes. Usual aging may be considered to be the culturally defined biologic and psychological losses with age that vary with degrees of pathology. Normal aging is that associated with nonpathological longitudinal changes in biologic function between 35 to 100 years of age. Ideal aging is that situation where biologic capacity is optimized for overall function with exercise, nutrition, and other factors in the absence of pathology.

Reduction in the levels of superoxide dismutase, caused by progressive loss of expression of its gene with age, may account for many of the age-related declines in physiologic function. It has been shown that fruit flies endowed with increased longevity had higher levels of superoxide dismutase activity in their cells (14). Mechanisms for reducing free radical damage in cells can also be found in the activity of dietary antioxidants such as vitamin E, vitamin A, vitamin C, and butylated hydroxytoluene (BHT) (14). Experiments have demonstrated that diets high in vitamin E

or BHT have the capacity to prolong the life span of mice and chickens (15). Whether similar modification of the diet will also prolong the life span of humans remains to be seen.

ENDOCRINE AND IMMUNE SYSTEMS

Maturation of reproductive organs is influenced by hormones with both cellular and genetic effects. Cellular factors that activate cell mitosis are mediated by a class of genes designated as proto-oncogenes in the normal state or oncogenes in the mutated condition. The proto-oncogenes are expressed early during cellular development and differentiation to allow control of functions that are expressed in the mature cell. Estrogens and androgens stimulate cell growth and function by modulating expression of the proto-oncogenes. This in turn promotes or suppresses growth-regulatory mechanisms within specific cells.

Aging is associated with the accumulation of somatic mutations in regulatory genes, leading to the loss of coordinated control of cell growth and function. Several genes known as tumor-suppressor genes can suppress the activity of the oncogenes that otherwise would cause mature cells to undergo abnormal mitosis resulting in tumors (16). During normal maturation, steroid hormones serve as activators for specific genes that stimulate mitosis and growth of reproductive organs. All the while, this is achieved by metabolic suppression of the action of tumor-suppressor genes so that cell proliferation can take place in a controlled manner. When hormone levels decline with age, the tumor-suppressor genes become active again unless they have mutated so that suppressor function is lost. These mutational changes probably account for the increased probability of tumors with advanced age.

The loss of a tumor-suppressor gene is, in fact, the most common somatic mutation of human cancers (17). The frequency of somatic mutations in oncogenes and tumor-suppressor genes increases with age as a result of exposures to mutagens including dietary mutagens, radiation, and transforming viruses such as papilloma virus, immunodeficiency virus (HIV) and T-cell lymphotropic virus (HTLV) (18). Such mutational events perturb the mitotic inhibition state of mature cells, allowing activation of mitotic factors from oncogenes.

CONCLUSION

Immune system cells such as T and B lymphocytes are regulated by specific hormones such as interleukin-1 (IL-1), interleukin-2 (IL-2), tumor necrosis factor, and interferon, all of which control proliferation and differentiation in lymphocytes in response to antigenic exposure. In those situations, where excessive stimulation of IL-2 secretion by T lymphocytes is caused by abnormal antigen signaling, the resultant stimulation of T cells may lead to activation of autoimmune responses found in age-related diseases such as arthritis (19, 20).

In summary, it appears that both aging and associated pathology result from the decline in homeostasis of factors that regulate cellular proliferation and maintenance. Future attempts to retard the cellular aging process will have to manipulate genes at many levels. A better understanding of aging versus disease will emerge from longitudinal studies of aging, a search for potentially mutable risk factors, and long-term dietary intervention studies in humans.

REFERENCES

1. Finch CE. Longevity, senescence and the genome. Chicago: University of Chicago Press, 1990:504.
2. Reichel W. The biology of aging. J Am Geriatr Soc 1966;14:431–446.
3. Rose MR. Evolutionary biology of aging. New York: Oxford University Press, 1991:130.
4. Goldstein S, Gallo JJ, Reichel W. Biologic theories of aging. Am Fam Physician 1989;40:195–200.
5. Hayflick L. The limited in vitro lifetime of human diploid cell strains. Exp Cell Res 1965;37:614–636.
6. Goldstein S, Reichel W. Physiological and biological aspects of aging. In: Reichel W, ed. Clinical aspects of aging. 2nd ed. Baltimore: Williams & Wilkins, 1983:511–517.
7. Levy MZ, Allsopp RC, Futcher AB, Greider CW, Harley CB. Telomere end-replication problem and cell aging. J Mol Biol 1992;225:951–960.
8. Moyzis RK. The human telomere. Sci Am 1991; 265:48–55.
9. Hagberg JM. Effect of training on the decline of VO₂max with aging. Fed Proc 1987;46:1830–1833.
10. Buskirk ER, Hodgson JL. Age and aerobic power: the rate of change in men and women. Fed Proc 1987;46:1824–1829.
11. Tockman MS. The effects of age on the lung. In: Abrams WB, Beckow R, eds. Merck manual of geriatrics. Rahway: Merck, 1990:423–432.
12. Shock NW. The science of gerontology. In: Jeffers EC, Council on Gerontology, Proc. Seminars 1959–61. Durham: Duke University Press, 1962:123–140.
13. Shock NW, Greulich RC, Andres R, et al. Normal human aging: the Baltimore longitudinal study of aging. Washington, DC: U.S. Government Printing Office, 1984:174–179.
14. Rusting RL. Why do we age? Sci Am 1992;267:130–141.
15. Young VR. Diet as a modulator of aging and longevity. Fed Proc 1979;38:1994–2000.
16. Aaronson SA. Growth factors and cancer. Science 1991;254:1146–1153.
17. Weinberg RA. Tumor suppressor genes. Science 1991;254:1138–1146.
18. Hausen H. Viruses in human cancers. Science 1991; 254:1167–1173.
19. Johnson HM, Russell JK, Pontzer CH. Superantigens in human disease. Sci Am 1992;266:92–101.
20. Miller RA. Gerontology as oncology. Cancer 1991; 68:2496–2501.

46/ The Elderly and Their Families

James G. O'Brien, Jacob Climo

As our population ages into the 21st century, more people are experiencing longer relationships within their families. By the 1980s, it was already clear that resources were needed to buttress health care and social supports to enable more elderly to continue living at home, preferably with their families, rather than being institutionalized. Along with the basic goal of improving health care to prolong life itself, a corollary arose that successful aging increasingly means paying attention to sustaining a satisfying quality of personal life and social relationships.

Today in America, more adult children are responsible as caregivers for disabled and infirm elderly parents for longer periods of time and for a wider variety of illnesses than ever before in our history (1). In this rapidly changing social environment, the family remains the single most important support in the lives of noninstitutionalized aging Americans and the single most important outside support for those in institutions.

The elderly population of the United States is currently in a period of transition. Today, 12% of the population is aged 65 or older. By the year 2025, 20% of the population will be aged 65 or older (2). The changes in composition of the American population will not only encompass quantitative differences, but qualitative differences as well. A low fertility rate, high divorce rate, and the return of women to the work force have conjoined to change the structure of the family and its ability to deal with the needs of an elderly population. In addition, a great deal of uncertainty surrounds the projected changes. The average life span is predicted to increase, but the amount of the increase is unknown. Furthermore, the condition of those individuals experiencing greater longevity cannot be predicted: individuals living longer in independence and good health may substantially add to society's well-being; increased morbidity of the aged may pose an intolerable burden on the health care system. These questions and others add to the uncertainty about the future of American elderly.

As of 1986, an average of 77% of people over age 65 and 55% of people over age 85 described themselves as independent in the activities of daily living (ADLs) (3). Whites reported their health status as excellent or very good more often than did blacks (3). 16.1% of men and 8.3% of women over age 65 were still in the work force, and a large percentage of persons over age 55 reported a desire to remain in the work force, at least in part-time positions, beyond retirement age if allowed to do so (4).

This chapter presents a series of clinical case studies in which older adults and their familial relationships are described in the context of a clinical practice from the perspective of a primary care physician.

WELL-ADAPTED FAMILY

Mr. and Mrs. RT, a retired couple in their 70s, have lived for 35 years in their own house. They enjoy an adequate income from Mr. T's pension, Social Security, personal savings, and 30 acres of farmland inherited from Mrs. T's family. Mrs. T taught school for 3 years but became a housewife after her first child was born. They have two married daughters with families of their own and an unmarried son. One daughter, her husband, and three children live within a 10-minute drive. The second daughter, her husband, and child live in Los Angeles. Their unmarried son lives in Chicago.

Mrs. T, aged 72, enjoys relatively good health. She has degenerative joint disease involving hips and knees with mild discomfort with minimal effect on mobility managed with nonsteroidals. In addition, her hypertension is controlled with a diuretic. She was recently counseled for prolonged grief following the death of her sister but is now in good spirits.

Mr. T is 76 and in fair health. Seven years ago he had a myocardial infarction. He has stable angina and type II diabetes mellitus. Both conditions are controlled, by nitrates and oral hypoglycemic agents, respectively. He restricts sodium, sugar, and fats in his diet and exercises daily. A year ago he had a cataract extraction and lens implant. He wears a hearing aid to compensate for hearing loss. At the urging of his daughter and wife he no longer drives at night. But he is unwilling to give up driving completely.

Both Ts are active in their community and enjoy a wide network of relatives and school friends, and participate in social activities outside their home. The Ts also maintain frequent and satisfying ties to their children and grandchildren. When Mrs. T was grieving her sister's death, her family was patient and sympathetic; their supportive attitude helped her over her crisis. The T's see their nearby daughter and her children once or twice a week and speak with them on the phone frequently. They also talk regularly to their distant children and enjoy their visits; their son usually comes two or three times a year from Chicago, but it is increasingly difficult and expensive for their daughter in Los Angeles to visit more than once a year.

Periodically Mr. T suggests selling the house and relocating to a retirement community in a more pleasant climate, probably California to be closer to their other daughter and grandchildren. Mrs. T acknowledges that housekeeping is becoming more difficult and that a warmer climate and proximity to her daughter and grandchildren in Los Angeles is more desirable. But she is reluctant to leave her nearby daughter and grandchildren, her old circle of friends and relatives, and her emotional attachment to the area where she has lived most of her life.

Several examples of prevention appear in the sketch of the T family. Mr. T exercises regularly and watches his diet to prevent further heart disease and maintain good physical and mental health. He has also agreed to limit his driving in a way that minimizes the likelihood of accidents. Since driving is often an important source of individual independence and self-esteem, many elderly men and women are reluctant to stop driving. Yet current thinking suggests that many people can continue driving if they are willing to accept certain limitations such as daytime driving, driving only on certain streets, or driving when traffic is light. In many cases, restricted driving can retain an individual's sense of independence while preventing accidents.

Mr. and Mrs. T continue to debate the issue of relocating to California. A small yet increasing number of retired Americans migrate seasonally or permanently to national amenity areas such as California, Arizona, and Florida, which are known for their pleasant climates and desirable retirement lifestyle communities (5, 6). Although only 5% of all Americans move to another state for retirement, such amenity migrations are increasingly common among healthy, active people who seek to improve the quality of their lives and can afford to live all or part of the year in another location (2). When aging parents discuss moving, adult children's reactions reveal their perceptions of their parents' ability to live and make decisions independently. The Ts' strong family orientation appears as a theme in this debate in which the pull to be closer to one daughter and grandchildren in California is offset by the desire to remain near the other daughter and grandchildren in Michigan.

Living as a couple is one of the most satisfying and successful arrangements for the elderly because it can provide for both emotional and social and instrumental needs of the partners. A growing awareness of increasing difficulty keeping house or the anticipation of an increasing need for services may motivate an elderly couple or widow to move to a retirement center that provides domestic services, health care, safety, and an attractive social environment. Such discussion may be regarded as anticipatory preparation for the eventual late-life moves. To the extent that aging parents can discuss anticipated changes openly with their families, they may prevent the trauma of unexpected rapid and dramatic changes.

Somewhere around 10 million elderly parents live too far away from their adult children for frequent face-to-face relationships. Despite the limitations of geographical separations, such individuals in general remain in close contact and maintain strong bonds of affection through regular telephone communications, seasonal visits, and assistance in a health crisis (6).

Increasingly, distant family members wish to be more involved in decision making and assisting their disabled and infirm elderly parents. With the recent development and diffusion of high technologies such as video phones in the home, this trend will flourish. Distant relatives can become involved in their family member's health regimen and provide important assistance in everyday living through communication networks with health care professionals. Of course many domestic services must be performed by someone nearby. An important part of the T's routine involves regular contacts with their children and grandchildren. For most people maintaining social networks and emotional bonds to family, friends, and community is basic to the physical and mental health.

Both Mr. and Mrs. T exemplify the most effective treatment of chronic conditions: self-management of their illnesses at home in consultation with their physician. For example, when Mrs. T experienced prolonged grief over her sister's death, her physician referred her to counseling, and her family rallied to provide sympathy and support. The Ts have also developed advanced directives and have designated their oldest daughter as having Durable Power of Attorney (DPOA). Advanced directives are a means of extending competent adults' right to make decisions after they become unable to express their desires concerning medical treatment; and discussing their implementation before they are needed is a critical part of preventive care. (Advanced directives are discussed in Chapters 61 and 62.)

FAMILY WITH EXCESSIVE CAREGIVER BURDEN

Mrs. S is an 89-year-old widow. Until last year, she was living alone in a senior high-rise apartment. Following a significant stroke, she moved into her daughter's home and currently is living with her daughter, son-in-law, and teenage granddaughter, who is retarded.

Mrs. S's health is poor. She has atrial fibrillation and congestive heart failure. Although her stroke left no paralysis, it has affected her ability to swallow. She suffers from recurrent aspiration pneumonia, which has resulted in frequent emergency room visits and sometimes brief hospitalizations. In addition to these difficulties, she has degenerative arthritis and needs a walker to get around. She has macular degeneration and is unable to read.

Annette, the daughter she lives with, is the designated caregiver. Annette works full time as a cashier in a local supermarket; her husband works as a mechanic for a large automobile corporation, and her daughter attends a special school. Annette calls the doctor's office quite frequently for trivial problems and brings her mother to the emergency room, sometimes inappropriately.

Mrs. S's sons are peripheral to her everyday life. Her second daughter claims that her mother's increasing need for domestic services and health care are overwhelming her sister. Though she would like to help more, she doesn't know how to supplement her sister's involvement and experiences guilt. In the meantime, she observes that her sister, Annette, is burning out.

Today, almost three quarters of all elderly Americans live with a spouse in conjugal units (40%) or alone (35%). An important minority still live with their own aging parents or their adult children in nuclear, two-generation-household family units (12%) and/or with their parents, children, and grandchildren in extended, three-generational family households (6%).

The bulk of care of the elderly is provided by informal networks of family and friends with almost three-fourths of the care provided by women (7). Spousal caregivers "provide the bulk of the care required by their impaired partner" (8). While there has been a decrease in the number of parents and adult children living together, data show that over one-half of the children coresiding with elderly parents do so to benefit themselves (9).

Caregiving is composed of two components: personal burden to the caretaker, such as loss of independence and limited personal activity, and interpersonal burden, such as difficulties dealing with the behaviors of the elderly person (10). "Daughters and wives were more likely to report such limitations than sons and husbands" (11). Caregivers who quit work to provide care were more likely to be less healthy (9). Overall, social isolation increases with progressive frailty of the elderly person, and social network becomes a major factor in caregiver reactions to the burden of caregiving (9).

After age 85, elderly women continue to outnumber men 5 to 2 (12), but the proportion of widows is expected to decrease as men continue to gain in life expectancy. One of two major changes in the elderly population is the delineation of "women in the middle," women experiencing three or more simultaneous life roles such as child rearing, labor force participation, and caring for frail or disabled parents (13). Since women assume more caregiving responsibilities in the family, the proportion of women in this situation grows with the elderly population.

A second change is the substantial growth in numbers of men without children or strong family ties. Today, most divorced men remarry, and most men are married when they die. However, because of the increased divorce rate, lower fertility rates, and a tendency of divorced males not to develop substantial ties with their children, many men will enter old age and disability without the traditional source of care, the family (14).

The S case calls attention to the frequent problem of deciding when to set limits on a multigenerational living situation in which one adult child has major caregiving responsibilities for a disabled parent. Given the erratic nature of many chronic illnesses and the intense desire of many patients to get better, adult children and families often invest tremendous efforts to maintain the parent as a viable family member, even when the quality of life for everyone involved is deteriorating steadily as a result of overwhelming demands. Especially in families where institutionalization is seen as tantamount to abandonment, adult children are often willing to make sacrifices far beyond their capacity to provide effective health and domestic care.

In the turbulent atmosphere of providing daily needs for her mother, who increasingly needs more care than the daughter can provide, the family seems unable to effectively address planning for Mrs. S's future needs. The frequent telephone calls to the office may signal a cry for help. Similarly, the frequent unnecessary trips to the emergency room should result in some open discussion with the physician about expectations and the type of care that enhances quality of life.

A decision about institutionalization is probably one of the most difficult that elderly individuals and their families struggle with. Sometimes, there is a prior commitment by the children to never place the parent in a nursing home. Often, the physician is called upon to counsel or mediate some of these difficult situations in which the caregiver's family is overwhelmed and trying to maintain a parent at home when it is clear that care needs can only be met in an institutional setting. Not infrequently, the decision to place somebody in an institution has less to do with the constellation of symptoms and problems of the patient than with the continuing capacity of the family to provide care. On occasion, the physician can suggest other alternatives including adult foster care or a respite setting as an intermediate step that families can take that is less stigmatizing. This clearly constitutes a situation where the physician can bolster and support the family.

Conversely, the physician may be the only advocate to appropriately suggest maintenance of older adults in their homes when families are attempting to institutionalize them prematurely. Clearly, this is an equally distressing situation for the physician to have to cope with.

UNCOOPERATIVE FAMILY OF A FRAIL ELDER

Mrs. B, a widow for many years, in her late 60s, recently moved to Milwaukee from New York State with her 41-year-old son, his wife, and their teenaged daughter. Her son had not been successful in real estate and made a major midlife career change to enter law school in Wisconsin. There the family rented two apartments in the same building, with plans to build a house with a mother-in-law suite. After an unsuccessful year in law school, the son became manager of the housing complex they were living in. He later bought a house, but his remodeling plans ignored any need to relocate his mother.

Mrs. B was in frail health. She suffered from hypertension, arthritis, and cirrhosis of the liver; on an early visit she admitted she was a recovering alcoholic. In addition, she suffered from anxiety attacks. Mrs. B was capable of basic self-care and managed her own finances but depended on her son and daughter-in-law for shopping, transportation, and social supports.

The family generally, and Mrs. B in particular, did not make a satisfactory adjustment to the community. After 4 years, they had few friends and virtually no social involvements. Relationships within the family were also poor. Mrs. B was openly critical of her son and daughter-in-law's discipline of her granddaughter. Mrs. B did not get along with her daughter-in-law; when the daughter-in-law transported her to the doctor's office, she would leave her, never speak to the doctor, and only return when summoned from the office.

Mrs. B was a difficult patient. Periodically she would ask the doctor why she wasn't being referred to specialists for her arthritis or liver. Yet, when referred, she would refuse to go. She contracted with the physician for a limited supply of Valium for her anxiety. After 1 week of upper respiratory symptoms, she telephoned for a refill on Valium and for a cough medicine that had worked the previous year. One day later she died suddenly.

Following her death, the family was threatening and intimidating; they also revealed some disturbing information. First, they wanted to know why she died suddenly and blamed the physician when he said he wasn't sure. The daughter-in-law claimed that Mrs. B had been having fainting spells, which "I'm sure she told you about. Couldn't you have done some cardiac tests with a dye?" they asked. The physician agreed to an autopsy, but ultimately the family changed their minds. At the funeral home, which was attended by virtually no one, the son volunteered to the physician that he had been providing his mother with beer for many years. The physician's attendance at the funeral home allowed an open discussion that otherwise would not have occurred.

This is an isolated family that uprooted itself and made a poor adjustment to the new community. The son and daughter-in-law were apparently uninvolved in their mother's health care but enabled her alcoholism and possibly frightened her by planning to leave her in the apartment when they moved to their home.

This is a particularly difficult situation for the physician to deal with, and the potential is great for the physician to become a scapegoat for any bad outcome, given the family dynamics. The survivors are probably angry, perhaps feeling guilt and remorse yet unwilling at this stage to acknowledge their role in contributing to the patient's problems. Certainly they enabled the continuation of her alcoholism and failed to inform the physicians of her continued drinking, knowing full well that she was also consuming Valium.

Alcoholism among the elderly population constitutes a major problem and may be even less likely to be detected in this age group than in younger individuals. Many older adults are less likely to have work obligations and may not be visited or called on at night, which may lead to decreased detection of the problem. Many of the symptoms and signs of alcoholism may be attributed to aging, such as hypertension, falling, insomnia, and confusion (15). Most physicians have a low index of suspicion when dealing with elderly patients who don't fit the stereotype.

Sometimes the physician can only be as good as he is allowed to be by patient and family. The physician in this situation is disadvantaged by not knowing the family situation. They never asked him to make a home visit, and he had very limited opportunity to engage other family members in any discussion regarding the patient. Similarly, the patient was adamant in her refusal to acknowledge she was drinking.

FAMILY OF A FRAIL ELDER

Mr. S. is a 95-year-old African American male who lives with his wife of 70 years, whose age is 89. They live in a well-maintained neighborhood. Mr. S is amazingly well preserved despite some chronic problems including peripheral vascular disease, angina pectoris, hiatus hernia, and macular degeneration. Mr. S's primary complaints relate to fatigue, discomfort in his legs, and progressive reduction in his ability to be independent. Mr. S has recently refused hospitalization when he presented with a bout of tachycardia. He wants to die at home and be cared for in that setting.

He has accumulated approximately 150 pack-years of smoking. He is independent in all ADLs and is dependent in transportation. He is a retired General Motors worker, financially quite comfortable, with excellent health insurance in addition

to his Medicare. He is the dominant figure in this family and makes all of the critical decisions.

Mrs. S has hypertension, degenerative arthritis, peptic ulcer disease, and 3 years ago was diagnosed with transitional cell carcinoma of the bladder. She refused all treatment at the time of diagnosis, but wanted assurances that her physician would not be offended by this decision and would continue to take care of her. She is functional in all ADLs and instrumental activities of daily living (IADLs) with the exception of transportation (she has never driven). Both are cognitively intact.

The Ss have four sons; the three who live in the region are supportive but rarely help transport the parents to the office. This is usually done by a person they acknowledge as their daughter who actually is not their biologic daughter, a woman in her early 40s, Bobby. She is the advocate, broker, and coordinator for their personal and health care without any official sanction such as durable power. Bobby is the primary person to whom, in addition to the patients, the physician can explain complicated information. Typically she is the person who initiates contact with the office. Bobby is concerned about how much additional care she can provide. It appears that to maintain the S family at home the combined efforts of the children will also be required. The physician is willing to perform home visits, and the family certainly have resources to purchase supplemental care in the home.

This case is instructive in that it uses a non–family member to communicate, even though the patients are cognitively intact and children are present in the area. It is evident that Bobby is a vital component of this family and assumes responsibility for effective communication. For the physician, she is often the person to relay concerns regarding treatments, diagnostic studies, and personal issues. Her roles are multiple; she also assists with coordination, compliance, appropriate nutrition, and transportation and communicates with the other children. The physician has to support her in that role and have some sense of when she is taking on too much and is becoming overburdened. So although Mr. and Mrs. S are frail, they function independently with autonomy in their own home as a result of the superb although atypical support system.

American society is characterized by great diversity in aging, health, and behavior resulting from elderly racial and ethnic minorities, including the so-called white or European ethnic groups. In 1980, over 2.5 million people or about 10% of the 65 and over population were nonwhites. Moreover, the elderly nonwhite minority populations have been growing faster than the elderly white population. By 2025, at least 15% and perhaps 20% of American elderly will be nonwhite; the largest minority population will be Hispanic followed by African Americans (16). Ethnic and racial minorities are more likely to be poor, lack pensions, and to report poorer health status (18).

A recent demographic study found that elderly African Americans who lacked contact with family members had a risk of death 2.1 times higher than elderly African Americans who had contact with a family member (17). At the same time, Johnson and Barer's (18) recent behavior research reveals that black families have developed mechanisms for preventing social isolation and meeting their social needs: they often extend their kinship networks through the creation of "fictive kin," unrelated people within the family network who take on obligations and instrumental and affectional ties similar to those of conventional kin (19, 20).

FAMILY OF A PATIENT WITH ALZHEIMER'S DISEASE OR RELATED DISORDER

Mrs. G is a 78-year-old white female who recently lost her husband to cancer. She was living in a retirement community in Florida. With the death of her husband, she was struggling to manage on her own. She was unable to manage her checking account and had gotten lost on one occasion when driving her car. Subsequently, she was evaluated at the request of her daughter, Diane, and was determined to have early Alzheimer's disease. Diane decided the mother should come and live with her.

The transition proved to be much more difficult than Diane had predicted, as exposure to a new environment caused her mother to be more confused, staying awake most of the night looking for the bathroom or some of her old friends. Diane is employed at a middle-management level at a local hospital in a particularly demanding job that often necessitates early morning or late evening meetings. Diane discovered that her mother needed more supervision during the day than she had originally planned.

She is currently managing by having her mother attend a senior day-care center 2 days per week. This requires Diane to drive her mother there and pick her up, which, given Diane's work hours, is quite difficult to accomplish. On the other 3 days, Diane has a caregiver who spends time with her mother, but the cost of this is already straining a limited budget. She was expe-

riencing difficulties in accessing her mother's checking and savings account to pay for some of the necessary services because often her mother was unwilling to write a check. Simultaneously, she is trying to better understand the disease and what the future holds for her mother regarding treatment programs such as available experimental drugs. She also wants some assurances that the diagnosis of Alzheimer's disease is secure and does not represent some other, treatable, condition such as depression.

Chronic disease is a predominant feature in old age. Over 80% of individuals over age 65 have at least one chronic disease. This does not imply that there is an accompanying functional impairment. Chronic disease is irreversible, has both physical and emotional consequences, and may have social and economic features that intrude on all aspects of living. Usually, when there is functional decline resulting from chronic illness, families are involved in some aspect of care, from oversight responsibilities to direct provision of care. Nowhere is this more evident than in a chronic disease represented by progressive dementia.

It is quite challenging for the physician to deal with patients with dementia and their families. The family may be in denial and may need reality orientation from the physician. Secondly, physicians are usually taught to expect a cure when they treat a disease. Yet, successful treatment of elderly patients with chronic conditions requires long-term involvement and attention to helping the patient maintain a satisfying quality of life.

The approach is more one of palliation, with small gains and gradual decline being the norm. The small gains in improvement may be of enormous significance to an older adult. These need to be viewed, and accepted, as equivalent to a cure in acute disease. It is equally important in these situations to focus on autonomy, independence, and quality-of-life issues.

As for Mrs. G, depending on the resources in the community, her personal physician in collaboration with perhaps a social worker and a nurse should be able to provide a comprehensive evaluation and assist with the development of a management plan for her. The primary care physician may also be aware of a multidisciplinary geriatric assessment program in the area that would provide consultation and help respond to the changing care demands, including physical, mental, social, economic and functional needs.

Diane may be helped by participating in a local Alzheimer's support group, perhaps becoming informed through reasonable readings that would be of help to her, such as *The 36 Hour Day* (21).

Additional in-home services may be available on a voluntary basis. Other important issues that Diane will need assistance with include being designated Durable Power of Attorney and trying to better understand her mother's preferences regarding some advanced directives.

People are living longer in families. Longer life in families can mean many things: either good health and a high quality of life surrounded by loved family members and support or, alternatively, dependency, chronic illness, disability, and a family setting that provides little support and may even contribute to suffering and loneliness. Today, families have fewer adult children, who frequently have increasing responsibilities caring for elderly family members with chronic illness and disability. This chapter has described a series of family care studies to illustrate common problems and strengths. By working with physicians and health care professionals, families can maximize their potential as healthy environments for elderly members.

REFERENCES

1. Brody EM. Parent care as a normative family stress. Gerontologist 1985;25:19–29.
2. Morrison PA. Demographic factors reshaping ties to family and place. Res Aging 1990;12(4):399–408.
3. Cohen RA, Van Nostrand JP, Furner SE. Highlights from health data on older Americans, United States, 1992. National Center for Health Statistics, series no. 27.
4. Juster FT, Suzman R, Soldo B, et al. Health and Retirement Study. Gaithersburg, MD: National Institute on Aging, National Institutes of Health, 1993.
5. Litwak E, Longino CF. Migration patterns among the elderly: a developmental perspective. Gerontologist 1987;27(3):266–272.
6. Climo J. Distant parents. New Brunswick, NJ: Rutgers Press, 1992.
7. Collins C, Stommel M, Kind S, Given CW. Assessment of the attitudes of family caregivers toward community services. Gerontologist 1991;31(6):756–761.
8. Pruchno RA. The effects of help patterns on the mental health of spouse caregivers. Res Aging 1990;12(1):57–71.
9. Crimmins EM, Ingegneri DG. Interaction and living arrangements of older parents and their children. Res Aging 1990;12(1):3–35.
10. Miller B, McFall S. Caregiver burden and the continuum of care. Res Aging 1992;14(3):376–398.
11. Miller B, Montgomery A. Family caregivers and limitations in social activities. Res Aging 1990;12(1):72–93.
12. Fowles DG. A profile of older Americans, 1992. Washington, DC: The Program Resources Department, American Association of Retired Persons (AARP) and the Administration on Aging (AoA), U.S. Department of Health and Human Services, 1992.
13. Spitze G, Logan J. More evidence on women (and men) in the middle. Res Aging 1990;12(2):182–198.
14. Goldscheider FK. The aging of the gender revolution. Res Aging 1990;12(4):531–545.
15. Adams WL, Yuan Z, Barboriak JJ, Rimm AA. Alcohol-related hospitalizations of elderly people: prevalence and geographic variation in the United States. JAMA 1993;270(10):1222–1225.
16. Harper MS. Minority aging. Rockville, MD: U.S. Department of Health and Human Services, Public Health Service, Health Resources and Services Administration, DHHS Publication HRS-P-DV 90–4, 1990.
17. Bryant S, Rakowski W. Predictors of mortality among elderly African-Americans. Res Aging 1992;14(1):50–60.
18. Johnson CL, Barer BH. Families and networks among older inner-city blacks. Gerontologist 1990;30:726–733.
19. Sussman MG. The family life of old people. In: Binstock P, Shanas E, eds. Handbook of aging and the social sciences. New York: Van Nostrand Reinhold, 1976:218–239.
20. MacRae H. Fictive kin as a component of the social networks of older people. Res Aging 1992;14(2):226–247.
21. Mace NL, Rabins PU. The thirty-six hour day: a family guide to caring for persons with Alzheimer's disease, related dementing illnesses and memory loss in later life. Baltimore: Johns Hopkins University Press, 1982.

47/ The Mistreatment of Older Adults

Joan Yesner, Brian Merrick, James G. O'Brien

Elder abuse and neglect, defined as acts of commission or omission that harm or threaten to harm an older person, is not a new phenomenon. However, it was only in the 1980s that elder abuse became an issue of national concern. Beginning with child abuse in the 1960s and spouse abuse in the 1970s, family violence in all its forms has become the subject of the daily news.

In the 1990s, several efforts have been directed at defining and clarifying the issue at the federal level. These include the Elder Abuse Task Force of the U.S. Department of Health and Human Services; the National Institute on Elder Abuse, and the National Aging Resource Center on Elder Abuse, both funded by the Administration on Aging; and the Joint Commission on Accreditation of Healthcare Organizations. All 50 states now have adult protective service organizations that serve adults involved in abusive or neglectful situations.

The American Medical Association (AMA) published guidelines in 1992 for the diagnosis and treatment of elder abuse and neglect. The AMA guidelines emphasize the important role of physicians, noting that well-established relationships with older adults and their families allow family physicians, internists, and psychiatrists a vantage point to recognize abuse and prevent catastrophes. In settings such as offices and hospital emergency rooms or institutions such as nursing homes, physicians need to be prepared to respond to abusive situations.

The purpose of this chapter is to provide an overview of the mistreatment of older adults, in both community and institutional settings. The challenges of screening, detection, assessment, and intervention are explored, emphasizing the importance of the collaboration of the primary care physician with a multidisciplinary team or with other individuals.

FACTS ABOUT ELDER MISTREATMENT

DEFINITIONS

The mistreatment of older adults includes intentional or unintentional infliction of harm or deprivation of care. There have been numerous attempts to classify forms of mistreatment; most include the basic categories of physical abuse, neglect by a caretaker to meet the needs of an older person, emotional or psychological abuse, and financial exploitation.

PREVALENCE

It is difficult to know the exact extent of elder mistreatment, as there are no national prevalence data. Localized studies have used varying definitions and have relied largely on various agency reports. The most quoted study, a community-based, cross-sectional study done by Pillemer and Finkelhor in 1988, reported that 32 of 1000 older adults experienced mistreatment after reaching age 65 (1); these data suggest a national prevalence rate of 2 to 5%.

PHYSICIAN'S ROLE

For the physician concerned with the well-being and safety of patients, elder mistreatment can not be ignored as a serious health issue. Since different states have different reporting requirements, it is essential that the physician be familiar with the local laws.

According to researchers, physicians have been slower than other health professionals to address family violence. Barriers to recognizing and intervening in situations of elder mistreatment include ageist societal views that certain functional decline and loss of quality of life is inevitable in aging; a lack of time necessary for the physical evaluation and sufficient history taking with the older patient, family, and other caregivers; and lack of reimbursement for intensive assessments. Ideally, a multidisciplinary geriatric team approach should be used for the assessment so that complex issues can be more effectively addressed.

RISK FACTORS

Risk factors for elder mistreatment have been based on a few causal theories that are not clearly substantiated by clinical data. Explanations include recurrent cycles of family violence; the caregiver's personal problems (drug or alcohol addiction, severe mental illness); functional impairment of dependent older adults, which increases their vulnerability and risk for abuse or neglect; and stress caused by lack of financial resources or community services. Dependence of the perpetrator on the older person and social isolation are other factors to consider. Elder mistreatment occurs among men and women of all economic, ethnic, and racial groups; several forms of elder mistreatment can occur at the same time. It is important to remember the controversial nature of the theories and risk factors and, in general, to be alert and take nothing for granted.

ASSESSMENT

Screening for elder abuse and neglect should be routinely incorporated into practice, whether in the office, institutional, or home settings (Fig. 47.1). Four components are essential to a complete assessment of suspected elder mistreatment: a history from the patient, a history from the suspected abuser, a comprehensive physical examination, and tests to confirm findings. Table 47.1 lists warning signs that should alert the physician to possible mistreatment.

PATIENT HISTORY

The AMA guidelines and other protocols emphasize the importance of interviewing the older patient in privacy, separate from any family member or staff. They suggest moving from general questions to more specific questions such as, "Has anyone ever scolded or threatened you?" (2). The older adult must have adequate time to respond and must not feel hurried or judged. (Often adults suffering from mistreatment feel guilty and blame themselves.) Gentle pursuit of any indications of mistreatment is necessary to determine if the person is safe and to explore how the person feels about and copes with the situation. Sensitivity to cultural differences in use of body language and verbal responsiveness or to barriers to understanding caused by language differences or sensory impairments is always essential. Knowledge about the financial resources available to the person will be useful information in later planning or collaborating on interventions. Table 47.2 lists questions that would be useful in interviewing older patients.

HISTORY FROM THE POTENTIAL ABUSER

Interviewing the potential abuser, also separate from the older patient and staff, is an important part of the assessment. In addition, interactions between the patient and potential abuser should be observed for expressions of anger or fear or attempts to avoid proximity. Table 47.3 offers questions useful in interviewing potential abusers.

COMPREHENSIVE PHYSICAL EXAMINATION

The physician should conduct a comprehensive physical examination to document indicators of abuse or neglect. Inconsistent explanations for physical findings such as weight loss, fractures, skin breakdown, or others mentioned in Table 47.1, should be noted. Functional abilities should be checked to uncover any other injuries or fractures. The patient's cognitive status should be assessed using a test such as the Mini-Mental State Examination. The capacity to understand and make decisions is a crucial issue, as later interventions will depend on whether or not the person is determined to be clinically capable of making decsions and exercising informed consent.

TESTS

Further tests to confirm medical findings may be needed to clarify suspicious findings. Documentation in the medical record must be comprehensive and include the patient's own words and photographs or drawings, since the record could be used as evidence in later legal proceedings.

If the time needed for a thorough evaluation is not available to the physician, other professionals, such as a multidisciplinary geriatric assessment team can be a valuable resource. If the patient is receiving community services or home health care, the social workers or nurses involved should become part of the data gathering and management process as well and form an informal team.

INTERVENTION

The central issues in effective intervention by the physician are ensuring immediate medical care and patient safety, notifying the appropriate authorities, and participating in the plan to provide services and care. Hospitalization to treat injuries or clarify the cause of a "failure to thrive" diagnosis is the surest way to guarantee care and safety, but sometimes the patient is unwilling to be hospitalized or cannot make decisions because of cognitive impairment. In this circumstance, guardianship may need to be pursued.

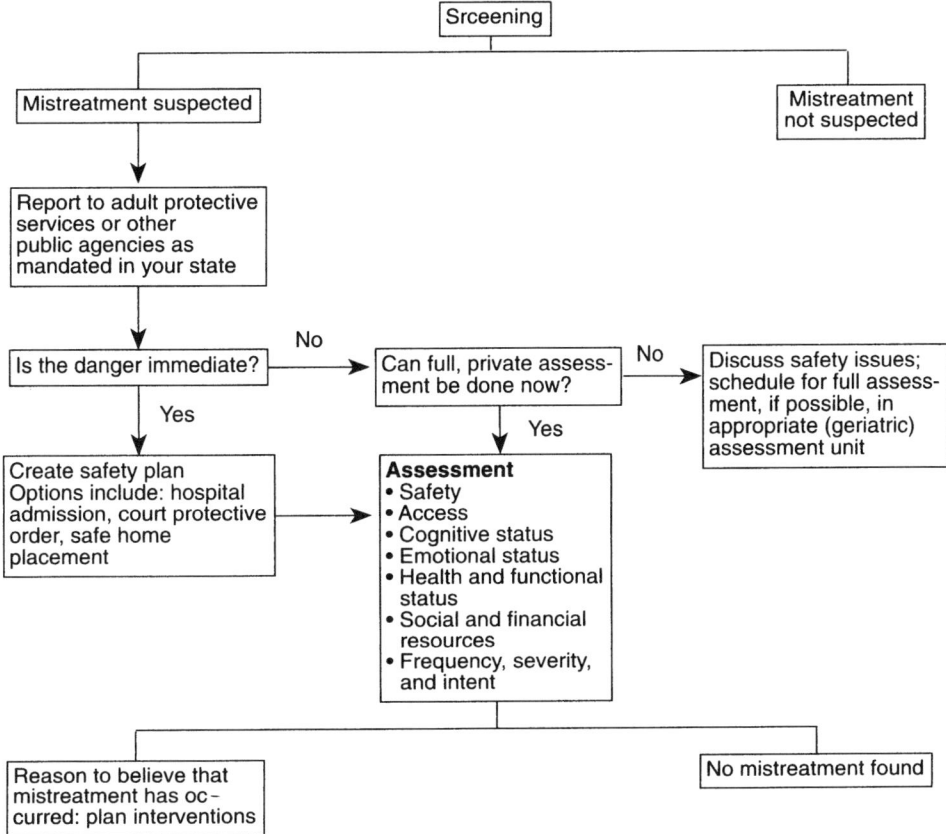

Figure 47.1   Screening and assessment for elder abuse and neglect should be based on an algorithm such as this one, developed and recommended by the American Medical Association. (Adapted with permission from AMA Dept. of Mental Health. Diagnostic and Treatment Guidelines on elder abuse and neglect. Chicago, 1992.)

REPORTING

Most states have laws that require certain professionals, including physicians, to report abuse and neglect of people over 60. Mandatory reporting is controversial because there have been concerns about the adult's right to privacy and self-determination. Despite this controversy, mandated reporters, such as physicians, nurses, psychologists, social workers, other health care professionals, and lawyers, have a legal obligation and ethical responsibility to report, and there are usually fines as penalties for not reporting.

Once the physician has determined sufficient suspicion of abuse or neglect (referred to as reasonable cause), a report to the local protective service agency should be made (usually verbally first, then on a standard form). The phone numbers of the Adult Protective Services hotline and local Area Agency on Aging should be easily available in hospitals and physicians' offices. State statutes defining elder mistreatment usually determine which agencies are designated for receiving and investigating reports. It is the task of the agency responsible for receiving the report to determine if abuse or neglect can be substantiated. Statistically, physicians are the least likely of all mandated reporters to file reports, but it is the physician who may be in a position to detect abuse early and prevent escalation.

AVAILABLE SERVICES

The five most common services offered by Adult Protective Services Agencies are case management, homemaking, legal interventions, counseling, and medical treatments and supplies (4). Availability of services may vary greatly in different regions. Adult Protective Service social workers can obtain court orders for protective care if an older adult lacks the capacity to understand or make reasonable decisions.

Table 47.1
Warning Signs of Possible Elder Mistreatment

History
  Pattern of "physician hopping"
  Unexplained delay in seeking treatment
  Previous unexplained injuries or injuries inconsistent
    with medical findings
  Previous reports of injuries similar to the current ones
  Conflicting accounts between patient and potential
    abuser

Physical findings
  Fractures, falls, dislocations
  Evidence of physical restraint
  Bruises, hematomas, welts, lacerations, abrasions,
    punctures
  Burns of unusual shape or in unusual locations
  Injuries that are bilateral, clustered, or in various
    stages of healing
  Evidence of overmedication or undermedication
  Unexplained sexually transmitted disease or genital
    infection
  Pain, itching, bruising, or bleeding in genital area
  Signs of poor personal hygiene, decubitus ulcers, de-
    hydration, malnutrition
  Inadequate or inappropriate clothing
  Absence of needed eyeglasses, hearing aids, dentures,
    prostheses
  Poor ambulation indicating hidden injuries or sexual
    assault
  Evidence of substance abuse in patient or caregiver

Clinical observations
  Signs of withdrawal, depression, agitation, low self-
    esteem
  Infantile behavior
  Mental status changes from previous exam
  Evidence of sleep disorder or deprivation
  Ambivalence, resignation, fearfulness toward care-
    giver or family members
  Substandard care despite adequate financial re-
    sources
  Confusion over, or lack of knowledge of, financial sit-
    uation
  Sudden transfer of assets to a family member
  Sudden inability to meet financial needs
  Caregiver refuses to let patient see physician alone
  Unusual behavior patterns between patient and care-
    giver

Adapted with permission from AMA Dept. of Mental Health.
Diagnostic and treatment guidelines on elder abuse and neglect.
Chicago, 1992; The Mount Sinai Victim Services Agency Elder
Abuse Project. Elder mistreatment guidelines for health care
professionals: detection, assessment and intervention. New
York, 1988; The Harborview Medical Center Department of So-
cial Work. Protocol for identification and assessment of elder
mistreatment. Seattle, 1992; Beth Israel Hospital Elder Abuse/
Neglect Protocol. Boston, 1991; and Bloom JS, Ansell P, Bloom
MN. Detecting elder abuse: a guide for physicians. Geriatrics
1969;44:40–56.

Table 47.2
**Screening Questions for Possible Victims of
Abuse and Neglect**

Has anyone at home ever hurt you?
Has anyone ever touched you without your consent?
Has anyone ever forced you to do something against
  your will?
Has anyone ever taken anything of yours without asking
  your permission?
Has anyone ever scolded or threatened you?
Have you ever signed any documents you didn't under-
  stand?
Are you afraid of anyone at home?
Are you alone a lot?
Has anyone ever failed to help you take care of yourself
  when you needed help?
Have you ever been tied or locked in a room?
Have you ever had to wait long periods of time for food
  or medication?
Do you have enough money to get the things you need?
After food and essentials, is any money left over for you
  to do some of the things you like to do?
If you don't have enough money, is it because someone
  is taking it?

Adapted with permission from AMA Dept. of Mental Health.
Diagnostic and treatment guidelines on elder abuse and neglect.
Chicago, 1992; and The Mount Sinai Victim Services Agency
Elder Abuse Project. Elder mistreatment guidelines for health
care professionals: detection, assessment and intervention. New
York, 1988.

ELDER MISTREATMENT IN INSTITUTIONS

Although uniform national prevalence data are
lacking, elder mistreatment occurs in a wide array of institutional settings, such as nursing
homes, board-and-care homes, or assisted living
facilities. The more common forms include sexual
abuse, medical neglect, and theft of personal
items (4).

National standards for care in nursing homes
are mandated by the 1987 Omnibus Budget Reconciliation Act effective since October 1990. This
law enunciates a set of residents' rights, which
include participation in health care decisions,
safeguards against inappropriate use of chemical
or physical restraints, access to a personal physician and to advocates such as Long Term Care
Ombudsmen, and the right to be free from abuse
or involuntary seclusion.

Older residents in institutions are typically
frail, chronically ill, and cognitively impaired,
thus requiring much assistance or supervision (6).
These needs, as well as social isolation and lack
of visitors, increase the potential for abuse. Ageism and societal ignorance about quality care in

Table 47.3.
Screening Questions for Possible Abusers

What would you like me to know about the patient?
What is his (her) medical condition?
What kind of care (including medicines) does he (she) require?
How involved are you with the patient's daily activities and care?
What do you expect the patient to do for himself (herself)?
What does he (she) expect you to do for him (her)?
Please describe your typical day.
Who helps you with the patient's care?
What responsibilities do you have outside the home?
Who owns the house you live in?
If you help the patient to pay the bills, how do you do so?
Is the patient's Social Security check deposited directly in the bank?

You may need to ask questions to follow up on particular findings

You know those bruises on (name patient's body part); how do you suppose he (she) got them?
The patient seems rather undernourished and thin; how do you suppose he (she) got this way?
Have you ever felt so frustrated with the patient that you pushed him (her) a little harder than you expected to?
Did you ever hit or slap him (her)?
Have there been times when you've yelled at or threatened him (her)?

Adapted with permission from the Harborview Medical Center, Department of Social Work. Protocol for identification and assessment of elder mistreatment. Seattle, 1992.

institutions may further exacerbate the potential for elder mistreatment.

Physicians have an important role in identifying, treating, and preventing abuse and neglect in institutions. They may be the one person other than regular staff who sees the older resident on a regular basis.

When abuse is suspected, state regulations dictate how reporting is done and investigations are conducted. The State Long Term Care Ombudsman Program established by the Older Americans Act provides advocates who investigate complaints by residents and often are in a position to uncover abuse. This mandated program has potential for improving interventions, and there is congressional support for increasing its authority.

REFERENCES

1. Pillemer K, Finkelhor D. The prevalence of elder abuse: a random sample survey. Gerontologist 1988; 28:51–57.
2. American Medical Association. Diagnostic and treatment guidelines on elder abuse and neglect. Chicago, 1992.
3. Tatara T. Elder abuse in the United States: an issue paper. Washington, DC: National Aging Resource Center on Elder Abuse, 1990.
4. Anetzberger GJ, Lachs MS, O'Brien J, Pillemer KA, Tomita SK. Elder mistreatment: a call for help. Patient Care 1993;June 15:93–130.

48/ Demographic Aspects of Aging

Current And Future Trends

William Rakowski, Deborah N. Pearlman

The American population is growing older. Not only are people living longer, but the absolute number and proportion of people over 65 are increasing dramatically. Much attention has recently been focused on the future growth of the older population, with the message that the aging of the U.S. population will increase both the utilization of health services and related costs. While the trend toward an aging population is indisputable, any assumption that the population of 32 million persons over 65 consists of a homogeneous group is inaccurate. Generalizations are necessary for public policy, but on a clinical level they belie the enormous heterogeneity found in the elderly with regard to their health and functioning (1, 2).

In this chapter we focus on those demographic and health characteristics of the elderly that appear to influence health service utilization and the characteristics of older patients who might comprise a primary care physician's practice. Although a substantial proportion of older people have illnesses and functional limitations, only a subgroup makes consistently high use of both physician and hospital services. Diversity within the older population will influence health services utilization and related costs, as well as the mix of patients seen in physicians' daily practice, well into the twenty-first century.

AN AGING POPULATION

People age 65 and older now constitute the fastest growing segment of the population. In 1900, older people comprised 4% of the U.S. population; today they represent over 12%. Projections prepared by the U.S. Bureau of the Census show that the elderly population will expand far more rapidly than the rest of the population. The ranks of the elderly are projected to increase at

least through the year 2030, when approximately 22% of the population will be 65 and older (3). Put another way, over the next 40 years the population age 65 and older is expected to double, from 32.2 million today to 64.4 million in 2030 (4).

Future growth in the number of elderly reflects the aging of the "baby-boom" generation—those born between 1946 and 1962. Between 2010 and 2020, the baby boomers will cause a rapid increase in the number of people age 65 and older and a comparable increase, beginning in 2030, in the 85-and-over age group (4). This rise in the median age of the U.S. population is a historic demographic event (5).

Increasing longevity has also contributed to the extraordinary size of the older population. The triumph over acute and infectious diseases of early childhood, evident since the first half of the twentieth century, has meant that larger proportions of people have survived to old age (6). Although this impressive decline in mortality appeared to plateau in the 1960s, mortality is again declining, especially among those at advanced ages. More importantly, improvements in life expectancy, even at advanced ages, are projected to continue well into the next century (7).

DIFFERENCES WITHIN THE OLDER POPULATION

AGE

The now well-known expression "the graying of America" refers both to the spectacular change in the size of the elderly population and to the striking growth in the population age 85 and older in particular. This latter group, the "oldest old," are the fastest growing segment of the United States. In 1990, people 85 and older represented only 1% of the total population and 12.6% of the over-65 population; by 2030 they will represent

5% of the total population and 22% of the over-65 population (3). This trend has evident implications for health care providers. Physicians can expect to see many more very old and frail elderly people in their clinical practices. At the same time, persons age 75 and older are diverse in demographic and health characteristics. Even older patients with identical diagnoses and functional limitations may require different treatment plans.

RACE AND ETHNICITY

Race and ethnicity are another source of diversity within the older population. Although the elderly are predominately white—about 86%, nationally—in recent years the minority population of elderly has been growing faster than whites, a trend that is expected to continue as the percentage climbs from 14% now to about 20% by the year 2010 (8, 9). This growth reflects the higher fertility rates among black and Hispanic populations relative to the white population. For example, between 1990 and 2030, the population of older whites will grow by 92%, compared with 247% for older blacks and 395% for older Hispanics (3). Nevertheless, the proportion of white elderly relative to people of other races will still be higher, because blacks and other racial minorities continue to die more frequently than whites from cancer, heart disease, and cerebrovascular diseases and are more likely than whites to suffer from and die of chronic disabilities (10, 11). The higher rate of morbidity and mortality among blacks reflects long-standing disparities in education, employment, and income—disparities that limit access to and use of health care.

Even though race is an important factor in determining life expectancy, for reasons not well understood, by age 75 black mortality rates are lower than those of comparably aged whites (12). One explanation for the black-white mortality crossover is that black Americans who survive middle age may have better coping resources or even a hardier and more resilient biology in later life than whites. Blacks who survive to old age appear to have informal sources of support within their families and communities that help them cope better than whites with stressful health situations (2).

SEX

A person's chance of surviving to old age is strongly related to his or her sex. For men, life expectancy at birth is now 72 years, compared with 79 years for women. By 2030, life expectancy for men will rise by 3.4 years, while another 3.3 years will be added for women. The gender gap in life expectancy is somewhat smaller for those who survive to age 65. Elderly men who turn 65 can expect to live another 15 years; elderly women can expect to live an additional 19.4 years. Largely because of the longer survival of women, the oldest-old population is primarily female. For example, in 1989 the ratio of men to women between the ages of 65 and 69 was 84 men for every 100 women; however, among those age 85 plus, the ratio was only 39 men for every 100 women (3).

Is the gap in life expectancy between women and men decreasing? This is the subject of considerable debate. Some demographers argue that the gender gap in life expectancy appears to be narrowing slightly; for example, the gender gap in life expectancy at birth was 6.9 years in 1987, compared with 7.7 years in 1970 (3). Others disagree and see no significant change in the ratio of women to men well into the next century. Gender differences in life expectancy have great significance. The continued improvement in the mortality rates of men will affect the demographic characteristics of future cohorts of older persons and, equally important, the number of years older women will live alone (4). However, there will have to be many years of consistent gains by men. Women can still expect to outlive men for the foreseeable future.

GEOGRAPHIC DISTRIBUTION

Extensive regional variations exist in the distribution of those age 65 and older. Not surprisingly, Florida has the highest proportion of elderly (over 17%). In 1989, about 52% of the population 65 and older lived in nine states—California, New York, Florida, Pennsylvania, Texas, Illinois, Ohio, Michigan, and New Jersey (3, 9). These states should continue to experience a higher than average demand for health care and rapid increases in health care costs well into the middle of the next century unless cost-control efforts are successful. Yet it is several smaller and rural states—such as Rhode Island (14.8%), Arkansas (14.8%), West Virginia (14.6%), Connecticut (13.6%), and Maine (13.4%)—that have relatively high percentages of people 65+ (3). Physicians in these states may face even more demands for geriatric care.

Residential migration is more common among the young elderly than the oldest-old. Older people who move to another state tend to be married, affluent, and relatively healthy. Today's elderly generally remain in the communities where they have spent most of their adult lives. As a result of such "aging in place," communities with high percentages of older people also have a disproportionately high number of elderly who are very old, widowed, and in poor health; consequently, these communities contain relatively higher concentrations of older people with costly health care needs.

HEALTH STATUS
PERSONAL HEALTH HABITS

Most older people view their health positively, although the poor elderly are twice as likely as elderly with moderate to high incomes to report health problems (12). In general, the elderly watch their day-to-day health. Older people have lower rates of smoking and drinking than the nonelderly. They are more likely than other adults to have a regular source of medical care, in part because 95% of the noninstitutionalized elderly are covered by Medicare hospital and physician insurance (3). On the other hand, the elderly are far less likely to exercise regularly and often have less health care knowledge than younger persons.

Perhaps the best-studied influences on health and longevity are behavioral risk factors, such as smoking and physical exercise. Despite these associations, geriatric practice routinely presents an inherently perplexing situation. That is, people with high-risk lifestyle practices are, by definition, less likely to survive into old age. At the same time, every clinical practice includes some very old patients who are long-time smokers and drinkers, persons with seemingly risk-inducing diets, and those who do not exercise. Indeed, certain lifestyle behaviors may have less impact on morbidity and mortality in later life than in middle age, because of the multiple competing risks that produce higher mortality. However, there is increasing recognition that many traditional risk factors in middle age continue to be associated with heightened risk in those over age 70 (13).

These findings are important for geriatrics because they underscore that prevention efforts aimed at older populations are worthwhile and can significantly decrease the risk of death, even in the sixth and seventh decades of life (13). We recognize that physicians' attempts to change high-risk behaviors in some older patients may encounter resistance or failure. These persons know, after all, that they are the survivors of their birth cohort. It is just a short step for them to infer that they must be "doing something right," and many people are comfortable with this as a justification for their actions. Many older persons have lived longer than they ever expected to live, so

that the future-oriented rationales of prevention have less salience for them. However, techniques to change lifestyle are being tested, and becoming more effective, with older persons.

MORTALITY

As previously noted, death rates for the elderly have declined dramatically over the past several decades. These declines have varied by age, gender, and race; the declines being greatest for people 65 to 84 years of age, relative to those age 85 and over; for older women; and for older whites, regardless of gender.

What diseases are the leading causes of death among the elderly? Heart disease leads all other illnesses as the major cause of mortality in old age, accounting for 40% of all deaths among people age 65 and older. Cancer, the second leading cause of death among the elderly, accounts for 21% of all deaths in this age group, but death rates from lung cancer are rising. The third leading cause of death, stroke, accounts for only 8% of all deaths among those over age 65 (3).

Although heart disease remains the leading cause of poor health and of death in old age, in recent years there has been a marked decrease in death rates for heart disease, the decrease being greatest for white males and least for black females (14). The reasons for this dramatic change are unclear. Better control of hypertension may explain some of the decline. Dietary changes, along with improvements in the diagnosis and treatment of patients with heart and vascular problems may also be related (3, 15).

MORBIDITY

Of equal importance with the number of years lived in old age is the healthfulness of those later years. One measure of health status is the prevalence of disease and disability in old age. Currently, four out of five persons age 65 and older have at least one chronic condition, and multiple disabling conditions are commonplace, especially among older women. The most frequently reported chronic conditions are arthritis, hypertension, sensory impairments (e.g., hearing and visual loss), and heart disease. Together, these four conditions account for 60% of older people's health problems (7, 8). At the same time, no one condition is reported by more than half of the population aged 65 and older.

The prevalence and types of chronic conditions reported by the elderly vary by age, sex, and race. The risk of chronic illness increases rapidly with age. Organic mental disorders, for example, affect nearly half of those age 85 and older and are one of the principal reasons for nursing home placement (3). Some diseases, such as arthritis, diabetes, and osteoporosis, are more common among older women, while coronary heart disease and sensory impairments (e.g., visual and hearing) are more common among older men (13, 16). Older blacks generally have poorer health status than older whites and are more likely than their white peers to suffer from hypertension, diabetes, arthritis, and glaucoma (3, 12). Conversely, younger elderly have a relatively lower burden of chronic conditions and a higher prevalence of acute conditions than the oldest old.

DISABILITY

Despite major medical advances in the treatment of heart disease, cancer, and stroke, less progress has been made in treating the chronic nonfatal diseases of old age. For many people over age 65, nonfatal diseases such as osteoporosis and dementia lead to dependency and disability. Those persons who lose some capacity for self-care often require a range of medical, social, and long-term care services—all of which contribute to the high cost of the health care system (7) and to the hidden cost of demands placed upon informal helpers.

The distinction between illness (the biologic or physical aberrance) and disability (the practical impact of that illness on daily life) is extremely important. Most elderly people with chronic illness are not limited in activities of daily living (ADLs), such as dressing, bathing, eating, and getting to and using the toilet. Limitations in instrumental activities of daily living (IADLs), such as managing money, shopping, paying bills, doing light housekeeping, using the telephone, and getting around in the community, may be more evident (4). Moreover, even among the elderly with functional limitations, the number and severity of ADL and IADL limitations varies greatly. Among the oldest-old, for whom the prevalence of chronic conditions and functional limitations are greatest, there is enormous heterogeneity in functional status and improvement in functioning is possible (16). Of course, for the elderly in already fragile health, illness is more likely to result in permanent disability.

The optimistic message is that although the risk of functional disability increases rapidly after age 65, most people not in nursing homes report few functional limitations caused by illness. In 1987, approximately 13% of the community-residing elderly population needed help with ADLs. A slightly higher proportion of people age 65 and older (17.5%) experienced limitations in IADLs. The most frequently reported ADL problems involved bathing (9%) and walking (8%); limitations in eating and using the toilet were reported less frequently. Problems with getting around outside (13.5%) and shopping (11%) were the most frequently reported IADL difficulties (3). As many physicians know, ADL and IADL limitations often compromise quality of life and indicate a need for long-term care, but these percentages illustrate that most older persons do not suffer from these problems.

Age differences with regard to functional limitations are dramatic. While 10% of persons age 65 to 69 were disabled in 1987, this was true of 57% of those age 85 and over. Similarly, 3% of persons age 80 to 84 were severely disabled—that is, they had four or more ADL impairments—while 9% of those age 85 and over had such difficulties (3). Across a wide variety of studies, multiple impairments are found to be a significant predictor of becoming institutionalized. However, people age 85 and older generally enter nursing homes at lower levels of impairment than people age 65 to 74, because the oldest-old are less likely than the young-old to have family and friends to turn to for help in maintaining independent living. The oldest-old also may have fewer financial resources to deal with illness or impairment. In contrast, the young-old generally enter nursing homes because of serious functional impairments (16).

Also striking are gender differences in disability. More women than men report ADL and IADL limitations, and these differences become more pronounced with age. For example, in 1987, 6.5% of women 65 to 69 and 5% of men in this age-group had at least one ADL limitation. Among those age 85 and older, however, 38% of women and 26% of men had such limitations. What accounts for the gender differences in disability with increasing age? The answer lies in the medical conditions that cause long-term disability. Whereas men are more likely to suffer from and die of chronic disabling diseases, such as cancer and stroke, women often survive for many years with a disabling condition (16). Therefore, although women tend to outlive men, they also tend to do so at the cost of having functional limitations.

To summarize, the association between chronic illness, disability, and severe functional impairment with advancing age is understandable, even as new medical technologies postpone the onset of functional problems later in life. From a public policy perspective, however, the greater prevalence of functional problems among blacks and Hispanics, compared with non-Hispanic whites, suggests racial disparities in access to, and utilization of, health services, which may be amenable to change.

SOCIOECONOMIC CHARACTERISTICS

MARITAL STATUS AND LIVING ARRANGEMENTS

Among the biggest differences between women and men at the older ages is marital status. Most older men (75%) remain married until they die; nearly half (49%) of older women over age 65 are widowed, with blacks more likely to be widowed than whites and Hispanics. Likewise, living arrangements differ significantly by sex: older men typically reside with their wives; older women commonly live alone (41%) (3).

The living arrangements of minority elderly individuals diverge somewhat from the patterns observed among whites in old age. Many minority elderly have experienced a lifetime of inadequate economic resources and health problems that have necessitated reliance on extended kin for support (17). Thus, black and Hispanic elderly are much less likely to live alone than whites and are more likely to live with relatives than whites (10, 17). Nevertheless, providers should not assume that these higher rates of living together are completely voluntary or that they occur without stress or cost to the coresidents.

FAMILY CARE

The major source of assistance to older people with ADL or IADL limitations is unpaid help. Nationally, about three-quarters of disabled older persons living in the community receive all their care from family and friends (i.e., informal care). Only about 5% of the community-dwelling disabled elderly rely solely on formal or professional care (18). An older person's living arrangements are an important predictor of the type and amount of informal care received and also of risk of institutionalization. Elderly persons living with a spouse receive substantially more care than those living with others or those living alone. Spouses give greater amounts of assistance, for longer periods of time, than other informal caregivers and paid helpers (19, 20).

The disabled elderly living alone are also more likely to use formal services and to enter nursing homes than are those living with others. This situation presents a challenge for physicians, since most frail older persons want to remain at home

for as long as possible. Physicians may find it useful to monitor changes in both who provides help to a disabled patient and the caregiver's needs so that they are aware of nonmedical factors that might affect a patient's ability to cope with disability.

The low fertility and marriage rates, coupled with the high divorce rates of the baby-boom generation, have raised concerns about future patterns of informal care and nursing home use. On the one hand, baby boomers will have fewer family members to depend on than their parents did. As noted earlier, having support available from family members is one of the most critical factors in preventing or delaying nursing home placement. Also, as life expectancy increases, more elderly disabled people may be cared for by adult children who are themselves past retirement age—and the aging of an adult child is another factor associated with nursing home placement. On the other hand, if the number of elderly able and willing to purchase in-home services increases significantly or if it becomes more common for family members other than adult children to bring an elderly disabled relative to live with them, the percentage of the nursing home population may not increase substantially. A rapid increase in the size of the nursing home population would not be surprising, however, in light of the anticipated increase in the proportion of people 85 + with chronic health problems (4).

INCOME

In recent years, the economic status of the elderly has improved, with poverty rates among those 65 and older declining from 25% in 1968 to 12.4% in 1986. Since 1982, the rate of poverty has remained lower among the elderly than for the rest of the population. These gains reflect the increased labor force participation of women, increases in the number of workers spending a full working career covered under Social Security and private pension plans, and automatic cost-of-living adjustments in Social Security payments. If the benefits of noncash programs such as Medicare and Medicaid are counted as income, the rate of poverty among the elderly is even lower (21). Adding noncash benefits in computing household income is highly debated as being only partly accurate, however, because it does not take into account that most long-term care services are not covered by Medicare anyway and that persons must "spend down" most of their assets as a condition for Medicaid eligibility (21).

Across-the-board improvements in older people's incomes, such as increased Social Security benefits, have not improved the standard of living of all senior citizens. While it is true that most of the elderly are no longer poor, the elderly are much more likely than other adults to have incomes just above the poverty level. In 1989, 8% of the elderly had incomes 125 to 150% of the poverty level; only 4% of adults under age 65 had incomes that fell in this range (3).

At the same time, elderly poverty persists among racial minorities (blacks, 31%; Hispanics, 21%), women (14%), people living alone (22%), and people with less than a high school diploma (21%), again underscoring that the elderly are a heterogenous group (3). Poverty rates are also higher in rural than in metropolitan areas, but in all residence areas, elderly women have higher poverty rates than elderly men (22). Other groups with high poverty rates within the older population are the oldest-old, the ill, and the disabled. Aged black women living alone have the highest poverty rates: 60% had incomes below the poverty level in 1989 (3).

This picture is not expected to improve dramatically over the next 40 years. Although real incomes of the elderly are expected to rise between 1990 and 2030, subgroups of the elderly—racial minorities, unmarried women, the very old, and those with ADL limitations—will continue to fall into the lower end of the income distribution through 2030. Thus, the elderly most at risk financially today—very old unmarried women with ADL limitations—are the subgroup of the elderly most likely to be poor in 2030 (4). This group will be the least able to purchase long-term care services that might facilitate independent living in the community and the most likely to move in with others or be in nursing homes.

It is often said that older persons live on "fixed incomes." In addition to the implication that fixed incomes are more subject to erosion by inflation, equally important is that fixed incomes cannot be used to make up for the drains on savings and other resources that can accompany illness. Health care providers must keep in mind that older persons are well aware of that risk and the accompanying threat of loss of independence.

HEALTH TRANSITIONS

In the past, professionals and laypersons alike have most often viewed aging in terms of losses. Death remains the one inevitable event of adulthood, and most persons experience a period of one or more illnesses in the years before dying. Death is rarely so sudden that there is no evidence of prior illness. While the incidence and prevalence of illness clearly does increase with advancing age, the traditional flaw in this approach has been expecting physical impairments to occur by a certain age. In effect, successive age-bands (65–69, 70–74, 75–79, etc.) are expected to show steady decrement, with most persons in the age-band showing the pattern (e.g., heterogeneity within an age-band is not great).

While many physiologic functions do show progressive losses with advancing age—notably hearing, vision, renal function, glucose tolerance, systolic blood pressure, bone density, pulmonary function, immune function, and sympathetic nervous system activity—these losses are not so very closely tied to particular age-bands (23). Some older people show minimal physiologic loss or none at all when compared with their peers. Certainly genetics influences the aging process, but aging is influenced by many other factors—people's attitudes about illness; their use of health care; and psychosocial factors, including lifestyle factors, health practices, and access to social support (6).

Research on "transitions," among the newer areas of health-related investigations, will certainly become more prominent because of its explicit focus on the potential for improvement in addition to decline. Analysis of the National Long Term Care Surveys (NLTCS) designed to measure the 1982, 1984, and 1989 prevalence of chronic disability in the elderly suggests that the proportion of older people with initial functional loss did in fact show long-term functional improvements. In particular, the percentage of persons age 65 and older who were mildly disabled (only IADLs) and severely disabled (five to six ADLs) in 1982 decreased significantly in 1989. Still, more people in 1989 had three or more ADL impairments than in 1982—the criteria often used as a threshold for determining eligibility for publicly financed home care and medical services. The increase in the moderately disabled population reflected upward shifts in the age structure, but the disabled population increased less than the 65+ population, which indicates slightly better health in the aggregate (24).

Current research is also challenging the notion that cognitive impairment is unidirectional, solely in the direction of decline. A series of studies conducted on persons with progressively deteriorating Alzheimer's disease found that some undesirable behaviors (e.g., wandering) were eliminated or attenuated by teaching caregivers behavior management skills or by redesigning the home environment (6).

Increasing diversity in later life raises an important question for physicians: What are the determinants of functional change? Functional improvement is more likely under certain conditions: when the loss has been recent, when the impairment is not severe, and when the individual's overall level of functioning is high. Age, sex, and race are related to the loss of functioning but not to the likelihood of regaining functioning. Functional loss is more likely for blacks, the very old, persons in poor health, those who have arthritis, and those who have suffered a stroke. Many individuals experience both directions of change at the same time—improvement in the ability to perform some ADL and IADL tasks and deterioration in the ability to perform others (25). Physicians who do not take into account that some of their disabled patients can regain functioning may misrepresent the long-term prognosis of their aged patients.

Specific recommendations for treatment from this literature are not yet warranted, but findings provide a measure of optimism for primary care physicians and for older adults. One of the fundamental conundrums of gerontology and geriatrics is resolving the knowledge of inevitable death (usually preceded by illness and functional decline) with the continuing search to prolong life and good health "for as long as possible."

USE OF HEALTH CARE SERVICES

Although the older population is heterogenous, the health care system in the United States has evolved on the assumption that older people are disproportionately high users of health care services. While this is true on a population level, it does not characterize all individuals. Mossey and colleagues (26) point out that only a small subgroup of the elderly make extensive use of health services. Who are these high users? Among community-residing elderly, high use of physician services is associated with chronic and acute health problems (e.g., coronary heart disease, cancer, and stroke), activity limitations, poor self-rated health, not being cognitively impaired, being female, and urban residence (26). Nursing home entry is more likely for older persons with multiple chronic conditions and mental impairment, although some demographic, psychosocial, and environmental factors also increase the risk of becoming institutionalized (27). For example, the lifetime risk of ever being in a nursing home is somewhat higher for women (42%) than for men (32%) (28).

Perhaps the most important finding from research on older people's health service use is that chronological age is not as significant a predictor of health care use as might be expected. High users of health care are not necessarily those who survive past age 75 or even 85 but rather the small proportion of older individuals with chronic and progressively disabling diseases (26, 29). Wolinsky and Arnold (29) take this point one step further, arguing that health status is the most important determinant of health service use and that all other factors, including age per se, contribute little to our understanding of health service use among the elderly population as a whole or among heavy users (27). What are the important implications of these research findings for physicians? In light of today's debate on restructuring the U.S. health care system, physicians will be under increasing pressure to find the most appropriate and cost-effective care for their severely ill patients who have high health care costs. Furthermore, physicians will have more alternatives to match services more closely to the needs of their remarkably diverse older patients.

CONCLUSION

In a country where tens of millions of persons are already age 65 or older, and where millions more will turn 65 in the next few years, diversity is one of the few certainties. Many of the older population's sociodemographic characteristics have not shifted dramatically in the past 25 years. Women still have longer life expectancy but report more functional impairment than men. Heart disease, cancer, and stroke are still the three leading causes of death. Risk of nursing home placement increases progressively with advancing age. The reality of living on a fixed income poses threats to the financial security of elderly households, and living just above the poverty line tempers the decrease that has occurred in the percentage of persons age 65 and over who live below the poverty line. Some of the largest risks are faced by older women, members of racial minority groups, and those who live alone.

These realities cannot and must not be ignored. Older adults are still an at-risk population, and traditionally disadvantaged groups continue to have relatively greater disadvantaged status in older adulthood. Primary care physicians and other professionals must always be alert for problems, even though a "problem focus" is often not pleasant. The difficult medical, personal, and family situations encountered in geriatric care will always exist, and considering the increase in the sheer numbers of older persons in coming years, these situations will become, if anything, more common. At some point, the huge numbers of older persons will bring a corresponding rise in the number of persons with health problems and the related need for health and social services—certainly a concern for primary care physicians with a geriatric practice. When there are 40 or 50 million persons aged 65 and over, even a 3% incidence rate will denote 1.2 to 1.5 million persons for whatever problem is being studied. Such numbers will demand attention, even when spread across 50 states and thousands of primary care providers.

Nonetheless, progress is being made, and there can be reason for both the physician and the older patient to be optimistic. Efforts to maintain good health and functional status are likely to be rewarded. Although health status is most often viewed as an outcome (i.e., by looking at rates of mortality, morbidity, and disability), it is also a powerful personal resource or predisposing factor that influences how readily people can adapt to difficult situations or avail themselves of opportunities. Increasing numbers of persons will be entering older adulthood in robust health, with a prospect of staying in good health for many more years. There will be increasingly more "well elderly" with the material, financial, and health status resources that can be applied to continued maintenance of good health and function.

REFERENCES

1. Dannefer D. Differential gerontology and the stratified life course: concept and methodological issues. In: Maddox GL, Lawton MP, eds. Annual review of gerontology and geriatrics, vol 8: varieties of aging. New York: Springer, 1988:3–36.
2. Berkman LF. The changing and heterogeneous nature of aging and longevity: A social and biomedical perspective. In: Maddox GL, Lawton MP, eds. Annual review of gerontology and geriatrics, vol 8: varieties of aging. New York: Springer, 1988:37–68.
3. U.S. Senate Special Committee on Aging. Aging America: trends and projections. Washington, DC: U.S. Department of Health and Human Services, 1991.
4. Zedlewksi SR, Barnes RO, Burt MR, McBride TD, Meyer JA. The needs of the elderly in the 21st century. Washington, DC: Urban Institute Press, 1990.
5. Siegel JS, Davidson M. Demographic and socioeconomic aspects of aging in the United States. Current Population Reports 1984; series P-23: no. 138.
6. Abeles RP, Ory MG. Aging, health, and behavior. ICPSR Bull 1991;(Sep):1–5.
7. Cassel CK, Rudberg MA, Olshansky SJ. The price of success: health care in an aging society. Health Affairs 1992;(Summer):87–99.
8. Soldo BJ, Agree EM. America's elderly. Popul Bull 1988;43(3):5–45.
9. Anonymous. Geographic profile of the aged. Stat Bull Metrop Ins Co 1993;74(1):2–9.
10. Butler RN, Hyer K. The aging populace. J Health Care Poor Underserved 1990;1:156–168.
11. Rogers RG. Living and dying in the U.S.A.: sociodemographic determinants of death among blacks and whites. Demography 1992;29:287–303.
12. Estes CL, Rundall TG. Social characteristics, social structure, and health in the aging population. In: Ory MG, Abeles RP, Lipman PD, eds. Aging, health and behavior. Newbury Park, CA: Sage, 1992:299–325.
13. Kaplan GA, Haan MN. Is there a role for prevention among the elderly? Epidemiological evidence from the Alameda County Study. In: Ory MG, Bond K, eds. Aging and health care: social science and policy perspectives. New York: Routledge, 1989:27–51.
14. Soldo BJ, Manton KG. Demographic challenges for sociodemographic planning. Socio-economic Planning Sci 1985;19:227–247.
15. Manton KG. The dynamics of population aging: demography and policy analysis. Milbank Q 1991; 69(2):309–339.
16. Manton KG. Planning long-term care for heterogeneous populations. In: Maddox GL, Lawton MP, eds. Annual review of gerontology and geriatrics, vol 8: varieties of aging. New York: Springer, 1988:217–255.
17. Burr JA, Mitchell JE. The living arrangements of unmarried elderly hispanic females. Demography 1992 29(1):93–112.
18. Doty P. Family care of the elderly: the role of public policy. Milbank Q 1986;64:34–75.
19. Horowitz A. Family caregiving to the frail elderly. In: Eisdorfer C, ed. Annual review of gerontology and geriatrics, vol 5. New York: Springer, 1985:194–246.
20. Tennstedt S, McKinlay JB. Informal care for frail older persons. In: Ory MG, Bond K, eds. Aging and health care: social science and policy perspectives. New York: Routledge, 1989:145–166.
21. Moon M. The economic situation of older Americans: emerging wealth and continuing hardship. In: Maddox GL, Lawton MP, eds. Annual review of gerontology and geriatrics, vol 8: varieties of aging. New York: Springer, 1988:102–131.
22. McLaughlin DK, Jensen L. Poverty among older Americans: the plight of nonmetropolitan elders. J Gerontol 1993;48:S44–54.
23. Rowe JW, Kahn RL. Human aging: usual and successful. Science 1987;237:143–149.
24. Manton KG, Corder L, Stallard E. Changes in the use of personal assistance and special equipment form 1982 to 1989: results from the 1982 and 1989 NLTCS. Gerontologist 1993;33:168–176.
25. Crimmins EM, Saito Y. Getting better and getting worse: transitions in functional status among older Americans. J Aging Health 1993;5:3–36.
26. Mossey JM, Havens B, Wolinsky FD. The consistency of formal health care utilization: physician and hospital utilization. In: Ory MG, Bond K, eds. Aging and health care: social science and policy perspectives. New York: Routledge, 1989:81–98.
27. Wan TH. The behavioral model of health care utilization by older people. In: Ory MG, Bond K, eds. Aging and health care: social science and policy perspectives. New York: Routledge, 1989:52–77.
28. Kemper P, Murtaugh CM. Lifetime use of nursing home care. N Engl J Med 1991;324:595–600.
29. Wolinsky FD, Arnold CL. A different perspective on health and health service utilization. In: Maddox GL, Lawton MP, eds. Annual review of gerontology and geriatrics, vol 8: varieties of aging. New York: Springer, 1988:71–101.

49/ Health Care Economics

David S. Greer, Vincent Mor

The economics of health care for the elderly population of the United States can usefully be divided into the pre- and post-Medicare eras. Medicare, the predominant insurer of care for the elderly, was enacted into law as part of the Social Security Amendments of 1965 (Title XVIII). Medicaid, hastily added to that legislation as Title XIX, created an additional joint federal-state program for medical assistance to the needy, including the elderly.

Prior to the 1965 Social Security legislation, support for medical care for Americans aged 65 and older was fragmented, highly variable both geographically and demographically, and frequently inadequate. The proportion of the U.S. population that was elderly had risen rapidly throughout the 20th century, particularly those at the upper end of the age scale. Most were women, frequently unmarried or widowed and living alone, and their distribution was uneven. At midcentury, the elderly population was increasing in educational level and political sophistication as well as size, and rapid advances in mass communication enabled them to better organize and develop national consensus on their needs. Life expectancy was rising and with it, the incidence of chronic disease and the need for medical care.

The cost of medical care in the United States was also rising at an accelerated rate at midcentury. In the 1950s and early 1960s, the medical care index rose at twice the rate of the consumer price index, largely because of increased use and inflation of the cost of hospital care. Annual per capita gross expenditures by noninstitutionalized elderly were twice that for those under age 65 ($177 vs. $86 in 1958), and the spread was wider if institutionalized individuals, more frequent among the elderly, were included.

Health insurance coverage among the elderly was inadequate. In 1957, less than 40% had some form of voluntary health insurance, with most policies deficient in benefit structure. A survey of the hospital insurance coverage of the elderly in the years 1958 to 1960 revealed that only 30.3% of persons over age 65 and 20.2% of those over 75 had insurance that would cover as much as three-quarters of their hospital bill. With incomes below the "modest but adequate" level established by the Bureau of Labor Statistics, most elderly could not pay for needed hospitalization or even less-expensive out-patient care.

A variety of municipal, county, state, and voluntary initiatives existed to fill the gaps in the "nonsystem" of care, but the results were generally unsatisfactory to both the needy recipients and the providers of care. In the early 1960s, consensus developed on the need for federal support, at least to augment the efforts of the existing support mechanisms. Some saw an opportunity, at last, to overcome the long-standing opposition by conservative forces to a national system of comprehensive coverage, and this did become possible for the elderly in 1965 as part of the Great Society Program of President Lyndon Johnson.

The legislative history of Medicare has been described as a "long overture" (1). It began in 1912 when Theodore Roosevelt, running for president, proposed the adoption of comprehensive national health insurance. The ensuing debate extended sporadically for almost half a century, with the opposition led by the American Medical Association, joined by those opposed generally to federal social support programs.

The depression of the 1930s awakened interest in federal health insurance as part of the initial Social Security legislation. Subsequent proposals, in 1939 by Senator Wagner of New York; in 1943 by Senators Wagner, Murray, and Dingell; in 1948 by President Harry Truman; and in 1951 by Oscar Ewing, the head of the Federal Security Agency, failed to overcome the opposition. The Ewing proposal, focused on the elderly, created a political opportunity and a constituency for President Johnson that ultimately culminated in the passage of Medicare and Medicaid legislation as part of the Social Security Amendments of 1965.

The complex structure, limited benefits, and provider payment policies of Medicare are in part attributable to the influence of a variety of political and legislative factors and factions that had their roots in the long debate over national health insurance.

MEDICARE: A THREE-PART PROGRAM

The Social Security legislation of 1965 created three programs of support for the medical care of the elderly: basic protection against the costs of hospital and related care, sometimes called "part A Medicare"; a voluntary supplementary program covering the cost of doctors' services and a number of other items and services not covered by the basic program ("part B"); and a joint federal-state program for medical assistance to the needy, not restricted to but including the elderly ("Medicaid"). Only the Medicaid program is means-tested, i.e., restricted to economically disadvantaged individuals.

The hospital insurance program, part A, is largely financed out of taxes paid by employers, employees, and the self-employed, in association with existing federal retirement programs. With varying deductibles and copayments by beneficiaries (which have risen steadily over the years), part A pays for room and board, nursing, medication, and the standard medical/social services delivered in hospitals and, with considerable limitation, in extended care facilities. Limited home health service benefits are also included, primarily part-time nursing care and physical, occupational, and speech therapy after hospital discharge.

Unlike part A, the part B program is voluntary and is funded by enrollee premium payments, supplemented by federal appropriations. Both the premiums and the deductibles have risen progressively since the initial $3.00 and $50.00, respectively. (In 1993, $36.60 and $100.00). The copayment requirement has remained at 20%, but the rapid rise in "reasonable, prevailing and customary" physician fees allowed by Medicare and the ability of physicians to establish charges above Medicare-approved fees have limited the financial protection afforded by part B. While over 10 states have instituted (and the federal government has encouraged) mandatory assignment in which part B providers cannot bill for the unpaid balance of their bill ("balance billing"), where such legislation is not in place, elders' actual copayment may be as high as half the bill, depending on the providers' charge. Part B covers physician services (partially) and a variety of other services

not covered by part A, such as additional home health visits, outpatient diagnostic radiologic and laboratory tests, ambulance, and various supplies and ancillary services rendered outside of hospitals.

In spite of the fact that over 98% of Medicare beneficiaries are enrolled in part B, the limitations of the Medicare program and rapidly escalating health care costs have made it necessary for many elderly to acquire supplementary insurance. For those below income and asset standards (set at disparate levels by the various states), the Medicaid program may provide benefits; these benefits, however, are often inadequate to ensure access to quality care. As of 1991, 65% of all Medicare beneficiaries have some form of supplemental private insurance coverage, although in some cases this may be disease-specific policies with limited coverage. A large and growing proportion of the elderly, not eligible for Medicaid and/or desiring more adequate coverage, purchase supplementary insurance from private sources.

POST-MEDICARE ERA

COST ESCALATION

In a large, complex, and dynamic enterprise like the U.S. health care "nonsystem," it is impossible to attribute change to any one factor. However, accelerated change did follow the initiation of the Medicare program in 1965. Cost escalation was immediate; during the period 1960–65, the per capita personal health care bill increased about 7% annually; increases after Medicare and Medicaid were appreciably higher than 7% and were dramatically high for the elderly, 20.2% in the fiscal year 1967 and 20.9% in 1968. From 1966 to 1975, the per capita health care expenditure for those under age 65 rose from $155 to $375, while for those 65 and over they rose from $445 to $1,360. In less than a decade the elderly were paying more for their health care out-of-pocket than they did before Medicare and Medicaid were adopted, despite the large proportional increase paid from public sources (from 29.8% in 1966 to 65.6% in 1975) (2).

The rapid rise in total medical care costs for the elderly has continued. Health care inflation in general has consistently outpaced overall inflation (3), and the cost of caring for older Americans has risen faster than that for those under age 65. In 1966, Medicare made a total of $1 billion in benefits payments; in 1990 it was $105 billion. Part A copayments, deductibles, and Part B premiums have all risen at least tenfold since the program began (4). Furthermore, the out-of-pocket cost to the elderly has continued to rise faster than their average income—in 1975 enrollees paid 4.2% of their income for health care, while in 1990 this figure was 5.7%. Figure 49.1 contrasts total national health care expenditures and Medicare expenditures from 1975 to 1990. As is evident, between 1975 and 1985 growth in Medicare spending outpaced national expenditures; this difference leveled off over the last years of the decade.

EXPENDITURES

Repeated efforts to contain the rapidly rising cost of health care in the United States have had limited success. Hospital utilization review, prospective payment of hospitals (the Diagnosis Related Group (DRG) system), and, more recently, reimbursement of physicians using a "Resource Based Relative Value Scale" (RBRVS) have thus far failed to bring either total health care or Medicare cost inflation down to the level of inflation of the general economy. Currently, the cost of health care to all payers stands at approximately $900 billion, 14% of the gross national product and, by far, the largest in the world; and coverage remains inadequate.

Medicare is primarily an acute care program; almost two-thirds of its expenditures goes to hospitals. Physician services account for about 25% of Medicare costs, again mostly for in-patient care. Skilled nursing facilities and home health care programs receive a minuscule, although rapidly growing, portion of Medicare expenditures (Fig. 49.2). Costs for disabled persons and patients with end-stage renal disease, many of whom are not elderly, have risen more rapidly than costs for the aged but remain a small fraction of the total cost.

A small subset of the aged population accounts for a large amount of the cost; in 1986 (the last year for which these figures are available) enrollees costing $15,000 or more represented only 3.1% of all aged persons enrolled but accounted for 38.0% of all Medicare reimbursements for the aged; contrarily, another 43.3% of aged enrollees cost less than $1000 each and accounted for only 5.5% of Medicare reimbursements for the aged (5).

Health Expenditures in Billions by Year: Medicare and Total

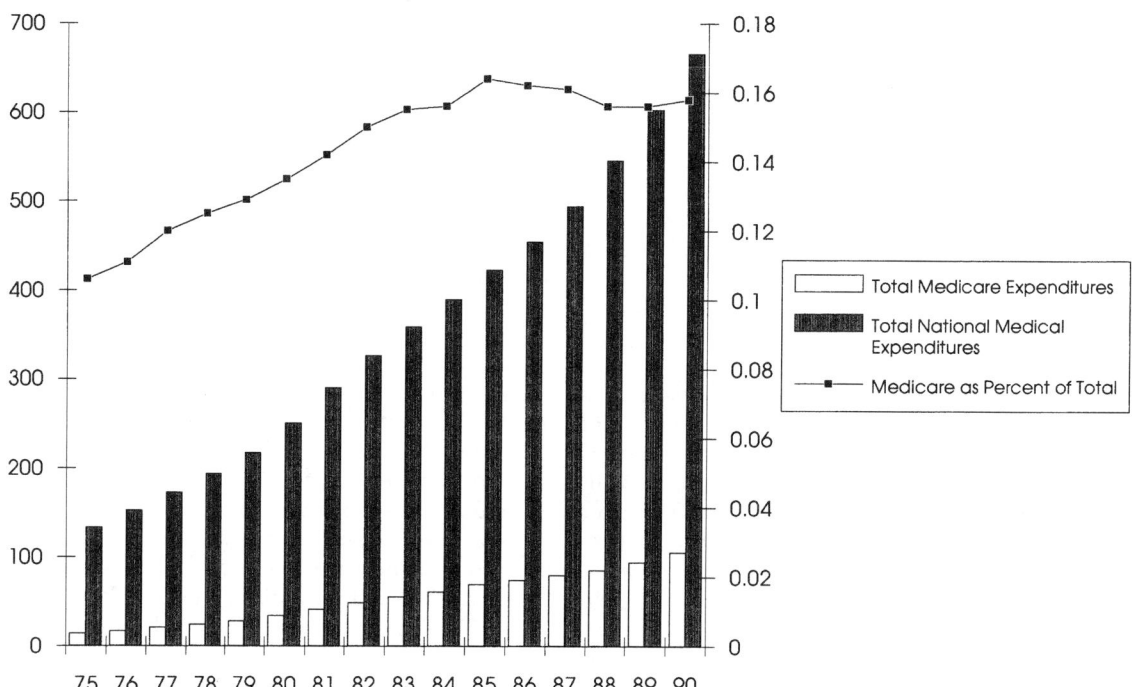

Figure 49.1   Health expenditures in billions by year: Medicare and total. (Source: Health Care Financing Administration, Bureau of Data Management and Strategy: Office of Statistics and Data Management.)

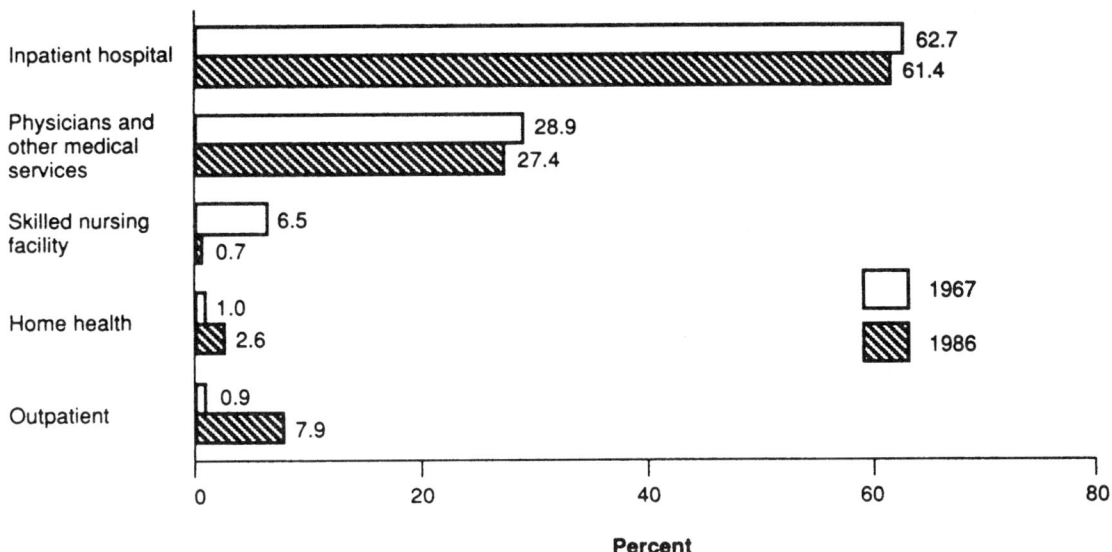

Figure 49.2 Percentage distribution of Medicare reimbursements, by type of service, calendar years 1967 and 1986. (Data from Anonymous. Health Care Financing Program Statistics: Medicare and Medicaid data book, 1990. Washington, DC: U.S. Department of Health and Human Services, 1990:19.)

Furthermore, throughout the history of the Medicare program, a disproportionate share of annual expenditures is allocated to individuals who die in that year (6).

IMPACT

What has this massive expenditure bought? Access to care for the elderly appears to have improved; for example, hospital discharges for the overall population declined from 109.1 per 1000 in 1964 to 93.4 in 1988 but increased for those over 65 from 190 in 1964 to 259.7 in 1988. Physician visits and surgery rates among the elderly have also risen (7). Possible overuse has replaced underuse as a dominant concern in the post-Medicare period.

It is impossible to assess the precise relationship between access to care and health status. Certainly, the health of many Americans, including the elderly, has improved since 1965, but improved health care benefit programs like Medicare are only one variable in a complex equation. While some have argued that longevity increases among the elderly during the 1970s and 1980s are attributable to increased access to medical care, there has been no concrete evidence for this assertion (8). Recent increasing interest in outcome research may provide better data on the impact of improved access to care on health status, but at present, it is impossible to determine what the dramatic increase in expenditure by both government and private sources has bought for patients and the population at large. Providers of care and insurers have experienced sharply increasing incomes but at the price of increased bureaucratic intrusion and loss of professional autonomy.

MEDICAID

Medicaid began as a stopgap program to consolidate and rationalize the many different state and county health and welfare programs serving the elderly and poor prior to 1965. Medicaid is partially federally supported and state administered; it pays for the medical care of certain low-income individuals and families. Over the years, the states have had considerable discretion on who and what is covered by Medicaid. Additionally, the states' levels of participation have changed over the years, as have federal mandates regarding coverage and services. Presently, states must cover low-income families with children who receive Aid to Families with Dependent Children (AFDC) and low-income aged and disabled persons. Participating states must offer certain basic services such as hospital and outpatient care, selected diagnostic testing, physicians' services and skilled nursing facility care. The program is jointly financed by the state and federal governments, the amount of the federal share ranging from 50 to 80%, depending upon the state's per capita income (5).

Since Medicare was not intended to fully meet the long-term care needs of the aged population, over the years Medicaid has paid a progressively larger share of all long-term care costs for the aged, which have taken an increasing percentage of the total Medicaid budget. For example, in 1986 when only 13.9% of all Medicaid recipients were aged, the aged accounted for 36.8% of all Medicaid expenditures, largely payment for long-term care services. Figure 49.3 shows the changes in Medicaid payments allocated to long-term care, hospital care, and all other payments between 1974 and 1986. In 1986 Medicaid paid $12.5 billion for nursing home services and an additional $1.3 billion for home health services. In many states, Medicaid recipients over 65 consumed nearly one-half of all payments.

Medicaid pays about half the cost of nursing home care in the U.S.; most of the rest is paid for privately. Over the past decade there has been concern about nursing home residents "spending down" their assets to qualify for Medicaid. For those with spouses still living in the community, asset "spend-down" may lead to the impoverishment of the spouse. Empirical studies have consistently shown, however, that only a relatively small proportion (less than 10%) of all those admitted to nursing homes as "private pay" become Medicaid eligible (i.e., have spent down) before they are discharged or die, unless they spend 3 or more years in the home, which is only a minority of all admissions (9, 10). Since assets and income

that are "excused" from consideration in determining the financial eligibility of older persons for Medicaid vary from state to state, admission to a facility across a state line may have substantial implications. To address this and to reduce the burden of spousal impoverishment, in the late 1980s the value of commonly held assets that could be protected for the community-living spouse was increased substantially in all states. To date, there is no empirical evidence about whether the rate of spend-down is increasing, although most pundits feel that it is.

Most states also have expanded home and community service programs to encourage the treatment of older, frail Medicaid recipients outside of the hospital and nursing home setting. Personal care attendants, home care services, extended home health aide care, and case management are services frequently reimbursed by Medicaid. Some states have been particularly aggressive about expanding their service options because the federal government pays for at least half of all approved services. In general, those states that have made a major investment in home and community care feel that it can help reduce their future nursing home costs. Unfortunately, there is little evidence for this assumption; contrarily, some studies indicate that such supplemental services do not reduce nursing home use or total health care costs (11, 12).

Medicaid expenditures on the aged are reaching crisis proportions. In spite of a recently man-

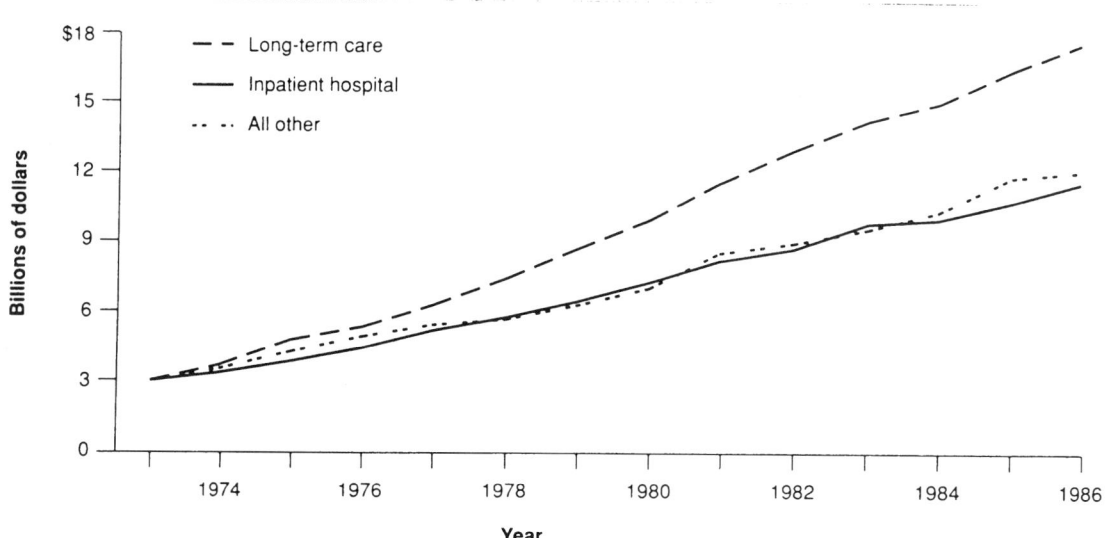

Figure 49.3   Medicaid payments for long-term care, inpatient hospital, and all other services: fiscal years 1973–86. (Data from Anonymous. Health Care Financing Program Statistics: Medicare and Medicaid data book, 1990. Washington, DC: U.S. Department of Health and Human Services, 1990:24.)

dated expansion of eligibility for previously un-covered low-income families, most states spend more of their Medicaid matching funds on the eld-erly and nursing home services than any other category. In the debate on national health care reform, many states are considering revamping their Medicaid programs to reduce the share that goes to the long-term care needs of the elderly. A major issue of intergenerational equity has arisen in this debate as the elderly are increasingly viewed by the population at large as wealthier than the average American. This perception is a radical change from the reality that shaped the policy debate prior to and during the passage of Medicare in 1965, and it may shape the nature of future policies. Indeed, in 1966, 28% of persons 65 and over lived below the poverty line; since 1985 a smaller proportion of the elderly than of all Americans are under the poverty line; this is par-ticularly true of households headed by white males and of married women (4).

FAMILY CARE PAYMENTS

The emphasis on care for the frail elderly at home has prompted considerable discussion about the role of the family in providing health-related and supportive care for elders in the community. One key factor predicting nursing home place-ment is the absence of a supportive family. In rec-ognition of this, many have advocated making the family an explicit partner in the long-term care-provider network by reimbursing them for their efforts to prevent nursing home placement. The rationale for this is that were the individual in the nursing home, Medicaid would be paying for the care; if the individual remains in the community, the family members bear a good deal of the bur-den.

During the 1980s, several states began dem-onstration projects to explore the feasibility and economics of making payments to family caregiv-ers (13). Since it is against Medicaid regulations to use Medicaid funds to pay related caregivers, these programs were financed by state funds and supplementation of basic Supplemental Security Income payments. In 1990, 35 states permitted payments to family caregivers and covered serv-ices that family members might provide. Pay-ments to relatives are usually restricted to the care of frail elders at risk of institutionalization and in many cases exclude certain kinds of rela-tionships. Fifteen states exclude payments to a spouse, four exclude adult children, and five states do not pay adult siblings. The recent ex-pansion of Medicaid-covered services through

demonstrations or "federal waiver" of coverage and service limits has apparently led to a reduc-tion in the availability of state-sponsored family payment programs (13). In general, the research suggests that compensation of family caregivers is an underused long-term-care financing option that could have enormous implications for future health care costs.

MEDICARE SUPPLEMENTAL INSURANCE

As with most traditional indemnity health in-surance policies, Medicare covers only part of el-ders' medical expenditures. Since copayments for physician and hospital care can be quite high, a large market for "supplemental coverage" has emerged, often sold by the Blue Cross and Blue Shield insurers, who serve as the Medicare fiscal intermediaries in many parts of the country. A 1991 survey of Medicare beneficiaries asked over 15,000 respondents whether they have and how they pay for supplemental coverage. Figure 49.4 presents these data, revealing that one-third of Medicare beneficiaries had supplemental cover-age from an employer-sponsored retirement plan, and another 42% purchased coverage privately or in combination with an employer-covered plan. Only 11.4% of beneficiaries had no supplemental coverage; 11.9% were dually eligible for both Med-icare and Medicaid.

Although the major carriers of supplemental health insurance offer several types of plans, many smaller insurers have entered the market, offering specialty products that in some cases have a very poor ratio of premiums paid to expen-ditures. In the late 1980s, several scandals prompted an investigation that resulted in legis-lation mandating a standardization of supple-mental coverage policies. Since 1991, Medicare ben-eficiaries' choices of supplemental coverage have been greatly simplified (14).

LONG-TERM CARE INSURANCE

In view of the enormous health care costs in-curred by older persons residing in long-term care facilities or requiring extensive long-term care services at home, it is not surprising that a mar-ket for private long-term care insurance has de-veloped over the last decade (15, 16). Advocates for private health insurance have often opposed those in the public sector who have proposed pro-gressive expansion of the Medicare and Medicaid programs in the long-term care area. The conflict has been both philosophical and political. Politi-cally, adoption of public coverage for long-term care, such as was proposed by the Pepper Com-

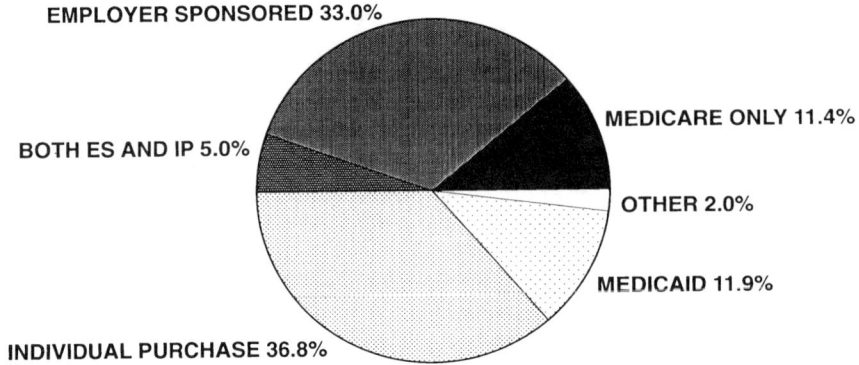

Figure 49.4   Supplemental health insurance for Medicare elderly, 1991. (Data from Anonymous. Medicare Current Beneficiary Survey, Round One Data. Health Care Financing Administration, Department of Health and Human Services: Office of National Health Statistics.)

mission (15), is not feasible given the huge cost. Furthermore, expansion of publicly financed services reduces the private insurance market for long-term care which, given the chance, should respond to individual buyers' concerns about their risk of incurring catastrophic long-term care costs.

According to Leutz and his colleagues, almost all of the 1.1 million long-term care insurance policies sold by 1988 were individual indemnity plans. While there has been some expansion of group plans used to indemnify the population of residents in continuing care retirement communities (CCRC), these constitute only a minority of arrangements. Most policies focus on nursing home care, although increasingly plans have been adding home care provisions which are "traded off" for nursing home covered days. Policy prices increase in relation to the age of the beneficiary at the time of policy purchase and most policies require a pre-purchase physical to adjust for the applicant's risk of needing services in the very near future.

Since the emergence of private long-term care insurance, there has been concern about the fiscal viability of some insurers and the benefits of the insurance to the policyholders. The General Accounting Office (an arm of Congress) has undertaken several investigations of the long-term-care insurance market, most recently in the summer of 1993 (17). They concluded that an average of 20% of long-term-care insurance policies lapse during the first year of ownership. The report also notes that commissions on the sales of long-term-care policies were higher than comparable industry standards, at least partly because the product was viewed "hard to sell." Such reports, as well as earlier exposes that revealed that some compa-

nies offering long-term care insurance were not financially sound and would find it difficult to meet their obligations, reinforced public skepticism about such policies. While the numbers of such policies sold have been growing over the years, it is likely that long-term care insurance will continue to be a "hard sell" for some time.

FUTURE PROSPECTS

As this is being written, the United States is debating yet another program to nationalize its medical care nonsystem and, particularly, to control its costs. Total medical expenditures in 1993 were about $900 billion, 14% of the gross domestic product. By far the most costly in the world, the American nonsystem nevertheless fails to insure some 37 million Americans and provides inadequate support for millions more. Many of the country's economic problems have been attributed to the diversion of resources into medical care.

A massive restructuring of the American medical service system has been proposed by the Clinton administration. Consistent with the nation's culture and values, the proposal relies heavily on free market forces to produce the desired result, coverage of the total population by a high-quality, cost-effective system of care. Individuals and groups are to be joined in large, regional purchasing cooperatives, called Health Care Alliances, which will purchase health care packages from competing vendors. The system is to be financed by employer contributions and government subsidization of the unemployed and/or indigent; individuals may share a small part of the costs. The Medicare program is to continue as a separate entity, somewhat expanded, but able to participate in the new system for supplemental coverage. The federal government will establish standard benefit packages that must be included in all alliance-vendor contracts, and it may also establish cost ceilings, either as a global national cap on total health care expenditures or as limitations on premium price increases.

The Clinton administration plan has aroused once again the traditional opponents of national health care systems and cost constraints. Prolonged national debate is inevitable, pitting public sector attempts to organize and control against private interests, e.g., the "medical industrial complex," private insurers, and professionals who have profited from the laissez-faire approach to medical care delivery. Superimposed on these contending factions is the distrust of central control and authority of the American public at large. Americans value their freedom, individual and entrepreneurial, even when freedom produces suboptimal social outcomes. History, the power of the opposing forces, and American sentiment seem likely to coalesce into potent resistance that will divert, if not destroy, this latest attempt to nationalize the health care delivery system of the United States. The outcome is, therefore, in doubt. Health care for the elderly, although temporarily insulated from the reform movement, is likely to be swept up by the turbulence in the national system.

REFERENCES

1. Blumenthal D, Schlesinger M, Brown-Drumheller P. Renewing the promise—medicare and reform. New York: Oxford University Press, 1988.
2. Gornick M. Ten years of Medicare: impact on the covered population. Social Security Bulletin. Washington, DC: Social Security Board, July 1976.
3. Friedman E. Medicare and Medicaid at 25. Hospitals 1990;64:38–54.
4. 1991 Green Book. Washington, DC: USGPO, 1991; May 7:134–135.
5. Health Care Financing Program Statistics: Medicare and Medicaid Data Book, 1990. Washington, DC: U.S. Department of Health and Human Services, 1990.
6. Lubitz JD, Riley GF. Trends in Medicare payments in the last year of life. N Engl J Med 1993;328:1092–1096.
7. Waldo DR, Lazenby HC. Demographic characteristics and health care use and expenditures by the aged in the United States: 1977–1984. Health Care Financing Review 1984;6(1):1–29.
8. Scitovsky AA. Medical care in the last twelve months of life: the relation between age, functional status, and medical care expenditures. Milbank Q 1989;66:640–660.
9. Mor V, Intrator O, Laliberte L. Factors affecting conversion rates to Medicaid among new admissions to nursing homes. Health Serv Res 1993:28(1):1–25.
10. Adams E, Meiners M, Burwell B. Asset spenddown in nursing homes: methods and insights. Med Care 1993;31(1):1–23.
11. Weissert W. Seven reasons why it is so difficult to make community-based long-term care cost-effective. Health Serv Res 1985;20(4):423–433.
12. Weissert W, Cready C. Toward a model for improved targeting of aged at risk of institutionalization. Health Serv Res 1989;24(4):485–510.
13. Linsk NL, Keigher SM, Simon-Rusinowitz L, England SE. Wages for caring: compensating family care of the Elderly. New York: Praeger, 1992.
14. Anonymous. Medigap insurance: insurers whose loss ratios did not meet federal minimum standards in 1988–89 (GAO/HRD-92–54). Washington, DC: U.S. General Accounting Office, Human Resources Division, Feb 1992.
15. Leutz W, Capitman J, MacAdam M, Abrahams R. Care for frail elders. Westport, CT: Auburn House, 1992.
16. Wallack SS. Recent trends in financing long-term care. Health Care Financing Rev 1988;(suppl):97–102.
17. Anonymous. Long-term care insurance: high percentage of policyholders drop policies (GAO/HRD-93–129). Washington, DC: U.S. General Accounting Office, Human Resources Division, Aug 1993.

50/ Retirement

Patricia Lanoie Blanchette, Gilbert L. Wergowske, Renee Hollison

Some guys in this business slow down, retire and take it easy. A couple of months later, they're dead.
—*Lee Iacocca, Chairman, Chrysler Corporation.*

Because retirement is such a prominent life event, it sometimes becomes a rationalization for subsequent changes in health. Though convenient, this spurious explanation discounts the effects of years of unrecognized or untreated illness (1). Our cultural ideology venerating work as one's main source of identity and self-worth reinforces the fallacy (2). While the life change associated with retirement is stressful, only a few suffer serious physical or emotional illness as a result. Most research in this area suggests that retirement does not contribute significantly to morbidity or mortality. Yet the myth is perpetuated in individual anecdotes and misinterpretations of research findings in the lay press (3–5).

Only in recent decades and in developed countries has retirement become possible. In much of the Third World, people still work until physical incapacity or death. The arbitrary selection of age 65 for retirement is a decision attributed to the government of Kaiser Wilhelm II (1888–1941). Since the average life expectancy at birth in Germany was then 63 years, their government pension fund was not overburdened. With life expectancy at birth in the United States now approaching 75 years in men and exceeding 78 years in women, the average worker can expect to spend approximately 19 or more years in retirement (6). Additionally, important changes in the gender of the work force have begun. Both life expectancy and gender are having a substantial impact on the financial and social costs of retirement.

Social problems are cyclically redefined under economic pressures to reduce the cost of their solutions. Mandatory retirement in the past was considered a socially acceptable way of contracting the labor force to accommodate the needs of the economy and a simple and legal means for employers to reduce costs by eliminating their most

expensive workers (7, 8). However, proponents of mandatory retirement failed to take into account the increasing years of healthy and productive life expectancy and the enormous costs of providing health care and retirement benefits to a rapidly growing number of older people. We are now seeing people retiring as a matter of choice and going into other types of productive work.

The term *retirement* is ambiguous. It can refer to the cessation of a long working or professional career, usually associated with advanced age. The term can also mean terminating one specific job to be entitled to "retirement" benefits. Military personnel, for example, may receive a pension after 20 or 30 years of service but continue to work full-time for other employers for another 20 or 30 years.

PHYSICAL HEALTH AND RETIREMENT

An increase in the use of health care services during 2 years before retirement has been observed, suggesting that ill health precipitates retirement (9–12). However, despite established myth, the converse does not appear to be true. Most published studies of health status following retirement indicate that retirement per se is not associated with either immediate or long-term effects on physical or general health, nor is it strongly associated with increased use of health care services. No clinically significant change in blood pressure or cholesterol levels in retirees was found in the Veterans' Administration Normative Aging Study (13). No change in health attributable to retirement was found in a study of steel workers retired because of the sudden and unexpected closing of their plants (14). No increase in mortality was found among workers at a Norwegian fish cannery who retired as a result of plant closure, compared with workers at a similar factory that remained open, although a 10% increase in subsequent time on disability pension was seen in the first group for the first 10 years of observation (15).

In some studies, people who retired in poor health actually improved after retirement (16–18), but this may be a false perception caused by reduction in job stress and role demands (19). Actual health does not always correspond to perceived health, and perceptions may change as adjustment to retirement progresses. Differences in physical and general health between working and retired people are better explained by reasons for retirement, including occupational diseases, and by lifelong preparation and expectations (12, 20).

Four of every five community-based people aged 65 or older have at least one chronic health condition (21). Although not all of these conditions compromise functional capacity, ill health is the primary self-reported reason given for early retirement, particularly among blue collar workers (22). When work-limiting ill health is cited as the primary reason for retirement, especially early retirement, the probability of death within 2 years of retirement is increased by about 4% (23). Such declines in perceived health state, which start 1 to 6 years before retirement, are not attributable to the life change event per se, but rather to the underlying chronic condition (24).

Aside from retirement for ill health, several other factors appear to influence health beyond retirement. Limitation of functional capacity was the leading predictor of poor health and mortality in the 1991 New Beneficiary Survey of the Social Security Administration (25). The number of health conditions and the presence of circulatory and respiratory conditions also indicated increased mortality. Among demographic features, increased age, male gender, unmarried status, low income, and low education predicted increased mortality. In a study of 627 retired Parisian men and women, high job mobility appeared to be associated with the number of health conditions present after retirement, especially for women and nonprofessional workers (26). High job mobility has also been associated with an increase in cardiovascular diseases (27).

MENTAL HEALTH AND RETIREMENT

Mental health problems are the most important reasons for early retirement, eclipsing both physical health problems and economic concerns (28). Retirement is itself a potentially stressful life event, but research results concerning its effects on mental health are contradictory. Overall, it appears that mental difficulties caused by re-

tirement are not particularly serious and that the number of people in whom serious disturbances occur is small (29). Related factors, such as low income, adversely affect the mental health of some retired people (30). Retirement specifically for reasons of poor mental health may be more common than is currently recognized (28), and this group of retirees would not be expected to thrive.

Each retirement must be considered individually, in the full complexity of the physical, psychological, social, and economic milieu of the person affected. Many factors affect the acceptance and course of retirement. The degree of insecurity and emotional disturbance that accompanies retirement depends on the retiree's personal goals and past losses (31) and interpretation of the professional and economic change. Thus, the stronger the preretirement work-oriented urge, the higher the predictability of postretirement obstacles to overcome (24).

VOLUNTARY VERSUS INVOLUNTARY RETIREMENT

Many people are not highly satisfied with their jobs and will leave the work force voluntarily as soon as they feel financially secure (6, 32). This accounts for almost half of retired persons. Voluntary retirement is more often associated with more time spent in preretirement leisure activities and preretirement planning. Both serve to lessen the adverse impact of lifestyle changes (12, 33–36).

Involuntary retirement most often results from health problems. Decline in health accounts for 25 to 35% of all retirements (37, 38). Other causes of involuntary retirement include compulsory age retirement and job closings. Retirements associated with job closings often come with inadequate notice to allow for preparation. Surprisingly, most people seem to adjust to the new circumstances and, after a period of adjustment, manage fairly well (39). The three most common factors for maladjustment are a feeling of economic deprivation, difficulty in keeping occupied, and retirement in poor health (40).

SUCCESSFUL RETIREMENT

Continuing participation in some type of work is a predictor of positive adjustment to retirement. For some, this may be an entirely new profession or pursuit. For others, it may simply be a change of focus. Nearly half of all retirees reduce work time gradually. The time spent in partial retirement often exceeds 5 years. Only 30% of retirees exit the labor force in a single transition, and about half of the members of this group eventually return to work (41). In keeping with the rapid pace of technology and the changing work environment, some have predicted a lifelong pattern of changes in work activities interspersed with periods of retraining as the norm for the future.

Volunteering in community activities is one way to keep occupied and maintain social contact. For the most part, persons who were active in the community before retirement continue their activity, and those who were not active remain inactive. However, certain demographic characteristics may help identify which of these inactive retirees may be recruited to volunteer projects. These include involvement in religious activities, level of education, and satisfaction with their neighborhood (42). Retired men do more household maintenance and paid work outside the home, while retired women do more housework, child care in the home, caregiving outside the home, and volunteer activities (43).

A strong marital relationship and religious beliefs and activities may diminish retirement-related depression. However, women may experience more frequent sadness because they are more likely to have many friends and to feel the pain of losses experienced by others. Conversely, men may be lonelier because they have more difficulty forming and keeping close friendships (16, 29, 44).

COMMON PROBLEMS IN RETIREMENT

One of the most common stresses of retirement is a concern over financial security and a vulnerability to financial abuse. Although the current average number of years spent in retirement is 19, this number continues to increase every year as life expectancy is increasing. We are rapidly approaching a time when the number of years in retirement equals the number of work years. Yet many workers have only a vague idea about their retirement needs and benefits. The early and middle work years are filled with the pressing needs of establishing a family and a home and providing for the education of children. The physician providing counseling with regard to preventive medicine should remember to advise a patient to get competent financial advice early to prepare for retirement. It is a misconception to think that the need for income is substantially reduced in retirement. While some may have paid off mortgages or reside with family, others may need to continue to pay the increasing costs of food, rent, utilities,

and maintenance. Additionally, new types of expenses may ensue, such as the need to purchase more services and a desire to travel to stay in touch with family. Social Security was not designed to be the sole source of support in retirement, yet only 30% of private sector retirees are now getting pension benefits (45), and individuals are not preparing adequately for retirement, as indicated by a drop of up to 50% in income-to-needs ratios after 8 years of retirement (46). As the retired population continues to grow, early preparation for retirement will become essential to maintain the nation's ability to care for those who are truly disadvantaged.

Loneliness, perhaps the most destructive accompaniment of aging, can be exacerbated by retirement. The resulting boredom and frustration can lead to a range of limiting illnesses, which may be psychosomatic, but are nevertheless physiologically factual (47). It is apparent, however, that loneliness is one factor that may be ameliorated with thoughtful intervention. In the longitudinal follow-up of the men in the Normative Aging Study, retirement per se produced no apparent effect on quantitative or qualitative social support (48). In another study, most retirees reported a slight decline in the quantity of social supports, compared with workers, but the quality of their interactions increased (49).

Retirees should think long and hard before deciding to distance themselves from their families and lifelong friends by moving into retirement communities many thousands of miles away. This has become an increasing phenomenon, especially for younger retirees for whom the distance may be easily enough traversed. However, as age increases and traveling becomes more cumbersome, many retirees find that their network of newer friends and acquaintances does not compensate for their loss of close contact with their families and hometowns. Loneliness may prevail.

Deafness contributes to the feeling of social isolation, and the affected person often fails to recognize the need for treatment. Unlike the blind whose disability may increase physical touch, deaf people may be socially ostracized because of the sheer difficulty in communicating with them or because of a mistaken impression that they are confused or demented (47). A formal hearing examination should be part of the evaluation for anyone doing poorly in retirement.

Widowhood or the loss of a lifelong partner is one of the most common and significant events that occur during retirement. For the employed person, the need to get back to work and the daily structure provided by a job may help in adjustment and in resolution of the grieving period. For the retired person, this structure and social support network may be lacking, and the loss felt even more acutely.

GENDER DIFFERENCES IN RETIREMENT

Much of what is known about adjustment to retirement is derived from the retirement experiences of men. With an increasing number of women in the work force, information about possible gender differences becomes increasingly important. For example, because of differential life expectancies, women are more likely to become widowed after retirement. Women more than men retire in response to the needs of others, such as illness of a spouse or other family member. In one study, women reported a greater number of stressful life events in the period prior to retirement. Further, their adaptation to retirement was more affected than that of men by the experience of life events. Women both before and after retirement appear to be more affected by crises in their social networks, because they are more likely than men to be called upon to provide support and because they are more likely to become emotionally involved than men (50).

PHYSICIANS' ROLE IN PREPARING PATIENTS FOR RETIREMENT

Physicians providing primary care should take an interest in advising their patients how to prepare for retirement. Although this would seem to be mainly a social concern, it is common for patients to ask the advice of their trusted physicians about such things as ability to work, proposed moves, and the choice to live with or apart from their children. Ignoring the social issues until they become medical issues is costly, ineffective, and wasteful.

The optimal time to start preparing for retirement precedes the first day of employment. It begins with learning good work and social habits, education, training and retraining for employment, and preventive health care, including the avoidance of occupational injuries and diseases. Mental and physical health problems must be identified and addressed in a timely manner. Financial preparation must begin early. A variety of both career and leisure interests should be encouraged.

SUMMARY

The belief that retirement directly precipitates sudden death and catastrophic life events is a myth. Quite often, failing health accelerates the decision to retire. The causes for retirement and preretirement planning play substantial roles in predicting successful adjustment to this major life change. The current pattern of long years of work followed by long years of retirement may be shifting to a new paradigm of periods of work followed by retraining for different types of work throughout a person's life. Successful retirement is associated with strong marital relationships, friendships, religious activities, leisure interests, and financial security. Common problems in retirement include loneliness and depression, widowhood, poor health, and deafness. Many of the problems may be ameliorated with proper planning, preventive medicine, and timely intervention. Physicians have an important role to play as trusted and knowledgeable advisors.

REFERENCES

1. Brim OG, Ryff CD. On the properties of life events. In: Balts PB, Brim OG, eds. Life-span development and behavior, vol 3. New York: Academic Press, 1980.
2. Ekerdt DJ. Why the notion persists that retirement harms health. Gerontologist 1987;27(4):454–457.
3. Casscells W, Evans D, DeSilva R, et al. Retirement and coronary mortality. Lancet 1980;1:1288–1289.
4. CBS Evening News, Transcript 12, November 13, 1979.
5. Gonzales ER. Retiring may predispose to fatal heart attack. JAMA 1980;243:13–14.
6. Portnoi VA. The natural history of retirement. JAMA 1981;245:1752–1754.
7. O'Connor J. The fiscal crisis of the state. New York: St. Martin's, 1973.
8. Minkler M. Research on the health effects of retirement: an uncertain legacy. J Health Soc Behav 1981;22:117–130.
9. Soghikian K, Midanik LT, Polen MR, Ransom LJ. The effect of retirement on health services utilization: the Kaiser Permanente Retirement Study. J Gerontol 1991;46(6):S353–360.
10. Crawford MP. Retirement as a psycho-social crisis. J Psychosom Res 1972;16:375–380.
11. Wan T. Stressful life events. Social support networks and gerontological health. A prospective study. Lexington, MA: Lexington Books, 1982.
12. Salokangas RKR, Joukamaa M. Physical and mental health changes in retirement age. Psychother Psychosom 1991;55:100–107.
13. Ekerdt DJ, Sparrow D, Glynn RJ, Bosse R. Change in blood pressure and total cholesterol with retirement. Am J Epidemiol 1984;120:64–71.
14. Gillanders WR, Buss TF, Wingard E, Gemmel D. Long-term health impacts of forced early retirement among steelworkers. J Fam Pract 1991;32:401–405.
15. Westin S. The structure of a factory closure: individual responses to job-loss and unemployment in a 10-year controlled follow-up study. Soc Sci Med 1990;31(12):1301–1311.
16. Tyhurst JS, Salk L, Kennedy M. Mortality, morbidity and retirement. Am J Public Health 1957; 47:1434–1444.

17. Ryser C, Sheldon A. Retirement and health. J Am Geriatr Soc 1969;17:180–190.
18. Martin S, Doran A. Evidence concerning the relationship between health and retirement. Sociol Rev 1966;14:329–340.
19. Ekerdt DJ, Bosse R, LoCastro JS. Claims that retirement improves health. J Gerontol 1983; 38(2):231–236.
20. Chau N, Bertrand JP, Mur JM, et al. Mortality in retired coke oven plant workers. Br J Ind Med 1993; 50(2):127–135.
21. National Center for Health Statistics. Unpublished data reported in U.S. Senate, Select Committee on Aging. "Aging America: Trends and Projections." Washington, DC, 1984.
22. Shanas E. Health adjustment in retirement. Gerontologist 1970;10:19–21.
23. Boaz RF, Muller CF. The validity of health limitations as a reason for deciding to retire. Health Serv Res 1990;25(2):361–386.
24. Kremer Y. The association between health and retirement: self-health assessment of Israeli retirees. Soc Sci Med 1985;20(1):61–66.
25. Iams HM, McCoy JL. Predictors of mortality among newly retired workers. Soc Security Bull 1991; 54(3):2–10.
26. Iwatsubo Y, Derriennic F, Cassou B. Relation between job mobility during working life and health state after retirement: a cross sectional study of 627 subjects living in the Paris area. Br J Ind Med 1991; 48(11):721–728.
27. Syme SL, Borhani NO, Buechlet RW. Cultural mobility and coronary heart disease in an urban area. Am J Epidemiol 1966;82:334–346.
28. Mitchell JM, Anderson KH. Mental health and the labor force participation of older workers. Inquiry 1989;26(2):262–267.
29. Salokangas RKR, Mattila V, Joukamaa M. Intimacy and mental disorder in late middle age. Acta Psychiatr Scand 1988;78(5):555–560.
30. Abramson JH, Ritter M, Golfin J, Kark JD. Work-health relationships in middle-aged and elderly residents of a Jerusalem community. Soc Sci Med 1992; 34(7):747–755.
31. Rapkin BD, Fischer K. Personal goals of older adults: issues in assessment and prediction. Psychol Aging 1992;7(1):127–137.
32. Henretta JC, Chan CG, O'Rand AM. Retirement reason versus retirement process: examining the reasons for retirement typology. J Gerontol 1992; 47(1):S1–7.
33. Abel BJ, Hayslip B. Locus of control and retirement planning. J Gerontol 1987;42(2):165–167.
34. Broderick T, Glazer B. Leisure participation and the retirement process. Am J Occup Ther 1983; 37(1):15–22.
35. Braithwaite VA, Gibson DM, Bosly-Craft R. An exploratory study of poor adjustment styles among retirees. Soc Sci Med 1986;23(5):493–499.
36. Broderick T, Glazer B. Leisure participation and the retirement process. Am J Occup Ther 1983; 37(1):15–22.
37. Parnes HS, Crowley JE, Haurin RJ, et al. Retirement among American men. Lexington, MA: DC Heath, 1985.
38. Sherman SR. Reported reasons retired workers left their last job: Findings from the new beneficiary survey. Soc Security Bull 1985;48(11):22–30.
39. Portnoi VA. Postretirement depression: myth or reality. Compr Ther 1983;9(7):31–37.
40. Thompson WE, Streib GF, Kosa J. The effect of retirement on personal adjustment: a panel analysis. J Gerontol 1960;15:165–169.
41. Elder GH, Pavalko EK. Work careers in men's later years: transitions, trajectories, and historical change. J Gerontol 1993;48(4):S180–191.
42. Okun MA. Predictors of volunteer status in a retirement community. Int J Aging Hum Dev 1993; 36(1):57–74.
43. Danigelis NL, McIntosh BR. Resources and the productive activity of elders: Race and gender and contexts. J Gerontol 1993;48(4):S192–203.
44. Koenig HG, Cohen HJ, Blazer DG, et al. Religious coping and depression among elderly, hospitalized medically ill men. Am J Psychiatry 1992;149(12): 1693–1700.
45. Reno VP. The role of pensions in retirement income. In: Pensions in a changing economy. Washington, DC: Employee Benefit Research Institute, 1993:19–32.
46. Burkhauser RV, Duncan GJ. Life events, public policy and the economic vulnerability of children and the elderly. In: Palmer JL, Smeeding T, Torrey BB, eds. The vulnerable. Washington, DC: Urban Institute Press, 1988.
47. Brooke N. The effects of retirement. Aust Fam Physician 1980;9(8):576–578.
48. Bosse R, Aldwin CM, Levenson MR, Spiro A III, Mroczek DK. Change in social support after retirement: longitudinal findings from the Normative Aging Study. J Gerontol 1993;48(4):210–217.
49. Bosse R, Aldwin CM, Levenson MR, Workman-Daniels K, Ekerdt DJ. Differences in social support among retirees and workers: findings from the Normative Aging Study. Psychol Aging 1990;5:41–47.
50. Szinovacz M, Washo C. Gender differences in exposure to Life events and adaptation to retirement. J Gerontol 1992;47(4):191–196.

51/ Competence

Brian Merrick, Joan Yesner

The ability to maintain and act upon a set of personal values consistent with an ongoing self-concept is one of the major challenges involved in the process of growing old. Physical, emotional, cognitive, and financial changes associated with aging can pose a serious threat to the level of functioning of the older person.

The determination of the older person's capacity to function from both the clinical and legal points of view is assuming increasing importance. It is necessary to clarify distinctions between *competence*, a legal term, and *capacity*, a clinical term, in examining implications for living arrangements and medical decision making.

It is estimated that 23% of those 65 to 74 and 45% of those over 85 have difficulties managing activities of daily living (ADLs) and that these figures will increase by 31% over the next 20 years (1). As older adults have the highest prevalence of cognitive impairment, the significant growth rate predicted for this segment of the population has obvious implications for clinicians working with this group (1).

A major responsibility of health care professionals working with older people is an accurate evaluation of the various facets of functional capacity. There are two major pitfalls to be avoided: (a) an underestimation of ability to manage (often based on ageist assumptions that to be old is to be disabled and suffering), resulting in a violation of personal autonomy, and (b) a disregard for significant deficits that do result in serious risk to health and/or safety.

DISTINCTIONS BETWEEN COMPETENCE AND CAPACITY

Although the term *competence* is broadly used to connote decision-making ability, it is important to understand that *competence* is a legal term and to differentiate between the clinical assessment of capacity to understand and make decisions and the legal determination by a judge that someone is incompetent. A person is assumed to be com-petent unless determined otherwise in a court of law. The legal concept of competence has traditionally been a global, all-or-nothing one arrived at in a static fashion within a limited context. The focus has been primarily on ability to comprehend information and make related decisions: "As a result of traditions of case law and wordings of statutes, competence is commonly conceptualized as an entirely cognitive capacity by attorneys and judges" (2).

There are two areas in which physicians play a central role in evaluating the capacity of the older person. The most obvious one is in capacity for medical decision making. The other is in helping to determine the degree to which independent living remains possible in the face of increasing impairments. Balancing respect for autonomy with the responsibility for provision of adequate care can often be difficult when faced with what appear to be very bad, even life-threatening decisions by some older patients. However, it is when a patient *refuses* a treatment that the physician has determined to be in the patient's best interest that the patient's capacity may be questioned. The physician, if overly protective, is open to charges of paternalism and, if too laissez-faire, to accusations of neglect. As a result, there is less reliance on the opinion of the physician alone and an increased need to involve other health care professionals—nurses, social workers, psychologists, physical and occupational therapists—as team members in the assessment process.

RELATIONSHIP TO INFORMED CONSENT

The requirements for establishing informed consent (discussed in Chapter 59) are closely related to the principles involved in determining capacity. Key elements are access to adequate information, the ability to understand it, and the ability to make a *voluntary* decision. A formal transfer of authority to make decisions is required to pursue a course of action that is involuntary for the older patient.

In the context of the requirements of informed consent, it is essential to understand that there has been an evolution in the conceptualization of how capacity is to be assessed: "Labels or diagnoses of physical and mental disability may provide no meaningful indication of a person's ability to function autonomously . . . newest definitions eliminate the emphasis on labels and replace it with objective standards . . . focus[ing] on actual behavior and specific functional abilities" (2).

Clinical reality reflects the need for a much broader, more complex understanding of the capacity to make decisions, which must encompass such things as the person's current functioning, the process of decision making, the content of the decision, and stability of the decision over time. In addition and just as important, clinical assessments of capacity should be related to a specific task or decision. We rarely judge a person unable to function in *all* spheres of life. A definition of capacity based on these concepts might look something like this: An ability to understand and process information, make decisions, and carry out related tasks in a manner consistent with and protective of a set of values demonstrated over a period of time. This implies that judgment has not been impaired by cognitive dysfunction, overwhelming emotional distress, or physical illness.

ASSESSMENT OF FUNCTIONAL CAPACITY

MENTAL STATUS EXAMINATION

A basic tool used in evaluating decision-making capacity is a mental status examination (MSE) that routinely includes assessment of level of orientation, memory function, abstract reasoning, judgment, thought content and processes, affect, and mood and inspection of visible behavior (see Chapter 2). Neuropsychological testing is often important in sorting out an inconclusive or confusing result of the MSE.

PSYCHIATRIC CONSULTATION

Consultation by a psychiatrist is helpful if there appear to be questions about judgment and perception relating to a present psychiatric disorder or history of one. Although it is frequently assumed that an evaluation by a psychiatrist is a necessary part of assessing capacity, it is not required by the legal system. However, a geropsychiatrist can be extremely helpful as a specialist who has developed skills in communicating with and evaluating cognitively and/or psychologically impaired older people. A potential weakness of a psychiatric consultation is that it is typically a

"one-shot deal," which may not provide a broad enough set of observations to fairly gauge capacity.

COMPLETE MEDICAL EXAMINATION

The importance of an adequate medical workup to discover any treatable causes of clouded judgment cannot be overstated. It would be difficult to think of another aspect of responsible and ethical medical care more fundamental in treating older patients than preservation of cognitive status.

IMPORTANCE OF MULTIDISCIPLINARY ASSESSMENT

From financial and time-management standpoints, it may be difficult for physicians to see working as part of a team as an efficient way to practice. But multidisciplinary teamwork is the only way to gather the necessary data to create the comprehensive biopsychosocial framework essential for an accurate assessment of capacity to function. In addition, involving several team members with different perspectives helps to reduce the potential pitfall of value-laden judgments about what constitutes rational decision making, a problem often mentioned as endemic to evaluation of capacity (3). Discussions among team members comparing the various elements of the older person's situation constitute an extremely important strategy in developing a balanced approach.

The assessment process involves background, observations over a period of time, and an approach that maximizes opportunities for the older person to try to make sense of the current situation. It is necessary to frame evaluative questions in a way that is suited to the older individual's sense of the world and to know how this person manages tasks and decisions on a daily basis. It is obviously beyond the ability of a single health care professional, in terms of time, energy, and expertise, to compile and manage this much information in an effective way. The multidisciplinary team structure is very well suited to such a task.

Team members, on the basis of their areas of expertise, are responsible for gathering information covering all of the different spheres of life to be considered when assessing capacity. In addition to the components of the standard medical workup, these spheres include a thorough social history (including values history) and a complete functional assessment. It is necessary to know the characteristics of the older person's home situation and how each ADL is managed.

Contact must be made with family members and/or other supports because they can provide an essential perspective based on direct daily observation over time. The older person may have informally transferred certain aspects of decision making to someone else who, under these circumstances, may need to be consulted by the clinicians.

The team approach is indispensable in evaluating the capacity of older persons who appear fairly intact cognitively but have a history of making decisions that functionally put them at substantial risk, a position that appears inconsistent with their values over time. In this situation, a determination about capacity cannot be made without a thorough social history and functional assessment.

When older persons exhibit symptoms of moderate to severe dementia that are not found to have a reversible cause, they are not capable of making most informed decisions. But if the person is not well known to the primary care or attending physician and there are no family members or surrogate decision makers, it may be very important to have the benefit of information (including a values history) gathered by other professionals working with the patient to respect wishes about medical care.

Another situation involving medical decision making requiring an excellent history gathered by the team approach is one in which an older person is making a decision that clearly goes against previously expressed wishes, and the recent change of mind seems to be the result of new cognitive impairment.

CASE EXAMPLE

A hospitalized 77-year-old woman with diabetes and multiple physical impairments, who lived alone with no family support and maximal services through community agencies, steadfastly refused nursing home placement despite many hospital admissions and extreme, ongoing instability in her medical condition. She clearly had the capacity to make such a decision, although it appeared to be a very bad one to the health care professionals working with her. The patient maintained that she would consider placement only if and when she needed kidney dialysis, because then she would no longer be safe at home. But even after dialysis was started, she continued to refuse placement.

The turning point in this situation occurred when the multidisciplinary team determined that the patient no longer had the capacity to make such a decision. The occasional waxing and waning deterioration

of her mental status secondary to the dialysis was considered in this determination. However, the most important factor was that she had consistently indicated that she wanted to be safe, yet even when told by professionals that this would be impossible at home, she insisted upon returning. She had clearly lost the capacity to understand the implications of an important decision about her health and living situation. The team contacted the legal department of the hospital and provided a medical certificate and affidavits, resulting in the court appointing an attorney as guardian and subsequent nursing home placement.

Generally speaking, a formal attempt to assess decision-making capacity is initiated when there is a real question about a decision, action, or behavior by an older person, and there is some reason to believe, because of dementia, confusion, disorientation, emotional lability, extreme inconsistency, or extreme denial, that thinking and judgment may be impaired. In clinical practice, it is almost always the decisions that disagree with the health care providers' recommendations that trigger a formal assessment of decision-making capacity.

This raises an interesting philosophical issue: If an older person appears to lack capacity to make a certain decision, doesn't that mean that agreement or disagreement is irrelevant because of the incapacity? Because the health care providers' ethical responsibility is to act in the best interests of the patient, "there is little practical purpose in challenging the decision-making capacity when the physician thinks that [the patient's] decision is in her best interests . . . the plan of care would be the same as if the patient were regarded as capable" (4).

With acknowledgment that patients have variable levels of capacity for decision making, which reflects clinical reality, it is important to try to identify the most equitable and accurate method for evaluating different types of decisions. The concept of a sliding scale has been proposed, basing the thoroughness of evaluation of capacity on the level of seriousness of the potential consequences of the decision in question: "A patient might need only a low level of capacity to consent to a procedure with substantial, highly probable benefits and minimal, low-probability risk, but a high level of capacity to refuse the same treatment" (4). The level of capacity required for decision making varies with "the extent and probability of risk, with the extent and probability of benefit, and with consent or refusal" (4). The greatest weakness in this concept appears to be in defining "low" and "high" levels of capacity. As there are no clear standards, there is a real potential for basing this judgment solely on the values of the individual clinician.

LEGAL RESPONSES TO INCAPACITY

It may be necessary to pursue a legal solution when an older person's decision-making capacity has been clinically determined to be impaired. The legal options available cover a wide range of situations in which there is a transfer of decision-making authority to a surrogate. Such transfers can be done voluntarily through legal agreements that do not require a decision. A basic principle underlying any such transfer is that of choosing the least restrictive alternative, that is, the one that would maintain maximum autonomy for the person despite the loss of capacity to function fully.

DECISIONS ABOUT MEDICAL CARE

In terms of medical decision making specifically, the recent trend toward increased use of advance directives and health care agents represents a significant move to encourage people to determine surrogate decision makers in advance of need. When these mechanisms are in place, much of the uncertainty and complexity of determining the wishes of incapacitated older people about their medical care is alleviated. For this reason, patients routinely should be encouraged to make these designations while they still have the capacity to do so. However, legal intervention through the court system may be indicated for decisions about medical care or living arrangements when (a) incapacity is significant with no surrogate available; (b) capacity is in doubt and the decision is important; (c) there is intense disagreement between the surrogate's opinion and the patient's known wishes and/or the physician's view; (d) the choice of surrogate is questionable; or (e) there is strong disagreement among family members about decision making in a situation in which the older person lacks capacity (5).

OTHER LEGAL OPTIONS FOR TRANSFERS OF AUTHORITY

Legal methods of formalizing voluntary transfers of decision making include power-of-attorney, durable power-of-attorney (which remains valid after loss of capacity), representative payee for management of Social Security and other government retirement income, and (as noted earlier) advance directives appointing a surrogate agent to make medical decisions if the older person becomes unable to do so. These options do not require a court process yet provide for a surrogate decision maker to manage important issues in health care or in financial matters.

Another, extremely restrictive, option is involuntary commitment, which is short-term and used only in a situation involving a mental health crisis in which confinement in a protected environment is seen as the only way to offer sufficient protection and treatment. The process for effecting commitment varies from state to state.

The most restrictive legal option is guardianship, which generally entails a total transfer of authority, including decisions about medical care, living situation, and finances on a long-term basis. Conservatorship is one form of limited guardianship that is somewhat less restrictive, transferring total control of the estate and finances only. Some states have provisions for public guardianship. Agencies are empowered to act as guardians in this circumstance. The decision by the judge is based on evidence presented by those petitioning the court for an involuntary transfer of decision-making authority. The petition includes information provided by a physician, who may be asked to sign a medical certificate and may include affidavits by the physician and other health care professionals working with the older person. The petition may be initiated through the legal department of a health care system or facility or may follow a referral to a community agency that provides adult protective services (see Chapter 47).

Adult protective services are a system of programs and services for older people living in the community. The goal of the services is to enable the older person to remain living safely at home, avoiding mistreatment by others. Agencies that provide adult protective services can petition a court for protective orders that ensure treatment or other care to those deemed incompetent. After the petition is filed, a hearing notice is issued to the subject of the petition. An examination of the evidence by the court may include interviews with petitioners or a home visit by a court-appointed individual. The probate court appoints a guardian (usually family member or attorney) as a substitute decision-maker for a person who falls into a certain category (such as mental illness, old age, developmental disability) and thus has been determined to be functionally impaired (incapacitated) (6). The person deemed incompetent is the ward. The trend to reform guardianship laws is toward limited guardianship that grants powers for the time necessary to provide for the demonstrated needs of the ward (7).

CONCLUSION

Assessing the functional capacity of an older person is a key task for a physician as decisions rise about health care and even about living arrangements. To ensure the most complete functional assessment, the physician should become a leader in a multidisciplinary process that uses the expertise of psychiatrist, social workers, nurses, rehabilitation therapists, and other professionals as well as the insight and experience of family members and friends. Once the older person is evaluated and found to be clinically incapacitated, surrogate decision-makers are used. Recourse to a court process to determine legal incompetence and to appoint a surrogate decision-maker should be pursued only if no other surrogate is available or there are serious unresolved issues or conflicts among the health care providers and others involved in the situation.

REFERENCES

1. Smyder MA. Aging and decision-making capacity. Generations 1993;17:51–56.
2. Hommel PA, Wang L, Bergman J. Trends in guardianship reform: implications for the medical and legal professions. Law Med Health Care 1990;18:213–226.
3. Beauchamp TL, Childress JF. Principles of biomedical ethics. 2nd ed. New York: Oxford University Press, 1983.
4. Lo B. Assessing decision-making capacity. Law Med Health Care 1990;18:193–201.
5. Anonymous. Making patient care decisions. American Hospital Association report of the Special Committee on Biomedical Ethics, 1985:12–13.
6. Kapp MB. Geriatrics and the law. New York: Springer, 1992:116.

52/ Housing for the Elderly

Marjorie Harvey Glassman

"Don't even mention a nursing home for me." Seventy-five-year-old Mr. K was adamant about returning home to his small apartment, a handicapped unit in elderly public housing. Mr. K was scheduled to be discharged from the hospital in 1 week. There had been some improvement in his functional status, but a combination of postpolio syndrome and cardiac problems made transfer from wheelchair to bed and toilet potentially unsafe. Hospital staff were considering nursing home placement. The previous combination of a 2-hour a day homemaker/personal care attendant was considered insufficient to meet his needs and ensure safety. His income was too low to purchase more services, and his only relative, an 83-year-old brother, was homebound with chronic obstructive lung disease. Mr. K was attached to the apartment he had lived in for 20 years, the view of the courtyard from his window, and the friendly neighbors in the community room. Forcing him into a nursing home would result in severe psychological trauma for this fiercely independent man.

Mr. K lived in a community where there was a wide range of housing options such as congregate housing, continuing care retirement communities, assisted living facilities, board-and-care homes, and foster care. However, Mr. K was facing the same dilemma affecting many frail, disabled elders. Low functional status and low income made him ineligible for any housing alternative other than a nursing home.

Mr. K, however, was able to remain in his own apartment through a special new state program that put on-site supportive services in specific housing projects. The hospital discharge planning department kept a detailed resource file that described a new program that provided both home care services and assistive living services for low-income elders over 65 whose disability was so severe that that they would be assessed as eligible for nursing home placement.

The discharge planner, the community case manager, and Mr. K worked out a schedule with time intervals between 8:00 AM and 8:00 PM. An aide came in at 8:00 PM to help Mr. K get out of bed and dress. She assisted with personal care and prepared breakfast. She then left to assist other tenants and returned at specific times during the day to assist with other tasks such as toileting. Mr. K also received Meals on Wheels, nursing care, and transportation. He attended an adult day health center three times a week. Emergency services were available for him on a 24-hour basis.

In an AARP study, 86% of older people questioned wanted to continue living in their own homes. This is up from 78% in an 1984 study (1). However, housing problems related to affordability, adaptability, and availability of assistive services may result in relocation. Trauma associated with relocation can be difficult for older persons whose identity and sense of community are rooted in their own homes. Atchley summarized older people's attitudes toward their homes as being more than a place to live. The elder's home is a symbol of independence, a focal point for family gatherings, a source of pleasant memories and a major symbol of one's status, which becomes more important as people grow older (2).

The purpose of this chapter is first to discuss ways that older people may remain in their own homes to "age in place." Housing is one of the most important factors in the quality of life of older people and should be an integral part of treatment planning for mentally and physically disabled elders. Most older people want to remain in their own homes and fear the possibility of nursing home placement. Information on reducing housing costs, home modification, and securing services is included. The chapter also provides a brief description of housing options available to older people and how they differ on the continuum of independent to dependent living. The role of the health professional and the clinical aspects of decision making for appropriate living arrangements for mentally and physically disabled elders is discussed. A consistent theme in the chapter is the importance of self-determination for older people in making choices about housing.

AGING IN PLACE

State and federal policies since the 1980s have encouraged "aging in place," with additional funding for alternatives to nursing placement and stricter guidelines requiring a proven need for skilled nursing services for admission to Medicare- and Medicaid-financed nursing homes. The results have been very positive for some elders, such as Mr. K, who would have been unsafe living at home without the extra services that he is receiving. Federal policy beginning in 1986 permitted payment for either skilled nursing home care or home care (through a waiver) for low-income disabled elders. The Medicaid Home and Community Options Act of 1991 offered both home care services and assistive living services for Medicaid-eligible people over 65 whose disability was so severe that they would be assessed as eligible for nursing home placement. The Nursing Home Reform Act of 1987 under the Omnibus Reconciliation Act (3) stipulated 10 sites for programs similar to the one described for Mr. K but containing more home medical services. Many states are also taking the initiative to establish similar programs with financial guidelines less strict than those based on medicaid eligibility.

These programs are not widespread, and many older people are threatened with involuntary relocation and nursing home placement because they lack the funds to pay for privately financed home services or home modifications. While insufficient income is a major risk for placement of older people, other risk factors include lack of family or friends to provide care, needs that are so great that the older person requires a great deal of supervision, or living in areas where few services are available. Many times information about resources is not easily available, and health professionals do not know how to access resource information.

REDUCING HOUSING COSTS

Older people are frequently unaware of ways they can reduce housing costs, so many of these government sponsored programs to reduce housing costs are underutilized. Most states have subsidized programs to help low-income elderly with the costs of heating and other utility bills. These programs may be open to home owners as well as renters. Free or low-cost energy audits and weatherization program are widely available. Information about these programs is available from local utility programs, local councils on aging, or state departments of aging.

Most local governments have a mechanism to reduce or eliminate property tax for income-eligible older people. One method is through a deduction of part of the value of the house. Another program is tax deferral, where no tax is paid until the house is sold or the owner dies and the tax owed is a lien on the estate. Information about property tax abatements is available from the local assessor's office.

Most homeowners age 65 and over own their homes free and clear. Home equity conversion is a method to tap into the homeowner's equity, to supplement their income, and if necessary to pay for home repairs, home modifications, and health services. This type of loan is also known as reverse mortgage or sale/lease back loan; a lump sum or monthly tax-free payments are made to the borrowers. The loan is paid when the house is sold or the person dies (3). There are home equity conversion loans sponsored by the state and federal governments, as well as by banks. Information about this type of loan is available through the state department of aging. Home equity conversion loans are complicated and require expert counseling to understand their advantages and liabilities. It is essential to use a reputable real estate attorney, particularly if the loan is through a private program.

HOME MODIFICATION

Physically disabled older people may become "prisoners" in their own homes and in danger from accidents until their homes can be made safe and free of architectural barriers. Hazardous areas of the house include thresholds where people can trip, doorways too narrow for wheelchair accessibility, and interior and exterior stairs. Exterior stairs can be a major barrier for disabled elders. Replacing exterior steps with ramps can be very expensive and not always architecturally possible. One choice for two-story homes is to relocate the bedroom and bathroom to the first floor. Bathrooms also have potential safety problems. Toilets with raised seats, grab bars, tub seats and mats, and clearance for wheelchair accessibility are some of the adaptations that are possible. When older people relocate, it is important to choose new housing that is free of architectural barriers as insurance, in case they are disabled in the future.

There are no prescribed formulas for home adaptations. Occupational therapists and physical therapists have the professional expertise to determine the most appropriate types of home modifications. The American Cancer Society, Multiple Sclerosis Society, and Muscular Dystrophy Association all offer printed materials on home adaptation and referral to nonprofit organizations providing home modifications. The IRS considers this type of permanent home change as a medical expense. The Veterans Administration offers low-interest loans to veterans. Many area agencies on aging have low-cost nonprofit home repair and adaptation programs. Home equity loans may be used to finance home modification.

IN-HOME SUPPORTIVE SERVICES

The availability of homemaker/home health aide services may become the decisive factor in whether a frail older person can remain at home. Low-income disabled elders who are dependent in several activities of daily living may qualify for free or low-cost home care. However, except for a few specialized programs, home care is rationed, with services restricted to 2 to 4 hours once or twice a week for elders who meet income and disability requirements. Higher-income elders will have to pay for their own homemakers and personal care attendants. Only affluent elders can afford to hire 24-hour care.

Limited homemaker/home health aide services are available under Medicare programs for elders recovering from a major illness. This is true regardless of income but is subject to utilization review and is not intended as a mechanism to aid elders who require custodial rather than acute care.

Most elders prefer paid home care services rather than family or friends. However, studies have shown that most home care services are provided by family and friends and that the amount of service provided is higher for lower-income than higher-income elders (2). It is important to assess the strength of the family and informal social network when making the choice between remaining at home or nursing home placement. One of the advantages of remaining in the same neighborhood or building for the elderly may be relationships with neighbors who are willing to provide assistance.

HOSPITALIZATION

Many older people have adverse reactions to hospitalization. Separated from their familiar surroundings and with a heightened state of anxiety, they become more easily confused and disoriented. The sequelae to many illnesses and medical procedures, particularly prostate problems, heart conditions, pneumonia, and surgery, may leave elderly people in agitated, depressed states in which they appear incompetent. During hospital stays, it is easy to make inappropriate plans, such as nursing home placements, that lead to irreversible life decisions (4). When competency is a question in discharge planning, a team evalua-

tion can be helpful, with a medical assessment for drug reactions, nutritional deficiency, psychiatric disorders, hearing and vision loss, and other medical problems. The occupational therapist can evaluate activities of daily living in the hospital setting as well as during a home visit with the patient. The social worker can meet with the family to obtain a history of the patient's functioning before hospitalization. It is also helpful to contact community professionals who may have worked with the patient. Patients with adverse reactions to hospitalization often need extra help for several weeks after discharge. Families and community professionals are often willing to provide the extra help if they understand the situation.

HOUSING OPTIONS

While most older people want to remain in their own homes, many find they have to reevaluate their housing needs and wants. Older people do not tend to do advance planning for their retirement and housing choices, so many decisions may be made in a time of crisis. Housing decisions can become complicated with financial limitations, death of a spouse, illness, or physical disability. Younger elders may be motivated to change housing for a better climate and lifestyle. As the person grows older, a major concern may be fear of nursing home placement. Frail and disabled older people who in the past would have entered a nursing home are now denied admission if they do not require 24-hour skilled nursing care and can have their needs met in a less restrictive environment.

There is no standard terminology from state to state on housing options, particularly for a new category called "assistive living." The following descriptions of housing options are on a continuum from low-service and supervision in independent living to the board-and-care home, which is the step before nursing home placement (Fig. 52.1). It is important to use community resources to learn local housing options and to encourage family and individuals to visit potential housing options.

On the independence side of the continuum are private homes and apartment or single-room-occupancy dwellings. Public or subsidized housing is also considered independent living but may include on-site supportive services.

The next level is congregate living, which is best for people who need only minimal assistance with activities of daily living. Residents have their own apartments but may take one or more meals in a common dining room. There may be a part-

Continuum of Housing Options

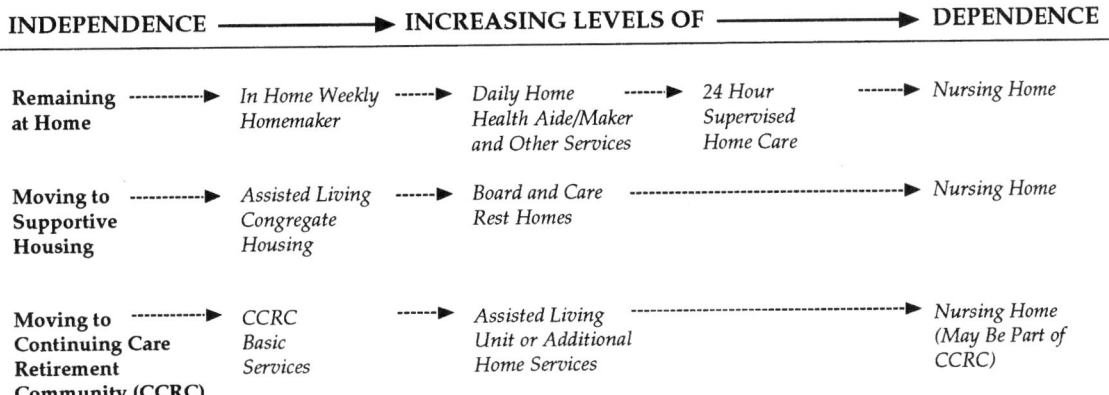

Figure 52.1.   Continuum of housing options.

time activity director or social service coordinator, and transportation. Housekeeping and linens are usually available, and there is a 24-hour emergency response system. Residents should be in generally good health, but they may use walkers or wheelchairs. They should be able to perform most activities of daily living independently. There is a wide range of cost for congregate housing: at the lower end of the scale are federal, state, and locally subsidized programs that charge a portion of the Social Security or Supplemental Security income benefits.

Assisted living is a new term that is used to describe a special type of community housing that offers more personal care and supervision than congregate housing. It is designed for a group of older people with more physical and cognitive problems than are suitable for a congregate living facility. Assisted living may also be referred to as a catered living facility or a residential care facility. Assisted living facilities are not necessarily licensed, although there is a move to set standards and establish licensure. Assisted living models are diverse. Some are freestanding, while others are attached to a continuing care retirement community or nursing home. The term "assisted living" has also been used to describe a package of intensive supportive services such as those provided for Mr. K. in the first case illustration.

Overlap on the continuum from independence to dependent living exists between board-and-care homes and assisted living facilities. Both provide help with personal needs as well as 24-hour custodial supervision. Neither are equivalent to a nursing home, which provides skilled nursing care around the clock. Board-and-care establish-

ments may also be called rest homes, retirement centers, and homes for the aged. Some boarding houses, adult group and foster care homes are also called board-and-care facilities. The wide variety of living arrangements has made all these variations difficult to license. The term "assisted living" is preferred by private pay homes, established for wealthy elders. The term board-and-care refers to the lower end of the market, although some centers also cater to a luxury market. Lower-priced board-and-care facilities usually have a number of people living on public assistance.

Continuing care retirement communities (CCRC) are designed to cover the space between independent living, assisted living, and skilled nursing care. These three services are usually arranged on the same campus. There is an up-front fee or purchase of the apartment and then ongoing monthly charges. Residents enter these facilities with a view that there is a guarantee they will be taken care of for life, no matter what level of care is needed. Residents are provided with meals, housecleaning, transportation, and recreational and educational activities.

The variety and intensity of care varies by CCRC model. Almost all require that the person must be in good physical condition to be accepted. In some facilities, residents purchase insurance and pay the same monthly fee whether they are in the independent living unit or the nursing care facility. Others offer a partial prepayment arrangement for a specific number of days or a reduced per diem rate. Some only guarantee the availability of the nursing home care and residents pay on a fee-for-service basis. All continuing care communities should be thoroughly investigated for their financial viability and the exact health care benefits residents can expect to receive. Some also have exclusions from coverage for residents who develop Alzheimer's disease and related dementias or other specific chronic illnesses.

Other housing options for older people include shared housing, either in their own home or in the home of a friend or roommate. There are also accessory apartments, for example, an apartment that can be built in their own home or an in-law suite that can be built in a family home.

ECHO housing (elder cottage housing opportunities) consists of a small but separate living unit constructed or moved to the same lot as a large home. ECHO housing has been used by adult children as a way of offering support and proximity to aging parents, while preserving independence and privacy. This type of house is more adaptable to rural or semirural areas. It has been more popular in England and Australia than in the United States. Government funds are not available for ECHO housing, and units have to conform to local zoning regulations.

HOUSING FOR THE MENTALLY ILL ELDER

Homelessness is a major problem for mentally ill elders, who may be at risk living in a shelter as well as on the streets. Safe housing designed to meet their needs should be a prime objective in treatment planning for the chronically mentally ill. When mental hospitals were first closed down, many elders were transferred to nursing homes or rest homes. These arrangements were beneficial for frail and disabled elders in need of skilled nursing, but many older people were inappropriately placed in a restrictive environment that offered neither active treatment nor case management.

The Nursing Home Reform Act of 1987 (OBRA 87) addresses issues of care for the mentally ill elder. OBRA 87 included the requirement for preadmission screening and annual resident reviews (PASARR). The assessment determines whether the individual is seriously mentally ill, is in need of active psychiatric treatment, has skilled nursing care needs, or could benefit from a more independent setting. Thus there has been a move away from institutional care to community housing for these elders.

At the same time Housing and Urban Development (HUD) has enforced rules against discrimination of mentally ill elders. One of the HUD standards is that there must be "reasonable accommodation" for mentally ill elders in the building that HUD subsidizes. This has meant that a history of mental illness or eccentricity of speech, manners, or behavior that does not harm others, cannot be grounds for denying mentally ill elders subsidized housing. Most mentally ill elders are good tenants if they are placed in appropriate housing with adequate supports.

Some mentally ill elders may have behavioral problems that are associated with a severe functional or organic mental disorder that may interfere with tenancy. These include violent, threatening behavior particularly with guns and knives; inability to meet minimum sanitary standards in caring for self and apartment; waking other tenants with loud noises in the middle of the night; and inability to manage money and pay the rent. Board-and-care or rest homes have been used as housing for mentally ill elders. These homes however rarely have the necessary resources for care of violent older people.

Supervised psychiatric halfway houses can be helpful but are in very short supply, with long waiting lists. Many state departments of mental health have specialized services for locating appropriate housing for the mentally ill.

Clinical case management is helpful in preventing eviction and monitoring medication for the chronic schizophrenic, manic depressive, or dual diagnostic alcoholic. However, chronic delusional disorders are difficult to manage if the elder refuses medication and has repeated episodes of violence as shown in the next case study.

Miss A, a 70-year-old woman, was known to every agency in the city. She appeared well groomed and articulate, so people were eager to help her find housing. However, within a few weeks of finding a new room, she would accuse the landlord or neighbors of being whores or pimps or plotting to kill her. She disturbed everyone with screaming and banging on doors at night. After a period of homelessness and a short stay in a rest home, she was again homeless and displayed behavioral problems at the shelter. She was placed in elderly public housing. Within a few weeks she was banging on doors and threatening tenants. She began to walk the hallways at night, waving a large kitchen knife. Eviction proceedings were started. Miss A fought the eviction but lost the case. She was hospitalized in the state hospital, where she did very well on the structured life and medication. She was not considered disturbed enough to be placed in a supervised halfway house. Miss A found a new subsidized apartment, and again she manifested the same behavior. When she waved the knife, the police came and brought her back to the hospital. She was eventually placed in a psychiatric halfway house, and with careful monitoring and medication, she is doing well.

There is also the marginal older person who may have a psychiatric history earlier in life but now lives a stable but isolated lifestyle on public assistance. This is the group of elders who may live in the old welfare hotels or in single-occupancy rooms (SROs). Unfortunately the supply of SROs and inexpensive residential hotels has sharply declined with the gentrification of the city, resulting in homelessness for this very fragile older population who are at high risk for relocation trauma.

ALCOHOLISM

Alcoholic elderly also used to seek housing in the poorer areas of a city where there were SROs. Those who were evicted because of behavioral problems lived on the streets or in shelters. The decline of SROs and public housing discrimination against applicants with an alcoholism history have added to homelessness. This provided little incentive for the homeless alcoholic to attain sobriety. HUD regulations no longer allow discrimination against subsidized housing applicants who have had problems with alcoholism but indicate they are seeking treatment.

Housing that offers an environment where drinking is discouraged can be a therapeutic choice for both active and recovering alcoholics. The Boston, Massachusetts Housing Authority has a Peer Advocate Alcoholism Program that provides alcohol education, outreach, intervention to help elderly tenants accept treatment, and support groups. The program sponsored alcohol education for all tenants and was instrumental in gaining tenant support for a ban on public drinking in community rooms, buildings, entrances, and hallways. This stopped afternoon "tea parties" and drinking that was such a major part of tenant interaction. Tenants did not have to drink to be a part of the group. When the ban went into effect, there was a marked decline in alcoholism problems in the buildings.

Most alcoholic tenants can be motivated to accept treatment and maintain sobriety if their drinking behavior becomes grounds for eviction. There is usually no penalty for alcoholics who quietly drink in their own apartments. However, public drinking, loud aggressive behavior, not paying rent, destruction of property, or urinating in inappropriate places can bring on an eviction proceeding for the alcoholic tenant. One of the key methods of helping the acting-out alcoholic tenant is the use of contracts that require the tenant to accept an alcohol rehabilitation program with follow-up or be evicted. This type of intervention has proved successful, but because of the chronic nature of alcoholism, contracts and rehabilitation programs may have to be repeated. In one of the

smaller subsidized buildings, monitoring is so careful that a tenant who walks into the building in an intoxicated state will receive a letter from the building manager within 1 hour and may be in an inpatient treatment program by that evening.

CONCLUSION

This chapter has reviewed housing choice as an important part of therapeutic planning for the mentally and physically disabled older person. The major focus has been placed on resources that can enable the older person to "age in place." Through reducing housing costs and monthly payments, older people may be able to afford more of the in-home supportive services and home modifications that can allow them to remain safely in their own homes.

A housing typology is difficult to describe because different terminology is used throughout the country. Continuing care retirement communities have to be evaluated on an individual basis for long-term care benefits. Housing options for elders are frequently described on a continuum from independent living to facilities that meet the needs of dependent elders. Older people however do not usually use a continuum of increasingly dependent facilities and nursing homes. Nursing home placement is frequently made from an independent living situation.

Relocation is very difficult for older people, particularly when the move is involuntary or when they enter a nursing home. The research on the effects of relocation has not produced any consistent answers about whether or not relocation increases probability of death or worsens illness; however, it is clear that older people are upset at the prospect of relocation (2) and may require counseling to adapt to new living arrangements.

Older people rarely seek advice about housing choice (1) and are at a disadvantage when a crisis requires housing change. The multitude of housing types and benefit programs makes it difficult for the health professional to assist older persons in deciding on housing choices that will meet their needs. Access to current information on housing resources and benefits is an essential part of housing counseling. Housing information and referral is available in each state on three different levels. Every state has a department or division of aging as well as regional area agencies on aging who have housing information. Local governments also have councils on aging that have an information component. These telephone numbers can be found by calling state government offices or by using the federal elder care information number, the Eldercare Locator at 1-800-677-1116. Local government is helpful on ways to reduce property taxes. Local councils on aging are also good sources of community information as well as informal resources that are not officially listed.

Physicians are no longer solely responsible for making decisions on nursing home placement for their patients. Admission to Medicaid- and Medicare-approved nursing homes must now be approved by a state-mandated interdisciplinary team. Only those elders who require skilled nursing care on a 24-hour basis are eligible. The state team will frequently provide information and referral for alternative housing choices.

Physicians, patients, families, significant others, and available community resources should work together to develop a housing plan that will maximize independence with safety for the older person.

REFERENCES

1. American Association of Retired Persons (AARP). Understanding senior housing for the 1990s. Washington, DC: AARP, 1990.
2. Atchley RC. Social forces and aging, 6th ed. Belmont, CA: Wadsworth, 1991.
3. Forrest R, Forrest MB. Retirement living; a guide to housing alternatives. New York: Facts on File, 1991.
4. Glassman M. Misdiagnosis of senile dementia: denial of care to the elderly. Social Work 1980;25(4):288–292.

53/ Community Options for Elderly Patients

David L. Rabin, Patricia P. Barry

A characteristic of many Americans is the high value they place on independence and personal autonomy. The stated preference of 84% of U.S. residents over age 55 is to remain in their current homes as they age, and never move (1). This tendency, sometimes referred to as "aging in place," is threatened late in life when physical frailty, combined with the high cost of health care, restricts choices available to older persons requiring long-term care. The desire of the older person to remain autonomous is frustrated by societal concerns about the cost of providing community and personal health care and the resulting societal preference for institutional, rather than community-based, long-term care.

The term *long-term* care refers to the medical and other services needed to attain and maintain optimal physical, social, and psychological function by frail and dependent persons with chronic impairments. This chapter describes the statutory, fiscal, and social environment within which newer community options for long-term care of the elderly are being developed, emphasizing those not discussed in detail in other chapters. The focus is on the range of community-based services currently available to support the temporarily and permanently disabled elderly population.

Since the extent of public funding for elderly community care is a function of state and local governments' choices among competing priorities, physicians have an important local role to play in making people aware of the need for community personal care and housing services. Similarly, physicians can encourage voluntary efforts to provide money and services to the elderly, since impaired elderly patients often cannot effectively advocate for themselves. In clinical practice, care of the elderly should include discussions with elderly patients about the need to plan for the likelihood of impairment. Physicians should be knowledgeable about available services for care of the elderly and should refer patients to social workers and agencies who can plan for and manage community services for them.

COMMUNITY-BASED LONG-TERM CARE: AN OVERVIEW

Sustaining the frail elderly in the community is one of the greatest challenges facing our society. There are many elderly who have health and personal care needs that are unmet. An estimated 4.4 million persons over age 70 who are living in the community have at least one functional disability—difficulty with bathing, dressing, eating, transferring, i.e., activities of daily living (ADLs)—58% of these impaired individuals received no help from either paid or unpaid sources (2).

Since physical impairment, functional disability, and an increasing need for personal care are predictable and likely accompaniments of old age and social isolation, older people, particularly those living alone, can plan for the likelihood of disability by moving to more sheltered environments where personal care is available. Many factors need to be considered in developing care plans for the elderly. They include personal preference, cost containment, changes in family structure, increased availability of medical technology, issues of generational equity, greater personal wealth, and access to long-term care institutions. While community-based options provide alternatives to short-term institutional care, thereby reducing the risks of permanent institutionalization and impoverishment, they are infrequently discussed by physicians with their elderly patients.

Although the variety of community-based services has expanded in recent years, the family remains the primary source of caretaking for the elderly. An estimated 70% of the care of impaired elderly is provided exclusively by an informal network of relatives and friends (3). Family/friend care is preferred for many reasons; it is more personal, acceptable, continuously available, adaptable, and perhaps most significantly, it is less costly. In some cases, such care may help avoid, or at least postpone, expensive institutional care.

Increased longevity of the elderly may diminish the ability of those closest to the older person—typically a spouse and children—to provide care. This is particularly the case for women, most of whom outlive their spouses and may live alone for long periods. The isolation of elderly women is compounded by trends toward smaller families and by the tendency for grown children to move away from parents. Grown children, both sons and daughters, may be working and unable to devote sufficient time to caretaking. In cases in which parents are age 85 or older, their children may be retired, living on fixed incomes, and in poor health themselves. Each of these factors alone complicates the provision of family care for older people and increases the need to supplement this care. Care by friends also tends to be unstable, particularly as these caretakers are likely to be elderly and therefore are themselves at risk of impairment.

FINANCING COMMUNITY-BASED LONG-TERM CARE

Since the inception of the federal Medicare and federal-state Medicaid programs in 1965, government policy has tended to favor reimbursement for institutional care over home- or community-based health services for the elderly. In contrast to the acute-care focus of Medicare, the Medicaid program provides comprehensive coverage, including long-term care, for the medically indigent. As the rising cost of long-term care threatens more elderly and their families, interest in publicly financed long-term care coverage for the disabled, regardless of income, has broadened (though not yet to the point of forging a national consensus). The reluctance to create new public programs for long-term care stems in part from the concern that providing federal dollars for custodial and preventive care may create demand for services that are now provided by family members.

Elderly who must pay out of pocket for custodial services rapidly deplete their accumulated savings. Once impoverished, they become eligible for Medicaid, which for some elderly means depending on welfare after a lifetime of financial independence. To preserve accumulated assets of the elderly, many families have encouraged older members to transfer assets to the younger generation to qualify for Medicaid coverage for institutional care. Provisions in the Fiscal Year 1994 Omnibus Budget Reconciliation Act make this practice more difficult, as Medicaid eligibility is delayed for individuals who dispose of their assets for less than fair market value within a period of up to 36 months prior to applying for Medicaid or entering an institution. This new law is designed to encourage families to use some of the elderly's assets for community-based services to postpone the need for state-sponsored institutional care.

Medicaid covers long-term care services, including nursing home care and medically related home care. In some states, Medicaid also pays for personal care services. In an attempt to encourage experimentation with community-based programs, two Medicaid waiver programs (Sections 2176 and 1915 (c-d)) permit states to offer community-based long-term care services in lieu of institutional care—in some cases without imposing the strict income limits on recipients. Eligibility for program services varies widely among and within states.

THE OLDER AMERICANS ACT AND OTHER STATE AND LOCAL PROGRAMS

The Older Americans Act (OAA), through its designated Regional Area Agencies on Aging, distributes federal funds to states to provide local services for persons ages 60 and above. Local Offices on Aging provide information and referral services to elderly clients with a variety of social and health needs. Voluntary and municipal agencies apply for OAA funding to provide a variety of services, including home-delivered meals (Meals-on-Wheels), personal care assistance, transportation, adult day-care, and case management. Unlike Medicaid, the OAA may serve persons of any income level, although by statute it must target services for persons with the "greatest social or economic need." In 1987, Congress approved a special funding category within the OAA for in-home care for the frail elderly.

Federal funds from the Social Security Act's Social Services Block Grant program help states to support a variety of services for older persons, including homemaker/home health services, case management services, transportation, and nutritional assistance. Like the OAA, this block grant program does not limit services by income, although in practice, most services are targeted at low-income populations.

While both the OAA and the Social Services Block Grant provide vital services to significant numbers of elderly Americans, there are gaps in coverage. The specific array and extent of services available is determined by local activities of government in cooperation with voluntary and proprietary agencies. This results in wide variation of service availability among localities. Few impaired elderly or their families can acquire the knowledge necessary to effectively organize community services for themselves. Because of the complexity of the existing systems that provide care to the elderly, the ever-changing needs of the impaired elderly, and the variable eligibility rules for particular services, physicians should refer impaired patients to agencies providing case management.

LONG-TERM CARE INSURANCE

There is a growing, but still modest, market for private long-term care insurance. Currently, 135 companies sell this type of coverage (4). Long-term care insurance typically covers nursing home care (skilled, intermediate, and custodial care) and home health care. Initially, long-term care insurance favored coverage for institutional care; however, customer preference for in-home care has led to increased coverage for home care services. Long-term care policies may also include benefits for community-based care, such as adult day-care or respite care.

Despite estimates that 30 to 40% of the elderly population could afford long-term care insurance, only 4% of the population over age 65 had policies in 1990 (5, 6). Reasons that may account for the limited popularity of these policies include lack of public understanding of the risks and expenses associated with long-term care and complex policies that are difficult to evaluate. Despite these drawbacks, this relatively new insurance product continues to evolve and could provide protection for significant portions of the population. It is in the physician's and patient's interest to consider long-term care insurance during the early years of aging when premiums are less costly.

HOME- AND COMMUNITY-BASED LONG-TERM CARE SERVICES

From a medical perspective, long-term care services include those necessary to prevent avoidable deterioration of health, treat acute exacerbations of chronic illness, restore optimal function, and maintain independence to the extent possible. To attain these goals, community-based long-term care should include preventive, diagnostic, therapeutic, rehabilitative, supportive, and health-maintenance services. As people age, their ability to care for themselves is likely to change. The more people plan and adjust to this likelihood of increasing disability by moving to more protective residential environments, the greater the possibility that they will maintain independence throughout their lives. The next section describes the major housing, social, and medical services available to assist elderly living in the community.

SUPPORTIVE HOUSING

There is a wide range of housing options for the older person who becomes impaired or who loses a caretaker. Older persons may renovate their homes to accommodate their impaired status. Typical modifications include replacing doorknobs and faucets with more easily manipulated lever handles, installing grab rails in the bathroom and other parts of the house, and widening doorways and adding ramps in stairways to accommodate wheelchairs. Some communities provide modest grants for modifications; others sponsor programs where members of the building trades donate or offer maintenance services to elderly homeowners at reduced prices.

Personal security becomes more important as a person ages. Burglar alarms and smoke detectors are particularly important additions to homes where an impaired individual lives. Many companies use the telephone to provide safety monitoring services to the elderly. Access is provided either by means of a continuous telephone monitoring system or through daily (or more frequent) telephone calls from the agency to individuals living alone. An example of the continuous monitoring system is the Lifeline device. The older person wears or carries a beeper-type device in the home, which can be used to summon help in the event of a fall or other emergency.

Emerging technology allows patients to be monitored at home by means of wristwatch-size computers that will transmit vital signs such as blood pressure, electrocardiogram pulse, temperature and other important data directly to a central location in a hospital or agency. Patients can be continually assessed without need for direct contact with health professionals—providing increased assurance for vulnerable elderly at home.

Living independently does not necessarily mean living alone. As an example, low- to moderate-income individuals might rent an apartment in a home for the aged, many of which are run by churches and other voluntary agencies, or may qualify for placement in low-income public housing for the elderly. Many of these residences become centers for recreation and socialization and prevent the social isolation that frequently burdens older persons who live alone.

For those who are no longer able to manage routine personal-care functions, there are a number of alternatives to institutionalization. Of increasing importance are the various types of "assisted living" facilities. The American Association of Retired Persons (AARP) defines assisted living as "any group residential program that is not licensed as a nursing home, that provides personal care to persons with need for assistance in the activities of daily living (ADL), and that can respond to unscheduled needs for assistance that might arise" (6). Assistive living settings include board-and-care homes with additional services, residential care units run by nursing homes, congregate housing settings, and mid-level services in Continuing Care Retirement communities. Ideally, residential care should offer alternatives to institutionalization by meeting the varied needs of the disabled elderly population.

Congregate care facilities typically provide meals, housekeeping, and some type of personal and/or medical assistance for elderly residents. They are designed to provide a secure and socially stimulating environment. Board-and-care homes, sheltered housing, and adult foster care are among the many terms used to describe these types of housing arrangements, and there is wide variation in the availability and type of services offered. A recent survey found there are 32,000 licensed congregate care homes operating nationwide under 25 different titles—estimates of unlicensed homes range from 28,000 to 100,000 (7).

Of particular interest among supportive housing arrangements are Continuing Care Retirement Communities (CCRCs), of which the Life Care model is an example. CCRCs typically require a substantial lump-sum investment (ranging from $34,000 to $95,000 for a one-bedroom unit), for which the purchaser receives access to on-premises social and medical services (8). In some cases a nursing home is located on the premises. Some CCRCs include payment for supportive services in the initial purchase contract; however, the trend in recent years has been to provide services on a fee-for-service basis. In addition to the initial investment, there is usually a monthly maintenance fee comparable to condominium fees. There was rapid increase in the development of such communities in the 1980s—a trend that has slowed in recent years. While a number of proprietary groups entered the CCRC market in the 1980s, nonprofits continue to dominate. Because of cost, this comprehensive housing option may be applicable to only a small proportion of the elderly. However, elderly with substantial capital in a home may be able to transfer equity through the sale of the home.

CARE COORDINATION/CASE MANAGEMENT

The care coordination/case management component of long-term care, providing organization and integration, consists of patient assessment, determination of needs, care planning, resource management, coordination, monitoring, and periodic reassessment, usually in cooperation with a multidisciplinary team of care providers. The care coordinator/case manager acts as an advocate for the patient and provides the link between the patient and family and appropriate community services, facilitating and supporting informal support systems and coordinating the efficient use of services to provide effective and quality care. Although the physician is important in directing overall medical care, few have the personal resources or the inclination to be case managers, thus the need is fulfilled by other health professionals. The most difficult task for the case manager is to balance the needs of the patient with the "gatekeeping" necessary to manage resources.

The first step in evaluation and planning for the long-term health care of elderly persons is to obtain and organize information regarding performance of ADLs, physical health, mental health, socioeconomic resources, and the environment, using the coordinated multidimensional, multidisciplinary approach referred to as geriatric assessment. In 1988, the National Institutes of Health sponsored a Consensus Development Conference on Geriatric Assessment Methods for Clinical Decision-making (9). The consensus statement issued by the conference noted that the goals of assessment are to improve diagnostic accuracy, guide the selection of interventions to restore or preserve health, recommend an optimal environment, predict outcomes, and monitor clinical change. These are often interdependent, so that diagnostic accuracy leads to appropriate interventions and better use of available services, resulting in improved level of function and optimal placement. Geriatric assessment can (and should) be performed in many different clinical settings, both institutional and community, including hospitals, nursing homes, physician offices, clinics, and the patient's home. Geriatric assessment units have been established in many such settings and have been effective in identifying new diagnoses, reducing the number of prescribed medications, improving placement, and reducing use of hospital services over time (10).

The Consensus Statement notes the particular importance of targeting assessment to those persons most likely to benefit, especially those who are "frail" but not terminally ill and those at critical transition points in long-term care. In addition, it is essential to link assessment with care management and follow-up services to implement the recommendations. Geriatric assessment is thus a process involving referral, collection of information, assessment, development, and implementation of a care plan, with periodic reassessment and modification of that plan.

HOME CARE

Home care has been defined as "the provision of equipment and services to the patient in the home for the purpose of restoring and maintaining his or her maximal level of comfort, function, and health" (11). Home care encompasses the spectrum of health and social services that may be provided in the home and thus includes health services such as physician house calls, visiting nurses, and other skilled care, as well as social support services such as homemaking, chore services, and meals. Home *health* care is more narrowly defined as the provision of health care services in the home. Home care may be a substitute for either acute hospital care or long-term institutional care or may reduce length of stay in either setting. Home care may substitute for ambulatory care for persons who are homebound or cannot be transported and can be preventive, diagnostic, therapeutic, rehabilitative, and long-term care.

Prevention in the home setting includes traditional medical interventions as well as home safety considerations, assistive equipment, and attention to family relationships, education, and counseling. Diagnostic home visits can provide important information. Ramsdell found that home visits by physicians and/or geriatric nurse specialists resulted in identification of problems not detected by primary care physicians in office visits, most often in the areas of psychobehavioral difficulties (38.3%), safety (35.7%), caregiver issues (33.8%), and even new medical problems (30%) (12). Koenig noted the following indicators for diagnostic home visits: multiple medical problems, mobility problems, falls, interacting chronic illness and psychosocial problems, poor therapeutic response, "difficult" chronically ill patients, terminal illness, caregiver "burnout," suspected abuse, refusal of office visits, and bereavement (13). The "stepwise" diagnostic approach, involving careful serial testing and therapeutic trials, is often more suitable for the controlled, supportive home environment. Increasing availability of sophisticated diagnostic equipment such as x-rays and laboratory services has improved the ability to provide appropriate diagnosis in the home.

Active treatment and rehabilitation can be provided successfully in the home setting. Sophisticated equipment designed and produced for use in the home is available, including intravenous products and ventilators. In most communities, skilled therapy can be provided, including nursing; physical, occupational, and speech therapy; respiratory therapy; and counseling, among others. The enhanced benefit of being at home and the support of family members contribute to successful outcomes for many patients.

Hospice care of the terminally ill patient is optimally provided in the home, where the goals of comfort, care, and choice are most compatible with a supportive family, friends, and environment. Over the past two decades, the hospice movement, which began in reaction to overtreatment of dying patients, has become an accepted part of the continuum of community-based care that can be provided for the elderly. Hospice care is now reimbursed by Medicare Part A for persons with less than 6 months' expected survival for whom further treatment is not desired or is futile. Referral should be made after discussion with the patient and family; some states require the presence of a caregiver in the home. Guidelines are available for pain control and other comfort measures, and counseling is provided in addition to medical, nursing, social work, and home health services. Hospice patients may be seen in the physician's office as long as this is feasible; physician home visits are an essential component of the later stages of hospice care (14).

Medical and supportive care for chronically ill and functionally disabled patients can be provided in the home, as an alternative to long-term institutional care, if patients are not socially isolated. A study of long-term home care use in East Boston by those over age 65 found that those age 85 or above were 12 times more likely to enter home care. The strongest predictors were being homebound, needing help with one or more ADLs, being dependent in functional health areas, scoring increased errors on mental status, and having no involvement with social groups (15).

The cost-effectiveness of home care remains controversial. A recent study at Boston University found that comprehensive case-managed home care of 197 elderly, eligible for admission to a skilled nursing home, resulted in increased hospital admissions (and Medicare costs), decreased nursing home admissions (and Medicaid costs), and decreased overall costs (16). A randomized controlled study of a VA Hospital-Based Home Care (HBHC) program, for those with two or more ADL impairments or terminal illness, found that although functional status did not improve, both in-hospital and net per person health costs were significantly lower in the HBHC patients, primarily because of fewer acute-care admissions (17). ADL dependencies are strong predictors of the use of long-term care resources, including institutionalization as well as home health care.

Blazer notes that the cost of home care services increases markedly with increasing impairment (18). Since institutional care costs increase only marginally with level of impairment, the result is a "break even" point in home care, with home care for the very impaired being considerably more expensive than institutional care. This creates the social dilemma of tension between individual preference for home care and societal interest in minimizing expenses.

The physician's role in home care can range from authorizing home health care services to participating in house calls, which (as noted) may provide valuable information regarding the suitability of home care and the appropriateness of the home situation. Burton noted the advantages of physician house calls, including service for patients with limited mobility, convenience and comfort, the ability to assess important nonmedical factors, improved physician-patient relationships, and increased understanding and effectiveness in relating to other health care professionals providing care in the home (19). He also noted the disadvantages of overuse by patients and families, lack of efficiency, inadequate reimbursement, and inadequate access to technology.

The AMA Council on Scientific Affairs has recommended that a growing proportion of health care, especially long-term care, should best and most appropriately be provided in the home setting and that physicians must fulfill their essential role as members of the home health team (20).

ADULT DAY-CARE

Adult day-care, also called "adult day health care," is designed to meet the needs of functionally impaired adults in a community setting, with group interaction and planned programs not usually available in the home. Adult day health care centers (ADHCs) provide nursing, social, and a combination of other services, which may include rehabilitation; health maintenance; functional, social, and recreational activities; and a hot meal. ADHCs may be hospital or nursing-home based or free-standing, usually nonprofit, and often subsidized by public or philanthropic funds. Clients may attend from 1 to 5 days per week; special transportation may be provided within a limited

geographic area but is often expensive and requires special equipment. Programs for the day care of demented persons are available in many communities; these may provide valuable respite for families and enable impaired elderly to remain at home.

The number of ADHCs has increased significantly over the past 20 years, and this growth is expected to continue. Day-care programs vary significantly in the type of service provided, objectives, staffing, characteristics of clients, and cost of care. A recent study indicated that many programs are underfunded and underused (21).

The effectiveness of day care has not been well studied. The Department of Veterans Affairs (DVA) Adult Day Health Care (ADHC) programs have been the subject of a recent randomized controlled trial to determine their effectiveness; results have not yet been reported. A randomized controlled trial of a Canadian geriatric day hospital that offered interdisciplinary assessment and rehabilitation services, including hospital-based services such as laboratory and diagnostic facilities, failed to show improved outcomes (functional status and quality of life) for the day hospital group compared with outcomes from "otherwise excellent geriatric outpatient care" (22). San Francisco's On Lok program is a successful working model of capitated, risk-based acute and long-term community care of vulnerable elderly, with a strong emphasis on day health care. The Program of All-inclusive Care for the Elderly (PACE) consists of eight sites that replicate the On Lok model and are currently being evaluated (23).

RESPITE CARE

Respite services provide temporary relief for caregivers, often in an institutional setting, and thus support maintenance of frail elderly in the community. Short stays (usually up to several weeks) in nursing homes provide opportunities for family vacations, trips, and even elective health care procedures or hospitalizations. The DVA has urged the development of inpatient respite care programs at DVA Medical Centers. In the community, Medicaid may provide coverage to eligible persons, and some states have subsidized respite programs. However, in general, the cost of this care, equivalent to nursing home care, is the responsibility of the family.

In addition to respite care, some skilled nursing facilities allow admissions for geriatric assessment and rehabilitation on a short-term basis, which may improve the elderly person's function and potential for remaining in the community. At this time, funding is not usually available except in those DVA medical centers that offer this service.

PUBLIC POLICY ISSUES

Finucane and Burton note that studies of community-based long-term care programs have generally failed to demonstrate an effect on mortality, likelihood of nursing home admission, or functional status (24). Such programs do, however, appear to increase use of inpatient and ambulatory services and health care costs. These findings may result from failure to appropriately target those elderly most at risk for nursing home admission, such as those with increased age, dementia, dependency in ADLs, lack of spouse or child, female sex, and poverty. Effects on quality of life and patient and family satisfaction are difficult to measure and often omitted from studies.

Although the cost-effectiveness of community-based long-term care is problematic, it is clear that the alternative to such programs—institutional care for all frail and dependent elderly—is neither feasible, desirable, nor affordable. In the United States, the lack of an organized health care system and an unstable social service system has resulted in a fragmented, "band-aid" approach to care of the vulnerable elderly, rather than the development of a comprehensive continuum of resources providing services at many levels of care. Under a more integrated system, services could be targeted to the specific needs of certain elderly, as identified by geriatric assessment. The ability to move flexibly from one level of care to another would then depend upon the needs of the individual person. A broad-based financial support system that permits flexible and varied programs is essential, since financing for only one or two types of services will result in inappropriate referral to and overuse of these funded programs, as has been the case in the past.

Adequate reimbursement for physician care in the community setting must also be provided and should take into account the complexity and time-consuming nature of such care. Physicians must increase their involvement in community-based care and their familiarity with services available in their own communities. Since they often serve as the "gatekeepers," failure to make appropriate referrals may result in inadequate access for their patients and in unnecessary institutional care. Establishing relationships with visiting nurses, social service agencies, and case manager services simplifies the provision of information and coordination of care for the frail and dependent elderly and helps to maintain their quality of life as long as possible.

Physician advocacy regarding need for long-term care services can assure local service availability; more importantly, counseling and referral can provide patients with the optimal available services. Anticipating long-term care needs, which can best be done by the physician, can assure the use of social and housing alternatives rather than medical services.

Acknowledgment. We appreciate the assistance of Catherine Sullivan, M.P.A., in the preparation of this manuscript and coordination among the authors and editor.

REFERENCES

1. Anonymous. Understanding senior housing for the 1990's. Washington, DC: American Association of Retired Persons, 1993:42.
2. Anonymous. Aging in America. US Dept. of Health and Human Services, DHHS publ. no. (FCoA) 91–28001, 1991:160.
3. US Bipartisan Commission on Comprehensive Health Care. A call for action (final report). Washington, DC: US Government Printing Office, 1990:97.
4. Cohen MA, Kuman N, McGuire T, Wallack SS. Financing long-term care: a practical mix of public and private. J Health Polit Policy Law 1992; 17(30):403–423.
5. Coronel SA. Long-term care insurance in 1991. Washington, DC: Health Insurance Association of America, 1993:6.
6. Kane RA, Wilson KB, Clemmer E. Assisted living in the United States: a new paradigm for residential care for frail older persons? Washington, DC: American Association of Retired Persons, 1993:xi.
7. Hawes C, Wildfire JB, Lux LJ, Clemmer E. The regulation of board and care homes: results of a survey in the 50 states and the District of Columbia. Washington, DC: American Association of Retired Persons, 1993:3,4,22.
8. Anonymous. Continuing care retirement communities: an industry in action (vol 1). Washington, DC: American Association of Homes for the Aging, 1991:25.
9. Consensus Development Panel, Solomon D, chairman. National Institutes of Health Consensus Development Conference statement: geriatric assessment methods for clinical decision-making. J Am Geriatr Soc 1988;36:342–347.
10. Rubenstein LZ. Geriatric assessment: an overview of its impacts. Clin Geriatr Med 1987;3(1):1–15.
11. AMA Council on Scientific Affairs. Home care in the 1990s. JAMA 1990;263:1241–1244.
12. Ramsdell JW, Swart JA, Jackson JE, Renvall M. The yield of a home visit in the assessment of geriatric patients. J Am Geriatr Soc 1989;37:17–24.
13. Koenig H. The physician and home care of the elderly patient. Gerontol Geriatr Educ 1986;7:15–24.
14. Rhymes JA. Home hospice care. Clin Geriatr Med 1991;7(4):803–816.
15. Branch LG, Wetle TT, Scherr PA, et al. A prospective study of incident comprehensive medical home

care use among the elderly. Am J Public Health 1988;78:255–259.

16. Steel K. Home care for the elderly: the new institution. Arch Intern Med 1991;151:439–442.

17. Cummings JE, Hughes SL, Weaver FM, et al. Cost-effectiveness of Veterans Administration hospital-based home care. Arch Intern Med 1990;150:1274–1280.

18. Blazer D. Home health care: house calls revisited. Am J Public Health 1988;78:238–239.

19. Burton JR. The house call: an important service for the frail elderly. J Am Geriatr Soc 1985;33:291–293.

20. AMA Council on Scientific Affairs. Educating physicians in home health care. JAMA 1991;265:769–771.

21. Conrad KJ, Hanrahan P, Hughes SL. Survey of adult day care in the United States: national and regional findings. Res Aging 1990;12:36–56.

22. Eagle DJ, Guyatt GH, Patterson C, Turpie I, Sackett B, Singer J. Effectiveness of a geriatric day hospital. Can Med Assoc J 1991:144:699–704.

23. Kane RL, Illston LH, Miller NA. Qualitative analysis of the Program for All-inclusive Care of the Elderly. Gerontologist 1992;32:771–780.

24. Finucane TE, Burton JR. Community-based long-term care: the dilemma of quality and cost. In: Hazzard WR, Andres R, Bierman EL, Blass JP, eds. Principles of geriatrics and gerontology. 2nd ed. New York: McGraw-Hill, 1989.

54/ Medical Direction and Medical Care in Nursing Facilities

Steven A. Levenson

THE PRIMARY CARE PHYSICIAN ROLE GENERALLY AND IN NURSING FACILITY CARE

Most nursing facility (NF) attending physicians and medical directors are primary care family physicians and internists. They are part-time players in the NF, lacking the time or inclination to become intimately familiar with the intricacies of long-term care or its underlying laws and regulations. They may read journals and attend Continuing Medical Education conferences about geriatrics and long-term care, but they are not and do not intend to become geriatricians. Nevertheless, they are mostly interested in filling these roles appropriately and in doing a good job. What they ask most often is "What is expected of me?" and "What does it mean to do a good job, and by what standards?"

Thus, this chapter focuses on trying to answer these and other questions asked frequently by primary care physicians serving in the nation's NFs as attending physicians and medical directors. The chapter's theme is that primary care physicians can be excellent attending physicians and medical directors, but they need to understand and adhere to certain essential principles to do so.

In this chapter, the term *nursing facility* is used instead of the more traditional *nursing home* for two reasons. First, the Omnibus Budget Reconciliation Act of 1987 (OBRA '87) regulations (see below) use *nursing facility* as a more comprehensive term. Secondly, many such facilities are now serving a broader role than traditional custodial care.

Like everyone else in the NF, the long-term care (LTC) physician is primarily a problem solver, not just a diagnostician and disease manager. Work and practice in the NF involves a continuous series of problems and issues that must be identified, defined, and evaluated before a solution can be reached. For the attending physician, those problems relate to their patients' symptoms, illnesses, and condition changes. For the medical director, those problems relate not just to individual patients but to the bigger picture of the systems and processes within which everyone, including the physicians, must operate.

For example, in a typical week in a typical NF, at least one resident will fall several times; another resident will fall and at first show no signs of injury but hours or days later be found to have a fracture; a family member will complain about the care a relative is receiving; several residents will have fevers but be unable to give any history; one or more residents will become physically aggressive or very restless; one or more demented residents will become delirious; numerous abnormal laboratory test results will come back and be reported to physicians; some nurses will call physicians to notify them of condition changes without having all pertinent information needed to decide what to do; one or more physicians will be late in making a scheduled visit; several physicians will argue with several nurses about the reason for calling them or the orders they have given; thousands of doses of medications will be administered; several residents will die; one or more residents (or their families) will refuse treatment for a life-threatening condition; one or more residents will suddenly stop eating or drinking; a number of physicians, nurses, social workers, dietitians, and therapists will pass information on to each other; several new assessments and care plans will be created and several others will be updated; and at least one plumbing crisis will occur.

The basically well elderly with occasional acute problems and those elderly with occasional minor flare-ups of otherwise stable chronic conditions have needs similar to those of younger adults. Few individuals in either of these categories are found in NFs.

Most NF residents are the truly "frail" elderly. They have a combination of underlying variables, including chronic illnesses, impairments or dysfunctions resulting from preexisting conditions, acute episodic illness of varying duration and severity, medication regimen, personal values and wishes, effects of "normal" aging, family wishes, physician prescribing choices, and life expectancy. In many individuals, especially toward the end of life, these conditions tend to wax and wane regularly (1).

Studies confirm that acute problems occur frequently and unpredictably among NF residents. A high level of nursing and medical skill is needed to define them correctly and manage them effectively. NFs are already handling many of these problems, thus contradicting "the stereotype that care for the chronically ill inevitably means custodial care and lack of specific diagnostics and treatment" (2).

In every case, a problem presents itself. Before an effective solution can be obtained, the problem must be defined correctly. For example, an agitated resident may have become so because of being pushed by another resident. Thus, the apparent problem may be that the resident is agitated, but the underlying cause is provocation that would probably agitate almost anyone. Or, the resident who stops eating may have done so because of an acute illness, increasing confusion due to medications, or impending death.

Often, neither the exact nature of the problem, its cause, or its solution are readily apparent. The physician is often informed of the situation and asked in some way to help define and solve the problem. A significant part of such care management is exercising judgment as to whether and to what degree aggressive medical attention is warranted. New problems continuously arise to supplant those that have been resolved.

Thus, LTC medical practice represents a challenge to correctly define and solve constantly occurring problems. How or why the physician may get involved in any situation varies widely and is often unclear to the physician. Typically, such involvement is secondary to a nonphysician's assessment and conclusions in the physician's absence that a problem exists and requires medical involvement.

For example, a nurse may have to call a physician because a fall occurs or because a test result is abnormal, yet no action is needed. Sometimes, the nurse may not need an order, but the physician assumes one is being requested. One physician may object to being called for a persistent fever of 103°F, while another may be annoyed about not being called for an upper respiratory

infection and fever of 100°F, which only later evolves into pneumonia.

Of all the steps in the problem-solving process, defining the problem correctly is often more difficult than finding a solution. For example, once it is recognized that a patient's acute confusional state is caused by medications, it is simple to stop the offending medication. However, it is often very difficult to get a physician to agree to consider this possibility and be willing to take the advice of a nurse or pharmacist and taper or stop the medication.

Above all else, successful LTC physicians and medical directors are good problem solvers. They appear to understand that the physician plays a vital, but not primary, role in defining, analyzing, and solving these problems in the NF in conjunction with many other disciplines and individuals. The less successful physicians do not appear to understand this role or may focus too much on the medical treatments or on their traditional physician orientation as self-reliant diagnosticians and treatment prescribers and their traditional prerogatives to give orders and expect them to be followed.

GIVING HIGH-QUALITY CARE

In any area, there are four possible relationships between what is done and the way in which it is done. The right thing may be done right, the wrong thing may be done right, the right thing may be done wrong, and the wrong thing may be done wrong. In the NF, all of these happen.

The ultimate goal of any health care setting is to give quality care. This means doing the right thing in the right way consistently, effectively, and efficiently. To do the right thing, one must understand what that is and how to do it. In long-term care, a variety of opinions exist about the right things and about the right ways to do them. Some of these opinions are supported by consensus, some by research, some by regulation, and a lot by habit or personal inclination.

To do the right thing in individual cases presupposes defining the problem correctly. Thus, providing quality care invariably depends on effective problem solving as discussed above. Both the medical director and the attending physicians have vital roles in helping define the realities of care, generally and in specific cases. The medical director must (a) clearly understand and help physicians and the facility define the care correctly, (b) help establish a system to provide the care, which includes the physicians in appropriate context, and (c) establish systems to monitor and improve the care (3).

GOALS OF CARE

LTC practice is not simply downsized hospital care. While acute care invariably involves managing a serious or life-threatening acute illness or injury, long-term care often involves treating diseases and dysfunctions, but always in a broader context that is patient-specific, system-specific, and institution-specific. The patient-specific context concerns the individuals' overall conditions and prognoses and their wishes and values. The system-specific context involves the demands and expectations on the LTC system (e.g., as defined by the OBRA '87 requirements). Institution-specific care concerns a facility's staffing, programs, services, and management and leadership objectives, policies, and procedures.

Thus, the attending physician should recognize that decisions about medical care and treatment must consider one or more of these. The major determinant of service needs for the LTC patient is level of function, not diagnosis. The NF should understand that information provided to physicians about a situation or problem (or requests for the physician to "do something") must include a broader explanation of the context of the information, so that physicians can coordinate their interpretation of that situation with that of the nurse or other individuals. Thus, another medical director's role is to help the facility understand these perspectives and help them provide the proper context for information.

There is no better example of this than the management of behavior. Until the advent of the OBRA '87 requirements, behavioral, cognitive, emotional, and mood disturbances were typically considered medical problems. Nurses called physicians, describing symptoms (agitation, delusions, etc.), and physicians usually prescribed psychoactive medications. Because neither the nurses nor the physicians typically defined the problem precisely or investigated the cause, the symptomatic treatment often failed to fix the problem. Furthermore, the undesirable side effects of psychoactive medications and restraints led to significant morbidity and mortality. Since OBRA implementation, there has been much more emphasis on identifying causes, finding alternative approaches to managing behavior disturbances, or simply learning to tolerate more of it without trying to suppress it.

OBRA REGULATIONS

The current regulatory and legal climate in the NF is the result of processes occurring over many years. The original Medicare and Medicaid regulations took effect in 1974, establishing "Conditions of Participation" that facilities would have to meet to qualify for federal reimbursement. Over the next decade, many problems with NF care were identified, and concerns were raised about the quality, consistency, and rational foundation for much of the care.

Physicians were largely oblivious to these issues, seeing their roles as limited to treating medical illnesses. There was very inconsistent application of such concepts as a comprehensive problem-oriented assessment, interdisciplinary review to determine potentially treatable problems, and effectively distinguishing treatable acute illness from the symptoms of normal aging or chronic conditions. Many potentially treatable medical conditions such as acute infections and adverse medication side effects were going unidentified and unmanaged, leading to considerable morbidity and mortality.

In the early 1980s, a series of court cases addressed the question of whether the entire survey process was capable of detecting the real problems of NFs and holding facilities accountable. The existing survey process was considered too predictable, process oriented, and irrelevant to the real care issues.

In 1986, the Senate Special Committee on Aging heard testimony about many common care-related problems in NFs such as inconsistent assessments, inadequate care planning, insufficient medical attention, too many medications (especially psychoactive medications) of questionable benefit prescribed per patient, and inadequate follow-up after a diagnosis was made or a treatment instituted (4). Soon afterward, the Institute of Medicine (IOM) released its report on improving NF care (5). This report's recommendations were incorporated into the law that led to extensive changes in the NF survey process and the OBRA '87 regulations governing care expectations.

Years after the OBRA '87 requirements have become law, many physicians remain puzzled by them. Though they have often not yet read them, many physicians remain convinced that these regulations severely limit their prerogatives to practice effective medicine in their patients' best interest. Both attending physicians and medical directors may resist feedback and suggestions based on other disciplines' (consultant pharmacists, nurses, etc.) concerns or reviews, claiming that people are trying to "practice medicine without a license."

Contrary to such attitudes, the OBRA '87 requirements are largely built upon a logical progression of ideas, based in turn on the realities of the changing elderly population and the growing understanding of geriatric medicine. Table 54.1 summarizes these "messages" of OBRA and their rationale. It is vital that physicians, nurses, administrators, and other care providers understand these essential themes.

The medical director has an indispensable role in helping the facility management and care providers understand the clinical relevance of many of these requirements and their consistency with current knowledge in the field. Those who fail to understand these concepts may fail to provide the care as it needs to be given, often because they see the process as a test of wills between themselves and the "government regulators" trying to tell them how to practice. The resident's care should not be held hostage in such a tug-of-war. The medical director must often exert considerable influence to overcome such attitudes and keep the physicians focused on providing good-quality care that will ultimately meet regulatory expectations.

Underlying these regulations is the idea that NF residents have certain rights, involving both their personal care and their health care. Facilities must meet their residents' personal and health care needs, including typical problems of institutionalized frail elderly such as pressure sores, functional and behavioral problems, and adequate nutrition and hydration.

Thus, relevant attending physician roles include appropriate assessments, making correct diagnoses, and prescribing appropriate treatments. But there is more to physician support than just good medical care. Like all care providers, physicians must consider the broader context of the care as discussed above. The LTC physician must be part of an interdisciplinary approach that includes the patient, family, and other health professionals in the decision-making processes.

There is no better example of this than the management of ethical issues, discussed at length elsewhere in this book. Many elderly individuals have strong feelings about limiting the extent and duration of their care when they reach the point that medical interventions are not significantly preserving or improving their quality of life. More individuals have been making advance directives, such as durable powers of attorney. The ethics decision-making process must be bidirectional. The attending physician has an important role in evaluating the condition and prognosis, deciding whether potentially treatable conditions exist, describing the treatment options, and explaining those options to patients, their families, and the facility staff. The patient-centered direction includes determining decision-making capacity,

clarifying the patient's values and wishes (either directly, by inference through discussion with the family, or by reviewing advance directives or other written statements), reviewing the treatment options, and selecting a course of action from those options. The physician may be the only one authorized to write the orders to implement those choices, but that differs from having the authority to choose the treatment course unilaterally.

THE PHYSICIAN AND CARE PLANNING

After assessing the resident, every facility must create an individualized care plan. The term *care planning* describes a process by which caregivers determine the goals of an individual's care and the methods to meet those goals. Care plans allow all those involved with the care of the patient to have some input. A care plan typically includes, among other things, medical goals, functional goals, short- and long-term goals, what to do in an emergency (e.g., intubation, antibiotics, use of emergency rooms), and appropriate nutritional and psychosocial support.

Attending physicians in NFs are rarely present for the actual discussion of the care plan but have an important role in assuring that the care plan is realistic, consistent, and pertinent to the medical problems and their related functional or psychosocial deficits. Physicians can help by determining physical, mental, and functional status appropriately and by ordering further treatments and assessments of potentially treatable conditions or dysfunctions. The physician should also at least review the care plan periodically as it relates to the medical orders.

In summary, physician support should be both medical (directly referable to the treatment of medical conditions) and nonmedical (referable to personal care and quality of life), as summarized in Table 54.2.

THE ATTENDING PHYSICIAN'S VITAL ROLE IN REGULATORY COMPLIANCE

Three recurring themes of the OBRA '87 regulations are particularly relevant to physician responsibilities. They are

- What are the "highest practicable" levels of function?
- What is "medically necessary"?
- When are negative outcomes "medically unavoidable"?

HIGHEST PRACTICABLE FUNCTION

Symptoms and dysfunctions in the frail elderly may be due to normal aging, acute illness, exac-

Table 54.1
Essential "Messages" of the OBRA '87 Regulations[a]

Rationale	Message
The residents of nursing facilities are a changing population, representing many of the most frail elderly	Therefore, they have rights, including the right to a reasonable quality of life, within the limits imposed by their irreversible underlying impairments (Resident Rights section)
Quality of life has both psychosocial and biologic components; there are five ways in which biology typically affects quality of life: "normal" aging, functional and behavioral limitations, acute illness, chronic conditions, and iatrogenic illness (such as medication complications)	Therefore, while not all problems of this population will respond to medical intervention, only a systematic assessment, interpreted according to some rational guidelines, can help reveal which of the above factors—alone or in combination—are the reason for an individual's problems, complaints, or symptoms (MDS and RAP requirement) Therefore, an effective medical care plan (the orders) and nonmedical interdisciplinary care plan depend on a search for causes, and consideration of alternative explanations for findings (Quality of Care requirements)
If the problem is determined to be medical, it may or may not be treatable by available medical modalities, or it may only be treatable to a certain extent; if treatable, the next question is whether it should be treated and to what extent	Therefore, decisions about whether and to what extent to treat an individual depends in part on the relative risks and benefits of the treatment, the ultimate impact of the treatment on quality of life, and the wishes of the resident or family (Resident Rights requirements)
If a treatment is then given and the resident's condition changes, it may change because of the treatment or despite it	Therefore, there is no way to know which is true without periodically reassessing whether the problem still exists and for how long the treatment needs to continue (Unnecessary Drugs requirements)
If there is a medical problem, the physicians should provide timely intervention according to accepted standards of care for the frail elderly	Therefore, there should be some physician services that help meet these expectations (Physician Services requirements)
A broad interdisciplinary effort is needed to provide and oversee the care	Therefore, an effective, consistent process should exist to ensure that the above things happen effectively and consistently and that the clinical care is monitored and reviewed to ensure that they are done properly (Administrative, Quality Assurance, and Medical Director requirements)

[a]From Levenson SA. Medical direction in long-term care. 2nd ed. Durham, NC: Carolina Academic Press, 1993. With permission.

erbations of chronic conditions, medications, or some combination of these. Physicians must use their expertise to help decide realistically the highest practicable level achievable for a given individual. To do this, they must gather appropriate data, including their own assessment and a review of the assessments of other disciplines; rule out potentially treatable conditions or problems; and then consider the possible nonmedical means of attaining that improvement.

Physicians are not expected or required to treat all symptoms or laboratory abnormalities or to correct irreversible functional impairments. However, there is an expectation that what is treatable will be treated if it can somehow help improve function and quality of life and if treating it is consistent with an individual's overall condition, prognosis, and values.

MEDICALLY NECESSARY

Another key role is deciding which treatments and medications are medically necessary. Medical necessity means that a treatment or medication is pertinent to a specific condition or problem, that it is the least risky among reasonable alternatives, that there is some thought as to whether the treatment continues to be required over time,

Table 54.2
Medical and Nonmedical Support by NF Physicians[a]

Medical Support	Nonmedical support
Accurate medical assessments, including careful definition and description of problems and diagnoses	Help the patient gain appropriate access to the right LTC programs and services
Evaluate current condition and a realistic prognosis	Help individuals find and remain in the least restrictive setting compatible with their condition and needs
Help establish realistic care goals based on the assessment and conclusions regarding condition and prognosis	Support the different members of the interdisciplinary team
Write medical orders consistent with these conclusions and goals	Interpret essential medical information for patients, families, and other team members to help them provide quality personal care and handle clinical, ethical, social, psychological, and functional problems
Manage chronic illnesses to maximize function and personal comfort	Help patients and families have realistic expectations of what long-term health care can offer
Manage acute illness as aggressively as indicated by an individual's goals, condition, and prognosis	Be aware of the wishes and needs of a patient or family, and consider these in medical decision making
Ensure adequate, timely follow up of the benefits or complications of medications and treatments	Help maximize a person's autonomy and function within the limits imposed by their condition
Modify medication and treatment orders in line with such assessments	
Provide clear, complete, and timely documentation of the reasons for various medical decisions	

[a]Modified from Levenson SA. Medical direction in long-term care. 2nd ed. Durham, NC: Carolina Academic Press, 1993.

and that attention is paid to any side effects or complications.

For example, the nurses and physician should first discuss options other than restraints or psychoactive medications to deal with the commonly occurring behavioral, cognitive, and mood disturbances found in many NF residents. If they decide that restraints or medications are needed, they should document explicitly how and why they reached that conclusion, so that outsiders reviewing the record can see their line of reasoning. If they cannot offer a reasonable justification, they should reconsider their choice. Thus, documentation not only demonstrates how decisions were made but also forces providers to think through what they are doing and why they are doing it. The ultimate justification for any medical or nursing intervention should always be to stabilize or improve function and to enhance quality of life.

If the caregivers decide to use restraints or psychoactive medications, they should reevaluate the resident periodically to see if the problem persists. If it persists, they should consider whether the treatment is appropriate or might need to be changed. If it stabilizes or resolves, they should consider whether the medication or treatment is still needed or if it could be tapered or discontinued. Often, the only way they can know this is to try.

MEDICALLY UNAVOIDABLE

Many negative outcomes occur in NF residents. They may get sicker despite treatment, have complications of acute illnesses, or die.

The OBRA '87 regulations stress that complications and negative results should be medically unavoidable; that is, they occur despite appropriate management, not because of inappropriate management or indifference. Physicians have a vital role in ensuring and demonstrating that negative outcomes are medically unavoidable. There are two important ways to fulfill this role: (a) help ensure that problems are not overlooked, but are assessed and managed in a timely fashion, and (b) document the reasoning behind decisions to treat or not to treat various conditions and abnormalities, to communicate the fact that they cared and made an effort, rather than ignored problems.

Other things that attending physicians can do to help improve the care and at the same time improve regulatory compliance include following pertinent policies and procedures; providing effective, responsible, cooperative alternative medical coverage when they are unavailable; seeking possible care problems and reporting them to the medical director; making timely required visits and visits for acute interim illness; and writing medical orders that minimize possibilities for error, misinterpretation, drug incompatibilities, and therapeutic duplication.

Physicians cannot anticipate and detect all possible problems and complications in their NF patients, because they are present only occasionally and the problems arise so frequently. Therefore, they must rely upon information provided them by the nurses, consultant pharmacists, and other caregivers. This does not mean the physician must agree with their conclusions or must respond to all such reports by doing something. Rather, this interdisciplinary approach is essential to effective care and requires dismantling traditional barriers to communication and sharply defined boundaries about what each discipline can or must do. Such boundaries and the fear of crossing them have often led to problems falling through the cracks and the subsequent appearance of negligent care.

Medical directors have a vital role in reinforcing appropriate attitudes among attending physicians. These include acknowledging the professionalism of other disciplines, accepting information willingly from them, and working collaboratively to define issues and determine whether they can or should be treated. Even a modest amount of interest and participation by physicians in NFs can make a considerable difference in the attitudes of the facility and other caregivers and their success in providing better quality care.

With the medical director's help and support, attending physicians should learn and use a systematic approach to fulfilling their functions, as illustrated in Table 54.2.

THE MEDICAL DIRECTOR ROLE

Careful assessment reveals the many forces and individuals that influence the care in LTC facilities. Most (nurses, physicians, administrators) work in the facility; other important influences (laws, regulations, surveyors) are external to the care system, although sometimes present in the facility (3).

Fulfilling the medical director's role requires some knowledge of geriatric medicine. But clinical knowledge must be balanced by administrative and leadership functions that help the medical care fit into the context of the LTC system. Doing these things requires the ability and desire to work with other physicians, facility residents, families, administrators, and other caregivers to ensure that appropriate, effective systems and processes are established to meet these clinical and regulatory requirements and to help solve and prevent problems effectively. The problems are not just clinical; they also relate to improving employee and professional morale and attitudes, improving the efficiency and consistency of the care, and to preventing problems and reducing risk. Again, that is why a good primary care physician can be an effective medical director and why a fully trained geriatrician may not do the job as well.

Thus, the traditional approach to medical direction—a sporadic advisory role oriented toward paper compliance—must yield to a more professional, visible, intervention-oriented, teaching role. For example, it is not enough for the medical director to attend committee meetings. Instead, these meetings should be used for effective interdisciplinary discussion of problems and coordinated attempts to solve and prevent them. When the consultant pharmacist provides information about the number of facility residents taking psychoactive medications, then the medical director should consider whether such use is appropriate and how the physicians might be educated to reduce the dosage, frequency, and duration of the neuroleptics they prescribe. When findings are presented about the incidence of pressure sores, the medical director should consider whether the attending physicians have been working with the nurses effectively to notice pressure sores in their early stages and to intervene aggressively before they evolve further. While other individuals might help with some of the medical director's administrative and paperwork responsibilities, they cannot substitute for rational authority and leadership by example.

THE MEDICAL DIRECTOR'S FUNCTIONS AND TASKS

Primary care physicians naturally want to know how they can provide these services efficiently as well as effectively. In part, the answer lies in taking an organized approach to the job (Table 54.3).

Recent discussions among medical directors have helped clarify functions and tasks in much greater depth. In 1988, a group of medical directors from around the United States met and reached a consensus about nine broad functions of medical directors (see Table 54.4), which included nine major functions and well over 100 different tasks (6, 7).

No medical director will perform all these activities. Each physician must create an individualized job description by matching a facility's needs with these potential functions. However, there are certain things all medical directors should do. These include organizing the medical staff sufficiently to ensure adequate, timely coverage; helping prevent and solve clinical problems effectively; overseeing the medical care and giving feedback to the attending physicians about how they are doing; and ensuring that clinical policies, procedures, and practices in the facility are appropriate and consistent with good geriatric medical care.

A few studies exist concerning the characteristics and activities of medical directors (8). They are usually primary care internists or family physicians who provide part-time medical direction to between one and three facilities. Generally, their activities may be divided into (*a*) routine tasks,

such as care reviews and general rounds, and (*b*) episodic tasks, such as family meetings, committee meetings, consultation in problem cases, and investigation of unexpected serious incidents. Most medical directors at least make rounds, review incident reports, review policies, review and try to correct problems with care, and communicate with the administrator and the director of nursing (DON).

Based on experience and on the few existing time analyses, it is fair to conclude that fulfilling the medical director's role will require about 4 to 8 hours of time per week per 100 facility beds (3). The time needed will be at the high end of this scale if the physician must organize and implement systems and policies and totally organize or reorganize the medical staff. The time requirement will decrease as the physician can shift to ongoing management and oversight of the care in an effectively operating system that minimizes crises and prevents problems.

Physicians serving as medical directors should consider themselves—and should be considered by the facility administration—to be part of the facility's leadership as well as the management. A key component of such leadership is to transmit appropriate attitudes and values to the physicians and to the other facility staff. An interested, enthusiastic, supportive medical director can help improve the attitudes and the care in a facility. In contrast, the unenthusiastic, uninterested physi-

Table 54.3
Steps to Fulfilling the Medical Director Role[a]

Understand the job
Assess the facility
Create a job description and service agreement
Clarify legal responsibilities and liabilities
Establish key relationships
Organize the medical staff
Create policies and procedures, and standards for care
Evaluate and improve systems for communicating and managing information
Oversee and evaluate the care
Help implement measures to solve problems and improve the care

[a]Modified from Levenson SA. Medical direction in long-term care. 2nd ed. Durham, NC: Carolina Academic Press, 1993.

Table 54.4
Major Medical Director Functions[a]

Participate in administrative decision making and recommend and approve policies and procedures
Organize and coordinate physician services and services of other professionals as they relate to patient care
Participate in the process to ensure the appropriateness and quality of medical and medically related care
Participate in the development and conduct of education programs
Help articulate the facility's mission to the community and represent the facility in the community
Participate in the surveillance and promotion of the health, welfare, and safety of employees
Acquire, maintain, and apply knowledge of social, regulatory, political, and economic factors that relate to patient care services
Provide medical leadership for research and development activities in geriatrics and long-term care
Participate in establishing policies and procedures for ensuring that the rights of individuals are respected

[a]Adapted from Pattee JJ, Altemeier TM. Results of a consensus conference on the role of the nursing home medical director. Ann Med Direction 1991;1(1):5–11.

cian can have a correspondingly negative effect on the other physicians and on the morale and attitudes of the whole facility.

THE PHYSICIANS AND THE NURSING STAFF

In any NF, the physicians will work most closely with the nursing staff, and the medical director will work closely with the DON in a number of care-related areas. Thus, it is appropriate to review the roles and responsibilities of these individuals, since many of them overlap physician roles and must be coordinated effectively.

The director of nursing is typically a registered nurse (RN) with some training or background in geriatrics and long-term care. Like the medical director, the DON is responsible to the administrator. However, the DON oversees what is usually the largest department, with a diverse group of individuals ranging from other RNs to a rapidly changing collection of nursing assistants. The DON is responsible for overseeing nursing care, representing the nurses' perspective in facility-wide meetings and problem-solving discussions, implementing federal and state regulations, overseeing nursing staff performance, creating pertinent policies and procedures, proposing and implementing pertinent services and programs, creating education and training programs for nursing staff, and dealing with individual cases, health department citations, and assorted problems and complaints.

Most NFs are staffed primarily by licensed practical (vocational) nurses and nursing assistants, under the supervision of an RN. The nursing assistants give most of the personal care (toileting, bathing, dressing, bed changing, etc.), and the nurses deliver both clinical and personal care. This may include assisting with activities of daily living, assessing condition changes, giving medications, and monitoring vital signs. Typically, the nurses—like the physicians—vary in their background, knowledge, training, skills, and experience. Some have a background primarily in acute care with little actual LTC experience, while others have a significant LTC background but little experience in the high-technology world of modern acute care.

To provide the most effective care possible in the NF, the physicians and nurses must collaborate closely and circumvent traditional communications barriers and rigid role definitions. Medical care does not mean just physician care. There are shared responsibilities in each step of the clinical problem-solving process, from problem definition, to adjusting the care plan and treatment

on the basis of observed responses, to the treatment regimen. Table 54.5 illustrates some of the shared roles in defining problems and choosing management options.

The medical director and DON have a major responsibility to work with the administrator and other department heads to establish and use a systematic approach to care. For example, many different disciplines (dietitians, physical therapists, social workers, nurses, etc.) assess residents, evaluate some aspect of their care management, and recommend new or modified treatments. This information must be communicated and coordinated effectively, so that there is ultimately one overall care plan with multiple components, not multiple care plans from different perspectives. A nursing assistant may be the first to recognize a significant condition change, and a physician may be the one to notice that the nurses have not been documenting observations of potential adverse reactions to psychoactive medications.

Similarly, problems that arise are typically interdisciplinary; that is, they result from the action or omission of several disciplines or individuals. For example, the failure to carry out a consultant's recommendation to order a test or to change a diet may be the result of something not done or misunderstood by a physician, nurse, dietitian, ward clerk, or the kitchen, or several of them together. Thus, the medical director and DON have special responsibility to support and enforce the interdisciplinary approach to defining problems and determining causes. They should avoid and discourage the traditional territoriality that leads to problems in NF residents being overlooked until an acute medical emergency finally occurs.

Table 54.5
Examples of Relative Roles of Physicians and Nurses in Various Aspects of Resident Care[a]

Responsibility	Nurses	Physicians
Recognize condition change	+ + +	+ + +
Define the problem precisely	+ + +	+ + +
Determine the cause(s) of the problem	+ + +	+ + +
Ascertain options for managing the problem	+ +	+ + +
Determine resident/family wishes related to care management	+ + +	+ +
Assess response to treatment	+ + +	+ + +

[a]Modified from Levenson SA. Medical direction in long-term care. 2nd ed. Durham, NC: Carolina Academic Press, 1993.

AN EFFECTIVE CARE SYSTEM

Related to this, another important leadership function of the medical director is to help ensure that a facility has the attitudes, systems, support, and staff to create and use an effective care system. This is needed to deal with the increasing demands on NFs to provide more medical care on-site instead of transferring residents to acute hospitals and because many NFs are starting to provide more intensive, short-term medical and rehabilitative care, often referred to as subacute care. Often, such care is being provided in a specialized unit within the skilled facility. Besides treating infections, dehydration, pneumonias, and electrolyte imbalance, more facilities are also offering ventilator care, total parenteral nutrition, wound management and extensive ulcer care, postoperative care, and intensive rehabilitation therapies after fractures, prolonged illness, or surgery.

Subacute care is a hybrid of acute and long-term care. Not only must the clinical care be technically proficient, but many of the issues of quality of life, family involvement, functional restoration, and treatment limitations found in traditional NF care are highly relevant. Thus, the attending physicians and medical director in the NF must help ensure that subacute and acute services are more like enhanced long-term care than they are downsized hospital care.

The medical director will need to advise facilities about essential items such as contractual radiology services, off-site laboratories, and transfer agreements with local hospitals. Also, the medical director will need to work with the nurses and attending physicians to develop and use effective protocols for identifying, defining, and triaging the symptoms, condition changes, and clinical problems that occur in short-stay patients.

QUALITY ASSURANCE ROLES

The OBRA '87 regulations require physician participation on a NF Quality Assurance (QA) committee. To do this appropriately, a medical director should understand the quality assurance process and the concepts and principles of continuous quality improvement (CQI) (9). CQI is the conceptual foundation for effective systems and processes in any health care facility to ensure that direct caregivers have the systems and support they need so they can provide the care that the patients require (10).

A successful medical QA program requires that the medical director and attending physicians identify important aspects of care and establish or adopt appropriate policies, medical care standards, and quality indicators. The medical director must help establish a system for reviewing the care and its documentation, evaluating the significance of the information that is collected, deciding on areas for change and improvement, giving the physicians feedback about how to change their practices and improve the care, and following up to determine whether changes are durable and effectively improve the care (11).

Successful LTC practice depends not only on having information but also on being able to understand what it means and what to do about it. In performing all their functions, medical directors have crucial roles as educators. These educational functions may be divided into providing information and interpreting that information.

Medical directors should be reviewing and communicating information from the geriatrics and general medical literature. Teaching opportunities also occur while making rounds; when attending committee meetings; when answering questions asked by staff, patients, and families; during periodic meetings with administrators, directors of nursing, and other key department heads; and in contacts with attending physicians to discuss issues related to the care of specific patients.

The role of physicians in long-term care is stronger and growing steadily. More interested, dedicated attending physicians and medical directors are needed. However, more physicians are providing effective medical direction, and more state medical director associations have been taking active, vigorous roles in improving the care in facilities and helping change the regulatory climate and attitudes towards LTC providers. The successes of these individuals and their facilities offer lessons for the entire LTC industry and the disciplines, including physicians, working within them. Meeting the demands of the future will require that physicians, administrators, regulators, nurses and others heed these examples and apply them more widely.

REFERENCES

1. Ouslander JG. Medical care in the nursing home. JAMA 1989;262:2582–2590.
2. Bernardini B, Meinecke C, Zaccarini C, et al. Adverse clinical events in dependent long-term nursing home residents. J Am Geriatr Soc 1993;41:105–111.
3. Levenson SA. Medical direction in long-term care: a guidebook for the future. 2nd ed. Durham, NC: Carolina Academic Press, 1993.
4. Senate Special Committee on Aging. Staff report. Nursing home care: the unfinished agenda. May 21, 1986.
5. Institute of Medicine. Improving the quality of care in nursing homes. Committee on Nursing Home

Regulations. Washington, DC: National Academy Press, 1986.

6. Pattee JJ, Altemeier TM. Results of a consensus conference on the role of the nursing home medical director. Ann Med Direction 1991;1(1):5–11.

7. Pattee JJ, Otteson O. Medical direction in the nursing home. Minneapolis: Northridge Press, 1991.

8. Katz P, Karuza J, Parker M, et al. 1992; A national survey of medical directors. J Med Direction 1992; 2:81–94.

9. Kritchevsky SB, Simmons BP. Continuous quality improvement: concepts and applications for physician care. JAMA 1991;266:1817–1823.

10. Levenson SA. The medical director and continuous quality improvement. J Med Direction 1992; 2(2):67–75.

11. Joint Commission on Accreditation of Healthcare Organizations. Quality improvement in long term care. Oak Brook, IL: JCAHO, 1992.

55/ Sexuality in Older Adults

Elizabeth A. Alexander, April L. Allison

With sexuality so at the heart of human experience throughout adolescent and young adult years, it is, in a way, surprising that as people mature they are expected not only to become less sexually active but also to lose all interest in sexuality. The societal norm, too often internalized by those who are aging, is that—with the exception of occasional "dirty old men"—aging is invariably associated with asexuality.

SEXUAL INTEREST AND ACTIVITY

Most of the studies done on sexual functioning have reflected societal biases about sexual activity in older people and consequently have excluded significant numbers of patients above the age of 65. The Kinsey study, in which thousands of men and women were interviewed, included only 31 women and 48 men over 65. Most of the older patients in Masters and Johnson's widely quoted work were in their 50s and 60s, with few of the small sample being over 65, and the Hite report, which included 1066 women, had only 6 women in their 70s (3). Other biases include a tendency to study populations that are married, that include only higher socioeconomic classes, and that are Caucasian. Despite the limitations of published research on sexuality and aging, studies to date show that many people indicate sexual interest and activity into their 70s, with health status and availability of a partner most often being the limiting factors on expression of sexuality (4). Not surprisingly, the level of sexual activity and interest for healthy married partners is positively correlated with the couple's earlier experience of sexuality within their relationship.

Availability of a partner generally means of a marital partner, and research to date indicates that most sexual activity among the elderly is within the context of marriage. Elderly women looking for a male partner find few eligible men available, since women have a life span approximately 7 years longer than that of men, compounded by the fact that women tend to marry

men who are older than they are (3). There is speculation that this gender gap may narrow in the coming years (5), but at the current time, compliance with societal norms limiting sexual expression to the context of marriage severely constrains the possibilities of an older woman finding a sanctioned sexual partner.

Both men and women are more likely to be married with spouse present if they are white than if they are of another ethnic group, although the gap lessens with age. As early as age group 55 to 64, fully 27.3% of black women and 24.8% of American Indian women have been widowed (6). Since most research focuses on the white elderly, there are few data on how the single elderly meet their needs for intimacy in differing ethnic or cultural environments.

EXTERNAL BARRIERS TO SEXUAL INTIMACY

While health status and availability of a partner may be the most common reasons for a decrease or cessation of sexual activity, there are other common barriers to a full expression of physical intimacy in old age. These include social stigma on sexual activity among the old. According to traditional social mores, desirability is linked to a youthful appearance, and the equation of desirability and maturity is incomprehensible to some. It may be tolerated when a man of wealth and status marries a young wife and/or fathers children in his old age, but similar behavior by a man of modest means or by a woman of any social class is too often considered reprehensible and disgusting.

External barriers to the development of an intimate sexual relationship in old age can also include the disapproval of adult children for a variety of reasons. An adult child may cling to the memory of the deceased parent and not be willing to accept that the surviving parent would take a new spouse. The adult child may try to prevent a courtship in an attempt to preserve an inheritance. It may be that the child shares the societal perception that old people should not behave sexually.

There may be institutional barriers to intimacy, whether marital or between single adults. This could include a lack of privacy and autonomy while living with adult children or it could result from nursing home regulations and the lack of privacy intrinsic in such institutional settings. While these barriers are restrictive for older heterosexual couples, gay or lesbian residents of nursing homes find even more constraints and social sanctions when they attempt to develop intimate relationships.

In addition to the disadvantageous sex ratio discussed above, heterosexual women face other substantial obstacles to the development of an intimate relationship. These include the persistent double standard regarding sexual activity outside of marriage for men and women and prevalent norms against an older woman marrying a younger man. An older man, on the other hand, is more likely to be limited by physiologic constraints on his sexual performance than by a lack of potential partners (as discussed below).

INTERNALIZED BARRIERS TO SEXUAL INTIMACY

There is often no clear demarcation indicating where the external constraints of societal norms and structures end and where an individual's internalized constraints begin. Many older adults believe that they are, in fact, unattractive because they are old. Some have self-expectations about their role in society as they age, seeing themselves as "retired" from sexual roles in much the same way that they have retired from their occupational or their parenting roles (7). Men often link their self-esteem to their occupational performance, and the loss of that occupational role can affect sexual performance.

For some, religious interpretations of the role of sexual intercourse can prohibit the development of a purely pleasurable or intimate relationship. If the participants are well past childbearing age, there may be dubious moral authority for them to simply enjoy their sexuality.

PHYSIOLOGIC CHANGES WITH AGING

As people age, the physiologic changes that affect sexual activity are gradual and often reflect the baseline status of vascular, hormonal, and neurologic health. When men and women have had satisfying sexual relationships in earlier years, they are less apt to have problems with the normal physiologic changes that occur with aging.

Kaplan divides the physiology of the sexual response cycle into three phases: desire phase, in which the "end organ" is the brain; arousal phase, in which the "end organ" is the vascular system; and orgasmic phase, in which the "end organ" is the spinal cord and muscular structures of the perineal floor that contract during orgasm (8). Normal changes in sexual response that occur with aging are outlined in Table 55.1 for both men and women, by phase of the sexual response cycle. Generally, the changes are ones of degree and timing, and they are gradual over time.

When older patients present with sexual concerns, it is useful to consider which phase of the response cycle is affected, as drugs and disease processes affect sexual response differently. Tables 55.2 and 55.3 list some of the categories of medications and illnesses (with common examples), and the phase(s) of the sexual response cycle affected. With aging, the impact of drugs and disease is magnified, so that many drugs or illnesses that may not have affected sexual expression in younger years do so more commonly as a person becomes older. Another useful way to think about the changes in sexual response that occur with aging is to consider that the progression of sexual arousal from desire phase through orgasm is extended and that the amount of "physiologic protection" against modifying influences, such as drugs or disease, may be reduced. In older people, there are more likely to be several factors that modify sexual response, so that the combination of disease processes, drugs, and normal changes of aging interact to affect a person's sexual experience.

ASSESSMENT AND SCREENING

It is important to ask about physical, sexual, and emotional intimacy in the course of routine care of older adults. Too often, physicians are influenced by the cultural bias that assumes sexual expression is normal in the young and unusual if not distasteful in elderly patients. Silence about this topic on the part of physicians reflects either discomfort with the idea of older persons being sexual people, embarrassment about asking, or a lack of knowledge about what to ask or how best to inquire. In routine care, when a patient does not express concerns about sexual issues, one can simply inquire about social and emotional intimacy (the quality of the relationship, if any), whether a patient still enjoys sexual activity with a partner, whether a patient feels comfortable using self-stimulation (masturbation) for sexual pleasure and release of tension, and whether a

Table 55.1
Effects on Sexual Response of Physiologic Changes Related to Aging[a]

	Women	Men
Desire phase	Affected most by illness in self or partner, relationship problems, cultural expectations, and self-esteem issues with aging; desire for sexual contact may decrease somewhat with aging in women, but this is variable	Interval for desired frequency of sexual contact increases with aging; desire affected most by illness, performance anxiety, and relationship problems; testosterone decreases slowly from age 55 on, affecting libido
Arousal phase (vascular phase)	Less increase in breast size; less skin flush; reduced elasticity of vaginal walls; decreased vaginal lubrication; more bladder and urethral irritation; less muscle tension in arousal phase	Longer time for arousal[b]; erections less firm; testosterone decrease; sperm production gradually declines after age 40; testes elevate toward perineum more slowly and less; ejaculatory control improves
Orgasmic phase (muscular phase)	Orgasmic response may be less intense with fewer contractions; ability to have multiple orgasms may decrease with aging	Ejaculatory control improves; force of muscular contractions perceived as less; fewer contractions per orgasm; volume of ejaculate decreased
Postorgasmic phase	May have a refractory period in which immediate arousal is more difficult.	Physiologically extended refractory period, in which another erection and orgasm is more difficult to achieve

[a]Information taken from Rykken DE. Sex in the later years. In: Silverman P, ed. The elderly as modern pioneers. Bloomington: Indiana University Press, 1987; Theienhaus OJ. Practical overview of sexual function and advancing age. Geriatrics 1988;43:63–67; and Mooradian AD, Greiff V. Sexuality in older women. Arch Intern Med 1990;150:1033–1038.
[b]Three seconds at age 18 from arousal to firm erection; 18–20 seconds at age 45 from arousal to erection; often more than 5 minutes at age 75 from arousal to erection.

patient has questions or concerns about any changes in sexual functioning. Often, both older and younger patients are hesitant to bring up concerns about sexual and physical intimacy; thus, they may need the encouragement and prompting of such specific questions to be able to talk about the subject.

ASSESSMENT OF PRESENTING PROBLEMS

When a patient expresses concerns about sexual functioning, the physician needs to ask about several historical issues. Table 55.4 lists the most critical pieces of information that the physician needs to make an accurate diagnosis and help the patient consider ways of approaching the problem. The most common concerns that people over 60 express about their sexual functioning are lack of desire, concerns about changes in erectile function, "retarded" ejaculation or longer time to trigger orgasm, painful intercourse, and lack of a partner or setting available for expression of sexual and physical intimacy.

Probably the best way to get an accurate assessment of problems in an ongoing sexual relationship is to ask the patient or the couple to describe what typically happens in a sexual encounter. This will allow the provider to assess what phase of the sexual response cycle is affected, to understand the impact of the problem on the person or the couple, and to know some of the things the couple has done or not done to deal with the concern. Such a specific description also avoids the pitfall of accepting a patient's diagnosis or label, since such a self-diagnosis may have very different meanings to the patient and to the physician.

DIFFERENCES IN PRESENTING SEXUAL PROBLEMS IN OLDER PATIENTS

Unlike younger couples with sexual difficulties, marital discord is less commonly an important diagnostic consideration in older couples who seek help with sexual concerns. By age 60, couples who have had longstanding marital distress that has affected a sexual relationship either have adopted a resigned truce about this issue (often being sexually abstinent) and thus do not request help, or the issue is quite apparent as a longstanding problem. Psychosexual causes of sexual dysfunction in the elderly do occur, with depression, lack of a partner, lack of privacy, and alcoholism being by far the most common. Organic causes of sexual dysfunction become more common with aging, although there may be a secondary psychological component that is added to the organic problem. This secondary phenomenon often oc-

Table 55.2
Common Medication Effects on Sexual Functioning in the Elderly[a]

Drug Category	Example	Phase(s) Affected	Alternatives
Antihypertensives—diuretics	Thiazides	Arousal phase	Consider Ca channel blocker, more pleasuring in arousal phase
Antihypertensives—centrally acting drugs	Clonidine, methyldopa	Arousal phase	Same as above
Antihypertensive drugs—β-blockers	Propranolol	Desire phase, arousal phase	Same as above
Antihypertensives—ACE inhibitors	Captopril	Arousal phase	Same as above
Antipsychotic drugs	Thorazine, Thiothixene, haloperidol	Desire phase; arousal phase; priapism, retrograde ejaculation	
Antianxiety	Diazepam	Desire phase; orgasm	Consider Buspar, decrease medications slowly
Anticholinergic	Atropine, hydroxyzine	Arousal phase; desire phase	More emphasis on pleasuring
Estrogen	Premarin	Arousal phase (improves lubrication, decreases pain)	Topical estrogen a choice for those who cannot take oral estrogens
Progestins	Provera	Desire phase (may decrease libido)	Use cyclic instead of daily dosing if side effects
H-2 receptor antagonists	Cimetidine	Desire phase, arousal phase	Consider alternatives to H-2 blockers
Narcotics	Codeine, Demerol	Desire phase, arousal phase, orgasm	Timing of medication may be important, related to timing of sexual activity
Sedatives	Alcohol, barbiturates	Desire phase, arousal phase, orgasm	Recognize and treat addictions
Other	Digitalis	Desire phase, arousal phase	Treat performance anxiety, reassure fears about cardiac arrest during sex
Tricyclic antidepressants	Imipramine, amitriptyline	Desire phase, arousal phase, delayed muscular phase	Consider Prozac, Zoloft
Other antidepressants	Trazadone, MAO inhibitors	Priapism, arousal phase, orgasm	Consider Prozac, Zoloft

[a]Information taken from Drugs that cause sexual dysfunction: an update. Med Lett Drugs Ther 1992;34:73–78; Kaplan HS. The new sex therapy: active treatment of sexual dysfunctions. New York: Brunner/Mazel, 1974:86–103; and Halvorsen JG, Metz ME. Sexual dysfunction, part 1: classification, etiology, and pathogenesis. J Am Board Fam Pract 1992;5:51–61.

Table 55.3
Information Needed for Assessment

Historical information
- Timing of onset of symptoms (gradual or sudden)
- Masturbatory history
- Phase of response cycle most affected
- Marital or relationship history
- Previous sexual functioning
- Setting limitations for sexual intimacy
- Desired outcome (what the individual or couple would consider to be an improvement)

Physical examination data
- Evidence of organic brain changes
- Integrity of spinal cord
- Bulbocavernosus reflex
- Perianal sensation
- Tone of external anal sphincter
- Testicular size
- Vaginal lubrication/atrophy
- Clitoral size
- Varicocele
- Penile pulses/peripheral pulses
- Evidence of other cardiac disease
- General muscle tone

Laboratory testing
- HbAIC
- LH, FSH
- Thyroid profile
- Liver enzymes
- Prolactin
- Serum testosterone (bioavailable testosterone & total testosterone)

Consider, based on history
- Doppler study of penile blood pressure (compared with brachial arterial pressure)
- Nocturnal penile tumescence study (usually not useful in elderly men) (19)

curs with patients who become discouraged or upset about changes in sexual functioning when they have previously enjoyed good sexual relationships. Changes in health status or body alterations can also cause concerns about whether it is possible or desirable to maintain ongoing sexual relationships.

TREATMENT CONSIDERATIONS

Treatment should depend upon the patient's or the couple's goals for themselves, rather than on some professional assessment of what is best or "normal." Setting these goals may involve education about what is possible (for instance, if a medication that is affecting sexual expression is necessary, discussion of ways to adapt to the change

may be important), including education about normal changes that do not mean the end of sexual functioning.

Helpful solutions often do not mean "cures" or returning the patient to a level of sexual functioning characteristic of a much younger person, but expansion of "repertoire" so that new and different options for physical and sexual expression are incorporated. For instance, a complaint of retarded ejaculation may be turned into a positive symptom, with a man and his partner learning to enjoy the prolonged period of sexual arousal and pleasuring prior to orgasm. In the course of dealing with sexual concerns that result from aging, illness, or medication, couples often improve communication about giving and receiving physical pleasure, with positive effects on sexual functioning. Table 55.4 lists the most common sexual concerns in the older population, with relevant diagnostic and therapeutic considerations.

SPECIFIC ISSUES IN THERAPY

In men above age 60 who have difficulty developing or maintaining an erection, at least part of the cause is almost always organic, with vascular disease predominantly the cause of erectile dysfunction in older men. However, in this culture, most men who experience difficulties with erection also have a secondary psychological component that adds to the problem and is generally quite treatable. It is reasonable to work toward removing the "performance anxiety" of erectile dysfunction before considering surgical or medical interventions.

Bibliotherapy is often a resource that can be extremely helpful to physicians in understanding and dealing with problems related to erectile dysfunction. *The New Male Sexuality* by Bernie Zilbergeld is helpful for patients concerned about erectile problems and offers sound advice and concrete suggestions for removing the secondary psychological component (9).

In considering other treatment options for erectile dysfunction, whether one chooses to consider surgical implants (either semirigid rod or inflatable prostheses), the use of injectable papaverine/phentolamine/prostaglandin E_1 into the corpora cavernosa or the use of sublingual testosterone shortly before sexual activity should be based on a thorough assessment of the type and amount of physiologic impairment (surgical, venous, arterial, neurogenic, psychogenic, or medication-induced), the goals of the patient and his partner, and the risks attentive to each therapeutic modality.

Table 55.4
Common Sexual Concerns of Aging

Concern	Diagnostic Consideration	Treatment Options
Erectile dysfunction	Consider vascular disease, medication side effect, and magnitude of secondary psychogenic effect	Use bibliotherapy (9); consider, depending on amount of psychogenic component, injectable papverine, testosterone, implants occasionally, negative-pressure penile orthotics
Painful intercourse, women	Document estrogen deficiency, document adequate stimulation in arousal phase	Consider either oral estrogens, topical vaginal estrogen, or both
Decreased libido	Consider depression, chronic illness (including alcoholism), medication effect, decreased androgens in both men and women, stress, perception of self as unattractive with aging, secondary to erectile dysfunction in men, and marital discord	Treatment depends on cause of decreased libido; occasional sublingual or systemic androgens appropriate
Absence of partner	Assess other needs for physical and emotional nurturance, masturbation as acceptable outlet, and strategies to increase social support	Increase social contact and support, consider self-stimulation for sexual release and pleasure

Implants of several types do allow penetration but do not change the ability to reach orgasm or the perceptual experience of sexual arousal (10). Temporary vacuum-type penile condoms that create a negative pressure are the least invasive of orthotic penile aids, have very few side effects, and are most appropriate for men with venous or neurogenic impotence (11). Recently, studies of injectable papaverine/phentolamine into the corpora cavernosa have suggested that one of the benefits is a long-term return to improved physiologic functioning, perhaps by removal of the secondary psychological component that occurs when men are able to stop worrying about their ability to have erections. Testosterone may be useful in men with low or low-normal serum testosterone levels, and again, the secondary benefit in terms of removal of the psychological effect may have long-term benefits. Injectable testosterone in long-acting forms may have more risk to the cardiovascular system than short-acting sublingual forms, while having significantly less hepatotoxicity (12); the cardiovascular side effects of prescribing testosterone must be considered in men with vascular disease. Penile revascularization surgery has met with only limited success, and is not considered a good option in treatment of impotence (11).

In women who complain of painful intercourse and who have vaginal atrophy, either oral estrogen (with progestin, if uterus is still present) or topical estrogen (or both) helps the vaginal atrophy that results in discomfort and inadequate lubrication during sexual arousal. Topical vaginal estrogen is absorbed somewhat, but certainly less so than oral estrogens, so for those women with a contraindication to estrogen replacement therapy, topical estrogen is a safer choice.

For older women who have been in previous heterosexual partnerships and are without partners or the likelihood of having male partners, physicians may wish to explore with them the use of fantasy, masturbation, and inclusion of friendships and companionship to meet the emotional and physical needs for nurturance that all people have into old age.

CONCLUSION

Although there may be a combination of physical and cultural constraints to the development of sexual intimacy among older people, the transitions that accompany aging can, in fact, be used to afford new possibilities for intimacy among older adults. These possibilities include the development of new definitions of sexuality, with an emphasis on pleasuring and sensuality rather than on orgasmic potential.

Changing roles, with retirement and with children leaving the home, can provide an opportunity for increased intimacy as gender role differentiation eases. Along with these changing roles is often a longing for redefinition, for rebirth that may manifest itself in various ways (7). It may be in a desire to see the world, to become politically active, or to discover greater spiritual depth. It may also manifest itself in a turning toward relationship.

Datan and Rodeheaver (7) refer to the development of existential love, rather than generational love, as perhaps the most important maturational change that can increase intimacy. They say of existential love that "the capacity to cherish the present moment is one of the greatest gifts of maturity." This discovery of existential love, coupled with an openness to sensuality and loving touch, can help patients redefine sexual expression as they age.

REFERENCES

1. Robinson PK. The sociological perspective. In: Weg RB, ed. Sexuality in the later years: roles and behavior. New York: Academic Press, 1983.
2. Brubaker TH. An overview of family relationships in later life. In: Brubaker TH. Family relationships in later life. 2nd ed. Beverly Hills, CA: Sage Publications, 1990.
3. Rykken DE. Sex in the later years. In: Silverman P, ed. The elderly as modern pioneers. Bloomington: Indiana University Press, 1987.
4. Ade-Ridder L. Sexuality and marital quality among older married couples. In: Brubaker TH, ed. Family relationships in later life. 2nd ed. Newbury Park: Sage Publications, 1990:48–67.
5. Goldberg L. A gerontology for the 21st century. In: Butler RN, Kiikuni K, eds. Who is responsible for my old age. New York: Springer, 1993:110–117.
6. Barresi CM, Hunt K. The unmarried elderly: age, sex, and ethnicity. In: Brubaker TH, ed. Family relationships in later life. 2nd ed. Newbury Park: Sage Publications, 1990:169–192.
7. Datan N, Rodeheaver D. Beyond generativity: toward a sensuality of later life. In: Weg RB, ed. Sexuality in the later years: roles and behavior. New York: Academic Press, 1983.
8. Kaplan HS. The evaluation of sexual disorders: psychological and medical aspects. New York, Brunner/Mazel, 1983.
9. Zilbergeld B. The new male sexuality. New York: Bantam Books, 1992.
10. Benson RC. An updated approach to correcting impotence in elderly men. Geriatrics 1985;40:87–102.
11. Mulligan T, Katz PG. Urologic considerations in geriatric erectile failure. Clin Geriatr Med 1991; 7:73–84.
12. Rousseau P. Impotence in elderly men. Postgrad Med 1988;83:212–219.
13. Theienhaus OJ. Practical overview of sexual function and advancing age. Geriatrics 1988;43:63–67.
14. Mooradian AD, Greiff V. Sexuality in older women. Arch Intern Med 1990;150:1033–1038.
15. Anonymous. Drugs that cause sexual dysfunction: an update. Med Lett Drugs Ther 1992;34:73–78.
16. Kaplan HS. The new sex therapy: active treatment of sexual dysfunctions. New York: Brunner/Mazel, 1974:86–103.
17. Halvorsen JG, Metz ME. Sexual dysfunction, part 1: classification, etiology, and pathogenesis. J Am Board Fam Pract 1992;5:51–61.
18. Starr BD. Sexuality and aging. Annu Rev Gerontol Geriatr 1985;5:97–126.
19. Kaiser FE. Sexuality and impotence in the aging man. Clin Geriatr Med 1991;7:63–72.

56/ Accidents in the Elderly Population

Michael S. Vernon

Despite advances in accident prevention, which have resulted in a decline in the accidental death rate over the past 30 years, accidents remain a common cause of death and disability in the older population. Accidents are the seventh leading cause of death in the population age 65 to 84 and surpass diabetes mellitus as the sixth most common cause in those over age 85 (1). The incidence of accident-related death increases with each decade after age 65 (Fig. 56.1).

Falls, motor vehicle accidents, fires, choking, and poisoning are the major causes of accidental death in the elderly, claiming thousands of lives annually (Fig. 56.2). Most nonvehicular accidents occur in the home. Long-term care facilities and hospitals are the sites of less than 10% of such deaths.

In addition to the mortality caused by accidents, there is a notable effect on quality of life from accident-induced injury. The best example is hip fractures caused by falls. Not only does the injury directly impair functional capacity, but the fear of falling again often results in restricted activity, whether imposed by the person who fell or by family members. Sometimes the concern for injury may even result in placing the elderly person in an institution. Fear of an automobile accident also may result in restricted activity. Independence in our society is closely linked to the ability to drive an automobile. Accident-induced fear of driving could seriously affect an older person's level of independence.

Accidents such as falls may be markers for an overall deterioration in health status of an older adult. Accidental injuries that reduce mobility and functional ability may begin a cascade of consequences, eventually leading to death from other illnesses.

Research into the causes and prevention of accidents leads to insights on interventions to decrease the impact of accidents in the elderly population. Incorporating this knowledge into everyday practice to assess a patient's risk of accidental injury or death can help determine strategies to reduce this risk.

FALLS

Each year one-third of community-dwelling elderly persons over age 65 fall (3). The proportion increases to about half by age 80. About half of those fall more than once. Each year more than half the ambulatory residents of extended care facilities fall. The seriousness of falls in the older population is more than just a matter of frequency; the frail elderly are much more likely to suffer serious injury (4).

Falls are the leading cause of accidental death in the population over age 65, accounting for 8900 deaths in 1988 (2). The number of deaths annually from falls peaks around age 85. Falls are both a marker for and a cause of short-term adverse health outcomes. Only about one-half of the elderly admitted to a hospital after a fall are alive a year later. Recurrent falls are frequently cited as one reason for admission of previously independent elderly individuals to nursing homes.

Fortunately, most falls do not produce serious injury. About 5% of falls result in a fracture or hospitalization, and fewer than 1% result in a hip fracture (5). More common fractures are those of the humerus, wrist, and pelvis. Soft tissue injuries such as hemarthroses, sprains, dislocations, and bruises often require medical attention.

The impact of hip fractures on an older person's health and function is well documented. The impact of other fractures from falls has not been described. Beyond the morbidity and mortality associated with falls is another factor that adversely affects the quality of life of the older person who falls. Fear of falling may cause a restriction of activities, either self-imposed or imposed by caregivers. Half of those who fall report being afraid of falling, and one in four admit to limiting essential activities of daily living in the home (6). Families frequently cite recurrent falling as one reason for admission to nursing homes. Unfortu-

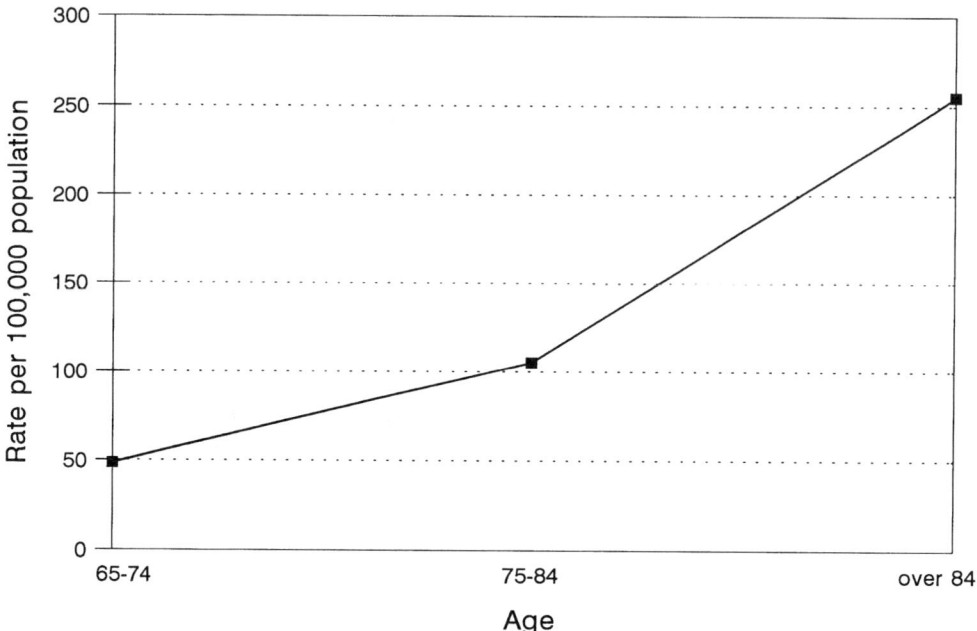

Figure 56.1.   1989 accidental death rate. (Adapted from Statistical Abstract of the United States, 1992.)

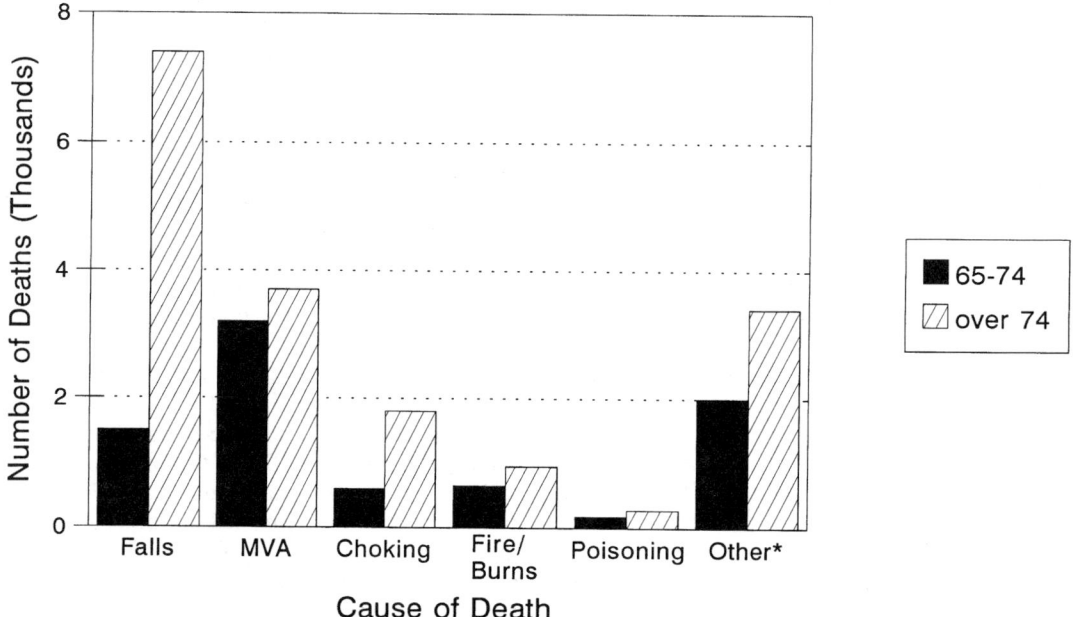

Figure 56.2.   1988 accidental deaths. *Includes medical/surgical complications, air/water transport, machinery, excessive cold. (Adapted from Accident Facts, 1989 edition. Chicago: National Safety Council.)

nately, restraints remain the primary preventive measure for frequent falls in nursing homes. Although the efficacy of restraints in preventing fall-related injury remains controversial, there is little doubt that the use of restraints has a negative impact on an older person's dignity.

CAUSES OF FALLS

Falls result from a complex interaction of intrinsic and environmental factors (3, 7, 8). About 40% of falls involve some type of interaction with an environmental hazard. About 5% result from an overwhelming hazard. A similar small percentage result from an overwhelming intrinsic event, such as a stroke or syncopal episode. Another 10% are related to acute medical illness, such as pneumonia or congestive heart failure, although some would classify these as multifactorial.

Attempts to devise uniform classifications for the causes of falls in the elderly has proven difficult. The interactions of the elderly person, activity, and environmental factors may vary with each event.

Intrinsic Risk Factors

The intrinsic risk factors that predispose the older individual to falling are comprised of multiple diseases and disabilities superimposed on the physiologic changes of aging. Maintaining an upright posture and ambulating are complex acts requiring the integration of a number of systems. Dysfunction in one system may affect the functioning of other systems, further increasing the risk of falling.

Within the nervous system, conditions affecting the central integrative function, the special senses, and peripheral sensory function can contribute to falls (9, 10). With normal aging, reaction time is slowed, primarily because of prolonged integrative function in the central nervous system. Diseases that impair this central sensory integration and response, such as Parkinson's disease, stroke, or dementia, have been associated with an increased incidence of falls (11).

Vision is also an important factor in balance and ambulation (12, 13). With normal aging there is a decrease in the amount of light transmitted to the retina. Light-dark adaptation is slowed, glare is less well tolerated, and both near and peripheral vision decline. Cataracts, glaucoma, and diabetic retinopathy can intensify these limitations. Bifocal lenses may heighten the risk of falls in circumstances such as descending stairs.

Whether presbycusis is accompanied by an age-related change in vestibular function is unclear. However, a number of conditions common in the elderly are well known to affect balance. Benign positional vertigo is common in the elderly, as is exposure to aminoglycosides, furosemide, and other ototoxic agents.

Proprioception appears to decline with age; one out of three elderly patients has a clinically detectable abnormality of position sense. There is evidence that the cervical spine serves an important role in maintaining balance. Proprioceptive abnormalities resulting from cervical spondylosis due to underlying arthritis may affect the elderly person's balance.

Conditions affecting the musculoskeletal system, especially the lower extremities, may impair stability and increase the likelihood of falling. Some elderly patients have a weakness in ankle dorsiflexion, which could explain their propensity to fall over backward with minimal displacement (13). Other common conditions affecting the muscles and joints, such as myopathies, strokes with hemiparesis, and arthritis, also may contribute to the risk of falling. Osteoarthritis of the knees often results in quadriceps weakness, and weakness of the hip musculature and quadriceps is a significant factor in falls. Foot disorders, such as hammertoes, bunions, painful calluses, and nail deformities, can pose significant problems in gait, particularly when they are compounded by inappropriate footwear.

A number of other conditions have been implicated as causative factors in falls. Several age-related physiologic changes predispose the elderly to orthostatic hypotension. The use of medications such as diuretics, antihypertensives, and antidepressants may contribute to orthostasis. Diseases resulting in abnormalities of autonomic nervous system function, such as diabetes mellitus and Parkinson's disease, can also lead to orthostasis. Even though this disorder is less common than previously thought and its role as a cause of falls is disputed, it should be considered as a contributing factor when the fall occurs while changing from a lying or sitting position to a standing position or occurs postprandially (14).

Medications play a significant role in falls among the elderly. Most frequently implicated are benzodiazepines (particularly the long-acting ones), antidepressants, and phenothiazines (15, 16). Other medications, such as diuretics, antihypertensives, and cardiac medications, may also play a role. Recent studies have failed to show an association of alcohol consumption with falls and injury (17). These studies may have been limited, however, by the use of self-report of alcohol consumption and underrepresentation of heavy drinkers in the study population (18). The role of alcohol in recurrent falls remains under study. One in ten elderly persons suffers from depression, which has been associated with an increased risk of falls independent of the effect of medication. The increased risk may be due to a lack of attention to environmental hazards, a decline in general health associated with depression, or a desire to injure oneself.

Finally, cardiorespiratory diseases, metabolic disorders, or other systemic illnesses may compromise the complex functions responsible for stability. Medications used to treat these conditions may further increase the risk of falling.

Activity

Most falls among both community and institutionalized elderly occur during routine daily activities that involve only mild to moderate displacement. Modest regular physical activity might be assumed to increase strength, endurance, coordination, and balance, thereby reducing the chance of falling. However, this higher level of activity results in an increased number of opportunities to fall and thus a higher rate of falls (3).

Environmental Factors

Most falls by community-dwelling elderly occur in the home, and about half of such falls involve an environmental hazard (3, 6, 8, 19). Approximately 10% of falls involve stairs, usually because they are poorly lighted or not equipped with handrails or because of visual impairment or bifocal lenses. Descending stairs appears to be more difficult, especially for elderly women, than ascending stairs. Most falls in the home are caused by tripping. Pets, furniture, electrical cords, and even grandchildren have been implicated. Other frequently cited household hazards include slippery floors, loose throw rugs, doorway thresholds, and slippery bathtubs. Finally, because visual-perceptual problems are common in the elderly, distracting optical patterns on stairs, escalators, and floors may also pose a threat.

EVALUATION

The purpose of evaluation is to identify risk factors that can be modified. Because the likelihood of falling increases with the number of risk factors, correcting even a few disabilities could significantly reduce the risk of falling (20). A careful history, a complete medical examination, and an assessment of gait and balance are the key elements. Because falls are a common, yet underreported, problem in the elderly, clinicians should ask about falls as part of the routine review of systems (21, 22).

Patients may be vague about the history. They may say that they "tripped over something" or "just went down." Additional history from a third party is helpful, but usually it is more available in the hospital or nursing home than in the home. Clinicians should elicit information about what the patient was doing at the time of the fall and any associated symptoms that might have preceded or followed the fall. Specific questions are useful: Did the fall occur following a change in position from sitting to standing? Did the patient experience dizziness or syncope at the time of the fall? Was there associated pain or weakness in one or both extremities? Finally, the clinician should perform a careful review of medications, with special attention to drugs associated with falls (i.e., benzodiazepines, antidepressants, and phenothiazines). A general medical history will identify chronic diseases, such as diabetes, Parkinson's disease, or arthritis, that increase the likelihood of falling.

The complete physical examination should give special emphasis to the neurologic and musculoskeletal systems. Although the relationship between postural hypotension and falls remains controversial, supine and standing blood pressure at 1 and 5 minutes should be measured.

The neurologic examination should include a formal assessment of the patient's mental status using an instrument such as the Folstein Mini-Mental State Examination, a test of visual acuity, and an evaluation of lower extremity strength and sensation, including touch, proprioception, and position sense. Increased muscle tone or cogwheeling should be noted. Cerebellar function should also be tested.

The musculoskeletal system should be examined for conditions such as arthritis of the hip or knees or foot problems, which could hinder ambulation. The remainder of the physical examination should identify systemic diseases that could compromise a function of the systems involved in gait.

Balance and gait should be assessed by using a series of maneuvers that replicate the usual tasks required in the activities of daily living. Two simple tests of balance and gait are easily administered in the office. The "get up and go" test and the performance-oriented assessment of mobility involve observing position changes and common maneuvers such as reaching up, turning, and bending over (23). Gait is observed for initiation, step height, length, continuity and symmetry, speed, path deviation, and turning. This is accomplished by having the patient get up from a chair, walk a distance at a usual rapid pace, and return to the examiner. At that time balance may be assessed by observing the patient react to an external nudge, stand with eyes closed, reach up, bend over, and turn the neck from side to side. After the patient completes these maneuvers, the examiner observes the patient sitting down in the chair without using the hands. If the patient uses an assistive device such as a cane, the assessment should be done with and without the aid. The assistive device should be evaluated for proper function and safety.

The role of laboratory and diagnostic studies has not been rigorously assessed. Generally recommended are complete blood count, electrolytes, glucose, BUN, creatinine, urinalysis, and thyroid function tests, with further testing as indicated by the history and physical examination (24). A chest x-ray and resting electrocardiogram may be reserved for those in whom a cardiopulmonary problem is suspected. Patients with syncope and palpitations or pulse irregularities warrant Holter monitoring, but it should not be a routine part of the diagnostic workup (25). Electronystagmography may be helpful in cases of true vertigo.

Typically this evaluation will reveal multiple risk factors potentially contributing to the fall. Once they have been identified, a systematic approach to modifying risk factors should begin. As they are resolved, new factors may emerge, creating the need for continual reassessment of risks for falling.

PREVENTION

Interventions aimed at reducing fall-related injury should address patient, environment, and activities. To date, carefully controlled prospective studies assessing the impact of such intervention are lacking. However, such studies are under way as a part of Frailty Injuries: Cooperative Studies of Intervention Techniques (FICSIT) (26). Eight clinical trials using different interventions address physical frailty and strategies for injury prevention. Until results of the trials are available, it is reasonable to attempt to reduce the number of contributing risk factors without creating new ones. For example, the treatment of depression, a known risk factor for falls, should be weighed against the use of tricyclic antidepressants, another known risk factor. The use of a cane or walker may be helpful at times, but such devices may also contribute to falls if used incorrectly.

A number of home hazard checklists have been developed to help older persons make their homes safer. Many hazards can be eliminated by proper lighting, hand rails and grab bars, nonslippery floor surfaces, and removal of obstacles. High-risk areas such as bathrooms and stairs deserve special attention. However, older persons often are reluctant to make even small changes in their environment. Careful education with follow-up by a home health nurse, physical therapist, or occupational therapist can help improve compliance with recommendations.

Patients should also be counseled to avoid clearly hazardous and probably unnecessary activities such as climbing on ladders, stools, or chairs, or walking on icy surfaces. On the other hand, activities that lead to improved strength, flexibility, and endurance, such as regular exercising and climbing stairs, should be encouraged. It is important for the patient to try to achieve a balance between excessive concern about falls and the need to maintain mobility and functional independence.

MOTOR VEHICLE ACCIDENTS

Elderly drivers account for a minority of injuries from motor vehicle accidents. Drivers over age 65 do, however, have a higher crash rate per miles driven than does the general population. The rate of involvement in a fatal accident per 100,000 drivers is lowest for the age group 65 to 74; for those over 75, the rate is about equal to that of the age group 25 to 34 (2). The low rate is mainly due to the fact that older drivers drive fewer miles. When the fatality rate is adjusted for miles driven, 70-year-old drivers have three times the rate of fatal accidents that 20-year-olds have. As the population ages, the increase in older drivers likely will result in an increased number of accidents. In 1988, motor vehicle accidents accounted for 6900 deaths in persons over age 65, making them the second leading cause of accidental death in older Americans.

The increase in frequency of motor vehicle accidents probably results from a combination of the normal physiologic changes that occur with aging and the chronic medical conditions that are prevalent in this population. Medications with central nervous system effects, including benzodiazepines, tricyclic antidepressants, and antihistamines, have the potential to impair driving ability and are commonly used in this population (27).

A number of physiologic and pathological changes associated with increased age result in a decline in vision as one ages. Visual acuity, visual field, and night vision all decline, and light-dark adaptation is delayed (28). Over age 65, visual acuity becomes significantly poorer under conditions of low light (29). Other more complex visual perceptual tasks important in driving are also affected by age: visual processing speed, light sensitivity, dynamic vision, near vision, and visual search (28). The decline leads to problems for older drivers in assessing vehicle velocity, reacting to unexpected vehicles, and reading signs (30, 31). Older drivers also have more difficulty dividing their attention between two tasks, which has been shown to affect lane tracking and the accuracy of visual analysis (32).

Visual perceptual changes interact closely with cognitive function. Visual attention and mental status may account for as much as 20% of the increased accident rate among older drivers (33). Among persons with dementia of the Alzheimer's type, performance on information-processing measures, specifically the switching of specific attention, divided attention, and sustained attention, are impaired in the early stages of the disease and may contribute to the increased accident risk (34). These persons have almost 5 times the number of accidents of persons without Alzheimer's dementia, and 18 times more accidents per miles driven (35). In a group of patients referred to a geriatric assessment center, 40% of the drivers were diagnosed as having Alzheimer's dementia (36). In another group of dementia patients, the mean duration of driving after onset of disease was 28.6 months (37). Patients with a clinical diagnosis of Alzheimer's dementia drove significantly longer than those with other dementia syndromes. Of the 93 patients driving at the time of the study, 21 reported motor vehicle accidents in the preceding 6 months.

In a study of the effects of age on motor function, participants were found to initiate and execute movements more slowly and with less precision as they aged (38). Specific medical conditions such as hip disease also affect driving ability. Multiple conditions that impair activities of daily living also may adversely affect driving ability.

Despite these changes, road test skills appear to be well preserved in the healthy elderly population (39). However, the relationship between road test performance and accident rates has not been established. Further studies are needed to assess road test performance by elderly persons with single or multiple medical impairments and to determine correlations between road test performance and motor vehicle accidents (40).

PEDESTRIAN ACCIDENTS

Of the 6900 deaths from motor vehicle accidents in 1988, about 2000 involved pedestrians. Almost twice as many pedestrian deaths occurred in those over 75 as did in the age group 65 to 74.

Despite the observation that older pedestrians are the safest age group at intersections, standing the farthest away from traffic, appreciating the greater risk of injury at night, and exercising appropriate safety precautions, most vehicular pedestrian deaths occur at intersections (41). Decreased walking speed, combined with the older person's difficulty in judging vehicle velocity, may play a role. Only 5% of the elderly over age 70 can walk quickly enough to successfully cross many intersections controlled by traffic lights. Decreased peripheral vision and hearing, along with an increased reaction time, may also contribute. An investigation of traffic-related injuries to the elderly found that about half the injuries resulted from falls with no vehicular involvement (42). Many of the falls involved ice and snow, but high curbs also presented a problem. These nonvehicular hazards may distract the individual from attending to traffic. Rates of injury are also higher in areas that have substantial business and commercial traffic.

DRIVER-RELATED ACCIDENTS

Elderly occupants of motor vehicles in accidents accounted for almost 5000 deaths in 1988. Over 90% occurred during the daytime and more than 90% involved two or more vehicles. Over 60% occurred at intersections, where timed perceptual decisions are crucial. When the elderly are involved in a vehicular accident they are at increased risk of injury and death, despite the fact that they tend to drive larger cars and thus presumably have greater protection in an accident. This suggests that older individuals are more susceptible to injury in an accident.

FIRES AND BURNS

When death from complications of medical and surgical procedures is excluded, death from fire is the fourth leading cause of accidental death in people over age 65. Sixteen hundred deaths from fire and burns occurred among the elderly in 1988. Most deaths were among those over age 75 (Fig. 56.2). About 90% of these occurred in the home. Flame burns account for most burns in the elderly, with scalds representing about 20% of burn injuries (43). Burn rates for men tend to decrease with age, but they remain relatively constant for women. However, the mortality rate is still higher with advancing age, despite recent improvements in survival from burns. The elderly account for 12% of the overall population, but almost 30% of fire deaths (44). Older blacks have five times the residential fire death rate of whites, and men have a higher rate than women. Because of decreases partly resulting from recent regulations requiring fire-resistant clothing for infants and young children, 80% of deaths from burning clothing are in the elderly. In fact, 27% of the female patients admitted to one burn center had been burned by clothing ignited during cooking (45).

Baux's formula, which equates burn mortality with the additive factors of burn surface area and patient age, was reaffirmed as recently as 1984, despite recent improvements in the survival of elderly burn patients (46). However, early aggressive surgical treatment in one burn center improved survival from 37 to 52% over 10 years (47). The hospital length of stay of surviving patients was reduced by almost half. Another center reported an 80% overall survival rate for elderly burn patients and a 67% rate for patients over age 75 (48). In this group, mortality rate correlated with patient age, burn size, presence of inhalation injury, number of complications of care, and fluid resuscitation requirements, but not with the number of preexisting medical problems. Aggressive surgical intervention was also used in this group, although others have questioned this approach.

On the basis of mortality data alone, aggressive care for elderly patients with burn injuries appears justified. But what about the quality of life following discharge? Studies of older burn victims have shown that most survivors return home, although about half require some assistance (49). About one-fourth of those over age 75 require admission to a nursing home following discharge from a burn center, but only about 5% overall require institutionalization (50, 51). There is no difference in death rates between survivors and the normal population (52).

Prevention of fire and burn injuries requires an appreciation of the factors that may predispose the elderly to injury and death. In residential fires, the elderly are prone to mental and physical conditions that impair ability to escape. Problems with vision, hearing, cognition, and mobility all may contribute. Burns from clothing fires may occur more frequently because of a decline in overall physical condition, decreased sense of smell, ar-

thritic hands, a weak grasp, and decreased reaction time. Many elderly have difficulty dropping to the floor and rolling, which is the recommended maneuver for extinguishing burning clothes. Although the elderly realize the potential for tap-water scald burns in their homes, few believe that exposure to hot-only tap water at temperatures common in many homes could cause a scald burn in 30 seconds or less. Furthermore, in one study, previous victims of tap-water scald burns had not lowered the settings of their hot water thermostats (53).

Cigarette smoking and excessive alcohol consumption play a well-recognized role in residential fires. Fifteen percent of those over 65 smoke, and 12% consume more than five alcoholic drinks per day (1). Continued efforts to increase smoking cessation and promote responsible alcohol use will, in addition to promoting overall health, result in a decrease in burn injuries. The use of fire-resistant upholstery and bed linens is increasing. Making fire-resistant clothing available to older persons as well as to infants would also be helpful. The development of a self-extinguishing cigarette is technically feasible but unlikely, given the current financial state of the tobacco industry.

By 1985, 74% of U.S. homes had smoke detectors, but the homes of older people and the poor were less likely to have them. Households without smoke detectors have a 50% higher risk of fire-related fatality than homes with smoke detectors. The early warning provided by a smoke detector may be especially important to an older individual with impaired mobility.

Other preventive measures include lowering the hot water temperature to less than 120°F, preferably to about 110°F; using cook stoves with front- or side-mounted controls; using microwave ovens instead of stoves; keeping fire extinguishers conveniently located and charged; ensuring that elderly persons are familiar with the use of fire extinguishers, have an escape plan in the event of fire, and practice fire drills regularly.

POISONING

Poisoning is a significant problem in the elderly population, accounting for over 500 deaths per year, or 13% of all poisoning deaths in the United States. Most result from medications, and most are unintentional (54). Confusion, dementia, mistaken identity of medications, and placing medicines in a container with an incorrect label all may contribute to this problem. The elderly are more vulnerable to toxicity and death from drugs because of changes in pharmacokinetics related to changes in body composition and renal and hepatic functioning. Underlying diseases, especially cardiovascular disease, also increase the risk of death from medication overdose. The elderly tend to be on multiple medications, both prescription and over-the-counter drugs. Errors in taking medicines increase when three or more are prescribed.

Cardiovascular drugs account for about 40% of the deaths from medications, three times the frequency of the next category, analgesics, antipyretics, and antirheumatics (1). Other implicated agents are oral hypoglycemics, psychotherapeutics, and theophylline. In addition to death, adverse consequences of medication use include falls, accidents, confusion, and hospital admissions.

Physicians should spend adequate time counseling their older patients about use of medicines. Patients should be cautioned not to place medicine in a container other than the one in which it was dispensed, with the exception of organized daily dispenser systems. Medicines should be stored separately from household cleaners and chemicals. The physician should assess the literacy status of the older patient and take extra time to explain instructions to those who have difficulty reading. Large-type labels should be used on prescription bottles. In addition to carefully explaining drug effects, side effects, and precautions, the physician should frequently question the patient about adverse effects. Monitoring drug levels is important, especially digitalis levels and prothrombin times for patients on warfarin. Patients should be encouraged to bring their medicines to each office visit for review, and attempts should be made to discontinue medications whenever possible.

CHOKING

Accidental ingestion or inhalation of objects or food resulting in suffocation from obstructed respiratory passages is a common, but little studied, problem in the elderly. Twenty-four hundred elderly patients choked to death in 1988. About 200 fatal choking incidents occur each year in nursing homes and extended care facilities (55).

A number of factors may contribute to death by choking in the older population. Cognitive impairment, swallowing disorders from cerebrovascular accidents or Parkinson's disease, and ill-fitting or absent dentures all may play a role (56). The use of psychotropic medications or alcohol may increase the risk of aspiration. In long-term care facilities, inadequate supervision during mealtime may result in aspiration of food. It is important that staff in such facilities be trained in appropriate first aid such as the Heimlich maneuver. Further study of this significant cause of mortality in the elderly is needed.

REFERENCES

1. Statistical abstract of the United States, 1992. 110th ed. Washington, DC: U.S. Department of Commerce, 1992.
2. Accident facts, 1989 edition. Chicago: National Safety Council.
3. Tinetti ME, Speechley M, Ginter SF. Risk factors for falls among elderly persons living in the community. N Engl J Med 1988;319(26):1701–1707.
4. Sattin RW, Huber DAL, DeVito CA, et al. The incidence of fall injury events among the elderly in a defined population. Am J Epidemiol 1990;131:1028–1037.
5. Nevitt MC, Cummings SR, Hudes ES. Risk factors for injurious falls: a prospective study. J Gerontol Med Sci 1991;46(5):M164–170.
6. Nevitt MC, Cummings SR, Kidd S, Black D. Risk factors for recurrent nonsyncopal falls: a prospective study. JAMA 1989;261(18):2663–2668.
7. Lipsitz LA, Jonsson PV, Kelly MM, Koestner JS. Causes and correlates of recurrent falls in ambulatory frail elderly. J Gerontol Med Sci 1991;46(4):M114–122.
8. Robbins AS, Rubenstein LZ, Josephson KR, Schulman BL, Osterweil D, Fine G. Predictors of falls among elderly people: results of two population-based studies. Arch Intern Med 1989;149:1628–1633.
9. Masdeu JC, Wolfson L, Lantos G, et al. Brain white-matter changes in the elderly prone to falling. Arch Neurol 1989;46:1292–1296.
10. Richardson JK, Ching C, Hurvitz ED. The relationship between electromyographically documented peripheral neuropathy and falls. J Am Geriatr Soc 1992;40:1008–1012.
11. Koller WC, Glatt S, Vetere-Overfield B, Hassanein R. Falls and Parkinson's disease. Clin Neuropharmacol 1989;12(2):98–105.
12. Felson DT, Anderson JJ, Hannan MT, Milton RC, Wilson PWF, Kiel DP. Impaired vision and hip fracture: the Framingham Study. J Am Geriatr Soc 1989;37:495–500.
13. Lord SR, Clark RD, Webster IW. Physiological factors associated with falls in an elderly population. J Am Geriatr Soc 1991;39:1194–1200.
14. Jonsson PV, Lipsitz LA, Kelley M, Koestner J. Hypotensive responses to common daily activities in institutionalized elderly: a potential risk for recurrent falls. Arch Intern Med 1990;150:1518–1524.
15. Kerman M, Mulvihill M. The role of medication in falls among the elderly in a long-term care facility. Mt Sinai J Med 1990;57(6):343–347.
16. Sorock GS, Shimkin EE. Benzodiazepine sedatives and the risk of falling in a community-dwelling elderly cohort. Arch Intern Med 1988;148:2441–2444.
17. Nelson DE, Sattin RW, Langlois JA, DeVito CA, Stevens JA. Alcohol as a risk factor for fall injury events among elderly persons living in the community. J Am Geriatr Soc 1992;40:658–661.
18. Carson JE. Alcohol use and falls. [editorial]. J Am Geriatr Soc 1993;41(3):346.

19. DeVito CA, Lambert DA, Sattin RW, Bacchelli S, Ros A, Rodriguez JG. Fall injuries among the elderly. J Am Geriatr Soc 1988;36:1029–1035.
20. Rubenstein LZ, Robbins AS, Josephson KR, Schulman BL, Osterweil D. The value of assessing falls in an elderly population: a randomized clinical trial. Ann Intern Med 1990;113(4):308–316.
21. Campbell AJ, Borrie MJ, Spears GF, Jackson SL, Brown JS, Fitzgerald JL. Circumstances and consequences of falls experienced by a community population 70 years and over during a prospective study. Age Ageing 1990;19:136–141.
22. Cummings SR, Nevitt MC, Kidd S. Forgetting falls: the limited accuracy of recall of falls in the elderly. J Am Geriatr Soc 1988;36:613–616.
23. Tinetti ME, Williams TF, Mayewski R. Fall risk index of elderly patients based on number of chronic disabilities. Am J Med 1986;80:429–434.
24. Rubenstein LZ, Robbins AS, Schulman BL, Rosado J, Osterweil D, Josephson KR. Falls and instability in the elderly. J Am Geriatr Soc 1988;36:266–278.
25. Rosado JA, Rubenstein LZ, Robbins AS, Heng MK, Schulman BL, Josephson KR. The value of Holter monitoring in evaluating the elderly patient who falls. J Am Geriatr Soc 1989;37:430–434.
26. Ory MB, Schechtman KB, Miller JP, et al. Frailty and injuries in later life: the Ficsit Trials. J Am Geriatr Soc 1993;41:283–296.
27. Ray WA, Gurwitz J, Decker MD, Kennedy DL. Medications and the safety of the older driver: is there a basis for concern? Hum Factors 1992;34(1):33–47.
28. Klein R. Age-related eye disease, visual impairment and driving in the elderly. Hum Factors 1991;33(5):521–525.
29. Sturr JF, Kline GE, Taub HA. Performance of young and older drivers on a Static Acuity Test under photopic and mesopic luminance conditions. Hum Factors 1990;32(1):1–8.
30. Kline DW, Kline TJ, Fozard JL, Kosnik W, Schieber F, Sekuler R. Vision, aging, and driving: the problems of older drivers. J Gerontol 1992;47(1):P27–34.
31. Scialfa CT, Guzy LT, Leibowitz HW, Garvey PM, Tyrrell RA. Age differences in estimating vehicle velocity. Psychol Aging 1991;6(1):60–66.
32. Brouwer WH, Waterink W, Van Wolffelaar PC, Rothengatter T. Divided attention in experienced young and older drivers: lane tracking and visual analysis in a dynamic driving simulator. Hum Factors 1991;33(5):573–582.
33. Owsley C, Ball K, Sloane ME, Roenker DL, Bruni JR. Visual/cognitive correlates of vehicle accidents in older drivers. Psychol Aging 1991;6(3):403–415.
34. Parasuraman R, Nestor PG. Attention and driving skills in aging and Alzheimer's disease. Hum Factors 1991;33(5):539–557.
35. Dubinsky RM, Williamson A, Gray CS, Glatt SL. Driving in Alzheimer's disease. J Am Geriatr Soc 1992;40:1112–1116.
36. Carr D, Jackson T, Alquire P. Characteristics of an elderly driving population referred to a geriatric assessment center. J Am Geriatr Soc 1990;38(10):1145–1150.
37. Gilley DW, Wilson RS, Bennett DA, et al. Cessation of driving and unsafe motor vehicle operation by dementia patients. Arch Intern Med 1991;151(5):941–946.
38. Stelmach GE, Nahom A. Cognitive-motor abilities of the elderly driver. Hum Factors 1992;34(1):53–65.
39. Carr D, Jackson TW, Madden DJ, Cohen HJ. The effect of age on driving skills. J Am Geriatr Soc 1992;40(6):567–573.
40. Carr D, Schmader K, Bergman C, et al. A multidisciplinary approach in the evaluation of demented drivers referred to geriatric assessment centers. J Am Geriatr Soc 1991;39:1132–1136.
41. Harrell WA. Perception of risk and curb standing at street corners by older pedestrian. Percept Mot Skills 1990;70(3 Pt 2):1363–1366.
42. Sjogren H, Bjornstig U. Injuries to the elderly in the traffic environment. Accid Anal Prev 1991;23(1):77–86.
43. Ostrow LB, Bongard FS, Sacks ST, McGuire A, Trunkey DD. Burns in the elderly. Am Fam Physician 1987;35(1):149–154.
44. Gulaid JA, Sacks JJ, Sattin RW. Deaths from residential fires among older people, United States, 1984. J Am Geriatr Soc 1989;37:331–334.
45. Turner DG, Leman CJ, Jordan MH. Cooking-related burn injuries in the elderly: preventing the "granny gown" burn. J Burn Care Rehabil 1989;10(4):356–359.
46. Jerrard DA, Cappadoro K. Burns in the elderly patient. Emerg Med Clin North Am 1990;8(2):421–428.
47. Slater AL, Slater H, Goldfarb IW. Effect of aggressive surgical treatment in older patients with burns. J Burn Care Rehabil 1989;10(6):527–530.
48. Saffle JR, Larson CM, Sullivan J, Shelby J. The continuing challenge of burn care in the elderly. Surgery 1990;108(3):534–543.
49. Larson CM, Saffle JR, Sullivan J. Lifestyle adjustments in elderly patients after burn injury. J Burn Care Rehabil 1992;13(1):48–52.
50. Hammond J, Ward CG. Burns in octogenarians. South Med J 1991;84(11):1316–1319.
51. Keys TC, Moresi JM, Deitch EA. Thermal injury in the elderly. The limited need for nursing home care. J Burn Care Rehabil 1989;10(5):494–531.
52. Manktelow A, Meyer AA, Herzog SR, Peterson HD. Analysis of life expectancy and living status of elderly patients surviving a burn injury. J Trauma 1989;29(2):203–207.
53. Adams LE, Purdue GF, Hunt JL. Tap-water scald burns. Awareness is not the problem. J Burn Care Rehabil 1991;12(1):91–95.
54. Klein-Schwartz W, Oderda GM. Poisoning in the elderly. Epidemiological, clinical and management considerations. Drugs Aging 1991;1(1):67–89.
55. Saunders LD, Green M, Doebbert G, Pearson MA, Kizer KW. Mortality from unintentional injuries in California, 1985. West J Med 1989 Apr;150:478–483.
56. Ekberg O, Feinberg M. Clinical and demographic data in 75 patients with near-fatal choking episodes. Dysphagia 1992;7(4):205–208.

57/ Iatrogenic Disease in the Elderly

Patricia P. Barry

Iatrogenic illness is an important cause of morbidity and mortality in the elderly; in many studies comparing young and old, older patients are at increased risk, although age alone is not always a risk factor. Most studies have been surveys of either hospital admissions or inpatient occurrences, and little information is available about outpatient iatrogenic events that do not result in hospitalization.

In-hospital care of the elderly has been found to be a common setting for iatrogenic disorders. As early as 1965, Reichel (1) reviewed complications of the care of 500 elderly hospitalized patients over a 7-month period, finding that 146 of them suffered 193 adverse reactions and 44 intercurrent infections. In 502 general medical patients reviewed by Gillick et al. (2), the incidence of complications, unrelated to disease but simply due to hospitalization, was 15%; 52% of the complications were due to an intervention. Steel et al. (3) documented 497 iatrogenic events in 36% of 815 admissions to a general medical service at a teaching hospital. Risk factors associated with complications included increased age, poor condition, increased numbers of drugs, admission from an institution, and increased length of stay.

A 1982 study (4) compared 174 patients over age 65 with 48 patients under age 65 on both medical and surgical wards of a VA Hospital. The complication rate for the elderly was 45%, compared with 29% for patients under 65. Although more complications were found among medical patients than surgical patients, the medical patients were more seriously ill. Patients with more illness tended to have more complications, but even among less seriously ill patients, the complication rate was high. The most common cause of complications was drugs; compared with younger patients, older patients had more infection, trauma, drug reactions, and psychological problems. The rate of procedure-related complications was the same in both old and young; psychiatric decompensation occurred in nearly 20% of medical patients over the age of 65. A more recent study (5) reviewed the causes of iatrogenesis in a group of 120 medical service patients older than 65 with long lengths of stay, admitted for acute myocardial infarction, congestive heart failure, and pneumonia. Some 216 complications occurred in 70 patients, most commonly due to therapeutic interventions. Risk factors for iatrogenesis were low functional and cognitive status, probably markers for poor reserves.

Hospital admissions due to iatrogenic complications of outpatient care are not uncommon. A 1974 prospective study (6) found a 2.9% incidence of admission to a medical service as a result of drug-induced illness. A 1980 Scottish study (7) of 1998 admissions to 42 geriatric medicine departments found that 209 patients had experienced adverse reactions to prescribed drugs, which contributed to their hospital admission. More recently, a 1986 study (8) of all admissions to the medical service of a teaching hospital revealed that 45 out of 834 admissions resulted from iatrogenic causes. Medications were responsible for 35 admissions; 9 admissions were procedure-related. Age alone did not appear to be a risk factor in this study.

Nevertheless, the elderly are at increased risk of iatrogenic disease. In the Harvard Medical Practice Study (9), physicians reviewed over 30,000 medical charts from 1984 in New York State and found that adverse events occurred in 3.7% of the hospitalizations, 27.6% of which were due to negligence. Rates of adverse events rose significantly with age, and although patients over the age of 64 comprised 27% of the admissions, they suffered 43% of all the adverse events. Older patients were also at greater risk for adverse effects caused by negligence. A further analysis of these data (10) revealed that the most common types of adverse event in the elderly were complications of drug treatment, followed by nonoperative therapeutic mishaps, late surgical complications, and wound infections. In addition, fractures

556

and falls occurred at a much higher rate in the elderly. These findings are consistent with more complicated illness and greater fragility of the elderly patients. Increased prevalence of disease necessitates more diagnostic and therapeutic interventions, including more medications. Atypical presentations of disease may require more extensive diagnostic evaluations to elucidate the underlying cause.

Iatrogenic complications of medical care may be conveniently remembered as the four "T's": tests, treatment, trauma, and "troubles" (11).

TESTS

Procedure-related complications are common in all studies; cardiac catheterization has been found to have a 15% complication rate (12); and in one study (3), it was the second most common cause of iatrogenic disorders, surpassed only by drugs. Complication rates for other procedures include 19% for thoracentesis and 25% for bronchoscopy (12). Angiography has been noted to have a 12% complication rate, most often acute renal failure (13).

In addition to those procedures already noted, preparation for barium enemas, colonoscopy, or intravenous pyelograms may cause dehydration; intravenous pyelograms may also result in allergic reactions to dye or even acute renal failure. Indeed almost any invasive diagnostic procedure can result in complications in an elderly person. Methodical consideration of the following questions may avoid unnecessary tests and thereby help reduce the risk of iatrogenesis:

1. Is the test needed to make or rule out a diagnosis?
2. If so, is it the least invasive test available?
3. Will the result change the treatment of the patient?
4. If so, do I know how to interpret the result?

Appropriate interpretation of test results requires a knowledge of the characteristics of both the test and the disease. Although sensitivity and specificity are terms often used to describe the accuracy of tests, these two parameters are calculated by using the test in a population in which the disease status is *known,* with sensitivity indicating the percentage of patients with the disease who have a positive test and specificity indicating the percentage of patients without the disease who have a negative test. In an individual patient, however, the disease status is *unknown.* The ability of the test to diagnose disease in this case depends also upon the pretest probability of the disease in the patient, or the prevalence of the disease in a similar population of patients. The positive predictive value is the percentage of patients with a positive test who have the disease; the negative predictive value is the percentage of patients with a negative test who do not have the disease (14).

The predictive value (and usefulness) of a test changes markedly when the pretest probability of disease is altered, a critical consideration when one is deciding whether or not to order a specific test on an individual patient whose disease status is unknown. Positive tests are most useful when probability is high; when it is very low, most positive tests will be false positives. Negative tests are most useful when probability is low; when it is very high, most negative tests will be false negatives. Understanding the usefulness and predictive value of specific tests is essential to avoid costly unnecessary tests and the associated risk of iatrogenesis. The use of sequential tests, with the choice of each test dependent upon the results of a previous one, can improve the predictive values and is preferable to a broad "shotgun" approach.

TREATMENT

Adverse drug reactions (ADRs) are the chief cause of iatrogenic disorders reported for elderly patients in most studies. The risk of ADRs appears to be associated with the number of medications taken (polypharmacy) and other patient-specific physiologic and functional characteristics, such as number and severity of illnesses, rather than with age alone (15). The elderly consume over 25% of all medications, but they have been excluded from many clinical drug trials (16); thus insufficient prescribing information is available regarding the effects of many drugs, especially in the frail elderly person with multiple chronic conditions.

In addition, most studies have surveyed hospital admissions or inpatient populations, and few data are available on ADRs in outpatients in community settings. Elderly outpatients have been reported as less likely to comply with drug regimens; again, this is more likely to reflect numbers of medications and complexity of schedules than patient age (17).

Finally, although frail elderly persons residing in institutions have the highest use of medications, prevention of ADRs in this population has not been adequately studied (18). Physicians should know about the need for lower doses of some medications in the elderly, the potential for changes in pharmacodynamics and pharmacokinetics in older persons and the subsequent effect on prescribing, and the need to avoid drugs with known toxic effects, and reduce numbers of medications whenever possible.

Treatment problems also include invasive therapy of other types, including surgery. In Steel's study (3), intravenous treatment caused 34 of 497 complications, including thrombosis, extravasation, infection, and enforced immobility. Indwelling bladder catheters resulted in trauma and infection in 10 patients. Nasogastric tubes can be associated with aspiration, trauma, and the need for restraints and immobility.

In particular, nosocomial infections, which develop in institutional settings, are a serious complication of treatment in the elderly. Older patients may have longer hospital stays, because of increased prevalence and severity of illness, and thus are at increased risk of acquiring infection as well as having an increased rate of infection per hospital day. In the nursing home, the most common nosocomial infections are urinary tract infections, pneumonia, and soft tissue infection (19). Urinary tract infections are most common, with bladder catheterization as the major risk factor in both hospitals and nursing homes. At present, no reliable methods are known to prevent infection in catheterized patients; thus catheterization should be avoided if at all possible. Infection with *Clostridium difficile* results from broad-spectrum antibiotic treatment and transmission by hospital and nursing home personnel from infected patients (19).

Determination of the effects of age on the risk of adverse outcomes of surgery is complicated by difficulty in evaluation of the surgical literature (20). Published studies often combine age groups over 65, fail to identify risk factors other than age, do not have a comparison group, and are confounded by cohort effects. Comparison of different studies reveals inconsistent definitions of comorbid conditions and disease criteria, categories of age groups, and types of procedures, and failure to account for important changes in surgical technique. Better studies are needed, using appropriate methods; meanwhile, age is most likely to be a "marker" for serious underlying disease, which should be explicitly identified and evaluated as a risk factor for morbidity and mortality. Important risk factors include cardiac and pulmonary disease, malnutrition, dementia, emergency surgery, and lack of experience of the surgical team. Evidence at present is unconvincing that age alone should be used to make decisions regarding the appropriateness of surgical procedures.

Consideration of the following questions may encourage the use of appropriate treatment and decrease the risk of iatrogenic illness:

1. Is the treatment absolutely necessary and likely to benefit the patient?
2. If so, is it the safest available?
3. Is it acceptable to the patient?
4. Once instituted, is it being administered appropriately?
5. Is it effective?
6. Do the benefits appear to outweigh the risks?

TRAUMA

Trauma is chiefly due to accidents and falls. Catchen (21) reviewed 1 year at Bellevue Hospital Center, during which there were 954 accidents (33 accidents per 10,000 patient days), 392 of which occurred in patients over the age of 65. Twenty-three percent of the patients incurred 44% of the accidents, thus there were many "repeaters." Most common were falls from bed, comprising 36% of these accidents, chiefly occurring in the evening or at night, often as the patient was attempting to get in or out of bed or was sleeping with the bed rails *up*. Twenty-eight percent of the falls were from wheelchairs, often caused by failure to lock the wheels of the chair during a transfer. Twenty-nine percent of all accidents in these patients occurred during their first week of hospitalization. However, the long-stay patients had cumulative effects, so that as their length of stay increased their risk of accidents increased. The patients with organic brain syndromes or stroke were most likely to have repeat falls; patients at risk also included those who were unattended, sedated, or restrained and those who were in bed with side rails *up*. These findings confirm results of earlier studies, and the author notes the need for safer beds and wheelchairs and training for patients in their use. Catchen also points out the particular danger of falls in the first week of hospitalization and the need for special care of elderly patients with reduced muscular and/or mental function.

Osterweil's recent review of environmental hazards in the institutional setting (22) also notes the high risk of falls for newly admitted patients and the more severe falls occurring when patients climb over rails or footboards. These risks have been reduced by careful orientation and specific fall-reduction programs as well as by the use of fall sensor devices. The use of adjustable beds that can be lowered to 19 inches or less from the floor may also reduce the risk of falls during transfers.

FUNCTIONAL DECLINE ("TROUBLES")

Physicians frequently do not consider activities of daily living as a factor in patient care or discharge planning and do not realize how hospitalization influences the patient's ability to function. This category of iatrogenesis, although not always included in studies, is common and important. Many elderly persons suffer complications not directly related to the illness or treatment, but caused by hospitalization and bed rest (23), including immobility, malnourishment, confusion, constipation, incontinence, and urinary retention.

Elderly patients are at particular risk for immobility and its well-known complications: atelectasis, pneumonia, pressure sores, thrombosis, weakness, decreased confidence, and prolonged hospitalization. Consequences of immobility include decreased range of motion and flexibility of joints, especially of the hip, knee, and ankle; loss of muscle strength and endurance, especially of the antigravity muscles; and loss of bone mass and strength (24). In addition, immobilization leads to detrimental effects on the cardiovascular system, including increased venous return and orthostatic hypotension; compromised respiratory function, including impaired clearance; and negative nitrogen balance (24). Adequate mobilization must begin as soon as possible and may require encouragement by the staff. Early ambulation, with assistance if necessary, should be emphasized; physical therapy may be essential. Adequate pain medication, appropriate assistive devices (canes, walkers, trapezes, handrails), a safe environment, lack of restraints, and minimal sedation are equally important in encouraging older patients to be active.

Elderly people may have diminished nutritional reserves because of illness such as cancer or other chronic disease. Diagnostic procedures that require fasting may worsen their nutritional status; anorexia, dietary restrictions, pain and anxiety may limit intake as well. Nutritional assessment and supplementation may be necessary. Strict low-sodium, low-fat, or diabetic diets may be unwarranted as well as unpalatable to elderly patients. Provision of a liberalized diet, appropriate for dentition, including food from home if possible, mobilization, and assistance with eating may be required. Medications should be reviewed, with particular attention to those causing anorexia and gastric distress, such as digoxin, aminophylline, or nonsteroidal analgesics.

Urinary and bowel function may be affected by treatment. Elderly surgical patients may develop acute urinary retention postoperatively, exacerbated by anticholinergic medication. Insertion of an indwelling catheter is often a routine procedure, but it may result in urinary incontinence or retention following removal. The use of intermittent, instead of indwelling, catheterization in patients with temporary urinary retention should be encouraged.

In many hospitalized elderly, in an unfamiliar environment and with restraints and barriers present, functional urinary incontinence may occur (23). Decreased intestinal motility, lack of fiber, medication effects, and decreased mobility may lead to constipation and fecal impaction (24), which may not be recognized until just before discharge. Decreased sedation, increased mobility, critical review of medications (particularly narcotics and anticholinergic drugs), elimination of catheters, and adequate fluids and bulk in the diet should be routine management for elderly patients during convalescence.

Development of an acute confusional state is common in hospitalized elderly. Risk factors include sight and hearing loss, medications, and the unfamiliar hospital environment. Sometimes, "unmasking" of a mild dementia may be a contributing factor. Physicians must encourage frequent orientation, attention to oxygenation and cerebral perfusion, review of drug therapy, and only minimal restraints. Adequate sensory stimulation, increased socialization with family, and attention by staff may help to minimize problems with cognition. Patients should always be provided with their glasses and hearing aids.

Prevention of iatrogenic disorders remains principally the responsibility of the physician. Understanding the specific risks and the general categories in which problems are most likely to occur will enable the physician to consider carefully the diagnostic and treatment alternatives and "above all, do no harm" to patients of all ages.

REFERENCES

1. Reichel W. Complications in the care of five hundred elderly hospitalized patients. J Am Geriatr Soc 1965;13:973–981.
2. Gillick MR, Serrell NA, Gillick LS. Adverse consequences of hospitalization in the elderly. Soc Sci Med 1982;16:1033–1038.
3. Steel K, Gertman PM, Crescenzi C, Anderson J. Iatrogenic illness on a general medical service at a university hospital. N Engl J Med 1981;304:638–642.
4. Jahnigen D, Hannon C, Laxson L, LaForce FM. Iatrogenic disease in hospitalized elderly veterans. J Am Geriatr Soc 1982;30:387.
5. LeFevre F, Feinglass J, Potts S, et al. Iatrogenic complications in high-risk, elderly patients. Arch Intern Med 1992;152:2074–2080.

6. Caranasos GJ, Stewart RB, Cluff LE. Drug-induced illness leading to hospitalization. JAMA 1974; 228:713–717.

7. Williamson J, Chopin JM. Adverse reactions to prescribed drugs in the elderly: a multicentre investigation. Age Aging 1980;9:73–80.

8. Lakshmanan MC, Hershey CO, Breslau D. Hospital admissions caused by iatrogenic disease. Arch Intern Med 1986;146:1931–1934.

9. Brennan TA, Leape LL, Laird NM, et al. Incidence of adverse events and negligence in hospitalized patients: results of the Harvard Medical Practice Study I. N Engl J Med 1991;324:370–376.

10. Leape LL, Brennan TA, Laird NM, et al. The nature of adverse events in hospitalized patients: results of the Harvard Medical Practice Study II. N Engl J Med 1991;324:377–384.

11. Barry PP. Iatrogenic disorders in the elderly: preventive techniques. Geriatrics 1986;41(9):42–47.

12. Schroeder SA, Marton KI, Strom BL. Frequency and morbidity of invasive procedures. Report of a pilot study from two teaching hospitals. Arch Intern Med 1978;138:1809–1811.

13. Swartz RD, Rubin JE, Leeming BW, Silva P. Renal failure following major angiography. Am J Med 1978;65:31–37.

14. Riegelman RK, Hirsch RP. Studying a study and testing a test. 2nd ed. Boston: Little, Brown, & Co, 1989:151–163.

15. Gurwitz JH, Avorn J. The ambiguous relation between aging and adverse drug reactions. Ann Intern Med 1991;114:956–966.

16. Gurwitz JH, Col NF, Avorn J. The exclusion of the elderly and women from clinical trials in acute myocardial infarction. JAMA 1992;268:1092–1096.

17. Darnell JC, Murray MD, Martz BL, Weinberger M. Medication use by ambulatory elderly. An in-home survey. J Am Geriatr Soc 1986;34:1–4.

18. Beers MH, Ouslander JG, Rollingher I, et al. Explicit criteria for determining inappropriate medication use in nursing home residents. Arch Intern Med 1991;151;1825–1832.

19. Norman D. Nosocomial infections. In: Gorbein MJ, Bishop J, Beers MH, et al., Grand rounds: iatrogenic illness in hospitalized elderly people. J Am Geriatr Soc 1992;40:1031–1042.

20. Gorbein MJ. Surgical complications in elderly patients. In: Gorbein MJ, Bishop J, Beers MH, et al., Grand rounds: iatrogenic illness in hospitalized elderly people. J Am Geriatr Soc 1992;40:1031–1042.

21. Catchen H. Repeaters: inpatient accidents among the hospitalized elderly. Gerontologist 1983;23:273–276.

22. Osterweil D. Environmental hazards in the institutional setting. In: Gorbein MJ, Bishop J, Beers MH, et al. Grand rounds: iatrogenic illness in hospitalized elderly people. J Am Geriatr Soc 1992;40:1031–1042.

23. Creditor MC. Hazards of hospitalization of the elderly. Ann Intern Med 1993;118:219–223.

24. Mobily PR, Kelley LS. Iatrogenesis in the elderly: factors of immobility. J Gerontol Nurs 1991;17:5–10.

58/ Management of the Dying Patient

Ian Maddocks

"Dying is coming home." This is an appropriate phrase with which to introduce a discussion about hospice care in the U.S.A. (1). Hospice programs offer to those dying of cancer not only a hope of freedom from pain and undignified discomfort but also an opportunity to remain in familiar surroundings for the final stage of the life journey. Home care appeals to client families because the usual alternatives, acute hospital care or a nursing home, are increasingly recognized as either inappropriately expensive, intrusive, and isolating or insufficiently resourced to meet the special needs of dying patients and their families. For the elderly who are dying, however, the option of home care may be less often available. The relevance of the hospice model, warmly applauded for what it has achieved for cancer sufferers, is less certain in its wider application to the increasing numbers of dying elderly persons.

HOSPICE CARE

EVOLUTION

During the 1960s, acute hospital technology directed at diagnosis, intervention, and cure often led to neglect of the dying. In their concentration on disease, exponents of that technology often tended to ignore important dimensions of patient comfort. Focusing on the individual patient, they neglected the wider human context of family and friends; immersed in the excitements of acute medicine and seduced by the power and effectiveness of their new investigative tools and restorative procedures, they neglected simple measures promoting the well-being of those beyond cure. But sensitive observers of this scene, some of them physicians but others having a more detached view, called for care that was patient- and family-centered, meeting needs as they could be expressed by the dying patient, and providing comprehensive and continuous attention to comfort in all its modalities: physical, emotional, and spiritual (2, 3). Further, the public was gaining increasing confidence in expressing a general concern about inappropriate doctor-driven medical technologies. It was time for a revolution, and "hospice" was its slogan.

The rapidity with which the idea of hospice found sympathetic expression in many parts of the English-speaking world testified to an underlying common tradition in culture and in medicine in those countries. The medieval hospice, a refuge for travelers and a resting place for the poor and the sick, was a powerful image within the history of the Christian church. Charity, the imperative to do good works and to provide for the poor, still exercised a powerful influence within medicine, though increasingly obscured by the dictates of economic rationalism and cost-benefit analysis. In countries drawing on a different tradition (Russia or Japan, for example) hospice was less popular, partly because it has not been usual in those countries to inform patients that they have cancer or that death is imminent.

DEFINITION AND NAME

The word *hospice* has not appealed to everyone, and *palliative care* or *terminal care* are alternative terms for these programs. Of the three, *palliative care* or *palliative medicine* has found widest acceptance in established medicine, being used in major textbooks and post-graduate courses.

The World Health Organization has developed this definition of palliative care (with a particular emphasis on cancer (4):

The total active care of patients whose disease is not responsive to curative treatment. Control of pain, of other symptoms and of psychological, social and spiritual problems is paramount. The goal of palliative care is achievement of the best possible quality of life for patients and their families. Many aspects of palliative care are also applicable earlier in the course of the illness in conjunction with anticancer treatment. Palliative care:

- affirms life and regards dying as a normal process;
- neither hastens nor postpones death;
- provides relief from pain and other distressing symptoms;
- integrates the psychological and spiritual aspects of patient care;
- offers a support system to help patients live as actively as possible until death; and
- offers a support system to help the family cope during the patient's illness and their own bereavement.

MODELS FOR CARE DELIVERY

The first tentative examples of a different way of caring for the dying were either homely refuges offering a high standard of nursing care in a domestic setting very unlike a hospital (for example, the pioneering St. Joseph's in Dublin, established by Mary Aikenhead in her own home in the middle of the 19th century) or mobile support programs for delivering excellent care in the patient's own home (such as the service for dying children established by Martinson (5) or the outreach programs initiated by the Macmillan nurses in Britain (6)). Each was a way of releasing dying persons from the oppressive grip of active acute medicine and of facilitating dignified and comprehensive attention to needs recognized by patients and families.

Other pioneers, similarly dissatisfied with existing services, sought change within the bastions of acute care and established hospice wards in major hospitals or provided a consultancy service that encouraged, on the hospital wards, a high standard of symptom control, family counseling, and family involvement in care, seeking to pilot and implement institutional routines and structures more appropriate for dying individuals (7, 8).

A COMPREHENSIVE PROGRAM FOR CARE

An ideal palliative care program will incorporate all of these models of care provision, linking them into a network that once having accepted responsibility for an individual, remains accessible and supportive wherever care is being offered, accompanies the patient and the family throughout the final journey and also beyond the time of death, and takes responsibility for bereavement support of family members.

A single palliative care team will link the elements of the network, being accorded status in the hospitals where advanced disease has been treated and now is recognized as needing palliative management, but also deploy its members into homes, and be able to offer inpatient care in a specialized facility or "hospice." In each situa-

tion it will work closely with other professional care providers and will seek to involve family members or important friends in care decisions. This model, facilitating a networking among diverse health professionals, has been widely promoted and implemented in Australia and is relevant to any palliative care program that seeks to be comprehensive (Fig. 58.1) (9).

The components of the palliative care team will vary with the emphasis of each service and each locality. Usually it will include

- Readily available medical assessment and follow-up consultation by physicians experienced in palliative medicine. In the United States, physicians exercise important gatekeeper roles, certifying that a patient is eligible for hospice care through having a terminal illness; but opportunity in the United States to claim recognized status as a specialist in the discipline has been limited. In the U.K. and Australia, where training programs and specialist certification in palliative medicine are well accepted, the specialty occupies a place similar to that of other medical specialties (10).
- Nursing consultation and support. Palliative care appeals to dedicated nurses as the kind of nursing they aspired to undertake when joining the profession. It involves intimate one-to-one patient support and a high level of interaction with family members, valued as offering closer and more continuing relationships than is possible in busy acute care ward situations. It also often involves autonomous nursing practice with a high level of decision making and clinical responsibility, especially in home care, and so is a popular service for the dedicated nurse practitioner.
- Social workers, physiotherapists, occupational therapists, psychologists, pastoral care workers, bereavement counselors, music therapists, and art therapists occupy quite central roles in some programs but are absent from others.
- Volunteers are more consistently involved. "Hospices are the only Medicare-supported programs required to use volunteers" (1); at least 5% of the hours required for patient care must be contributed by unpaid helpers. In 1990, it was estimated that 5 million hours were donated by hospice volunteers in the U.S. In the program in which I work in Australia, we estimate that volunteers contribute approximately 25% of the hours of service offered to clients and families.

TEAMWORK

A team structure is vitally important. Care must be offered around the clock, and no one individual can work for 24 hours, nor has any single professional all the necessary skills. There is value in sending two team members on home visits; one may get to chat with the family while another examines and discusses care with the patient. Clearly directed staff meetings are essential

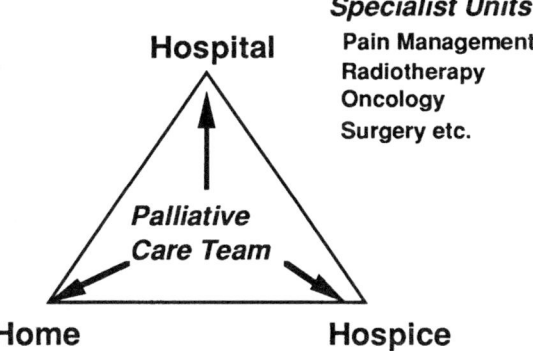

Figure 58.1. The network of palliative care. A model common in Australia, with a single multidisciplinary team overseeing care at many sites throughout the terminal illness (From Maddocks I. Changing concepts in palliative care. Med J Aust 1990;152:535–539, with permission.)

for mutual support and for adequate "hand-over." Staff continuity is important for maintaining communication both within the team and with the other providers in the various sites of care. A good reputation for a hospice team and effective education of other professionals stem primarily from their acknowledgment of good work done with particular cases.

ENTRY CRITERIA: ONLY CANCER?

Palliative care programs do not pretend to undertake the management of every dying patient. Most will demand some certified opinion of a limited life expectancy. This requirement promotes the inclusion of advanced cancer and effectively excludes many dependent and suffering individuals with a more open-ended prognosis. In a sense, those who have terminal cancer are fortunate; they will readily qualify for the expert care that is offered. The arteriopath with painful legs or amputated limbs, the stroke victim unable to move or express himself, or the demented very elderly patient will be more likely to languish in a nursing home where there is significantly less professional or volunteer support.

The judgment of prognosis, even in advanced cancer, is notoriously uncertain, but in the U.S., a physician is required to offer certification of less than 6-months expected survival to qualify a patient for admission to a program.

Other requirements for a hospice program to receive Medicare certification are (1)

- 24-hour staffing
- Medical and nursing care
- Home health services
- Access to inpatient care
- Social work services
- Counseling, including bereavement counseling
- Medications, medical supplies and durable medical equipment
- Physical, occupational and speech therapy

FUNDING

It is common for communities to enthusiastically raise capital funds for the building of a hospice unit and then experience difficulty in maintaining its operation without government support. The Medicare support provided in the U.S., limited to a fixed daily sum for a specified period, forces community teams to be very careful in their use of expensive inpatient resources. In Britain, also, funding for hospice construction and operation has often been as dependent upon large charitable foundations (e.g., the Macmillan Fund) as upon government grants. The National Health Service there allows family practitioners and visiting nurses to provide home support without costs of individual services needing to be counted. A salaried service is the rule in Australia, and some comprehensive hospice programs are fully funded as integral parts of the national health service.

THE CONTRIBUTION OF FAMILIES

In addition to receiving generous community and government support, hospice patients are often able to rely upon an intense commitment to care by family members. In middle age, death from cancer constitutes a higher proportion of all deaths than it does in old age; the loss of the younger person is generally felt more keenly and arouses wide public sympathy; there are more family members and friends available to help; and it will not need to be for long, since death comes relatively quickly. By contrast, the death of a very elderly person is better accepted by the family and may be actively wished for by that person; there are few living friends; families may have become accustomed to separation by the old one receiving care in a nursing home. The sense of responsibility and sadness therefore is lessened.

Death from cancer can be predicted, and preparations made. Families are strongly motivated to do what they can to minimize suffering, and they can make an estimate and a commitment to the time, effort, and finance of providing care; mobilizing family members (often scattered widely and carrying major professional or personal responsibilities) to provide support for the anticipated duration of life. Spouses, children, or friends sometimes can shoulder a major burden of care when it will not be for long; and they are encouraged to this effort because the approach of death is being played out with a tragic emotion that compels their attention.

In many instances, however, it will not be possible for family members to provide adequate care without skilled assistance and support. Few modern families can call upon the human resources or experienced skills that extended households or stable villages once provided almost universally. In these times, even an elderly woman may never have been called upon to nurse a dying relative, and many younger adults have never seen a dead body. Family structures are unstable; family members spread widely to distant locations. So a hospice team must try to instill confidence and teach skills to support those family members who can provide care and will sometimes itself substitute for the extended family.

THE DYING ELDERLY

Dying is coming home? Not for all, and particularly often, not for the elderly. "Home" for the elderly is often a small unit in a residential institution, a hostel room, or a nursing home bed. The ideal of death at home in one's own bed, surrounded by family, can less often be achieved as age increases.

There are important factors other than age that determine where death will overtake an elderly individual:

The Availability of Beds. Increasingly, hospital beds are becoming more jealously preserved for narrowly defined "acute care," with an emphasis on those diseases that attract best remuneration under a case-mix classification. Hospitals have become places for treatment rather than for care, and dying attracts a frugal funding. Concurrently, in many places, admission to a nursing home must satisfy a rigorous assessment of need. In consequence, care at home has assumed much greater importance, and where hospice beds are available, they will usually be fully occupied. Death also has become more likely to occur in a nursing home, terminating a period of admission shorter than was formerly the rule.

Gender. Males, who die younger than females, have a greater opportunity to die at home, partly because there is often a surviving spouse to maintain care, whereas elderly females are more often forced to accept institutional care.

Cause of Death. Sudden death often occurs at home; acute illness causing death leads to admission to an acute hospital; cancer (with its more predictable prognosis) qualifies for a hospice program. The dependency and uncertain prognosis associated with stroke or dementia tends to encourage admission to a nursing home.

Socioeconomic Status. More affluent families can afford the additional home supports that are necessary to maintain care.

DYING AND PALLIATIVE CARE FOR THE ELDERLY

In providing care for a dying elderly person, therefore, these differences are to be expected:

1. Family support is less available. An older person has outlived spouse and friends; the children are distant and caught up in their own responsibilities. Local, national, and cultural sociologic factors will play an important part. In Britain, for example, very elderly women are less likely to be married because of the slaughter of their potential spouses in World War I.
2. The elderly patient is more likely to face death in a nursing home, hostel, or retirement institution. The degree to which such facilities readily access skilled medical opinion, the amount of nursing care that they can provide, and the stimulus and encouragement that their environments and staff are able to offer, all vary greatly. The common fear of an elderly person of being "put into a home" may have been framed in a crueler past, but remains sadly appropriate in many instances.
3. Symptoms are different. It is important to counter the perception that dying is a painless process for the elderly; indeed pain prevalence has been de-

scribed as increasing with age (11). While many symptoms are just as prevalent among the dying elderly as are described in younger dying patients, others are more common: confusion, incontinence, difficulty with sight and hearing, dizziness, and persistent cough (Fig. 58.2) (12).

4. Ability to function in the usual home situation is already reduced, and the greater discomfort or frailty caused by a terminal illness exaggerates dependence. The home of an elderly person may more often lack modern conveniences such as a telephone or washing machine, and difficulty caused by stairs or distance to the toilet is more common. Simple tasks such as fastening clothing or cutting toenails become formidable impediments to self-care.

5. Death is accepted or even sought by patients. One report suggests that the suicide rate among those over 65 is twice the average for adults (13). The elderly are less inclined to fear death itself but fear being a burden to others; their own death makes sense to them. Also they are less inclined to accept the counsel of the young (which includes many caregivers).

6. There is a lack of responsiveness by medical and nursing services to the discomforts and anxieties of the elderly. Eliciting an account of symptoms takes longer, sorting out what needs to be done to improve comfort is more complex, involving the patient in decision making calls for a level of patience and persistence that many professionals feel too pressured to provide.

7. Pathologies, and therefore symptoms, are multiple. The management of cancer or other disease with a definite limited prognosis or with major and immediate symptoms to address is often complicated by diabetes, arthritis, emphysema, osteoporosis, or vascular disease.

8. Multiple medications often have been prescribed, of which many (e.g., diuretics, sedatives) can be withdrawn with benefit in the terminal phase of life.

9. Dementia is common and inhibits communication, making it difficult to assess wishes or to provide the spiritual and emotional support that is regarded as central to good palliative care. Cognitive impairment sharpens the ethical issues of palliative care. Demented patients are discounted more than those with cancer—they are less likely to attract the interest of care providers (14).

10. Counseling and bereavement care for the elderly spouse constitute a special challenge. The whole world of the elderly spouse focuses on the one who is dying or has died, and short-term psychotherapy is ineffective; the elderly mourner needs long-term contact (15).

ISSUES IN PROGRAM DELIVERY

Comprehensive and effective palliative care will attend to a wide range of responsibilities:

1. Efficient management
2. Symptom control
3. Education and training, especially of volunteers, but also of a wide range of health professionals
4. Research

MANAGEMENT

There will rarely be enough resources to fulfill all the requests for home support or inpatient hospice care. Staff who are dedicated to palliative care are tempted to extend themselves, and it is important to involve other professional care providers whenever possible and to use every opportunity to recruit and support family and friend helpers. Criteria for admission to inpatient care, in particular, must be appropriate to the responsibilities faced and the resources available. Pro-

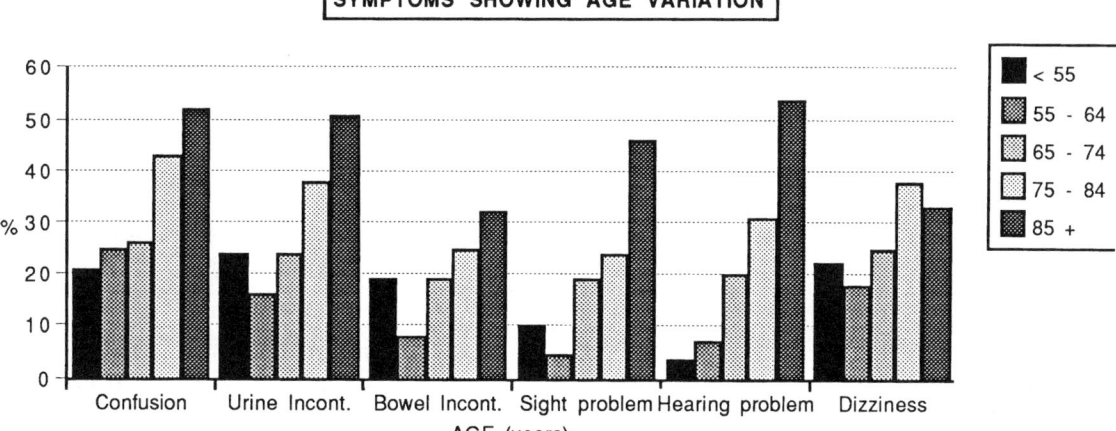

Figure 58.2. Common symptoms in the dying aged, showing variation with age in 800 deaths (From Cartwright A. Dying when you're old. Age Ageing 1993;22:425–430, with permission.)

viding consultant support for other physicians will often be the most economic use of expertise. A particular problem for the elderly who are dying in nursing homes may be the functional separation of such facilities from the specialist skills of modern medicine. For a dying elderly patient with a complex problem of pain or confusion, it may prove difficult to obtain appropriate opinion.

Fund raising is often an important part of the work of those who direct and administer palliative care programs. Much goodwill and considerable generosity are generated among client families, and it is also usual for whole communities to regard palliative care as deserving of support.

There is an opportunity not yet grasped, however, to bring to bear the appeal and compassion so readily lent to the dying young upon the harsher realities of death for the elderly. The very aged who are dying do not receive comparable attention from the medical community, the health care systems, or the public, yet their discomforts—physical, emotional and spiritual—are in no way less.

SYMPTOM CONTROL IN CANCER

The symptoms experienced by dying persons can include any that are recognized in clinical care, and relief calls for a broad experience of medicine, but particular emphasis focuses on some specific discomforts:

Pain

The following tenets are widely accepted as basic to good palliative care practice:

1. Accept a patient's account of pain, while acknowledging and distinguishing the many physical, emotional, and spiritual factors that may contribute to it. Pain pathology includes:

    a. Inflammation around tumor deposits, for which antiinflammatory drugs such as aspirin or non-steroidal antiinflammatory drugs (ibuprofen, naproxen, indomethacin) or the free use of corticosteroids (dexamethasone 4 to 16 mg daily) will be appropriate.
    b. Mechanical pressure that stimulates specialized nerve endings, causing pain for which minor analgesics such as acetaminophen, codeine and propoxyphene hydrochloride, or opioids will be necessary.
    c. Skeletal muscle spasm, benefiting by treatment with diazepam or muscle relaxants such as baclofen (Lioresal) or cyclobenzaprine (Flexeril); smooth muscle spasm for which oral or infused scopolamine may be useful.

    d. Nerve trunk irritation (neuropathic pain) which often responds inadequately to conventional analgesics, including opioids, but is helped by agents that stabilize nerve membranes and are commonly used in other situations: the antiarrhythmics lidocaine (up to 2 g by continuous subcutaneous infusion daily) or mexiletine (100 to 200 mg three times a day orally); anticonvulsants such as phenytoin or valproate; tricyclic antidepressants such as amitriptyline.

Drug therapy will therefore be guided by a comprehensive assessment of the underlying pathology, and will involve combinations of analgesics and adjuvant medications. Reassurance, and the encouragement of relaxation, sleep and peace of mind offer as much or more than drug therapies.

2. Offer pain medications according to simple rules (16).

    a. By the ladder: freely increasing dose and analgesic strength of medication in response to the degree of pain
    b. By mouth: using the simplest appropriate methods of administration
    c. By the clock: aiming to prevent pain by administering any analgesic regularly and before pain returns; adding to a baseline regimen orders for additional "breakthrough" doses

3. Recognize no upper limit for opioid dose apart from what is necessitated by side effects.
4. Ignore any risk of addiction as irrelevant and inappropriate in suffering persons close to death.
5. Prescribe in advance for common side effects: nausea and constipation with opioids, for example.
6. Recognize impairment of renal and hepatic function as one factor making elderly patients more prone to confusion or other toxic effects precipitated by medications.
7. Be aware of the many physical and emotional factors that lower pain threshold (fear, sleeplessness, anxiety, anger, irritability, despair, etc.). Seek to reduce them through careful attention to the life story, personality, and human context of the individual patient, and explore appropriate innovative measures to lessen isolation and facilitate acceptance, relaxation, and good humor.
8. Remain alert to new or innovative measures for the relief of pain that responds poorly to conventional therapy.

The use of epidural or intrathecal opioids, local anesthetics, or other drugs, for example, often allows small doses to be effective while avoiding systemic side effects (17). Continuous subcutaneous infusion of opioids provides very steady pain relief (18); other commonly used adjuvants by the same route include metoclopramide (Reglan) (20 to 80 mg over 24 hours) or haloperidol (Haldol) (5 to 15 mg over 24 hours) for nausea, midazolam (Versed) (10 to 45 mg over 24 hours) or haloperidol for restlessness or confusion, lidocaine (1 to 2 g over 24 hours) for neuropathic pain, and ketamine (200 to 500 mg over 24 hours) for opioid-resistant pain.

The use of ketamine by intravenous bolus allows excellent analgesia for short-term procedures such as daily hygiene of a patient with severe pain on movement; other measures for such "incident" pain include short-acting buccal opioids such as fentanyl or buprenorphine, and inhaled nitrous oxide–oxygen.

Fentanyl skin patches provide steady pain relief over 48 hours and are ideal for home use, but they will usually need to be accompanied by some breakthrough orders, since the pain stimulus from cancer often varies greatly over 24 hours.

Restlessness and Confusion

A common ideal for "the good death" is that the dying person will remain alert and symptom-free through to the final moments of farewell. This is not common; more often there are periods of intermittent discomfort, drowsiness, and confusion, slowly "winding down" over a variable length of time during which communication and responsiveness is progressively lost. Confusion is a common cause of admission to a hospice (19).

There are many causes of restlessness and confusion—medication (especially opioids and corticosteroids), pain, hypoxia, anxiety, psychosis, hypercalcemia and other metabolic disturbances, and cerebral metastases should all be considered. When morphine causes hallucinations or aggressive behavior or frank confusion, a different opioid (oxycodone by mouth or suppository, or fentanyl by patch or subcutaneous infusion) may prove to be much better tolerated. Sometimes there is a tension between increasing medication to relieve symptoms and reducing medication to maintain alertness. Discussion with families to clarify issues and expectations is an essential part of care.

Subcutaneous haloperidol (Haldol) or midazolam (Versed) offer a fairly predictable means for controlling terminal restlessness, and doses may need to be titrated to quite high levels to relieve symptoms. There is some risk that a person sedated in this way may continue to experience emotional distress, feeling aware but "locked in" and unable to express discomfort. Therefore simple ancillary measures such as adequate light, soothing music, and companionship should not be ignored.

Gastrointestinal Problems

Nausea, vomiting, anorexia, and constipation are common associations of advanced cancer and its management. Constipation should be guarded against by prescribing a laxative regimen with every use of opioids, and the rectal examination for impacted feces is a mandatory part of routine assessment. Opioids often cause nausea, and an antiemetic drug should be available.

In palliative care, established bowel obstruction is a particular difficulty. The acute medicine response of "drip and suck" with intravenous line and nasogastric aspiration usually is inappropriate; corticosteroids may sometimes relieve obstruction due to inflammatory adhesions, percutaneous endoscopic venting gastrostomy relieves nausea and vomiting without the discomfort of the nasogastric tube, and subcutaneous saline infusions will relieve thirst, as will regular attention to mouth toilets using a soothing weak solution of sodium bicarbonate. Subcutaneous infusions of scopolamine or octreotide will reduce bowel secretion (20).

Weakness, Wasting, and Weight Loss

The finding of *cachexin*, a substance present in the blood of cancer patients whose tissues waste rapidly, and its identification as closely related to tumor necrosis factor offers a possible mechanism for the muscle wasting and weakness that is common in cancer. So far, however, no effective antidote has been found. Megestrol acetate or corticosteroids may be suggested on empirical grounds to encourage short-term improvement in appetite and weight, but responses are not consistent and are rarely prolonged (21). More important is the provision of appropriate equipment and advice to encourage mobility and everyday comfort in the face of increasing weakness. Common-sense advice and encouragement to provide easily swallowed, nourishing, and attractive small portions of favorite foods are more appropriate than efforts at parenteral nutrition. Forcing fluids upon a very weak and drowsy individual may constitute harassment, and a continuous subcutaneous saline infusion (1 L over 24 hours) will be more comfortable and will prevent thirst.

Incontinence

A major source of embarrassment and distress, incontinence calls for attentive nursing with frequent toileting, use of absorbent pads, condom drainage, or use of a catheter.

Pressure Ulcers

Skin ulceration is a constant risk in the weak, wasted, and dependent, especially in the presence of incontinence. The use of soft foam overlays, sheepskins, water chairs, and mattresses to lessen the pressure on prominent body parts, together with regular turning and attention to skin surfaces with protection of early erosions, should make it possible to avoid uncomfortable ulcers in the dying as readily as in long-term geriatric patients.

Psychological Discomfort

That fear of the unknown which death entails, and fear of the process of dying, whether it will involve additional suffering, is almost universal. Anger is a common response to the threat of inevitable death, and anticipatory grief extends through close family and friends. Care providers need to be ready to reflect feelings honestly when the patient indicates a need to address the realities of the terminal state. Anxiolytic medications and antidepressants have a place in treatment, but open exchange and the sharing of fears and hopes must not be neglected. Requests for euthanasia are not framed only in despair, but may be a logical outcome of a wish not to be a burden and source of worry to others. Again, honest responses about what can and cannot be done to smooth the path of dying, with a promise to do nothing to unnecessarily prolong the course of the condition, will often lead to a quiet acceptance of the natural process.

EDUCATION

Dying, like birth, is a universal experience, and its causative pathologies are legion. Whether either birth or death should become the professional province of one narrow class of health care specialists is a question that most persons would answer in the negative. Education in the discipline of palliative care must become part of the preparation of every worker in health care but will be particularly emphasized in the preparation of community nurses, family physicians, and internists who engage in oncology practice. Conferences of these practitioners increasingly include sessions to discuss innovations and review current practice in palliative medicine. The discipline's first multiauthor text, the *Oxford Textbook of Palliative Medicine* (22), did not appear until 1993, but many more succinct works have appeared since Dame Cicely Saunders first presented her pioneering experience in 1967 (3). In a

number of centers there are well-founded postgraduate award courses and specialist training programs (23).

Community education is a further responsibility of palliative care teams and may go hand-in-hand with fund raising, the building of public awareness of hospice and palliative care programs, and the encouragement of greater confidence among families and individuals to confront the threat of death, so that gradually we may modify the charge that western civilization is "death-denying." Volunteers, who often join a program after a personal experience of care for a dying relative or friend, make a major contribution to a quiet "demythologizing" of the widespread awe of death.

RESEARCH

Palliative care has brought to medicine a change in attitudes to dying patients and has demonstrated new structures for the delivery of health care, breaking down long-established professional hierarchies in its effective multidisciplinary teams, and transcending the traditional boundaries that divide hospital and community practice. Few services, however, have laboratory facilities or budgets that support intensive research efforts.

Recent academic appointments in the discipline, however, particularly in the United Kingdom and Australia, promise increasing attention to the many areas awaiting further research, including topics as diverse as the clarifying of symptom categories, opioid metabolism, and the prevention of pathologic grief. Case series for randomized trials are difficult to attain because of rapidly changing clinical status, but anecdotal reports of the good effect of one or another innovative therapy can be convincing if they approach the trial of treatment with adequate attention to blinded observation of the effect of therapeutic agent and placebo.

A FUTURE FOR PALLIATIVE CARE?

Greater numbers of frail elderly persons challenge nearly all societies to consider urgently the ways in which their care can be accomplished with appropriate dignity and adequate comfort. It will not be necessary or desirable to extend existing palliative care programs so that these programs accept responsibility for all dying elderly individuals. While great emphasis has been placed on death at home in the pursuit of sensitive and appropriate care and in the hope of reducing costs, it is equally important to improve the process of dying in institutions: by assisting them to be more responsive to the needs of dying patients and their families; by ensuring that their staff receive adequate education in the new insights and techniques of symptom control and emotional support; and by advocating for a greater recognition of the very great numbers of older persons who will need good palliative care in the coming years, with a call for greater support for their care from medicine, from government, and from the wider community.

The lessons that palliative care programs have learned in home care or in hospital-based teams must become a stimulus for improving interest in, and resources for, good comprehensive palliative care in every site where people die, and not for cancer only, but for all causes of death.

REFERENCES

1. Harvard Medical School Health Publications Group. Dying with dignity. Harvard Health Lett (Special suppl) 1993;1(6):9–12.
2. Hinton J. Mental and physical distress in the dying. Q J Med 1963;32:1–21.
3. Saunders CM. The management of terminal disease. London: London Hospital Medical Publications, 1967.
4. World Health Organization. Cancer pain relief and palliative care. Technical report series 804. Geneva, WHO, 1990.
5. Martinson IM. Dying children at home. Nurs Times 1980;76:129–132.
6. Clench P. The development of home care services in the United Kingdom. In: Spilling R, ed. Terminal care at home. Oxford: Oxford University Press, 1986:19–34.
7. Mount BM. The problem of caring for the dying in a general hospital: the palliative care unit as a possible solution. Can Med Assoc J 1976;115:119–121.
8. O'Neill WM, O'Connor P, Latimer EJ. Hospital palliative care services: three models in three countries. J Symptom Pain Manage 1992;7:406–413.
9. Maddocks I. Changing concepts in palliative care. Med J Aust 1990;152:535–539.
10. Ford G. Specialist medical training in the UK. Palliat Med 1988;2:147–152.
11. Rapin CH. The mechanism of pain memory in the elderly. J Palliat Care 1991;7:48–50.
12. Cartwright A. Dying when you're old. Age Ageing 1993;22:425–430.
13. Ley DCH. The elderly and palliative care. J Palliat Care 1989;5:43–54.
14. Ryan DP, Carson MG, Zorzitto ML. The First International Conference on Palliative Care in the Elderly: an overview. J Palliat Care 1989;5:40–42.
15. Benbow SM, Quinn A. Dementia, grief and dying. Palliat Med 1990;4:87–92.
16. Twycross RG. Opioid analgesics in cancer pain—current practice and controversies. Cancer Surv 1988;7:29–53.
17. Cherry DA, Gourlay GKJ. The spinal administration of opioids in the treatment of acute and chronic pain: bolus dose, continuous infusion, intraventricular administration and implanted delivery systems. Palliat Med 1987;1:89–106.
18. Maddocks I. Subcutaneous administration of fluid and drugs in palliative care. Aust J Hosp Pharm 1992;22:181–184.
19. Briggs PG. Who needs a hospice? Med J Aust 1992; 156:417–420.
20. Faisinger RI, Spachynski K, Hanson J, Bruera E. Symptom control in terminal patients with malignant bowel obstruction. J Pain Symptom Manage 1994;9:12–18.
21. Regnard C, Mannix K. Weakness and fatigue in advanced cancer—a flow diagram. Palliat Med 1992; 6:253–256.
22. Doyle D, Hanks GWC, Macdonald N, eds. Oxford book of palliative medicine. 1st ed. Oxford: Oxford University Press, 1993.
23. Maddocks I. Postgraduate courses and awards in palliative care. Palliat Med 1992;6:269–271.

Commentary
James G. O'Brien

This chapter is being highlighted as an exceptional chapter that provides a comprehensive view of palliative care. It focuses in particular on the unique challenges posed by the dying elderly. This approach introduces realism to the phenomenon of dying and clearly identifies the need to move beyond expected sequenced approaches that may not always occur and to appreciate that difficulties may arise. Certainly these occur with greater frequency in the elderly, including confusion, incontinence, and comorbid conditions. Other complicating factors include the older adult who is living alone, perhaps not in his or her own home, but in fact much more likely to die in a hospital or nursing home. The chapter provides excellent solutions for responding to these challenges.

The author contributes a national perspective from other countries with more advanced systems of care, which exposes some of the obstacles that need to be addressed in this country if we ever hope to integrate palliative care principles into mainstream practice. In terms of developing a comprehensive and compassionate program for the dying patient, the author shares with us a vision of essential or critical elements of an ideal system of palliative care.

SECTION III

Ethical Issues in the Elderly Patient

59/ Preventive Ethics in Geriatric Practice

Laurence B. McCullough, Jill A. Rhymes, Thomas A. Teasdale,
Nancy L. Wilson

Every physician who treats older persons is well aware of the many ethical issues that physicians, patients, families, institutions, and society confront in the care of elderly patients. These range from such dramatic "four-alarm" issues as physician-assisted suicide (1–5) and the withholding of nutrition from terminally ill patients (1, 2), through less dramatic but still very stressful issues such as long-term care decision making, (6) to quotidian issues such as whether elders should continue to drive their own cars or how special diets should be addressed in the nursing home (7). These and the many other ethical issues and conflicts that occur in geriatric practice continue to receive a great deal of attention in the literature.

This literature focuses almost entirely on the resolution of ethical conflict in the care of geriatric patients. As a consequence, the prevention of ethical conflict in geriatric practice has been neglected—in the literature and therefore as a clinical skill. Ethical conflicts are intellectually engaging, especially the "four-alarm" ones; but they are also stressful for physicians, patients, families, and institutions to confront and seek to resolve. It will be far better for all these parties—the physician in particular—to prevent ethical conflicts more effectively than is presently the case. The purpose of the four chapters in this section of the book is to introduce the physician to ethically justified, clinically applicable strategies of preventive ethics in geriatric practice generally and especially in long-term-care decision making, in advance directive decision making, and in the use of an adjunct to advance directives, the "Values History."

This chapter begins with a definition of ethics and of its basic concepts and terms. These serve as the basis for consideration of the two main topics of this chapter: preventive ethics in the physician-patient relationship and preventive ethics for dealing with health care institutions. Because of their importance and prominence in the geri-

atrics literature, ethical issues in health care policy affecting the elderly and ethical issues in research with elderly subjects are also considered.

ETHICS: DEFINITION, CONCEPTS, AND TERMS

ETHICS

Ethics is the disciplined study of morality. Descriptive ethics studies actual moral beliefs and practices of individuals, institutions, and society on the basis of both quantitative and qualitative methodologies of the social sciences (8). Normative ethics concerns what morality ought to be. The chapters in this section are concerned with normative ethics (henceforth, simply "ethics") in the context of health care. Normative ethics in the context of health care has come to be known as bioethics (9).

Bioethics in geriatric practice, a subspecialty of both geriatrics and bioethics, concerns what morality ought to be for the physician-patient relationship, for health care institutions, and for society in matters of health care policy. This chapter focuses mainly on the first two, with particular attention to preventive ethics strategies in geriatric practice.

BEHAVIOR AND CHARACTER

Morality concerns the beliefs and practices of people about behavior and character toward other people, institutions, society, other life forms, and inanimate objects. Ethics inquires into ethically justified behavior, asking, What ought we to do? What ought we not do?

Ethics is also concerned with ethically justified character: whether we are disposed or not disposed to be concerned with the interests of others and to act for the sake of their interests rather than always our own. Character is an especially important consideration for the morality of physicians and health care professionals. Character is addressed in terms of the virtues and vices (10). Virtues are those traits of character that blunt mere self-interest so that one can see, and routinely act to protect and promote, the interests of others. Vices are those traits of character that unleash mere self-interest, so that one ignores or even fails to see the interests of others, much less protect and promote them. Ethics asks about character, What character traits ought to be cultivated as virtues?, What character traits ought to be avoided as vices? The virtues important to medicine are discussed below.

MANAGING MORAL PLURALISM

The United States is perhaps the most pluralistic society in the world. There are many sources of morality in such a society, including law, historical experience and traditions, religious beliefs, professional education and training, personal experience, professional consensus, authorities and experts, and institutional policies and practices.

Sometimes, the disagreement among these sources of morality runs very deep, as it does, for example, on the subject of physician-assisted suicide. The competition among these sources of morality grows even more pronounced for bioethics in an international context. Within and across nations there is a striking variety of views on bioethical issues (11).

Ethical Analysis and Argument: The Basic Tools of Ethics and Bioethics

Because of the actual and potential disagreement among the many sources of morality in a pluralistic society, no one or combination of them can be the source of morality upon which ethics and bioethics could reliably be based (12). Bioethics requires methodologies that seek to transcend these competing sources of morality. Over the centuries the discipline of philosophy has developed well-tested and reliable methodologies for attempting to achieve this ambitious goal. These philosophical methodologies are ethical analysis and argument, the basic tools of ethics and bioethics.

Intellectual Criteria for Ethical Analysis and Argument

Ethics relies on ethical analysis and argument that proceed according to intellectual criteria for rigorous thought and judgment and requires that one submit to the intellectual discipline required by such criteria. That discipline requires going where ethical analysis and argument take one,

not where "gut" feelings or personal opinion take one. "Gut" feelings and decisions based on them should not be confused with ethics. On the basis of disciplined ethical analysis and argument, one can develop accounts of what morality ought to be that can command respect from all, regardless of what particular sources of morality shape or influence each individual. The criteria that must be applied are clarity, consistency, coherence, applicability, and adequacy.

Clarity requires that basic concepts and terms are given clear meanings and that relevant distinctions are drawn. Consistency requires that after terms are clarified, they are used with the same meaning throughout an argument. Consistency also applies to argument and requires that reasoning not violate logical rules and be free of contradiction. Coherence also applies to argument and requires that premises fit together into a related set that as a whole produces the conclusion. Bioethics is not an "ivory tower" enterprise. On the contrary, bioethics must be applicable to the actual clinical and social situations that prompt moral concerns on the part of physicians, patients, families, institutions, and society. Bioethics must also display adequacy in that ethical analysis and argument and their results must be applicable in the future, especially in the prevention of ethical problems and conflicts.

Competing Accounts

Bioethics can sometimes produce more than one rigorous account of what morality in geriatric health care ought to be. This is especially the case for issues of considerable controversy such as physician-assisted suicide. After all, given the competing sources of morality in our society and internationally, it should not surprise anyone that thoughtful reflection will yield more than one intellectually rigorous and reliable account of what morality ought to be for a particular issue or conflict, e.g., withholding nutrition from a terminally ill patient. From a clinical point of view, this feature of bioethics should be seen as an advantage. Clinical experience teaches that prevention and management strategies for conflictual situations may not work; the world does not always cooperate with well-thought-out attempts to manage it. It is therefore very useful to have already identified ethically justified strategies so that if the first one fails, others will be at hand. The basic approach of this and the next three chapters is to develop preventive ethics and management strategies that emphasize a flexible, practical approach to ethical issues that the physician will confront in the care of elderly patients.

That there can be competing, well-made ethical analyses and arguments and clinical ethical judgments suggests that the results of bioethics are rarely final, marked by certainty, and immune to all possible criticism. It is far more often the case that the results of bioethics are less than certain. In this respect, ethical reasoning is like clinical reasoning. The latter is far more frequently marked by differing degrees of probability than it is by certainty. Nonetheless, when they are well made, rigorous clinical reasoning and judgments are reliable in the sense that physicians, patients, institutions, and society may act on them with a degree of confidence. So too for well-made clinical ethical judgments. This and the next three chapters aim to provide the physician with clinical strategies for preventive ethics and managing ethical issues and conflicts that are based on well-made clinical ethical judgments.

PREVENTIVE ETHICS IN THE PHYSICIAN-PATIENT RELATIONSHIP

THE OBLIGATION TO PROTECT AND PROMOTE THE PATIENT'S INTERESTS

The physician-patient relationship as a moral relationship is other-directed, from the physician to the patient (for the most part) and from the patient to the physician. The physician's concern ought to be directed primarily to the patient's interests rather than primarily to the physician's own interests. Indeed, it has been a staple of the history of Western medical ethics that the physician's primary ethical obligation is to protect and promote the patient's interests and that this obligation is constitutive of the physician's character (13). Preventive ethics in geriatric practice therefore begins with the virtues of physicians that make the obligation to protect and promote the patient's interests a way of life for physicians (14).

FOUR FUNDAMENTAL VIRTUES

Four virtues seem fundamental to the physician-patient relationship (15). These virtues (a) direct the physician's attention primarily to the patient's interests and, as a rule, secondarily to the physician's interests and (b) move the physician to act to protect and promote the patient's interests.

Two virtues seem essential to the first of these two tasks. The first virtue is *self-effacement*, the willingness routinely to put aside differences that should not count in the care of patients. Otherwise, the physician's own interests become the physician's primary focus of concern, and the patient's interests slip from view. The second virtue is *self-sacrifice*, the willingness to risk one's other relationships, health, and even life that are threatened in and by the care of patients. Self-effacement and self-sacrifice blunt the physician's understandable inclination to focus on himself or herself in favor of focusing on the interests of the patient.

Two virtues seem essential to the second of the two tasks of the virtues in the physician-patient relationship. *Compassion* is the willingness to acknowledge and to relieve the suffering and distress of others. Compassion thus has an intellectual component, the capacity to identify clinically when a patient is in pain, suffering, or distressed. Compassion also has a motivating component; it moves the physician to relieve the pain, suffering, and distress of the patient. *Integrity* is the willingness to form rigorous, well-made clinical ethical judgments about how to protect and promote the interests of others. This is crucial in medicine, because of the enormous power that physicians can wield in the care of patients (16). Integrity therefore requires the physician to act within and not exceed the competencies of medicine to protect and promote the patient's interests. Integrity is also the source of satisfaction that comes from practicing medicine with a commitment to excellence. Compassion and integrity together move the physician to protect and promote the patient's interests.

The moral demands of these virtues are not absolute, i.e., without limits. For example, it is not at all clear that integrity and compassion require the physician to administer cardiopulmonary resuscitation when the probability of mortality is very high and there is a high probability of serious harm to the patient during (multiple rib fractures) and after resuscitation (admission to a critical care unit for weeks with loss of cognitive function followed by death). Indeed, the practice of resuscitating all patients may involve physicians acting in ways that contradict the obligations generated by the virtues of integrity (to avoid futile intervention) and compassion (to avoid unnecessary pain and suffering).

The obligations generated by the virtues can also be limited by the legitimate self-interests of physicians. Legitimate self-interests are those interests that physicians are ethically justified in taking into account and sometimes wanting to protect. Legitimate self-interest—a controversial category in contemporary bioethics (17)—includes three sorts of interests: (a) the requisites for providing good patient care, e.g., adequate rest, time to study and reflect; (b) the obligations that physicians owe to the nonpatients in their lives, e.g., spouse, children, friends; and (c) those activities beyond medicine in which the physician finds meaning and the possibility for as coherent a life as conditions in the late 20th century permit. Unless a compelling case can be made for them, other forms of self-interest of physicians should be regarded as mere self-interest.

The virtues may come into conflict with each other, as shown in an ethical analysis of physician-assisted suicide. It is a clinical reality that some—usually *rare*—treatments for pain for seriously ill or dying patients are effective only at the price of compromise in the patient's quality of life that the patient reasonably judges to be unacceptable. One form of suffering, serious pain that threatens the patient's dignity and humanity, is traded for another, obtunded consciousness and the sundering of relationships that make the patient's life meaningful. Compassion requires the physician to acknowledge the patient's unavoidable suffering in such circumstances and to relieve it. The only means of relief seem to be those that will cause the patient to die quickly, from a cause other than the illness. It seems therefore an ethical obligation for the physician, on the basis of the virtue of compassion, to provide the means for such patients to commit suicide. This obligation would seem to include administering the means directly for patients who are physically unable to do so for themselves but are competent to request such assistance. At the same time, medicine is defined in part by its general life-preserving orientation. Assisted suicide seems to contradict this general orientation and so may constitute a threat to the integrity of medicine. Thus, compassion and integrity lead to a potential conflict of obligations to patients with intractable pain.

THE ETHICAL PRINCIPLES OF BENEFICENCE AND RESPECT FOR AUTONOMY IN CLINICAL JUDGMENT AND PRACTICE

The four fundamental virtues of the physician ground the ethical obligation to protect and promote the interests of the patient. What does it mean to protect and promote a particular patient's interests? This question is addressed by the ethical principles of beneficence and respect for autonomy. These two principles are based on two perspectives on the interests of the patient: (a) that of medicine, translated into clinical ethical judgment by the ethical principle of beneficence; and (b) that of the patient, translated into clinical ethical judgment by the ethical principle of respect for autonomy (18).

The Principle of Beneficence

The ethical principle of beneficence requires that the physician produce a greater balance of goods over harms for the patient, *as those goods and harms are understood from a rigorous clinical perspective*. This is the most ancient of all the ethical principles of bioethics (19).

Beneficence emphasizes acting for the benefit of the patient as the primary consideration, not avoiding harm. That is, *primum non nocere*, or "first, do no harm," is not the primary meaning of the principle of beneficence. "First, do no harm" occurs nowhere in the Hippocratic texts, for example. Indeed, its historical origins remain unknown. If "First, do no harm," a version of the ethical principle of nonmaleficence (13), were a first principle of bioethics, modern medicine would have to cease its work. Virtually none of what medicine offers patients, especially frail geriatric patients, is free of harm. Because medicine is fundamentally oriented to benefiting patients *on balance*, beneficence is the primary ethical principle, with nonmaleficence a limiting principle. That is, when physicians are doing only harm to the patient, which can sometimes happen, they ought to cease doing so.

The principle of beneficence requires the physician to do the following. First, the physician identifies which goods can realistically be sought and which harms can realistically be avoided for the patient by the physician. These can be identified on the basis of the competencies of the health care professions: the prevention of premature or unnecessary death and the prevention, cure, or at least amelioration of disease, injury, handicap, and unnecessary pain and suffering. Death is premature when it occurs before life expectancy, adjusted for underlying irreversible morbidity. Death is unnecessary when it can be prevented at an ethically justified cost in terms of iatrogenic pain, suffering, injury, disease, or handicap. Pain and suffering become unnecessary when they do not result in the achievement of any of the other goods of beneficence. Unnecessary pain and suffering are harms to be avoided.

Second, the physician forms rigorous clinical ethical judgments about which courses of intervention or nonintervention are reliably expected to produce a greater balance of goods over harms and thus protect and promote the interests of the patient to some reasonable degree. Usually, beneficence-based clinical judgment identifies a variety or sometimes a continuum of responses that protect and promote the patient's interests. Thus, one should beware of the phrase "best interests," where this is taken to mean that beneficence-based clinical judgment routinely identifies the only response that is in the patient's interest. One of the principal sources of paternalism in the clinical setting is failing to see that there are justified alternatives. For example, hospital admission of a patient with mild pneumonia gives the patient a setting in which treatment and monitoring occur with greater reliability than at home, but there are risks to hospitalization (e.g., disorientation or other infections). Treating such a condition on an out-patient basis avoids the risks of hospitalization, although at the possible risk of managing the patient's problem in a less structured setting.

The limits of beneficence-based clinical judgment are crucial for understanding religiously based objections by patients to certain forms of medical interventions, e.g., the refusal of blood products by Jehovah's Witnesses. Members of this faith value their health and life, but they value more their steadfast obedience to God's commands, which they understand to include the prohibition of blood products. Medicine cannot speak to whether this hierarchy of values is reasonable because a scientifically based, secular profession can claim no competence in theological matters (20). Failure to appreciate the limits of beneficence-based clinical ethical judgment sets up the unwitting physician for egregious forms of paternalism, e.g., waiting until a Jehovah's Witness patient who has refused blood products lapses into unconsciousness and then administering them.

The Principle of Respect for Autonomy

The ethical principle of respect for autonomy requires the physician to act in such a way that the consequences for the patient of the physician's behavior are reliably expected to be a greater balance of goods over harms, *as those goods and harms are understood from the patient's perspective.* That is, we each bring our own values and beliefs to being a patient and can form preferences on the basis of those values and beliefs. This is as true of geriatric patients as it is of any other age group of adult patients. Respect for autonomy translates the patients' perspectives on their interests into clinical ethical judgment.

To employ the principle of respect for autonomy reliably in clinical ethical judgment, the physician first provides an adequate amount of information to the patient—or to the surrogate of patients not capable of making their own decisions—about the patient's condition, about all alternatives for its management (including watch-

ful waiting), and about the benefits and risks of each management strategy, including watchful waiting. It is important that the physician attempt to identify and correct mistaken beliefs of the patient about these matters.

Second, the physician elicits from the patient—or the patient's surrogate—values and beliefs of the patient relevant to evaluating the patient's condition and alternative management strategies. That is, the patient needs to understand relevant clinical information cognitively (in terms of the consequences of various management strategies) and evaluatively (in terms of the worth or importance of those consequences for the patient on the basis of his or her values) (21). As with beneficence-based clinical judgment, the goal is to identify the full range or continuum of management strategies that reasonably protect and promote the interests of the patient on the basis of that patient's (or surrogate's) values-based evaluation.

INFORMED CONSENT AS A PREVENTIVE ETHICS STRATEGY

When the principles of beneficence and respect for autonomy are properly used in clinical judgment and practice, clinical decision making becomes a shared process of negotiating care management strategies on the basis of the common ground created by striving to identify *all* beneficence-based and autonomy-based management strategies. This should be the goal of a meaningful informed consent process, one that eschews the largely meaningless, bureaucratic ritual epitomized in the request "go get the consent" (22). When this occurs, informed consent is neglected as the basic clinical strategy of preventive ethics in geriatric practice. A meaningful informed consent process creates a common ground between beneficence-based and autonomy-based clinical ethical judgment.

The authors propose a nine-step informed consent process (23) (Table 59.1). Although this number of steps may appear burdensome at first, they are necessary for creating synergy rather than conflict between beneficence-based and autonomy-based clinical judgment. These steps begin with the recognition that the geriatric patient needs enough knowledge to participate meaningfully in the informed consent process and that the patient may need or welcome assistance in this process. These steps also distinguish cognitive understanding from evaluative understanding (21).

Table 59.1
The Informed Consent Process

1. **The Patient's Understanding.** The physician initiates the process by eliciting from patients what they believe about their condition, its diagnosis, alternatives available for managing it, and the prognosis under each alternative.

2. **The Patient's Fund of Knowledge.** In a respectful and supportive fashion, the physician corrects factual errors or incompleteness in the patient's fund of knowledge. (This does not require that the patient be provided a complete medical education.)

3. **The Physician's Judgment.** The physician provides and explains his or her clinical judgment about the patient's condition and available management strategies (including watchful waiting).

4. **Cognitive Understanding.** The physician works with patients, as needed or requested, to help them develop as complete as possible a picture of their condition and available management strategies (including watchful waiting).

5. **The Patient's Values.** The physician works with patients, as needed or requested, to help them identify their relevant values and beliefs.

6. **Evaluative Understanding.** The physician, as needed or requested, helps patients in a *nondirective* fashion to evaluate alternative management strategies in terms of their values and beliefs.

7. **Value-Based Preferences.** Patients are asked to identify which alternatives are consistent with their values and beliefs, to express value-based preferences.

8. **The Physician's Recommendation.** The physician makes a recommendation, based on the clinical judgment already expressed in step 3 and the patient's preferences expressed in step 7.

9. **The Management Plan.** A mutual decision about managing the patient's condition is reached.

The Obligations of Patients in the Informed Consent Process

Approaching informed consent as a meaningful decision making process assumes that the physician-patient relationship is a genuine partnership between the two parties (24). At the very least, this implies some mutuality of obligations. In short, patients have obligations, too. The obligations of patients to their physicians were a staple in the history of medical ethics until early in the 20th century (25). Only recently has this subject begun to receive attention again (26, 27).

The informed consent process set out above refers explicitly to the patient's cognitive and evaluative understandings of his or her condition and alternatives for managing it. At the very least, this requires that the patient attend to what the physician has to say. Moreover, when matters are serious—as they are when the patient's beneficence-based or autonomy-based interests can be harmed in far-reaching and irreversible ways— the patient owes the physician serious attention and due consideration of the benefits and risks of alternative management strategies. That is, the patient owes it to the physician to be serious when matters are serious, as they are, for example, in cases of chronic debilitating diseases, life-threatening events, and terminal illnesses.

Therefore, morality in the physician-patient relationship should involve a genuine partnership, a mutuality of obligations, and the physician's commitment to strategies that prevent ethical conflict from occurring and managing it when it does. The nine-step informed consent process can be used to prevent ethical conflict by reaching mutually agreed-upon decisions, complemented by a willingness to negotiate to manage ethical conflict. This process can also be used for conditional consent for situations that might occur. For example, the primary geriatrician might explain to a patient with pulmonary problems what a bronchoscopy would involve should one be judged useful by a consulting pulmonologist. Conditional consent strengthens the subsequent informed consent process by improving the patient's fund of knowledge and providing the patient with an opportunity to begin to think in advance about interventions that might be offered.

Informed Consent with and for Patients with Diminished Decision-making Capacity

Patients with diminished decision-making capacities pose special challenges to the physician in geriatric practice, given the significant rates of dementing disorders and other factors that can adversely affect an elderly patient's decision-making capacity (e.g., disorientation caused by hospitalization). Decision-making capacity may fluctuate over time—a clinical phenomenon that is well appreciated in geriatrics.

The patient should be presumed to be capable of participating in the informed consent process. The presence of a disease that may reduce decision-making capacity should not be taken as conclusive evidence that the patient cannot participate in the informed consent process. Clinical signs of variably reduced decision-making capacity should alert the physician to the fact that the patient may require extra assistance in the steps described above, especially the "Cognitive Understanding," "The Patient's Values," and "Evaluative Understanding" steps. That assistance should be undertaken, in the attempt to ameliorate reduced decision-making capacity. The informed consent process itself should be used as an evaluation tool with patients of reduced decision-making capacity. This approach provides patients with the opportunity to show themselves capable of participating in the informed consent process, especially by exercising evaluative understanding.

If the patient cannot participate, even with vigorous assistance from the physician, especially in the "Cognitive Understanding," "The Patient's Values," and "Evaluative Understanding" steps, then the patient can reliably be regarded in clinical ethical judgment to have reduced decision-making capacity to the point where someone else must now make decisions for the patient. An adequate attempt has been made to reverse reduced decision-making capacity and that attempt has failed to benefit the patient by bringing the patient up to a threshold of substantial autonomy.

Two Standards for Surrogate Decision Making. Two standards have been proposed as guidelines for making decisions for patients with irreversibly reduced decision-making capacity. The first is that the surrogate decision maker should, so far as possible, make the decision that the patient would have made were the patient still able to do so. This approach to surrogate decision making is called "substituted judgment" (28) (See Table 59.2.) Prior attempts to elicit the patient's values and beliefs in "The Patient's Values" step can be a valuable adjunct to this process.

The surrogate decision maker should be taken through the nine steps of the informed consent process. During "The Patient's Values" step, the surrogate should be asked to identify the patient's values and beliefs, and in the "Evaluative Understanding" and "Value-Based Preferences" steps, to identify all of the alternatives consistent with the patient's values and beliefs. The surrogate should then and only then be asked which alternative is preferable. Failure to carry out the "Evaluative Understanding" and "Value-Based Preferences" steps sets up the physician for conflict if the surrogate's preferred alternative is reliably thought to be unreasonable to the physician. The chances that this will occur are greatly reduced by first asking the surrogate to identify all alternatives consistent with the patient's values and beliefs and then asking the surrogate for a preference.

A second standard of surrogate decision making applies when neither the surrogate nor anyone else knows what the patient's relevant values and beliefs are. The surrogate decision maker should then be asked to make a decision that seems most in accord with a reasonable perspective in the patient's interests, the "best interests" standard (28) (See Table 59.2). Again, to prevent ethical conflict, the surrogate decision maker should be asked to identify all reasonable alternatives in the "Evaluative Understanding" and "Value-Based Preferences" steps and to seriously consider the physician's recommendation made in "The Management Plan" step.

The basic clinical strategy of preventive ethics in geriatric practice should by now be clear. Physicians should seek always to avoid "either/or" decisions in the thinking of patients, surrogate decision makers, and themselves. Physicians should ask themselves whether the patient's (or surrogate's) preference expressed in the "Evaluative Understanding" and "Value-Based Preferences" steps is reasonable in beneficence-based clinical judgment and assume the burden of proving that it is not. In short, clinical ethical judgment that is preventive ethics–oriented habitually seeks to create common moral ground with patients and surrogate decision makers. (See Table 59.3.)

PREVENTIVE ETHICS IN DEALING WITH HEALTH CARE INSTITUTIONS

The physician-patient relationship is now affected by institutional third parties that own or manage the resources consumed in the care of pa-

Table 59.2
Two Standards for Surrogate Decision Making

In *Superintendent of Belchertown v. Saikewicz* (373 Mass. 728. 370 N.E.2d 417, 1977) the Supreme Judicial Court of Massachusetts articulated the substituted judgment standard of decision making for incompetent patients. Mr. Saikewicz was a 67-year-old profoundly mentally retarded resident of the Belchertown State School who had been diagnosed with myeloblastic monocytic leukemia. A guardian ad litem for Mr. Saikewicz had recommended against chemotherapy because the pain and suffering that he would experience would outweigh any benefit that chemotherapy might confer. The court decided the case on the basis of "how the right of an incompetent person to decline treatment might best be exercised so as to give the fullest possible expression to the character and circumstances of that individual." That is, the surrogate decision maker was to take Mr. Saikewicz's perspective on this decision, imagining for a moment that Mr. Saikewicz was competent to make his own decision.

In *In the Matter of Storar* (52 N.Y.2d 363, N.Y.S.2d 266, 420 N.E.2d 64, 1981) (certiorari denied by U.S. Supreme Court) the Court of Appeals of New York (that state's highest court) articulated the best interests standard of surrogate decision making. Mr. Storar was a 52-year-old profoundly retarded man living in the Newark Development Center who was diagnosed with cancer of the bladder. His mother was appointed his legal guardian and requested radiation therapy, which was administered for 6 weeks. At this point, Mr. Storar's physicians judged his bladder cancer to be terminal. Blood transfusions were administered, but eventually Mrs. Storar requested that they be discontinued because of the discomfort and resistance that Mr. Storar displayed. The court held that because he was never competent, Mr. Storar was more like a child than an adult and that therefore someone else had to decide what his best interests were in terms of the benefit to be gained from blood transfusions and the burdens that this intervention imposed on him.

Table 59.3
An Example of Preventive Ethics in Geriatric Practice

A 68-year-old male patient was suffering from wet gangrene in his left foot, secondary to poor vascularization, a complication of his multiple-year history of diabetes mellitus. The patient had resisted surgical management because, as a Jehovah's Witness, he wanted to avoid the need for blood products. His team negotiated with him a plan of vigorous intravenous antibiotic therapy, which failed to improve his condition. He was now at risk for systemic infection and death, facts of which he was fully aware. When presented with the option of surgical management, the patient indicated that this would be acceptable provided that no blood products were administered.

His request caused consternation among some members of his team, and the patient was told that surgery could not be done safely without blood products, at which point the patient refused the surgery and asked that antibiotic treatment continue. The medical student on the team took it upon herself to ask the chief surgical resident if surgery without blood products was a reasonable alternative. The chief resident thought that surgery without blood products certainly implied higher risk, but not high enough to be regarded as unreasonable. The patient would have to understand that the surgery would be performed as quickly as possible, that blood products would not be administered, and that his refusal of blood products would probably increase his risk of both death and postoperative morbidity. The student took this information back to her team and then to patient, who consented to surgery without blood products. The surgery (below-the-knee amputation) was successful, and the patient was discharged for rehabilitation and preparation for a prosthesis.

---

tients. These resources are no longer owned solely by patients and their physicians, but by others: employers or former employers of patients and patients' spouses and governmental entities. Medicare and Medicaid are major government payers for medical care and long-term care, respectively, for geriatric patients. Privately and publicly owned resources are managed by both private and public institutions of health care. Moreover, providers of health care, including both physicians and institutions, increasingly subsidize the health care of patients (e.g., by completing and submitting paperwork for Medicare beneficiaries).

Further changes can be expected with health reform. These changes, which will continue to result in a complex pattern of ownership and management of health care resources, have an important ethical implication: Neither the physician nor the patient has an overriding right to the use of privately and publicly owned health care resources. There are limits on the use of health care resources and considerable dispute about where those limits should be set.

THE PRINCIPLE OF JUSTICE

Disputes about the management of health care resources are analyzed and managed clinically under the ethical principle of *justice*. Justice requires individuals and institutions to render to each individual what is due that individual. The problem is determining what counts as "due" someone. There are competing ethical theories of justice in Western philosophy, no one of which can claim final authority or supremacy over the others (the fond hopes of advocates of particular philosophical theories of justice notwithstanding).

Two important distinctions can be made and applied in the clinical setting to guide the physician's response to the institutional management of resources at the bedside. The first distinction is between *substantive justice* and *procedural justice*. Substantive justice concerns what the outcome of the distribution process ought to be, i.e., *who* ought to get *what* as due to him or her. Procedural justice concerns the distribution process itself, i.e., how the decision-making *process* about scarce resources ought to be conducted so that it is fair. There is far more agreement among philosophical theories of justice about procedural justice than about substantive justice. Basically, procedural justice requires that the interests of all affected parties be considered in decisions about managing institutional resources (see Table 59.4).

The second distinction is between horizontal and vertical distribution of resources. Horizontal distribution concerns universal access to some basic, decent minimum of health care resources (14). Current health care policy debates about a right to health care involve the horizontal distribution of health care resources (see next section).

Vertical distribution of health care resources concerns bedside decision about access to different levels of intensity of intervention. It is at this level that there are debates in the clinical setting about how much to provide for a particular patient, knowing that providing high-intensity care for that patient may well distort both vertical and horizontal distribution of resources, thus affecting the interests of other patients, institutions, payers, and society. The rationing of health care resources involves setting limits on the vertical distribution of those resources.

Bedside Vertical Distribution of Health Care Resources

Recently, E. Haavi Morreim has made a proposal for the bedside vertical distribution of health care resources. Morreim argues that a standard of medical expertise (about what resources are required to protect and promote the patient's interest) should be distinguished from a standard of resource use (what resources are actually available to protect and promote the patient's interest) (29). The physician can be held to a standard of expertise of beneficence-based judgment about the interests of patients, Morreim argues, independently of whether resources are available to implement such clinical judgment. By contrast, she argues, the physician cannot be required to confiscate resources not owned by either the physician or the patient. Physicians can and ought to be held to a standard of reasonable advocacy for vertical distribution of resources for their patients. "My patient always comes first," just won't do anymore, argues Morreim. Advocacy for resources is now more complex and must take into account the legitimate interests of institutions, their moral fiduciary obligations to patients, and the obligations of patients.

Reasonable Advocacy for the Patient

This advocacy and responses to it occur without the benefit of a well-articulated, publicly debated and supported national policy to guide decision making about rationing of vertical distribution of health care resources. Nonetheless, it is possible to provide a conceptual framework for such decision making and, on this basis, to propose an advocacy process. The conceptual framework has three main components: the legitimate interests of institutions; the moral fiduciary obligations of institutions; and the obligations of patients.

The Legitimate Interests of Institutions. A new issue in bioethics in recent years concerns the legitimate interests of institutional owners and managers of health care resources concerning the use of such resources. Institutions are not ethically obligated in all cases to risk harm to their legitimate interests in the care of partic-

Table 59.4
An Example of Procedural Justice

The State of Oregon faced the reality of having to ration health care resources for Medicaid recipients in Oregon. An elaborate decision-making process was established, a key feature of which were "town meetings" around the state in which citizens and organizations were free to participate. This process aimed at taking account of the interests of all affected parties to decisions about how best to allocate limited Medicaid funds to meet health care needs of Medicaid recipients.

ular patients. The legitimate interests of institutions include such matters as fiscal stability, paying suppliers, meeting payrolls, and conforming with environmental protection laws. Not all of an institution's interests are legitimate, however. Legitimate interests are those that can be shown in ethical analysis and argument to be essential to fulfilling the institution's mission.

The Moral Fiduciary Obligations of Institutions. Institutions that provide health care have beneficence-based and autonomy-based obligations to their patients. Provider institutions such as clinics and hospitals ought to be understood to be bound by an obligation to protect and promote the interests of their patients, just as physicians are. Like physicians, both voluntary and for-profit provider institutions ought to be considered the moral fiduciaries of their patients. They should primarily be concerned with the interests of patients and only secondarily with their own legitimate interests. A central ethical issue in the management of health care institutions concerns how to prevent and manage ethical conflicts between the institution's moral fiduciary obligations to its patients and its legitimate interests (e.g., fiscal stability).

The Obligations of Patients. Patients have ethical obligations in the allocation of institutional resources, although this topic has received little attention in the literature on justice and health care. These obligations have two sources.

The first source is found in the distinction between what might be called the "negative" and "positive" exercises of autonomy, or "negative" and "positive" rights (30). Negative rights are understood in ethical theory to be rights to be left alone, especially when no one else's legitimate interests are placed at risk by doing so. Respect for autonomy is strongest in the case of such negative rights, creating a very heavy burden of proof for paternalism, i.e., interfering with negative rights for purely beneficence-based reasons. Positive rights are understood in ethical theory to be claims on others for their resources or resources held in common in society. Most of the resources consumed in health care are not owned by the patient. Thus, a patient's positive right to institutional resources, even when it is exercised as the outcome of the informed consent process, is properly subject to limits. That is, institutions and society have legitimate interests in the ownership and management of health care resources that limit the positive exercise of the patient's autonomy to consume those resources. The patient,

therefore, has an ethical obligation to take account of and respect those legitimate interests.

The second source of patients' obligations is found in what the authors term the obligations of the "prudent saver." Americans have created a patchwork of private entitlements (through private health insurance) and public entitlements (Medicare, Medicaid, VA, military medicine, Champus, city and county hospitals and clinics) to health care in the United States. None of these entitlements, however, is an entitlement to *everything*. Both public and private insurance plans include covered and noncovered benefits, as well as deductibles and copayments. In short, patients are expected to pay some of the costs of health care. This assumes that geriatric patients have been prudent savers for uncovered health care costs.

This is a difficult obligation to fulfill for many elderly individuals, especially those with modest or fixed incomes and little or no savings, perhaps because they lived from paycheck to paycheck for many years. It may be unrealistic to think of such individuals—and many tens of thousands are Medicare beneficiaries and qualified veterans—as prudent savers. Yet they come into the care of physicians and institutions who then have fiduciary beneficence-based obligations to them. It may not be fair to physicians and institutions to expect them to subsidize health care for those who were not prudent savers. Yet, as fiduciaries of patients, physicians and institutions have an ethical obligation to provide adequate care, care that at least meets beneficence-based clinical judgment about what is in the patient's interest.

FOUR STEPS OF REASONABLE ADVOCACY AS A PREVENTIVE ETHICS STRATEGY

Preventive ethics strategies in dealing with health care institutions must take into account such matters of substantive justice as the vertical distribution of institutional resources, the legitimate interests of the institution, the moral fiduciary obligations of the institution, and the patient's obligations to the institution, including whether patients should be regarded as having fulfilled their obligations as prudent savers. In response to this moral complexity, we propose a preventive ethics strategy that draws on Morreim's proposal that the physician act as a reasonable advocate for the patient. Four steps are involved in fulfilling this preventive ethics strategy (Table 59.5).

First, reasonable advocacy requires that the physician be able to demonstrate on the basis of

Table 59.5
Reasonable Advocacy as Preventive Ethics Strategy

1. Demonstrate that a management plan is in the patient's interest.

2. Identify how the institution's legitimate interests will be affected and ethically justify those risks.

3. Do not claim "My patient always comes first."

4. Challenge overly restrictive institutional policies.

the informed consent process that a proposed management plan is in the patient's interest and is reliably expected to produce the expected benefits for the patient. The patient has no positive right to intervention that is not expected to be beneficial, and the institution has no moral fiduciary obligation to provide it.

Second, reasonable advocacy requires that the physician identify how the institution's legitimate interests will be affected and argue that risks to those interests are ethically justified in a particular case. The latter condition is more readily satisfied when the outcome of nonintervention for the patient in beneficence-based clinical judgment (not autonomy-based clinical judgment) is very grave (e.g., failure to prevent unnecessary death or permanent, serious disability). This aspect of reasonable advocacy presumes that the institution in question has a clear understanding of its legitimate interests. This is usually not the case, however. Thus, a crucial element of preventive ethics in dealing with health care institutions is to foment ongoing discussion within the institution about its mission and legitimate interests.

Third, reasonable advocacy does not include the simple assertion that "My patient always comes first." At one time in the history of medical ethics, provider institutions were understood in terms of the "purest beneficence" in their obligation to expend resources on their patients (31). Institutions' legitimate interests and the sometimes enormous expense of contemporary medicine and medical technology make "My patient always comes first" an ethically irresponsible assertion.

Fourth, the physician should challenge institutional policy that prohibits ever risking the legitimate interests of the institution. When institutions prohibit *any* risk, they, in effect, put their moral fiduciary obligations systematically in second place to their economic and other interests. They may be free to do so, but only if they explicitly abandon their mission as a moral fiduciary of

patients. In short, part of preventive ethics in dealing with provider institutions is to call them back constantly to their moral fiduciary obligations, especially for patients who were not able to be prudent savers. Doing so creates the common moral ground for negotiating vertical access for one's patients to institutional resources.

ETHICAL ISSUES IN GERIATRIC HEALTH CARE POLICY

The main ethical issues in health care policy for geriatric patients concern horizontal and vertical allocation of resources. There is now a voluminous literature on the subject of allocation of geriatric health care resources. There is also growing awareness among practicing physicians about ethical issues in geriatric health care policy (32). These issues are at some remove from the clinical setting of geriatric practice, but decisions about them by federal, state, and local governments will have both direct and indirect impact on geriatric practice.

Any discussion of geriatric health care policy must begin by acknowledging that the elderly enjoy a statutory entitlement to largely hospital-based, physician-oriented services. At the same time, it is important to underscore that Medicare does not meet the health care needs of all older Americans. Older Americans and their families bear considerable cost for Medicare-reimbursed services and for services that Medicare is not designed to cover (e.g., family-provided home care and custodial care). Medicare and Medicaid payments for long-term care also provide a large indirect subsidy to children and grandchildren of elders who might as a matter of moral—not legal—obligation have to divert monetary resources from their own interests and needs to pay for hospital and physician services. The elderly are, in short, an advantaged population when it comes to medical care (33) as are, indirectly, their children. Only qualified veterans enjoy a comparable advantage. Elderly qualified veterans are thus especially advantaged.

Much of the ethical debate has centered on whether horizontal and vertical access to health care resources can be justifiably limited on the basis of age. The most prominent recent arguments have been advanced by Daniel Callahan (34) and Norman Daniels (35). Callahan argues in favor of the view that there is a natural life span (early 80s) and that medicine should confine itself to helping people achieve this natural life span. For patients in their 80s, the goal of medicine should be to prevent and manage suffering. Thus, on the basis of age, greatly limiting vertical distribution of health care resources is ethically justified (34). Daniels argues against the view that the allocation of resources pits older generations against younger ones. Rather, we should be concerned about what health care resources should be available at each stage of our lives. To achieve justice-based equality over a "prudential life span," age-based rationing of health care resources would be ethically justified (35).

Marshall Kapp has astutely pointed out that age-based discrimination against the access of elders to health care resources is a curious worry about a government that already discriminates in favor of age and that pays for already generous medical services to the elderly, compared with other government programs (36). The arguments of those such as Callahan and Daniels tend to ignore political realities. This failure to make ethics applicable to the political process calls into question the applicability of their arguments that discrimination on the basis of age is ethically justified. Their arguments, however, help to underscore the apparent unravelling of public support for the Medicare program. There are indeed well-made arguments, on the basis of substantive justice, that question age-based preferences for the elderly.

Nancy Jecker has raised an important issue, namely, the disproportionate effect on women of attempts to limit access to health care on the basis of age (37). These effects, she argues, must be analyzed under the principle of justice in the larger context of a pattern of ethically questionable gender-based discriminatory practices in our society. The inequalities that might be caused by age-based rationing would be even greater for women than men, such inequalities would not provide overall social benefit, and women are already a disadvantaged and vulnerable group and so should receive priority in a justice-based approach to rationing health care.

Debates about geriatric health care policy—the rationing of vertical distribution of resources in particular—and the political resolution of those debates must be understood in light of a fact about the history of Western political philosophy. There are competing accounts of substantive justice in the history of Western philosophy and no convergence on a single, final theory of substantive justice. There are several important implications of this history.

Proposals about what geriatric patients should receive as a matter of substantive justice require ethical analysis and argument. Simple advocacy for the elderly should not expect to command in-

tellectual respect. Physicians can contribute to this debate an informed clinical perspective on the outcomes of various proposals for the vertical distribution of resources for geriatric patients. Any political resolution of debates about substantive justice in geriatric health care will be fragile. This is because a political resolution will vote into law one or more but not all views on substantive justice. The "losing" positions will not have their intellectual force diminished one iota, and their voices will continue to be heard in the ethical debate. As experience is gained with a particular public policy, support for that policy can be expected to weaken. This is happening with Medicare and, to a lesser extent, with Social Security. As citizens, physicians can take a preventive ethics posture toward the formation of health care policy affecting geriatric practice. Physicians need to be attentive to public debates, contribute to them and to the formulation of political resolutions, and be prepared to keep their shoulders to the wheel, for this is a never-ending task. The problems are chronic and inherently controversial; they can at best be managed well, but not solved once and for all.

ETHICAL ISSUES IN RESEARCH WITH ELDERLY SUBJECTS

The final issue addressed in this chapter is research with elderly subjects. There is already a considerable consensus (and a body of law reflecting that consensus) on the ethics of research with human subjects. Because of the abuse of human subjects of research by governments, including the United States, and by institutions and investigators, present federal regulations of human subjects research place very strong emphasis on respect for the autonomy of the research subject, strict requirements of informed consent, the need to justify the research on scientific grounds, and the need to protect vulnerable populations from more than minimal risk.

This understandable caution poses ethical challenges for researchers in geriatric medicine and health care, particularly for research on patients with diminished decision-making capacity, those who have lost decision-making capacity, and nursing home residents. There is a compelling need for increased scientific knowledge and clinical skills to care for the ever-growing numbers of such patients. Yet such patients often cannot meaningfully consent or consent at all to participation in research, and they are often vulnerable by reason of frailty compounded by life in the "total institution" of the nursing home.

Greg Sachs and Christine Cassel have argued that despite these problems, appropriate guidelines for the protection of elderly subjects of human research can be devised (38). These guidelines must address informed consent for research on elders with impaired cognition, with special attention to the range of impairments potential research subjects exhibit; the protection of residents of long-term care facilities from exploitation; and the subtle devaluing of older people in calls, such as Callahan's (34), to ration health care—and, in effect, research monies—on the basis of age. The physician's preventive ethics posture toward research with elderly subjects is to work with institutions (hospitals, nursing homes, community agencies) to develop policies that address these matters.

CONCLUSION

This chapter has emphasized and set out in some detail a preventive ethics approach to the care of geriatric patients. Ethical conflicts may be intellectually engaging to discuss, but they are stressful for physicians, patients, patients' families, institutions, and society. Applying the clinical skills of preventive ethics in geriatric practice can help to prevent these stressful events, thus improving the quality of geriatric care.

Acknowledgment. The authors wish to acknowledge the research assistance provided by George Khushf, Ph.D., in the preparation of this chapter.

REFERENCES

1. AGS Public Policy Committee. Voluntary active euthanasia. J Am Geriatr Soc 1991;39:826.
2. American Medical Association, Council on Ethical and Judicial Affairs. Decisions near the end of life. In: Code of medical ethics reports of the council on ethical and judicial affairs of the American Medical Association. Chicago: American Medical Association 1991:49–63.
3. Teno J, Lynn J. Voluntary active euthanasia: the individual case and public policy. J Am Geriatric Soc 1991; 39:827–830.
4. Jecker NS. Giving death a hand: when the dying and the doctor stand in a special relationship. J Am Geriatr Soc 1991; 39:833–835.
5. Watts DT, Howell T. Assisted suicide is not voluntary active euthanasia. J Am Geriatr Soc 1992; 40:1043–1046.
6. McCullough LB, Wilson N, eds. Ethical and conceptual issues in long-term care decision making. Baltimore: Johns Hopkins University Press, 1994.
7. Kane RA, Caplan AL, eds. Ethical issues in the everyday life of nursing home residents. New York: Springer, 1990.
8. McCullough LB, Wilson NL, Teasdale TA, Kolpakchi AL, Skelly JR. Mapping personal, familial, and professional values in long-term care decisions. Gerontologist 1993;33:324–332.
9. Reich WT, ed. Encyclopedia of bioethics. 2nd ed. New York: Macmillan, 1995.
10. Pence G. Virtue theory. In: Singer P, ed. A companion to ethics. Cambridge, Massachusetts: Basil Blackwell, 1991:249–258.
11. Lustig BA, Brody BA, Engelhardt HT Jr, McCullough LB, eds. Regional developments in bioethics: 1989–1991, Bioethics Yearbook II. Dordrecht, The Netherlands: Kluwer Academic Publishers, 1992.
12. Engelhardt HT Jr. The foundations of bioethics. New York: Oxford University Press, 1986.
13. Beauchamp TL, Childress JF. Principles of biomedical ethics, 3rd ed. New York: Oxford University Press, 1986.
14. McCullough LB, Chervenak FA. Ethics in obstetrics and gynecology. New York: Oxford University Press, 1994.
15. McCullough LB. The physician's virtues and legitimate self-interest in the physician-patient contract. Mount Sinai J Med 1993;60:11–14.
16. Brody H. The healer's power. New Haven: Yale University Press, 1992.
17. Pellegrino ED, Thomasma DL. The virtues in medical practice. New York: Oxford University Press, 1994.
18. Beauchamp TL, McCullough LB. Medical ethics: the moral responsibilities of physicians. Englewood Cliffs, NJ: Prentice-Hall, 1984.
19. Baker R. The history of medical ethics. In: Bynum WF, Porter R, eds. Encyclopedia of the history of medicine. London: Routledge, 1994:848–883.
20. Engelhardt HT Jr. Bioethics and secular humanism: the search for a common morality. Philadelphia: Trinity Press International, 1991.
21. White BC. Competence to consent. Dordrecht, The Netherlands: Kluwer Academic Publishers, 1994.
22. Wear S. Informed consent: physician beneficence and patient autonomy. Dordrecht: The Netherlands: Kluwer Academic Publishers, 1992.
23. McCullough LB. An ethical model for improving the physician-patient relationship. Inquiry 1989; 25:454–465.
24. Veatch RM. The patient as partner. Bloomington: Indiana University Press, 1987.
25. American Medical Association. Code of medical ethics. Proceedings from the national convention 1846–1847. Chicago: American Medical Association, 1848:83–106.
26. Benjamin M. Lay obligations in professional relations. J Med Phil 1982;10:83–105.
27. Meyer MJ. Patients' duties. J Med Phil 1992; 17:541–555.
28. Brock D, Buchanan A. Deciding for others. Cambridge, England: Cambridge University Press, 1989.
29. Morreim EH. Balancing act: the new medical ethics of medicine's new economics. Dordrecht, The Netherlands: Kluwer Academic Publishers, 1992.
30. McCullough LB, Chervenak FA. Limits on refusing treatment. Hastings Cent Rep 1991;21:12–18.
31. Percival T. Medical ethics. Baltimore: Williams & Wilkins, 1927.
32. Williams ME, Connolly NK. What practicing physicians in North Carolina rate as their most challenging geriatric medicine concerns. J Am Geriatr Soc 1990;38:1230–1234.

33. Feder J. Health care and the disadvantaged: the elderly. J Health Politics 1990;15:259–269.
34. Callahan D. Setting limits: medical goods in an aging society. New York: Simon & Schuster, 1987.
35. Daniels N. Am I my parents' keeper? An essay on justice between the young and the old. New York: Oxford University Press, 1988.
36. Kapp MJ. Rationing health care: will it be necessary? Can it be done without age or disability discrimination? Issues Law Med 1989;5:337–366.
37. Jecker N. Age-based rationing and women. JAMA 1991;266:3012–3015.
38. Sachs GA, Cassel CK. Biomedical research involving older human subjects. Law Med Health Care 1990;18:234–243.

60/ Long-Term-Care Decision Making

Laurence B. McCullough, Jill A. Rhymes, Nancy L. Wilson,
Thomas A. Teasdale

Long-term care has been defined as a "range of services that address the health, personal care, and social needs of individuals who lack some capacity for self-care" (1). Long-term-care decision making is occasioned by physical, mental, or social changes that result in a loss of function so that the elder, family members, friends, or physician believes that the services of others are required to supplant the loss of self-sufficiency (2). Long-term-care decisions thus concern nearly all aspects of a person's daily life (3, 4). Often multiple decisions must be made over time. Family members are usually intimately involved and play multiple roles, including those of caregiver and decision maker (5). The physician is not involved when long-term-care decision making is accomplished by the dyad of elder and family member, e.g., for the elder to move in with a family member after the death of a spouse (6, 7). The physician frequently becomes involved after the elder and family members are well into the decision making process (e.g., after an acute event such as a fall). This decision-making process operates under many constraints, including personal finances, limits on family members' ability or willingness to provide care, public regulations, and the bureaucracies of public and private institutions that deliver or administer services (8, 9).

Physical, social, or mental changes that prompt the long-term-care decision making process obviously can have ethically significant consequences (10). The purpose of this chapter is to provide the physician with a values-oriented approach to informed consent as a preventive ethics strategy in long-term-care decision making.

First, the authors provide an ethical analysis of long-term care, to identify how it differs from acute care. Second, the physician's role in long-term-care decision making is discussed, with an emphasis on the physician as a good-faith mediator of a values-laden informed consent process. Third, empirical research concerning the values of participants in long-term-care decision making and the ethical implications of this research are considered. Fourth, an informed consent process is described that adapts the preventive ethics strategy of Chapter 59 to the context of long-term-care decision making. Fifth, long-term-care decision making within the nursing home context is discussed. Sixth, long-term-care decision making regarding elders with dementias is considered.

ETHICALLY DISTINCTIVE FEATURES OF LONG-TERM CARE

Long-term care differs significantly from acute care. Brian Hofland notes that acute care typically involves well-defined problems as well as well-defined alternatives for managing them, whereas long-term care is more ambiguous, with problems less well defined and alternatives therefore more resistant to clear definition (11). Acute care involves problems that are typically clearcut. The acute-care patient has or is thought to have an anatomic or physiologic abnormality (e.g., a fractured hip or congestive heart failure of a specific stage). Pathophysiology is the province of the health care professions, medicine in particular. Thus, a built-in feature of acute care is that the physician—rather than the patient—possesses the intellectual basis for naming the patient's problem. This dependence on physicians to name our problems when we are patients in acute care settings is one of the sources of the power of physicians over patients. This power is usually not shared with the patient (12).

This power is exercised in an institutional context in which resources for the diagnosis and management of acute care problems are organized and made available for physicians to use in the care of patients. Physicians, not patients, control access to these resources, another source of the physician's power in the acute care setting. The physician's power is exercised within a hierarchical structure, in which the physician writes orders that other professionals or technologists then carry out. Physicians recommend management strategies to patients, even strongly, but physicians no longer issue orders to patients, to which compliance is to be "prompt and implicit," as was expected in 19th century American medical ethics (13).

An important implication of the physician's role in the acute care setting, especially in the hospital setting, is that patients experience dependence on their physicians. As one court has put it, patients experience an "abject dependence" on their physicians (14). This kind of dependence causes a loss of power by the patient, to which the informed consent process can be understood as a response to enhance the patient's autonomy.

In summary, in the acute care setting, the physician possesses the power to name the problem. The physician is thus the chief ontologist, undertaking diagnostic workups to place the patient's reality into the correct pathophysiologic category. (Ontology is the philosophical study of basic categories of reality.) The patient cannot perform this role, because the patient lacks the relevant knowledge. The physician controls access to institutional resources and so enjoys significant power. The informed consent process and, increasingly, third-party payers and managers function as significant counterweights to the physician's power. The patients' pathophysiology and the response of physicians and health care institutions to it have significant implications for patients in other spheres of their lives and for others in their lives, but these are implications of acute care.

Long-term care differs sharply in all three respects. First, the elders may not be patients at all. They are usually living in some community setting, getting along more or less well enough with their lives. The physical, mental, or social changes that are occurring may not be seen as problems by the elder, even though family members or the physician may see them as problems. In short, there is no chief ontologist in long-term-care decision making. For example, an older woman living alone may regard herself as quite capable of taking care of herself, yet her daughter notices that her mother's nutritional status seems to be deteriorating. *Competing realities*—for *both* the elder's problem and for the caregivers' problem(s)—constitute the defining feature of long-term-care decision making. Competing realities are a major source of ethical conflict within that process. Moreover, even when the reality is agreed upon, its significance may not be. For ex-

ample, an elder and family members may disagree about how risky it is for the elder, who is recovering from the effects of a severe fall at home, to continue to live at home alone.

Second, the resources that might be marshalled in response to a situation that is agreed to be a problem are not under the sole control of the physician. This is because most of the resources consumed in long-term care in the United States are those of the so-called informal caregivers, the elder's moral intimates: spouses, children, step-children, in-laws, neighbors, and friends. These individuals do not stand in hierarchical relationships to the elder, nor the elder to them. As Nancy Jecker has pointed out, their relationships constitute tangled and often inchoate webs of obligations (15). Moreover, the informal caregivers do not stand in hierarchical relationships to physicians or institutions that deliver formal long-term care services. In short, no one issues orders to anyone (except in institutional settings such as the nursing home). Requests, compromise, and negotiation are the tools of decision making in long-term care (16). The exercise of autonomy in this context is less dramatic than it is in end-of-life decisions (see Chapters 59 and 61). Rather, the physician's concern should be with the everyday exercise of autonomy (17) and with the potentially corrosive effect on autonomy of nursing home routine (18).

Third, the psychosocial spheres of the elder's life are an essential part of long-term-care decision making, not an implication of that process. This is because the elder's problem, while it may be occasioned by mental or physical change, is also occasioned just as often by social change (e.g., the death of a spouse or a child being transferred out of town). Loss of self-sufficiency is frequently a social phenomenon in the lives of elders and their moral intimates, not a medical one. Relocating to receive care or accepting assistance with daily tasks may have a profound effect on an elder's self-identity and opportunity to perform cherished social roles.

In summary, long-term-care decision making involves competing realities and competing interpretations of realities. There can be disagreement about whether multiple mental or physical or social changes that reduce self-sufficiency in activities of daily living have occurred and, when they have occurred, whether they should count as problems. There is no chief ontologist, even when the elder is a patient. The power to name the problem is thus contested, not settled as it is in the acute care setting. Second, the power to command resources in response to a long-term care problem (once it is agreed to be such) is widely diffused among the elder, informal and formal caregivers, and institutions. Because of the large role that they play, informal caregivers are a major long-term-care resource and important decision makers with the elder and the physician. The obligations of family members and their legitimate interests are essential to deciding whether they ought to serve as such a resource. Third, long-term care is inherently biopsychosocial in nature. Indeed, long-term-care decision making—with its competing realities, essentially temporal character, and shifting cast of participants—may best exemplify the biopsychosocial model in health care and social services.

THE PHYSICIAN'S ROLE IN LONG-TERM-CARE DECISION MAKING

The physician has several roles in this complex decision-making context. In their research, the authors have identified a number of roles played by the physician in long-term-care decision making (Table 60.1). For present purposes the most important of these roles is the *good-faith mediator* of a decision-making process that is often already well along by the time that the physician becomes involved in it.

A good-faith mediator resists being an unquestioning advocate for any one party in long-term-care decision making. In particular, the physician should be wary of being enlisted by family members in carrying out decisions in which the elder was not involved. At the same time, being an uncritical advocate of the elder's autonomy overlooks legitimate limits that family members may want to place on their caregiving role and responsibilities.

VALUES IN LONG-TERM-CARE DECISION MAKING

In short, long-term-care decision making is a complex and unavoidably *value-laden* process. Indeed, the process is mainly about negotiating the practical implications of each participant's value commitments, commitments of which he or she (the physician included) may be unaware. The physician's preventive ethics role is to bring these values to the surface, in the search for common ground, because the search for a common ground of shared values is the defining feature of preventive ethics in clinical practice. That is, long-term-care decision making ought to be a process in which the evaluative understanding (the assessment of alternatives on the basis of one's values) of each party is as explicit as possible. The alternative can be an emotionally wrenching or even guilt-laden and therefore potentially divisive dispute between elders and family members over alternatives, such as whether the elder stays at home or goes to the nursing home. Focusing on alternatives in the absence of participants' underlying values sets up those participants for ethical conflict by obscuring from their view their potential common ground of shared values. This outcome is a disservice to elders and their families. Recent research into the values of participants in long-term-care decision making indicates that informed consent aimed at a common ground of values as the basis for long-term-care decision making is a realistic, practical clinical goal for the physician.

Table 60.1
Roles of the Physician in Long-Term-Care Decision Making

Physician-educator	
Formal caregiver	Provide medical care and plan appropriate diagnostic tests and clinical management
Educator	Communicate diagnoses and prognoses; discuss care needs; provide information about long-term-care resources in the community
Gatekeeper	Authorize access to appropriate agencies, payment schemes, etc.
Counselor	
Counselor	Counsel elder and family via nondirective assistance with decisions
Historian	Remember and remind elder and family of elder's course, previous decisions, and results of those decisions
Mediator	As neutral party, seek win-win outcome to prevent and manage ethical conflict between elder and family and between elder/family and community agencies and institutions
Advocate	
Advocate	Advocate for management that is reliably judged to be in the elder's interest medically
Surrogate	Stand-in for other participants in decision making when necessary
Lawgiver	Direct a course of action

This research has emphasized the importance of values in long-term-care decision making. One focus has been on what the values, beliefs, and behavior of people ought to be (i.e., on normative ethics). This focus has led, for example, to concern for the implications of the ethical principle of respect for autonomy (19, 20). Normative studies have also been concerned with the values held by family members, particularly the value of filial obligation, which is the obligation of adult children to care for their frail elderly parents or parents-in-law (15, 21). A second focus of research on long-term-care decision making has been on descriptive ethics, empirical studies of the values of elders and family members (22–26) and of the values held by health care professionals (28–30).

A recent empirical study mapped the self-reported values of the three most common participants in the long-term-care decision making process: elders, involved family members, and health care professionals (30). In mapping these personal, familial, and professional values, three questions were addressed:

1. What values do participants in long-term-care decision making report retrospectively as relevant to the process? These values constitute a "values map" for long-term-care decision making.
2. How frequently are various values reported by elders, family members, and health care professionals as relevant to the long-term-care decision making process?
3. How common and how different are the values held by elders, involved family members, and health care professionals?

Older people who had changed their living situation and/or had started receiving help with personal care because their capacity for self-care was reduced were identified. Equivalent numbers of persons who had made one of five different care arrangements during the preceding month were included: (a) remained at home with the addition of paid help; (b) moved in with a relative or acquaintance to receive help; (c) began attending adult day-care; (d) entered a congregate housing setting with services; or (e) entered a nursing home. These settings were chosen to reflect the fact that most functionally disabled elders with long-term care needs do not live in institutional settings. Older people who had made changes for reasons not related to functional needs were excluded, as were those with significant cognitive or communication problems. The total sample analyzed consisted of 23 interview sets: 24 elders (including one married couple), 23 family members,

and 13 professionals for a total of 60 interviews subjected to qualitative data analysis.

The sampled elders' ages ranged from 70 to 94, which is consistent with those of a long-term care population. The elders were predominantly Caucasian (96%) and included an equal number of men and women. Their mean educational level was high, and a substantial percentage were in the middle- or high-income range. They most often identified a family member (82.6%) and someone of another generation (82.6%) as most involved in their decision. The long-term-care decisions carried out ranged proportionately over a wide range of alternatives, most of them in community-based settings.

The 23 family members or friends ranged widely in age, their mean age (57) reflecting this caregiving population (31). Before the decision was made, all but 4 of them had been providing either direct assistance or financial help to the older person. Clearly, changes in elder care or residence would influence the lives of these family members or friends.

The professionals included both medical and social service practitioners who were experienced in geriatric and long-term care. In contrast to the elders, most family members, friends, and professionals reported previous personal experience with long-term-care decision making.

A semistructured instrument was used, to standardize the interview process and provide interviewers with questions useful in probing for additional information. Data analysis obeyed accepted methods of qualitative investigation (32), beginning with a descriptive analysis of the respondents, followed by content analysis of the interview transcripts. Large numbers of specific values were identified for elders (348), family members and friends (398), and professionals (241). These were consolidated in two further steps: grouping into "generic" values and grouping into "categories" of values. The goal was to produce a clinically useful values map that represented the respondents values.

This process of qualitative analysis resulted in a values map of manageable size that includes generic values and categories of generic values of elders (Table 60.2), family members or friends (Table 60.3), and professionals (Table 60.4). As the tables show, the generic values are broad in scope, ranging from the general to the quite specific. For elders, generic values range from "to maintain self-image" to "to be safe from personal and property crime." For family members or friends, generic values range from "to prepare for elder's future" to "to minimize job conflict for me."

Table 60.2
Values Map for Elders[a]

Categories and Generic Values[b]	Frequency[c]
Environment	22
To maintain personal privacy	9
To have a pleasant living environ-ment	8
To be in a stimulating environment	7
To have mobility	7
To be in a familiar setting	6
To be at home	6
To have convenient services	5
To be in a personable setting	4
To have enough living space	3
Self-identity	18
To be independent (in control)	11
To be self-sufficient (carry out my decisions)	8
To minimize personal burden	6
To maintain self-image	6
To maintain continuity with the past	5
To avoid negative personal feelings	4
To be treated with respect	4
To be responsible for others	3
Relationship	17
To have company	8
To be with acquaintances	6
To be with people like me	5
To be with family	5
To have likable help	5
To please others	4
To be alone	1
Care	16
To have reliable care	6
To have housekeeping help	6
To receive needed personal care	5
To have regular meals provided	4
To receive immediate help	2
Health	15
To have health care	15
To be healthy	3
Caregiver burden	11
To avoid burdening others	11
Finances	10
To have financial security	6
To have financial independence	5
Security	6
To be prepared for the future	5
To be safe from personal and prop-erty crime	3

[a]From McCullough LB, Wilson NL, Teasdale TA, Kolpakchi AL, Skelly JR. Mapping personal, familial, and professional values in long-term care decisions. Gerontologist 1993;33:324–332. With permission.
[b]Twenty-four elders were actually interviewed, but the group included one married couple, who were treated as one interview.
[c]Number expressing the category or generic value at least once.

For professionals, generic values range from "for elder to be independent" to "to get physical therapy or rehabilitation for elder." The values map reflects multiple decisions that involve all aspects of a person's daily life for a long time.

Both generic values and categories of generic values exhibited commonalities and differences. For the sample as a whole, 31 (86%) of the elders' generic values were also identified by family members or friends; 42 (82%) of family members' or friends' generic values were also identified by the elders. Of the professionals' generic values, 25 (66%) were also identified by both elders and family members or friends, and 7 (19%) were identified by either elders or family members or friends.

This study was subject to several limitations. Because it was retrospective, the results might be influenced by recall bias or the avoidance of cognitive dissonance. The values expressed, especially those of the elder and family members, may have been influenced by the fact that both parties were interviewed after they had accumulated some experience with the long-term-care decision they had made. Thus it cannot be determined whether the commonalities of generic values and categories of generic values were functions of the long-term-care decision-making process or something that participants bring to the process. Nonetheless, the high rates of commonality strongly support a preventive ethics approach to long-term-care decision making. Although the sample is large for a qualitative study (60 interviews), it does not represent all participants in long-term-care decision making, because its size is limited to 23 decisions and because it lacks racial and economic diversity.

Two observations about the general features of the values map are in order. First, when one compares the top three categories (by frequency of response) of generic values for each group of respondents, some interesting differences emerge. For elders, these top-listed values concern environment, self-identity, and relationship. For family or friends, they are care, security, and psychological well-being. For professionals, the values are care, physical health, and a tie between relationship and psychological well-being. Given the high percentage of physicians among the professionals, their emphasis on health-related values was not surprising. The lower frequency of these values among elders and family members or friends may reflect either an assumption that health concerns had already been addressed adequately or a priority of other values. These data suggest both a potential for conflict among competing values and considerable commonality of values, particularly

Table 60.3
Values Map for Family Members/Friends[a]

Categories and Generic Values	Frequency[b]
Care	21
To meet elder's care needs	16
To have supervision for elder	11
To have meals for elder	9
To provide high-quality care for elder	7
To avoid nursing home for elder	7
To provide personal care for elder	4
To provide housekeeping help for elder	3
To have care that is convenient for elder	1
Security	18
For elder to be safe	13
To prepare for elder's future	7
To protect elder from inadequate family-given care	1
For me to be in a low-crime environment	1
Psychological well-being	16
For elder to be happy	7
For elder to be active	7
To continue things as they are for elder	5
To provide emotional and mental support for elder	5
For elder to be in a stimulating environment	4
To preserve elder's quality of life	1
Caregiver burden	15
To avoid general burdens on myself	9
To avoid emotional burdens or worries for myself	7
To minimize job conflict for me	5
To reduce burden on other family members	4
To avoid life-style changes for me	3
To maintain my own freedom/independence	3
To avoid physical and health burdens on myself	2
To maintain my privacy	1
Relationship	15
To ensure socialization and companionship for elder	8
To have elder near family and friends	6
To preserve marital relationship	5
To have others' support for decision	3
To minimize conflicts with elder	3
To fulfill my duties to persons other than elder or spouse	1

Table 60.3—continued
Values Map for Family Members/Friends[a]

Categories and Generic Values	Frequency[b]
Quality of environment	15
To keep elder in familiar surroundings	8
For elder to be in comfortable surroundings	4
To maintain elder's privacy	4
To have enough room for elder	3
To preserve elder's mobility	2
Elder respect	15
To respect elder's choices	13
For elder to be independent	8
To preserve elder's dignity	1
To preserve elder's rights	1
Health	14
To provide health care for elder	14
To preserve elder's life and health	2
Finances	14
To do what is financially affordable for self and elder	14
Caregiver benefits	5
To feel good about elder's situation	3
To have job satisfaction	1
To do what is financially gainful for me	1
Filial responsibilities	5
To fulfill my intergenerational duty to elder	5
To respect choices of parent other than elder	1
Elder identity	4
To meet religious needs of elder	2
To preserve elder's identity	2

[a]From McCullough LB, Wilson NL, Teasdale TA, Kolpakchi AL, Skelly JR. Mapping personal, familial, and professional values in long-term care decisions. Gerontologist 1993;33:324–332. With permission.
[b]Number expressing the category or generic value at least once.

between elders and their family members. A preventive ethics approach to long-term-care decision making seeks to avoid conflicts among competing values.

This study also indicates that the physician needs to remember that elders may have values and priorities of values for themselves in long-term-care decision making other than health-related values. Elders expressed values related to self-identity, for example, more often than values concerned with physical and mental health—in contrast to the frequency of health-related generic

Table 60.4
Values Map for Professionals[a]

Categories and Generic Values	Frequency[b]
Care	13
To have supervision for elder	7
To provide capable, quality care for elder	7
For elder to have meals/nutrition	6
To meet elder's general care needs	6
To meet elder's personal care needs	4
Health	13
To provide medical care for elder	6
For elder to be safe from threats to health	6
To get physical therapy or rehabilitation for elder	5
To maintain elder's health and physical function	4
Relationship	10
To have socialization and companionship for elder	6
To maintain elder's family relationships	3
To minimize conflicts between elder and caregiver	2
To minimize conflicts between elder and noncaregiver in family	2
Psychological well-being	10
To preserve elder's emotional and mental health	5
To maintain or increase elder's activity	5
To get stimulation for elder	4
For elder to be happy	3
Quality of environment	9
To keep elder at home, if possible	5
To have enough physical room for elder	2
To avoid negative aspects of nursing home	2
For elder to be comfortable	2
To reduce architectural barriers for health and safety reasons	2
Elder respect	9
To respect elder's preferences	6
For elder to be independent	5
To maintain elder's dignity	3
To respect elder's religion	1
Caregiver burden	9
To reduce caregiving burden on spouse	6
To reduce caregiving burden on adult children	3
To accommodate family caregiver concerns and wishes	3
To reduce caregiving burden on paid help	1

Table 60.4—continued
Values Map for Professionals[a]

Categories and Generic Values	Frequency[b]
Decision-making process	8
To have elder understand/accept decision (which may not be elder's)	5
To do what is feasible	4
To do what is professionally satisfying	2
To have elder involved in decision-making process	2
To activate agency/community help for elder	1
To involve family in decision making	1
Finances	3
To do what is financially affordable for elder	3

[a]From McCullough LB, Wilson NL, Teasdale TA, Kolpakchi AL, Skelly JR. Mapping personal, familial, and professional values in long-term care decisions. Gerontologist 1993;33:324–332. With permission.
[b]Number expressing the category or generic value at least once.

values expressed by the professionals. Balancing these may well be a central preventive ethics task of the long-term-care decision-making process.

THE INFORMED CONSENT PROCESS FOR LONG-TERM-CARE DECISION MAKING

The informed consent process described in Chapter 59 can be effectively adapted to long-term-care decision making. In implementing this process as a good-faith mediator, the physician should keep in mind the main implications of the preceding discussion.

First, the participants in long-term-care decision making may or may not agree on the elder's and the family's reality. The physician should try to have participants agree or reach as much agreement as possible on these realities. If that attempt fails, the decision-making process should proceed for each description of the elder's situation. Competing descriptions do not always mean different long-term care plans for the elder.

Second, physicians should appreciate that they can order only institutional, hierarchically organized resources. The family members and other involved informal caregivers are acting from a sense of obligation, tempered and limited by their legitimate interests—especially other obligations in their lives and their concern for their own family members (e.g., teenage children). Parties need to understand these realities as well.

Third, the elder and family members will be exercising their autonomy in an everyday, nondramatic fashion.(17) This will especially be true in the nursing home setting (18) (see next section).

Their values can be at stake, therefore, in subtle ways that need to be elicited.

Fourth, the nursing home has been frequently described as a "total institution." In particular, its corrosive effect on the autonomy of elders and the sense of obligation on the part of family members should not be underestimated (18).

Fifth, the inherently psychosocial nature of long-term-care decision making means that it is necessarily value-laden. Thus, the primary concern of the physician should be to assist elders and family members articulate their evaluative understanding and to express preferences for managing the elder's situation in terms of their values.

Sixth, the physician can expect that some values will be held in common by elders and their families, although their rankings of those values may differ. Physicians should also be wary of their own understandable tendency to give priority to health-related values. Elders and families may not do so.

With these considerations in mind, the long-term-care decision-making process can be undertaken with ethical justification in a step-wise manner that reflects the informed consent decision-making process described in Chapter 59. The goal is preventing the ethical conflict that can occur in the absence of an ethically justified, orderly approach to long-term-care decision making that explicitly includes identification of and reflection on values (Table 60.5).

LONG-TERM-CARE DECISION MAKING IN THE NURSING HOME

The preceding strategy can be used for the full range of long-term-care decisions, including nursing home placement as the outcome. After the elder and family have made a decision for the nursing home, the long-term-care decision-making process continues. This point is worth emphasizing for two reasons. First, as George Agich has pointed out, the elder's autonomy is very much at stake in the day-to-day decisions in nursing home life, because autonomy is expressed in these day-to-day decisions (17).

As Charles Lidz and his colleagues have documented, the nursing home as a "total institution" has corrosive effects on the elder's autonomy (18). In this setting, the physician is appropriately an advocate for the elder's autonomy, in the sense described in Chapter 59. A responsible advocate recognizes ethically justified limits on the exercise of an elder's autonomy when those limits are grounded in the institution's clear sense of its fiduciary obligations to the elder and its legitimate interests.

The day-to-day ethical issues in the life of nursing home residents have been discussed by Rosalie Kane and Arthur Caplan (9). The physician needs to be attentive to such mundane exercises of autonomy as phone privileges, roommate selection, and opportunity for spiritual growth. The physician should take advantage of the nursing home staff's day-to-day knowledge of the elder to identify what is important to the elder, especially those with dementing disorders and diseases. As Agich argues, ethically significant expressions of autonomy can still remain in the midst of dementia (e.g., going into a stairwell for peace and quiet) (17).

The physician should work with nursing home administrations to create an environment that is not so systematically corrosive of the elder's autonomy. Lidz and colleagues question nursing home policies that excessively favor considerations other than autonomy (18). For example, they point out that overconcern for bodily safety can lead to use of restraints that undermine autonomy, making the elder worse off. They suggest that patients with different cognitive abilities should not be routinely mixed together, since this erodes the abilities of those with the least cognitive loss. In short, the physician can enhance the elder's autonomy in the nursing home by obliging the nursing home to review whether its policies and practices enhance or undermine autonomy of residents.

LONG-TERM-CARE DECISION MAKING REGARDING ELDERS WITH DEMENTIA

Elders with mild and even moderate dementia may be capable of participating at a meaningful level in the informed consent process. As noted in Chapter 59, the best way to determine whether the elder with mild or moderate dementia can participate is to attempt the informed consent process as a trial. The same strategy should be used in long-term-care decision making regarding elders with dementia. They should not be presumed, by virtue of a diagnosis of dementia, to be incapable of participating in long-term-care decision making. An important area of future research in long-term-care decision making concerns the capacity of elders with dementia to participate in the decision-making process, especially in the identification and expression of their values and evaluative understanding.

When the elder cannot participate in the long-term-care decision-making process, the authors recommend that the substituted judgment standard (described in Chapter 59) be used to guide

Table 60.5
A Value-Based, Preventive Ethics Approach to Long-Term-Care Decision Making

1. **Defining the elder's reality**. The physician initiates the process by eliciting from the elder and from involved family members (of other informal caregivers) what they believe the elder's reality to be, the alternatives that are available to manage it, and the prognosis under each alternative.

   An attempt should be made to reach agreement on the reality of the elder's condition, a view that neither underestimates nor overestimates the elder's capacities and the care burden those capacities imply for family members.

2. **Participants' fund of knowledge**. In a respectful and supportive fashion the physician corrects factual errors or incompleteness in the elder's or family members' fund of knowledge by providing information directly or—importantly—linking them with knowledgeable professionals in the community.

   a. The elder and family members may sometimes not be aware of all long-term care services for which the elder is eligible.

   b. Sometimes family members have already steered the elder toward one alternative, and not informed the elder about other alternatives. Family members should be alerted in advance that the informed consent process requires the physician to provide the elder and them with a "level playing field" of information. This is one of the first duties of the physician as good-faith mediator.

3. **The physician's judgment**. Physicians provide and explain their clinical judgment about the elder's situation and available management strategies (including watchful waiting).

   a. The physician should give particular attention to the elder's functional capacities, how they might be improved or strengthened, and their long-term prognosis.

   b. The physician should emphasize that alternatives should be considered as trials. They may not work; the elder may not accept them; the family may not accept them; the elder's situation could change. Time limits for such trials and markers of success and failure should be established, if possible.

4. **Cognitive understanding**. The physician should work with the elder and the involved family members to help them develop as complete as possible a picture of the elder's situation and **all** of the available management strategies (including watchful waiting).

   Watchful waiting in this context includes a trial of the elder continuing with his or her present living arrangement with an agreement from the elder to a frank appraisal of the success of this strategy and its impact on family members.

5. **Participants' Values**. The physician works with the elder and family members, to help them identify their relevant values.

   The categories of values and generic values in Tables 60.2–60.4 may be mentioned to elders and family members who have difficulty in expressing their values. Some individuals do not have a powerful values-oriented vocabulary, and the physician must help them express their concerns in a meaningful fashion.

6. **Evaluative understanding**. The physician helps the elder and family members **in a nondirective** fashion to evaluate long-term care alternatives, including a trial of present arrangements, in terms of their values.

   a. As a good-faith mediator, the physician should not take sides in this process.

   b. As a good-faith mediator, the physician should listen for values held in common and for value differences and help elders and families appreciate both their commonalities and differences.

7. **Value-based preferences**. The elder and family members are asked to identify which long-term care arrangements are consistent with their values.

   The goal should be for both the elder and the family members to consider and identify all alternatives that are consistent with their values. Doing so maximizes the chance that an agreement can be reached.

8. **The physician's recommendation**. The physician makes a recommendation, based on the clinical judgment already expressed in step 3 and the elder's and family members' value-based preferences expressed in step 7.

   It is reasonable to expect the elder and family members to take account of the physician's judgment, either about the health-related aspects of each alternative or about areas in which agreement has emerged in the previous steps.

9. **The management plan**. A mutual decision about managing the patient's situation is reached.

   a. This may not occur. The elder and family members must then respect each other values, understand why they disagree, and seek to manage their disagreement.

   b. This nine-step process will need to be recycled as the elder's situation changes or if the arrangement is found not to be satisfactory to the elder or family members. Long-term-care decisions are seldom made once and for all.

decision making. The goal should be to identify the patient's relevant values for the patient, so that those values can shape the nine-step decision-making process described above. Family members are an important source of information about the elder's values. The physician's past experience and discussions with the elder may also help in identifying the elder's values.

Family members should be supported in the identification of reasonable limits on their obligation to provide long-term care for the elder. This is especially important with demented elders, given the considerable emotional, physical, and spiritual demands that caring for them can impose on their family members. Family members, especially frail spouses, siblings, or adult children, are not obligated to sacrifice themselves endlessly in the care of a loved one. The physician may with ethical justification recommend that family members consider limiting their obligations to provide care when the burden of caregiving has compromised the health status of family members.

Acknowledgment. The authors wish to acknowledge the research assistance provided by George Khushf in the preparation of this chapter.

REFERENCES

1. Kane RA, Kane RL. Values and long-term care. Lexington, MA: Lexington Books, 1982:4.
2. McCullough LB. Long-term care for the elderly: an ethical analysis. Soc Thought 1985;11:40–52.
3. Kane RA, Kane RL. Long-term care: principles, programs, and policies. New York: Springer, 1987.
4. Pelaez M, David D. Training professionals to enhance autonomy in long-term care. Gerontologist 1991;31:71 (suppl).
5. High D. A new myth about families of older people? Gerontologist 1991;31:611–618.
6. Gold DT, Late-life sibling relationships: does race affect typological distribution? Gerontologist 1990; 30:741–748.
7. Horowitz A, Silverstone BM, Reinhardt JP. A conceptual and empirical exploration of personal autonomy issues within family caregiving relationships. Gerontologist 1991;31:23–31.
8. Dunkle RE, Wykle ML, eds. Decision making in long-term care: factors in planning. New York: Springer, 1988.
9. Kane RA, Caplan A, eds. Ethical conflicts in the management of home care: the case manager's dilemma. New York: Springer, 1993.
10. McCullough LB, Wilson NL, eds. Ethical and conceptual dimensions of long-term care decision making. Baltimore: Johns Hopkins University Press, 1994.
11. Hofland B. Introduction. Generations 1990;14:5–8 (suppl).
12. Brody H. The healer's power. New Haven: Yale University Press, 1992.
13. American Medical Association. Code of medical ethics. Proceedings from the national convention 1846–1847. Chicago: American Medical Association, 1848:83–106.
14. Canterbury v. Spence 464 f. 2d 772, 785 (D.C. Cir. 1972).
15. Jecker N. The role of intimate others in medical decision making. Gerontologist 1990;30:65–71.
16. Moody HR. Ethics in an aging society. Baltimore: Johns Hopkins University Press, 1992.
17. Agich GJ. Autonomy in long-term care. New York: Oxford University Press, 1993.
18. Lidz CW, Fischer L, Arnold RM. The erosion of autonomy in long-term care. New York: Oxford University Press, 1992.
19. Collopy BJ. Autonomy in long-term care: some crucial distinctions. Gerontologist 1988;28:10–17 (suppl).
20. Collopy BJ. Ethical dimensions of autonomy in long-term care. Generations 1990;14:9–12 (suppl).
21. Selig S, Tomlinson T, Hickey T. Ethical dimensions of intergenerational reciprocity: implications for practice. Gerontologist 1991;31:624–630.
22. Wetle TT, Levkoff S, Wikel JC, Rosen A. Nursing home resident participation in medical decisions: perceptions and preferences. Gerontologist 1988; 28:32–38 (suppl).
23. Sabatino CP. Client rights, regulations and the autonomy of home care consumers. Generations 1990; 14:21–24 (suppl).
24. Wetle TT, Crabtree B. Balancing safety and autonomy: defining and living with acceptable risk. Gerontologist 1991;31:237 (abstr).
25. Kivnick HQ. Client values: perceptions, preferences, and what difference do they make? Gerontologist 1991;31:237 (abstr).
26. Farran CJ, Keane-Hagerty E, Salloway S, Kupfere S, Wilken C. Finding meaning: an alternative paradigm for Alzheimer's disease family caregivers. Gerontologist 1991;31:483–489.
27. Kane RA. Type and frequency of ethical issues facing publicly subsidized case managers in long-term care. Gerontologist 1991;31:237 (abstr).
28. Kaufman SR, Becker G. Content and boundaries of medicine in long-term care: Physicians talk about stroke. Gerontologist 1991;31:238–245.
29. Eustis NN, Fischer LR. Relationships between home care clients and their workers: implications for quality care. Gerontologist 1991;31:447–456.
30. McCullough LB, Wilson NL, Teasdale TA, Kolpakchi AL, Skelly JR. Mapping personal, familial, and professional values in long-term care decisions. Gerontologist 1993;33:324–332.
31. Stone RS, Catetera GL, Sangl J. Caregivers of frail elderly: a national profile. Gerontologist 1987; 27:616–626.
32. Patton MQ. Qualitative evaluation and research methods. 2nd ed. London: Sage Publications, 1990.

61/ Advance Directives

Laurence B. McCullough, David J. Doukas, Warren L. Holleman,
Rebecca B. Reilly

Most physicians who treat older patients know what advance directives are: the living will and the durable power of attorney for health care. While conceived and introduced into American medicine as legal instruments to effect and protect patient's choices about end-of-life care, advance directives can also serve as preventive ethics tools for the physician in geriatric practice caring for patients at the ends of their lives. This is particularly the case when advance directives are well understood by all parties: the physician; the patient; the patient's family; the physician's professional colleagues; and health care institutions, particularly hospitals and nursing homes. The purpose of this chapter is to provide the physician with an ethically justified, practical approach to the use of advance directives, which is designed to anticipate and prevent the ethical conflicts that can occur in association with them.

Accordingly, the legal development and ethical significance of the living will and durable power of attorney are explained first. Then some of the ethical conflicts that can be associated with advance directives are considered. Finally, a stepwise preventive ethics approach to advance directives in clinical practice is presented.

LEGAL DEVELOPMENT AND ETHICAL SIGNIFICANCE OF ADVANCE DIRECTIVES

Advance directives have become so commonplace in the thinking of most physicians, though not yet in their practices, that we sometimes forget the legal and ethical rationales for their invention (1). These origins are important to remember because they help the physician to appreciate both the power and the limitations of these legal documents.

THE LEGAL RIGHT OF SELF-DETERMINATION

The story begins at the turn of the century, in the common law of informed consent, which de-

veloped as part of malpractice law. In a landmark case decided by the highest court of the State of New York in 1914, *Schloendorff v. Society of New York Hospital* (2), Justice Cardozo applied the fundamental legal doctrine of self-determination to informed consent.

Every person of adult years and sound mind has the right to determine what shall be done to his body, and a surgeon who performs an operation without the patient's consent commits an assault.

The only exception that the New York Court of Appeals allowed was for emergencies: the patient's life is in immediate peril and there is no time in which to obtain consent. The point of informed consent as a legal requirement has been clear since *Schloendorff*. Each adult patient is presumed competent and as such has the right to control what is done or not done for him or her. Consent may be granted or withheld entirely according to the patient's values and preferences.

THE LEGAL RIGHT OF PRIVACY

The story continues with the well-known ruling of the United States Supreme Court on abortion in 1973. *Roe v. Wade* (3) and cases that preceded it established that there is a constitutional protection of privacy and that this constitutional protection extends to the physician-patient relationship. Privacy creates a zone or area of thought, speech, and behavior into which the government may not intrude unless there is compelling reason to do so. Privacy thus creates a zone of noninterference around the physician-patient relationship into which the state may not intrude without sufficiently compelling reasons. The burden of proof is on the state, because there is a presumption in favor of privacy. The state may, for example, intrude into privacy to protect life—of the individual (out of a paternalism known as *par-*

ens patriae, the state as one's parent) or of others (e.g., to protect them from serious harm).

The interest of the state in protecting life is based on the Fourteenth Amendment to the United States Constitution, which prohibits the taking of life, liberty, or property of persons without due process of law. The state may also intrude into privacy when criminal matters are at stake. (In *Roe* the Supreme Court found that the fetus is not a person in the meaning of the term in constitutional law and so is not accorded protection by the Fourteenth Amendment before viability. Hence, abortion before viability is a protected exercise of a privacy right by the pregnant woman in consultation with her physician.)

When the case of Ms. Karen Ann Quinlan, known as *In Re Quinlan* (4) reached the Supreme Court of New Jersey, the court had the tools of legal self-determination (expressed through informed consent) and of privacy with which to analyze and decide the case. Ms. Quinlan suffered two prolonged episodes of anoxia of unknown origin, was resuscitated by a rescue team, was hospitalized, and subsequently was in persistent vegetative state. Inasmuch as she was an adult, her father petitioned the court for guardianship of her person for the purpose of requesting that ventilatory support be discontinued. He understood that if his request were implemented, his daughter would most likely die rather than breathe on her own. The lower courts denied his request, but the Supreme Court of New Jersey granted it.

Portions of that court's reasoning are crucial for the physician to understand. The court first asked itself, in effect, if it could decide this case on the basis of informed consent and legal self-determination. If Ms. Quinlan had made statements in the past that effectively refused such things as ventilators later, then those earlier statements should bind her physicians in the present. That is, self-determination could be exercised in advance, in the form of informed refusal of life-prolonging intervention. In Ms. Quinlan's case the New Jersey court ruled that her prior statements were not specific enough to count as advance informed refusal. But the court implied that clear specific statements by competent adults in advance of becoming incompetent might indeed be binding.

The court then turned to the constitutional right of privacy, based on *Roe* and cases that had preceded it in the federal courts, as well as the New Jersey state constitution's provisions on the right to privacy. Three reasons for justified state intrusion into privacy were considered and rejected by the New Jersey Supreme Court.

The first was the state's legitimate interest in the preservation of life, based in the Fourteenth Amendment. Privacy would have to give way before an interest in the preservation of Ms. Quinlan's life. Did the state have such an interest? No, reasoned the court, because Ms. Quinlan's prognosis was very poor and her treatment was very invasive. Her prognosis was considered to be very poor because she was not expected to recover to a cognitive, sapient state. The treatment was considered to be very invasive because she was receiving 24-hour intensive nursing care, ventilatory support, intravenous antibiotics, a catheter, and a feeding tube.

The court's second consideration was the ethical integrity of medicine. Would it be an unconscionable violation of medical ethics to disconnect Ms. Quinlan's ventilator? No, the court reasoned, because there were already arguments in the medical literature that it is not the physician's ethical obligation to preserve life without exception.

The court's third consideration was whether discontinuation of her ventilator would involve either Ms. Quinlan's physicians or her hospital in criminal behavior. No, the court reasoned, because withdrawal of the ventilator would not constitute killing. Ms. Quinlan would die from irreversible respiratory failure secondary to massive, irreversible central nervous system injury. Thus, this is not a matter of suicide or homicide. (The court added that even if homicide were involved, it would not be unlawful given the collapse of the state's interest in preserving the life of a patient who is in persistent vegetative state.)

Ms. Quinlan's privacy rights thus prevailed in the court's reasoning. There was one remaining problem to address. She could not exercise those rights herself. To be meaningful, the court reasoned, her rights would have to be exercised *for* her, since they could not be exercised *by* her. Mr. Quinlan could play this role because he had shown himself convincingly to be a suitable guardian. The court makes no mention of whether Mr. Quinlan would do what his daughter would have wanted; the court satisfied itself only that Mr. Quinlan was trustworthy.

THE CONTRAST BETWEEN THE RIGHTS OF SELF-DETERMINATION AND PRIVACY

Here emerges a crucial dimension of the constitutional right of privacy. Each of us retains the right to privacy despite even the irreversible loss of the capacity to make our own decisions. Others can exercise our privacy rights for us, because they are trustworthy, not necessarily because they would exercise our privacy rights as we would.

By contrast, self-determination, as the basis for advance decision making about life-prolonging intervention, would require that others exercising my right exercise it as I would, or as close to what I would as possible. This distinction becomes clear in other cases such as *Satz v. Perlmutter* (5) in which the court affirmed the right of self-determination of any competent, adult patient to refuse any medical intervention, even if his or her life would end as a result. *Satz* makes it clear that self-determination is a far more powerful right than the right of privacy, because no interest of the state, presumably, is stronger than a citizen's legal right of self-determination. In summary, the common law of refusing intervention, even when death is expected to result from doing so, is based on an interesting admixture of privacy and self-determination.

THE LIVING WILL

The *Quinlan* case was followed rapidly by legislation to codify into statute a right to refuse in advance of a time when one was no longer competent to refuse life-prolonging intervention for terminal illness. California was the first to enact such legislation, in 1976, and now almost all states have such legislation. (6) These statutes are based on an amalgam—not well worked out in the statutes—of self-determination, privacy, and the state's interest in preserving life.

Self-determination is obviously the basis of an individual's projecting a decision to refuse medical intervention into the future as binding on physicians and institutions. But, the limitation to terminal illness of living will or natural death acts reflects a right to privacy tempered by the state's interest in the preservation of life. In addition, many states also exclude pregnant women from the applicability of living wills, a provision that clearly reflects an interest in preserving life. (To the authors' knowledge, no challenge to this limitation of the scope of the statute has been reported in those states.)

The state's interest in the preservation of life is even more obviously expressed in the provision for revocation of the living will. Typically, only competent adult patients may execute a living will but, statutes make no provision for *competently* revoking a living will. Anyone may revoke a living will at any time, e.g., by tearing it up or verbally negating it. This provision of living will statutes makes sense only on the assumption that the statute expresses the legislature's interest in preserving life when in doubt. As was stated in *Quinlan,* the state does have a legitimate interest in the preservation of life.

Living will laws also provide criminal and civil immunity for physicians and institutions who carry out a valid living will in which no malpractice occurs. To the authors' knowledge, there are no reported cases challenging this protection anywhere. This indicates very wide acceptance of living wills.

Living will legislation has evolved over the past 18 years. Initially, the definition of terminal illness in legislation applied to classic instances of terminal illness, such as terminal cancers. Ironically, the initial definitions of terminal illness did not include persistent vegetative states. Some states' definitions of terminal illness reflect this evolution toward a broader scope of diagnoses, and others some do not. Physicians should familiarize themselves with the definition of terminal illness in relevant statutes for their jurisdiction. The federal government recognizes the living will as well, in Veterans Affairs institutions. The VA policy includes persistent vegetative state as a terminal illness.

The living will, then, is an expression of informed refusal before the patient is terminally ill as defined by relevant statute (or VA policy) and has lost decision-making capacity. The latter is a clinical judgment, to be made according to prevailing standards of reasonable clinical judgment. No adjudication of incompetence by a court is required by living will statutes.

States vary according to whether the patient's declaration or living will must be written. In addition, states vary on whether a written or oral declaration must take a particular form. Almost all states allow the patient to list and attach explicit treatment preferences to a living will. In addition, most states provide for the exercise of the rights to refuse for patients without living wills, usually by family members listed by priority. Physicians should familiarize themselves with the provisions of the relevant statute and Veterans Affairs policies and procedures.

DURABLE POWER OF ATTORNEY FOR HEALTH CARE

As experience was gained with living wills, a concern arose that the scope of informed refusal that living wills sanctioned was not broad enough. There were clinical situations in which the patient was not necessarily terminally ill but was not competent, and it was questioned whether aggressive management is what the patient would have wanted. Usually the patient's wishes would be represented by family members. While it has long been customary to ask family members for permission in such cases, the legal sanctions for this custom were indeed scant.

For many years common and statutory law allowed for durable power of attorney. Power of attorney is the assignment of certain powers to others, e.g., to dispose of jointly owned property in the physical absence of one of the owners. Power of attorney does not persist beyond that individual's loss of decision-making capacity. A simple power of attorney is by definition not durable. Hence, the durable power of attorney was invented precisely to permit the conveyance of one's legal powers to another upon one's loss of capacity to make decisions. The durable power of attorney for health care permits the conveyance to another, the "agent," of one's powers to make health care decisions upon one's loss of decision-making capacity. As with living wills, the loss of decision-making capacity is a clinical judgment, to be made in accordance with prevailing standards of reasonable medical judgment. Adjudication of incompetence by a court is not required.

The legal rationale of durable powers of attorney is clearly founded in legal self-determination. Some states, however, have legislated limits on situations in which the agent may exercise powers of decision making, including pregnancy, involuntary admission to a psychiatric facility, and the authorization of electroconvulsive shock therapy. To the authors' knowledge, there is no reported case of legal challenge, especially for wrongful death, against a physician or hospital who has let a patient die subsequent to the decision by an agent holding a legally valid durable power of attorney.

THE LIVING WILL AND DURABLE POWER OF ATTORNEY FOR HEALTH CARE CONTRASTED

Notice that for a durable power of attorney to take effect, *only the loss of decision-making capacity* is required. There is no requirement, as there is in living wills, that the individual also be terminally ill.

There are other important differences between the living will and the durable power of attorney. The former can be used only to refuse life-prolonging intervention. The latter can be used just as informed consent can be used, either to *request* or to *refuse* any intervention. The living will stands alone as representative of the patient's preferences, whereas a durable power of attorney

is carried out by the patient's agent. The living will presupposes that the patient has adequate knowledge as to what is to be withheld. The agent holding durable power of attorney is supposed to know which alternatives are available to manage the patient's condition, as well as the patient's values and preferences (to the extent possible).

THE PATIENT SELF-DETERMINATION ACT

The final piece of the legal puzzle is the Patient Self-Determination Act of 1990, which took effect in December 1991 (6). A parallel policy for Veterans Affairs institutions took effect in 1992. This federal statute grew out of the case of Ms. Nancy Beth Cruzan of Missouri, decided by the United States Supreme Court in 1990 (7). Ms. Cruzan had been in a severe automobile accident that left her in a persistent vegetative state, supported by gastrostomy tube feedings. Her parents requested that this form of life support be discontinued, on the basis that this is not what Ms. Cruzan would have wanted, based on previous conversations with her.

The original trial court agreed that the state's clear and convincing standard of evidence (75% probability of correctness) was satisfied by the evidence introduced about Ms. Cruzan's prior statements. On appeal to the Missouri Supreme Court, this decision was reversed on the grounds that this evidentiary standard had not been met. The matter was appealed to the U.S. Supreme Court, challenging Missouri's evidentiary standard as an unconstitutional infringement on the rights to privacy and self-determination. A majority of the Court (expressed in several opinions) held that Missouri's evidentiary standard was not unconstitutional. One opinion adopted the legal right of informed refusal, "for the purposes of this case," an ambiguous endorsement of the doctrine of informed consent in these matters as it has developed in the common law of the various states.

The effect of the Court's ruling was that Missouri and the one other state with such a provision for clear and convincing evidence about prior statements and preferences at the time (New York) could retain that provision. The Supreme Court did not require the states to set such an evidentiary standard for evidence about the prior wishes of individuals without living wills or durable power of attorney. The case was reheard, her parents' original request was granted, and the attorney general of Missouri declined to appeal the new decision.

Senator John Danforth of Missouri introduced into the federal legislature the Patient Self-Determination Act in 1990, which was successfully attached to the Omnibus Budget Reconciliation Act of that year (8). This law aims to reduce the number of situations in which patients do not have advance directives by requiring HMOs and institutions that receive federal monies to notify their patients on admission (or enrollment in the case of HMOs) about their rights under relevant state law to execute an advance directive. The law also requires documentation of the patient's advance directives. In addition, patients are to be notified about their rights of informed consent generally. Finally, among other provisions, the law also requires hospitals to have policies on these matters, to notify patients that there are such policies, to provide information to patients about those policies, and to provide education to the professional staff and community of the institution about advance directives. Physicians should familiarize themselves with the policies and practices of the institutions in which they provide care to geriatric patients.

The physician should *not* assume that the Patient Self-Determination Act solves the problem of patients not having advance directives. The main weakness of this federal law is that discussions with newly admitted patients may be hindered by such factors as time constraints, distractions, disorientation, fear, pain, serious illness, or diminished cognitive capacity. Ironically, this law would not have helped Ms. Cruzan, because it will not help any patient who arrives at the emergency department of a hospital suffering from a loss of decision-making capacity. Physicians should assume that they bear significant responsibility for discussing advance directives with patients in the *outpatient* setting and for anticipating and seeking to prevent ethical conflicts that can arise in association with advance directives.

ETHICAL PROBLEMS WITH ADVANCE DIRECTIVES

Despite their many benefits, advance directives have highlighted and, in some instances, created a number of ethical problems for physicians, patients, and their families. These problems are now well enough understood that they can be anticipated and prevented in the clinical setting.

The first is that physicians are reluctant to ask patients their preferences regarding end-of-life care. This reluctance may be due to fears of offending the patient, time constraints, or the physician's own discomfort with the subject of death. Patients want to discuss these matters, but appear to be waiting for physicians to initiate the discussion. One study of patients who had not discussed end-of-life preferences with their physicians indicated that 68% wanted the physician to raise the issue, and that only 11% did not. In all age groups, most patients considered it important for physicians and patients to discuss this matter, regardless of the patient's health status (9–11).

A second problem is that patients may not realize that not having advance directives may be harmful to their interests. In the absence of advance directives, decisions might be made other than those the patient would have preferred. In addition, decisions might be made by persons other than those who know the patient well, whom the patient trusts, or who have the patient's interests at heart. The patient's family sometimes disagrees over how aggressively to manage the patient's condition. Sometimes there are no family members available. In these situations the physician must make a judgment, which can be difficult to do with confidence when the physician is not acquainted with the patient's values and preferences. In one study in which patients were asked their preferences regarding end-of-life care and in which their physicians were then interviewed to determine whether the physicians could predict which treatments their patients preferred, the physician's accuracy was no greater than chance would have predicted. This result is particularly alarming, given that the overwhelming majority of patients (90%) predicted that their wishes would be represented accurately by their physicians (12).

Third, the living will lacks specificity. Typically, statutes refer to the withdrawal of mechanical or other artificial means of support. Linda and Ezekiel Emanuel have proposed the "Medical Directive" (13) and the "Health Care Directive" (14) to address this problem. These documents, however, involve multiple scenarios and many decisions. The clinical applicability of such documents is limited by their cumbersome and complicated nature. Doubts have also been raised about their empirical adequacy (15). These points, in the authors' judgment, are well taken: the lack of specificity must be addressed, without abandoning utility and simplicity.

Fourth, proxy decision-makers vary in their ability to reflect accurately the patient's preferences. Researchers presenting decision-making scenarios to patients and their proxies found that, in many of the scenarios, almost as many proxies got it wrong as got it right (9, 10, 16, 17). The physician should advise the patient to select individual(s) who know the patient well and who have the equanimity, wisdom, and courage to make appropriate decisions in stressful situations. (Incidentally, the physician should also advise the patient to pick one or two alternate agents for durable power of attorney for health care, should the first-named agent not be available.) Concordance between proxy decision-makers and the patient's prior preferences should not be assumed by the physician.

One reason that the proxy often does not know the patient's wishes is that the patient did not discuss the matter with the proxy or provide written instructions. A fifth ethical problem raised by advance directives, then, is how aggressively the physician should attempt to persuade patients to communicate to the proxy their preferences, beliefs, and values regarding suffering, pain, death, and end-of-life care. In some cases the patient might decline to provide instructions out of trust and deference to the agent named to make decisions. This is certainly a valid exercise of the patient's autonomy. Patients might not provide instruction because they do not want to address the questions involved, preferring to leave these matters to the agents they identified. Finally, the patient might not provide instruction because the institution's forms do not provide space for doing so. Many standard documents used to designate durable power of attorney for health care contain space for instructions, but this space can be very limited. The Veterans Affairs policy provides an entire form specifically for this purpose.

Sixth, patients may write instructions or make oral statements in association with a living will or durable power of attorney that strike the physician as unreasonable, inappropriate, or involving the physician in substandard care. These may be requests either for treatment or against treatment. Aggressive management does not make sense in all cases any more than nonaggressive management does. A particularly troublesome situation is caused when the patient's agent requests that "everything be done" for a patient who has suffered severe and irreversible brain damage. To respond accordingly would require the physician to provide care that conferred no benefit and perhaps only harm on the patient, and certainly a harm to other patients who might have benefitted from more appropriate use of scarce medical resources.

This was precisely the situation confronted by the physicians caring for Ms. Helga Wanglie (18, 19), who elected to seek resolution through the hospital ethics committee and—unsuccessfully—the court in response to a request from the patient's husband that everything be done. Such solutions seldom satisfy any of the parties involved.

It is far better to address these problems with patients before they lose their capacity to decide, before medical crises arise, and before ethical conflicts become refractory. The physician should review the patient's living will and instructions to the patient's agent and, if any unreasonable or inappropriate requests are found, discuss them with the patient without delay. Such discussion might reveal that the request is rooted in the patient's anxiety, depression, guilt, religious fear, financial uncertainty, or a failure in the physician-patient relationship such as miscommunication or mistrust. If the physician addresses these underlying problems preventively—in a way consistent with respect for the patient's autonomy—the patient may be persuaded to alter the inappropriate request.

Seventh, patients and their families sometimes overstate what their religious convictions require of them in preventing death. The Western religious traditions, which include Judaism, Christianity, and Islam, view human life as sacred and view failure to show reverence for human life as the most egregious of sins. Thus, in the Western religious traditions there is a strong taboo against suicide. In Dante's *Inferno* (canto XIII), for example, people who committed suicide are considered worse than murderers, worse even than serpents. Some patients and families feel obligated to insist on aggressive management until the moment of death, believing that doing anything less might be a form of suicide. The physician can help terminally ill patients and their families by reminding them of the limits of medical science and of human life as well. Failing to "do everything" is not the equivalent of suicide or murder in those cases where nothing medically can be done to extend life or where extending life only artificially prolongs the moment of death. Refusals to accept death at this stage might be rooted less in religious factors than in psychological factors such as denial or guilt or in misunderstandings caused by the physician's failure to communicate that death is imminent. The physician who addresses these factors preventively will have a greater success in preparing patients and their families to face death. If religious objections persist, however, the physician should consider consulting the patient's religious adviser, who can address the patient's religious fears about death and attempt to clear up theological misperceptions about the "sinfulness" of accepting death. Such consultations sometimes reveal that the religious adviser has misunderstood the seriousness of the patient's illness and has been inappropriately advising the patient to "fight" the illness.

Once the physician and religious adviser are on the same clinical page, there is much greater likelihood that they can together help the patient and the patient's family face death.

Eighth, the physician's professional colleagues may have difficulty with particular strategies for permitting patients to die, the withdrawal of nutritional support in particular. Some take the view that withdrawal of nutritional support is tantamount to murder and suicide, that the cause of death becomes starvation rather than the illness itself, and that nutrition and hydration are not medicines that the physician prescribes to persons in their capacity as patients but rather are sustenance that patients should receive by virtue of their humanity. Justice Scalia articulated such a view in the *Cruzan* decision (7), and Ms. Quinlan's parents expressed a similar view in their decision to continue providing nutrition to their daughter after withdrawing her from ventilatory support, despite receiving the "permission" of Roman Catholic theologians to withhold nutrition and fluids (20). The courts that have examined this matter, however, have uniformly ruled that nutritional support is the same as any other nursing or medical intervention and that its withdrawal is, like that of a ventilator, not a killing—thus extending the reasoning of the *Quinlan* court (21–23).

The ninth ethical problem is that the patient's family members and loved ones may have objections to the patient's decisions as expressed in advance directives. The worst time for conflicts about such matters is after the patient has lost decision-making capacity. It is far better to help patients identify and deal with potential problems within their family before those decisions are to be implemented, and give the family time either to accept them or—at the very least—respect them. If this approach fails, however, the physician is obliged to honor the patient's living will, despite the objections of the family. The authors have, unfortunately, encountered situations in which the physician shirked this responsibility. The express wishes of the patient are to be respected by all parties, and the physician has an important role in educating family members, particularly by setting an example of respect for the patient's wishes and encouraging and expecting recalcitrant family members to follow the example.

Tenth, an advance directive is not a physician's order. When advance directives apply, they need to be translated directly into physician's orders that reflect and implement the patient's preferences. These orders should be explicit, compre-hensive, and well-publicized among appropriate professional staff and colleagues: No professional caring for the patient should have any doubt about just what is and is not to be done when life-threatening events occur.

The eleventh is that the physician's obligations do not end with writing orders for nonaggressive management. There are substantive ethical obligations to the dying and their families. The patient is owed appropriate management of pain, symptoms, suffering, and respect for dignity. The family is owed assurance and support that the patient's wishes are being carried out and that, therefore, everything that ought to have been done was indeed done and done in a professional and caring manner. In this way, family members are given good memories of their loved one to sustain them in their loss.

The twelfth problem involves misconceptions that patients, families, and some physicians can have about the applicability of living wills to reversible illness and injuries in which death is not imminent. Some persons may be afraid to sign a living will for fear that aggressive management might be withheld in acute, nonterminal situations. The physician should assure such patients that the living will applies only to terminally ill patients. On the other hand, some patients might make too strong and general a statement such as "I don't want ever to be put on machines." The physician should inform such patients that there are situations in which a trial of mechanical support could save their life and return them to their previous state of health and quality of life or something close to these.

A thirteenth problem involves the potential for abuse by proxy decision-makers and other family members or friends who might inappropriately benefit from a premature death or a prolonged life. For example, family members have been known to request that patients in a persistent vegetative state be kept on life supports, not to benefit the patient but to benefit themselves, for example, from continuing to receive pension checks. The physician should be willing to challenge proxy decision-makers who appear to be acting from interests other than those of the patient. If individual confrontations fail to achieve results based on the patient's interests, then the physician should involve the institution's ethics committee and, if necessary, the courts. One safeguard against such abuse is that family members, potential heirs, and creditors are not allowed to witness the signing of the durable power of attorney for health care.

A PREVENTIVE ETHICS STRATEGY FOR ADVANCE DIRECTIVES

The thirteen potential ethical conflicts discussed above usually occur because the physician waits too long to involve the patient in decision making. Such decisions should be discussed in the outpatient setting, well in advance of hospitalization or admission to a nursing home. If the patient is willing, the family should also be involved, so that they will know, understand, respect, and support the patient's decisions. There are administrative steps that can encourage this process. In the clinic in which one of the authors (WH) serves as consultant, a letter explaining advance directives is given to all patients as they sign in with the receptionist (Table 61.1).

Advance directives are displayed in the waiting room, the nurses' station, and in the examining rooms. Records of conversations and copies of advance directives are part of the patients' charts.

For those patients who make it to the hospital or nursing home without advance directives, the response of the physician's institutions to the Patient Self-Determination Act should not be presumed to be sufficient. Discharge planning should be used as an additional setting in which decision making can be initiated, in anticipation of readmission. Discussion of advance directives with all geriatric patients—in the outpatient setting, at discharge planning, as well as at admission—should be regarded as the ethical standard of care. Too many ethical conflicts continue to occur because physicians are not initiating conversations with geriatric patients about advance directives. The primary clinical task, therefore, is to prevent such conflicts, particularly those discussed above.

The authors propose an eight-step preventive ethics strategy for advance directives (Table 61.2). This strategy is based on years of addressing ethical conflicts and recognizing that they are often preventable. These steps will take time, but they will be cost-beneficial in the time, stress, and ethical conflicts that they can prevent for the physician, for patients, for patients' families and loved ones, for institutions, and for society. In addition, they are likely to conserve financial and medical resources by reducing the amount of aggressive management provided to terminally ill patients.

First, the physician should explain that there are two forms of advance directives and that they serve different purposes and take effect under dif-

Table 61.1
Letter Concerning Advance Directives

Dear Patient:

On December 1, 1991 a new law, "The Patient Self-Determination Act," went into effect. Under that law, if you are admitted to a hospital for any reason, you will be asked if you have an "Advance Directive." If not, you will be provided information about advance directives and encouraged to write one. There are several types of advance directives, but the ones most commonly used are called "Durable Power of Attorney for Health Care" and "Living Will" (or, "Directive to Physicians").

A Durable Power of Attorney for Health Care enables you to specify in advance the person you wish to make medical decisions for you, should you become seriously ill and unable to communicate.

A Living Will ("Directive to Physicians") tells your doctors how you want to be treated should you lose your ability to communicate. If, for example, you suffered a severe stroke or a serious head injury from which you were not expected to recover, would you want to be kept alive on a breathing machine? Or would you prefer simply to be kept comfortable and allow nature to take its course? You can indicate such preferences through the use of Living Wills.

Thinking about these things is not easy, but the best way to assure that your wishes are honored is to express them in advance. As physicians at the Baylor Family Practice Center we encourage all patients, regardless of your age or health status, to take the time to consider advance directives. We suggest that, instead of waiting until you are admitted to a hospital, that you do it now. We hope you will discuss this matter with your loved ones and with your family physician at your next visit. *Materials are available from the brochure rack in the reception area or from your nurse.*

As your family physicians our goal has always been to serve you as best we can. You can help us serve you by expressing your wishes clearly.

Sincerely,

Your Baylor Family Physicians

Table 61.2
A Preventive Ethics Strategy for Advance Directives

1. Explain the different types of advance directives (living will and durable power of attorney for health care) and review completed patients' directives for inconsistencies or unreasonable preferences.
2. Describe interventions used to respond to life-threatening events.
3. Involve religious adviser when appropriate and with patient's consent.
4. Ask patients if anyone in their family might have problems with their preferences, and address family members' concerns.
5. Be wary of using the term withdrawing "care."
6. Ask where the patient keeps originals of advance directives, record directives in patient's chart, and distribute copies.
7. Ask yourself if any colleagues have objections to the patient's preferences and address colleagues' concerns.
8. When the advance directives apply clinically, write an order that expresses and implements the patient's preferences. These orders should always address pain and symptom relief and maintenance of dignity.

ferent conditions. The living will can be used by patients only to refuse treatment in advance of the time that they are both terminally ill (as defined in relevant state law or VA policy) and found in reasonable clinical judgment to have lost the capacity for making their own decisions. The physician should be clear with the patient about whether applicable law defines persistent vegetative state as a terminal illness. If it does not, the patient is well advised to consider executing a durable power of attorney explicitly to cover this possible outcome of disease or hospitalization.

The durable power of attorney for health care can be used by patients to assign to someone else (usually called the patient's "agent") the power to make decisions for them when, in reasonable clinical judgment, they have lost the capacity to make their own decisions. The patient need not also be terminally ill, as is the case for living wills. If relevant statutes exclude certain conditions or situations (e.g., electroshock convulsive therapy), these exclusions should be made clear to the patient.

The physician should review the patient's instructions on the durable power of attorney document. If these instructions are unclear or clearly unreasonable or difficult to implement, this should be explained, so that patients can clarify their intentions and preferences. For example, a request that everything be done may not make sense for a patient who is irreversibly dying despite aggressive management that results, on balance, only in unnecessary pain and suffering. Such an outcome is justifiably regarded as unreasonable in beneficence-based clinical ethical judgment and this should be explained to the patient. All alternatives should be reviewed so that the patient's preferences do not lead later to conflict with beneficence-based clinical ethical judgment. If the patient persists in providing instructions

that the physician finds unreasonable to the point of not being able in conscience to carry them out, the physician should refer the patient to a colleague willing to carry out those instructions and then withdraw from the patient's care.

Any conversations between the patient and the agent, to which the physician is witness, should be recorded in the patient's chart. This record can serve as an important reference point later, when particular decisions need to be made.

For patients who have executed a living will and durable power of attorney for health care, both documents should be reviewed for instructions that might lead to clinically contradictory courses. Potential conflicts (e.g., between having a living will and an instruction on the durable power of attorney to "do everything") should be pointed out, and the patient's preference for the management of such conflict elicited. The patient should be asked to draft new documents if necessary, and the physician should record such preferences in the patient's record.

Second, the patient should be provided with a frank description of the kinds of intervention that are used in aggressive management of life-threatening events, especially critical care interventions. The physician should briefly but accurately describe such interventions as intubation and support by mechanical ventilation, cardiopulmonary resuscitation, admission to the critical care unit, and the administration of medication, fluid, and nutrition by peripheral and central lines as well as nasogastric and PEG tubes. Both the short- and long-term consequences should be discussed, including the probability of implementing the patient's preferences given the patient's present and future expected health status. Patients with chronic diseases need to appreciate that life-threatening events usually accelerate the process of decline, and aggressive management followed by survival usually leaves the patient with a lower baseline than before the event.

It is especially important that the concept of trial of intervention be discussed with the patient. Increasingly, aggressive management is undertaken on a trial basis, to determine whether it will benefit the patient, and stopped if it becomes clear that it is no longer doing so. Recent research indicates that patients who want aggressive management accept the concept of a trial and prefer it over a strategy of always doing everything (25). In particular, the physician should explain to the patient and the patient's family that admission to the intensive care unit is a trial of intervention. Indeed, such a trial is usually necessary because it is still quite difficult to predict which patients will benefit from intensive care admission.

Third, many patients make health care decisions on the basis of their religious beliefs, traditions, and convictions (25). Patients often turn to religious advisers for help in making decisions about advance directives. When they do, the religious adviser should not be offering advice in a vacuum. With the patient's permission, therefore, the religious adviser should be provided with the information described in the previous two steps. In addition, the physician should be aware that most faith communities do not make it obligatory to resist death at all costs. Rather, moral theological views tend to recognize limits to what medicine can and should accomplish. Patients sometimes may not be aware of this and so may overestimate what their faith requires of them. If a patient or a religious adviser insists that his or her faith requires that everything be done, this should be discussed with them frankly, apprising them of the prospects of success and the cost in unnecessary morbidity, pain, and suffering to the patient and the patient's family of doing so. The religious adviser should be asked to consider carefully all of the clinical information that he or she now has and reconsider the advice earlier given to the patient or the patient's family.

Fourth, patients should be asked whether they anticipate that anyone in their family may have concerns, problems, or objections regarding the decisions in their advance directives. A patient, for example, may prefer to name an adult son or daughter as agent, rather than his or her spouse. The patient's spouse may be unaware of this preference. The physician should offer the patient the opportunity to meet with family members, so that these preferences and decisions can be explained. The physician can point out that family members have an ethical obligation to respect the patient's choices. Adult children, especially, need to be

made aware of and to avoid role reversal, taking over decision making as if the patient were now a child and the adult children were now parents of the patient.

Fifth, the physician should beware of ever using the language of withdrawing or withholding "care." *Caring* for patients, especially for patients who are dying, should never be withdrawn. All patients remain members of the moral community until their deaths. Caring for patients also includes diligent attention to, and management of, unnecessary pain and protection of the patient's dignity (26). The patient's suffering can be alleviated by addressing such symptoms as nausea, dyspnea, and shortness of breath.

Sixth, ask patients where they keep originals of their advance directives and who has copies. The physician—with the patient's consent—should be sure that there are copies of the patient's directives in the patient's office records, the hospital records, the nursing home's records, and with family members. In particular, the physician should be certain that the emergency department of the patient's hospital has copies of these directives.

Seventh, physicians should ask themselves and inquire among colleagues—especially nursing colleagues, as well as trainees—if any one has concerns, problems, or objections to the patient's advance directives. Some individuals may object to withdrawal or withholding of nutrition as a form of killing by starvation.

There are two responses to this sort of objection. If the patient is being supported by interventions in addition to nutritional support (e.g., a ventilator, antibiotics, or pressor drugs), one or more of these could be discontinued to allow the patient to die comfortably. This response is very useful in the case of patients on multiple life supports, because it does not require that colleagues participate in what they may judge in conscience to be killing by starvation. The second response applies when nutritional support is the main or sole intervention that is preventing the patient's death. This is frequently the case for patients in a persistent vegetative state. Not everyone accepts the explanation that death subsequent to discontinuation of nutritional support is caused by metabolic decline and immune system failure secondary to irreversible central nervous system injury or disease. As noted above, at least one member of the United States Supreme Court does not, namely, Justice Scalia in his opinion in *Cruzan*. Since there is no conclusive ethical argument that Justice Scalia and those who share his opinion are mistaken, this view should be regarded as reasonable and respected. Such a view, however, cannot be allowed to stand in the way of implementing advance directives, because there is no conclusive argument that withdrawal or withholding of nutrition must be regarded as killing by starvation in all cases. Individual clinicians with Justice Scalia's opinions must respect the patient's preference as also being reasonable, and in conscience they are free to withdraw from the patient's case, but they are not free to block the implementation of an advance directive.

Eighth, having undertaken the previous seven steps the physician is in a position to write an order that implements the patient's advance directive(s). The physician's orders should be comprehensive and clear. The goal is the following: no professional with responsibility for the patient, upon reading the orders, should be unclear or uncertain in any way about what should and should not be done in a life-threatening event. These orders should be readily accessible in the patient's chart, e.g., as a face sheet.

As noted above, there are serious beneficence-based and autonomy-based obligations to dying patients. Chief among these obligations are adequate pain and suffering control and maintenance of dignity. Hence, the physician's orders should in all cases address the management of the patient's pain, symptoms, and suffering and protection of dignity.

Seriously ill patients can tolerate high doses of analgesics, if the level is titrated appropriately (27, 28). Proper pain and symptom management has also been shown to reduce the risk of suicide among seriously ill patients (29). Proper titration of pain medication also minimizes the risk of mortality from aggressive pain and symptom management. Since the patient's death is acceptable in both beneficence-based and autonomy-based clinical judgment, however, risking mortality for the sake of adequate pain and symptom control does not violate beneficence-based clinical ethical judgment. Quality assurance mechanisms should be extended to cover review of pain and suffering management for dying patents, so that these matters can be addressed openly and with institutional sanction. Quality assurance in this matter is essential, given that physicians continue to undertreat pain, despite recent advances in pain management (28, 30).

VALUES AND ADVANCE DIRECTIVES

Executing an advance directive is a weighty matter. In effect, the patient is making decisions about how he or she will die and be remembered by loved ones. Such decisions are obviously freighted with religious beliefs and moral values. Recognition of the importance of discussing values related to advance directives has led investigators to develop an adjunct document known as the "Values History." Because of its clinical importance, the "Values History" is discussed separately, in Chapter 62.

Acknowledgment. The authors wish to acknowledge the research assistance provided by George Khushf, Ph.D., in the preparation of this chapter.

REFERENCES

1. President's Commission for the Study of Ethical Problems in Medicine and Biomedical and Behavioral Research. Deciding to forego life-sustaining treatment: a report on the ethical, medical, and legal issues in treatment decisions. Washington, DC: U.S. Government Printing Office, 1983.
2. Schloendorff v. Society of New York Hospital, 211 N.Y. 125, 126, 105 N.E. 92, 93 (1914).
3. Roe v. Wade, 410 United States Reports 113 (1973).
4. In re Quinlan, 70 NJ 10 (1976).
5. Satz v. Perlmutter, 362 S.2d 160 (Florida District Court of Appeals), 1978).
6. Wolf SM, Boyle P, Callahan D, Fins JJ, Jennings B, Nelson JL, et al. Sources of concern about the patient self-determination act. N Engl J Med 1991; 325:1666–1671.
7. Cruzan v. Director, Missouri Dept. of Health, 111 L Ed 2d 224, 110 SCT 2841 (1990).
8. The Patient Self-Determination Act. 42 U.S.C. Sections 1395 cc and 1396 a Supp. 1991.
9. Lo B, McLeod GA, Saika G. Patient attitudes to discussing life-sustaining treatment. Arch Intern Med 1986;146:1613–1615.
10. Emanuel LL, Barry MJ, Stoeckle JD, Ettelson LM, Emanuel EJ. Advance directives for medical care: a case for greater use. N Engl J Med 1991;324:889–895.
11. Edinger W, Smucker DR. Outpatients' attitudes regarding advance directives. J Fam Pract 1992; 35:650–653.
12. Seckler AB, Meier DE, Mulvihill M, Paris BEC. Substituted judgment: how accurate are proxy predictions? Ann Intern Med 1991;115:92–98.
13. Emanuel LL, Emanuel EJ. The medical directive: a new comprehensive advance care document. JAMA 1989;261:3288–3293.
14. Emanuel L. The health care directive: learning how to draft advance care documents. J Am Geriatr Soc 1991;39:1221–1228.
15. Sachs GA, Cassel CK. The medical directive. JAMA 1990;263:1069–1070.
16. Uhlmann RF, Pearlman RA, Cain KC. Physicians' and spouses' predictions of elderly patients' resuscitation preferences. J Gerontol: Med Sci 1988; 43:M115–M121.
17. Zweibel NR, Cassel CK. Treatment choices at the end of life: a comparison of decisions by older patients and their physician-selected proxies. Gerontologist 1989;29:615–621.
18. Miles SH. The case of Helga Wanglie: a new kind of "right to die" case. N Engl J Med 1991;325:511–515.
19. Rie MA. The limits of a wish. Hastings Cent Rep 1991;21:24–27.

20. Beauchamp TL, Childress JF. Principles of biomedical ethics. 3rd ed. New York: Oxford University Press, 1989:164.

21. In re Conroy, 486 A.2d 1209 (N.J. 1985).

22. Bouvia v. Superior Court, California Reporter, 225 Cal.Rptr. 297 (Cal.App.2 Dist.) (1986).

23. Brophy v. New England Sinai Hospital, Inc., 398 Mass. 417, 498 N.E.2d 626 (1986).

24. Reilly RB, Teasdale TA, McCullough LB. Option of trial in advance directives. Gerontologist 1992; 32:69 (Special Issue 2).

25. Grodin MA. Religious advance directives: the convergence of law, religion, medicine, and public health. Am J Public Health 1993;83:899–903.

26. Wanzer SH, Federman DD, Adelstein MD, Cassel CK, Cassem EH, Cranford RE, et al. The physician's responsibility toward hopelessly ill patients. N Engl J Med 1989;320:844–849.

27. Foley KM. Diagnosis and treatment of cancer pain. In: Holleb AI, Fink DJ, Murphy GP, eds. American Cancer Society textbook of clinical oncology. Atlanta: American Cancer Society, 1991:555–575.

28. Ogle KS, Warren D, Plumb JD. Pain management in advanced cancer. Prim Care 1992;19:793–805.

29. Foley KM. the relationship of pain and symptom management to patient requests for physician-assisted suicide. J Pain Symptom Manage 1991; 6:289–297.

30. Solomon MZ, O'Donnell L, Jennings B, Guilfoy V, Wolf SM, Nolan K, et al. Decisions near the end of life: professional views on life-sustaining treatments. Am J Public Health 1993;83:14–23.

62/ The Values History in Well Elder Care

David J. Doukas, Laurence B. McCullough

The living will and durable power of attorney for health care (DPA/HC) are two legally recognized advance directives that serve valuable functions. Unfortunately, as they are currently conceived and used, these documents pay insufficient attention to the patient's values that justify and give meaning to the patient's decisions in these documents. As a consequence, physicians and proxy decision-makers are not encouraged to elicit and discuss the patient's underlying values, which are useful in understanding the patient's decisions from the patient's point of view and in preventing ethical conflict in end-of-life care. To enhance the preventive ethics dimensions of advance directives, this chapter describes an innovative, supplementary advance directive instrument to the living will and the durable power of attorney for health care, the Values History (1–5).

In the language of ethics, advance directives are intended to enhance the autonomy of patients in making end-of-life decisions about medical interventions (see Chapters 60 and 61). Making such decisions on the basis of one's values is an essential component of patient autonomy (see Chapter 59). The Values History enhances the patient's autonomy in two important ways otherwise not addressed by the living will and DPA/HC. First, the Values History encourages and enables discourse between patient and physician about the patient's values regarding end-of-life treatment. Second, the Values History allows a step-wise informed consent process about individual treatment preferences that explicitly incorporates patient's values.

These two phases of advance directive information allow an important preventive ethics strategy regarding end-of-life care: the use of standard advance directives, complemented by a discussion of values and value-based preferences that can then be used in future circumstances of patient incapacity. The reasoning behind this strategy is that values do correlate with medical treatment preferences and that informed consent to these directives is deficient from the perspective of patient autonomy by not explicitly including discussion of the patient's values (1, 2).

SHORTCOMINGS OF ADVANCE DIRECTIVES AND THE PATIENT SELF-DETERMINATION ACT OF 1990

Following the United States Supreme Court decision in *Cruzan v. Director, Missouri Department of Health* in 1990, the U.S. Congress was prompted into legislative action to help facilitate and encourage patient education about advance directives (7). The Patient Self-Determination Act of 1990 (PSDA) requires all health care institutions that accept Medicare and Medicaid funding (e.g., hospitals, hospice, home health agencies, HMOs) to provide patients information about their rights regarding informed consent and refusal of care and advance directives under applicable state laws (8).

The PSDA includes both an educational component and an opportunity component. The educational component provides information to the patient about informed consent (and refusal), the living will, and the durable power of attorney for health care. The opportunity component provides the patient the occasion to sign a living will or DPA/HC while at a "teachable moment"—upon admission. While these advance directives may indeed be helpful to both patient and health care provider in understanding basic patient preferences toward life-sustaining care, the authors believe that they do not go far enough. In other words, the PSDA does not fully exploit its educational and opportunity components. Moreover, the PSDA does not remedy recognized problems with advance directives (1, 9).

As discussed in Chapter 61, the living will and DPA/HC serve important patient needs by allowing patients to make decisions prospectively about medical intervention, by requiring health provider and family compliance, and by being executable without the requirement of physician or attorney involvement. However, each of these advance directives have shortcomings that require some form of redress if health practitioners are to make sense of them. The living will is vague in elaborating or detailing which medical procedures the patient has refused (9, 10). Misinterpretation has been reported in the literature because of the living wills' lack of detail (9, 10). It is not surprising then that physician interpretation of living wills can affect their opinion on the document's validity in particular circumstances (10).

Likewise, the DPA/HC, while a helpful legal instrument in empowering an agent to make decisions for the patient when the patient lacks decisional capacity, may also fall short for the same reasons. The DPA/HC is limited by the extent to which the agent and patient confer about the patient's values and explicit treatment preferences (1, 11).

The living will and DPA/HC ask the patient to make decisions about end-of-life care without benefit of considering the values upon which such decisions are based. While the living will allows the patient to make a general statement about end-of-life care, explicit preferences (though often allowed by statute) are rarely elicited. Further, the values underlying those preferences may never be discussed.

Neither advance directive obliges the physician to work with the patient prospectively. In particular, the physician has no legal mandate to review the patient's values critical to what is obviously a value-laden decision-making process (12, 13). The PSDA does not require physician involvement in either the education or opportunity phases and applies only to one outpatient setting (the HMO). Indeed, under the PSDA, the physician need have no involvement in the patient's consideration or signing of a living will or DPA/HC. The questions that arise are

- Do patients understand what they have signed?
- Have the patients carefully explored their own values and preferences regarding end-of-life care?
- Have the patients considered how they want to control the circumstances of death?
- Have the patients discussed how they want to be remembered by relatives?
- Most importantly, can the physician write orders that reflect the patient's values?

THE VALUES HISTORY

The limitations of current advance directives led investigators to develop an explicitly value-based advance directive instrument called the

Values History (1–5). While appointing an agent or signing a living will are important first steps, they are not necessarily the most effective method for assuring that patients' autonomous choices will be respected when they are incapacitated in the future. The patients' values and beliefs serve as an important stepping stone for further understanding the basis upon which they executed these advance directives. These values can clarify the reasoning of these directives to the patient's family and physician, while also allowing for elaboration on the reasoning behind more specific treatment preferences. The Values History promotes patient autonomy by eliciting value-based data that can then be used in a myriad of future medical scenarios that cannot readily be addressed by means of a standard advance directive.

Documenting the patient's values helps to contextualize these preferences for future use (in the absence of a known illness). The values in the Values History have been evaluated and statistically correlated with the specific medical interventions in the instrument in several studies (6, 14, 15). In three different empirical studies, significant correlations have been found between patient values and the medical therapies that patients would wish to forgo if they were terminally ill. In a multigenerational study, individuals expressed concerns within their families about avoiding therapies that would burden their family members (14). Similarly, in an outpatient population, patients of all ages were highly concerned about the implications of all forms of end-of-life care in relation to the distress it would cause their families (6). In a study of HIV-infected men, concerns about perceived burden toward themselves as well as the need to be able to communicate with a physician who would implement their wishes was of paramount importance (15).

These findings support the claim that patient values can help the patient, the patient's family, and the physician better understand how to invoke the patient's specific directive preferences in future, unforeseen medical circumstances. This approach allows greater flexibility in the physician's response to the patient's future incapacity by heightening awareness of why patients would prefer or not prefer treatment modalities. These values can then assist the physician in writing orders when the need might later arise for them (in addition to the patient's expressed preferences in the Values History).

The Values History also differs from the living will and DPA/HC in that "trials of intervention" can be articulated for specific treatments (16). The patient can prospectively elect to have an intervention stopped either after a specific time or when reasonable medical judgment shows that it is not expected to benefit the patient and thus merely prolong the patient's dying. This concept of trials of intervention is important in critical care, replacing the "all or nothing" approach (17). Increasingly, aggressive management is undertaken in a trial to see whether it will benefit the patient. Recent research indicates that for those patients preferring aggressive management, the concept of a trial is preferred over the strategy of always doing something (18). Trials of intervention also create the possibility of finding common ground between the patient's values and the physician's values. Identifying a common ground of values is the core strategy of preventive ethics. In particular, patients should understand that admission to the intensive care unit is a trial of intervention used (in the absence of patient refusal) because it is difficult to predict who will benefit from such admission. Existing advance directives do not address this clinical reality, the Values History does. Hence, the Values History as as adjunct to advance directives has considerable clinical utility in preventing ethical conflicts.

THE COMPONENTS OF THE VALUES HISTORY

The Values History (Fig. 62.1) contains two parts: (a) an identification of values and (b) an articulation of advance directive preference statements based on the patient's values (1, 2). Almost all jurisdictions and Department of Veterans Affairs policy allow specific directive statements to be added to a living will, as well as the DPA/HC, when their intent is in concordance with the advance directive (the reader is directed to review state law and VA policy in this regard).

The values section begins the Values History by eliciting the patient's values regarding end-of-life care. This section contains two forms of value statements. Patients are first asked about their evaluation of future life in the context of length of life versus quality of life. This area of values is assessed because it is a fundamental trade-off that any advance directive must address. Patients are then asked to identify the end-of-life values that are most important to them. The reader is encouraged to discuss the patient's values at length to allow elaboration or the addition of other values that more completely reflect the individual's concerns or beliefs.

The directives section invites the patient to select specific treatment directives in light of those values and beliefs. The goal of this two-part approach is to encourage patient-physician discus-

sion on the use of medical treatments at the end of life, which in turn may help patients better understand their values (19). In turn, the physician can better respect the patient's autonomy by helping to remove constraints that could potentially hinder the informed consent process (19). Hence the values discourse helps clarify the patient's personal and value-based reasons for consenting to or refusing treatment and facilitates the health professional's understanding of these expressed values and preferences so that they can be later respected and implemented. These expressions can help both physicians and patients by removing ambiguities surrounding the living will and DPA/HC noted above, while also enhancing physician-patient conversation on end-of-life care. These two goals, when met, permit the health professional to write orders for the patient's health care on the basis of the patient's values.

The Values History's directive section begins with treatment preferences in acute care situations: consent for or refusal of cardiopulmonary resuscitation (CPR), ventilator use, and endotracheal tube use. Preferences regarding chronic care modalities follow, including those for use of intravenous fluids, enteral feeding tubes, and total parenteral nutrition, medication, and dialysis. During this part of the Values History process the physician explains the treatment modalities, their beneficial effects, short-term *and* long-term consequences, and possible harms in the context of terminal illness, irreversible coma, and persistent vegetative state. During conversations on discontinuing treatment, the patient should be reassured that the administration of medications for symptom relief (including treatment for pain, nausea, and shortness of breath) would not be withheld if required for comfort care, even if such therapy might involve an incremental increase of the risk of mortality.

For all of the above directives (except CPR), the patient may choose intervention, a trial of intervention (limited by time or medical judgment), or nonintervention. With the intervention of CPR, the patient may choose either a trial of intervention to determine medical effectiveness or nonintervention. With the other therapies, the patient may decide that after a set time trial attempting an intervention, if no benefit of the therapy is apparent, it should be discontinued. A time-limited trial is more concrete and explicit about the patient's preferences by setting specific parameters. Patients can instead decide to have a treatment continued so long as it benefits them in the physician's best medical judgment. Benefit-based trials require a significant level of trust between the

THE VALUES HISTORY[a]

Patient Name: _____

This Values History serves as a set of my specific value-based directives for various medical interventions. It is to be used in health care circumstances when I may be unable to voice my preferences. These directives shall be made a part of the medical record and used as supplementary to my living will and/or durable power of attorney for health care.

I. VALUES SECTION
There are several values important in decisions about terminal treatment and care. This section of the Values History invites you to identify your most important values.
A. Basic Life Values
Perhaps the most basic values in this context concern length of life versus quality of life. Which of the following two statements is the most important to you?
_____ 1. I want to live as long as possible, regardless of the quality of life that I experience.
_____ 2. I want to preserve a good quality of life, even if this means that I may not live as long.
B. Quality of Life Values
There are many values that help us to define for ourselves the quality of life that we want to live. The following list contains some that appear to be very important. Review this list (and feel free either to elaborate on it, or to add to it) and circle those values that are most important to your definition of quality of life.
 1. I want to maintain my capacity to think clearly.
 2. I want to feel safe and secure.
 3. I want to avoid unnecessary pain and suffering.
 4. I want to be treated with respect.
 5. I want to be treated with dignity when I can no longer speak for myself.
 6. I do not want to be an unnecessary burden on my family.
 7. I want to be able to make my own decisions.
 8. I want to experience a comfortable dying process.
 9. I want to be with my loved ones before I die.
10. I want to leave good memories of me to my loved ones.
11. I want to be treated in accord with my religious beliefs and traditions.
12. I want respect shown for my body after I die.
13. I want to help others by making a contribution to medical education and research.
14. Other values or clarification of values above:

II. DIRECTIVES SECTION
Some directives involve simple yes or no decisions. Others provide for the choice of a trial of intervention.
Initials/Date
_____ 1. I want to undergo cardiopulmonary resuscitation.
                 _____ TRIAL to determine effectiveness using reasonable medical judgment.
                 _____ NO
                 Why?
_____ 2. I want to be placed on a ventilator.
                 _____ YES
                 _____ TRIAL for the TIME PERIOD OF _____
                 _____ TRIAL to determine effectiveness using reasonable medical judgment.
                 _____ NO
                 Why?
_____ 3. I want to have an endotracheal tube used in order to perform items 1 and 2.
                 _____ YES
                 _____ TRIAL for the TIME PERIOD OF _____
                 _____ TRIAL to determine effectiveness using reasonable medical judgment.
                 _____ NO
                 Why?

_____ 4. I want to have total parenteral nutrition administered for my nutrition.
  _____ YES
  _____ TRIAL for the TIME PERIOD OF _____
  _____ TRIAL to determine effectiveness using reasonable medical judgment.
  _____ NO
  Why?

_____ 5. I want to have intravenous medication and hydration administered; regardless of my decision, I understand that intravenous hydration to alleviate discomfort or pain medication will not be withheld from me if I so request them.
  _____ YES
  _____ TRIAL for the TIME PERIOD OF _____
  _____ TRIAL to determine effectiveness using reasonable medical judgment.
  _____ NO
  Why?

_____ 6. I want to have all medications used for the treatment of my illness continued; regardless of my decision, I understand that pain medication will continue to be administered including narcotic medications.
  _____ YES
  _____ TRIAL for the TIME PERIOD OF _____
  _____ TRIAL to determine effectiveness using reasonable medical judgment.
  _____ NO
  Why?

_____ 7. I want to have nasogastric, gastrostomy or other enteral feeding tubes introduced and administered for my nutrition.
  _____ YES
  _____ TRIAL for the TIME PERIOD OF _____
  _____ TRIAL to determine effectiveness using reasonable medical judgment.
  _____ NO
  Why?

_____ 8. I want to be placed on a dialysis machine.
  _____ YES
  _____ TRIAL for the TIME PERIOD OF _____
  _____ TRIAL to determine effectiveness using reasonable medical judgment.
  _____ NO
  Why?

_____ 9. I want to have an autopsy done to determine the cause(s) of my death.
  _____ YES
  _____ NO
  Why?

_____ 10. I want to be admitted to the Intensive Care Unit for my medical care, if necessary.
  _____ YES
  _____ NO
  Why?

_____ 11. *For patients in long-term care facilities or receiving care at home who experience a life-threatening change in health status:* I want 911 called in case of a medical emergency.
  _____ YES
  _____ NO
  Why?

_____ 12. OTHER DIRECTIVES:

I consent to these directives after receiving honest disclosure of their implications, risks, and benefits by my physician, free from constraints and being of sound mind.

_____   _____
Signature   Date

_____
Witness

_____
Witness

13. PROXY NEGATION:
I request that the following persons NOT be allowed to make decisions on my behalf in the event of my disability or incapacity:

_____

_____

_____

_____   _____

Signature   Date

_____

Witness

_____

Witness

14. ORGAN DONATION:
Specific State Version Inserted Here
15. DURABLE POWER OF ATTORNEY FOR HEALTH CARE:
Specific State Version Inserted Here

[a]From Doukas D, McCullough L. The Values History: the evaluation of the patient's values and advance directives. J Fam Pract 1991;32(1):145–153.

patient and physician. The physician must allow adequate time for a therapy to benefit the patient before considering stopping it. The parameters the physician will use could usefully be discussed with the patient. However, benefit-based trials more accurately convey how the agent in a DPA/HC may approach intervention in an unforeseen future medical condition.

The Values History also offers several unique directives: autopsy, refusal of ICU care, a directive to exclude a specific decision making (because of differing values), and "Do not call 911" for patients in long-term care facilities or home care (20). The open directive at the end of the directive section allows the patient to add consent, refusal, or trials of intervention to other specific directives not otherwise addressed (e.g., specific types of surgery). The Values History concludes with the naming of a DPA/HC agent and organ donation.

SPECIAL CONSIDERATIONS

Formulating and implementing advance directive orders for patients in nursing homes, for patients electing to die at home, and for surgery involves special considerations and warrants further discussion. For nursing home patients, the order to "Do not call 911" avoids all forms of aggressive management in nursing homes without resuscitation equipment and personnel trained in its appropriate use.

This strategy may meet some institutional resistance, given the perception of the present reg-

ulatory environment of nursing homes in the United States. Some managers of nursing homes want to avoid all avoidable mortality in the nursing home and so may resist the "Do not call 911" order. The physician's response should be the following: (a) the regulations should not be interpreted to snuff out the last expression of the elder's autonomy; (b) there is no risk of lawsuit against the nursing home, given that the authors know of no reported lawsuits against physicians or hospitals that have implemented valid advance directives; (c) the nursing home can develop policies that respect and implement living wills, a process that will be self-educating for the institutions's personnel and leadership; (d) death subsequent to an advance directive implemented by a "Do not call 911" order is an acceptable form of mortality. To interpret present regulations as disallowing this outcome is to twist those regulations out of shape.

For patients receiving home health care, there have been other proposals about using "Do not call 911" orders (20). However, there are several potential difficulties with this strategy. First, orders are usually not written to be implemented by family members, but by professional colleagues and trainees. The physician does not stand in a hierarchical relationship of power with respect to the family members. Second, family members may justifiably place limits in their espousal and filial obligations, including the obligation to to care for the loved one dying at home (21). Some family members may reasonably judge the care burdens of doing so to be beyond their capacities, physical, emotional, or financial.

A patient does not have an unlimited, autonomy-based positive right to impose unreasonable care burdens on family members. Writing a "Do not call 911" order without a frank and mutually respectful discussion of the sense of family members' obligations and their thoughtful sense of limits on those obligations sets up the physician, the patient, and the patient's family for preventable ethical conflict. This conflict can be prevented in several ways. Family members need to be informed honestly about the care burdens involved and also about home services, such as hospice, for which the patient may qualify, which could reduce those burdens to a reasonable level. Family members also need to know that ambulance crews usually employ full resuscitation protocols for all rescues in response to 911 calls. Families can avoid this outcome by bringing the patient to the hospital before an emergency or perceived emergency. In addition, the physician can write orders that will address how the patient is to be managed once the patient reaches the emergency department of the hospital. The physician should work with colleagues in the emergency department and for hospital administration policies that will sanction such orders.

Patients for whom orders have been written to implement their advance directive(s) may require surgery. That is, in reliable beneficence-based clinical ethical judgment, surgery may reduce the patient's pain and suffering. The patient may be a reasonable risk for surgical management, albeit at high risk. From a surgical point of view, the problem with do not resuscitate orders remaining in effect during surgery is that administration of anesthesia or intraoperative technique can result in life-threatening events, from which the patient has a reasonable probability of recovering and then going on to enjoy the benefits of the surgery. It makes little or no sense in beneficence-based clinical ethical surgical judgment to let the patient die from reversible iatrogenic events when the patient is reliably expected to benefit from the surgery. This line of reasoning is sound in beneficence-based clinical ethical judgment and explains resistance among surgeons and anesthesiologists to maintaining do not resuscitate orders during surgery, despite autonomy-based arguments to the contrary. Surgical resistance to maintaining do not resuscitate orders during surgery could result in some patient not receiving surgery and experiencing worse pain and suffering than is necessary.

The preventive ethics strategy here is not surprising: negotiation with the surgical team. The physician should be prepared to present a clear statement of the patient's problem and why the operation is reliably expected to be effective in addressing that problem. The physician and the surgical team should undertake frank appraisal of the patient's surgical risk. The physician should also negotiate with the surgical team to determine when the physician's orders for nonaggressive management of life-threatening events will again take effect. The physician needs to be aware of surgeons' understandable sensitivities about surgical mortality rates. The physician and the surgical colleagues should work with their institutions and payers to ensure that death subsequent to surgery and reinstatement of the physician's orders for nonaggressive management of life threatening events is an acceptable form of postoperative mortality.

METHOD OF USE

A Values History can be implemented in seven steps. [See Table 62.1.]. The family can be part of this process when the patient consents to their involvement. The patient's family, and specifically the DPA/HC agent, should receive a copy of the completed Values History. Any misunderstandings should be clarified at the meeting of family members, agent, patient, and physician. Such discussions of the patient's values and end-of-life preferences would help in avoiding future difficulties should the patient become unable to communicate. These conversations between patient and family would facilitate the resolution of conflicts on health care goals for the patient.

The authors believe that a Values History can be completed by a patient over several visits. This has two advantages over precipitous consent to other advance directive instruments in less than half an hour (22, 23). The Values History is intended to be used in a reflective and introspective process by the patient, so that decisions are made thoughtfully and meaningfully. With discussion occurring over time, the physician can distribute the time required for these discussions during several medical visits (as many physicians are concerned about the lack of insurance or Medicare reimbursement for such counseling). Values statements would be discussed during initial visits, with specific treatment directives discussed subsequently.

These discussions enhance patient autonomy, while also helping to prevent future attempts by family members and others to interfere with implementing the patient's preferences. The authors urge that the completed Values History be reviewed with the patient periodically (every 6 to 12 months), especially if there is a significant deterioration in the patient's health status. In this way, changes in values or preferences that may occur over time can be documented, as well as discussed. Orders could then be updated as necessary.

1. Upon patient execution of either, or both, the living will and DPA/HC (as part of well elder care), the physician should discuss the quality of life versus length of life that is a built-in feature of aggressive medical management.
2. The physician reviews the values section of the Values History to have the patient consider and express priority for length versus quality of life.
3. The physician proceeds to review the patients' quality-of-life values with them and requests that they select those most important to them, while exploring other alternative patient values as well.
4. Using the patient's values as a framework, the patient and physician discuss the various therapeutic options in the directive section, especially in exploring "why" a therapy is accepted or refused.
5. The physician helps facilitate the consent process by
   a. Framing the process in relation to known patient values.
   b. Exploring other values that may emerge in the process.
   c. Clarifying for the patient inconsistencies between values and directives in a nonpaternalistic fashion, by removing reversible constraints to consent.
   d. Framing treatment options in terms of known patient conditions and diseases as well as high-risk activities and genetic propensities.
6. Other specific advance directive preferences concerning surgery and calling 911 from home or the nursing home should be discussed.
7. The directives individually should be initialed and dated. The complete Values History should be signed by the patient, dated, and witnessed, with *copies* placed in the medical chart (i.e., doctor's office, hospice, or extended care facility). The original should be placed in a readily available place in the patient's home (known to family and friends).

CONCLUSION

The Values History is a clinical tool intended to be used in conjunction with the legally recognized advance directives, the living will and the DPA/HC. The authors propose that the Values History better respects the patient's autonomy than either of these advance directives without the adjunct of the Values History. The Values History is therefore a powerful supplementary document that can add clarity and meaning to these advance directives, while also facilitating patient conversation on end-of-life care with family and physicians. In the Values History, physicians have a tool of considerable power to better understand their patients' values and preferences regarding end-of-life care.

Acknowledgment. The authors wish to acknowledge the assistance of Rebecca Reilly, M.D., in the preparation of this manuscript.

REFERENCES

1. Doukas DJ, Reichel W. Planning for uncertainty: a guide to living wills and other advance directives for health care. Baltimore: Johns Hopkins University Press, 1993.
2. Doukas DJ, McCullough LB. The Values History: the evaluation of the patient's values and advance directives. J Fam Pract 1991;32:145–153.
3. Doukas DJ, McCullough LB. Assessing the Values History of the aged patient regarding critical and chronic care. In: Gallo J, Reichel W, Andersen L, eds. Handbook of geriatric assessment. Rockville, MD: Aspen, 1988:111–124.
4. Doukas DJ, Lipson S, McCullough LB. Value history. In: Reichel W, ed. Clinical aspects of aging. 3rd ed. Baltimore: Williams & Wilkins, 1989:615–616.
5. Doukas DJ, McCullough LB. Truthtelling and confidentiality in the aged patient. In: Reichel W, ed. Clinical aspects of aging. 3rd ed. Baltimore: Williams & Wilkins, 1989:609–615.
6. Doukas DJ, Gorenflo DW. Analyzing the Values History: an evaluation of patient medical values and advance directives. J Clin Ethics 1993;4:41–45.
7. Doukas DJ, Brody H. After the Cruzan case: the primary care physician and the use of advance directives. J Am Board Fam Physicians 1992;2:201–205.
8. Omnibus Budget Reconciliation Act of 1990. Pub L. no. 101–508 §§4206, 4751.
9. Wolf SM, Boyle P, Callahan D, Fins JJ, et al. Sources of concern about the patient self-determination act. N Engl J Med 1991;325:1666–1671.
10. Eisendrath S, Jonsen A. The living will—help or hindrance? JAMA 1983;249:2054–2058.
11. Wanzer S, Adelstein J, Cranford R, et al. The physician's responsibility toward hopelessly ill patients. N Engl J Med 1984;310:955–959.
12. Emanuel EJ. A review of the ethical and legal aspects of terminating medical care. Am J Med 1988; 84:291–301.
13. Tomlinson T, Howe K, Notman M, Rossmiller D. An empirical study of proxy consent for elderly persons. Gerontologist 1990;30:54–64.
14. Doukas DJ, Antonucci TA, Gorenflo DW. A multi-generational assessment of values and advance directives. Ethics Behav 1992;2:51–59.
15. Doukas DJ, Gorenflo DW, Venkateswaran R. Understanding patients' values. (letter) J Clin Ethics 1993;4:199–200.
16. Wear S. Anticipatory ethical decision-making: the role of the primary care physician. HMO Pract 1989; 3:41–46.
17. Civetta J, Taylor R, Kirby R, eds. Critical care. Philadelphia, JB Lippincott, 1988.

18. Reilly R, Teasdale T, McCullough LB. Option of trial in advance directives. Gerontologist 1992;32:69 (Special Issue 2).

19. Ackerman T. Why doctors should intervene. Hastings Center Rep 1982;14–17.

20. Stollerman G. Decisions to leave home. (editorial) J Am Geriatr Soc 1988;36:375–376.

21. Jecker NS. The role of intimate others in medical decision making. Gerontologist 1990;30:65–71.

22. Scissors K. Advance directives for medical care. (letter) N Engl J Med 1991;325:1255.

23. Forrow L, Gogel E, Thomas E. Advance directives for medical care. (letter) N Engl J Med 1991; 325:1255.

Index

Page numbers in *italics* denote figures; those followed by "t" denote tables.

Absorption of drugs, 41–42
Abstinence syndromes, 138
Abuse. *See* Elder abuse and neglect
Accidents. *See* Trauma
Acetabular fractures, 349–350
Acetazolamide, 434t, 435
Acetohexamide, 55
Acetyl-L-carnitine, 59
Achalasia, 198–199
Achilles tendon, 361, 362
α-1-Acid glycoprotein, 43
Acid-base balance, 257
Acne rosacea, 383, 446–447
Acquired immune deficiency syndrome (AIDS). *See* Human immunodeficiency virus infection
Acromioclavicular joint arthritis, 315
Actinic keratosis, 389–390, *390*
of eyelid, 427–428
Activities of daily living, 16t, 16–17, 24, 31, 187, 464, 476
assessment of, 188, 524
instrumental, 17–19, 18t
limitations in, 491, 493, 509, 521
preoperative evaluation of, 410
Acute phase response, 157
Acyclovir, 208
Addison's disease, 258, 370
Adenoviral conjunctivitis, 429
Adhesive capsulitis of shoulder, 340
Adrenal changes with aging, 369–370
Adrenocorticotropic hormone, 366, 369–370
Adult children of elderly persons. *See also* Family
as caregivers, 4–5, 476–479
communication with, 5
decision making by, 7
developmentally disabled, 163
emotional separation from parents, 12–13
geographic separation from parents, 4–5, 477
Adult day-care, 153, 526
Adult protective services, 485, 512
Adult respiratory distress syndrome, 212
Advance directives, 13, 33, 512, 597–607, 609–610
ethical problems with, 601–603
legal development of, 597–601
contrast between living will and durable power of attorney for health care, 600
contrast between rights of self-determination and privacy, 598–599
durable power of attorney for health care, 599–600
living will, 599
Patient Self-Determination Act, 13, 600–601, 609–610
right of privacy, 597–598

right of self-determination, 597
for nursing home patients, 614
for patients receiving home health care, 614–615
preventive ethics strategy for, 604t–605t, 604–607
shortcomings of, 609–610
for surgery patients, 615
values and, 607, 610–616. *See also* Values History
Adverse drug reactions, 44, 557
African-Americans. *See* Black elders
Age spots, 387–388
Aging
adverse drug reactions and, 44
cognitive decline with, 142
definition of, 8
demographics of, 488–495
effect on lipid and lipoprotein levels, 247
nutrition and, 224
physiologic changes with, 8, 472–475, 473t. *See also* Physiology of aging
successful, 463–470. *See also* Psychosocial epidemiology
"Aging in place," 490, 514–516, 521
Agnogenic myeloid metaplasia, 403
α₂-Agonists, 434, 434t
β-Agonists, 111, 112
Aid to Families with Dependent Children, 499
Akathisia, 181–182
Akinesia, 180
Albumin binding, 43
Albuterol, 111
Alcohol abuse, 6, 133–139, 480
counseling about, 33
diagnosis of, 133, 136–137
falls due to, 549–550
hospitalization related to, 65
housing for persons with, 519
myopathy induced by, 322
natural history of, 133–134
nutrition and, 235, 239
prevalence of, 133
residential fires and, 553
sexual dysfunction due to, 543t
treatment of, 137–139
Alcoholics Anonymous, 139
Aldosteronism, 370
Allergic conjunctivitis, 429
Allergic dermatitis, 381
Alprazolam, 56t
Alteplase, 53
Alzheimer's Association, 152
Alzheimer's disease, 7, 142, 145, 146, 155–159
aluminum and other trace elements in, 158
biological aspects of, 155–157

619